THE CANNABIS ENCYCLOPEDIA
*The Definitive Guide to Cultivation &
Consumption of Medical Marijuana*

Published by Van Patten Publishing, USA
Cover design: Wendover Brown, Christopher Valdés, Ricki Jaeckel
Cover image by Toni13: 'Pakistan Chitral Kush' from CannaBioGen
Back-cover images: Lochfoot (www.lochfootphoto.com) and Christopher Valdés (www.valdudes.com)
Artwork: Christopher Valdés, Emiliano Villani
Book design and layout: Ricki Jaeckel

Primary photographers
(Listed in descending order by number of images that appear in the book)

Jorge Cervantes	Christopher Valdés	Hugo Martinez	María Garcia
Mel Frank	Nomaad	Todd McCormick	
Justin McIvor	Doobie Duck	Chimera	
Toni13	Hash Marihuana & Hemp Museum	Mitch Connor	
Alex (Gato)	(Amsterdam and Barcelona)	Joop Dumay	

Contributors: Fred Gardner, Dr. John McPartland, Mel Frank, Samantha Miller (Pure Analytics), Toni13, and Marc (Carbon Active)

Technical editors: Ralph B., Theo Tekstra (Gavita Holland), Samantha Miller (Pure Analytics)
Copy editor: Linda Meyer

The Cannabis Encyclopedia – Trade Paper	The Cannabis Encyclopedia – Hardcover	The Cannabis Encyclopedia – Limited Edition
10-digit ISBN: 1-878823-34-5	10-digit ISBN: 1-878823-39-6	10-digit ISBN: 1-878823-26-4
13-digit ISBN: 978-1-878823-34-2	13-digit ISBN: 978-1-878823-39-7	13-digit ISBN: 978-1-878823-26-7

First Printing
10 9 8 7 6 5 4 3 2 1

Printed in China

For wholesale orders:
USA /Canada: Homestead Book Co., www.homesteadbook.com, tel: +1-800-426-6777
Quick Distribution: qdcb@sbcglobal.net, tel: +1-510-527-7036
Ingram Books: www.ingrambook.com
Europe: Van Patten Editorial, S.L., info@vanpattenpublishing.com
Holland: Kulu Trading, www.kulutrading.com, tel: +31-356-93-22-66
UK: AVALON Wholesale, LTD, www.freedombooks.co.uk, tel: +44 (0) 23-9283-2383 or +44 (0) 23-9278-0600

Check www.vanpattenpublishing.com for a complete list of our distributors.

Page 19, Cannabinoid Receptor Illustration Reprinted by permission from Macmillan Publishers Ltd: NAT. NEUROSCIENCE, Greuter BA, Brasnjo, G., Malenka RC. Postsynaptic TRPV1 Triggers cell type-specific long-term depression in the nucleus accumbens. 2010; 13:1519-1525. © 2012

This book is dedicated to my mother, Esther J. Van Patten; my father, Dr. C. R. Van Patten; my brother, C. R. (Bob) Van Patten Jr.; and my wife's mother, Simona Cervantes, all of whom could have benefited from medicinal cannabis.

CONTENTS

Note: This table of contents has been pared down to represent the book's main categories. Individual chapters start with a detailed table of contents and include page numbers.

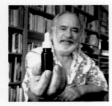
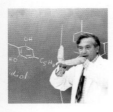
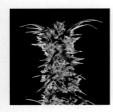
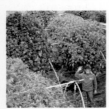
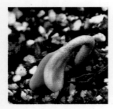
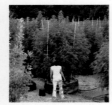

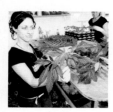
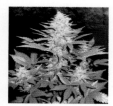
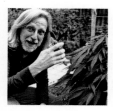
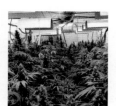
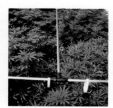
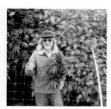
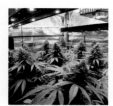

Part 3 | Advanced Medical Cannabis Horticulture

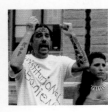
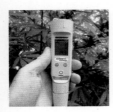
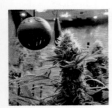
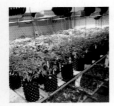
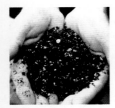
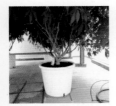
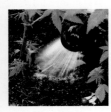

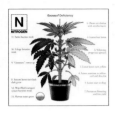
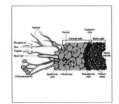
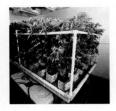
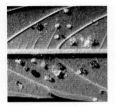
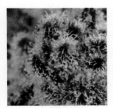
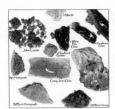
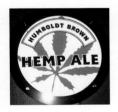

INTRODUCTION

CANNABIS IS A UNIQUE PLANT—medicinal, industrial, and intoxicating—a plant with natural defenses against the axe, fire, and intense political and legal control. Every day we see news articles and television reports about how the civilized world deals with cannabis. Media outlets focus on medical cannabis dispensaries, the doctors who prescribe cannabis, and the patients and gardeners who produce it, frequently centering on the *illegal* production. The equation is often driven by politicians and others who have ignored science and wield cannabis as a means to divide and control populations. However, cannabis has a natural and evolutional defense that started long before man cut the first tree and before fire burned the first leaf. Natural survival laws ensure that cannabis will be here long after man-made laws are gone.

Medical patients, caregivers, and recreational cannabis gardeners are often caught in a quagmire. On one side lie man-made local and federal laws; on the other side Mother Nature. This unfortunate plant prohibition is based on ignorance and fear. Charles Darwin was so fearful of hypnosis in relation to the Theory of Evolution that he waited until nearly the end of his life to publish the *Origin of Species*. To change, societies suffer as Darwin suffered. No matter how much our growth is arrested, it cannot stop the evolution of a species.

Fortunately we live in the 21st century and draconian laws about cannabis are disappearing. The beginning to the end of cannabis prohibition is in sight. Medical cannabis and scientific research are promoting social acceptance. Colorado and Washington state (in the USA) and Uruguay have legalized recreational cannabis, and many other countries have decriminalized or tolerate use and cultivation. The tsunami of social change, mainstream acceptance, and legalization of cannabis is upon us. We will all be gardening in peace soon.

About the Encyclopedia
The Cannabis Encyclopedia is the sequel to *Marijuana Horticulture: The Indoor/Outdoor Medical Grower's Bible*. One wonderful night six years ago, Michka, our French publisher (www.mamaedicions.com) and I were discussing my sixth rewriting of the "cannabis bible." After describing the extent of my new work, she said, "It sounds like an encyclopedia." After our meeting *The Cannabis Encyclopedia* took on new dimensions and research. It is an excellent sequel that is completely updated and expanded. We changed to an 8.5 × 11-inch (21.6 × 27.9 cm) format with three columns to save space and paper, and the new book contains more than twice the information of *Marijuana Horticulture*, including 2,000 all-new color images.

This book is a compilation of more than 30 years of personal cannabis research and collaboration. Within its pages you will find the experience of thousands of cannabis gardeners, editors, and writers from several continents.

Gathering information today is much easier than it was 30 years ago, when I started writing, but sorting the wheat from the chaff is difficult. The information needed to be verified, so I called upon well-educated scientists and horticulturists with expertise in specific areas—soil, lighting, nutrients, greenhouses, cannabinoids, and so forth. With the addition of new chapters—*Medical Cannabis*, *Measuring Cannabinoids*, *Medical Cannabis Varieties*, *Medicinal Concentrates & Tinctures*, and *Cooking with Medicinal Cannabis*—plus the complete rewriting of all the original chapters, the book had grown into *The Cannabis Encyclopedia*.

Many people from many different countries helped me research this work; their names are listed under "Contributors" in the back of the book.

Influence of the Internet
Today the organic nature of the Internet is used to spread both information and seeds. The Internet has linked cannabis gardeners around the world, and prohibition has helped us forge a unique bond to understand and promote cannabis.

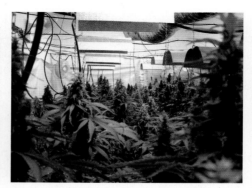

Growing a nice medical cannabis garden in your backyard is easy. But it was not always possible in California. Today medical cannabis is legal in more than 20 states in the USA and in many other parts of the world.

Intensive indoor cannabis gardens are very popular where prohibition dominates. Ironically, indoor gardeners grow 4 to 6 intensive crops a year. Producing multiple generations annually gives breeders a big advantage when developing new varieties.

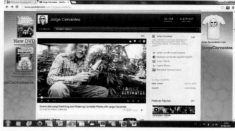

To find information on everything related to medical cannabis—growing, breeding, harvesting, making concentrates, cooking, and more—use your Internet browser to search for "medical cannabis" or "Jorge Cervantes" on Internet forums, Facebook, Instagram, and YouTube.

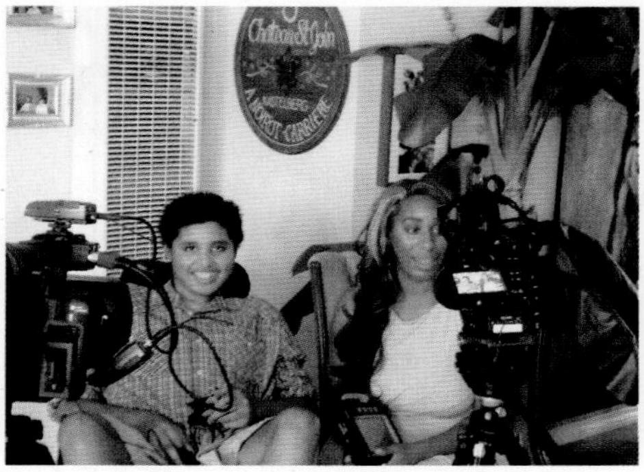

Keen knowledge of cannabinoid profiles and genetic qualities is essential to grow the best medical cannabis. Cannabis has changed Joey Perez's (left) life as attested to by his mother Mieko who runs the Unconventional Foundation for Autism (http://www.uf4a.org/).

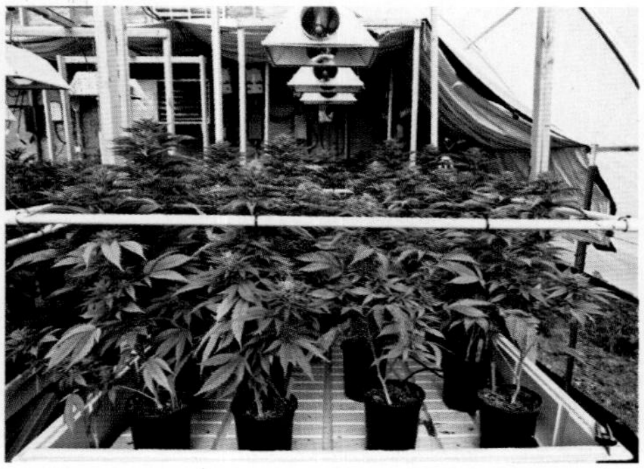

Setting up an indoor, outdoor, or greenhouse garden is easy when you have all the necessary information at your fingertips.

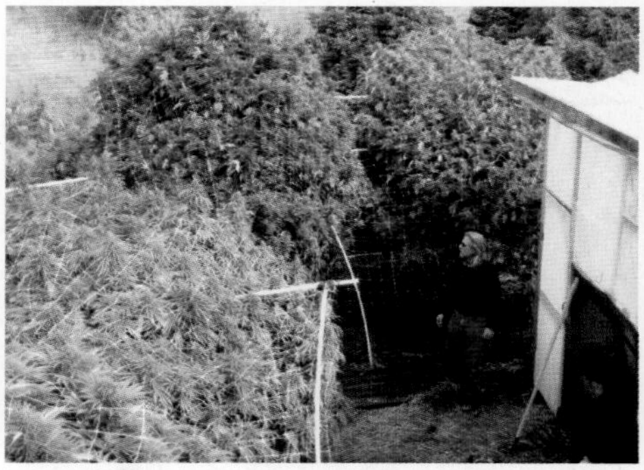

Everyone can grow big plants with the proper knowledge. All you need is great organic soil, plenty of sunshine and an eight-month growing season.

Information and high-quality cannabis seeds are available via the Internet to all gardeners, wherever they may be.

Facebook, Instagram, YouTube, etc., have linked us all—patients, caregivers, gardens, manufacturers, and retailers. This new wave of easy, instant communication will continue to help catapult the cannabis industry; the organic nature of the Internet confirms natural laws.

Social media has linked us together, creating unknown volumes of information. Combine social media with the changing attitude about cannabis, and new synergistic phenomena takes place. The exponential amount of information about cannabis overwhelms prohibitionists, and causes the fears and paranoia of the past to disappear. This phenomenon is happening all around the world!

Breaking all barriers, the Internet has made it is virtually impossible for information about cannabis to be suppressed. Unlike a book, a digital signal is difficult to stop at borders. The Internet is a conglomeration of all of us, and collectively we are smarter than any individual or government organization.

On www.marijuanagrowing.com you will find a complete forum for every chapter in this book. Visit the forums to discuss the contents of *The Cannabis Encyclopedia* and to ask questions of Jorge and other experienced gardeners. Check out the *Organics* forum, the *Marijuana Infirmary*, and the *Medical Cannabis* forum, among others. Feel free to add more information in your forum posts. Share cooking tips and recipes, as well as photos and videos of your gardens.

How to Use this Book

The full table of contents is separated into five sections. The first page of each chapter contains a detailed chapter table of contents.

Part 1 covers medicinal cannabis, measuring cannabinoids, and the botanical classification of cannabis and various medical varieties. This section is written for the lay person who wants to understand the scientific detail behind medical cannabis, including CBD-rich varieties.

Part 2 delves into the life cycle of cannabis and details each phase of growth—from germination to harvest, drying, and curing. This basic section is designed for all gardeners. It takes an in-depth look at garden rooms, greenhouses, and outdoor cultivation. Four case studies are included in chapter 13.

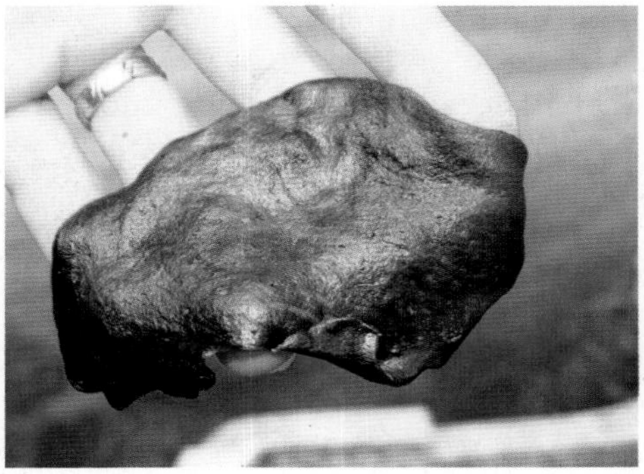

Cannabinoids are found in oil-base resin that is separated from water-base foliage and flowers. The "resin" is collected and pressed into hashish (above) or separated with a solvent into oils and other concentrates.

Part 3 is for advanced gardeners wanting to learn essential facts. Experts will find detailed answers to specific questions—preserving the sanctuary, meters, air, water, soil, nutrients, additives, container gardens and hydroponics, diseases and pests, and basic breeding.

Part 4 is essential for medical patients and caregivers, and is perfect for gardeners with big crops. Post-harvest subjects such as concentrates, tinctures, and extracts are explained in detail. And the simple science of cooking for consumption is clearly presented.

Part 5 contains an appendix (abbreviations used in this book), a 30-year history of Jorge's cannabis career, and a detailed index.

Jorge's Wish for You

The Cannabis Encyclopedia provides the accurate information you need to cultivate and responsibly consume the best medicinal and recreational cannabis imaginable. All that is needed now is your desire for excellent health and above all your tender loving care to grow the absolute best cannabis possible!

—Jorge

FOREWORD

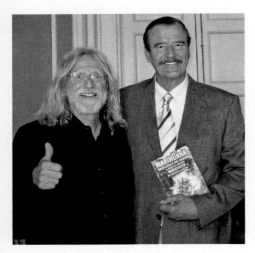

George F. Van Patten and Vicente Fox Quesada, president of Mexico (2000–2006), pose for a photo at the 2013 press conference hosted by Steven DeAngelo (Harborside Health Center) that announced the Symposium Mexico-USA on the Legalization and Medical Use of Cannabis.

I met George Van Patten on July 8, 2013, in San Francisco, California, during the press conference that announced the *Symposium Mexico-USA on the Legalization and Medical Use of Cannabis*, held at the Fox Center. (*http://centrofox.org.mx/en*).

On that occasion, George gave me the fifth edition of his book *Marijuana Horticulture: The Indoor/Outdoor Medical Grower's Bible* (2006), published under his pseudonym, Jorge Cervantes. Specialists consider this work to be a comprehensive treatise; some of them, including George, call it the bible for cannabis production, since it covers all forms of indoor and outdoor cultivation of this medicinal plant.

George shared that when he was updating the sixth edition of *Marijuana Horticulture*—adding more than twice the original text and a thousand more images—his French publisher, Michka, remarked that the revised content resembled a true encyclopedia.

The inclusion of new and important studies, as well as multimedia elements and information technologies for consultation purposes, resulted in the book that you have in your hands: *The Cannabis Encyclopedia: The Definitive Guide to Cultivation & Consumption of Medical Marijuana.*

The Cannabis Encyclopedia incorporates and condenses information that is difficult to find, representing valuable research and the modern culture of this ancient plant. George's purpose today, like that of the eighteenth-century French encyclopedists in their time, is to arrange in a consistent and systematic way the current knowledge on a given topic.

Scientific arguments dispel many prohibition myths and antiquated beliefs about cannabis, affirming that we are indeed in the process of facing the final frontier, an unstoppable new paradigm: the legalization of cannabis.

Prohibition does not work. Prohibition generates temptations. Prohibition kills. The dramatic world war on drugs, in which tens of thousands of young people have been killed, is proof that prohibition has failed. These people were not born criminals; they were not genetically predisposed toward criminality. And yet, because of flawed public policy, disinformation, a lack of education, and a lack of better economic incentives and opportunities, they became victims of an insane war against an enemy we can never defeat with prohibition.

With its social contribution of information and knowledge, *The Cannabis Encyclopedia* allows us to affirm that there is no turning back; the legalization of cannabis—the freedom to choose—is inevitable. The question essentially revolves around the issue of freedom of choice versus prohibition.

We are all created equal and free. It follows, then, that if we are created this way, we must be allowed the freedom to determine what is best for ourselves, to decide our own behavior, and to act responsibly, as long as we do not detrimentally affect the rights of others.

Mexico is not a significant producer or consumer of drugs; however, because of its unique geography—between drug-producing countries to the south and a giant drug-consuming country to the north—it is caught in a permanent war from which it must exit.

The United States has demonstrated a total inability to enforce its own laws and prevent the importation and distribution of drugs within its own territory. One is left to wonder how this has occurred—how mass quantities of drugs can easily cross the border from Mexico into the United States, where they are sold in every corner of the country. I wonder who launders the money and buys the weapons and ammunition in the United States. Who brings the proceeds back to Mexico to bribe police, public officials, even members of the army? Estimates indicate that about 2,000 weapons enter Mexico illegally from the United States every day (Small Arms Survey, 2011, Graduate Institute of International Development Studies, Geneva, Switzerland), a figure that could surely have increased in recent years.

If countries were to adopt a regulatory policy in conjunction with the decriminalization of drugs, they would have money (through taxes) to operate educational, regulatory, and informative initiatives, and citizens would not have to shoulder an immense burden—the cost of the war on drugs.

In his book, *Drogas: Prohibición o legalización (Drugs: Prohibition or Legalization)* (Colombia, Editorial Debate, 2013), former president of Colombia Ernesto Samper Pizano asserts, "There are 300 million consumers of different drugs in the world, and legalizing the use of marijuana would solve 60 percent of the drug problem in the world . . . It is no secret that marijuana is less harmful than alcohol in terms of

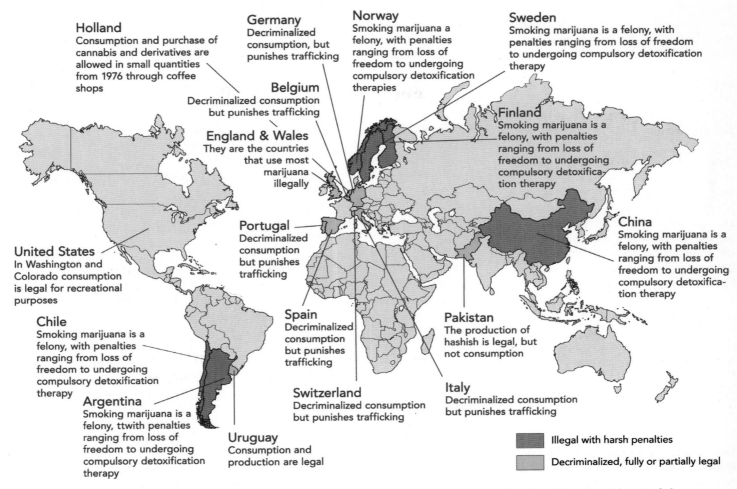

Holland
Consumption and purchase of cannabis and derivatives are allowed in small quantities from 1976 through coffee shops

Germany
Decriminalized consumption, but punishes trafficking

Norway
Smoking marijuana a felony, with penalties ranging from loss of freedom to undergoing compulsory detoxification therapies

Sweden
Smoking marijuana is a felony, with penalties ranging from loss of freedom to undergoing compulsory detoxification therapy

Belgium
Decriminalized consumption but punishes trafficking

England & Wales
They are the countries that use most marijuana illegally

Finland
Smoking marijuana is a felony, with penalties ranging from loss of freedom to undergoing compulsory detoxification therapy

China
Smoking marijuana is a felony, with penalties ranging from loss of freedom to undergoing compulsory detoxification therapy

Portugal
Decriminalized consumption but punishes trafficking

United States
In Washington and Colorado consumption is legal for recreational purposes

Chile
Smoking marijuana is a felony, with penalties ranging from loss of freedom to undergoing compulsory detoxification therapy

Spain
Decriminalized consumption but punishes trafficking

Pakistan
The production of hashish is legal, but not consumption

Argentina
Smoking marijuana is a felony, ttwith penalties ranging from loss of freedom to undergoing compulsory detoxification therapy

Switzerland
Decriminalized consumption but punishes trafficking

Italy
Decriminalized consumption but punishes trafficking

Uruguay
Consumption and production are legal

Illegal with harsh penalties

Decriminalized, fully or partially legal

Source: Sandra Sánchez, www.sinembargo.mx. Periodismo digital con rigor. Mexico, August 4, 2013. Translated from Spanish to English.

health; no one has died from a cannabis overdose."

In this new paradigm, taking responsibility for one's own health would mean consuming cannabis in a responsible and controlled manner, the same way that society currently establishes its expectation for responsible tobacco and alcohol use.

The public opinion in favor of cannabis legalization outweighs the approval of government prohibitionist policies. The trend is well established and, like many other prohibitions, this one must eventually give way to the freedom of choice exercised in an educated and responsible manner.

Doctors, specialists, entrepreneurs, activists, opinion leaders, journalists, legislators, members of congress, experts, and public officials who have attended seminars and conferences held in the Americas, Europe, and Latin America on the legalization and medical use of cannabis insist on discussing the legalization of marijuana beyond any ideologies, and to destigmatize the research for medical use. Even Secretary General of the Organization of American States, José Miguel Insulza, declared his "sympathy [with] the emergence of alternative drug policies, like the recent move toward the legalization of marijuana in Uruguay or the debate to regulate it in Mexico."

Internationally recognized institutions such as the Global Commission on Drug Policy and the Cato Institute; Mexican academic institutions such as the Universidad Nacional Autónoma de México (UNAM); and hemispheric leaders, presidents, and former presidents of several countries are in favor of a paradigm shift regarding the fight against drug trafficking, after more than four decades of poor results using prohibition to eradicate violence and drug use.

According to a survey by the Pew Research Center in March 2013, for the first time in more than four decades of surveys on the issue, a majority of Americans are in favor of legalizing the recreational use of cannabis. According to the national survey, 52 percent say that cannabis use should be legalized, while 45 percent say it should not. The support for cannabis legalization has increased by 11 points since 2010. The change is even more dramatic since the late 1960s. In a 1969 survey conducted by Gallup, only 12 percent were in favor of legalizing cannabis, while 84 percent were opposed to it.

In the USA, twenty-one states and Washington, DC, have approved medical use of cannabis, and the approval of recreational use is being discussed in other states, as has already happened in Colorado and Washington state. In Canada, some regulations concerning cannabis usage have been publicly issued. The Netherlands and Portugal have already accomplished legalization, and consumption is not penalized in Mexico.

While in the United States, Uruguay, and Spain, specifically the City of Barcelona, the legalization of marijuana progresses, in Mexico such initiatives are very slow. Our country is slow to act and, above all, the fundamental issue of prohibition remains unsolved, which does not prevent the 40 deaths per day caused by the drug cartels.

Mexico has had a late start in the process of cannabis legalization, and the response has not been as expeditious as necessary. Prompt action is required to reduce violence, achieve peace and harmony, and improve our country's damaged image abroad.

In Mexico, some local and federal legislators are vigorously pushing these initiatives. They have studied the subject, visited other countries, had contact with George Van Patten, and observed the experiences of the United States, the Netherlands, Portugal, and Australia, among others.

However, the federal government of Mexico and the government of the Federal District (Mexico City) are not progressive. They are on the defensive, resistant to change, and are perceived as hesitant and indifferent—but the legalization process is already irreversible.

Legalizing cannabis is the way out of the trap in which we find ourselves. This option provides substantial benefits:

- Separation of violence and crime from the health issue
- Reduction of consumption, as happened in Portugal after legalization
- Substantial reduction of revenues for the drug cartels
- Making funds available to governments for education and to prevent violence
- Allocation of time and resources to address other widespread forms of criminality
- Education to decide and exercise our freedom responsibly

- Rescue of thousands of young people—the future of every country—who walk the wrong direction into a life of crime
- Promotion of economic growth and the creation of opportunities for countries to move forward and not watch others pass them by

The time has come for the governments of our countries and the governments all over the world to act and govern as the great president Abraham Lincoln envisioned [in the Gettysburg Address]: "That this nation, under God, shall have a new birth of freedom and that government of the people, by the people, for the people, shall not perish from the earth."

When this monumental change happens, there will be a better world of harmony and peace for all.

The freedom of choice and decision is ours; let us exercise it.

—Vicente Fox Quesada, President of Mexico (2000–2006) and President of the Fox Center (http://centrofox.org.mx/en)

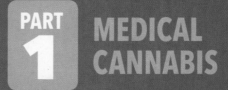

PART 1 **MEDICAL CANNABIS**

1 MEDICAL CANNABIS

*by Fred Gardner and
Dr. John McPartland*

WE CAN ONLY IMAGINE how people, countless thousands of years ago, discovered that a certain plant had healing properties. Maybe a woman was gathering seeds for food when a painful period began. As she stripped the seeds out of the plant's flower tops, a sticky resin coated her hands. She gnawed a bit of the gummy substance. Soon afterward, she started feeling better.

Her friends confirmed that this was indeed a cramp-reducing plant. They began growing it on purpose. When their tribe moved on, they brought seeds to put in the ground at their next settlement. Similar discoveries must have been made many times in many groups. People came to realize that the seeds were nourishing, the resin was pain-reducing, and the stalk provided fiber for ropes and nets.

Here and there tribes began intentionally growing this especially useful plant. The specifics are lost in the mists of history, but the plant abides and is now known to botanists as *Cannabis*. (The Latin name for the plant is italicized, and cannabis, the product made from the plant, is not.)

Cannabis evolved long before humans did, but because no one has found *Cannabis* macrofossils in rocks, it is hard to say when. Two DNA studies estimate that *Cannabis* evolved either 21 or 27.8 million years ago. Fossilized pollen identified as *Cannabis* dates to 787,000 years ago in southern Siberia.

Younger pollen, about 125,000 years old, has been extracted from a Siberian bog. Neanderthal bones from the same date were found in a cave 30 miles away. Some time after *Homo sapiens* migrated into the area 40,000 years ago, we forged a partnership with the plant.

"Hemp followed man naturally," wrote Nicolai Vavilov, the great Russian plant scientist, "keeping near his dwelling places, settling on rubbish and everywhere the soil was manured." Hemp's "camp follower" image was popularized by Edgar Anderson, a well-known botanist at Harvard University and the Missouri Botanical Garden.

At some point people began selecting the plants with the features they appreciated for cultivation—tall stalks, big oily seeds, or healing, psychoactive resin. Vavilov, Anderson, Carl Sauer, Andrew Sherratt, and Carl Sagan have linked the origins of agriculture to our ancestors' efforts to grow more useful *Cannabis*. Sauer proposed that agriculture was developed by people living in fishing communities alongside rivers and lakes (the habitat of "ditchweed") who began cultivating the plants as a source of fishing lines and nets. Nobody knows the exact where and when.

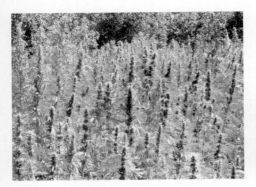

Cannabis growing in the Rif Mountains, Morocco

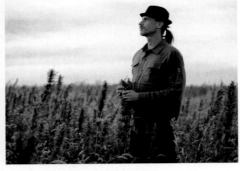

Conservationist and hemp activist David Bronner, president of Dr. Bronner's Magic Soaps, inspects a field of industrial hemp in Colorado, 2013. See www.drbronner.com for more information.

Classification

Swedish botanist Carl Linnaeus formally described *Cannabis sativa* in 1753. Thirty-two years later Jean-Baptiste Lamarck identified *Cannabis indica* as a second species. Experts continue to debate whether they should be classified as separate species or as separate varieties of one species. Extant populations of a possible third species, *Cannabis ruderalis*, may be a wild-type relic that descended from the ancestor of *C. sativa*.

Then came *That '70s Show*, when *Cannabis* taxonomy became embroiled in the US legal system. The ethnobotanist Richard Evans Schultes, a defense witness, asserted that narcotics laws referred to *C. sativa*, whereas the accused possessed *C. indica*, which was statutorily overlooked and technically legal. Ernest Small, a taxonomic botanist, argued for a single species on behalf of the plaintiffs.

Unfortunately, Schultes and his colleague Loren Anderson made subtle shifts in *Cannabis* taxonomy that departed from the original concepts of Linnaeus and Lamarck. They included drug plants as well as fiber-type plants within *C. sativa*. (We now know that the drug plants are rich in 9-tetrahydrocannabinol or THC, and the fiber-type plants are rich in cannabidiol or CBD.) Linnaeus's *C. sativa* specimens were examined by William Stern in 1974 and found to be "old cultivated hemp stock of northern Europe"—rope, not dope—CBD-dominant plants.

Schultes and Anderson delimited *C. indica* to plants that Schultes saw in Afghanistan. Thus they characterized "*indica*" as short, densely-branched plants with broad leaflets, and "*sativa*" along the lines of Lamarck's species—tall, laxly branched, with narrow leaflets. They spawned the vernacular taxonomy of "*sativa*" and "*indica*" that is in use to this day. With burgeoning interest in high-CBD plants, some of which are *C. sativa* in the Linnaean sense, the vernacular taxonomy has become truly muddled.

Botanist Karl Hillig segregates these populations: *C. sativa* represents CBD-dominant plants from Europe, either cultivated (*C. sativa* hemp biotype) or wild-type (*C. sativa* feral biotype).

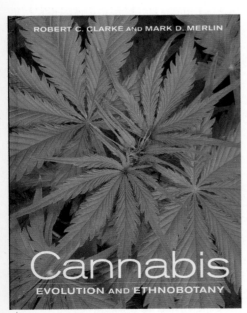

Robert Clarke and Mark Merlin's book Cannabis Evolution and Ethnobotany

C. indica represents THC-dominant plants from Asia, either Lamarck's plants from India—*C. indica* NLD ("narrow leaflet diameter," known as "*sativa*" in the vernacular) or plants from Afghanistan—*C. indica* WLD ("wild leaflet diameter," the vernacular "*indica*").

Naturalists Robert Clarke and Mark Merlin adopted Hillig's system and expanded it. Examining the worldwide distribution of *Cannabis* plants—wild, cultivated, and feral (once cultivated, again wild)—these experts conclude that:

Narrow-leaf hemp, *C. sativa*, subspecies *sativa*, was cultivated predominantly in Europe.

Broad-leaf hemp, *C. indica*, subspecies *chinensis*, was cultivated in China, Korea, Japan, and Southeast Asia.

Narrow-leaf drug plants, *C. indica*, subspecies *indica*, were cultivated in South and Southeast Asia and the Middle East.

Broad-leaf drug plants, *C. indica*, subspecies *afghanica*, were cultivated in Northern Afghanistan and Pakistan.

Note that the widespread interbreeding and hybridization of narrow- and broad-leafletted plants has made the application of these terms botanically imprecise in many cases.

Medical Use before the Modern Era

All the famous Old-World cradles of civilization put cannabis to medical use—China, Mesopotamia, Greece, India, and maybe Egypt. The Scythians, a tribe of migrants who inhaled cannabis-infused steam for ritual purposes, migrated out of their Siberian homeland around 800 BC. They lacked a written language, but their word for *Cannabis* has been reconstructed as *kanab, kanap, konaba,* or *kannabis*. The Scythians influenced civilizations in China, India, and Mesopotamia at the cusp of history.

Physician and historian Ethan Russo has visited a tomb in the Yánghai burial ground that contained nearly a kilo of cannabis. It was crudely manicured—flowering tops, leaves, and seeds, and no stems. The grave did not contain hemp fiber. It dates to 766–416 BCE. Scythians are buried nearby. Yánghǎi lies in the Turpan Basin, now part of China.

The ancient Chinese knew cannabis as "má." Their pictogram for má represents two plants hung upside down to dry. Combining má with the character yào (drug) means "narcotic" or "anaesthetic."

The legendary physician Shénnóng writes extensively about má in his Daoist-flavored medical text, Shénnóng Běn Cǎo Jīng (also known as Pen Ts'ao Ching). He warned, "Taking much of it may make one behold ghosts and frenetically run about. Protracted taking may enable one to communicate with the spirit and make the body light." Shénnóng supposedly lived about 4000 years ago, but the man's legendary existence went unmentioned until about 130 BCE.

The Scythians entered history when they invaded Mesopotamia during the reign of King Sargon II (722–705 BCE). After the Scythians invaded Assyria, a new word appeared in Neo-Assyrian cuneiform. The word, which means "hemp," transliterates as qunubu or qunnabu. The word appears in contexts that hint of use by shamans, which strengthens the Scythian connection.

Herodotus, the Greek "father of history," wrote extensively about the Scythians around 440 BCE. Herodotus coins the

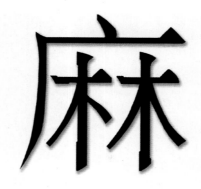

The Chinese pictogram "má" represents cannabis—two plants hung upside down to dry.

word xávvaßiç from a word he adopted from the Scythians. He described them using xávvaßiç for cordage and cloth, and vaporizing xávvaßiç in small tents.

In India there are more than 50 words for Cannabis and cannabis products. Archeologists working in the Ganges River basin have unearthed Cannabis seeds from at least 1300 BCE. The Atharvaveda, compiled around 900 BCE, gives the name bhǎnga to a plant that many experts believe is Cannabis. These dates preceded the arrival of the Scythians, whose earliest presence in the Hindu Kush may date to the 7th century BCE.

Siddhārtha Gautama (ca. 563–483 BCE), the Buddha of our historic era, was an Indo-Scythian. He supposedly subsisted on one hemp seed per day during his six steps of asceticism. Practitioners of Ayurvedic medicine, India's traditional system, recommend the herb to counter pain, insomnia, and loss of appetite.

The Egyptian hieroglyph šmšmt has been interpreted as Cannabis. The word appears in the Pyramid Texts of 2350 BCE, "the cords (or ropes) of the šmšmt plant." However, flax and not hemp was the primary fiber crop of ancient Egypt. Other authors interpret šmšmt as Corchorus olitorius, a fibrous herb whose leaves are eaten and used medicinally in Egypt. The word also resembles šmšm, the Arabic word for sesame. Good evidence of Cannabis in Egypt begins in the Roman era.

Noted Polish anthropologist Sara Benet (neé Benetowa) argues that kaneh

bosm (qānēh bośem) is Cannabis in the Old Testament, Exodus 30:22–25. The word is usually translated as "aromatic cane." Moses used kaneh bosm for a sacred anointing oil. Benetowa notes "the astonishing resemblance" between Semitic kanbos and the Scythian word for Cannabis. But the Book of Exodus was composed around the 8th or 9th century BCE, and the Scythians did not invade the Land of Israel until 630 BCE. By then the Israelites had already been scattered and exiled by the Assyrians.

Cannabis is not native to the Fertile Crescent. Kanbos, which also transliterated ḳanbūs or qannabbôs, first appears in Mishnah, written in the 1st century BC.

Given the evidence that cannabis products were widely used to treat illnesses in the ancient world, the real mystery is why it fell out of favor—a historical phenomenon that Ethan Russo dubbed "Cannabis interruptus." Seeking an explanation, Russo cited "the perishable nature" of the historical record, and "humanity's propensity toward constant warfare, invasion, and cultural conflict."

It's as if prohibitionists have always existed in every society, and from time to time they prevail over the physicians and patients who have put cannabis products to good use. One theory is that in many cultures, members of the priestly class viewed psychoactive plants as a threat to their role as proper intermediaries between the material and spiritual realms. They didn't want people having visions and creative insights without their supervision. In modern times, prohibition of cannabis has provided an effective method of social control—a mechanism for funding and arming the police and a marker for disobedience among the citizenry.

The pattern of cannabis proving medically useful but getting banned continued in various parts of the world throughout the Middle Ages. In Islamic Egypt, according to Russo, "While many derided its psychoactive effects on the basis of a ban on intoxicants in Muslim sharia law, a begrudging acknowledgment was frequently made of its abundant medical attributes."

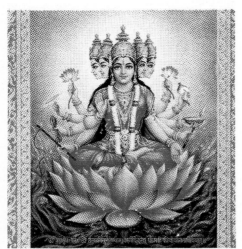

LET US TAKE HIGHER   Phone : 13863

EDEN HASHISH CENTRE
Oldest & Favourite Shop In Town Serving You
The Best Nepalese Hash & Ganja

Hindu deity Shiva has long been associated with cannabis.

An Egyptian king imposed a prohibition in the 13th century, but by the time Napoleon invaded Egypt in 1798, use of the herb was widespread and the French saw fit to impose a ban of their own. Thirty years later a French physician, Aubert-Roche, reported that during an outbreak of plague in Alexandria, cannabis alleviated fever, agitation, pain, bronchitis, and insomnia. And so the pendulum kept swinging between proscription and prescription.

Cannabis in the Medical Literature

England, like France, discovered medical cannabis via its colonies. The news was imparted by a brilliant Irish-born, Edinburgh-educated physician named William Brooke O'Shaughnessy. The British East India Company sent O'Shaughnessy to Calcutta in the 1830s. He was a young star, having already won accolades for devising an effective treatment for cholera—electrolyte replacement therapy—which would give rise to intravenous drug delivery.

In India, O'Shaughnessy observed that doctors were using "gunjah" extracts to treat a wide range of medical problems, including some for which Western medicine had no useful treatments. He studied the relevant literature, conducted animal studies, and tested the effects of cannabis on himself before treating

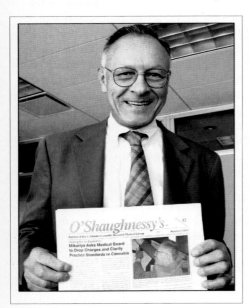

Dr. Tod Mikuriya holds the first issue of O'Shaughnessy's, *which he cofounded with Fred Gardner.*

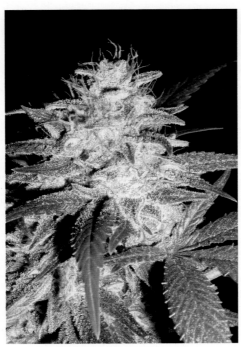

'Sensi Star' is a Cannabis afghanica *variety with a high THC content.*

patients. In 1839 O'Shaughnessy presented his findings in a paper published in the *Transactions of the Medical and Physical Society of Bengal*: "On the Preparations of the Indian Hemp, or Gunjah (*Cannabis Indica*)."

At a hospital in Calcutta, O'Shaughnessy treated patients with rheumatism, hydrophobia, cholera, tetanus, and epilepsy "in which a preparation of Hemp was employed with results which seem to me to warrant our anticipating from its more extensive and impartial use no inconsiderable addition to the resources of the physician."

O'Shaughnessy's cannabis preparation—an alcohol extract—alleviated the symptoms of all three rheumatism patients in his clinical trial. Cannabis saved the lives of the tetanus patients (though one died of gangrene), and spared the hydrophobia patients the terrible agonies associated with rabies. It reduced diarrhea in the cholera patient. And as for the baby girl who was seen at 40 days with "infantile convulsion," O'Shaughnessy reported, "The child is now in the enjoyment of robust health and has regained her natural plump and happy appearance." O'Shaughnessy thought

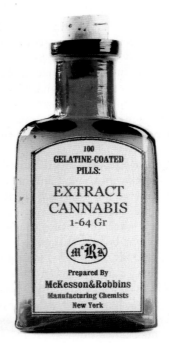

Gelatin-coated cannabis pills produced by McKesson & Robbins, one of the many US drug companies marketing cannabis extracts prior to prohibition in 1937

Indian hemp held greatest promise as an anticonvulsant.

In 1841 O'Shaughnessy returned to Great Britain carrying his message and, equally important, *C. indica* seeds of the narrow-leaf drug type. Plants of the narrow-leaf hemp type had been widely grown for fiber in Britain, but the narrow-leaf drug type was hitherto unavailable. Its arrival, and the publication in 1843 of O'Shaughnessy's findings and recipes in the *Provincial Medical Journal*, enabled chemists to produce potent tinctures for use as doctors and patients saw fit. Western medicine had come to employ cannabis.

"The use of cannabis derivatives for medicinal purposes spread rapidly throughout Western medicine," wrote Tod Mikuriya, MD, who collected and republished the early journal articles in *Marijuana: Medical Papers 1839–1972*. Prestigious physicians noted its benefits, including Johns Hopkins University's William Osler, who prescribed cannabis as the first-line treatment for migraine headaches.

Back in India the British government undertook large-scale studies to investigate "deleterious effects alleged to be produced by the abuse of ganja." In 1894 an exhaustive *Report of the Indian Hemp Drug Commission* concluded: "The general opinion seems to be that the evil effects of ganja have been exaggerated."

Prescriptions for cannabis-based medicines peaked between 1890 and 1920 in the United States. Factors in the declining market share included competition from new and inexpensive synthetic medicines such as aspirin, injectable opiates and barbiturates, and a growing disdain for "crude" herbs.

Above all was the problem of inconsistent potency. As explained by the *U.S. Dispensatory* for 1926, "Because of the great variability in the potency of different samples of cannabis it is well nigh impossible to approximate the proper dose of any individual sample except by clinical trial. Because of occasional unpleasant symptoms from unusually potent preparations, physicians have generally been overcautious in the quantities administered." In other words, inconsistent potency led to fear of overdose, which led to too-weak cannabis preparations! This helps explain why American consumers did not protest when the federal government banned "marihuana" in 1937.

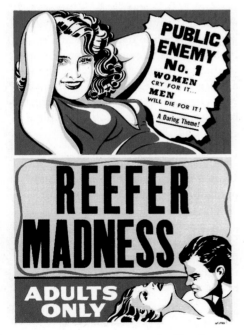

Reefer Madness is the name of a film that came to epitomize the propaganda campaign that led to federal marijuana prohibition in 1937.

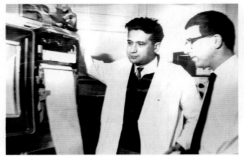

Pharmacologists Raphael Mechoulam (left) and Yechiel Gaoni worked out the exact molecular structure of THC and CBD and reported their findings in 1963 and 1964.

The only testimony against prohibition when Congress debated it came from William Woodward, MD, of the American Medical Association. Woodward argued, "The medicinal use of Cannabis, as you have been told, has decreased enormously. It is very seldom used . . . partially because of the uncertainty of the effects of the drug. That uncertainty has heretofore been attributed to variations in the potency of the preparations as coming from particular plants used . . . To say, however, as has been proposed here, that the use of the drug should be prevented by a prohibitive tax, loses sight of the fact that future investigation may show that there are substantial medical uses." How prescient!

In 1938 New York City Mayor Fiorello LaGuardia assigned the New York Academy of Medicine to investigate the claims on which federal marijuana prohibition was based. A blue-ribbon commission of scientists and physicians concluded that marijuana is not addictive and does not lead to insanity and violent crime. Copies of the "LaGuardia Commission Report" were bought up and destroyed by agents of the Federal Bureau of Narcotics.

The end of World War II was followed by almost two decades of demonization of marijuana and individuals who used it. But by the early 1960s, developments in science and society were causing cracks in the wall of prohibition. The precise molecular structures of THC and CBD were determined in 1964 by Israeli scientists Raphael Mechoulam and Y. Gaoni. That year in New York City, Bob Dylan shared marijuana with

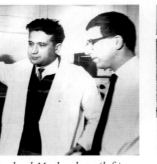

Dr. Mechoulam popularized the term "entourage effect" to describe how compounds in Cannabis work synergistically.

the Beatles, presaging an era in which millions of young people around the world—especially soldiers and students—would start smoking marijuana, evaluating its effects for themselves, and questioning the government's claims.

Anecdotal Evidence

Those who started smoking marijuana in social settings in the 1960s,'70s, and '80s were generally unaware that it had been widely prescribed as a medicine in the not-too-distant past. As Dr. Mikuriya put it, "It wasn't just marijuana that got prohibited, it was the truth about history."

Anecdotal reports of medical efficacy circulated. Seemingly everyone knew someone in the VA hospital who was using marijuana for spasticity, or had an aunt who made it through chemo thanks to the herb, or a friend who said it helped him sleep. But no physicians or researchers were tracking patients who used marijuana.

In 1990, in response to the AIDS epidemic, a Vietnam vet named Dennis Peron created the San Francisco Cannabis Buyers Club. The club provided a setting in which people who were using marijuana for medical purposes could compare notes and get a sense of their numbers. Mikuriya, seeing "a unique research opportunity," signed on as medical coordinator and began interviewing members about their conditions, patterns of marijuana use, and results.

Peron's remarkable club became the headquarters for activists working to

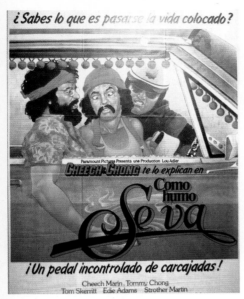

¿Sabes lo que es pasarse la vida colocado?

CHEECH-CHONG te lo explican en

Como humo Se va

¡Un pedal incontrolado de carcajadas!

Cheech Marin, Tommy Chong
Tom Skerritt, Edie Adams, Strother Martin

Cheech and Chong became icons for counterculture cannabis. Their movies and comedy routines made light of the supposed dangers associated with marijuana.

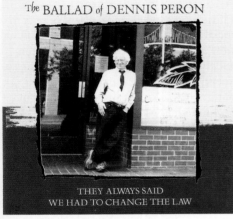

The BALLAD of DENNIS PERON

THEY ALWAYS SAID
WE HAD TO CHANGE THE LAW

Dennis Peron outside the San Francisco Cannabis Buyers Club at 1444 Market Street. In 1995 the club became the headquarters for activists planning California's medical marijuana initiative.

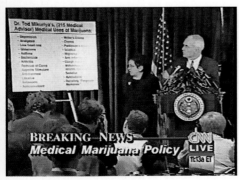

BREAKING NEWS
Medical Marijuana Policy

Clinton Administration officials led by Drug Czar Barry McCaffrey denounced Tod Mikuriya, MD, and threatened doctors who approved marijuana use by their patients after California voters passed Proposition 215 in November 1996.

legalize marijuana for medical use. They drafted "Proposition 215," a ballot measure that would allow patients with a doctor's approval to use cannabis medicinally. California voters passed Prop. 215 in November 1996 by a 56 to 44 percent margin—over the opposition of law enforcement and every elected official in the state, except for Terence Hallinan, district attorney of San Francisco.

At Dr. Mikuriya's urging, the new law had been written to cover not just patients suffering from a few grave conditions, but also those with "any other condition for which marijuana provides relief."

In December 1996, US drug czar Barry McCaffrey and Attorney General Janet Reno threatened to revoke prescription-writing licenses of California doctors who dared to approve marijuana use by patients. At a widely publicized press conference, McCaffrey pointed mockingly to a large chart entitled "Dr. Tod Mikuriya's (215 Medical Advisor) Medical Uses of Marijuana." McCaffrey said it was patently absurd that one drug could be effective in treating so many conditions. "This isn't medicine," he scoffed, "it's a Cheech and Chong show."

The American Civil Liberties Union and the reform group now known as the Drug Policy Alliance backed a suit by AIDS specialist Marcus Conant, MD, to prevent the government from carrying out its threat. The federal courts agreed with the plaintiffs that doctors and patients have a Constitutional right under the First Amendment to discuss marijuana as a treatment option.

The Endocannabinoid System

As the legal/political conflict was playing out, vindication for Mikuriya came from scientists studying how cannabis exerts its effects. In 1990— just as the Cannabis Buyers Club was forming in San Francisco—a group of scientists met in Crete and launched the International Cannabis Research Society. The "C word" in the group's name would be changed to "Cannabinoid" in 1998 because, as one researcher explained, "The field is moving away from the plant."

The ICRS members were mostly pharmacologists and biochemists employed at academic research centers. Almost all received or coveted funding from the US National Institute on Drug Abuse (NIDA), an agency whose stated goal for years has been to prove the harmfulness of marijuana. The scientists' Holy Grail was a drug that exerts the beneficial effects of cannabis without causing any psychoactivity.

In their search for such a drug, the researchers discovered the body's endocannabinoid signaling system— compounds made in the body that activate endogenous receptors that also respond to plant cannabinoids.

The predominant cannabinoids in *Cannabis* plants are CBD and THC. CBD, which is not psychoactive, predominates in hemp—plants bred for fiber and/or seed. CBD was identified in the early 1940s by Roger Adams, a University of Illinois chemist, but he did not work out its precise molecular structure.

After the discovery of endocannabinoids, CBD and THC were renamed "phytocannabinoids"—compounds found in the plant, almost all consisting of 21 carbon atoms in ring structures and side-chains, with atoms of hydrogen and oxygen attached at different points.

About 100 phytocannabinoids have been identified to date, including some biologically active ones that might have medical potential. (Some cannabinoids are fleetingly created when plant material is being analyzed, others are created by enzymes that metabolize the plant compounds.)

In addition to phytocannabinoids, the *Cannabis* plant biosynthesizes hundreds of chemical substances that are not unique to it, some of which are biologically active—including terpenes and flavonoids that provide smell, taste, and color. Three flavonoids have been found that are unique to *Cannabis*: cannflavin-A, -B, and -C.

Endogenous ("endo-") cannabinoids are made in our bodies for sending signals from one nerve cell to another. These compounds in animals preceded the plant cannabinoids in order of evolutionary appearance. Endocannabinoids and phytocannabinoids exert similar effects when tested on lab animals: reduction of pain, body temperature, spontaneous activity, and motor control.

Synthetic compounds that exert these effects are also classified as cannabinoids. In 1974, Eli Lilly produced nabilone, a synthetic form of THC that was marketed as Cesamet (and reintroduced years later as Nabilone). In the mid 1980s Pfizer produced a synthetic compound, CP-55940, which proved too psychoactive to market as a medicine. But unlike THC, which is not water-soluble and exerts a weak, fleeting effect, CP-55940 can be handled in aqueous solution, and binds long enough to reveal where in the body it acts. This was a great boon to research.

The existence of cannabinoid receptors in the brain was established in 1988 by William Devane working in the lab of Alynn Howlett at St. Louis University. The receptors are proteins embedded in cell membranes. Endocannabinoids or phytocannabinoids binding to them induce a cascade of molecular events within the cells.

These receptors, later dubbed CB1 receptors, are concentrated in the cerebellum and the basal ganglia (regions responsible for motor control, which may explain why marijuana reportedly eases muscle spasticity); in the hippocampus (storage of short-term memory); and in the limbic system (emotional control). Cannabinoids acting through the CB1 receptors play a role in the processes of reward, cognition, and pain perception, as well as motor control

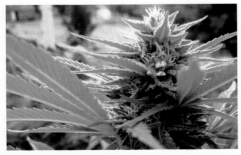

'Sour Tsunami', bred by Lawrence Ringo in Humboldt County, is a CBD-dominant variety. Ringo made stabilized seeds widely available to medical users..

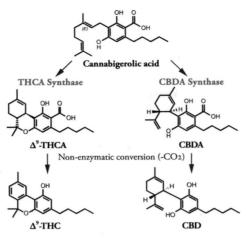

Plant cannabinoids have 21 carbon molecules with oxygen and hydrogen attached at various locations.

In 1992 a second cannabinoid receptor was found in cells of the spleen, white blood cells, and other "peripheral" areas of the body. The discovery of the CB2 receptor renewed hope that effective non-psychoactive drugs involving the immune system—not the brain or central nervous system—could be developed.

Also in '92, Devane and Lumir Hanas, working in Mechoulam's lab at Hebrew University in Jerusalem identified the first endogenous cannabinoid— a relatively simple molecule called N arachidonylethanolamine (AEA) They named it "anandamide" after the Sanskrit word for bliss. Anandamide works at the CB1 and CB2 receptors. Its effects are duplicated by THC. Also in Mechoulam's lab, in 1994, Shimon Ben-Shabat found a second endogenous cannabinoid , 2-AG (2 arachidonoylglycerol),which also binds to both the CB1 and CB2 receptors. Unlike anandamide, which is a relatively weak agonist, 2-AG is generally a full agonist at the CB1 receptor.

Anandamide and 2-AG are unusual neuromodulators in that they work by a process called "retrograde signaling." Conventional neurotransmitters—serotonin, dopamine, etc.— cross the gap (synapse) between a "presynapic" sending cell and a "postsyapic" receive cell. Endocannabinoids are made on demand in the postsynaptic neuron and sent back across the synapse to tell the sending cell to tone it down or speed it up.

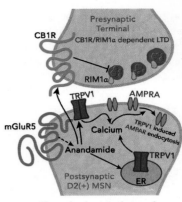

A nerve cell sends chemical signals across a gap - the synapse- to activate a receiving cell. Endocannabinoids are made of the membrane of the receiving cell and sent back across the synapse to adjust the rate of transmission.

Photo © 2012 Macmillan Publishers Ltd.

Anandamide and 2-AG restore balance— homeostasis—by inhibiting nerve cells firing too intensely and disinhibiting nerve cells firing too sluggishly. Think of a conductor facing an orchestra and directing the tempo and volume at which the instruments produce their sounds. The endocannabinoid system is the master tone-setter of the body.

Endocannabinoids send their stay-on-an-even-keel signals in systems that regulate appetite, movement, learning (and forgetting), perception of pain, immune response and inflammation, neuroprotection, and other vital processes.

The fact that endocannabinoid signaling is part and parcel of every physiological process explains why cannabinoid intake—inhaling cannabis vapor, for example—can benefit patients dealing with any of the symptoms and medical conditions on Tod Mikuriya's infamous list. The scientists have explained what he observed and reported!

At the 2013 meeting of the International Association for Cannabinoid Medicines, Raphael Mechoulam approvingly quoted a paper that concluded "modulating endocannabinoid activity may have therapeutic potential in almost all diseases affecting humans."

At each yearly meeting of the International Cannabinoid Research Society there has been increased emphasis on therapeutic applications and less on drug-abuse liability. Studies submitted for presentation at the 2014 meeting reflected renewed interest in the cannabis plant itself.

What the Doctors Have Learned

California's 1996 medical marijuana initiative did not create a record-keeping system because Dennis Peron and his coauthors did not want to generate a master list of cannabis users that federal prosecutors could consult if and when they chose to. So, for all the years since, a vast public health experiment has been conducted without any state agency tracking it.

In 2006, ten years after medical use had been legalized, Mikuriya surveyed 30 doctors who had attended meetings of the California Cannabis Research Medical Group (which he had organized in 2000). He published the results in *O'Shaughnessy's*, a journal he cofounded with one of us (Fred Gardner) in 2003.

Approximately 160,000 patients had been authorized to use the herb by the doctors surveyed. Unanimously, the doctors were struck by the extent to which cannabis enabled patients to reduce their intake of prescription and over-the-counter drugs. As Mikuriya put it: "Opioids, sedatives, NSAIDS, and SSRI antidepressants are commonly used in smaller amounts or discontinued. These are all drugs with serious adverse effects."

Dr. Robert Sullivan, one of the first MDs to offer cannabis consultations in Orange County, California, reported that his patients had cut down on "opiates, muscle relaxants, antidepressants, hypnotics (for sleep), anxiolytics, neurontin, anti-inflammatories, anti-migraine drugs, GI meds, prednisone (for asthma, arthritis)." Cannabis was proving to be the anti-drug.

Reports of cannabis-using pain patients reducing their opioid intake by 50 percent jibe perfectly with studies showing that lab animals need half the opioids to achieve pain relief when also treated with a cannabinoid. Is it any wonder that synthetic drug manufacturers see the medical use of cannabis as a threat to their profit margins?

What of the alleged adverse effects, including addiction, on which marijuana prohibition rests? Dr. Philip Denney said of the ten-year survey: "Virtually none reported by patients, except contacts with the legal system. Patients are able to easily stop using cannabis in order to pass drug tests or when traveling. Overdose from edible cannabis—an unpleasant drowsiness lasting six to eight hours—is rare and transient."

Dr. Frank Lucido responded that "decreased productivity" caused two patients to stop using cannabis. But, he added, "the overwhelming majority report that they are more productive when their symptoms are controlled with cannabis." Employers please take note.

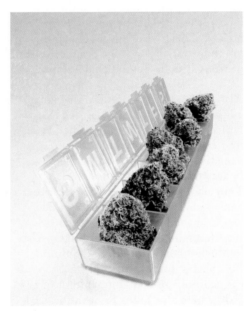

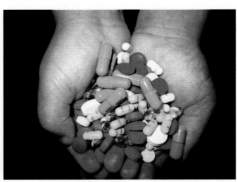

Cannabis flowers available at dispensaries have enabled patients in medical marijuana states to reduce or entirely stop use of synthetic pharmaceuticals that have adverse side-effects.

The CBD Era

The passage of Proposition 215 in California encouraged people around the world to press for access to medicinal cannabis. Multiple Sclerosis (MS) patients in England began lobbying the Health Ministry with increased urgency. In the spring of 1997, MS patients held a public meeting in London that caught the attention of pharmaceutical entrepreneur Geoffrey Guy, MD, who pledged to help them achieve their goal.

Guy observed that cannabis being used in England by MS patients and others reporting medical benefit contained substantial amounts of CBD as well as THC. The reduced psychoactivity of CBD-rich cannabis would be a key selling point when he pitched the Home Office his plan to produce a pharmaceutical-grade cannabis medicine. His company, GW Pharmaceuticals, was duly licensed to cultivate *Cannabis* for this purpose in the spring of 1998.

To achieve marketing approval, GW's extracts would have to be produced with near-perfect consistency and show safety and efficacy in clinical trials. Guy's first step had been to purchase the genetically diverse plant collection of Hortapharm, a Dutch firm founded in the 1980s by American ex-pats David Watson and Robert Clarke.

It was they who had the insight that CBD and compounds other than THC had significant effects. They traveled the globe collecting 'land-race' strains, some with substantial amounts of these previously disregarded 'minor' cannabinoids.' Watson and Clarke also understood that the terpenoids that give Cannabis varieties their aromas exerted effects when ingested.

GW set about growing thousands of plants in sophisticated glasshouses in the southeast of England. In addition to developing high-THC and high-CBD strains, GW grew plants rich in cannabichromene (CBC), cannabigerol (CBG) and tetrahydrocannabivarin (THCV) to test for medical effects. In recent years cannabidivarin (CBDV) has become a compound of interest to the company.

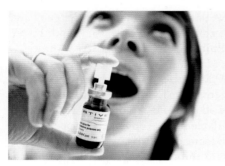

Sativex from GW Pharmaceuticals, a sub lingual cannabinoid spray, consists of approximately equal amounts of CBD and THC.

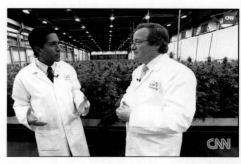

Drs. Sanjay Gupta and Geoffrey Guy at the GW Pharmaceuticals cultivation facility. GW is seeking FDA approval for Sativex (to treat intractable cancer pain) and Epidiolex (for pediatric epilepsies).

Harborside supplied the lab with a steady stream of samples to test for mold and to analyze for levels of THC, CBD, and CBN.

It turned out that CBD-rich cannabis was not as rare in California as experts had predicted. *O'Shaughnessy's* reported that about one in 600 samples brought to Steep Hill and other labs in 2009 held 4 percent or more CBD. ProjectCBD was created to report what doctors, patients, growers, and manufacturers were learning about CBD-rich medicines.

P.S. (Post Sanjay)

In August 2013, Sanjay Gupta, MD, narrated a documentary on CNN in which he acknowledged that we all had been "systematically miseducated" about marijuana. The show provided dramatic examples of cannabis exerting beneficial effects. Most memorable was the story of a five-year old, Charlotte Figi, afflicted with a severe form of epilepsy.

Charlotte's seizures had escalated as conventional treatments failed. Her mom in Colorado Springs and her dad, a Special Forces sergeant deployed to Afghanistan, did research online and

By 1999 GW was producing its flagship medicine, Sativex—a whole plant extract formulated for spraying under the tongue. Sativex contains approximately equal amounts of CBD and THC, plus trace amounts of all other compounds produced by the plant. GW initiated clinical trials and began providing Sativex and other cannabis extracts to researchers. Their findings, reported in journal articles and at conferences in the years that followed, suggested that CBD could ease symptoms of rheumatoid arthritis, diabetes, epilepsy, alcoholism, PTSD, antibiotic-resistant infections, and neurological disorders. CBD also demonstrated neuroprotective and anticancer effects. People using Sativex decreased their use of opiates and other pharmaceutical drugs. Sativex produced fewer and milder side effects than pure THC (Marinol).

In April 2005, Sativex won conditional approval from Health Canada as a treatment for pain in MS. The UK and some 20 other countries have approved Sativex for treatment of spasticity in MS. Sativex is currently undergoing clinical trials as a treatment for cancer pain in the USA and other countries.

For many years it was assumed that CBD had been bred down to trace levels in all *Cannabis* being grown in the USA for medical and recreational purposes. Because no analytic chemistry labs were testing cannabis samples, there was no way to assess cannabinoid content. This situation changed in the winter of 2008–2009 when Steve DeAngelo, director of Oakland's Harborside Health Center, encouraged two erstwhile growers, David Lampach and Addison DeMoura, to launch a lab, aptly named Steep Hill.

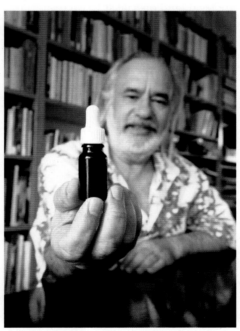

Wernard Bruining founded the first coffee shop in Amsterdam, Mellow Yellow, in 1972. Today he is the Dutch vanguard for medical cannabis. Visit his site, www.mediwiet.nl for more information.

Photo by Lika Bruining.

learned about cannabis as an anticonvulsant. Paige Figi obtained buds from dispensaries, and a friend taught her how to extract oil for Charlotte. A CBD-rich variety provided seizure relief, but Paige could not get resupplied.

In February 2012 she met Joel Stanley, who, with his brothers, grew marijuana for their own dispensaries and had a hemp strain that worked miraculously well for Charlotte. The Stanleys renamed their plant "Charlotte's Web" and offered to grow it in large quantities for the Figis and others in need. When Sanjay Gupta visited their greenhouse, one of the Stanley brothers pointed to a Charlotte's Web plant and claimed, "There's nothing like this in the world. This plant is 21 percent CBD and less than 1 percent THC."

Fortunately, there are other cannabis plants with CBD:THC ratios greater than 20:1, and they are being grown in California and other states where it is legal to do so. Nor is it clear that the higher the CBD-to-THC ratio, the more effective the medicine. There may be an optimal ratio for treating each illness and each individual. Terpenoid and flavonoid content will influence the effects of any given cannabis-based medicine. A challenging research opportunity presents itself to doctors and patients, growers and medicine makers.

The federal Farm Bill of 2014 legalized cultivation of "industrial hemp"containing 0.3 percent THC or less for research purposes. This enabled the Stanley Brothers to grow 36,000 Charlotte's Web plants—now bred to contain 30:1 CBD-to-THC—on 17 acres, and to

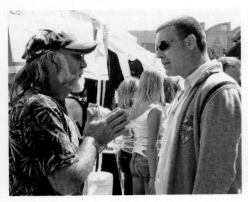

Lawrence Ringo (left) and Jaime Carion ('Cannatonic' breeder, Resin Seeds) at the High Times Medical Cannabis Cup in San Francisco. Nobody did more to expedite and expand the availability of CBD-rich plants for medical use than these two men.

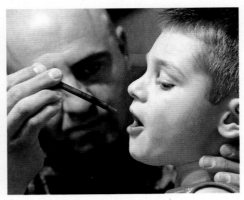

Jason David provided CBD-rich oil from Oakland's Harborside Health Center to his son Jayden, who achieved seizure relief. News of Jayden's improvement inspired Charlotte Figi's parents to seek CBD in Colorado. Photo from Braverman Productions.

now plan to grow plants in Uruguay and other foreign countries, and send the oil back to patients in the USA.

GW Pharmaceuticals is seeking FDA approval for Epidiolex, a CBD extract devoid of THC. Epidiolex was made available in 2014 to epilepsy specialists conducting Investigational New Drug (IND) programs at hospitals in the USA, involving some 200 children. More than half experienced significantly fewer and less severe seizures. About 15 percent were unhelped, and about 15 percent were seizure free. A similar pattern has been reported by Bonni Goldstein, MD, and Margaret Gedde, MD, physicians who treat hundreds of children using CBD-rich cannabis for epilepsy in Los Angeles and Colorado Springs, respectively.

redefine their extract as CW Hemp Oil. Several thousand hemp plants were also grown in Kentucky for medical use. "Industrial hemp" is providing more than food and fiber. A bill to remove CBD and hemp from the Controlled Substances Act has been introduced in Congress.

Hundreds of parents of children with epilepsy, cancer, and other serious illnesses have moved to Colorado in hopes of obtaining Charlotte's Web. A nonprofit called Realm of Caring, cofounded by Paige Figi, counsels families who are using the Stanley Brothers' product, maintains a waiting list of prospective clients, and acts as an educational resource. In 2014, eleven states passed bills legalizing cannabis containing minute amounts of THC. Prohibitionists see these so-called CBD-only bills siphoning support from bills that would legalize THC for medical

use (as happened in Florida in November 2014). Advocates see them as a first step toward more comprehensive legislation.

Numerous companies are producing and distributing cannabis-based medicines in the USA and overseas. The boldest sell CBD-rich products through the mail and online. Although CBD remains on Schedule One of the federal Controlled Substances Act, hemp food products containing less than 0.3 percent THC are legal (and on sale at Costco).

Federal regulators have not moved against companies importing medical products containing larger amounts of CBD extracted from hemp plants grown legally overseas. The Stanley Brothers—who were advised in 2014 against shipping Charlotte's Web Hemp Oil from Colorado to patients in other states—

Project CBD organizer Martin Lee says, "How ironic that the prohibition of cannabis, presented to Congress and a gullible public as a way to protect children from a deadly vice, is crumbling because children are in dire need of cannabis as medicine."

The doctors group organized by Tod Mikuriya in 2000, now known as the Society of Cannabis Clinicians, had more than 100 members as of June 2014. The SCC has been headed since 2009 by Jeffrey Hergenrather, MD, a founding member. "Doctors' and patients' understanding of how cannabis works has advanced significantly in recent years," he says. "Now it's time for the medical schools to acknowledge the endocannabinoid system."

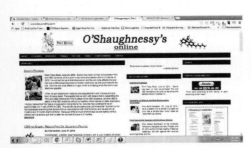

O'Shaughnessy's, online at www.beyondthc.com, covers the ongoing history of the medical marijuana movement.

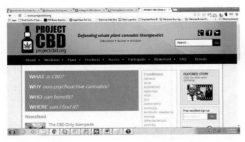

ProjectCBD.org reports on the availability of CBD and what scientists, doctors, patients, and growers are learning about it.

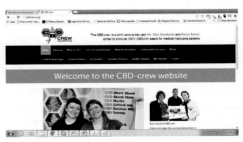

The CBD Crew, a partnership between Mr. Nice and Resin Seeds, produces CBD-rich varieties.

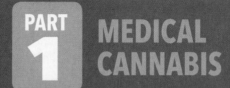

2 MEASURING CANNABINOIDS

By Samantha Miller, President and Chief Scientist of Pure Analytics Cannabis Laboratory

WITH THE RISE of the medical cannabis dispensary, several other types of businesses and service providers have evolved to help support their needs, including laboratories that test products for the medical cannabis industry. Prior to the existence of medical cannabis legalization, cannabis testing was restricted to analysis conducted as part of criminal investigation or within one of only a few research programs, such as the one at the University of Mississippi, overseen by Dr. Mahmoud ElSolhy, or, in Israel, that of Dr. Raphael Mechoulam, which perform government-sanctioned research.

Today the development and advancements of independent cannabis testing laboratories in states with medical and recreational cannabis legalization represent exciting progress both in the pursuit of medical-grade cannabis grown and processed to specified standards. Exciting, too, is the foundation of a powerful tool for the independent cannabis farmer to drive strategic breeding programs focused on isolating traits of interest and increasing potency in a predictive way using testing in the vegetative stage to assist selection of plants for breeding or growing. See "Cannabinoid Potency Testing as a Tool for the Farmer and Breeder," on page 29.

Several types of testing are performed by laboratories specializing in cannabis analytics to support the medical dispensary model, including cannabinoid potency testing; microbiological screening for molds, fungi, and bacteria; and pesticides testing that looks for residues of harmful

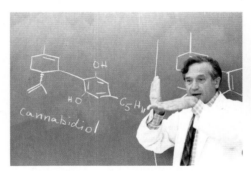

Dr. Mechoulam lecturing at the Hebrew University of Jerusalem

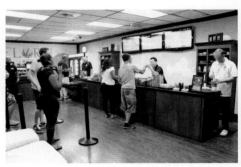

The medical cannabis dispensary, Florin Wellness Center (FWC), is doing a brisk business in this photo snapped by Paul Clemons.

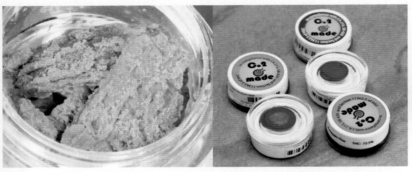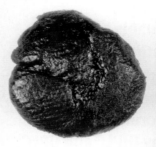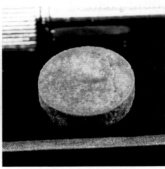

Various cannabis concentrates (left to right): wax, shatter, bubble-hash, and pressed kief (hash).

chemicals that may have been applied during the growth cycle. As testing services and legalized cannabis have proliferated and the marketplace of products has quickly evolved and changed, so have the offerings by cannabis laboratories. Many laboratories now offer testing for flavors and fragrance compounds (known as terpenes) contained in cannabis. The gravitation toward chemically extracted concentrates known as wax, shatter, dabs, and more has also resulted in the demand for specific services such as residual solvent testing and testing for toxic impurities found in low-grade butane, propane, and CO_2 gas often used to make wax. In regions where regulation is in keen focus, you will also find state-imposed requirements, such as in Nevada, mandating heavy-metals testing and residual fertilizer and nutrient testing.

The first US cannabis lab opened in Colorado. Many others quickly followed, the majority in California where the burgeoning dispensary market saw the proliferation of hundreds of dispensaries within a single city, almost overnight. The most common type of testing performed by cannabis laboratories is cannabinoid potency testing. Potency testing provides medical cannabis patients with important information on the active compounds in their cannabis. This can help them select the right cannabis for them based on their specific ailment, telling them which active compounds are present and their relative amounts. Cannabinoids commonly tested for include THC, THCA, CBD, CBDA, CBN, CBC, and CBG, and soon will include THCV and CBDV, thanks

to the efforts of chemical manufacturing companies supporting the specific needs of the cannabis testing industry.

American cannabis laboratories are limited in the cannabinoids they can legitimately include in their analysis, depending on which cannabinoids are available for purchase as certified reference standards from chemical standards companies in the USA. At the time of this book's publication, the cannabinoid reference standards available in the USA for use by analysts include: THC, THCA, CBD, CBDA, CBG, CBN, CBDV, and CBC. These reference standards are purified cannabinoids in solution, and are used to calibrate the equipment used to measure potency. These certified reference solutions are what allow the chemist to identify and quantify the cannabinoids present in an extract. When equipment is properly calibrated using certified reference standards, two different labs should be able to measure the same extracted cannabis and provide a similar result. Some cannabis labs choose to report on cannabinoids based on theoretical data rather than verification of identity and amount based on the use of a certified chemical reference standard. Such a practice may be acceptable in a research setting but it is not acceptable in a patient-oriented setting where service providers should be operating under the same standards "as if" they were being regulated by the federal government and their analyses "certified." However, in a crowded and highly competitive marketplace of service providers, many will "reach" to claim they can provide services or analyze for certain compounds such as exotic and rare cannabinoids that others cannot

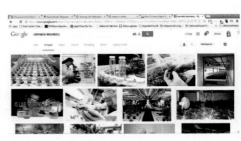

Finding a cannabis testing lab on the Internet requires research.

in an attempt to develop a competitive advantage in the cannabis-testing marketplace. If no one else is testing for a particular compound, there is likely a reason why, and the legitimacy of the analysis may be called into question. This leads us to the importance of selecting a service provider who can provide reliable and accurate results.

Selecting a Cannabis Laboratory

As dispensaries, patients, and farmers set out to choose the service provider who is right for them, it can quickly feel like wading through a confusing litany of opinions, marketing speak, and options. Having the facts at hand about testing processes and equipment relative to your own needs can help guide you to the best service provider for your needs.

Cannabinoid potency testing has been by far the most controversial during the infancy of the independent cannabis testing lab industry in the USA. It has led to many blind tests of service providers within a region by various groups either seeking to legitimize the testing process or rather to expose flaws in the practices of cannabis testing service providers. One such "ring test,"

COMPARISON OF GC AND HPLC OR UPLC

Gas Chromatography	High-Performance Liquid Chromatography or Ultra-High-Performance Chromatography
A low-pressure stream of gas helps move the compounds to the detector	A high-pressure stream of solvent helps move compounds to the detector
Detector destroys compounds	Detector usually doesn't destroy compounds
Cannot detect cannabinoid acids	Can detect cannabinoid acids
Analysis does NOT produce significant hazardous waste. Eco-friendly	Analysis produces a lot of hazardous solvent waste

published in *O'Shaughnessy's* journal of medical cannabis in 2011, was conducted by California NORML and included the cannabis labs offering services in the state of California at the time. The results from 10 laboratories were quite revealing and reinforced the fact that the use of certified reference materials is needed in order for lab-to-lab results to be in good agreement. Those labs who "made their own" chemical reference standards rather than purchasing certified ones were found to have results that deviated significantly from the rest of the pack, whereas good agreement was seen across a handful of labs. The test brought to light several basic principles that can act as a guide in evaluating a cannabis lab. Read the complete ring test on the web at www.projectcbd.org/RingTest.html#RingTest

Understanding testing processes and equipment can help guide you in choosing service providers and testing options best suited to your needs. Different service providers specialize in different types of samples and offer different analytical options. In the unregulated environment of cannabis testing at the time of this writing, there is no specified way to perform a particular type of analysis. This leads to a variety of different methods being used, making it confusing for the patient and farmer to interpret and understand how to compare results between service providers. Knowing a few key things can help guide you in the right direction.

The Potency Testing Process
The basic steps of the potency testing process that affect the accuracy and precision of the results are:
1. sampling
2. calibration of equipment
3. quality of chemical reference standards used
4. experience and expertise of the person performing the work

Sampling can be performed at several stages in the movement of cannabis from the farmer to the patient. The product may first be sampled at the farm and provided to a dispensary that then takes a sample to submit to the lab where the cannabis is finally sampled by the lab itself. Each step along the way—as well as the handling of the sample—can influence the final potency results and whether cannabinoids such as CBN (a degradation product) are present. At each point at which it is handled and sampled, the cannabis sample must be representative of the entire quantity of material it is selected from. For the farmer with several pounds of the same strain of cannabis, taking a representative sample means making a selection of buds of various sizes from various plants and various parts of the plant. A recommended sample size to submit to the lab is 0.25 to 1 gram (0.008–0.035 oz) per pound of material.

At the lab, the sample should be cut up or ground to homogenize it or make it uniform. A portion of this homogenized sample is weighed on very sensitive scales and then extracted with solvents such as methanol or isopropyl alcohol for analysis. Scales used to weigh samples should be calibrated regularly, and a dated log of those calibrations should

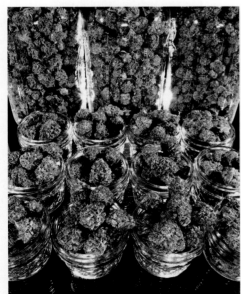

This harvest of 'Bubba Kush' buds measured from 13 to 19 percent THC. The samples were taken on different parts of the plants.

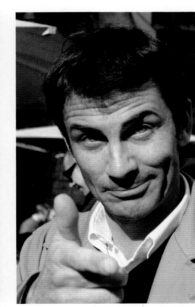

It takes more than good looks to operate scientific testing equipment.

GAS CHROMATOGRAPHY

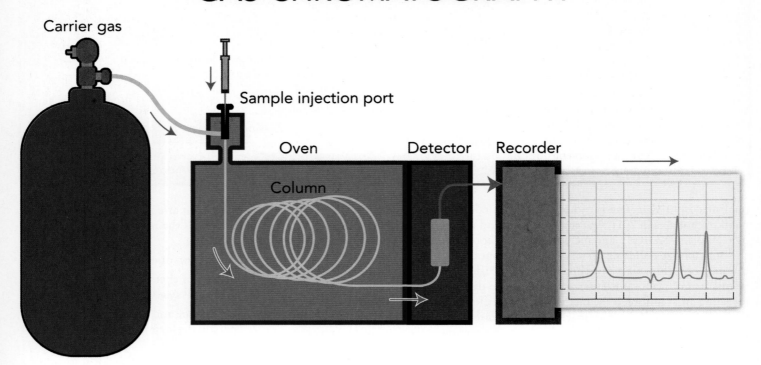

Carrier gas

Sample injection port

Oven

Detector

Recorder

Column

Sample path in a gas chromatograph

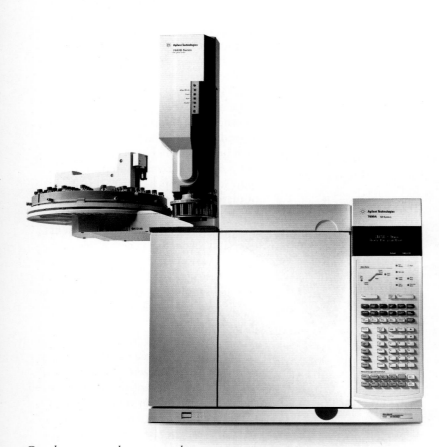

Gas chromatograph auto-sampler

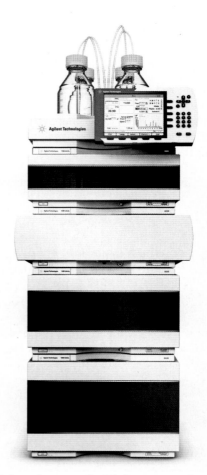

High-performance liquid chromatograph. (Ultra-high-performance liquid chromatographs have the same appearance.)

be kept. In some labs, samples are dried to zero moisture content before being weighed for analysis. Depending on how much moisture was in the plant material to begin with, this can greatly affect the results anywhere from 3 to 10 percent by weight. The extraction of the sample involves placing a measured amount of solvent in a vial with the weighed cannabis sample. Different laboratories use different solvents for their extraction. Not every solvent does a good job at completely extracting all the cannabinoids. Methanol, ethanol, and isopropanol are the best options for complete (also known as exhaustive) extraction, whereas acetone and hexane used by some service providers do not extract THC and CBD as completely. This incomplete extraction would cause an overall lowering of the potency results. After the addition of solvent, the extraction process can vary. Some may heat the sample to extract; others may sonicate using ultrasonic waves, or put in a shaker bath or table. Using an ultrasonic water bath is generally the best method for full extraction of cannabinoids. (Find a study of these solvent extraction issues at http://blog.restek.com/?p=3018.)

Depending on the type of sample being analyzed, one way of analyzing it may be more appropriate than another. Most potency and pesticide testing on cannabis samples involves analyzing the sample using some form of chromatography equipment. Two common types are gas chromatography (GC) and high-performance or ultra high-performance liquid chromatography (HPLC or UPLC). These pieces of instrumentation may be equipped with many different types of detectors. Some service providers claim to be superior based on their chosen equipment. Both types of instrumentation yield accurate and viable results when calibrated correctly and used by an experienced operator who can interpret and validate the data output.

Gas Chromatography (GC)

A gas chromatograph is a type of analytical instrumentation in which a low-pressure stream of compressed gas—often hydrogen or helium—pushes a sample from the injector to the detector of the instrument through a small-bore tube known as a column. The column in a gas chromatograph is a 15- to 30-meter length of fused silica tubing coated with various substances on the inside. These coatings and the length of the tubing cause the compounds to separate from one another in space and time as they travel through the column. In this way, samples reach the detector separately and can be measured individually. If an analysis is not performed correctly or is performed too quickly, two compounds may reach the detector at the same time and be measured as one compound, resulting in an erroneous reported result.

Gas chromatographs may be equipped with several types of detectors. The most common types of detectors for cannabis potency testing include FID (flame ionization detector), MS (mass spectrometers) and TCD (thermal conductivity detector). FIDs and MS detectors are the best choices for reliable cannabinoid analysis by GC. Pesticides analysis may include detectors such as ECD (electron capture detector), NPD (nitrogen-phosphorous detector), or PFPD (pulsed flame photometric detector).

In the case of all GC detector types, the sample extract that is injected into the instrument is often heated to temperatures between 302°F and 392°F (150°C–200°C). In order to vaporize the sample so that it may be moved from the injector onto the column by the stream of gas, the sample also is combusted when it reaches an FID detector. This sample vaporization will decarboxylate or activate any acidic cannabinoids as if they had been combusted or vaporized. In a mass spectrometer detector, the sample is ionized and fragmented in order to identify the compounds present. Sample vaporization makes gas chromatography the best option for analysis of cannabis samples meant for inhalation by combustion or vaporization. From an analytical perspective, this direct measurement of cannabinoids in their decarboxylated state best mimics the experience of the patient upon inhalation.

High-Performance and Ultra-High-Performance Liquid Chromatography (HPLC and UPLC)

High-performance and ultra-high-performance liquid chromatography are commonly referred to as HPLC and UPLC. The difference between HPLC and UPLC is the maximum pressure the instrumentation can withstand. UPLC instruments can analyze faster and still maintain accuracy in most cases as compared to HPLC. In HPLC and UPLC a high-pressure stream of solvent helps move compounds from the injector to the detector. As with GC, there are several types of detectors that are commonly used for cannabinoid analysis. UV-Vis (ultraviolet visible spectroscopy) detectors use wavelengths of light passing through the sample to measure what is there. Photodiode array (PDA) and fluorescence detectors use certain wavelengths of light to excite compounds in the detector, which are then measured as they emit photons of light falling back down to a less energetic state. HPLCs and UPLCs may also be equipped with MS detectors. These are generally a second detector in line after the PDA or UV-Vis detectors.

The measurement of cannabinoids in an HPLC or UPLC system can be conducted without vaporizing the sample using heat. As a result, analysis by HPLC or UPLC best mimics the mode of use for edible or ingestible samples. By not heating the sample during sample preparation or analysis, different cannabinoid information can be obtained to understand the properties of the sample as an ingestible form of cannabis. It is important to understand whether or not the cannabinoids are in their acidic form or decarboxylated form for the purposes of ingesting cannabis for therapeutic or recreational uses. THC-acid and CBD-acid have very different psycho-active and therapeutic properties as compared to decarboxylated THC and CBD. For example, THC-acid is non-intoxicating, while heated THC is very intoxicating when orally ingested in very small amounts. For example, one oral dose of THC is 15 mg. It is important to analyze orally ingestible samples by

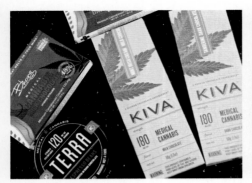

Cannabis edibles

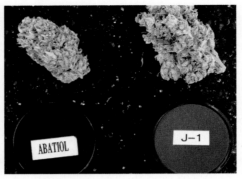

Two different cannabis buds have distinct cannabinoid profiles.

HPLC if you are unsure about whether or not the cannabinoids are decarboxylated and need to verify the content of an ingestible preparation. Many producers of ingestible cannabis preparations do not understand clearly the conditions for complete conversion of cannabinoid acids to THC and CBD, resulting in many cases of partially decarboxylated edibles and tinctures. In some cases it is important to verify that NO decarboxylation has occurred for those patients seeking to use a cannabinoid acid therapy program specifically avoiding the decarboxylated forms. You can learn more about considerations for oral ingestion of cannabinoids by visiting, www.purenalytics.net/blog.

One of the reasons it is important to restrict the use of HPLC and UPLC to specific samples where it is needed is due to the large amount of environmentally toxic hazardous waste that is produced as a result of performing analysis by HPLC. As described earlier, a high-pressure stream of solvent is used to move analyte from the injector to the detector. This stream of solvent is generally a mixture of acetonitrile and isopropyl alcohol. Its destiny is the hazardous waste bottle, so unnecessary HPLC analyses should be avoided in an effort to have low environmental impact, and use of this method restricted to ingestible samples where it is truly required. Some examples of ingestible samples include tinctures, juiced cannabis, edibles, and capsules.

Comparing Test Results – HPLC vs. GC

A second reason why HPLC and UPLC should not be used on samples meant for inhalation is that the results are not expressed in the form in which the cannabinoids will be consumed when heated and inhaled, the decarboxylated forms THC and CBD, and can give the perception of higher potency than the cannabis contains. For patients on a specific dosage regimen, it is important to be able to accurately calculate THC and CBD consumed. Results from HPLC and UPLC analysis will show THCA, THC, CBDA, and CBD in addition to other cannabinoids such as CBN and CBG. Many laboratories that use HPLC/UPLC for cannabinoid analysis of flowers express their final results as THC=THCA + THC in a sample. This can be confusing to the consumer because the THCA value is not properly mathematically converted to its equivalent amount of decarboxylated THC. THC is the form that will be experienced by the user when smoked or vaporized, thus the potency measure for cannabis intended for inhalation should be in the neutral or THC form rather than THCA because of this.

Expressing results as THC+THCA can cause the expression of "THC" results higher than what the user will experience with smoking or vaporizing because of the following considerations: THCA and CBDA are heavier molecules than THC and CBD. To express the total decarboxylated THC that a sample may have in it, you must first adjust the THCA value by multiplying THCA or CBDA by a factor of 0.88 to account for this difference in molecular weight. Understanding the conversions in the figure below can help you compare results that were generated by HPLC/UPLC and

GC. You should also consider whether or not the results are expressed on a dry-weight basis as well. You should know how the lab you are using calculates and reports results so you know if you have to perform any of the conversions noted below to make the results meaningful for the way you'll be using the cannabis.

To convert THCA to THC:
- Multiply the THCA value by 0.88%
- Example: 21% THCA × 0.88 = 18.5% THC

To convert THC to THCA:
- Multiply the THCA value by 1.14
- Example: 17% THC × 1.14 = 19.4% THCA

The same applies to CBDA and CBD

As you can see, depending on your sample type (flower, concentrate, edible, or tincture), one type of equipment may provide more meaningful results, depending on your use of cannabis.

- Cannabis for inhalation samples such as flowers and concentrates to be *smoked or vaporized* should be analyzed by GC
- Cannabis for oral *ingestion* should be analyzed by HPLC or UPLC if state of decarboxylation is unknown or unverified
- When evaluating test results, you should know if they are expressed in terms of:
  - Acid forms or decarboxylated forms
  - Dry weight or full moisture

Many patients and farmers wonder what results are typical and how the information varies by strain:

Potency Rating	THC Potency (% by weight)
mild	3–10
moderate	10–16
strong	17–20
very strong	21+

Typical THC results for cannabis flowers
- Ranges from mild to very strong
- Average: 16.5 percent

Potency Rating	CBD Potency (% by weight)
low	0–2
moderate	3–5
high	6–20

Typical CBD results for cannabis flowers

Often not found in significant amounts

Always accompanied by THC

CBD-rich: >4% CBD by weight

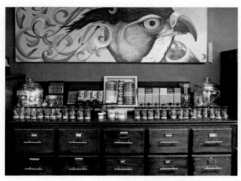
Medical cannabis dispensaries like the Abatin Wellness Center in Sacramento, California, are well stocked.

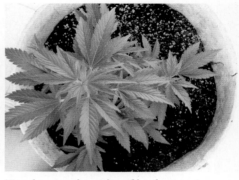
Test the cannabinoid profile of vegetative plants to see if they are candidates for a breeding program.

Alternate Methods of Potency Testing: Thin-Layer Chromatography (TLC)

Thin-layer chromatography tests measure the cannabinoid profile for up to 6 cannabinoids: THC, THCV, CBD, CBN, CBG, CBC, and their corresponding acids. The tests cost about $10 USD each and take some practice to perform with accuracy. The sample is prepared and mixed with a solvent. A selective dye detects the cannabinoid levels and shows them on blotter paper. The results are then interpreted and compared to a chart. Every cannabinoid reacts differently with the dye, resulting in distinctive colors. Please see www.marijuanagrowing.com and www.alpha-cat.org for more information on thin-layer chromatography.

A segment of service providers presents results from TLC (thin-layer chromatography) on what are often referred to as "test strips." In some cases, these test strips are promoted as being able to provide accurate potency results for cannabis. In general, without specialized equipment, test strips are only viable for use to tell whether or not certain cannabinoids are present, but not to tell how much is present (i.e., potency).

How Patients Can Use Potency Results

Patients are often faced with a dizzying array of options in a medical cannabis dispensary. Having accurate cannabinoid potency information can help patients select the best medicinal cannabis for their ailment or condition. Knowing a bit about the different effects and medical applications of various cannabinoids can help the patient have a successful and efficacious experience. THC is the main active ingredient in cannabis, responsible for some of the intoxicating effects of cannabis. THC is often used to treat pain, nausea, insomnia, and loss of appetite—among

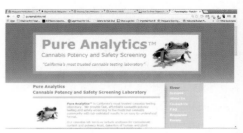
Pure Analytics developed a testing program to facilitate rapid high-CBD isolation.

many other ailments. CBD is the second most predominant cannabinoid and is considered a nonintoxicating ingredient in cannabis, although when consumed there are clear mood-altering effects for most. CBD provides relief from muscle spasms, seizures, and anxiety, is known to have antibacterial and anti-tumor activity, and prolongs the effects of THC. CBN is the degradation product of THC. The presence of CBN can indicate that a product is old or has not been stored properly. CBN forms when THC is exposed to UV light and oxygen over time. CBN does have some therapeutic properties and has been shown to lower heart rate and reduce convulsions. Cannabinoid acids such as THCA and CBDA have been reported by patients to provide relief from symptoms of spasticity and convulsions.

Cannabinoid Potency Testing as a Tool for the Farmer and Breeder

As the number of medical cannabis users remains on the rise, there is an ever-increasing demand for options with specific THC:CBD ratios. Likewise is the increasing demand for cannabis

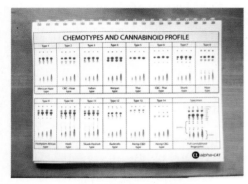
The cannabinoid profiles of 14 different varieties of cannabis are represented in this page of thin-layer chromatography tests.

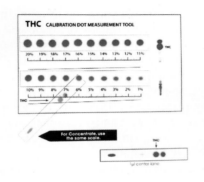
Once prepared and tested, the sample circles are measured with a plastic calibration measurement tool to discern cannabinoid levels.

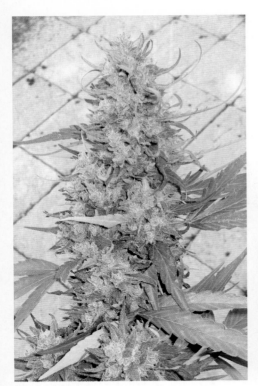

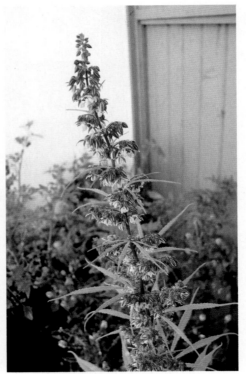

*Heavy-yielding, CBD-rich 'Cannatonic ×
Sour Tsunami' was developed using tests
provided by Pure Analytics.*

*Measure the cannabinoid content of male
plants before they bloom. Choose males with
desirable cannabinoid profiles for breeding
programs.*

with the highest potency levels, since
potency readily translates to the amount
of active compounds and the value of
the cannabis in the current marketplace.
The demand for cannabis with specific
THC:CBD ratios is often driven by a
population with a specific ailment or
disease. One such example gaining
notoriety at the moment concerns the
specific needs of children with a type
of epilepsy known as Dravet syndrome.
Reports of 400 to 800 seizures per day
have not been uncommon for these children, who also suffer from developmen-
tal, cognitive, and emotional issues. Des-
peration leads parents of these children
to pursue experimentation with cannabis
extracts as a treatment for their child's
condition. The type of cannabis required
by these children to reduce their seizures is almost entirely CBD with very
little THC. The preferred THC:CBD
ratio for most Dravet children being
medicated with cannabis is 1:20 or
greater. This type of cannabis was first
isolated and identified only about 4
years prior to publication of this book.
At that time there was only one known
plant and source. The miracle that this
particular type of cannabis represented

for the families of these children has
pushed CBD-rich cannabis toward the
mainstream, as illustrated in a CNN
documentary by Dr. Sanjay Gupta. As
a result, the demand for cannabis with
this specific THC:CBD ratio spiked.

Just as that first 1:20 strain (known as
ACDC) was first isolated, a technique
was developed in an independent cannabis lab in California based on preliminary research conducted by Pacifico
et al. in Italy that would allow the rapid
development and isolation of this rare
and now important type of cannabis.
The program was developed at Pure
Analytics for analyzing and interpreting
vegetative-stage cannabinoid data to
facilitate rapid high-CBD isolation, ratio
characterization, and CBD and THC
potency optimization, as well as the
prediction of absolute potency numbers
when plants are sampled within the correct stage of development. In the 2014
growing season alone, hundreds of 1:20
THC:CBD phenotypes were isolated
that were to be grown into plants and
made available on the medical cannabis market. This technique, when it is
performed properly and the data is inter-

preted correctly, can allow farmers to
have the crystal ball they always wanted,
to see what the flowers will produce
before they are formed.

With a vegetative-stage cannabinoid test
performed using the proprietary pro-
tocol developed by Pure Analytics Lab
in California a farmer may identify his
THC:CBD ratios early in the growth
cycle, identify plants with the highest
cannabinoid accumulation potential,
and obtain a prediction of final flower
potency. The farmer may determine
cannabinoid ratio in both males and
females, and these ratios will remain in
place through the full maturation and
flowering process of the plant. Meaning, a 1:20 cannabinoid ratio identified
in a two-week-old vegetative plant will
result in flowers with the same ratio of
THC:CBD. This technique also allows
identification of the seedlings with the
greatest cannabinoid accumulation
potential, enabling the farmer to identify
his most potent strains with desired
THC:CBD ratios while still in the vegetative stage. This is a powerful advance-
ment allowing cloning of both females
and males with desired traits in the vegetative stage to enable the strategic mass
breeding of genetically identical clones,
thus creating a more consistent resulting
seed population. For more information
on using vegetative-stage testing, visit
www.pureanalytics.net/blog.

Cannabis Safety Testing –
Pesticides, Microbiological
and Other Contaminants

While the testing of cannabinoids is
endlessly fascinating, other types of
cannabis testing are also meaningful to
the health and welfare of patients using
cannabis that they have not controlled
the production of. Many medical cannabis dispensaries test for various types
of contaminants that may be harmful to
patients. These include pesticides analysis and microbiological analysis, as well
as tests for chemical residues such as solvent, solvent impurities, heavy metals,
and nutrient residues. There are many
different ways to perform a given type
of analysis. For example, a pesticides
analysis may be performed by a variety
of different pieces of equipment.

TYPES OF INSTRUMENTATION SUITABLE FOR PESTICIDES ANALYSIS

Acronym for Equipment	Description
GC-FID	gas chromatography with flame ionization detection
GC-ECD	gas chromatography with electron capture detection
GC-MS	gas chromatography with mass spectrometer detection
GC-PFPD	gas chromatography with pulsed flame photometric detection
GC-NPD	gas chromatography with nitrogen phosphorous detection
HPLC or UPLC-UV-Vis	high- or ultra-high-performance liquid chromatography with UV-visual photometric detection
HPLC or UPLC-MS	high- or ultra-high-performance liquid chromatography with mass spectrometer detection
HPLC or UPLC-PDA	high- or ultra-high-performance liquid chromatography with photodiode array detection
HPLC or UPLC-FD	high- or ultra-high-performance liquid chromatography with fluorescence detection

For pesticides it is important that a chromatographic analysis is performed every time, and that the analysis is sensitive enough to be meaningful. There are "shortcuts" that are tempting to use because they are cheaper and faster, but they are not an adequate replacement for a full chromatographic analysis. The problem with shortcuts such as immunoassay screens or general screens using a mass spectrometer for detection is that they generally cannot achieve a detection limit that is truly meaningful relative to potential pesticide contamination. For example, if a contaminant can pose a health risk at 50 parts per billion or ug/kg, then a pesticide screen that can only detect contamination at higher levels such as 100 parts per million or mg/kg is not meaningful or particularly useful.

When comparing different approaches to pesticide analysis, you need to consider a few key areas:

5. Equipment used

6. Sensitivity of the method, also referred to as "detection limit"

7. Compounds analyzed for and reported on

8. Whether third-party-certified reference standards are used when identifying a positive hit

It is important to realize that not every type of equipment listed can see every pesticide that may have been used. Some detectors are very specific and some are more general. It follows that the more generalized the detector is, the more reduced its sensitivity to potential pesticide contamination will be. As noted earlier, unless specially configured, a mass spectrometer is not the best choice for pesticide-contamination detection due to its higher threshold of detection, meaning it likely can't see trace-level contamination. The use of mass spectrometer detection may also lead to bad habits in the lab. Pesticides analysis is not trivial, nor is it cheap to perform. To be done properly each class of pesticides should be analyzed and evaluated separately using the detector most sensitive to that class of compounds. For example, chlorinated pesticides should always be confirmed by GC-ECD (gas chromatography with electron capture detection) and phenoxyacid herbicides by HPLC-FD (high-performance liquid chromatography with fluorescence detection). They should also always be confirmed against certified reference material of the pesticide. Meaning, if myclobutanil is reported as present, myclobutanil purchased as a third-party-certified reference standard from a chemical company should have been analyzed along with the sample. If this was not done, the result was not validated. That leads us to an explanation of how the use of mass spectrometers can lead to bad habits in the lab.

Mass spectrometers are amazing pieces of equipment with immense capability to identify unknown compounds that may be in a mixture. Mass specs are equipped with access through their software to a powerful NIST (National Institute of Standards and Technology) database developed over the years by thousands of scientists who have submitted their data to the NIST. It allows one to run a search of the database relative to a datapoint from a mass spec analysis. The software searches the database and finds the closest match with a probability rating that it is a true result. This is acceptable for a preliminary identification of a contaminant but not a basis for reporting that the compound is present. It must be verified against the certified chemical standard for the same compound in order to be a legitimate result identifying a specific compound.

Here are some key questions to ask a service provider when learning about their pesticides analysis:

1. What type of equipment do you use to perform a pesticides analysis?

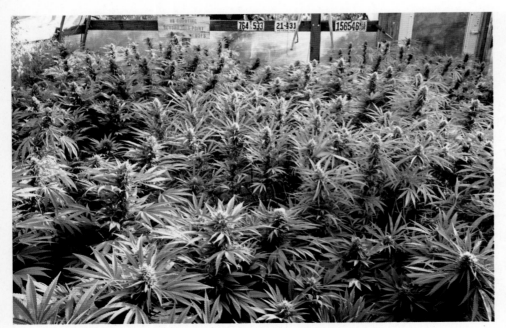

Growing organic medical cannabis is one of the best ways to avoid contaminated medicine.

coupled plasma mass spectrometer) and if done properly by defined methods offer a fairly reliable analysis. Nutrient residues may be analyzed by a variety of methods depending on what type of contamination is anticipated. ICP-MS and ion chromatography would be the two most likely approaches.

Focus on Safety – *Aspergillus* Contamination, Why It Matters

Aspergillus is a genus that consists of more than a few hundred mold species. It is found in most climates where cannabis grows. Some *Aspergillus* species can cause grave illness in animals—including humans. *Aspergillus fumigatus* and *A. flavus* are the most problematic because they produce aflatoxin, a toxin and carcinogen. Both species can contaminate cannabis—including edibles. *A. fumigatus* and *A. clavatus* species commonly cause allergic diseases. Other *Aspergillus* species frequently infect grain crops.

Pulmonary aspergillosis is usually caused by *A. fumigatus*, which results in paranasal sinus infection. The symptoms include cough, chest pain, fever, and breathlessness; these common symptoms make diagnosis difficult. Patients with asthma, cystic fibrosis, sinusitis, AIDS, weak immune systems, and weak lungs are susceptible, as are chemotherapy patients.

- *You want to hear "chromatograph" in the answer. At a minimum, all samples need a chromatography screen from one type of equipment listed on page 31. Note that not all equipment has the same sensitivity or can "see" the same compounds.*

2. Which compounds do you analyze for?
   - *They should be able to provide you a list of compounds they can detect. If a compound is not on their list, they won't "see" it in the analysis.*
   - *If the response is, "We test for everything," this may mean they are not using certified reference standards. This is the response that those performing a mass spec screen often provide. Not only are reference standards probably not being used, but it is unlikely that the detection limit is meaningful.*

3. What is your detection limit?
   - *You want to hear "parts per billion (ppb) range to low part per million (ppm) range." Detection may vary depending on which chemical it is.*
   - *This may also appear as µg/kg range to low mg/kg range.*

Microbiological analyses are also used to screen medical cannabis. The majority of service providers screen for mold and fungus contamination while others also screen for bacterial contamination, which becomes more meaningful relative to products intended for oral ingestion. Methods used to screen for microbiological contamination include microscopy, PCR analysis (polymerase chain reaction), plating and culturing with plates that can indicate classes of organisms, mycotoxin screens by TLC, and more. All but microscopy may provide false positives due to mishandling or cross-contamination of samples.

Analyses for heavy metals are usually performed using an ICP-MS (inductively

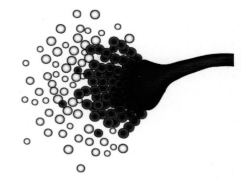

Aspergillus *mold*

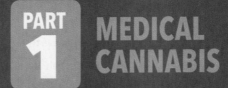

3

MEDICAL CANNABIS VARIETIES

IN 1753, CAROLUS LINNAEUS classified the plant kingdom for the Western World. In the process of doing so, Linnaeus classified and named the genus and species, *Cannabis sativa*. He concluded that the genus *Cannabis* has but one species, *sativa*. However, travel and communications were difficult in the 1750s, and Linnaeus was unaware of *C. indica* and *C. ruderalis*.

Kingdom: Plantae—all plants

Division: Magnoliopsida—magnolia class

Order: Rosales—nine families

Family: Cannabaceae—hemp family, flowering plants, about 170 species in about 11 genera

Genus: *Cannabis*—three species

Species: *indica*, *sativa*, and *ruderalis*

Varieties (misnomer of "strain"): infinite number of combinations

Here is a simple way to remember three important terms used often in this book:

Indica Sativa Ruderalis

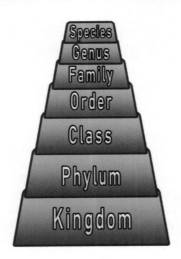

genus = last name
species = first name
variety = nickname

Qualities of Cannabis

1. Annual dioecious flowering herb
2. Imperfect flowers (dioecious) = male and female + intersex plants (aka hermaphrodites)
3. Produces cannabinoids that are concentrated in glandular trichomes which appear on foliage, primarily on floral clusters
4. Wind pollinated
5. "Short-day" plants except *C ruderalis*—equatorial varieties are possibly autoflowering and may be "day neutral"

Cannabis Varieties

Legally, all cannabis, whether rope or dope, is classified as *Cannabis sativa (C. sativa)*.* Regardless of origin, all cannabis is considered *C. sativa* under international law. However, according to *Hemp Diseases and Pests* authors Dr. J. M. McPartland, R. C. Clarke, and D. P. Watson, as well as CAB International, *Cannabis sativa* can be further classified as: *Cannabis sativa (= C. sativa var. sativa)*, *Cannabis indica (= C. sativa var. indica)*, *Cannabis ruderalis (= C. sativa var. spontanea)*, *Cannabis afghanica*

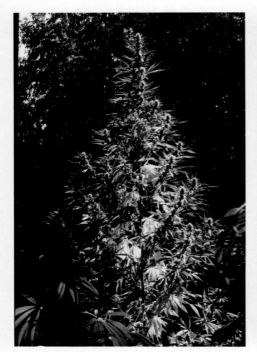

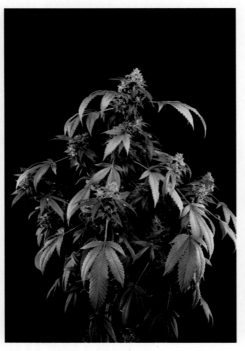

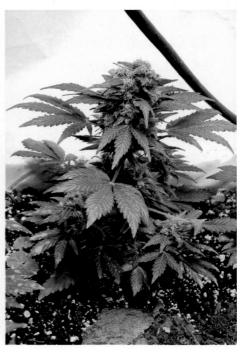

Cannabis sativa *plants tend to grow tall, with much space between internodes and narrow-blade leaves. Image by Mel Frank (MF).*

Cannabis indica *is shorter, conical in shape, and has relatively wide leaflets.*

Cannabis ruderalis *is generally short with few branches. It flowers after 3 to 5 weeks of growth, regardless of photoperiod.*

(= *C. sativa* var. *afghanica*). Each has a distinct growth pattern, look, smell, taste, etc. In this book, I have treated *C. afghanica* as a subspecies of *C. indica*. This is how it is classified by the majority of cannabis breeders and gardeners.

Cannabis sativa, C. indica, and *C. ruderalis* are most often bred together. Breeders cross the "varieties" together and select for desirable qualities in the offspring. See chapter 25, *Breeding*, for more information.

Medical cannabis gardeners grow varieties with different cannabinoid profiles. The cannabinoid profiles may change from plant to plant. Varieties with high levels of THC and CBD offer the most therapeutic value.

Cannabis sativa

Cannabis sativa (= *C. sativa* var. *sativa*) originated predominately in warmer to tropical climates of Asia, the Americas, and Africa. Each area of origin lends specific characteristics, but all *sativas* have the following general traits: tall, sometimes leggy stature with more distance between internodes than *C. indica*; a large sprawling root system,

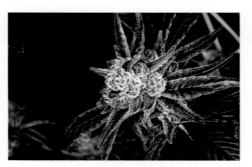

'Peyote Purple' from CannaBioGen is a good example of how C. indica *leaves can also be narrow.*

large narrow-bladed leaves that tend toward lighter shades of green; and somewhat sparse flowers, especially when grown indoors under lights or in low light conditions. Female flowers start at branch nodes and typically develop along the length of the stem and branches rather than clustering around branch nodes. Flower formation is slower and less dense than with *C. indica*. *C. sativa* flower buds enjoy more air circulation and are less prone to fungus.

Overall, *sativa* varieties bloom later than *indica* varieties. While good producers outdoors, often growing to 15 feet (4.6 m)

or taller, indoors pure *sativa* varieties often grow too tall too fast to be practical for grow-room cultivation. Some *sativa* varieties grow up to 10 feet in 3 months!

Central African *sativas*, including THC-potent 'Congolese', grow similarly to Colombian varieties with a tall leggy stature, often growing to more than 15 feet tall (4.6 m) with loosely packed buds.

South Africa has major seaports. Sailors brought *C. sativa* from many different places and planted it in South Africa. Consequently, the potency of South African cannabis can be very high or very low, and it can be short, tall, leggy, bushy, etc. The famous 'Durban Poison' yields pale-green, potent early buds and is the best-known South African variety.

Asian *sativas*, including Thai, Vietnamese, Laotian, Cambodian, and Nepalese, have diverse growth characteristics and vary significantly in potency. While Thai and other *sativas* from the area are often very potent, they are some of the most difficult to grow indoors and the slowest to mature. Thai varieties produce light, wispy buds after flowering for about

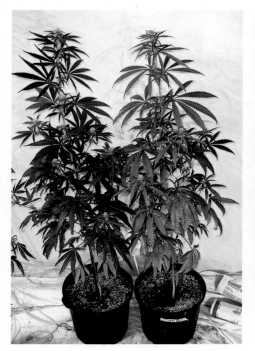

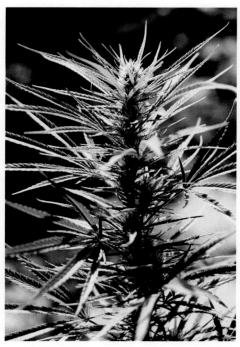

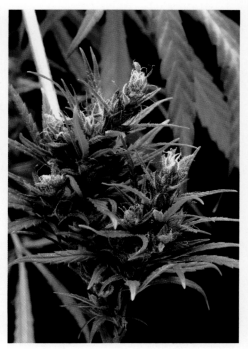

'Jamaican Grape' from Next Generation Seeds grows tall with more length between branch internodes.

Seeds from this Thai plant grown in 1976 came from a "Thai stick," a bud tied around a bamboo stick. (MF)

This South Indian landrace plant was part of a breeding program starting in 1977 by Mel Frank. (MF)

four months on plants with large, sprawling branches. Thai, Vietnamese, Cambodian, and Laotian *sativas* are more prone to grow into hermaphroditic adults.

Nepalese *sativas* can grow oversized leaves on tall, leggy plants that produce sparse, late-blooming buds, but other varieties from this region develop into short, compact plants that bloom earlier. Tetrahydrocannabinol (THC) production and potency is often quite high, but can also be second-rate.

Industrial hemp is *C. sativa*. The tall varieties produce the longest fibers for a wide range of industrial uses. Hemp, affectionately referred to as "rope," is often seeded and contains extremely low levels of THC and often very high levels of CBD.

Recreational *C. sativa* typically causes an energetic, cerebral, and inspiring effect, often followed by a desire to eat (especially sweet items)—aka "the munchies." Craving food is especially important for patients who suffer from nausea or lack of appetite while undergoing chemotherapy, HIV/AIDS treatment, and other procedures.

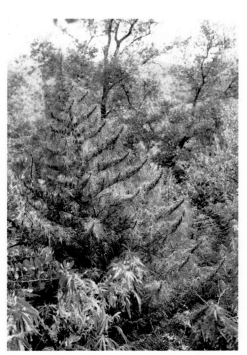

This large, robust Mexican sativa landrace was grown in 1978. (MF)

Mexican, Colombian, Thai, and Jamaican varieties can be very potent, with a high THC:CBD ratio that produces a soaring, energetic, "speedy" high. But potency can also be minimal, with low levels of THC. Most exported Colombian,

Mexican, Thai, and Jamaican cannabis is poorly treated throughout life and abused when dried and packaged. This abuse causes more rapid degradation of THC. Consequently, seeds from fair smoke are often more potent than the parent.

C. sativa varieties grown indoors have been crossbred with *C indica* to reduce their height and flowering time. *Sativa-indica* hybrids generally take a little longer to flower than pure *C. indica*.

Cannabis indica

Cannabis indica (= *C. sativa* var. *indica*) was classified by European botanist Jean-Baptiste de Lamarck in 1785 from samples he believed to be from India. Today scholars largely agree that *Cannabis indica L.* originated on the Asian subcontinent or maybe in present-day Afghanistan.

C. indica is popular among indoor, outdoor, and greenhouse gardeners and breeders for its squat, bushy growth; condensed root system; thick stout stems; broad leaves with wide blades; and dense, THC-laden, fat, heavy flowers. Typically, *indicas* grow a maximum of

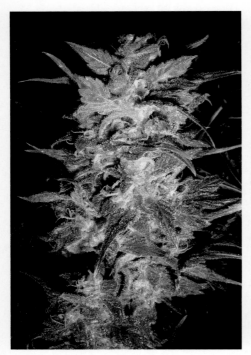

'Strawberry Cough' indica from Next Generation Seeds.

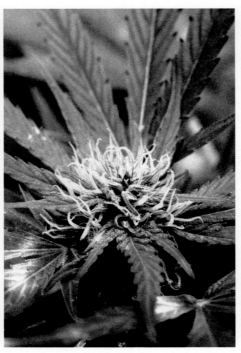

'Pink Afghani' × 'African #3' was an early Mel Frank hybrid, 1982. (MF)

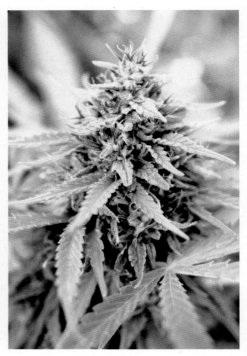

Original 'Afghani #1' from 1981 (MF)

6.5 feet (1.9 m) tall and produce more side branches than *sativas* do. Typically foliage is very dark green, and in some varieties, leaves around buds turn reddish to purple. Short, whitish stigmas may turn reddish to purple under natural sunlight. Flower formation starts around branch nodes, and thick clusters of buds develop. Dry flower weight is typically much heavier for *indicas* than *sativas*.

C. indica varieties generally contain a higher ratio of CBD:THC and often contain more CBN than *C. sativa* does. *Indicas* tend to produce more corporeal effects, often described as a more physical, relaxing, and even incapacitating "couch-lock" effect. Side effects such as dry mouth may also occur.

Some *indicas* have a distinctive odor similar to that of a skunk or cat urine, while others smell sweet and exotic. Heavily resin-laden plants tend to be the most fungus- and pest-resistant. Few *indicas* with heavy, dense, compact buds are resistant to gray (bud) mold.

Cannabis afghanica (= *C. sativa* var. *afghanica*) could be classified as a sub-species of *C. indica*. It originated near

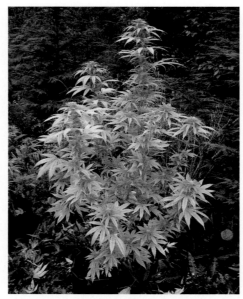

'BC Kush' from Next Generation Seeds shows classic short-and-squat growth.

present-day Afghanistan. It is quite short, seldom reaching 6 feet, with distinctive, broad, dark-green leaflets and leaves. Dense branching and short internodes, most often with long leaf stems (petioles), dominate the profile of *C. afghanica*. The most common examples of pure *C. afghanica* include the many different hash plants and Afghani

varieties. *C. afghanica* is cultivated exclusively for drugs with much of the resin being made into hashish. It is known for its high cannabinoid content. Many growers and breeders do not distinguish *C. afghanica* from *C. indica*, lumping them both into the *C. indica* category. 'Hash Plant', of which there are many, is one of the classic *C. afghanica* varieties.

Cannabis ruderalis

Cannabis ruderalis (= *C. sativa* var. *ruderalis*) (= *C. sativa* var. *spontanea*). Botanists disagree as to whether *C. ruderalis* qualifies as a separate species or subspecies. Russian botanist D. E. Janichevsky hypothesized in 1924 that *ruderalis* found in central Russia was *C. sativa* or a separate species, *C. sativa L.* var. *ruderalis* Janisch. In 1929 Nicolai Ivanovich Vavilov, a well-known plant explorer, named wild and feral populations of cannabis in Afghanistan *C. indica* Lam. var. *kafiristanica* Vav., and wild and feral populations found in Europe *C. sativa L.* var. *spontanea* Vav.

Ruderalis varieties are generally believed to have *C. indica* ancestors that acclimated to harsher climates. *C. ruderalis* is very short, from 1 to 2.5 feet (30.5–76.2 cm)

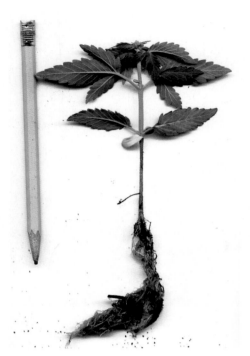

Seedling of the original 'Lowryder'.

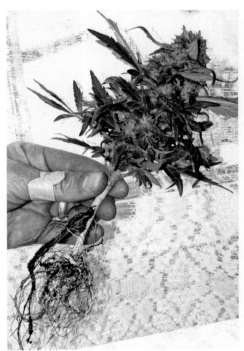

One of the first flower tops from 'Lowryder'.

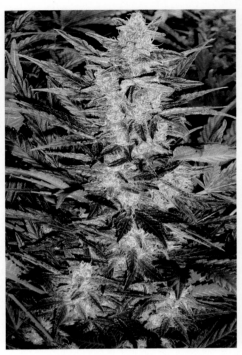

The next step in development was called 'Lowryder #2'.

tall at harvest and has a weedy, scrubby growth habit. Branching is sparse and leaves have wide blades similar to *C. indica* but are often a somewhat lighter shade of green. Stems are thick and sturdy. Flowers are small and moderately dense. Root systems are adequate to support small plants.

C. ruderalis is unique among cannabis, in that it flowers according to stage of maturity, typically after the fifth to seventh pair of internodes appear. *C ruderalis* crosses available today usually flower 21 to 30 days after planting seeds. Mature plants are ready for harvest in 70 to 110 days regardless of the photoperiod. *C. ruderalis* flowers and reproduces according to an individual plant's age, regardless of the photoperiod.

The word *ruderalis* comes from *ruderal*. In the plant kingdom, *ruderal* means "the first species to colonize land disturbed by humans or natural occurrences." *C. ruderalis* is native to Asia, Central Europe, and Russia, and adapted to the harsh environments found in these climates. It is adapted for life in extreme northern climates with short, 3-month growing seasons.

C. ruderalis varieties are crossed with *C. sativa* and *C. indica* varieties to incorporate the daylight neutral gene. Breeders are hybridizing plants with the autoflowering gene from *C. ruderalis* that incorporate qualities from *C. sativa* and *C. indica*: robust growth stature, large flowers, and cannabinoid profile. See "Autoflowering Feminized Cannabis," on page 38.

Feminized Cannabis

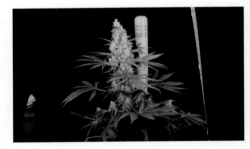

'Black Jack' from Sweet Seeds is a new variety, one of the many new feminized varieties released every year in Europe.

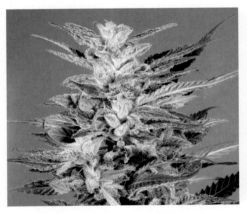

'Jorge's Diamonds' from Dutch Passion is a popular feminized variety. Cannabis seeds are available feminized or in female version only. Virtually any cross or variety can be feminized. See chapter 25, Breeding, for information on feminizing plants.

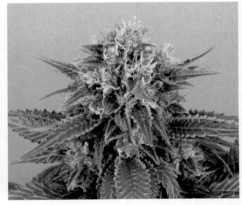

'Kalashnikova' from Royal Queen Seeds is another example of a new feminized variety from Europe.

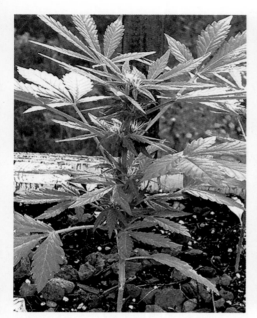

This 'Lowryder' female is just starting to flower.

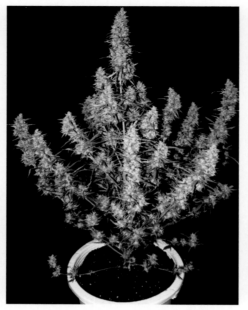

Autoflowering feminized 'Magnum' can be found at the Spanish company Hemp Trading (www.hemptrading.com).

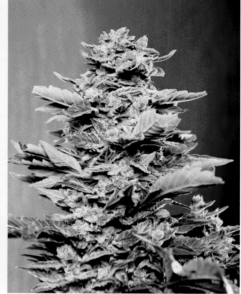

EZ Ryder is another auto-flowering variety developed by the Joint Doctor.

Autoflowering Feminized Cannabis

Autoflowering feminized cannabis plants were originally popularized by the Joint Doctor, a longtime cannabis gardener and breeder. These varieties have almost all the characteristics of regular cannabis varieties but they flower automatically. The autoflowering gene can be incorporated into daylight-sensitive cannabis plants that flower under a 12/12-hour day/night photoperiod so that they flower after 3 to 4 weeks of growth.

Indica-dominant varieties are very popular because they naturally flower early and the trait is easy to select. *Sativa*-dominant autoflowering plants are often called semi-autoflowering or super-autos because they start flowering after about 28 to 32 days of growth. These plants can grow to more than 5 feet (1.5 m) tall. At harvest (90 to 110 days after planting), super-autos yield up to 4 ounces (113.4 gm) of dried flower buds. The extra days of growth translate into higher yields. Original and smaller autoflowering seed flowers in about 21 days, matures into ripe buds in 55 to 85 days, and yields up to 2 ounces (56.7 gm).

Autoflowering cannabis is perfect for cool and cold climates with short growing seasons. Autoflowering and super-auto seeds grow easily outdoors in alpine and northern climates having short summers with very long days and short nights. The plants can be started indoors and moved outdoors after 3 weeks of growth. Autoflowering plants are also quite resistant to cold, diseases, and pests.

Outdoors in warm climates, gardeners can harvest 3 or more crops of autoflowering cannabis!

Super-autoflowering plants are mostly *sativa*, and grow bigger than original autoflowering plants, reaching 6.5 to 8 feet (2–2.4 m) under proper conditions. Super-autos share the other qualities of autoflowering plants flowering under any light regimen and can be feminized too. They differ in that Super-autos grow for up to 30 days before they initiate flowering. Plants grow bigger during a longer vegetative growth stage. Larger vegetative plants have more branches and foliage and produce more flower buds. Each super-auto plant can yield 3.5 to 9 ounces (99.2–255 gm) of dry flower buds when grown outdoors under the proper conditions. Plant super-autos in spring and summer. Harvest 90 to 100 days after seeds pop through the soil.

Stitch, a French breeder, started developing super-autos from Mexican and Guatemalan genetics in the late 1990s and continues to develop more varieties today. Look for 'Chaze' super-auto and other varieties.

Indica / Sativa Crosses

So many varieties are the result of just two original varieties—'Skunk #1' and 'Haze'. 'Skunk #1' is a fabulous plant. It was the first stable cannabis variety. These two plants are the cornerstones of modern cannabis breeding.

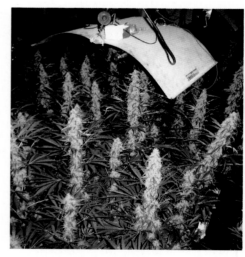

'Power Plant' from Dutch Passion

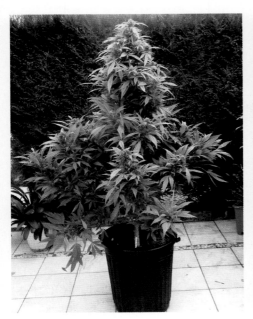

'Sensi Star' from Paradise Seeds

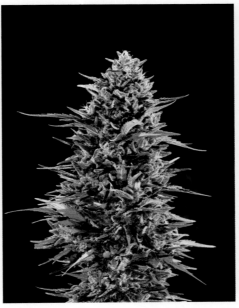

'Skunk #1' at peak resin production

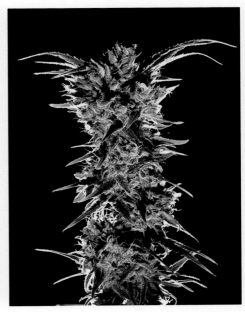

'Catatonic' from Resin Seeds is high in CBD.

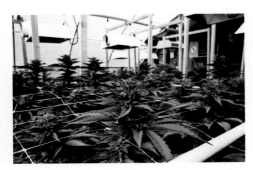

CBD-rich 'Harlequin' from SOHUM Seeds

High-CBD Varieties

About one out of 500 samples brought into California cannabis testing labs in 2012 had high levels of CBD. Cannabis can be selectively bred for high CBD levels. Several breeders have taken on the task, among them Jaime from Resin Seeds (Spain) and Lawrence Ringo from SOHUM Seeds (Southern Humboldt Seed Collective, California). Other breeders are hot on their trail, developing CBD-rich varieties as we speak.

High THC Varieties

There are many THC-rich varieties available to medical cannabis gardeners today. In fact, most of the varieties are loaded with THC-rich cannabinoids and can be grown well indoors, outdoors or in a greenhouse.

'Haze' has been my favorite variety since 1983 when Nevil, Founder of the Seed Bank in the Netherlands, gave me a big branch for my trip back to Amsterdam from the Cannabis Castle. This is my all-time favorite variety! This opinion is shared by countless cannabis aficionados. Developed in the early 1970s by the Haze Brothers in Central California, original 'Haze' was bred by crossing Colombian/Mexican hybrids during the first year. A South Indian male was crossed with the best Colombian/Mexican female offspring during the second year. The third year, the best

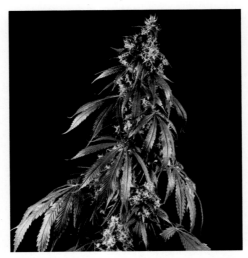

'Arjan's Haze' (The Greenhouse) is one of the many 'Haze'-based varieties available today.

females were crossed with an imported Thai male. Now there are many versions of the "Original Haze." Nevil's 'Haze' is one of the strongest I have seen.

A safe estimate is that 'Haze' is found in the genetics of 10 to 15 percent of cannabis varieties today.

'Haze' is often crossed with other varieties that ripen much quicker. Some of the favorite crosses include: 'Buddha' (Dutch Passion), 'Fuma con Diablos' (Flying Dutchmen), and 'Northern Lights #5' × 'Haze' (Sensi Seeds). Of course, there are many "Original Haze" varieties!

Taste—distinctive sweet and spicy, pine-lemony

High—clear, up, soaring, vivacious, animated

Potency—some varieties more potent than others

Genotype—*sativa*, Colombian, Mexican, Thai, and South Indian

Culture—difficult, long maturing, hyper-prone to overfertilization

Odor—Smell it once and you remember its distinctive odor forever!

Habit—long and lanky with wispy buds

Yield—low

Disease/pest resistance—very resistant to diseases and pests

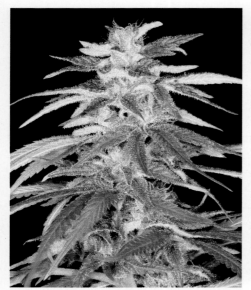

'Super Silver Haze' is one of the all-time favorites!

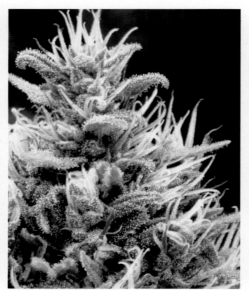

'Original Skunk #1' was developed by Sacred Seeds. (MF)

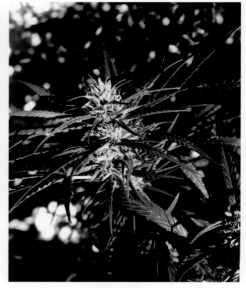

'Northern Lights' was one of the original, strong breeding plants.

Indoors—three months or more

Outdoors—harvest late-December through February

Ease to manicure—slow

Water hash quality/quantity from trim—good

'Skunk #1' is the ultimate classic! Nearly half of Dutch-grown seeds and Canadian varieties today have a portion of 'Skunk #1' genes. 'Skunk #1' was developed in 1978 by California-based Sacred Seeds. This single variety transformed cannabis breeding in the Netherlands and the rest of the world. It has been the winner of numerous harvest festivals, including the Cannabis Cup in Amsterdam. You cannot go wrong with this variety. Sensi Seeds registered the name, but you can find this variety at numerous seed banks, and there is a little bit of skunk in countless other varieties. This long history has made 'Skunk #1' (and most of its direct derivatives) one of the least-expensive varieties available.

'Skunk #1' is probably part of the genetics of 30 percent of the varieties available today.

Taste—skunky, sweet

High—soaring, cerebral

Potency—strong but able to function on it, low CBD

Genotype—'Colombian' *sativa*/'Afgani' *indica* × 'Acapulco Gold' Mexican *sativa*

Culture—easy to grow but sensitive to overfertilization

Odor—distinctive, skunky and sweet, strong but not overpowering

Habit—high flower:leaf ratio; thick long colas; prone to long internode space

Yield—very high

Disease/pest resistance—susceptible to mold during flowering

Indoors—50 to 70 days, many early-flowering varieties are available

Outdoors—mid October, excellent greenhouse crop

Ease to manicure—very easy

Water hash quality/quantity from trim—good

'Northern Lights' ('NL') was developed by "The Indian" on an island in the Pacific Northwest. He started with 11 seeds and named them 'NL #1', 'NL #2', etc. Of the plants, 'NL #5,' 'NL #8' and 'NL #1' were the best, in that order. Nevil shuttled clones back to Amsterdam from Seattle, Washington, in the mid 1980s. Today, 'NL #5' is the main variety of 'NL' in use by breeders. 'Northern Lights #5' is often crossed with other varieties such as 'Blueberry', 'Haze', 'Juicy Fruit', and 'Jack Herer'. Varieties are available from Sensi Seeds (who has

registered the Northern Lights name), Canadian Professionals, and Nirvana.

'Northern Lights #5' is an absolute must if you grow indoors. This potent, user-friendly plant is also very popular among commercial growers.

Taste—strong, full-bodied, sweet, piney, hashy

High—body stone, couch-lock,

Potency—very strong, great resin production

Genotype—predominately Afghan *indica*/Thai *sativa*, very stable

Culture—easy to grow, can be pushed with fertilizer

Odor—sweet piney

Habit—high flower:leaf ratio, compact buds, purple tinge to leaves as plant matures

Yield—very good, a favorite among commercial growers

Disease/pest resistance—somewhat resistant to thrips and spider mites, best to cross with *sativa*

Indoors—60 to 65 days

Outdoors—early October

Ease to manicure—easy and fast

Water hash quality/quantity from trim—good but low volume

PART 2 ESSENTIAL MEDICAL CANNABIS HORTICULTURE

4

CANNABIS LIFE CYCLE

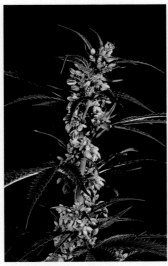

This male plant is laden with ripe male flowers that are packed with pollen. Cannabis is wind pollinated. Male plants release their pollen into the wind to pollinate nearby female plants. But pollen can also drift for several hundred miles when unobstructed. (MF)

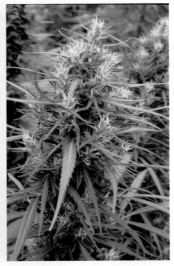

This female, thin-leaved sativa *is easily distinguished by the white fuzzy pairs of pistils protruding from each seed bract. The pistils catch male pollen that is ushered to fertilize the female ovary. (MF)*

UNDERSTANDING HOW cannabis naturally develops and completes its life cycle is fundamental to growing the best medicinal crop. Cannabis, whether cultivated indoors or out, has the same basic requirements for growth. It needs light, air, water, nutrients, a growing medium, and the proper environment to produce energy and to grow. Without any one of these essentials, growth stops and death soon results. Both indoors and outdoors, the light must be of the proper spectrum and intensity, and the air must be warm, arid, and rich in carbon dioxide. Water must be abundant but not excessive, and the growing medium must contain the proper levels of nutrients in an available form to sustain vigorous growth. When all these needs are in balance, cannabis plants will flourish on their own.

Innate Qualities of Cannabis

1. Cannabis is an annual plant, which means it completes its life cycle within one year or less.

2. Cannabis is dioecious, having both male and female plants. Mature female flowers contain more cannabinoids than males.

3. *Cannabis sativa* and *Cannabis indica* are "photoperiod determinate" plants; they require long nights to begin flowering. Flowering in *Cannabis ruderalis* is not triggered by the light cycle of long nights and short days. *C. ruderalis* flowers after 3–4 weeks of growth, regardless of the light schedule.

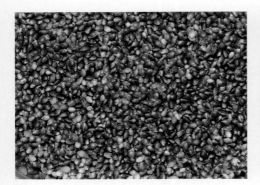

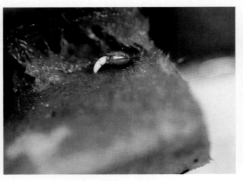

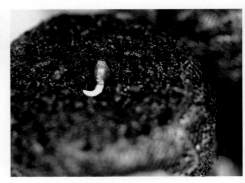

Seeds contain an exact genetic code to grow into strong, healthy cannabis plants with a rich cannabinoid profile. Seed selection is essential to produce a crop of cannabis with all the desired characteristics.

The initial white rootlet has just emerged from the seed.

The seed has germinated and the little white rootlet is growing rapidly. Now is the time to plant this sprouted seed.

Life Cycle of Cannabis

Cannabis is an annual plant; seeds planted in the spring will grow throughout the summer and flower in the fall. Cannabis typically is a dioecious species, meaning it has separate male and female plants. Plants with male flowers produce pollen, which is dispersed by the wind, and the female-flower-bearing plants will produce seeds when fertilized. The annual cycle starts all over again when the new generation of seeds sprouts the following year. In nature, cannabis goes through distinct growth stages: seedling, vegetative, pre-flower, and flower.

Seeds & Seedlings

Healthy seeds germinate 3 to 7 days after absorbing water from the medium, and transform into little sprouts. The seedling growth stage lasts about a month. During this first growth phase, seeds germinate, or sprout, establish a root system, grow a stem, and produce leaves to harvest sunlight and convert it into usable energy—a process known as photosynthesis.

Germination

During germination, moisture, heat, and oxygen activate the embryo within the durable outer coating of the seed. The embryo expands, nourished by a supply of food stored within the seed. Soon, the seed's coating splits, a white taproot grows downward, and a sprout's cotyledons (seed leaves) push upward in search of light.

Seedling Growth

The primary root (taproot) grows downward due to gravity and branches out, similar to the way the stem branches up and out aboveground. These secondary branching roots are called lateral roots, and produce tiny rootlets that draw in water and inorganic salts—the chemical nutrients required to sustain life. Roots also serve to anchor a plant in the growing medium and provide support for the growth above the soil. Seedlings should receive 16 to 24 hours of light to maintain vegetative growth. The seedling growth stage usually lasts 4–6 weeks, and most varieties will continue to vegetative growth as long as plants receive at least 16 hours of light every 24 hours.

Vegetative Growth

Cannabis will stay in the vegetative growth stage as long as it receives a minimum of 16 hours of light daily. As the plant grows above soil, its roots continue to fill the medium below the soil line. Cells in the root tips continue to divide and push farther and farther into the soil in search of more water and nutrients. Lateral root branches sprout, perpendicular to the primary roots, and then form thin root hairs that are also designed to harvest water and nutrients from the soil. If the soil dries out completely, these frail root hairs will desiccate and die. They are very delicate and are easily damaged or torn by klutzy hands if

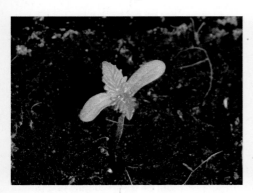

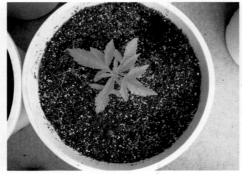

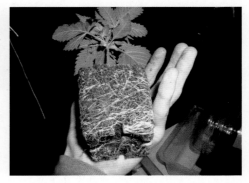

In a week to 10 days, a small seedling will break through the soil. The first rounded seed leaves give way to the first set of "true leaves" having the classic serrated edges.

The tender little seedling continues to grow. Leaves multiply, stem girth increases, and the tip continues upward toward the light.

In a few weeks seedlings have established root systems and have started the vegetative growth stage. Plants soon outgrow containers and must be transplanted.

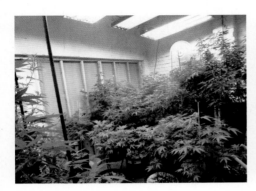

This indoor vegetative garden room is illuminated 18 hours a day, with 6 hours of darkness. This light regimen keeps plants in the vegetative growth cycle.

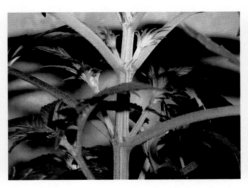

Stems must be stout to support heavy flower buds. The internodes on this plant's stems are growing close together. This is a desirable trait when cultivating indoors.

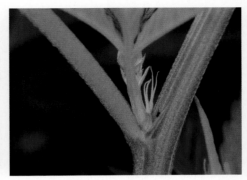

This female pre-flower appears about 4 to 5 branches down from the top of the plant, about 2 months after the seed sprouts. The white fuzzy hairs (female stigmas) show that this plant has designated sex and is a female.

exposed or moved roughly. Extreme care must be exercised during transplanting. A strong, healthy root system is essential for optimum growth.

Like the roots, the terminal growth shoot at the top of the plant also has cells that divide and multiply at its tip, called the meristem. These cells give rise to new auxiliary buds, which themselves become lateral leaves and shoots. The central, or apical, bud carries growth upward; side, or lateral, buds turn into branches or leaves. The vascular system, located within the main stem, transmits water and nutrients from the root system to the growing buds, leaves, and flowers where sugars are produced via photosynthesis and are then redistributed throughout the plant. This fluid flow takes place in specialized tissues called xylem and phloem; xylem bring nutrients and water to the sites of photosynthesis in the leaves, and phloem brings the resulting sugars to parts of the plant that do not undergo photosynthesis.

The stem also supports the plant with cellulose and lignin located within cell walls and structures along the stem. Outdoors, rain and wind push plants around, causing microtears in these tissues, which are repaired by the deposition of cellulose and lignin. These tissues together provide strength and make the stem strong and rigid. Indoors and in greenhouses, with no natural wind or rain present, cellulose and lignin production is often lower, so plants develop weak stems and may need to be staked up later, especially during flowering. To help build strong stems, make sure

to have adequate air movement in the grow-room or greenhouse environment.

Once green tissues are present in the seedling, the plant starts to manufacture food (carbohydrates) and produce energy from the sunlight and nutrients in the soil. This process is known as photosynthesis. Chlorophyll is the substance that gives plants their green color, and it is found in cellular structures called chloroplasts. Inside chloroplasts is where light energy, carbon dioxide (CO_2) taken from the air, and water and nutrients from the soil are converted into carbohydrates and oxygen. This process releases usable

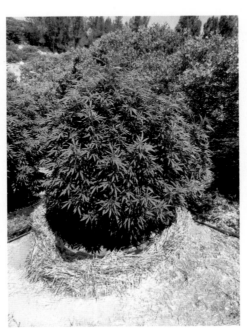

Vegetative growth outdoors is often much more profuse than indoors. It is difficult for artificial light and an artificial growing environment to compete with natural sunlight and Mother Nature.

energy and creates starches or sugars that are later used in the production of plant tissues and cellular components.

Tiny breathing pores called stomata are located on the underside of the leaf. Stomata are the entry point of CO_2 into the plant, where it is then used in photosynthesis. The stomata open and close to regulate the flow of moisture and oxygen from the leaf—both of which are waste products of photosynthesis. The stomata are very important to the plant's overall health and function.

Pre-flowering

Cannabis grown from seed typically begins to show early development of floral bud structures commonly known as pre-flowers. The vast majority of varieties begin to produce these immature sexual organs by the fourth or fifth week of vegetative growth. In some varietals, pre-flowers can be seen as early as the fourth node; however they generally appear between the fourth and sixth node from the bottom of the plant. Cannabis plants are normally either all male or all female, with each sex having its own distinct form of pre-flower. Use pre-flowers to identify the gender of the plants and separate the females for flower production. Female flowers are cultivated for their high cannabinoid content, and are therefore prized. Male plants have lower levels of cannabinoids (THC, CBD, CBN, etc.) and are not typically kept by cannabis cultivators. Male plants are normally removed and destroyed by growers, but can also be maintained and evaluated as potential breeding stock.

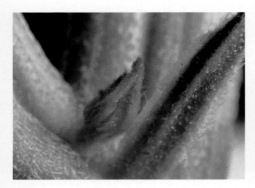

A tiny male pre-flower appears near the end of the natural vegetative growth cycle. The little shoot has all the characteristics of a male flower and will continue to grow and then manufacture and release male pollen. (MF)

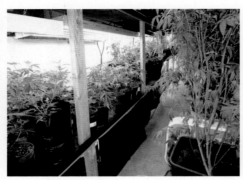

Mother plants are growing on the right in this garden; rooted clones in the vegetative growth stage are growing under T5 fluorescent lights on the left.

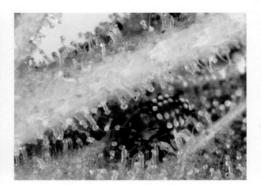

Insects and mites can become a big problem, especially on indoor and greenhouse crops. This aphid has found a new way to disguise itself. The translucent spots on its back look very similar to cannabis resin! (MF)

Indoor plants grown from seed are most often left in the vegetative growth stage for 4 to 6 weeks, or until they are a minimum of 12 to 18 inches (30–45 cm) tall, before being induced to flower. Smaller plants can be induced to flower, but this practice is typically not recommended for plants grown from seed and is more practical for crops grown from clones. Premature flowering of young plants from seed can cause sexual instability (intersex expression) in some varieties.

Flowering

Cannabis enters the flowering stage in the late-summer and early fall. As the nights become longer and days shorter, plants are signaled that their annual life cycle is beginning to come to an end, and the flowering stage begins. *C. sativa* and *indica* are photoperiod-determinate plants requiring longer nights and shorter days to induce flowering. *C. ruderalis* is not induced to flower by changes in light cycle and starts flowering when the plants reach 3 or 4 weeks of age, regardless of the light regimen.

Left unpollinated, female flowers develop without seeds, commonly known as "sinsemilla" from the Spanish *sin semilla*, or literally "without seed." Unfertilized female plants continue to produce flowers and become increasingly covered in resinous, glandular trichomes, which produce the essential oils that give cannabis its unique smells (terpenes), in addition to the medicinal compounds known as cannabinoids. Trichomes produce numerous plant

secondary metabolites, and recent studies show that some of the molecules produced in cannabis trichomes belong to families of compounds with proven antifungal, antimicrobial, and antibiotic properties. Genes that provide resistance to dehydration are also present, and in many species trichomes are known to inhibit insect movement. All of these factors support the hypothesized role of trichomes and their by-products providing protection from insects, fungi, UV light, and so forth, that might damage the developing seed within the female flower during gestation.

After weeks of heavy flower production, cannabinoid content and other secondary metabolite production peaks in the unfertilized sinsemilla flowers. This is the ideal moment for harvest; no new flowers are

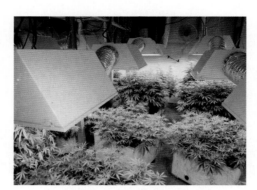

Small indoor plants typically yield from 1 to 4 ounces (30–120 gm). Outdoors and in greenhouses, cannabis is able to stay in the vegetative growth stage for several months and reach final heights of from 5 to 25 feet (1.5–8 m). Given an ideal environment, the longer vegetative period allows single plants to produce 5 to 10 pounds (2–5 kg) of cannabinoid-rich dried flowers.

being produced, and the unseeded floral clusters are at their maximum coverage of glandular trichomes rich in cannabinoids and other essential oils.

Male plants produce pollen, which is released into the wind and by chance lands upon the stigma of a nearby unpollinated female flower. The flower becomes fertilized, and the seed that will form the next generation begins to grow under the protective layer of trichomes found on the female bract. After shedding all the pollen from the staminate flower, male plants senesce and eventually die. The seeds in the female plant continue to mature for 3 to 6 weeks after fertilization. Once ripe, the seeds will split through the protective bract, and the female plant will also begin to senesce, leaving the seeds to fall to the ground.

Indoors, flowering can be induced in most commercial varieties of cannabis by providing 12 hours of uninterrupted darkness and 12 hours of light every 24 hours. Plants that developed in tropical regions often start flowering when given 12-hour days and nights, but flowering can continue for up to 20 weeks. Some growers who cultivate equatorial *sativa* varieties will increase the period of darkness to 13 hours and beyond, in an attempt to mimic the natural light cycle in the tropics.

Plant growth structure changes during flowering. New shoot and leaf growth slows and flowers begin to form. Cannabis has both male and female

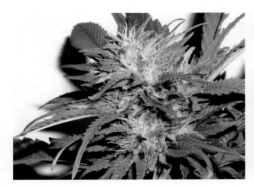

This cannabis flower appears to be frosted with cannabinoid-rich resin and will be ready to harvest in a couple of days. The cannabis varieties available today make growing a potent medical cannabis crop easy.

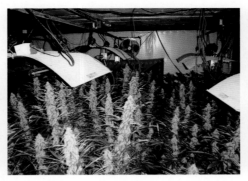

Some varieties such as 'Power Plant' produce big central buds very quickly.

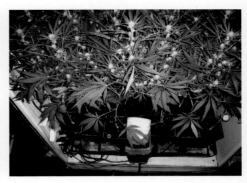

This garden has been flowering for 4 weeks. Small indoor gardens like this 40-inch-square (1 m²) garden are easy to set up. Note that this garden is being watered automatically and requires little maintenance.

plants. When both male and female flowers are in bloom, male flowers release pollen into the air that lands on female flowers, thereby fertilizing them. The male dies after producing and shedding all its pollen. Seeds form and grow within the female flowers. As the seeds are maturing, the female plant slowly senesces and dies. The mature seeds then fall to the ground and germinate naturally or are collected for planting next spring.

Mother Plants

Vigorous, healthy female plants known to produce high-quality flowers with desirable cannabinoid profiles make the best mother plants, although any plant deemed desirable can be made into a mother, or donor, plant. Mother plants are given 18 to 24 hours of light daily to ensure they stay in the vegetative growth stage. For vegetative reproduction, stem cuttings of shoots or branches are cut from mother plants and placed in

a growth medium to establish roots. The rooted stem cuttings are often called "clones," since the new plants share the exact genetic code of the mother plant and thus will grow identically when given the same environment. Cultivating several vigorous, healthy, insect-free mother plants is the key to having a consistent supply of all-female clones.

A single mother plant can supply a garden with hundreds of clones in a

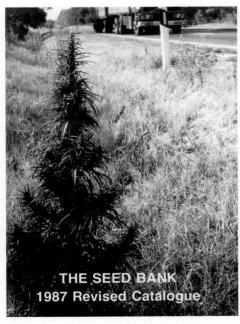

THE SEED BANK
1987 Revised Catalogue

This C. ruderalis plant was growing along the highway in Hungary in the mid-1980s, when Nevil, founder of the Seed Bank, snapped this photo. Breeders have been working with daylight-neutral ruderalis genetics for many decades. In the last few years ruderalis varieties have been crossed with "regular" varieties that impart a strong cannabinoid profile and harvest weight.

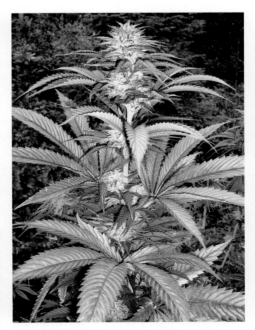

Genetics and temperature play a big role in purple-colored leaves. Some plants like this 'Purple Pineberry' are predisposed to turning color. When grown in cool weather the colors are more pronounced.

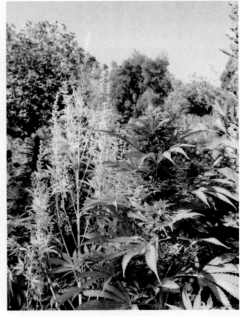

Male plants are normally removed from the garden so that they do not pollinate female plants. The male plant on the left is in full flower and spreading its pollen to all the female plants. Females will grow ripe seeds in 6 to 8 weeks.

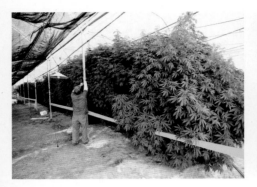

Mother plants can be maintained and grown for many months. These mother plants on a Mexican farm have been in the ground for almost a year!

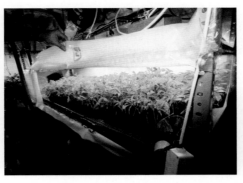

Once cut, clones are rooted under fluorescent light for about two weeks, until they develop a root system.

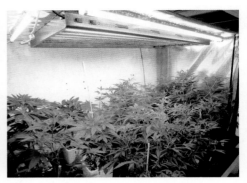

This indoor garden is growing under T5 fluorescent lights. The T5s are able to supply plenty of light for vegetative growth. The plants are in individual containers and are easy to move in the garden.

few short months. Indoors clones can be induced to flower as early as 6 to 12 inches (15–30 cm) tall, or can be grown until 3 feet (90 cm) or taller before being induced to flower. The identical "clones" are moved into the flowering room as soon as the previous crop is harvested. Outdoor gardeners grow clones indoors until they are about 2 feet tall (60 cm) before moving them outdoors or to a greenhouse for planting.

Clones

Branch tips are cut and rooted in a new medium to form stem cuttings or clones.

Clones take 10–20 days to grow a strong, healthy root system, but can begin to show roots in as short as 6 days. Clones are given 18–24 hours of light so they stay in the vegetative growth stage, and once the root system is established, clones are transplanted into larger containers. Indoors, clones grow for an additional 1–4 weeks or more in the vegetative growth stage before being induced to flower. Outdoors, clones are transplanted into large containers or Mother Earth, and they stay in the vegetative growth stage until nights grow long in the late summer, which induces them to flower.

Three Gardens

This section outlines 3 different gardens in 3 different locations: indoor, greenhouse, and outdoor. The examples show different planting and harvesting scenarios that use the natural advantages provided by each garden and the varieties grown. For more complete information about each type of garden, see chapters on *Garden Rooms*, *Case Studies*, *Outdoors*, and *Medical Cannabis Varieties*.

Indoor Gardens

Maintain mother plants and clones 18 to 24 hours of light daily. Induce

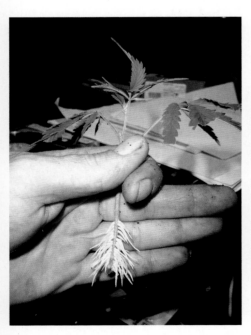

Branch tips are cut and rooted in rockwool cubes or other growing mediums. The cuttings grow roots in about 2 weeks and are then ready to plant.

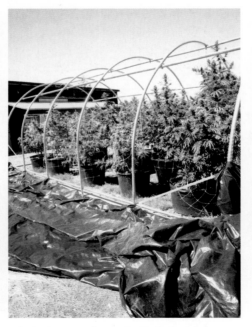

Black plastic is alongside this light deprivation greenhouse. Every day the black plastic is pulled over the greenhouse to black it out and create a total of 12 hours' darkness, which induces flowering in indica *and* sativa *varieties of cannabis.*

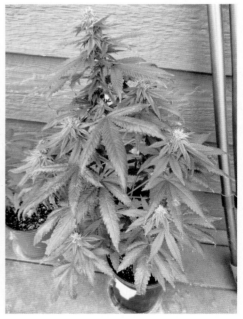

This autoflowering feminized seedling is an example of how a germinated seed can grow into a mature plant ready for harvest in just 70 days and receive 18 hours of daily light!

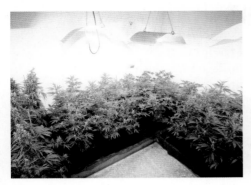

The garden on the right is about a week ahead of the garden on the left and will be harvested a week earlier.

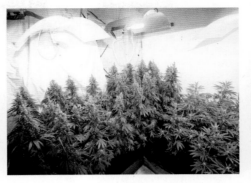

The plants on the left will be ready to harvest in about a week. The plants on the right are about 2 weeks into flowering and will be harvested in about 6 weeks.

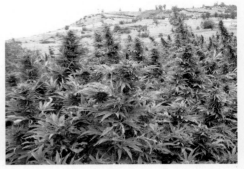

Plant a spring crop in warm climates. Diminished sunlight intensity produces smaller buds, about half to three-quarters as big as others. If plants get cold at night, growth slows.

vegetative plants to flower by providing 12 hours of uninterrupted darkness and 12 hours of light every 24 hours. Once the dark/light schedule has been set to 12 hours dark and 12 hours light, most varieties of cannabis will flower and can be harvested in 60 to 90 days.

First Harvest
Indoor Spring Crop – 90 days

January 1 – Move well-rooted 12- to 18-inch-tall (30–45 cm) female clones into room under 18 to 24 hours of light.

January 21 – Transplant clones into 3-gallon (11 L) containers.

January 30 – Induce flowering with 12-hour days and nights.

February 7 – Take cuttings and start the next crop of clones. Give clones 18 to 24 hours of light.

March 30 – Harvest first crop.

Second Harvest
Indoor Summer Crop – 90 days

April 1 – Move well-rooted female clones into room under 18 to 24 hours of light.

April 21 – Transplant clones into 3-gallon (11 L) containers.

April 30 – Induce flowering with 12-hour days and nights.

May 7 – Take cuttings and start the next crop of clones. Give clones 18 to 24 hours of light.

June 30 – Harvest first crop.

Third Harvest
Indoor Autumn Crop – 90 days

July 1 – Move well-rooted female clones into room under 18 to 24 hours of light.

July 21 – Transplant clones into 3-gallon (11 L) containers.

July 30 – Induce flowering with 12-hour days and nights.

August 7 – Take cuttings and start the next crop of clones. Give clones 18 to 24 hours of light.

September 30 – Harvest first crop.

Greenhouse Gardens
Greenhouse crops can be harvested 2 or more times a year, but most often greenhouses are planted in the spring and yield a single harvest in the fall. In cold climates, greenhouses must be heated. All greenhouses must be vented or cooled in warm weather. The

This Mexican greenhouse needs shade cloth and supplemental lighting at night to keep plants in the flowering growth stage. The days and nights are between 11 and 13 hours long all year round. This is the perfect photoperiod for flowering in cannabis.

basic harvest scenario below shows how to harvest 3 greenhouse crops every year.

First Harvest
Greenhouse Spring Crop – 90 days

March 1 – Move bushy, well-rooted 1- to 2-foot-tall (30–60 cm) clones and seedlings into greenhouse.

March 1 – Long 12-hour nights and short 12-hour days in spring signal cannabis to flower.

March 15 – Remove any male plants. To distinguish plants, look for male pre-flowers.

March 15 – Transplant clones and female seedlings into large containers.

April 15 – Darken greenhouse after 12 hours of daylight, until harvest.

May 30 – Harvest: The less-intense sunlight will make for smaller buds than harvests later in the season.

Second Harvest
Greenhouse Summer Crop – 90 days

June 1 – Move bushy, well-rooted 1- to 2-foot-tall (30–60 cm) clones and seedlings into greenhouse.

June 15 – Remove male plants; male pre-flowers distinguish male plants from females.

June 15 – Transplant clones and seedlings into larger containers.

July 1 – Induce flowering by blacking out (covering) greenhouse after 12 hours of light.

July 15 – Verify the gender of all plants. Remove any remaining males.

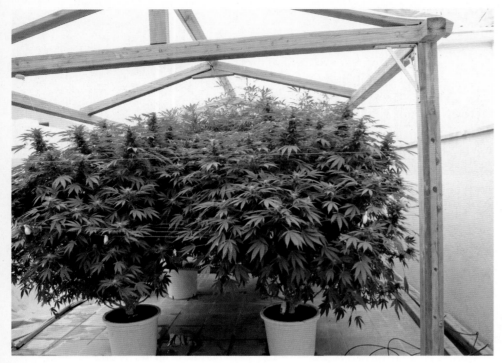

This small greenhouse protects flowering cannabis from regular rains and bad weather. It also keeps plants a little warmer at night. More regular irrigation is necessary when growing large plants in small containers.

August 1 – Maintain flowering by covering greenhouse after 12 hours of light until harvest.

August 30 – Harvest a heavy crop of top-quality medical cannabis flower buds that have received maximum levels of sunlight.

Third Harvest
Greenhouse Autumn Crop – 75 days

September 1 – Move bushy, well-rooted 1- to 2-foot-tall (30–60 cm) clones and seedlings into greenhouse.

September 15 – Long nights and short days of autumn signal cannabis to start flowering.

October 15 – Medical cannabis flowers develop but low light levels limit growth.

November 15 – Harvest smaller buds that have received less-intense fall sunlight.

Outdoor Gardens
Typically, outdoor gardens are planted in the spring and harvested in autumn. By applying information from this chapter, outdoor gardens can be harvested 2 or 3 times a year within moderate to temperate climates. Transplanting clones and seedlings and harvesting a single crop is all that is possible in cold climates with a growing season of 90 days. Extra care must also be taken to protect seedlings and clones from harsh weather.

First Harvest
Mild Climate Spring Crop – 90 days.

March 1 – Move bushy, well-rooted 1- to 2-foot tall clones and seedlings into a full-sun-heated greenhouse.

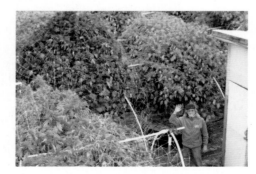

Spring-planted autumn crop – 210 days. A complete 7-month-long season will yield very big plants when grown properly. These 10-pound (4.5 kg) plants received full sun all day long and grew in outstanding organic soil.

March 1 – Long nights will induce cannabis to flower.

March 15 – Remove male plants; male flowers distinguish male plants.

March 15 – Transplant clones and female seedlings into large containers.

March 15 – Move outdoors in mild climates – may need to cover on cool nights.

April 15 – Darken plants after 12 hours of daylight if flowering slows.

May 30 – Harvest smaller buds that received less-intense spring sunlight.

Second Harvest
Mid-summer Crop – 70–75 days

May 1 – Start *ruderalis*-dominant (super-autoflowering feminized) variety indoors.

May 15 – Transplant autoflowering feminized variety to 3-gallon (11.3 L) containers.

May 21 – Transplant strong, healthy plants to outdoor garden.

June 1 – Female flowers are visible.

July 15 – Harvest 3 to 3.5 ounces (85–100 gm) of dried flower buds per plant.

Third Harvest
Pure *Indica/Sativa* and *Indica/Sativa* Crosses

March 1 – Plant clones and seedlings indoors.

May 1 – Move bushy 1- to 2-foot-tall clones and seedlings outdoors in temperate climates.

May 1 – Pre-flowers appear; remove male plants.

June 1 – Move bushy 1- to 2-foot-tall clones and seedlings outdoors in all climates.

August 1 – Flowers start to form; remove any "surprise" male plants.

September – Harvest a large crop from big plants.

5
SEEDS & SEEDLINGS

EXPONENTIAL GROWTH of seed selection and legal seed sales in the Netherlands, the United Kingdom, Canada, France, Switzerland, Spain, medical cannabis states in the USA, and many other countries, is making cannabis genetics more accessible than ever before. Most of the seeds (genetics) are available worldwide via Internet purveyors. Cannabis seeds are sold in every country

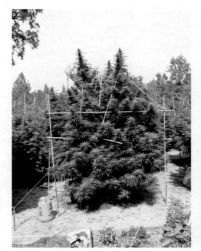

Cannabis seed varieties developed in California are often crossed by European breeders and sold to gardeners around the world.

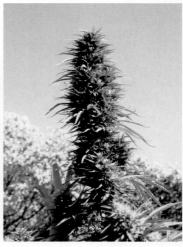

This Cannabis sativa *plant grown in 1976 originated in Colombia. (MF)*

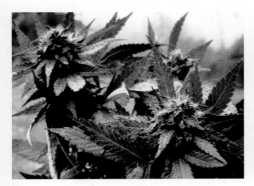

This 'Afghani' from 1979 is classified as Cannabis indica. *(MF)*

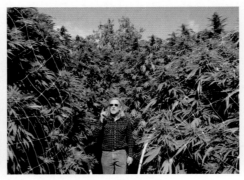

Regular cannabis plants are NOT feminized. Regular or naturally occurring cannabis plants are dioecious, having male plants and female plants.

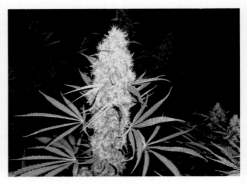

Feminized 'Power Plant'

on earth—some of which are illegal. Google "buy marijuana seeds" for an eye-opening example. See "Finding Seeds" on page 58 for more information.

There are thousands of varieties of cannabis. Most popular varieties include a combination of two or more of the following: *Cannabis sativa, Cannabis indica,* and *Cannabis ruderalis.* There are fewer pure *indica, sativa,* or *ruderalis* seeds available. The majority of seeds are bred to grow best indoors. Often indoor varieties are easy to acclimate to green-house climates. Fewer tried-and-true varieties are available for outdoors, but their number continues to grow.

Cannabis seeds available today are of 4 basic types:

1. **Natural** – produce separate male and female plants

   Mother Nature's original seeds

   Natural or "regular" seeds require 11 to 12 hours of light and 11–12 hours of darkness daily to flower. See chapter 8, *Flowering,* for more information on *indica* and *sativa* varieties.

2. **Feminized** – produce 99+ percent female plants. No male plants; male flowers occasionally occur.

   Female-only plants were first developed in India in 1982.*

   Feminized seeds require 12 hours of

light and 12 hours of darkness daily to flower.

All regular seeds can be feminized.

*Study by H. Y. Mohan Ram and R. Sett, Department of Botany, University of Delhi, Delhi (India) – "Induction of Fertile Male Flowers in Genetically Female *Cannabis sativa,* Plants by Silver Nitrate and Silver Thiosulphate Anionic Complex"

3. **Autoflowering** – ready for harvest 70–80 days after germination

   Seeds contain *C. ruderalis* genes mixed with *indica* and/or *sativa* genes.

   Autoflowering seeds flower regardless of light regimen. Autoflowering

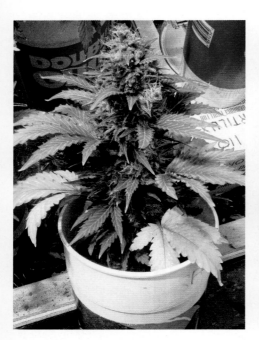

Cannabis ruderalis from the Joint Doctor

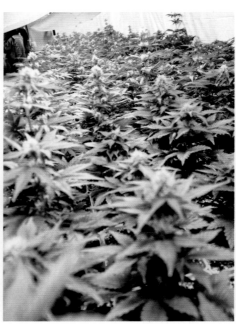

Autoflowering feminized 'Diesel' × 'Lowryder'

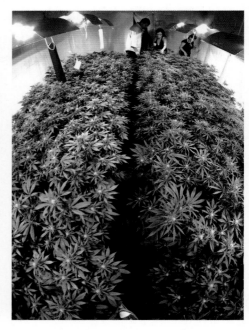

This beautiful roomful of F1 hybrid 'Bubblicious' plants is from Resin Seeds.

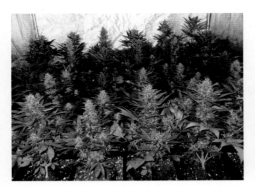

Ruderalis *cross*

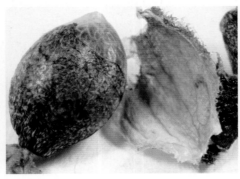

This seed contains the complete instructions (genetic codes) to grow a 'Jack Herer' plant. (MF)

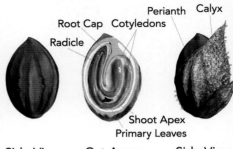

The cutaway drawing in the center shows how the seed will develop into different plant parts.

feminized seeds have been very popular in Europe since 2008, with the introduction of 'Lowryder II' genetics. Before that they were considered a novelty.

New autoflowering varieties are growing 3 to 4 feet (91–122 cm) tall.

Super-autoflowering varieties are growing 6 to 7 feet (183–213 cm) tall.

4. **Autoflowering Feminized** – produce 99+ percent female plants that flower and are ready for harvest 70 to 110 days after seed germination.

Seeds contain *C. ruderalis* genes mixed with *indica* and *sativa* genes.

Autoflowering feminized varieties flower after 3 to 4 weeks of growth, regardless of light regimen.

Super-autoflowering feminized varieties flower after 4 to 5 weeks of growth. They grow longer and bigger.

F1 hybrid seeds have "hybrid vigor." F1 hybrids grow faster and bigger than seeds of non-F1 hybrids. See chapter 25, *Breeding*, for more information on F1 hybrid plants.

Seeds

A seed contains all the genetic characteristics of a plant. The genetic code contained within a plant dictates whether it is regular, feminized, autoflowering, or autoflowering feminized. Seeds are the result of sexual propagation, and contain genes from each parent, male and female.* Some (intersex) plants, known as hermaphrodites, bear both male and female flowers on the same plant. The genes within a seed also dictate a plant's

size; disease- and pest resistance; root, stem, leaf, and flower production; cannabinoid levels; and many other traits. The genetic makeup of a seed is the single most important factor dictating how well a plant will grow under artificial light or natural sunlight and the levels of cannabinoids it will produce.

*See chapter 25, *Breeding*, for deviations from the above rule (i.e., in relation to intersex plants).

The genetic makeup of a seed is the single most important factor dictating how well a plant will grow under natural or artificial sunlight and the levels of cannabinoids it will produce.

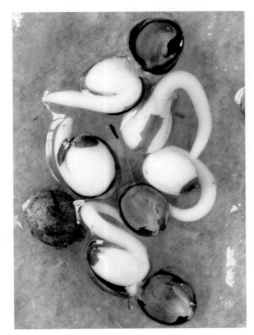

The outer shell of 'Skunk #1' seeds breaks away when germinating.

All seeds have the same basic requirements for germination and seedling growth. Strong healthy parents, proper breeding practices, and excellent care will yield strong seeds that germinate well. Strong seeds produce healthy plants and heavy harvests. Seeds stored under adverse conditions (hot, cold, or humid) or stored too long will germinate slowly and have a high rate of failure. Vigorous seeds initiate growth within a day or two. Some seeds take longer to germinate. Seeds that take longer than a month to germinate might always be slow and less productive.

The cask, or protective outer shell, on some seeds never properly seals, which allows moisture and air to penetrate. It also causes hormone concentrations to dissipate and make seeds less viable. Permeable seeds invite diseases and pests to move in. Such seeds are white, immature, fragile, and crush easily with slight pressure between finger and thumb. These are weak seeds that do not have enough strength to germinate and grow well.

A simple view of a seed exposes an embryo containing genes and a supply of food wrapped in a protective outer coating. Seeds range in size from small dark ones from tropical climates to huge seeds bred for hemp oil extraction. Mature seeds that are hard, beige to dark brown, and spotted or mottled have the highest germination rate. Soft, pale, or green seeds are usually immature and should be avoided. Immature seeds germinate poorly and often produce sickly plants. Healthy, fresh, dry, mature seeds less than a year old sprout quickly and grow robust plants.

SEED TYPE	ADVANTAGES	DISADVANTAGES
regular seeds	F1 hybrid vigor	not F1 hybrids – less vigor
	no diseases	slow to start
	easy transport	moisture/heat-sensitive
	small	easy to lose
	genetic expression	must cull males
feminized seeds	F1 hybrid vigor	not F1 hybrids – less vigor
	all female	possible intersex qualities
	use less space	expensive
	use less light	
autoflowering seeds	F1 hybrid vigor	not F1 hybrids – less vigor
	flower in 70+ days	could produce poorly
	flower in summer	must remove males
		difficult to clone effectively
autoflowering feminized seeds	F1 hybrid vigor	not F1 hybrids – less vigor
	flower in 70+ days	may produce poorly
	flower in summer	difficult to reproduce seeds
	99+% female	difficult to clone effectively

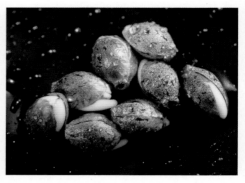

Strong, healthy seeds germinate quickly.

Seed Germination

Cannabis seeds need only water, heat, and air to break dormancy and germinate; they do not need extra hormones, fertilizers, or additives. Seeds sprout without light in a range of temperatures. Strong, viable, properly nurtured seeds germinate in 2 to 7 days. At germination, the outside protective shell of the seed splits, and a tiny, white sprout (radicle) pops out. This sprout is the root, or taproot. Cotyledon, or seed, leaves emerge on a stem from within the shell as they push upward in search of light.

Break dormancy: Put newly harvested seeds in the refrigerator for a week or two to simulate winter. Remove and germinate. Seeds will germinate more uniformly because they all come out of dormancy at the same time.

Timeline for germinating most seeds:

At 36 to 96 hours Water is absorbed, root tip (radicle) pops through outer shell and is visible.

At 10 to 14 days First roots and root hairs become visible.

At 21 to 30 days At least half of seeds are rooted by day 21. Seeds not rooted by day 30 will probably grow slowly.

Once seeds are rooted, cell growth accelerates; stem, foliage, and roots develop quickly. Seedlings develop into full vegetative growth within 4 to 6 weeks of germination.

Seeds are prompted to germinate by:

water

temperature

air (oxygen)

See chapter 25, *Breeding*, "Advantages/ Disadvantages" between seeds and clones.

Seedlings are less work to grow outdoors because branches are usually farther apart at first. Clones grow too densely from the bottom and require more pruning work.

Ten seeds from a reputable seed company germinate into about half female and half male* plants. Some plants will be small, and others will be strong, healthy, cannabinoid-potent females. Of these "super" females, one will be more robust and cannabinoid-potent than her siblings. This super female is selected to be the mother of future "super" clones.

*Scientific studies show a minimal weighting of averages that favor one sex or the other. This could be based on various factors including the external to the gene set and a phenotypic control of gene expression.

Normally all the seeds are germinated and planted. Males and weak plants are culled. The best female, or a clone of the female, is often retained as a mother plant. The mother can't be chosen until harvest. Two scenarios are possible: re-vegetation or taking cuttings from desirable females before they flower. This way, the plants grown out are big by the time the desirable female and corresponding clones are chosen for mother plants.

Plant 10 Regular Seeds:	50% male 50% female 25% weak 25% strong 10% = 1 strong "best" possibly "super" female mother						

| **Plant 10 Feminized Seeds:** | 99+% female
50% weak
50% strong
25% "best" with 1 "super" female mother | | | | | | |

| **Plant 10 Autoflowering Seeds:** | 50% male
50% female
25% weak
25% strong
5 female plants at harvest, no mothers | | | | | | |

| **Plant 10 Autoflowering Feminized Seeds:** | 99%+ female
50% or less weak
50% or more strong
10 female plants at harvest, no mothers | | | | | | |

Water

Soaking seeds in water allows moisture to penetrate the protective seed shell within minutes. Once inside, moisture continues to wick in to activate the dormant hormones. In a few days, hormones activate and send enough signals to produce an initial root tip. The white radicle (rootlet) emerges to bring a new plant into the world. Once a seed is moist, it must receive a constant flow of moisture to transport nutrients, hormones, and water so that it can carry on life processes. Some seeds need lots of moisture to wash out the dormancy hormones in the seed coat, and if they do not get enough moisture, they do not germinate. Conversely, too much water deprives the seed of oxygen, reducing its quality or destroying it. If fragile germinated seeds are allowed to suffer moisture stress now, seedling growth will be stunted. Soaking most seeds in water for 12 to 24 hours is all they need to initiate germination.

All the nourishment for a seed's initial growth requirement is pulled from the fleshy cotyledons, or seed leaves.

Water seedlings with low-EC (electrical conductivity) household tap water during the first week or two of life. Supplemental nutrients are unnecessary and if applied in excess can disrupt internal seed chemistry. Some gardeners prefer to germinate seeds using distilled or purified water that contains virtually no dissolved solids.

Temperature

Overall, cannabis seeds germinate in temperatures from 70°F–90°F (21°C–32°C) and grow best at 78°F (26°C). Temperatures below 70°F (21°C) and above 90°F (32°C) impair germination. Low temperatures delay germination. High temperatures upset seed chemistry causing poor germination. Seeds germinate best under the native conditions and temperature ranges where they were grown.

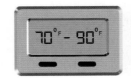 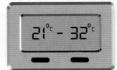

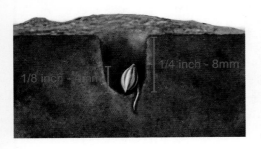

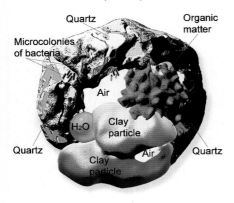

The complexity of soil

Seeds need oxygen from the air to germinate. Growing mediums that are too moist (soggy) will cut off oxygen supplies and the seeds will literally drown. Cannabis seeds germinate best when moisture is between 60 and 70 percent.

Air & Oxygen

Sow seeds twice as deep as the width of the seed. For example, 0.125-inch (3 mm) seeds should be planted 0.25 inches (6 mm) deep. Adequate oxygen is unavailable for seeds planted too deeply, and tender seedlings have insufficient stored energy to drive through deep layers of soil or crusty hard soil when sprouting.

Agricultural Astrology – Planting by the Moon

Ancient Babylonians and Egyptians planted and harvested based on moon phases in relation to geographic location. The premise is that plants grow better when planted during the appropriate moon phase.

Moon phases cause ocean tides to rise and fall. They also affect the rise and fall of moisture in soil and fluids inside plants. The moon phase influence is said to be the same indoors, outdoors, and in greenhouse-grown cannabis.

Cannabis gardeners who plant by the moon report faster-sprouting seeds that grow into vigorous plants. However, scientific evidence is lacking in regard to cannabis and other plants' relationship with agricultural astrology.

How to Germinate Seeds: Step-by-Step

Step One: Soak seeds overnight in a glass of plain water. They may float on the surface at first but should sink to the bottom in a few minutes. Make sure seeds get good and wet so that water penetrates the outer shell and growth is activated. Do not let seeds soak for more than 24 hours, or they might get too wet, suffer oxygen deprivation, and subsequently rot.

Step Two: Remove seeds from glass of water. Pour water out onto two paper (or cloth) towels on a dinner plate. Fold the towels over the seeds to cover them.

Step Three: Drain the water from the dinner plate by tipping it to the side.

Step Four: Place the seeds in a warm location (70°F–80°F [21°C–27°C]), making sure they are in darkness. Some gardeners go so far as to set the plate in a vertical position (so taproot grows downward). The seeds can also be set on a grate for drainage and air circulation.

Step Five: Check moisture level of towels several times a day, watering once or twice to keep them evenly moist. DO NOT LET THE TOWELS DRY OUT!

Germinate Hard-Shelled Seeds

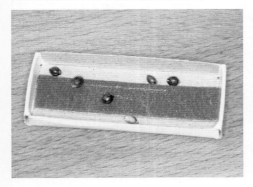

Set seeds in a matchbox with an emery board or sandpaper on the bottom.

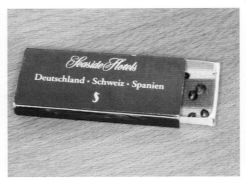

Close seeds inside the matchbox.

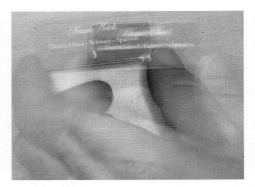

Shake matchbox for 10 to 15 seconds to scarify the seeds.

Some seeds have a very hard outer shell (testa) and are difficult to germinate. Such hard cases can be softened or scarified to allow water to penetrate.

To scarify, line a matchbox with a piece of fine-grain sandpaper or emery board. Put the seeds in the matchbox and shake for 10 to 15 seconds. Remove the seeds and make sure they have been scuffed a bit. Just a little scuffing will allow water to enter and set germination in motion.

Some gardeners soak their seeds in a 5 to 10 percent bleach solution to help dissolve the outer shell of the seed and speed germination. This practice can be overdone and is not necessary.

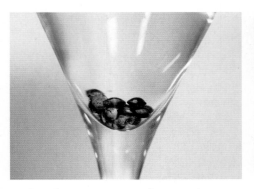

Soak seeds in water overnight to speed germination.

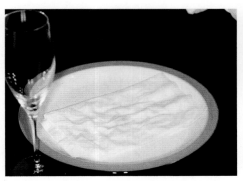

Keep seeds moist after soaking in water.

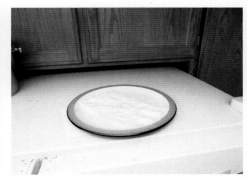

Remove excess water from plate.

Let excess water drain away freely. The paper or cloth towels will retain enough moisture to germinate the seeds in a few days. Each seed contains an adequate food supply for germination. Prevent fungal attacks by watering with a mild 2 percent bleach or organic fungicide solution.

Step Six: In a few days, seeds will sprout. Once seeds have sprouted and each seed's white rootlet is visible, use tweezers to carefully pick up the fragile, germinated seeds and plant them. Do not wait for the white rootlets to grow more than 0.25 inches (1 cm) before planting, or growth could slow. Plant each germinated seed with the white root tip pointing downward. Take care not to expose the tender rootlet to prolonged light and air. Cover germinated seeds with 0.25 to 0.5 inches (1–2 cm) of fine, moist planting medium. See "How to Plant Seeds: Step-by-Step."

Note: Overwatering and underwatering are the biggest obstacles most gardeners face when germinating seeds and growing seedlings. Keep the soil uniformly moist but not waterlogged. Do not let the growing medium's surface dry for long. Setting root cubes or planting flats on a grate allows good drainage. A shallow flat or planter with a heat pad underneath may require daily watering, while a deep, 1-gallon (3.8 L) pot will need watering every 3 days or more. A properly watered flat of rockwool cubes needs water every 3 to 5 days when sprouting seeds. When the growing medium's surface is dry (0.25 inches [1cm] deep), it is time to water. Remember,

there are few roots to absorb the water early in life, and they are very delicate.

Germinate Old or Stressed Seeds

Old seeds or seeds that have suffered temperature, humidity, or light stress (or all three) are less viable and may not germinate. Increase germination rates by using MS (Murashige and Skoog) media used for tissue culture, available via a few Internet-based retailers.

Once planted, germinating seeds can also be placed a few feet below an HID lamp to add dry heat while they are pushing up through the soil. The heat dries the substrate, which requires more

frequent watering. In cold rooms, place a heat pad or soil heating cables below growing medium to speed germination. Cannabis seeds germinate and sprout quickest when the soil temperature is from 78°F–80°F (25°C–27.5°C) and the air temperature is 72°F–74°F (22°C–23°C). Stems will stretch between internodes if temperatures exceed 85°F (29°C) for long.

How to Plant Seeds: Step-by-Step

Step One: Prepare fine soil planting medium, fine soilless mix, rockwool cube, Jiffy cube, etc., to receive seeds. Make sure all supplies are ready to go.

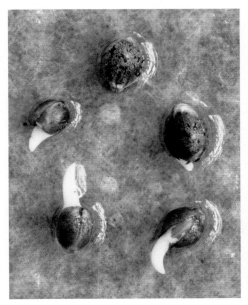

The rootlet on these germinated 'Skunk #1' seeds is the perfect length to transplant. At this point, fuzzy little root hairs have not yet developed. (MF)

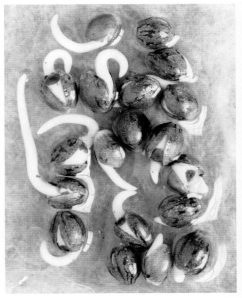

Rootlets on many of these sprouted 'Skunk #1' seeds are becoming too long for optimal planting. Once a rootlet gets a bit longer, small fuzzy root hairs start to grow, and planting disrupts their continued growth. (MF)

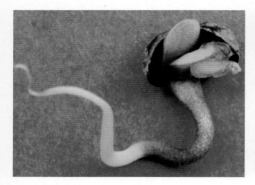

This germinated seed was allowed to dry out for a little more than an hour. Notice how the tip of the root has shriveled. This small oversight caused the resulting plant to have a very slow start in life.

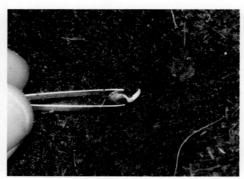

Carefully set a germinated seed into a pre-made hole in growing medium.

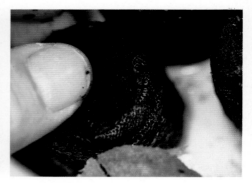

Press growing medium over planted seed to ensure complete contact.

Pre-drill planting holes in medium after saturating with water.

Step Two: When seeds have sprouted and the white sprout is visible, carefully pick up the fragile sprouts (with tweezers). Plant each seed in a pre-drilled hole in the growing medium or rooting cube, with the white root tip pointing down. Take care not to expose the tender rootlet to prolonged intense light or air.

Step Three: Cover the germinated seed with 0.25 inches (1 cm) of moist growing medium. Keep the medium evenly moist. Once the taproot sprouts, small fuzzy feeder roots will appear in 10 to 14 days.

Once a seed receives moisture, it must remain constantly moist. Moisture stress now will stunt or stop seedling growth. Dried or burned rootlet tips are the indicator of a good thing gone awry.

Soggy growing mediums cut oxygen supplies and cause seeds to drown. Planting seeds too deeply causes poor germination. Plant seeds twice as deep as the width of the seed.

Jiffy pellets expand when water is added. They make excellent pop-up pots to grow seedlings. They are also very easy to transplant.

Grow More Females from "Regular" Seed

Environmental factors that influence sex determination of cannabis take effect the moment seedlings have 3 pairs of true leaves (not counting cotyledons).* These factors include but are not limited to the following:

1. Increase the level of nitrogen to make more female plants. Lower the nitrogen level to create more male plants.
2. Increase the level of potassium to increase male tendencies. Lower the potassium level to encourage more female plants.
3. A higher nitrogen level and a lower potassium level for the first 2 weeks increases females.
4. Low temperatures increase the number of female plants. Warm temperatures make more male plants.
5. High humidity increases the number of female plants. Low humidity increases male plants.
6. Low moisture in the growing medium increases males.
7. More blue light increases the number of female plants. More red light increases male tendencies.
8. Fewer hours of daylight (e.g., 14 hours) increases the number of females. Longer days (e.g., 18 hours) make more male plants.
9. Stress: Any environmental stress tends to yield more male plants when growing from seed.

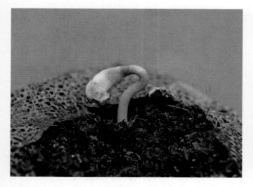

This germinated seed has pushed above the soil and started to grow toward the light.

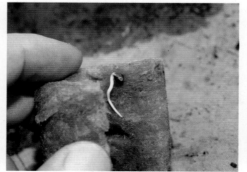

If planting in rockwool, make sure seed rootlet is at least 0.25 inches (1 cm) long. Newly germinated seeds can push or "heave" out of rockwool. The root pushes the seed out. This is why it is best to germinate seeds before putting them into the rockwool substrate.

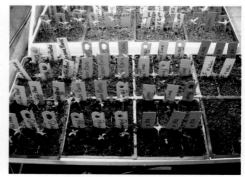

Color-coded labels make initial plant identification much easier.

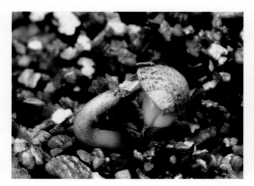

Germinated seeds break through soil and still carry the outer cask of the seed. (MF)

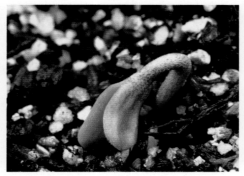

A germinated seed turns into a seedling when the rounded cotyledon leaves appear. Cotyledon leaves will sustain the seedling with nutrients throughout the next week or two. (MF)

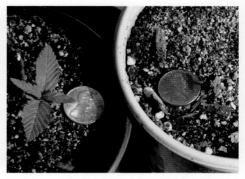

Strong seeds like the 'Skunk #1' on the left germinate quickly and grow up healthy. Weak seeds like the 'Cantaloupe Haze' on the right start slowly and might not grow as well. (MF)

*Henk, owner of Dutch Passion Seeds, www.dutch-passion.nl, was kind enough to allow us to adapt this information about environmental factors from his archives.

How to Help Ensure Female Seedlings

Ethylene diluted in water and sprayed on cannabis plants increases the number of female flowers and decreases the number of male flowers. To have the fullest effect, the hormone must be applied before pre-flowers appear. At this point plants are in the process of designating their sex, male or female.

Ripening fruit (especially bananas) releases a lot of ethylene. Several bunches of bananas can be set in a small, enclosed garden room containing the plants.

Large quantities of ethylene can be generated through the use of a catalytic generator, available from http://www.catalyticgenerators.com.

The spray releases a gaseous vapor of ethylene. Ethylene gas surrounds and overwhelms plants with the female hormone, promoting female tendencies. When enveloped in female hormone, cannabis plants designate sex and soon start producing female hormones, female pre-flowers, and, later, female flowers. See chapter 22, *Additives*, for more information on the hormone ethylene.

Note: Some of the products that release ethylene are plant growth regulators (PGRs). See chapter 22, *Additives*.

Note: Ethylene sprays can be phytotoxic when not diluted properly or when they are applied in hot weather.

Increase Yields

Treat seeds with carbon dioxide (CO_2) or ethylene before sowing to strengthen and increase root development, growth, budding, flowering, ripening, seed production, and overall yield.

Seedlings

When a seed sprouts, its white taproot emerges. Soon afterward the sprout breaks through the soil surface and a pair of cotyledons, also known as seed or seedling leaves, appears. The seed leaves spread out as the stem elongates. Within a few days, the first true leaves appear, and the little plant is now officially a seedling. This growth stage lasts for 3 to 6 weeks. During seedling growth, a root system grows rapidly, while green, aboveground growth is slow. Water and heat are critical at this point of development. The new, fragile root system is very small and requires a

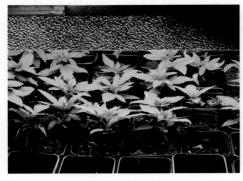

These strong seedlings are receiving 14 hours of light and 10 hours of darkness to promote more female plants.

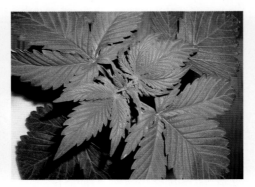

This 'Chronic' seedling is off to a healthy start in life.

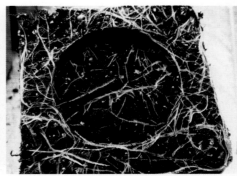

Plants soon outgrow their containers. Roots encircle the inside of smooth plastic containers. This seedling will be transplanted into a larger Smart Pot to promote root growth.

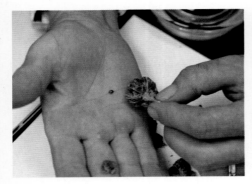

Occasionally a seed or two can be found in normally sinsemilla cannabis buds.

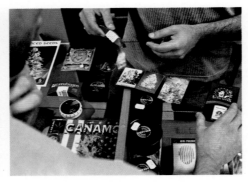

Retail cannabis seed sales are growing daily. This photo was snapped in Northwestern Spain at the Kaya Grow Shop in Vigo, Galicia.

foliage and root growth starts. Rapid growth aboveground is the most obvious signal that the vegetative growth stage is in process. Plants need more room to grow; transplanting into a larger container is essential to hasten development.

Finding Seeds
Medical Gardeners

Medical cannabis gardeners may have seeds from the plants they are growing. These dedicated gardeners usually know the variety well and can tell you many specific details about growing it, often reciting the qualities of the plant—taste, aroma, and medicinal benefits, etc.—by heart. Cultivate relationships with these expert medical gardeners!

Seeded Medical Cannabis

Containers of medical cannabis sometimes contain seeds. These seeds are often referred to as "bag seed." You will know more or less the taste, aroma, and medicinal qualities of the bud the seed came from. However, you will not know the growth characteristics of the plant, and the plant will probably not be

small but constant supply of water and warmth. Too much water will drown roots, often leading to root rot and damping-off. Lack of water will cause the infant root system to dry up.

As seedlings mature, some will grow fast and strong and appear healthy in general. A little soil heat now will help nurture small seedlings to a solid start. Other seeds will sprout slowly and be weak and leggy. Cull sickly plants, and focus attention on the remaining strong survivors. Seedlings should be big enough to thin out by the third to fifth week of growth. Thinning out seedlings is often very difficult for gardeners who pay exorbitant prices for a few seeds!

Seedlings need at least 14 hours of light daily. They require less-intense light now and grow well under fluorescent tubes for the first 3 to 4 weeks. CFL or HID light can also be used. Compact fluorescents should be 12 to 18 inches (30–45 cm) and the HID 3 to 4 feet (90–120 cm) above seedlings for best growth.

If not growing in rich organic soil or pre-fertilized mix, start feeding 2 to 4 weeks after seeds have sprouted. Some gardeners wait until leaves yellow to begin feeding. Use a mild quarter-strength solution.

Strong, rapid seedling growth is essential for strong, healthy plants and a bountiful harvest. Take special care to nurture seedlings so they get a good start on life. Any lack or excess of water, light, or temperature will stunt seed-

lings. Avoid high temperatures and low light levels, which cause lanky growth. The first 3 weeks of life for autoflowering and autoflowering feminized varieties are critical. These varieties grow for 70–80 days from seed. Without super strong growth during the first 21 days, yields are much lower.

The seedling stage is over after 3 to 4 weeks of growth. At this point rapid

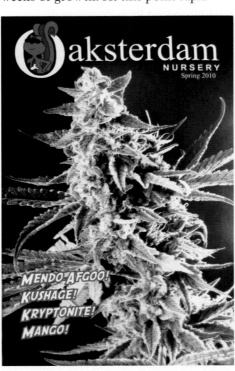

The Oaksterdam Nursery in the "Oaksterdam" district in Oakland, California, supplied medicinal cannabis seeds and clones to licensed caregivers and patients. A US government raid April 3, 2012, closed the facility. Before closing, more than 15,000 students graduated from Oaksterdam University.

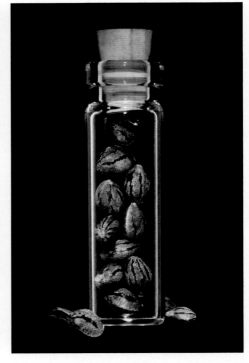

Ten 'Granddaddy Purple' seeds are stored in this clear vial. The cork breathes, allowing air to enter and exit. Such containers are perfect to store seeds for a few months, but not for the long term.

genetically stable. Such seeds could grow into magnificent plants and produce many cannabinoid-potent clones, but often these seeds will grow into plants that have only some desirable traits of the parents.

Medical Cannabis Dispensaries

Many medical cannabis clubs and dispensaries in California and other states where medical cannabis is legal sell seeds. Google "medical cannabis club," "medical marijuana dispensary," and so forth. Often the attendant at the dispensary knows the seed producer or breeder and may possess personal information on growing the seeds. This personal information will help gardeners and plants get off to a healthy start.

Legal Cannabis Seed Stores

Seeds are available at shops in many countries. Stores in Canada, Holland, Italy, Spain, Switzerland, United Kingdom, and a growing list of other countries sell seeds to the public via retail outlets. Find such seed stores at the websites listed in the magazines and cannabis fair guides. A personal conversation with knowledgeable, reputable seed merchants yields precise cultivation information. Ask many questions and request personal stories about favorite varieties.

Internet Seed Retailers

Internet cannabis seed purveyors offer the largest selection and best prices overall. Many medical cannabis gardeners do not have access to seeds at local stores, or the selection at local stores might be very limited.

Note: We do not advise ordering seeds via mail or courier service unless they are legal in your area and also legal to ship through the post. There are many seed sellers that advertise in magazines and on the Internet that send seeds anywhere worldwide. We advise to source medical seeds locally and legally.

Caution! Too often seed merchants do not tell the truth about their seed stock in this unregulated industry. They sell seeds that are not what they advertise them to be. Other companies receive payment and do not ship the seeds. It is easy to overcome such problems with a little homework.

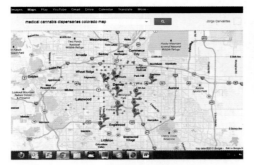

A simple Internet search will reveal many, many medical cannabis dispensaries in Southern California.

Much information is available online about cannabis seed companies and the varieties they offer.

Always check our Seed Bank Review Forum, http://www.marijuanagrowing. com/forumdisplay.php?39-Seed-Bank-Review-Forum, for current information on seed banks. Members make reviews and tell their experiences with many seed sellers.

Seed Quantities and Pricing

Seeds are generally sold in packages of 5, 10, and 15. Prices range from about $3 to $30 USD per seed. Often less expensive seeds are perfectly adequate for many gardeners' needs and desires. More expensive seeds are usually more stable, and extra care has been taken to produce them. Furthermore, expensive seeds are often winners of recent cannabis cups or are more difficult to produce.

Seeds	Cost Each	Cost 10 Seeds
regular	$50–$300	$5–$30
feminized	$100–$300	$10–$30
autoflowering	$5–$6	$50–$60
autoflowering feminized	$5–$10	$50–$100

Unless feminized, always purchase packages of 10 to 15 seeds, because the odds are that half of the seeds will be female and the other half male. Of the desired female seeds, some will show more desirable characteristics than others.

Always open the seed pack or inspect seeds visually before purchasing. Look for weak, moist, or damaged seeds. Growing lists of companies package

their seeds in hermetically sealed containers that also prevent tampering.

If you are not going to plant all the seeds in a sealed package at the same time, remove them from the sealed package and store in an airtight container in a cool, dark, dry, place. Keeping seeds dry is essential, or they might start to germinate. Place them in a small dark vial or film canister with a dry packet of silicone—the kind you find in electronics packages. Label the crush-proof container before you place the seeds inside.

Storing Seeds

Store seeds in a sealed, airtight, crush-proof container and include a packet of silicon crystals to absorb moisture. Store seeds in a cool, dark, dry place. Long-term seed storage is most successful at temperatures of 35°F–41°F (2°C–5°C). Replace silicon every 1 to 4 weeks to ensure that seeds stay dry. Place a max./min. thermometer in the refrigerator to record maximum and minimum temperatures and humidity. Make sure to label containers! Some seeds will remain viable for 5 years or longer when stored properly. When 50 percent of the stored seeds do not germinate, the average storage life is over. Seeds a year old or older often take longer to sprout and have a lower rate of germination.

Seed hormones—ABA, cytokinins, and gibberellins—are primed to respond to moisture, which is the first signal to germinate. Prevent moisture from signaling seeds to germinate by keeping them dry. Small amounts of moisture in

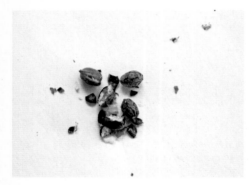

Always check seed packs for crushed or moist seeds or seeds that have started to sprout.

the form of condensation can give seeds a false start on germination and cause them to expend all their stored energy. If possible, avoid moisture levels above 5 percent to ensure viable seed when storing seed long term. Moisture levels above 5 percent will cause germination levels to decrease over time.

Seeds with a thin, outer protective shell never truly go dormant, because moisture and air are always present within. This moisture and air cause hormone levels to slowly dissipate. Such seeds do not store well for a long time.

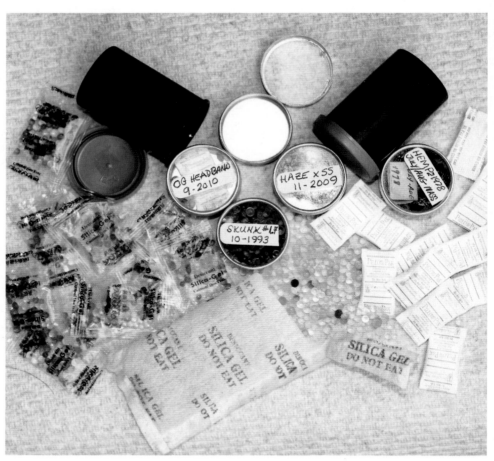

Store seeds in airtight containers along with a packet of silicon crystals to absorb moisture. Make sure to remove, dry, and replace silicon regularly. (MF)

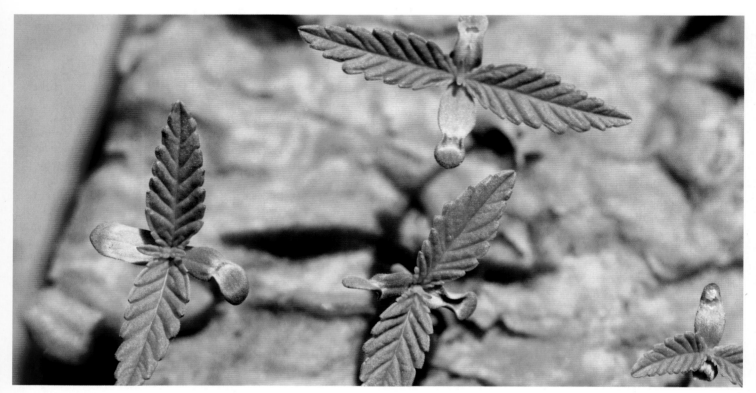

These 'Skunk#1' seeds were frozen for 16 years. Note some gray dead tissue on all embryonic leaves. Germination was over 90 percent, and survival was over 80 percent. (MF)

6

VEGETATIVE GROWTH

THE CANNABIS SEEDLING growth stage lasts for approximately 2 to 3 weeks, from seed germination to (strong) root set. Once a strong root system is established, foliage growth increases rapidly and seedlings enter the vegetative growth stage. When chlorophyll production is full speed ahead, a vegetative plant will produce as much green leafy foliage and root growth as is physically and genetically possible. Of course, growing conditions—CO_2, soil oxygen levels, nutrients, water, and so on—must not be limited and must be in the proper balance to be available for rapid uptake. Properly maintained, some varieties of medical cannabis will grow from half an inch to 2 inches per day. A plant stunted for any reason could require weeks to resume normal growth. A severely stunted plant may never fully recover.

A strong, unrestricted root system in a perfect rhizosphere (root zone) that is able to take in all necessary available nutrients is essential to robust growth. Unrestricted vegetative growth is the

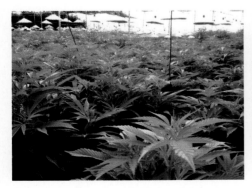

Strong vegetative growth is essential to a healthy harvest.

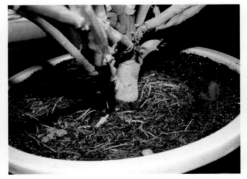

Growing large plants in relatively small containers, in this case a 5-gallon (19 L) pot, requires daily irrigation with a complete nutrient solution. A layer of mulch would keep roots from being exposed.

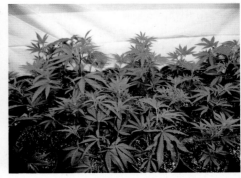

These plants will spend a short time in vegetative growth and will be subject to fewer problems.

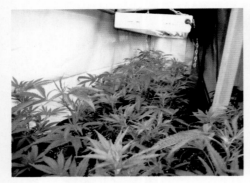

Vegetative growth in cannabis is maintained indoors, outdoors, and in greenhouses with 16 to 24 hours of light daily. Autoflowering (feminized) cannabis will flower according to chronological growth and is not affected by photoperiod.

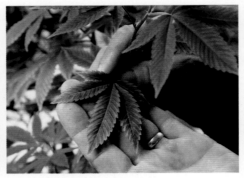

Multiple nutrient deficiencies, excesses, diseases, and pests become apparent during vegetative growth.

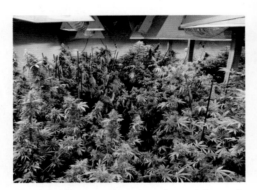

Cannabis flowers when given long nights and short days.

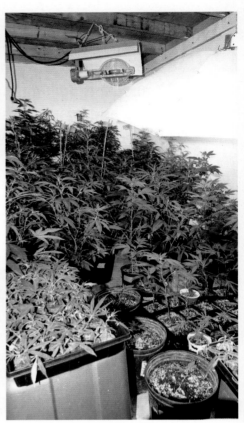

In this garden, mother plants and clones all grow under long 18-hour days with short 6-hour nights.

key to a healthy harvest. A plant's nutrient and water intake changes during vegetative growth. High levels of nitrogen are needed. Potassium, phosphorus, calcium, magnesium, sulfur, and trace elements are used at much faster rates. Transpiration is carried on at a more rapid rate, requiring more water. The larger a plant gets and the bigger its root system, the faster the soil will dry out. The key to strong vegetative growth and a heavy harvest is supplying plants with the perfect environment both aboveground and belowground.

During vegetative growth, plants need water and often need supplemental fertilizer too. Outdoor and greenhouse organic gardeners are able to build organic soil with bulk nutrients and amendments. Indoor gardeners usually need to add supplemental fertilizer. The garden will also need adequate air circulation and ventilation both day and night. Nutrient deficiencies that start during the first or second week of growth indoors usually show outward signs by the third to fifth week of growth. Nutrient deficiencies that start during the fourth or fifth week of growth outdoors and in greenhouses show visible outward symptoms during the sixth to eighth week of growth. Low-level nutrient imbalances can take longer to manifest, if ever.

Infestations of diseases and pests often flare as nutrient deficiencies progress. Many times new clones from another garden are already infested with spider mite eggs, powdery mildew, or root disease, with few outwardly visible signs.

Always quarantine and dip new clones and seedlings in an organic fungicide/insecticide/miticide before introducing them to the garden.

After 1 to 3 months of vegetative growth, nutrients have had a chance to build to toxic levels, and plants may show outward signs of deficiencies or excesses. Leaching containers will wash away water-soluble toxic nutrients. See chapter 21, *Nutrients*, for more information. Other problems—overwatering, underwatering, air circulation and ventilation, etc.—also occur now. See "Common Nutrient Problems" in chapter 21 for more information.

Cannabis will continue vegetative growth for a year or longer under an 18-hour photoperiod and a temperate climate. But sooner or later a genetic maximum is reached, causing cannabis to degenerate. *Indica* and *indica*-dominant varieties suffering stress from wintry conditions tend to flower regardless of hours of light, often producing more resin on stunted plants.

Indoors and in greenhouses, growth stages can be controlled with the light-and-dark cycle (photoperiod). It is the main stimulus to induce flowering. Give plants a 12-hour day and 12-hour night light schedule to induce flowering. Give plants 0 to 8 hours of darkness and 16 to 24 hours of light to retain vegetative growth. Controlling the photoperiod allows indoor and greenhouse horticulturists to control vegetative and flowering cycles. See chapter 17, *Light, Lamps & Electricity*, for more information on photoperiod control. Outdoor gardeners work with Mother Nature and harvest after long nights and short days in spring and autumn.

Once a plant's sex is determined, it can become a mother, clone, or breeding male and can be harvested or even rejuvenated (see chapter 8, *Flowering*).

Note: Plants show early male or female "pre-flowers" about the fourth week of vegetative growth. See "Pre-flowering" in chapter 8, *Flowering*.

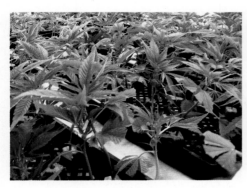

Clones are ready to transplant once new, green growth starts.

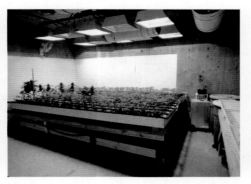

The clones in this perfect Trichome Technologies garden are easy to care for.

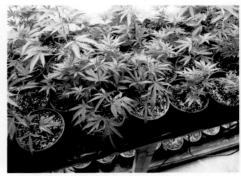

Fluorescent light is perfect for these recently transplanted clones. It gives them enough light to grow a strong root system and put on more green growth.

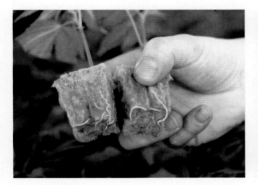

Good, strong roots must grow before cubes are ready to transplant.

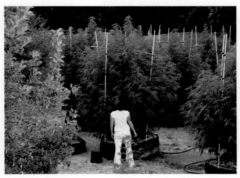

A long vegetative growth stage lets cannabis plants get big enough to grow an abundant crop of flower buds.

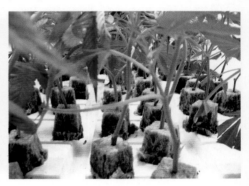

Rockwool rooting cubes provide ready-made containers to root and transplant clones.

Transplanting, pruning, bending, and trellising are all initiated when plants are in the vegetative growth stage. Information on these subjects follows.

Transplanting

When plants have outgrown their containers, they must be transplanted in order to continue rapid growth. Inhibited, cramped root systems grow sickly, stunted plants. Signs of rootbound plants include slow, weak growth. Severely rootbound plants tend to grow straight up with branches that painstakingly stretch beyond the sides of the pot. By the time you see these symptoms, the plant is rootbound. To check roots, remove a plant from its pot to see if roots are deeply matted on the bottom or circling the sides of the pot. When growing short plants that can be watered daily and reach full maturity in 70 to 90 days from clones or seedlings, there is little need for containers larger than approximately 3 to 5 gallons (11.4–19 L). Larger plants and mother plants will need a large pot if they are kept for more than 3 months.

Outdoors and in greenhouses, plants can grow much larger than indoors. Containers should be as big as possible to accommodate a large root mass. Big plants that produce 10 pounds (4.5 kg) of medical cannabis buds can be grown in 200- to 500-gallon (757–1893 L) containers.

Transplant into the same type or similar growing medium; otherwise, a water pressure differential (hydroscopic tension) develops between the different mediums, which slows fluid movement and root penetration. For example, when a rockwool block is transplanted into soil, it holds more water than the soil is able to hold. Roots migrate slowly into soil. Transplanting small rockwool cubes into soil works best. Each cube holds little water, and roots migrate into soil faster. Make sure to keep the soil evenly moist and the rockwool semimoist to promote root growth into the new medium.

Starting seeds and clones in root cubes or peat pots makes them easy to trans-

plant. Set the cube or peat pot in a hole in the growing medium, and ensure that the growing medium is in firm contact with it. Keep root cubes and substrates evenly moist after transplanting.

Transplanting is the second most traumatic experience after severing the stem during cloning. It requires special attention and manual dexterity. Tiny root hairs are incredibly delicate and easily destroyed by light, air, or clumsy hands. Roots grow in darkness, in a secure environment. When roots are taken out of contact with the soil or an aeroponic garden for long, they will quickly dry and die.

Transplanting should involve as little disturbance to the root system as possible. Water helps the soil pack around roots and keeps them from drying out. Roots need to be in constant contact with moist aerated soil in order to supply water, oxygen, and food to the plant. But, the fine line is that these tender roots also need air (oxygen) so they are able to absorb nutrients and water.

Dip Transplants in Miticide

Dip rooted clones and seedlings into a miticidal/fungicidal solution before transplanting. Stop diseases and pests before moving plants into a clean vegetative or flowering room. Mix a fungicidal/insecticidal/miticidal dip to disinfect clones before transplanting in the growing medium. Fill a container with low (5.0–6.0) pH water and add a natural fungicide such as hydrogen peroxide in a 3 percent solution. Or include a 10 percent mix of chlorine or vinegar. **Do not mix chlorine and vinegar! The resulting gas is hazardous!**

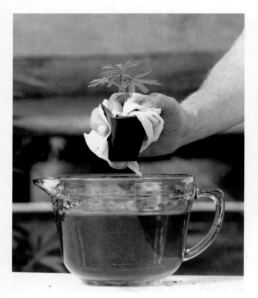

Mix the clone dip, and use a rag to cover and contain soil when dipping.

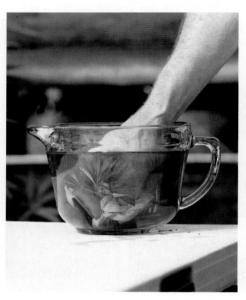

Submerge the entire clone in the dip to ensure liquid covers all foliage.

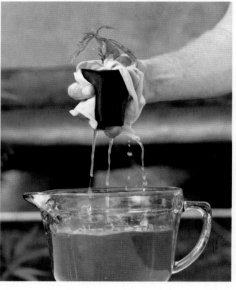

Remove the clone or seedling, and gently shake off excess dip before transplanting.

After transplanting, photosynthesis and chlorophyll production are slowed, as are water and nutrient absorption via roots. Transplant late in the day so transplanted plants will have all night to recover.

Transplants need subdued light so foliage can grow at the rate roots are able to supply water and nutrients. Give new transplants filtered, less-intense light for a couple of days. If there is a fluorescent lamp handy, move transplants under it for a couple of days before moving them back under the HID, or into a greenhouse or outdoors to harden-off.

Ideally, plants should be as healthy as possible before being traumatized by transplanting. But transplanting a sick, rootbound plant to a bigger container has cured more than one ailing plant. Once transplanted, cannabis requires low levels of nitrogen and potassium and increased quantities of phosphorus. Any product containing *Trichoderma* bacteria or mycorrhizal fungi will help ease transplant shock. Plants need a few days to settle in and re-establish a solid flow of fluids from the roots throughout the plant. When transplanted carefully and disturbed little, there will be no signs of transplant shock or wilt.

Cutting the bottom off a biodegradable fiber or paper container is a simple transplanting technique that disturbs roots very little. Simply cut the bottom half out of the pot and set the plant in the planting hole. Remove the above-ground part of the container so that it is not exposed to air. If exposed to air, it will take longer to biodegrade and thus will impair root growth.

For more information on self-pruning containers and pots that promote and

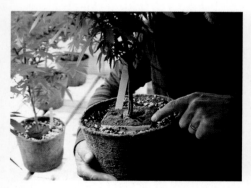

Always remove the plastic from rockwool cubes when transplanting!

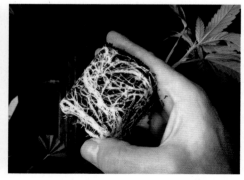

This plant is rootbound and in need of transplanting. Often such compressed roots have to be gently loosened before transplanting, so that they will grow outward and downward.

make a lot of roots, see chapter 19, *Containers*.

Seedlings and clones can also be transplanted directly into 3- to 5-gallon (11.4–19 L) pots, a system that requires fewer containers and involves less work and less possible plant stress. The larger volume of soil holds water and nutrients longer and requires less-frequent watering.

When clones and seedlings in 4-inch (10.2 cm) pots are transplanted directly into 5-gallon (19 L) containers, the roots grow down, out, and around the container walls and bottom. In fact, the majority of roots will grow out of the soil and form a layer behind the container wall that is subject to temperature extremes.

To encourage roots to develop a dense, compact system, transplant just before a plant has outgrown its container. Transplanting a well-rooted clone in a root cube into a 4-inch (10.2 cm) pot, and later transplanting the 4-inch (10.2 cm) pot into a 3-gallon (11.4 L) pot or grow bag causes roots to develop a more extensive system in a small ball of growing medium. Successful transplanting causes minimal stress. Many cannabis crops are in the ground for such a short time that bungled transplanting costs valuable recuperation time and loss in production.

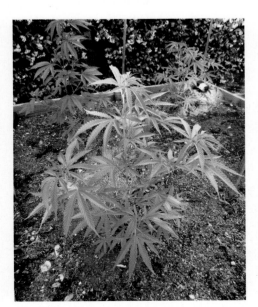
Transplant clones and seedlings into raised beds or containers.

Transplant clones and seedlings into raised beds and large containers or planter boxes or directly into 3-to-5-gallon (11.4–19 L) pots. If plants are allowed to grow 6 to 7 months in full sun, 1 or 2 plants will fill a 200-gallon (757 L) container outdoors. When growing for 3 to 4 months, containers can be 10 to 50 gallons (37.9–189.3 L) in size. Once plants start crowding and shading one another, bend stems outward and tie them to a trellis attached to the planter. Large planters require less maintenance than smaller containers or beds. The larger mass of soil retains water and nutrients much longer and more evenly. One downside is that all plants must receive the same water regimen and diet.

For more information on moving plants outdoors, see chapter 12, *Outdoors*.

Transplanting: Step-by-Step

Step One: The day before transplanting, water clones and seedlings with a half-strength mix of a product that contains *Trichoderma* bacteria and/or mycorrhizal fungi.

Step Two: Fill a 3-gallon (11.4 L) to 200-gallon (757 L) container with rich potting soil or soilless mix to within 2 inches (5.1 cm) of its top. Water the growing medium with a mild, quarter-strength organic nutrient tea or a salt-based hydroponic fertilizer solution until saturated and solution drains freely out the bottom.

Step Three: Carefully remove the root ball from the container. Place your hand over the top of the container with the stem between your fingers; turn the container upside down, and let the root ball slip out of the pot into your hand. Take special care at this point to keep the root ball in one integral piece.

Step Four: Carefully place the root ball in the prepared hole in the new container. Make sure the roots are growing downward, and the soil mass is level with or only a bit deeper than the new medium, slightly and firmly compressing (if necessary and possible) the entire new and old medium into a single unit.

Step Five: Backfill around the root ball. Gently but firmly place soil into contact

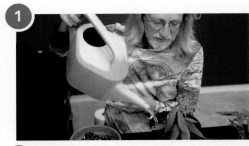
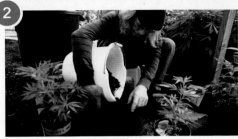
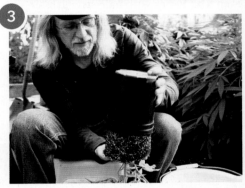
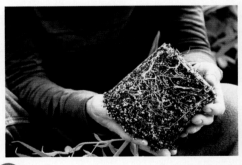
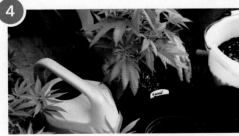
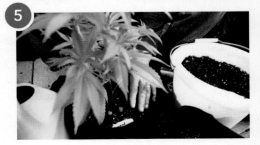

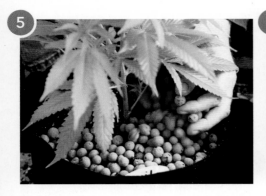

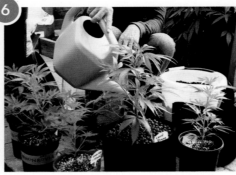

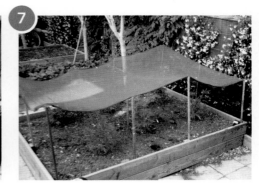

with root ball. Add a top layer of mulch to conserve moisture and protect the delicate layer of surface roots. In this case we used expanded clay pellets.

Step Six: Water with half-strength fertilizer containing *Trichoderma* bacteria and/or mycorrhizal fungus. Soil should be saturated—not waterlogged—and should drain freely. If rooting cube and new substrate are not identical, pay special attention to moisture levels. Let rockwool dry out enough so that roots penetrate new growing medium in search of moisture.

Step Seven: Place new transplants under fluorescent lamps on the perimeter of the HID garden, or under a screen to subdue sunlight outdoors or in a greenhouse for a couple of days. Once transplants look strong, move them under full light or into a greenhouse to harden-off.

Bending and Training

The goal of bending branches is to increase the number of bud sites per plant exposed to full intense sunlight or artificial light. More bud sites equates to more flower buds at harvest. The screen of green (SCROG) growing technique teaches gardeners to bend branches with the help of a horizontal trellis. Buds are bent out horizontally and produce more budding sites. In fact, a friend of mine published an excellent book for indoor medical gardeners: *Secrets of the West Coast Masters*, by Dru West (West Coast Masters, 2011). It is based on trellising

INDOOR CONTAINER SIZE

Plant Age	Container Size
1–3 weeks	root cube / soil block
2–6 weeks	4-inch (10.2 cm) pot
6–8 weeks	2-gallon (7.6 L) pot
2–3 months	3-gallon (11.4 L) pot
3–8 months	5-gallon (19 L) pot
6–18 months	10-gallon (38 L) pot

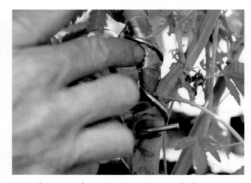

Use heavy aluminum wire to help support plants. This plant broke in the wind and was wrapped with duct tape. A piece of aluminum wire was wrapped around the branch to provide extra support while the plant recovered.

GREENHOUSE / OUTDOOR CONTAINER SIZE

Plant Age	Container Size
1–3 weeks	4-inch (10.2 cm) pot
3–6 weeks	1-3-gallon (4-11.4 L) pot
6–8 weeks	3-5-gallon (11.4-19 L) pot
2–3 months	5-10-gallon (19-38 L) pot
3–6 months	50-200-gallon (189.3-760 L) pot
6–9 months	50-500-gallon (189.3-1893 L) pot

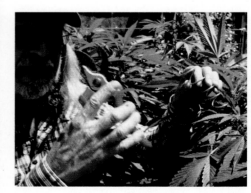

Wrap wire around a broomstick to form a coil. The pliable coil of wire is much easier to wrap around branches.

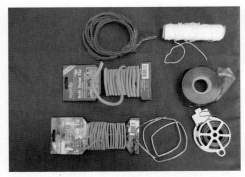

There are many tie-downs to use when bending. Favorite tie-downs include the green insulated wire (bottom left) and the plastic-covered wire (bottom right). Twine, string, and ribbon must be tied and are more tedious to use. I prefer to use insulated wire that does not cut into branches.

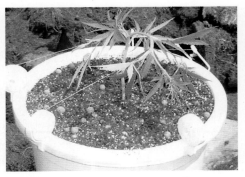

A 'Jack Herer' is growing in a 5-gallon (19 L) container in full sun on a walled balcony protected from the wind. The initial bending starts as soon as the clone (moved from indoors) is established in the container.

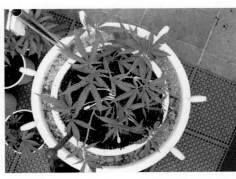

Directing the branches outward by bending them toward the edge of the container will encourage the plant to grow much wider so that all branches will develop bigger flower buds.

to increase the number of bud sites, thereby increasing production.

Pruning redirects growth hormones and affects plants more drastically than bending. Selective pruning and bending allow us to manipulate auxin hormone levels in branch and flower tips. Removing or bending a branch or branch tip causes hormonal balances to shift. Cutting the meristem (top growth tip) of a cannabis plant will diffuse auxins and cause greater concentrations in lower branch tips. Bending a growing tip changes hormone concentrations less than pruning does.

Bending is similar to pruning, in that it alters the flow of hormones. Bending efficiently neutralizes the effect of growth-inhibiting hormones and is much easier on plants than pruning. To bend, choose young, supple branches that are pliable. Lean a branch in the desired direction, and tie it in place. Young, supple branches can take a lot of

bending before they fold over or break. Even if a branch folds, tie it in place; if necessary, use a wooden splint. The stem will heal itself. Young, supple branches take bending much better than old, stiff ones. Bending branches horizontally will encourage buds to grow vertically toward the light. Each bud will turn into an impressive flower top because they all receive more light. A wooden planter box with a lattice trellis alongside or nylon net above makes great anchors to tie bent plants to.

When to Bend and Train Branches

Bend plants when branches are still supple enough to avoid injury. Especially on outdoor plants, branches lose pliability and become more rigid as they age. For best results, start bending plants before they are 12 inches (30.5 cm) tall so that branches have time to adjust hormone levels and grow evenly.

When grown in the vegetative stage for more than a month or two, plants may

need to be bent and trained over a longer season. Once plants enter the flowering stage, bending becomes increasingly more difficult. Bending is less fruitful after flowering plants initiate the last upward spurt of growth.

Wire ties, the kind used to close plastic bags, can be purchased at a nursery. Wire ties are either precut or cut to length by the gardener. Use these ties on small plants that need little direction. Wire ties are generally too small for larger plants and can cut into stems. Thicker ties made of plastic-coated electronic wire or telephone cable work well. They are fastened with a simple twist and stay rigid, leaving the stem room to grow. If applied too tightly around a stem (girdling), liquids cannot flow, and death could result. See "Trellises & Ties" on page 68.

Use grafting tape (or green plastic plant tape with no glue) to cover and support broken branches. A small stick can be

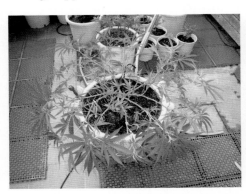

As the plant grows, its branches are bent further outward. The branches in the center of the plant will receive more light and will develop quickly.

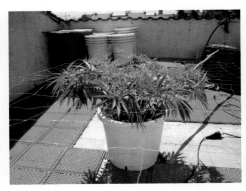

The foliage has grown and the bent plant is showing nice form. The large plastic netting will soon fill with foliage.

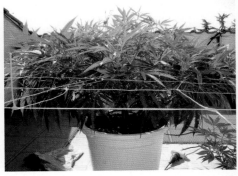

It is early summer, and the plant is well established. The larger trellis is accommodating the extra growth, and bending is continued.

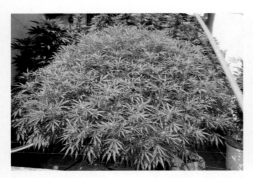

The plant is starting to bud up and has formed a huge canopy over the small container.

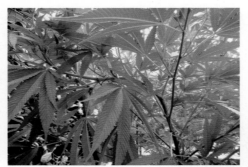

A plastic-coated wire tie was used to bend this branch down to keep it from growing over the 8-foot (2.4 m) fence.

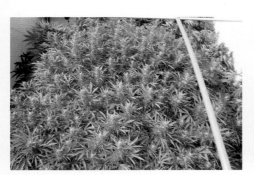

The plant is now in full bloom. It nearly fills a large part of the terrace, completely covering the plastic trellis visible earlier.

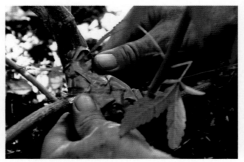

Duct tape can work well to repair broken branches.

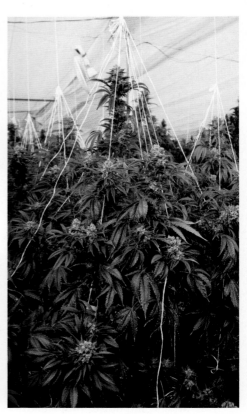

A pyramid of twine is suspended overhead to hold up bud-laden branches. These plants were started from seed normally grown indoors, and their branches are weak. The trellis helps keep the heavy branches upright.

used as a splint for extra support. It protects the wound and also holds broken branches in place. I used duct tape on this plant and was lucky, since the glue can cause issues. Duct tape also stretches and breathes with the plant.

Be gentle when bending branches, even though plants can take some abuse. Sometimes a crotch will separate or a branch will fold over, cutting off fluid flow. These mishaps are often easily fixed with a small wooden splint snugly secured with duct tape to support the split and broken stem. But sometimes a branch broken at a crotch cannot be repaired.

Gardeners also combine pruning and bending. It is easy to prune too much, but it is hard to overbend.

Trellises and Ties
Medical cannabis plants that grow more than 3 to 4 feet (91.4–122 cm) tall often need to be trellised so that weighty buds do not cause branches to break. Trellises serve to direct plant growth within a

given space, and take advantage of sunlight. Adequate trellising also keeps plants standing with minimal damage after rainstorms. Complicated, poorly planned trellises get in the way when maintaining a garden. Plan a simple, easy-to-use trellis. Some gardeners use bamboo stakes or a tomato cage anchored in containers. Raised-bed gardeners can build a frame to set up horizontal trellis netting over plants; branches full of flower buds grow through the netting.

Outdoor gardeners can set up hoop-house trellises over plants by covering the hoop house with 6-inch (15.2 cm) plastic netting, after using the same hoop house as a greenhouse. Branches grow through the trellis netting. If branches grow and start to droop after the first net is in place, wait until they are about 2 feet longer and throw another 6-inch (15.2 cm) net over the plants as a second trellis.

Building your own circular wire trellises is a good option for big plants. Large tomato baskets work well for medium-

size plants. Buy 3- to 6-foot-tall (122–182.9 cm) lengths of galvanized wire fence made from 6-inch (15.2 cm) squares. Form the fence into a big circle 3 to 4 feet (91.2–122 cm) in diameter. Cut and bend the ends of wire to connect the basket into a cylinder. The result will be a 6-foot-tall (182.9 cm) trellis that is 3 to 4 feet (91.2–122 cm) across. Set it over plants before they grow too big. Anchor the trellis in the ground with large staples or tent stakes.

Pruning
Pruning redirects growth hormones and affects plants more drastically than bending. Selective pruning allows gardeners to manipulate auxin hormone levels in branch and flower tips. Removing a branch or branch tip causes hormonal balances to shift. Cutting the meristem (top growth tip) of a cannabis plant will diffuse auxins and cause greater concentrations in lower branch tips.

Always use clean instruments when pruning. A straight razor, single-edge razor blade, a sharp pair of pruners or

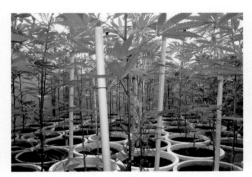
The 'Flo' plants in this garden are destined to grow outdoors. Lower branches and leaves will be stripped before transplanting deep in the soil.

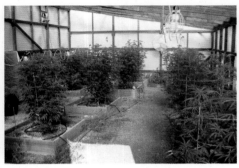
The plants in this greenhouse are trellised with large tomato cages. They will grow to fill the greenhouse and will soon need new trellises.

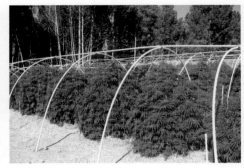
The plastic has been removed, and this hoop house is now a trellis for some very big plants. It is near the first of June, and these established plants are ready to grow!

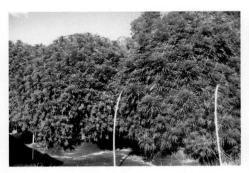
By August 20, the plants have grown through the first netting-trellis and a second netting-trellis has been applied over the top.

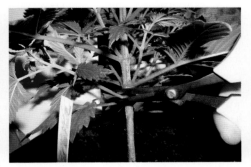
Prune lower growth that receives little or no light. These little branches produce small buds that are difficult to harvest.

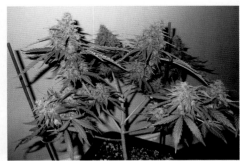
This short plant was pruned once by removing the meristem.

scissors—all work well for different applications. Sanitize clippers and blades between cuts by dipping in rubbing alcohol* or bleach, or flame with a torch. Use indoor pruners *only* in the indoor garden. Pruners used outdoors have everything from spider mites to fungus spores on them. If outdoor clippers must be used, dip them in rubbing alcohol, or flame with a butane torch to sterilize before making cuts. After pruning, the open wound invites diseases and pests. Wash your hands and tools before and after pruning. Make cuts at a 45-degree angle to discourage moisture from sitting on wounds.

*Alcohol works but it is not 100 percent effective, especially on spores and virus particles. A 10 percent bleach solution or a commercial sanitizer will work 100 percent of the time.

Avoid pruning for a month (or more) before inducing flowering. Since pruning diffuses floral hormones, flowering is retarded. If cannabis is pruned heavily 4 to 6 weeks before flowering, peak

maturation will be delayed for a week or longer. It takes a month or more for hormones to build up to pre-pruning concentrations.

Leave leaves alone! Removal of healthy leaves hacks up a healthy plant. Removing strong, healthy leaves DOES NOT make plants more productive, even though this practice supplies more light to small leaves and growing tips. Plants need all their leaves to produce the maximum amount of chlorophyll and food. Removing leaves slows chlorophyll production, stresses the plant, and stunts its growth. Stress is a growth inhibitor. Remove only dead leaves or leaves that are more than 50 percent damaged.

Remove sickly lower growth that receives little light. This weak growth is a ready environment for diseases and pests to attack. Removing shaded lower growth will also increase air circulation between and around plants.

Pruning all the branches or removing more than 20 to 30 percent of the foliage

in a short time frame may cause plants to suffer so much stress that harvest is diminished, especially if there is a short recovery time. However, growth and pruning also depend upon plant health, conditions, stem girth, and other variables.

Over time **pruning too much** may alter hormonal concentrations, causing spindly growth. This is often the case with mother plants that provide too many clones. Mother plants that are up to 12 months old provide the best clones. Many gardeners keep mothers for only 6 months.

Pruning outdoor plants early to mid-season does not affect harvest time. Hormones have a chance to relocate and stabilize before harvest. Pruning branch tips and the main growing shoot forces growth down to lower branches and may be necessary to keep plants under control in small gardens.

Prune plants when small to have the most effect on branching. Removing

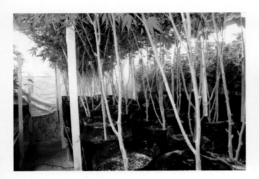

The plants in this garden were too tall when moved in from the vegetative room. They grew fast and the light was able to penetrate only the first 2 feet (61 cm) of foliage. Removing lower growth sends energy upward and increases air circulation below. Nonetheless, plants were growing too long under poor conditions. This is why lower leaves were removed and both time and resources were wasted.

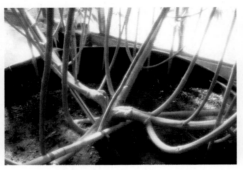

The main stem of this cannabis plant was split to form 4 branches. The wounds on each of the split branches heal and form 4 new "main" stems. This unique, labor-intensive pruning technique promotes the most growth and budding sites from a single cannabis plant. This technique is effective when plants are grown for 6 to 10 months and all other elements —soil, water, nutrients, light, etc., are kept at optimum levels to support the extra growth.

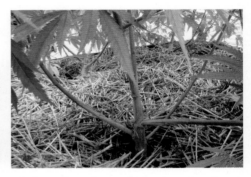

The lower branches on this outdoor plant have been removed because they receive little light and would produce spindly buds. Removing shaded, spindly lower growth increases air circulation and sends valuable growing energy to plant tips.

top growth early will leave a few lower branches to grow upward. Pruning top or side branches later in life will have less dramatic effects and affect hormonal balance less due to the abundance of foliage and hormones.

For the most part, pruning and removing weak spindly growth and dead leaves is all the pruning necessary. See "Remove Lower Branches," below.

An expert medical cannabis gardener from Humboldt County, California, has a unique pruning style for giant plants. The meristem is made to form a callus by cutting it—similar to the FIM technique. Once a callus forms at the tip of the meristem, it is split into 4 separate pieces. The 4 separate quarter-branches are splayed out at 90-degree angles and trellised. The insides of the stems heal rapidly, and branch shoots start growing upward.

Pruning Techniques
No Pruning
Not pruning has several advantages. Floral hormones are allowed to concentrate in tips of branches, causing flower buds to grow stronger and denser. Indoors, short, unpruned plants can be crammed into a small area. Crowded plants have less space to bush out laterally and tend to grow more upright. Clones are set into the flowering room after 1 to 30 days in the vegetative room.

Little clones are clustered together in 3-gallon (11.4 L) pots.

Many indoor gardeners do not prune at all, especially when growing a short clone crop that is only 2 to 3 feet (61–91.4 cm) tall. Short clone crops require no pruning to increase light to bottom leaves or to alter their profile. "No pruning" is the easiest and most productive method when growing short crops, but branches heavily laden with flower buds may need to be trellised.

Outdoors, not pruning is common. Gardeners in Northern California let plants grow to their potential and throw trellising netting over plants to support branches full of flower buds. Many short, stout plants that grow up to four feet (122 cm) tall and are not pruned do not need to be trellised.

Remove Lower Branches
Remove spindly branches and growth that is not collecting light energy, including dead and dying leaves. Removing weak, light-starved lower branches is common in outdoor, indoor, and greenhouse gardens alike. Pruning lower branches concentrates growth in upper branches. Cut lower branches off cleanly at the stem so no stub is left to rot and attract pests and diseases. If you must harvest a little medicinal cannabis early, removing a few lower branches will least diminish the harvest.

Pruning out spindly branches and growth inside plants opens up the interior and provides better air circulation. It also makes inspecting soil, plant stems, and irrigation fittings easier. This is a much better practice than removing all lower leaves.

Remove All but Four Main Branches
Remove the plant's meristem (central stem) just above the 4 lowest (main) branches. Removing the central leader concentrates the floral hormones in the 4 remaining branches. The resulting fewer branches will be stronger and will bear a larger quantity of dense, heavy flower buds. Remove the stem above the 4 main branches, but do not remove leaves on the main branches. Select plants with 3 sets of branch nodes about 6 weeks old and pinch or prune out the last set of nodes so that 2 sets of branches remain. Move plants

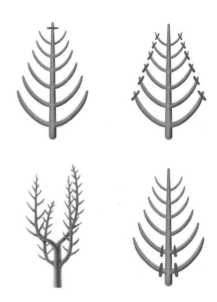

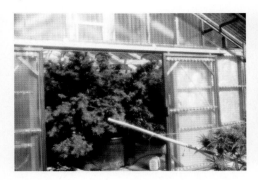

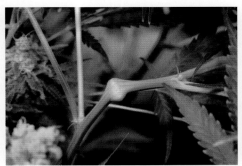

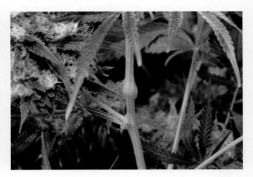

This humongous, pampered plant is growing in a 500-gallon (1893 L) container in a greenhouse. The two 1-gallon (3.8 L) containers on the right add perspective to this plant that has just started to bloom.

Bend or fold plant tips over to practice super-cropping. This practice sends energy down to lower branches.

Plants often heal, and the tip of the plant once again is able to orient growth upward.

into the flowering room or greenhouse when they are about 12 inches (30.5 cm) tall. To maintain a low garden profile, varieties that grow fast and tall, such as 'Critical Mass', 'Power Plant', and similarly robust bloomers, should be set in the flowering room or greenhouse when about 8 inches tall.

Establish a bud count before pinching because only the next lower 5 to 7 buds will actually break or open and grow properly. If the plant is 10 leaves or nodes taller, a soft pinch of only the meristem and 1 leaf, will probably give about 5 breaks. If the plant is 15 leaves or nodes tall, then a soft pinch will give the same results, but all high on the plant. A harder pinch, the top 3 to 5 nodes down, may cause 3 to 5 good branches to grow below. This is a slower process that can extend the maturation period but adjusts the height overall.

Pinching Branch Tips
Pinching back or pruning tops (branch tips) causes the 2 growing shoots just below the cut to grow bigger and stronger. The effect is echoed down the plant. Pinching back and pruning branch tips increases the number of budding sites. It diffuses floral hormones (auxins). At high concentrations, auxins prevent lateral buds from growing very quickly. Lower branches develop more rapidly when the top of the plant (terminal bud) is removed. The further the tip of the branch is from hormones, the less effect the auxins have.

To pinch back a branch tip, simply snip it off below the last set or two of leaves. Pinching off tender growth with your fingers helps seal the wound and is often less damaging to plants than cutting with scissors or pruners. When the main stem is pinched back, side and lower growth is stimulated. When all the tops are pinched back, lower growth is encouraged. Continually pinching back, as when taking clones from a mother, causes many more little branches to form below the pruned tips. Eventually, the plant is transformed into a hedge-like shape. Most gardeners do not pinch plants back, because it diminishes the yield of prime, dense flower tops; but it may not affect the overall dry weight. Promoting many small buds also requires more work when trimming harvested buds.

Super-Cropping
Super-cropping is a form of pinching back or pruning branch tips. Regardless of who coined the buzzword, there are several different versions of super-cropping used by cannabis gardeners.

FIM Technique

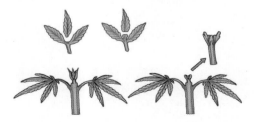

The drawing in the center and the close-up on the right show the FIM pruning technique—the bottom 10 percent of the bud remains intact. This is the key to FIM pruning.

The theory of super-cropping is that plants respond to impaired fluid flow by producing more cannabinoid-rich resin and compact female flowers. The branch is folded over, approximately 2 to 3 inches below the growing tip, creating a wound. Some gardeners swear by this practice, and there might be a morsel of truth in it.

Super-cropping can also incorporate FIM pruning, which is explained below. It can be combined with bending, too. Removing healthy leaves so that "budding sites receive more light" is also practiced by some super-croppers who claim higher production. See "Stress," on page 72, for more information.

FIM Technique
The FIM technique first appeared in print in the July 2000 issue of *High Times* magazine. According to the best information I could find, the technique was started by a gardener from South Carolina. He tried to pinch the tip of a plant and said, "F%&k, I missed!" (FIM) when he did not remove the entire bud as desired. Once the growing tip was pinched, or FIMed, the gardener left the plant to develop. Many different flowering tops formed as a result of this single pruning. According to some cannabis gardeners, this technique increases yield. However, my experience has been that it does not. FIM pruning also creates a small, dense flower top that is prone to disease.

Grafting
Little is known about grafting cannabis, and it is seldom practiced, which is

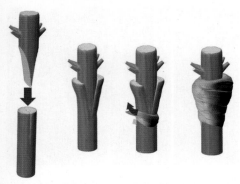

Cleft (or top wedge) graft

The top green part (scion) of one cannabis plant is grafted onto the rootstock. Sativa varieties are generally more disease-resistant than indica varieties. Grafting sativa rootstock onto indica varieties may help make plants more disease resistant.

why grafting commands a small place in the medicinal cannabis garden. Grafting cannabis will help solve drought and possible root-disease problems. Grafting an *indica* stock with a compact growth habit to a large *sativa* root system provides more nutrients for the aboveground plant. The resulting plant would be a drought-resistant super plant.

Most medical states in the USA impose a maximum number of plants we are able to grow. Grafting 3 or 4 different varieties onto 1 mother plant would help a gardener stay below mandatory plant maximums.

Yes, it is possible to graft cannabis rootstock onto a scion (branch) of hop species (*Humulus lupulus*). Hops, the female flower clusters from hop plants, are used in the production of beer. The plant will live; however, it will not produce more cannabinoids.

Stress

Cannabis grows best and produces most heavily when it is given a stable environment. Stressed plants are less productive than unstressed plants. Stress-induced traumas include withholding water, photoperiod fluctuation, low light intensity, ultraviolet light, nutrient toxicities and deficiencies, cold and hot soil, temperature extremes, mutilation, and any other weird stuff beyond ideal growth conditions. In addition, any overt applications of growth hormones

such as gibberellins, cytokinins, abscisic acid, ethylene, or colchicine cause stress. Stress can also cause female plants to produce male flowers and male plants to produce female flowers. See chapter 22, *Additives*, and chapter 25, *Breeding*, for more information on hormones and other agents.

Stress can cause plants to produce more resin, but it simultaneously causes odd and/or less growth. For example, Felix, a Swiss outdoor gardener, grew a field of cannabis at 900 feet elevation (274 m) and another at 4200 feet (1280 m). The upper field suffered stress because it was exposed to cooler temperatures and more ultraviolet radiation. Plants there produced about 25 percent more resin-packed THC than plants in the lower field. But, plants that grew at 900 feet elevation (274 m) yielded at least 25 percent or more dry weight than plants at 4200 feet (1280 m). Removing large green shade leaves allows more light to shine on smaller leaves, but it also causes growth to slow and harvest to diminish. Remove only leaves that are more than half damaged by pests or diseases. Often, partially yellow leaves green up once stress is eliminated.

How to Make Cannabis Plants Suffer Stress

1. Photoperiod fluctuation and then back to a 12-hour day/night photoperiod.

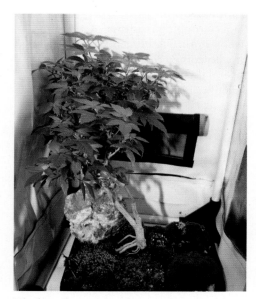

The branches on this "bonsai" plant have been pruned, as have the roots, so that it will grow slowly in this small container. The stressful environment keeps the plant small.

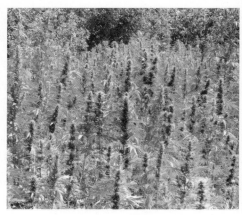

These plants—grown under stressful conditions in the Rif Mountains of Morocco—receive more intense UV light, limited nutrients, and little water.

2. Low light intensity (This may cause more male plants.)

3. Nutrient toxicities and deficiencies

4. Cold and hot growing mediums

5. Cold and hot ambient temperatures

6. Mutilation

7. Sex stress

8. Watering

9. Pathogens

10. Chemicals

11. Much more

Mutilating plants by breaking the trunk, driving a stake through stems, and otherwise torturing or slapping them around might increase resin production, but most often the resulting stress retards growth, causes other problems, and reduces overall production.

Withholding water may also cause more resin production, but it impairs growth and diminishes leaf, stem, and flower production. Water stress slows or stops clones from rooting. If clones have too many leaves and are too busy transpiring, root growth is very slow. Conversely, waterlogged rooting mediums harbor no air, and rooting is then slowed to a crawl.

Stress can also affect plants' sex. See chapter 25, *Breeding*, for more information.

PART 2 ESSENTIAL MEDICAL CANNABIS HORTICULTURE

7
CLONES & CLONING

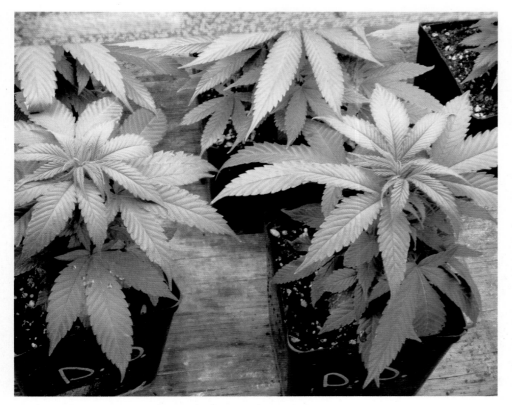

Healthy "clones" are the mainstay of most cannabis gardens.

MEDICAL CANNABIS can be reproduced (propagated) sexually or asexually. Seeds are the product of sexual propagation; stem cuttings (aka clones*) are the result of asexual or vegetative propagation. In its simplest form, taking a stem cutting involves cutting a growing branch or branch tip, placing the cut end into a growing medium, and keeping it moist until roots grow. Medical cannabis gardeners commonly refer to a "clone" as a branch of a cannabis plant that has been cut off and rooted.

*Technically, cloning is taking one cell of a plant and promoting its growth into a plant; it shares the same DNA and is effectively a copy of the donor (mother) plant.

Clones are taken from desirable females called mother plants. Once rooted, clones are transplanted and moved into an indoor vegetative room, greenhouse, or outdoors. Crops of clones are most often induced to flower with a 12/12-hour day/night schedule and harvested

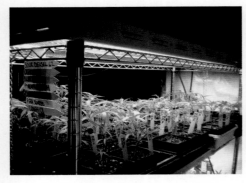

Well-illuminated, healthy clones are fast-growing, and develop more quickly than fungus and spider mites can reproduce. By the time such pests and problems take hold, healthy plants are well on their way to maturity.

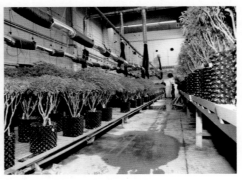

Strong, healthy, cannabinoid-potent females make good mothers. Weak plants that are susceptible to disease and pest attacks over time make poor mothers, even though they might exhibit strong genetic qualities. Such mothers tend to lose strength and often contract low levels of diseases that they pass on to clones.

CLONES

Advantages	Disadvantages
all female	can carry undetectable diseases
exact replica of mother	genetic instability maintained
consistent growth	not F1 hybrids—less vigor
less time to harvest than seeds	difficult for some gardeners to root
flower-ready (competent buds)	difficult to find locally and legally

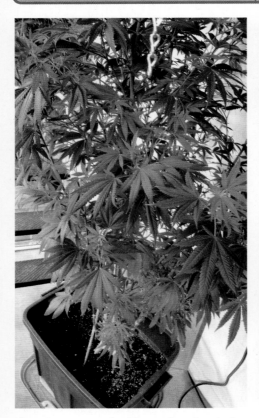

Growing a strong, healthy mother plant is the first step to producing strong, healthy cuttings.

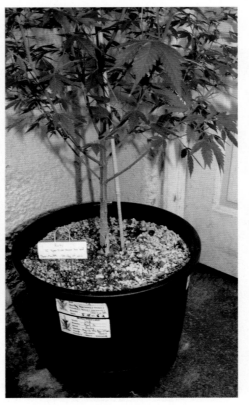

Label all mothers and corresponding clones.

about 2 months later. Short crops of clones in small containers are much easier to move and maintain than big plants in large containers, whether grown indoors, outdoors, or in a greenhouse.

Mother Plants

Mother plants are selected for desirable medicinal qualities. Cannabinoid and terpene content are more important than harvest weight. The most robust mother plants are taken from superior F1 hybrid females. See chapter 3, *Medical Cannabis Varieties*, for more information.

All cannabis plants can be cloned, regardless of age or growth stage. However, autoflowering plants complete their life cycle in less than 90 days and make very short-term mothers. It is time-consuming to re-vegetate plants that flowered before clones were taken. Clones taken from flowering plants root quickly but require a month or longer to revert to vegetative growth. See "Cloning a Flowering Female," on page 84.

Take clones from mother plants that are at least 2 months old. If taking clones from seedlings, wait until male or female pre-flowers are easily visible with the naked eye. Clones taken from female plants cloned before they have expressed sex may dawn male flowers or develop poorly when induced to flower with a 12/12-hour day/night photoperiod.

Mother plants are most resilient when grown from F1 hybrid seeds. Most often clones are taken from other clones. There are countless examples of gardeners who made clones of clones from the same variety more than 20 times. That is, clones (C-1) were taken from the original female grown from seed. These clones were grown in the vegetative stage, and clones (C-2) were taken from the first clones (C-1). Blooming was induced in (C-1) 2 weeks later and (C-2), grown in the vegetative stage. Then, clones (C-3) were taken from the second clones (C-2). This same growing technique is still going on with clones of clones well past (C-20) and there has been no apparent breakdown in the clone's potency or vigor. However, mothers that are weak may suffer stress or contract disease such as powdery mildew will produce weak clones. Weak and diseased mothers should be banished from the garden, container and all.

A female plant will reproduce 100 percent females, all exactly like the mother except for phenotype deviation*. When grown in the exact same environment, clones from the same mother usually look alike. But the same clones subjected to distinct environments in different garden rooms will often look different.

*Since we do not have enough research on cannabis, we must look at other plants for information. The Bradford pear for instance, arose from a genetic difference in the bud. The new shoot had better pears, and new trees were made from them. They are not always complete to form—older DNA that has been acted on, and an established phenotype. A true clone made from a single cell was used to make a big group, carry all identical but new DNA, and a cursory but malleable phenotype.

Once a plant grown from seed has designated sex (male or female), and it receives any other necessary trigger—temperature, light cycle, etc.—it is biologically "competent," ready to enter the flowering growth stage. See "Florigen" in chapter 8, *Flowering*, for more information.

Keep several mother plants in the vegetative growth stage for a consistent source of cloning stock. Start new mothers from seed every 6 to 12 months. Give

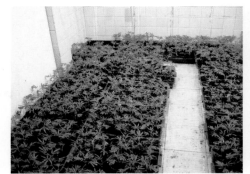

One or two large female plants can be the source of many clones!

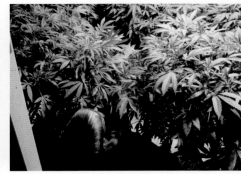

Richard Lee, founder of Oaksterdam University, inspects a roomful of mother plants.

mother plants 18 to 24 hours of light per day to maintain rapid growth.

Transplant old mother plants into the outdoor garden. Once mother plants are 6 to 12 months old they are usually potbound and prone to pest and disease attacks. Move old mother plants outdoors in the early spring for a spring crop, or plant them for a fall crop. Once mothers have hardened-off and acclimated to the outdoor climate, Mother Nature takes over!

Preparing to Clone

Cloning is the most traumatic incident cannabis plants can experience, aside from harvest. Clones go through an incredible transformation when they change from a severed green growing tip

to a rooted plant. Their entire chemistry changes; the stem that once grew leaves must now grow roots in order to survive. Clones are at their most fragile point in life just after being cut.

While rooting, clones require a minimum of nitrogen but increased levels of phosphorus to promote root growth. Sprays should be avoided during rooting, as they compound cloning stress. Given good instruction and a little experience, most gardeners achieve a consistent, 100 percent clone survival rate.

Large cuttings having large, starch-filled stems will grow roots more slowly than will small clones with small stems. The excess starch in moist substrate also attracts diseases. Thin-stemmed

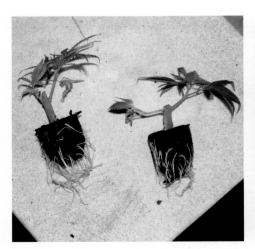

Weak mothers that are susceptible to disease and pest attacks make poor clones, even though they may initially exhibit strong genetic qualities.

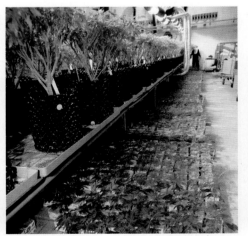

Clones below are exact genetic replicas of mother plants above. Each mother's cell carries a DNA blueprint of itself. Radiation, chemicals, disease, and poor cultural practices can damage this DNA. Unless damaged, the DNA remains intact.

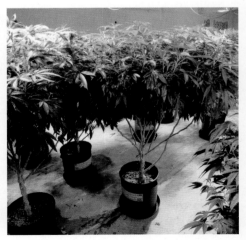

These mother plants provided hundreds of clones, and were finally moved outdoors and harvested in the fall.

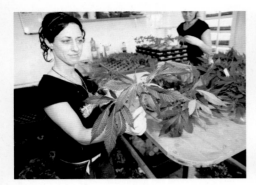
Big, healthy growth like this makes excellent clones.

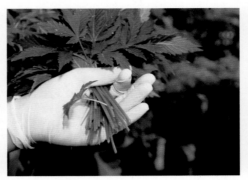
All of these stems were cut on an angle so that more interior stem surface is exposed. This is where many roots will grow.

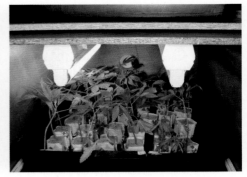
These clones were just taken and still need to get used to their new environment. When they grow roots, these clones will look much stronger.

clones have fewer reserves (accumulated starch), but they only need enough reserve energy to initiate root growth.

Small clones with a few leaves need less moisture and will root faster than big cuttings with many leaves. At first leaves contain moisture, but after a few days the stem is no longer able to supply enough moisture to the leaves, and the clone suffers stress. A small amount of leaf space is all that is necessary for photosynthesis to supply enough energy for root growth.

Integrity in Parents
1. Maintain 18-to-24-hour day photoperiod
2. Keep plants healthy
3. Grow for 6 to 12 months
4. Repot as needed

Easy-to-clone plants
Look for plants that dawn small (rootlet) nubs (primordia) near the base of the trunk. Such plants tend to strike roots exceptionally fast.

Most 'Skunk' and *indica* varieties grow roots easily.

Difficult-to-clone plants
Ruderalis crossed with *indica* or *sativa* varieties are autoflowering and do not make suitable mother plants.

Outdoor varieties with a slight tendency to pre-sex (designate sex) in an 18-hour photoperiod include: 'Early Girl', 'Early Skunk', and many others. Check with seed companies for details. But early flowering does not always exclude them as mother plants.

Clones taken from weak, leggy mother plants most often produce weak, leggy clones. Harvested plants that have been induced back into vegetative growth can also produce weak clones if not fully reverted.

Precautions
Clones root well within a slightly acidic pH range of 5.5 to 6.6. Aeroponic clone gardens normally do best with a pH of 5.4 to 5.6. Most diseases grow poorly below these pH levels. Always make sure there is plenty of air in the rooting medium to stimulate root growth.

Do not kill clones with kindness and fertilizer. At best, giving clones an excess dose of fertilizer causes rooting to be delayed. In fact, a dose of ammonium nitrate, a common salt-based fertilizer, will actually stop root hairs from growing.

Inexperienced gardeners and diseased plants cause most clone-rooting problems. Weak plants that lack vigor provide slow-rooting, weak clones. Poor growing conditions also affect the strength of clones.

See "Dip Plants in Miticide" in chapter 6, *Vegetative Growth*. Watch out for miticidal dips that coat leaves too heavily. The dip should cover well enough to protect plants with insecticidal and fungal properties, yet allow stomata to breathe.

If a spider mite infestation occurs, many gardeners destroy infested clones and start over with clean clones. Others spray with aerosol pyrethrum or another organic miticide. Remember, all pesticides—natural or not—are phytotoxic. Spraying cuttings is a bad idea in general,

AVERAGE ROOT GROWTH FOR CANNABIS CLONE

Action	Cut from Young	Cut from Old
cell division starts	day 4	day 6
first root nubs form	day 6	day 10
roots start to grow	day 7	day 20
enough roots to transplant	day 14	day 28

This table shows average times for roots to grow from the stem.
Note: Clones taken from younger growth root faster than those taken from older growth.

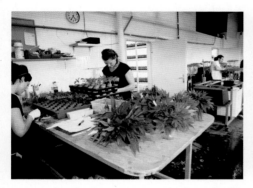

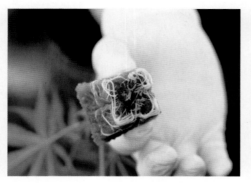

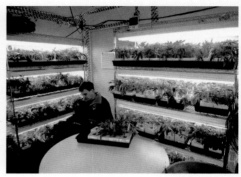

Keep a clean room! Leaves on the floor should be cleared away 3 or 4 times daily.

Transplant clones before they become rootbound!

Richard Lee, Oaksterdam University, inspects clones in a spotless clone room.

including antidesiccant sprays. Sprays clog stomata and can impair root growth in clones. If you must use sprays, use natural organic sprays, apply them when it is cool, and keep their use to a minimum. See "Sprays and Spraying" in chapter 24, *Diseases & Pests.*

The roots on this clone are circling the container and the roots near the center are already turning dark, signifying overwatering and pending death. Do not overwater clones. Keep the medium evenly moist but do not let it get soggy. Any kind of stress disrupts plants and slows rapid growth. Different mediums need distinct watering schedules. Rockwool holds water for a long time, while peat pellets need watering more often. Clones are tender; they have a small developing root system and need extra vigilance now.

Keep the cloning area clean. Do not take clones where fungus spores and diseases are hiding! *Pythium* flourishes in high temperatures and excessive moisture. Powdery mildews prefer cool moist conditions. Spider mites, whiteflies, and thrips love weak, tender clones. Remove infested clones from the cloning room. Cooler, humid conditions, 65°F to 78°F (18°C–25°C), inhibit most mite reproduction and avert infestations. But cool, humid conditions may increase chances of specific fungal attacks.

Root-Inducing Hormones
Root-inducing hormones may help speed cannabis root development. Most often, root-inducing hormones are used to help strike roots on woody plants that

are not for human consumption. Medical gardeners avoid dangerous synthetic rooting hormones (IBA and NAA*) altogether and wait a few days longer for roots to grow. Use an aero-cloner or deep water cloner (aka DWC or bubble cloner) to expedite root growth. Using just plain water under proper conditions, roots will strike on 80 to100 percent of clones only 1 to 3 days later than when hormones are employed. Root-inducing hormones also have less effect when all the conditions are just right and roots are naturally ready to grow.

*IBA (Indole-3-butyric acid, 3-indolebutyric acid, indolebutyric acid) is synthetic and classified by the EPA as an agricultural chemical and pesticide. It is also a mutagenic, able to cause mutation. NAA (1-naphthalenaecetic acid) is a synthetic product registered under the EPA as a pesticide.

Two main hormones stimulate undifferentiated growth: 1-naphthalenaecetic acid (NAA) and indolebutyric acid (IBA). Most commercial rooting hormones contain one or both of the synthetic ingredients IBA and NAA. Many root-inducing hormones also contain a fungicide to help prevent pathogens, including damping-off. Read the labels carefully for root-inducing hormones. When purchasing, search for value. Products contain different concentrations of IBA and NAA. Commercial products hold their ingredients in a powder, liquid, or gel form.

When the stem of a cutting develops roots, it must transform from produc-

ing green stem cells to manufacturing undifferentiated cells (callus) and, finally, to fabricating root cells. Once undifferentiated, cells quickly transform into root cells.

As soon as cuttings are taken, clones start dispatching natural rooting hormones to the wound; these hormones arrive in full force in about a week. The artificial rooting hormone fills the need until natural hormones take over. See chapter 22, *Additives*, for more information on root-inducing hormones.

NOTE: If exceeded in concentration or duration, IBA applications impair root formation

Rooting hormones are available in liquid, gel, or powder form. Liquid forms are easy to dilute. Gel-holding hormones are easy to keep consistent and are simple for novice gardeners to use. Powder forms are the choice of most professional gardeners because they are inexpensive, consistent, and cause no problems. Natural root-inducing products such as willow water are in liquid form and are used over the long term. Do not apply rooting liquids, gels, or powders, above soil line, or excess stem swelling could occur aboveground.

Liquid rooting hormones are easy to dilute and mix in different concentrations. Gardeners mix the most dilute concentration for softwood cuttings. Apply any rooting hormone containing IBA only once. Do not exceed concentration or dip duration. Give cuttings a

5- to 15-second dip in concentrated solutions of IBA and NAA. With a quick dip, stems evenly absorb the 500- to 20,000-ppm concentrated hormone.

Root-inducing gels are easy to use and most practical for small amounts of cuttings. Gels are not water-soluble. Once applied, gels hold and stay with the stem longer than liquids or powders. However, the cut end of a clone stem often develops fungal infections.

Rooting powders often contain mixture of talc and IBA and/or NAA and are less expensive than liquids or gels. Many professional cannabis gardeners prefer to make their cuttings with powder because it is so consistent and is easier to contain than liquids or gels. To avoid contamination, pour a small amount into a separate container, and throw away any excess.

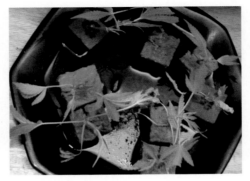

Damping-off (in this case, Botrytis cinerea) has infected these unhappy clones. They must be tossed out, and the clone area must be scrubbed down with bleach.

To apply, roll the moistened stem of the cutting in the powder. Apply a thick, even coat. Tap or lightly scrape excess powder off the cutting; excess hormones can hinder root growth. In the rooting

medium, make a hole bigger than the stem. If the hole is too small, the rooting powder gets scraped off upon insertion.

Some gardeners soak their cuttings in a dilute solution (20–200 ppm IBA and/or NAA) for 24 hours. But I have seen few gardeners use this time-consuming technique, and I am not sure if it is more beneficial than dipping stems.

Willow (tree) water induces roots. The substance in willow trees that promotes rooting is unknown, but repeated experiments have proven that willow water promotes about 20 percent more roots than plain water. This willow water can be mixed with commercial rooting hormones for improved results.

To make willow water rooting compound, find any willow tree and remove

Rooting Hormones

Hormex is an IBA-based powder available in 6 different strengths ranging from 1000 ppm to 45,000 ppm.

Rhizopon AA (Rhizopon B.V.) is an IBA powder is from Hortus USA, the world's largest company devoted to the research and manufacture of rooting

products. Products are available in both powder form and water-soluble tablets in strengths from 500 to 20,000 ppm.

To determine rooting hormone concentration, multiply the manufacturer's listed percentage by 10,000 (e.g., a product with 0.9 percent IBA contains 9000 ppm IBA.

Warning! Root-inducing hormone products containing IBA and IAA are not recommended for use with edible plants. Root-inducing hormones should not be used to grow medical cannabis. Read label carefully before deciding to use these or *any* products.

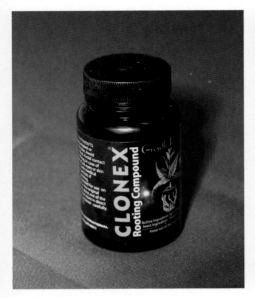

Clonex *cloning gel is a blend of vitamins, minerals, and antimicrobial agents, 0.3 percent (3000 ppm) IBA. Gel seals cutting tissues, thus reducing chance of infection and embolisms.*

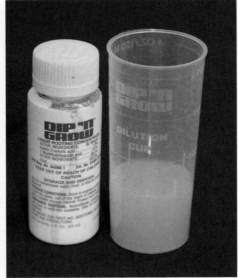

Dip-N-Grow *IBA, NAA, antibacterial. Cost is one penny per 100 cuttings.*

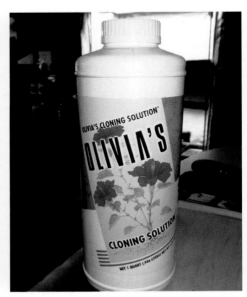

Olivia's rooting hormone is one of the many root-inducing hormones available today.

some of this year's branches that are about one and a half inches in diameter. Remove the leaves, and cut the branches into 1-inch lengths. Place 1-inch willow sticks on end, so that a lot of them fit in a water glass or quart jar. Fill the jar with water, and let it soak for 24 hours. After soaking, pour off the willow water, and use it for rooting hormone. Soak cannabis clones in the willow water for 24 hours, and then plant them in rooting medium. If using a commercial liquid rooting hormone, substitute the willow water in place of regular water in the mix.

Several commercial products contain *Trichoderma* bacteria or mycorrhizal fungi, both of which help plants grow bigger, stronger, and faster.

Coconut milk contains the cytokinin zeatin (see chapter 22, *Additives*) and encourages clone root growth. Mix equal parts coconut milk, grated coconut meat, and clean hot water in a blender and blend until smooth. Use to water clones.

Before Starting
Taking clones, or cuttings, is the most efficient, productive means of cannabis propagation for many indoor, green-house, and outdoor medical cannabis gardeners. Once desirable female plants

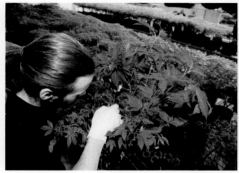

When taking clones, begin by choosing a strong, healthy, genetically desirable mother plant. Use a sharp, sterile blade to perform the actual cutting.

have been distinguished and selected, branch tips and branches can be cut and rooted.

Disinfect all tools and working surfaces to kill bacteria, fungi, viruses, and other diseases already present. Sterilize a sharp scissors, razor, or razor blade by dipping in alcohol, vinegar, or bleach (5 to 10 percent solution) or by heating with a torch. Wash your hands thoroughly beforehand. Make sure to have all cloning supplies within arm's reach—rooting cubes, rooting hormone, razor or scissors, humidity dome, etc.—before you start to take clones.

To avoid problems:
Keep the work area clean. Wash work surfaces and tools before starting.

Have grow medium ready.

Prepare mother plant in advance.

Take clones with clean (sterile) instruments.

Store cut clones in water.

Insert (stick) cutting in growing medium or aeroponics system.

Place clones under humidity dome/tent.

Carefully monitor grow medium moisture levels and humidity.

Watch for root growth.

Transplant when roots emerge from root cube or medium.

Harden-off by gradually exposing cuttings to their new environment.

Cloning: Step-by-Step
Step One: Choose a strong, healthy, desirable mother plant that is at least 2 months old. If a variety is difficult to clone, leach the soil with 2 gallons (7.6 L) of water for each gallon (3.8 L) of soil every morning for a week before taking clones. Drainage must be good. Or mist leaves heavily with plain water every morning. Both practices help wash out nitrogen. Do not fertilize mother plant while leaching the growing medium.

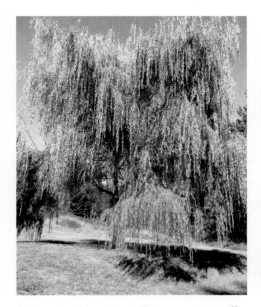

An extract of weeping willow tree water will promote rooting.

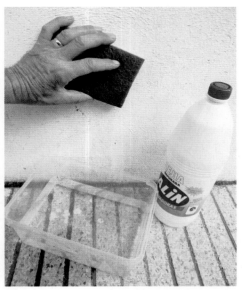

Mix a mild bleach solution to clean and disinfect all garden room surfaces.

Step Two: With a sharp, sterile blade, make a clean 45-degree cut across firm, healthy 0.125- to 0.25-inch-wide (approx. 3–6 mm) branches, 2 to 4 inches (5.1–10.2 cm) in length. Take care not to smash the end of the stem when

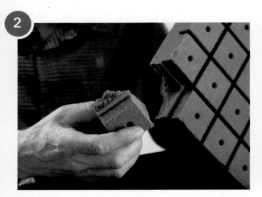

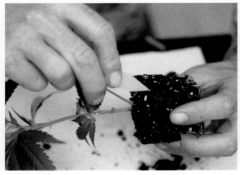

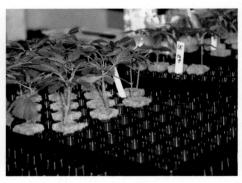

Oasis is a favorite of many gardeners.

Make sure to remove the plastic netting around Jiffy pellets before transplanting.

Rockwool cubes are super convenient, hold a lot of air when wet, and serve as a container.

making the cut. Trim off 2 or 3 sets of leaves and growth nodes so the stem can fit into the soil. There should be at least 2 sets of leaves above the soil line and 1 or 2 sets of trimmed nodes below the ground. When cutting, make the slice halfway between the sets of nodes. Immediately place the cut end in water. Store cut clones in water while cutting more clones.

Step Three: Oasis, Jiffy, and Rockwool rooting mediums are convenient and easy to maintain and transplant. All have different moisture- and air-holding abilities.

Place a tray containing rooting cubes or plugs into a standard nursery rooting flat or strong plastic tray. Fill rockwool tray with water having a pH of 5.5 to 6.5.

Fill small containers or nursery flats with fine perlite/vermiculite, soilless mix, or fine potting soil. Saturate the

substrate with water. If none exist, make holes through three-fourths of the rooting cube for inserting clone stems. Use an unsharpened pencil, a chopstick, or a nail to make a hole in the rooting medium—a little larger than the stem. The hole should stop about one-half inch (1.3 cm) from the bottom of the container to allow for root growth.

Step Four: Use a rooting hormone, and mix (if necessary) just before using. For liquids, use the dilution ratio for softwood cuttings. Swirl each cutting in the hormone solution for 5 to 10 seconds. Place each cutting in a hole in the rooting medium. Gently pack rooting medium around the stem. Gel and powder root hormones require no mixing; dip stems in gels as per instructions, or roll the stem in the powder. When planting, take special care to keep a solid layer of hormone gel or powder around the stem when gently packing soil into place.

Step Five: Lightly water until the surface is evenly moist. Keep cuttings evenly moist at all times! Clones have no roots to bring water to leaves. Water arrives from leaves and the cut stem until roots can supply it. If clones dry out they will wilt and die. Water as needed to keep growing medium evenly moist, but do not let substrate get soggy, or clone stems will soon contract pathogens, rot, and die.

Step Six: Clones root fastest with low levels of light for 18 to 24 hours daily. If clones must be placed under an HID, set them on the perimeter of the garden so they receive less-intense light, or shade them with a cloth or screen. A fluorescent tube 6 inches (15.2 cm) above clones or a 400-watt metal halide 4 to 6 feet (1.2–1.8 m) away supplies the perfect amount of light for clones to root. Cool white fluorescents (or a combination of warm white and cool white) are excellent for rooting clones.

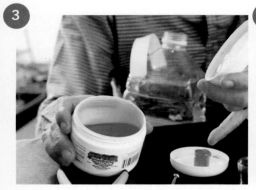

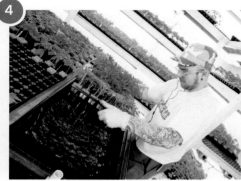

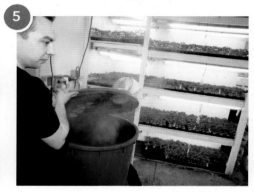

This rooting hormone gel is color-coded.

Watering a tray of clones is as easy as dipping them in a tank of nutrient solution.

A humidity generator releases moist air into the cloning room to increase the humidity to above 90 percent for the first few days after cloning.

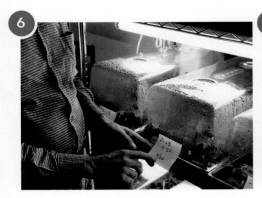

These clones were taken on August 20. The date was recorded on the Post-it note.

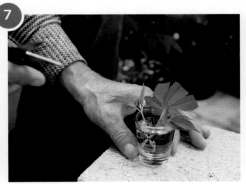

Cut clones can be held in a glass of water. Cutting leaves in half decreases the amount of fluids necessary to support life. Roots must regrow to support new life.

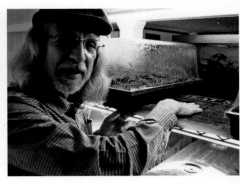

Heating pads add extra warmth in cool garden rooms.

Step Seven: Clones root fastest when humidity levels are 90 to 100 percent during the first 2 days and gradually reduced to 80 to 85 percent during the following week. A humidity tent will help keep humidity high. Purchase a premade cloning dome or construct a humidity tent out of plastic bags, rigid plastic, or glass. Remember to leave openings for air to flow in and out so little clones can breathe. If practical, mist clones several times a day as an alternative to the humidity tent. Remove any sick, rotting, or dead foliage.

Cut leaves in half to lower transpiration surface and to keep them from overlapping. Moisture that could foster fungus is often trapped between overlapping leaves. Keep grow medium evenly moist so there is enough moisture to keep tender cuttings alive.

Step Eight: Clones root faster when the growing medium is a few degrees warm-er than the ambient air temperature. A warmer substrate increases underground chemical activity, and lower air temperature slows transpiration. For best results, keep the rooting medium at 75°F to 80°F (23.9°C–26.7°C). Growing medium temperatures above 85°F (29.4°C) will cause damage. Keep the air temperature 5 to 10 degrees (Fahrenheit) cooler than the substrate. A warmer growing medium coupled with cooler ambient temperature slows diseases and conserves moisture. Misting clones with water also cools foliage and slows transpiration to help traumatized clones retain moisture unavailable from nonexistent roots. Put clones in a warm place to adjust air temperature, and use a heating pad, heating cables, or an incandescent lightbulb below rooting cuttings.

Step Nine: Some cuttings may wilt but then regain rigidity in a few days. Clones should look close to normal by the end of the week. Cuttings that are still wilted after seven days may suffer from pathogens such as rot and damping-off, or may root so slowly they never catch up with others. Cull sick clones. Put healthy, slow-rooting clones back into the cloning chamber to grow more roots.

Step Ten: In 1 to 3 weeks, cuttings should be rooted. Signals that they have rooted include: yellow leaf tips, roots growing out drain holes, and vertical growth of the clones. To check for root growth in flats or pots, carefully remove a root ball and clone to see if it has good root development. For best results, transplant clones when roots have just started to break through the growing medium. If you wait until a dense root system is growing out the sides and bottom of rooting cubes, some roots will be dead. Clones transplant best when roots have just started to grow beyond the walls of rooting cubes.

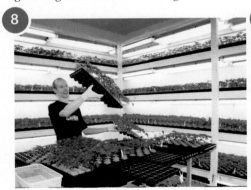

Clones are ready to transplant when roots show out the bottom of rooting flats.

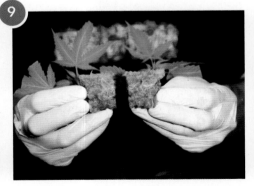

The roots on these clones are perfect for transplanting. They are white, strong, and healthy.

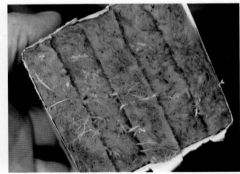

Note the tips of these roots are turning dark, signifying too much moisture and the beginning of rot. This clone must be transplanted immediately to avoid further rot.

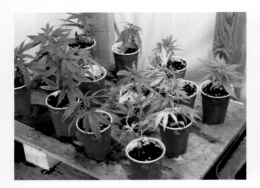

Cull sickly clones. Weak clones will always grow poorly and will often spread pests and diseases to the rest of the garden.

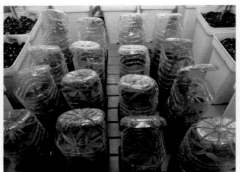

Individual clones can be covered with plastic containers to keep humidity high.

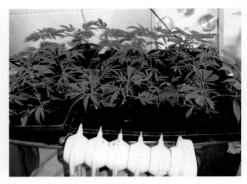

These well-cared-for clones have been transplanted to larger containers and have resumed growth. Soon each will be transplanted to its final container.

Caring for Clones

Cuttings always look strong and healthy right after you take them. About 5 or 6 days later, leaves may start to change color. Leaves stay small and often turn a deeper shade of green. After about a week, lower leaves may start to yellow if their nutrient levels dissipate.

A week after being taken, a clone's belowground stem will develop stubby callused roots called primordia. The primordia are semitransparent to white, and should look healthy. The clone will produce very little green growth during this process. Leaves and the severed stem now supply fluids for the clone. Once the root and vascular transport system is in place and working properly, roots are able to supply water and nutrients. Clones then start vegetative growth.

Any sign of slime, pests, or diseases means there are problems. Root damage due to lack of oxygen or overwatering will kill thin, hairlike roots. They will turn brown from rot or shrivel when dry. Once damaged, roots remain damaged. New roots must grow to replace damaged roots. Cull slow-growing clones that have damaged roots. Some gardeners let clones with desirable genetic qualities root longer and will transplant them when adequate roots develop.

Clone foliage can lose much of its protective waxy coating when pampered indoors. Now leaves and stems are very tender and supple. They will need to be transplanted and hardened-off before moving to another location.

Rooting clones need progressively more light as they grow. Move the light source closer to clones once roots form. Fertilize with a mild organic fertilizer solution when all clones have started vegetative growth.

Transplant only the strongest well-rooted clones. Slow-rooting clones should be kept in the cloning chamber or culled out. Do not move clones into bright light until they have fully developed root systems. Once transplanted, clones are ready to harden-off.

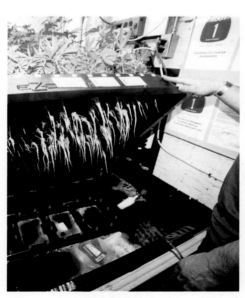

An aero-cloner consists of a chamber with small spray nozzles inside. The stems and roots are bathed in a 100 percent–humidity root zone environment. Water is pumped under pressure and atomized into the air or dispersed as a spray via nozzles. Clones strike roots nearly as well when water is not atomized. Clones root incredibly quickly in this system.

Harden-off strong clones by moving them into a brighter garden room. Make sure they have adequate air ventilation and circulation. Some gardeners "pre-grow" clones in a small vegetative room before introducing them to the flowering room or moving them into a greenhouse or a protected outdoor location.

Set up a vegetative pre-growing area that is lit with HID or bright compact fluorescent lighting for the rooted clones. Place them in this area to let them grow for the first week or two of vegetation.

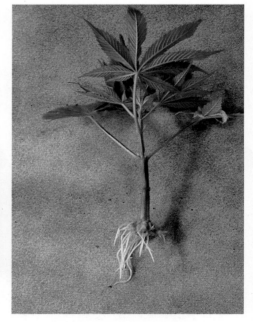

Strong, white roots on this clone have initiated from the callus on the cut stem.

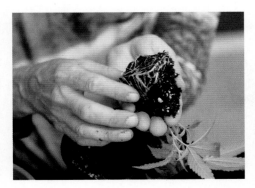

Transplant clone when roots have outgrown the container. This clone could have been transplanted a few days earlier.

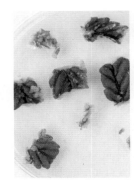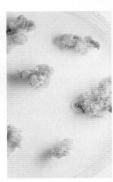

Left to right: Leaves are cut into small pieces and set in a specific agar solution where the green leafy growth changes to white callus – undifferentiated growth.

Callus (undifferentiated growth) has clearly formed and roots are ready to form.

perfect for gardeners wanting to produce many densely rooted cuttings quickly and efficiently. Cuttings grow a mass of roots in seven to ten days and can be transplanted into hydroponic growing mediums or soil. Aero-cloners are somewhat labor intensive. Clones must be taken, rooted, and transplanted—carefully. Producing clones for small gardens is best accomplished in rooting cubes.

Scraping the Stem

Always cut stems at a 45° angle when taking cuttings. Very lightly scraping away the outer layer of the stem to expose only the cambium layer below allows hormones to concentrate where roots start, and causes many roots to grow there. Splitting the clones' stem exposes more surface area to grow roots. Both practices increase the number of healthy roots, but rooting time is longer.

After the cutting has been trimmed and scraped, dip the bare stem into a rooting hormone. Now it is ready to "stick" into the substrate. First a heavy callus develops, from which prolific roots grow. Roots will take longer to strike, 10 to 14 days, but they will grow much more densely.

This area needs to be just big enough to accommodate plants from the time they are a few inches tall until they are about a foot tall and ready to be moved into the flowering room. Such a small room is a very efficient use of space, light, and electricity.

Cloning Techniques

Aero-cloner

Aeroponic cloners are the most efficient cloners I have seen. We built one about 30 years ago. Since then, several commercial models have become available. They are

Air Layering

Air layering is seldom used by medical cannabis gardeners, except with the most difficult-to-root clones. It is interesting but normally unnecessary. Cannabis cuttings strike roots easily. The classic book *Marijuana Botany*, by Robert C. Clarke, has a good section with accurate drawings on air layering.

Micropropagation

Micropropagation of cannabis is possible. This form of cannabis propagation is relatively simple in theory, but

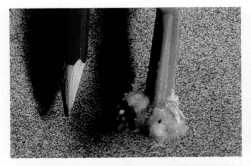

From top: Lightly scraping the stem causes a larger callus to form.

More roots grow from a large callus at the end of the stem.

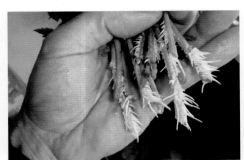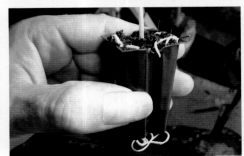

From top: The stems on these clones were scraped lightly before applying a root-inducing hormone.

This little clone has so many roots that they are growing out the top and bottom of the container!

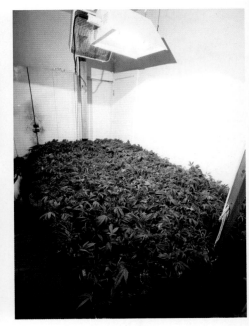

Root clones under fluorescent, CFL, or metal halide lights. This single 1000-watt metal halide is illuminating hundreds of clones.

application takes long-term perseverance, professional knowledge, and proper management. Micropropagation makes sense only if reproducing thousands of identical clones. For more information on micropropagation, see www.marijuanagrowing.com/.

Cloning for Sex

Determine plant sex accurately, 100 percent of the time, by "cloning for sex." To clone for sex, take two cuttings (in case one dies) from each parent plant in question. Use waterproof labels and an indelible marker to identify sets of clones and corresponding parents.

Keep parents under 18 to 24 hours of light. Give rooting clones a 12-hour light/dark regimen. Set them in a shady spot in the flowering room, set up a small 12-hour day/night cloning room or set them in a ventilated closet or under a light-tight cardboard box so they receive 12 hours of uninterrupted darkness.

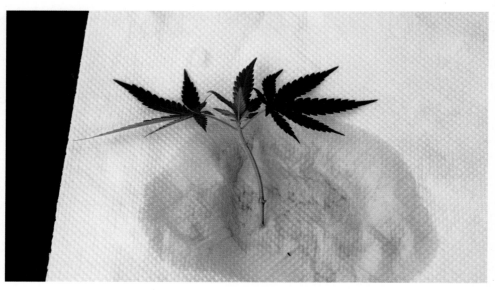
Wrap clones in a moist paper towel for storage and transport.

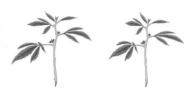

1. Make 2 cuttings

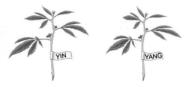

2. Label each cutting

12 Hours

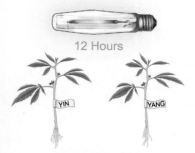

3. Give 12 hours of
light while rooting

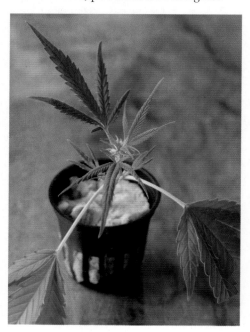

4. Cutting will determine
sex in 2-3 weeks

Unless there is a problem, clones will show sex within two weeks. Cull all males except those used for breeding. Take clones from desirable female plants. Let little females continue to flower.

Cloning a Flowering Female

Taking cuttings from flowering plants and inducing vegetative growth can take two months or longer. Females early in the flowering stage produce better cuttings, and their roots grow more quickly. Harvested plants are slower to revert back into vegetative growth. Once a plant reaches the senescence point, growth hormones have dissipated. Furthermore, powerful flowering hormones must be reversed, and rooting hormone signals must be sent. Now is the time to give plants 18 to 24 hours of light to signal them to revert to vegetative growth.

Weak rejuvenated clones often have irregular branching and occasionally flower prematurely or when suffering stress. Foliage and flower buds are more prone to pest and disease attacks too.

Weak favorite flowering harvested plants can be cloned, but results are not always the best. To clone a harvested female, cut from the lower green branches that have the most vegetative growth. Cut a 3-to-6-inch-long (7.6–315 cm) stem. Trim off flowers and lower leaves. Keep several green leaves and bud. If leaves have yellowed substantially or are diseased, survival chances diminish exponentially.

Storing Clones

To store cuttings for later use, wrap recently cut, trimmed, unrooted stems in a damp cloth or paper towel. Put the wrapped clones into a plastic bag and store in the refrigerator. On a daily basis, remove the water that condenses inside the bag in the cool refrigerator. Keep the temperature above 40°F (4.4°C). Temperatures below this level may cause plant cells to rupture. Cuttings should last in the refrigerator for about 3 weeks if they get out to have a daily dose of light.

8
FLOWERING

CANNABIS MUST FLOWER and produce seeds to successfully complete its annual life cycle. It is a dioecious plant, being either male (pollen producing) or female (ovule producing). However, intersex plants—mistakenly called hermaphrodite plants, with both male and female flowers—can also occur. Feminized seed that produces only female plants is also available.

In nature, cannabis flowers in the fall,* after the long, hot days of summer. The long nights and short days of autumn help signal cannabis to start flowering. (Plants are either "short-day" or "long-day." "Long-day" plants, including most varieties of cannabis, require short days and long nights to flower. For more information on this subject, see "Florigen," on page 86.) Plants are normally either male or female. Feminized seed that grows only female plants is also very popular. Cannabis produces male or female pre-flowers after 4 weeks of vegetative growth. For more information, see "Pre-flowering" in this chapter.

Cannabis ruderalis–dominant varieties flower after 3 to four weeks of growth, regardless of light/dark regimen. Plants with the "*ruderalis*" gene are called "autoflowering" varieties.

Growth patterns and chemistry change during flowering. Cannabinoid production slows at first and then accelerates; flower formation is rapid at first and then slows. Stems elongate; leaves grow progressively fewer blades. This tendency is more pronounced in *indica* varieties than in *sativas*. Nutrient needs change as growth stages change. Plants focus on flower production

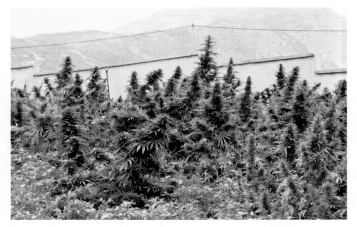

These plants are growing in Morocco. You can see the Rif Mountains in the background.

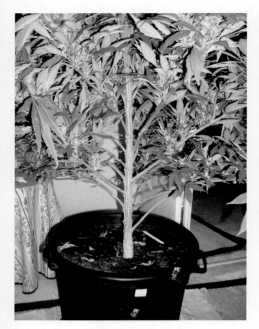

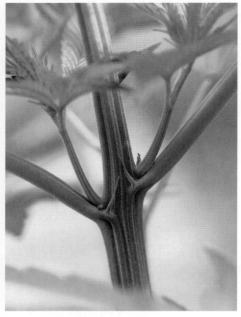

Phyllotaxy, the arrangement of leaves on the stem, changes when a plant enters the flowering stage. Branches are symmetrical lower on the plant, and will change to asymmetrical as flowering progresses.

Here is a close-up of asymmetrical growth—one of the first signs of flowering. (MF)

ual rather than immediate. The medium holds some elements but the cation sites readjust to equilibrium as necessary. The plant is vegetating when the light is changed to 12 hours. It will take 3 to 5 more days for preprogrammed leaf growth on the meristem to manifest. After several 12-hour nights, the cells in the meristem are reprogrammed to flower. At this point cells start looking for a different nutrient menu.

Cannabis is in vegetative growth during the transition to flowering and has vegetative nutrient needs. The same nutrients are required during growth and flowering, only the ratio between them changes. For the first few days this ratio may change from minute to minute, so we provide different ratios of nutrients during this time and plants are able to extract what they need. Careful monitoring of feeding will help plants always have a complete menu of nutrients.

Trichomes and Resin Glands

During flowering, cannabinoid-rich resin glands and other trichomes on foliage become clearly visible with the naked eye. The capitate-stalked glands that cover bracts and small bud-leaves interspersing the buds are the most important to medical cannabis gardeners. These glands account for more than half of all the THC contained in the plant.

Bulbous and sessile resin glands on the surfaces of all flowers, leaves, stalks, and branches, along with a small amount of THC present in interior cells, account for the balance of total THC. These large, stalked glands are our focus.

rather than vegetative growth. Green chlorophyll production, which requires much nitrogen, slows. Calcium, phosphorus, and potassium uptake increases to promote floral formation.

When flowering is initiated, organic cannabis gardeners change to a soluble flowering mix with less nitrogen. Gardeners that use chemical salt–based nutrients switch to a "super bloom" formula with less nitrogen and more calcium, potassium, and phosphorus. The fertilizer is added when flowering is

induced indoors. Both fertilizer regimens promote bigger flower buds.

Changing the ratio of nutrients during flowering does not mean that plants need no nitrogen. For example, there is a lag time in growing mediums' ability to hold fertility while other substrates hold nutrients for a very short time. This is why the fertilizer ratio should be changed after floral induction. The increase in floral nutrients necessary during flowering, most notably phosphorus (P) and potassium (K), is grad-

Florigen

Florigen (also known as "the flowering hormone") is the term used to describe the molecules that initiate and maintain flowering. Since the 1930s, biologists have believed that florigen is responsible for controlling flowering in plants, but it was not until August 2011 that a group of Japanese scientists discovered specific florigen hormone receptors. Florigen is synthesized in leaves and stimulated by environmental changes such as photoperiod and temperature.

Florigen is found at the apex of shoots where buds grow to induce flowering. It redirects vegetative stem apexes to become flowering stem apexes. The subject is quite complex and beyond the scope of this book. I started a thread about florigen on the forum at www.marijuanagrowing.com that encompasses further research and discussion.

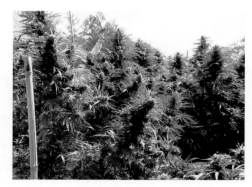

Florigen is the elusive hormone thought to be responsible for flowering.

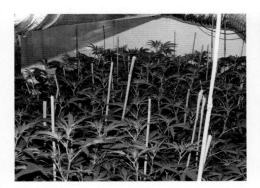

This crop was induced to flower with a 12/12-hour day/night photoperiod. The onset of flowering causes growth patterns, as well as chemistry, to change.

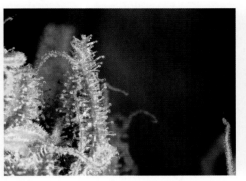

Pests and diseases would have a difficult time attacking this 'Chocolope' bud covered with resin glands.

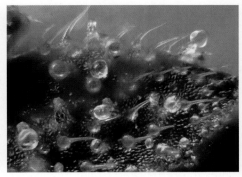

Pointy sessile resin glands (cystolith hairs) contain no cannabinoids, but the capitate-stalked resin glands with a ball on top are packed with cannabinoids. (MF)

Trichomes

Biologists hypothesize that trichomes evolved as a defense mechanism of the cannabis plant against a range of potential enemies. These adhesive sprouts form a protective layer against offensive insects and mites, preventing them from reaching the surface of the plant. The chemicals in the trichomes make cannabis less palatable to animals and can inhibit the growth of some types of fungus.

The protective trichomes also help insulate plants from desiccating wind and low humidity as well as forming a natural "sunscreen" to protect against UVB light rays.

Humans may have promoted heavier resin production through casual selective breeding.

"All mice are animals, but not all animals are mice. Similarly, all resin glands are trichomes, but not all trichomes are resin glands. *Trichome* is a general botanical term for any outgrowth of an epidermal cell. Trichomes can be scales, root hairs, glandular or nonglandular, single or multicellular, often hairlike growths. Cannabis has three kinds of resin glands (bulbous, capitate-sessile, and capitate-stalked) and several of non-resinous silica and carbonate warts and hairs, all called trichomes."
—*Mel Frank, Cannabis author, researcher, and photographer*

Nonglandular Trichomes

Nonglandular trichomes—cystolithic (sessile and cystolith glands [also known as plant hairs]) are common on many plants and do not produce cannabinoids. These trichomes have a pointed tip and are often long and hairlike. The waxy protective trichomes are most common on leaf undersides, petioles, and stems.

More common on some varieties than others, cystolithic trichomes are most abundant on outdoor plants. More cystolithic trichomes form on plants when they harden-off and are moved from indoors to outdoors. The glands exude insecticidal and miticidal substances to gum up pests' mouthparts and repel them, but they have no useful cannabinoids.

Bulbous Glands

Bulbous glands are the smallest glands, ranging in size from 15 to 30 micrometers. One to 4 cells constitute the "foot" and "stalk," and 1 to 4 cells make up the "head" of the gland. Head cells secrete a resin, believed to be cannabinoid-rich, along with related compounds that accumulate between the head cells and the cuticle. A nipple-like bulge may form on the membrane from the pressure of built-up resin as these glands mature. Look for bulbous glands scattered about on foliage surfaces.

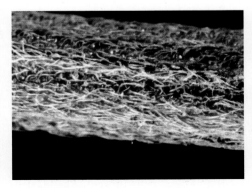

Cystolith hairs point in the direction of growing shoots. (MF)

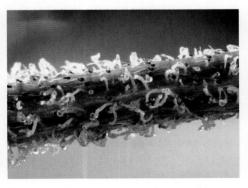

These cystolith hairs have mutated and lost their way. (MF)

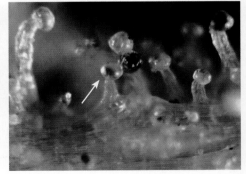

Bulbous glands sit on a base of a few cells located on foliage and flower buds. (MF)

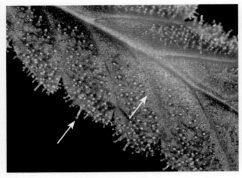

Capitate-sessile (bulbous glands) are visible near the center of the leaf. Capitate-stalked resin glands grow progressively taller and are clearly visible on the edges of this leaf of 'Blueberry × Sandstorm'.

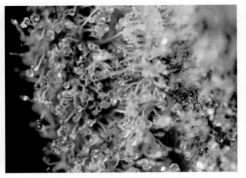

Long, thin stalks support the ball-like heads of capitate-stalked resin glands.

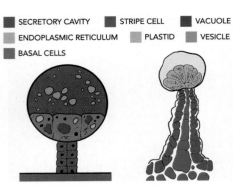

Capitate-stalked resin glands are full of chemical activity. This is where the majority of cannabinoids occur. Disc cells, and principally the secretory cavity, of the gland perform a key role in the physiology of secondary products. But these activities are not yet completely understood.

Capitate-Sessile Resin Glands

Capitate-sessile glands measure from 25 to 100 micrometers across the globular-shaped head or bulb. The bulb appears to lie flush on young and immature plants. One to 4 cells below the bulb is the beginning of a stalk that elongates and grows during flowering to transform the capitate-sessile gland into a capitate-stalked resin gland.

The globular head or ball is composed of 8 to 16 cells that form a dome. The specialized cells secrete a cannabinoid-rich resin that collects between the rosette, and its outer membrane appears spherical.

Capitate-Stalked Resin Glands

Capitate-stalked trichomes appear and become visible with the naked eye when flowers form. Use a 10X to 30X handheld lens to distinguish resin glands—bulbous, capitate-sessile, capitate-stalked, and nonglandular trichomes. Look for them on female flower bracts and new flower growth and surrounding foliage where they form heavily on the plant. The resin glands also tend to accumulate heavily on veins of lower leaf surfaces around flower buds. Cannabinoid-potent varieties typically contain higher concentrations of capitate-stalked resin glands.

Male plants and flowers contain smaller and lower concentrations of less-potent stalked glands than found on the female bracts. Male flowers typically have a row of large capitate-sessile glands along opposite sides of anthers.

Unless clearly visible on leaf surfaces, few cannabinoids are found on older leaves. Leaves around flower buds are much more densely populated with capitate-stalked resin glands rich in cannabinoids.

Capitate-stalked resin glands are composed of a stalk with a bulbous head. They look like a post with a knob, ball, or bulb at the top. They form mainly on flower buds and small leaves. The highest concentration of cannabinoids is located at the base of the bulbous resin head.

In the above illustration, disc cells are shown attached to foliage by stipe cells (red) and basal cells (green). The plastid (orange) in disc cells secrete lipoplasts where they synthesize lipophilic substances that accumulate and ultimately

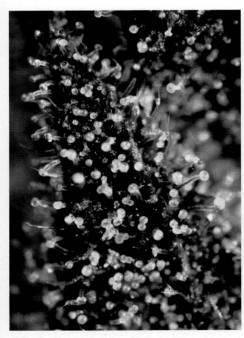

Look closely and you can see the pointy cystolithic, nonglandular trichomes alongside the more numerous capitate-stalked glandular trichomes.

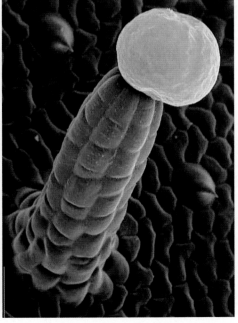

This electron scanning microscopic view at 370X of a single capitate-stalked resin gland allows us to distinguish individual cells. These 150- to 500-micrometer-tall resin glands are pretty tough when they are young and strong. But once they age they become more fragile.

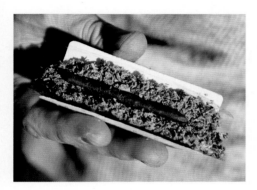

A "snake" of hash has been added to this cannabis cigarette or joint.

migrate and form BLUE vesicles. THC occurs in the top of the capitate-stalked resin gland. For more on this complex subject, see www.marijuanagrowing.com.

Cannabinoid Profile

Many cannabinoids (CBD), not just THC, have unique effects on brain functions, which in turn cause different effects on human cognition and psychiatric symptoms. Different levels of cannabinoids relative to one another produce different effects. As a result, measuring the "potency" of cannabis plants is problematic.

A very resinous plant could have low levels of THC and high levels of CBD. Or a plant with little resin could contain high levels of THC and low levels of CBD. Cannabinoid profile depends on the makeup of cannabinoids and other active ingredients. For example, resin consists of cannabinoids and other substances such as non-psychoactive resins like phenolic and terpenoid polymers, glycerides, and triterpenes. When resin is concentrated in kief or hashish, about a third is water-soluble plant material, another third is non-psychoactive resins, and the balance cannabinoids.

In many cannabis plants, THC may be only a very small percentage of the total cannabinoids. The remainder (5 to 10 percent) of the resin will be essential oils, sterols, fatty acids, and various hydrocarbons common to plants.

About 80 to 90 percent of the cannabinoids are synthesized and stored in microscopic resin glands that appear on the outer surfaces of all plant parts except the root and seed.

The arrangement and number (concentration) of resin glands vary somewhat with the particular strain examined. Marijuana varieties generally have more resin glands, and they are larger than resin glands on non-drug varieties.

Resins occasionally secrete through pores in the membrane of gland heads. Usually secretion occurs many weeks after stalked glands appear. The glands seem to empty their contents, leaving hollow spaces (vacuoles) in the stalk and head cells. After secretion, the glands cease to function and begin to degenerate. Gland heads, stalks, and trichomes become clumped together, and the whole flowering surface becomes a sticky mass. This is not necessarily desirable.

Small quantities of cannabinoids are present in the internal tissues of the plant. The bulk is found in small single cells (non-articulated laticifers) that elongate to form small, individual resin canals. The resin canals ramify the developing shoots, and penetrate the plant's conducting tissue (phloem). Minute clumps of resin found in the phloem are probably deposited by these resin canals. Other plant cells contain insignificant amounts of cannabinoids and probably a good 90 percent of the cannabinoids are localized in the resin glands.

Cannabinoid Production

More than 36 tons (79,366 pounds) per hectare (2.5 acres) of dry medical cannabis flower buds can be grown in successive or continual crops in a well-equipped greenhouse under controlled conditions. This works out to 9.92 pounds per 11.1 square feet (3.6 kg/m²) of greenhouse growing space per year.

The breakdown of the harvest consists of 9 tons of cannabinoids (about 66%) and essential oils (about 33 %) per hectare, 1.98 pounds per 11.1 square feet (900 gm/m²) per year.

* "Guidelines for Good Agricultural and Wild Collection Practices for

Medicinal and Aromatic Plants" (GACP-MAP) http://www.europam. net/documents/gacp/EUROPAM_ GACP_MAP_8.0.pdf

Terpenes and Essential Oils

Lightweight terpenes belong to a large group of unsaturated hydrocarbons, several of which can be extracted with steam distillation. The product, essential oil, holds aroma, flavor, and specific character.

Five essential oils, including the mono- and sesquiterpenes, alpha- and beta-pinene, limonene, mycene, and beta-phallandrene impart virtually all of the sweet, unique, minty, citrusy, etc., qualities found in odorless cannabinoids. The volatile oils enter the atmosphere and dissipate over time. This causes cannabis to lose much of its bouquet and flavor when stored.

Essential oils constitute 0.1 to 0.3 percent of the dry weight of a fresh marijuana sample—about 10 percent of the weight of the cannabinoids. For every 1000 grams of dry bud, from 1 to 3 grams of essential oil is extracted. Essential oils are predominately found inside heads

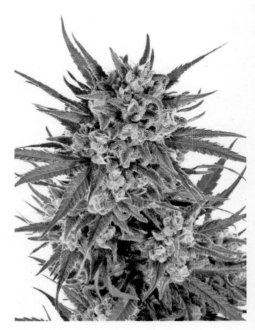

'Jack Herer' from Sensi Seeds consistently produces high levels of cannabinoids.

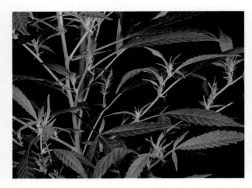

Small buds are developing on this 'Chocolope' clone 2 weeks after inducing flowering with a 12-hour photoperiod.

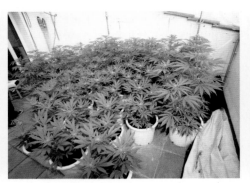

These little clones have just started to flower.

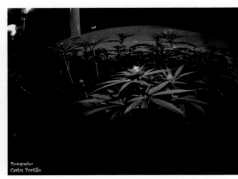

This garden is flowering under 12 hours of darkness and 12 hours of light every 24 hours.

resin glands, and they have been detected in the resin canals or laticifers.

The mix of essential oils is diverse in different samples of cannabis. Some scientists hypothesize that cannabis content and fragrance may be associated because essential oils are precursors or are related to the cannabinoids.

Indica, Sativa, and Ruderalis

Induce *sativa* and *indica* varieties and crosses to flower in greenhouses and indoors by giving plants more hours of total darkness and fewer hours of light.

Outdoors, cannabis will flower when it receives 12 hours or more of darkness daily. Give cannabis 12 hours of uninterrupted darkness and 12 hours of light to induce visible signs of flowering in about two weeks. This program is effective in all but the latest blooming pure *sativa* varieties.

Medicinal cannabis gardeners with a vegetative room illuminated 18 to 24 hours a day and a flowering room or greenhouse with 12-hour days and 12-hour nights, create environments that mimic the photoperiod in spring and

fall. With this simple combination a crop can be harvested every 6 to 10 weeks. In warm southern climates or with the help of artificial light, the harvest can last all year.

Plants show sex (male or female flowers,) during the pre-flowering stage, which actually occurs during vegetative growth (discussed on page 92). Once the sex of the plant is established, males, unless used for breeding, are harvested before they shed pollen, and females are coaxed into higher yields. Once the photoperiod is set, disrupting it can cause

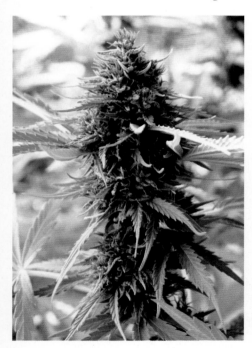

'Original Afghani #1' from 1978 had reddish stigmas, but more often this variety would have had white stigmas. (MF)

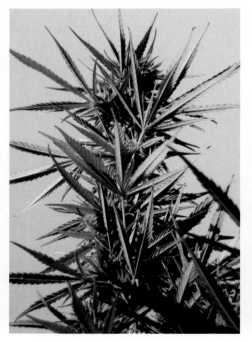

This pure sativa from Mexico shows classic long thin leaf blades. (MF)

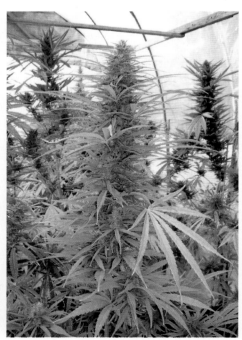

The tall 'Durban Poison' phenotype has large narrow-blade sativa leaves.

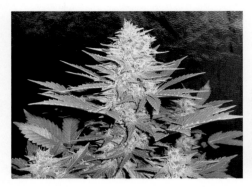

This autoflowering feminized plant was bred to be grown in a sea of green (SOG) garden.

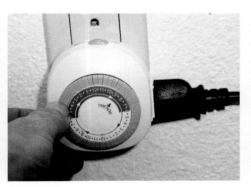

If the photoperiod bounces around, it causes plants to suffer stress. Make sure the timer works properly, and inspect it periodically.

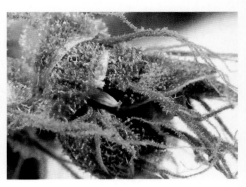

A tiny male flower can be seen on this female flower cluster. The male flower appeared late, when the female was overripe.

plants to suffer stress. If they suffer enough stress, intersex (hermaphrodite) tendencies increase. Water intake of flowering plants is usually somewhat less than in the vegetative stage. Adequate water during flowering is important for plants to carry on internal chemistry and cannabinoid production. Withholding water to "stress" a plant will actually stunt growth and diminish yield.

Pure *Cannabis sativa* has its origins in tropical regions. Tropical varieties are accustomed to 12 hours of sunlight and equal darkness all year round. The climate is such that they have a long and temperate growing season with leisurely and consistent growth. Super intense sunlight can be difficult for them to assimilate. Many tropical *sativa* varieties grow under the shade of the jungle canopy. Indoors, gardeners often give pure tropical *sativas* too much light. The result is even smaller and lighter flower buds. Lamps are set further away or use lower wattage bulbs that produce less intensity and heat. Plants do not get as hot and receive adequate light to grow big flower buds.

Give pure tropical *sativas* more darkness and less light to induce flowering—11 or 12 hours of light and 13 or 12 hours of darkness. Some gardeners go so far as to gradually decrease daylight hours to 10 daily with 14 hours or more of darkness. Such practices simulate native climates, which gives plants a chance to express their genetics. This technique will promote bigger flower buds.

Autoflowering *Cannabis ruderalis* varieties do not require long nights to flower. *C. ruderalis* starts to flower within a month of germinating. Many autoflowering *ruderalis* varieties are ready to harvest 70 days after planting and produce up to 4 ounces (112 gm) of dried medicinal flower buds when properly grown. European breeders have feminized many autoflowering varieties. To date, the top varieties produce 3 to 3.5 ounces (85–99.2 grams) in 70 to 80 days.

Different Flowering Light/Dark Schedules

1. 12/12—standard day/night schedule for most plants

2. 12/12—switch to 11/13 after 1 week and 10/14 after 2 weeks. This is the schedule for tropical *sativa* varieties like 'Haze'.

3. 12/12—flower for 3 weeks, then increase light to 11/13. Flowering is prolonged but harvest is increased.

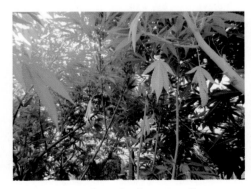

Do not remove large fan leaves to allow more intense light to reach small buds, or to stress the plants!

Note: Often *indica*-dominant varieties flower about the same.

4. 24 hours—flowering regime for daylight-neutral *C. ruderalis* crosses with *C. indica* and *C. sativa*.

Note: See "Photoperiod" in chapter 17, *Light, Lamps & Electricity*, for more detailed information on *indica*, *sativa*, and *ruderalis* varieties and flowering.

Stress and Sex

Bouncing the photoperiod around and dramatically raising or lowering temperature has the effect of producing more male plants. I recently spoke to a gardener who induced male flowers on a female plant by lowering the nighttime temperature (normally 70°F [21.1°C]) to 60°F (15.6°C) for 2 weeks.

Note: Each stimulus (temperature, photo period, etc.,) creates a climate that causes plants to suffer stress. And the stressful environment does not necessarily turn the entire plant male. Normally a few hard-to-spot male pollen sacks appear sporadically on a few branches. The most susceptible plants already have a predisposition to intersexuality.

To promote male or female plants during seedling growth, see "Grow More Females from 'Regular' Seed" in chapter 5, *Seeds & Seedlings*. The most dependable way to deduce sex is cloning for sex (see chapter 7, *Clones & Cloning*).

Large leaves are chockful of food for the plant. They are essential to plant health and vitality. Indoors and in greenhouses

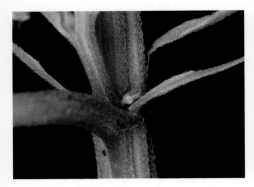

Male early pre-flowers are somewhat difficult to see with the naked eye. A small loupe may be necessary to see them properly. (MF)

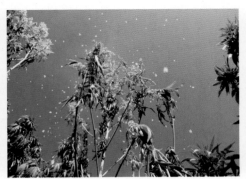

This fully mature male is shedding pollen into the wind.

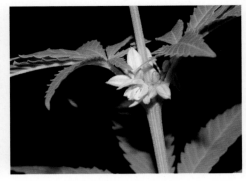

This male flower has dispersed all of its pollen. Other male flowers will open in the next few days and dispersing their pollen.

where the hours of darkness are controlled, cannabis flowers for 6 to 10 weeks or longer. This is a very short time. However, hacking off leaves and branch tips to initiate more budding sites can be somewhat effective. Most lower leaves supply the roots, while upper leaves supply energy to the top of the plant and promote flower growth. Remove only leaves that are more than 50 percent damaged by diseases, pests, and cultural practices (e.g., yellow leaves hanging straight down should be removed).

Pre-flowering

Pre-flowers are described by Robert Clarke in *Marijuana Botany* as "primordial." They are the first indication of a plant's sex. Pre-flowers grow at branch internodes, just behind the leaf spur, or stipule, around the fourth week of vegetative growth, when the plant is 6 to 8 weeks old. This is the point of sexual maturity and the first sign that a cannabis plant is preparing for flowering, its next stage in life.

You can see pre-flowers with the naked eye, but a using a 5X or 10X loupe or magnifier will make viewing and determining a plant's sex easier. You can accurately determine plant sex after 8 weeks, as soon as male and female flowers are identified. With this method, sex can be distinguished before inducing flowering indoors and in greenhouses. Outdoors, "sexing" plants is used to separate out unwanted males grown from seed.

Male Pre-flowering

Male pre-flowers are normally visible when plants are 6 to 8 weeks old, after the fourth week of vegetative growth. The pre-flowers emerge behind the stipule at the fourth to fifth branch internodes and generally do not turn into full flowers. However, male plants have been known to grow flowers after a long period of vegetative growth.

Always wait to induce flowering until after pre-flowers appear. Inducing flowering with 12 hours of uninterrupted darkness and 12 hours of light before pre-flowers develop will stress the plant. This stress could cause peculiar growth, and plants might develop intersex (hermaphrodite) characteristics. Inducing flowering before pre-flowers form will

Staminate Primordia

The red arrow shows where pre-flowers develop on both male and female plants. Staminate flowers are located at the node between the stipule and emerging branch.

not expedite flowering. In fact, growth will slow and flowering will occur at about the same time as if you had waited for pre-flowers to show.

Plants grown from seed under a 24/0 photoperiod will generally show pre-flowers after plants that are given an 18/6 day/night photoperiod. Once pre-flowers are distinguishable as male or female, plants can be induced to flower with a 12/12 day/night photoperiod.

Until you have plenty of experience, make sure seedlings have completely designated sex before removing them from the garden. Use a 5X or 10X loupe to identify pre-flowers. Once a male pre-flower appears, it will take about 10 days before it starts shedding pollen.

Male Flowering

The male (staminate) cannabis plant gets less attention because once gender shows, most cannabis gardeners remove all males to prevent pollination of females (pistillates). The goal is to have unpollinated females remain seedless (commonly called sinsemilla from the Spanish *sin semilla*, meaning "without seeds").

When flowering under natural sunlight or an induced 12/12 day/night photoperiod, male cannabis normally reaches maturity and flowers 1 to 2 weeks before females. However, male plants do not necessarily need a 12/12 day/night photoperiod to dawn flowers and shed pollen. Males can flower under long days and short nights as well, but produce

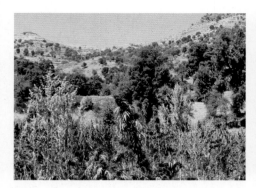

Male plants are generally taller than females. Males also die back before females.

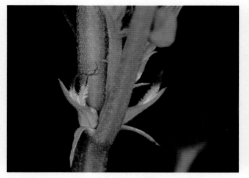

This pre-flower is fully mature, and the stigmas have died halfway.

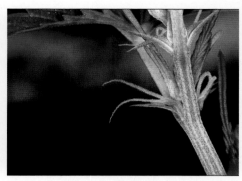

Pre-flower stigmas on this newly designated female are strong and healthy!

fewer and weaker flowers with less pollen. Once male flowers appear, pollen develops relatively quickly and can disperse in about 10 days. To avoid pollination problems, remove males as soon as they are distinguished. If growing male plants, isolate them from females, so females will not be pollinated.

Males continue flowering and shedding yellowish, dustlike pollen from bell-shaped pollen sacks well into the females' flowering stage, which ensures pollination. If you are making seeds, pollinating females too early, before females have developed many receptive female stigmas, will result in a small seed crop.

Males are usually taller than females and have stout stems, sporadic branching, and fewer leaves. In nature, wind and gravity carry pollen from male plants to fertilize (pollinate) receptive females. Male plants produce fewer flowers than

females, because one male plant can pollinate many females. Males also contain lower levels of cannabinoids.

Males plants fertilize (pollinate) females, causing females plants to level off THC production and start seed formation. Remove and destroy males, except those that have been selected and used for breeding, as soon as their sex has been determined. The instant they show sex, separate male plants used for breeding from females. Do not let them shed pollen. Unnoticed pollen sacks often form and open early or are hidden under foliage. If growing from seed, take special care to ferret out male flowers and plants. See chapter 9, *Harvest, Drying & Curing*, for information on removing males from the garden.

See chapter 25, *Breeding*, for complete information and detailed images of male flowers.

Female Pre-flowering

After several weeks of normal vegetative growth, plants grown from seed develop pre-flowers. This is when female flower formation initiates, and it is not contingent upon photoperiod. It occurs when a plant is old enough to show signs of sexual maturity, about the fourth week of vegetative growth, or 6 to 8 weeks from seed germination. The pre-flowers emerge behind the stipule about the fourth or fifth branch internodes.

A pre-flower looks like a regular female flower; most have a pair of white fuzzy stigmas. Stigmas normally form after the light-green seed bract of the pre-flower has formed. Wait until stigmas have fully formed to ensure that the plant is a female and not a male. The pre-flowering stage lasts from 1 to 2 weeks.

Plants grown from seed under an 18/6-hour day/night photoperiod will usually show pronounced pre-flowers before plants given a 24/0-hour day/night photoperiod. And under a 16/8-hour day/night regimen, pre-flowers show more quickly and are often more pronounced. As soon as you can distinguish pre-flowers as male or female, males can be culled and females can be induced to flower with a 12/12-hour day/night photoperiod in enclosed gardens.

Wait to induce flowering until pre-flowers have appeared. Inducing flowering with 12 hours of uninterrupted darkness and 12 hours of light before pre-flowers set will cause plant to suffer stress. Such stress could cause strange growth, even

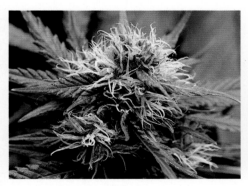

Be on the lookout for small male flowers that may suddenly appear on female plants. Such seemingly harmless male flowers carry viable pollen that will pollinate receptive females.

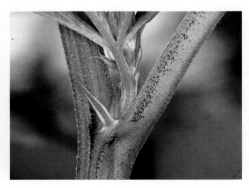

Tiny stigmas are just starting to emerge from this newly formed female pre-flower.

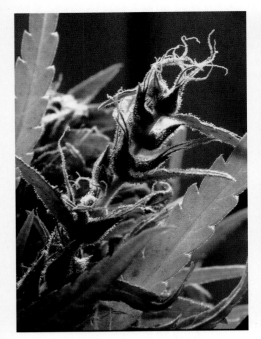

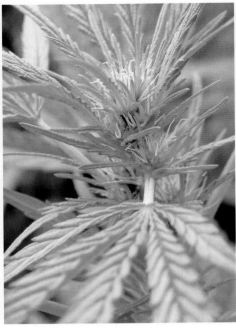

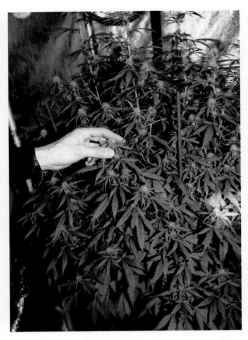

Distinct seed bracts with attached stigmas are easy to distinguish on this 1979 landrace variety from Thailand. (MF)

Flower buds are just starting to develop on this outdoor sativa-dominant plant. Notice that the distance between internodes decreases as stigmas appear and buds develop.

Tiny developing buds with stigmas cover this indoor crop in the Netherlands.

cause sex reversal. Inducing flowering before pre-flowers develop does not make plants flower faster; plants will flower at about the same time as if you had waited for pre-flowers to develop.

Female Flowering

Female cannabis is prized for heavy cannabinoid production and weighty flower yield. Ideal female, *indica*-dominant, indoor varieties grow squat and bushy with branches close together on the stem and dense foliage on branches. Outdoor and greenhouse varieties have a similar growth habit with a larger profile. Indoors most varieties show the first female flowers 1 to 3 weeks after inducing flowering with the 12-hour photoperiod. Outdoors, pre-flowers appear a few weeks after planting, and flowering is induced with an 11- to 13-hour day/night photoperiod.

High-quality marijuana consists entirely of female flower clusters; distinct clusters of female marijuana flowers are called buds. Female flowers are about 0.1 to 0.2 inches (2.5–5.1 mm) long and usually form in pairs. But you will see such pairing only in "running" buds most commonly seen in Southeast Asian varieties or on plants stretching for light.

More typically, flowers grow tightly together, forming egg-shaped or tear-drop-shaped clusters usually between 0.8 and 3 inches (2–7.6 cm) long; each cluster generally consists of between 30 and 150 densely packed flowers.

Clusters of flower buds (colas) develop rapidly for the first 4 or 5 weeks, after which they grow at a slower rate. Buds put on much of their harvest weight as they swell during the last 2 or 3 weeks of growth before harvest. Pure *sativas* originating in the tropics can flower for 4 months or longer! Once the ovule has

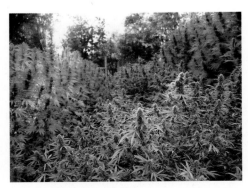

Outdoors in Northern California this sativa-indica cross has plenty of space and sunlight to grow to its fullest potential. Indoors, plants grow much smaller regardless of genetic background.

been fertilized by male pollen, seed bract formation and resin production slow, and seed growth starts.

White, fuzzy female stigmas are fertile as soon as they appear. Unfertilized, these flower buds will continue to develop as sinsemilla. Make sure to keep all male plants and male pollen away from female flowering plants. If female flowers are fertilized by male pollen, seeds will develop and other flower bud growth will slow or stop.

C. indica, C. sativa, and *C. ruderalis* all have different flowering habits. See "Sinsemilla Flowering" below for more information.

See chapter 25, *Breeding*, for complete information and detailed images of female cannabis flowers and "Seed-Crop Flowering"; see chapter 17, *Light, Lamps & Electricity*, for more information on photoperiod and flowering.

Sinsemilla Flowering

Sinsemilla (pronounced *sin-semiya*) is derived from two Spanish words: *sin*, which means without, and *semilla*, which means seed. Sinsemilla is the word that describes flowering female

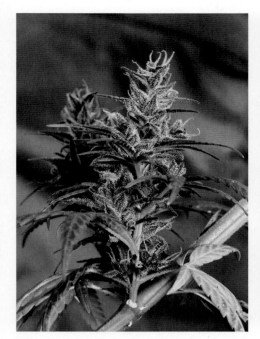

This Nigerian landrace flower bud has a wispy growth habit but is still boasts lots of cannabinoid-rich resin. (MF)

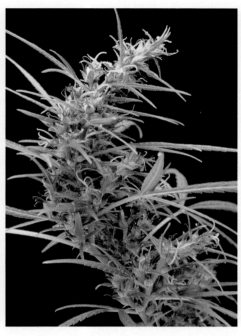

Sativa *flower buds like this South Indian bud grown in 1981 are much lighter and form more slowly than* indicas. *(MF)*

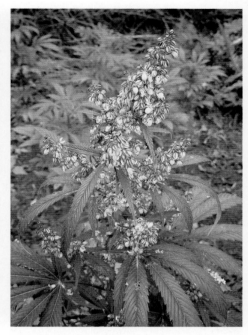

This beautiful 'Purple Pineberry' male plant is heavy with flowers that are just starting to release pollen.

cannabis tops that have not been fertilized by male pollen.

Highly prized medicinal sinsemilla flower buds are the most potent part of any variety, with a proportionately large volume of cannabinoids per flower bud. Unpollinated female plants continue to flower until bract formation and cannabinoid-rich resin production peak, 6 to 10 weeks after turning the lights to 12 hours indoors, inducing flowering in a light deprivation greenhouse or naturally flowering outdoors. During 6 to 10 weeks of flowering, seed bracts develop

and swell along the stem, yielding more and heavier flower buds than pollinated, seeded flowers.

Cannabis ruderalis flowers when it is chronologically ready, after about 3 weeks of growth. Many growers report best results with a 20-hour light and 4-hour dark period. Most European seed companies have developed autoflowering-feminized crosses of cannabis *ruderalis × indica × sativa*. Productive varieties produce 3 to 4 ounces (85–113.4 gm) of dried cannabis flower buds with each 70- to 80-day crop from seed.

Make any female cannabis plant sinsemilla by removing male plants as soon as they are identified. Removing males virtually guarantees that male pollen will not fertilize succulent female stigmas. Be aware, however, that pollen dispersed from wild or cultivated male cannabis plants could also be floating in the air. Or sometimes a few early grains of pollen are shed by premature male plants that have not been culled. And sometimes an intersex plant with a few male flowers will sprout on a predominately female plant. Read about intersexuality in chapter 25, *Breeding*.

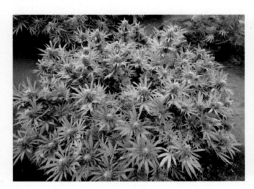

Indica-*dominant 'Shooting Star' from Hammerhead Genetics shows a completely different growth habit when cultivated outdoors.*

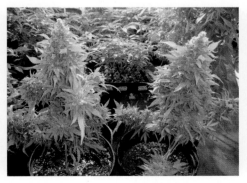

This crop of 'Bonkers' with a very strong indica *influence grows well indoors and in greenhouses.*

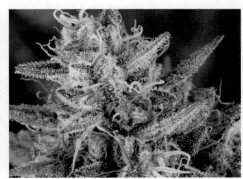

'Matanuska Tundra' is predominately indica *and developed in the Matanuska-Susitna (Mat-su) Valley in Alaska, in conjunction with Sagarmatha Seeds.*

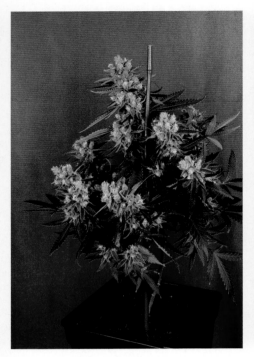

'Grapefruit' from DNA Genetics is a high-yielding sativa with a sweet taste.

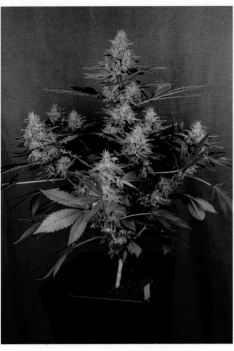

'NYC Diesel' is a sativa-dominant variety from Soma Seeds.

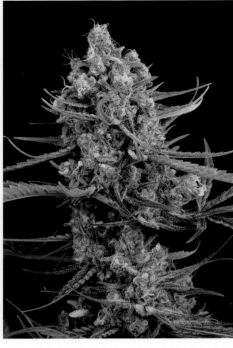

'Chocolope' from DNA Genetics is 95 percent sativa with 'OG Chocolate Thai' × 'Cannaloupe Haze' pedigree.

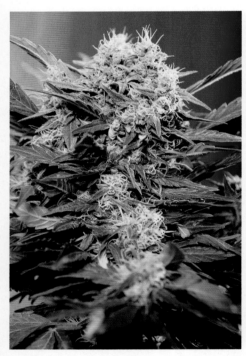

Daylight-neutral 'Lowryder' was crossed with regular 'Chronic' to yield this autoflowering variety.

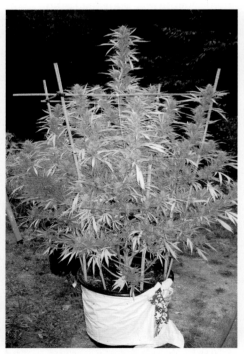

This super-auto (super-autoflowering) variety, 'Super Stinky', was developed by Stitch, a French breeder. Such varieties flower after 30+ days, grow to 5 feet (1.5 m), and perform well outdoors.

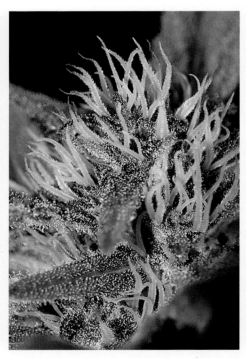

Purple colors in buds tend to show toward the end of harvest. This bud has a few weeks to go before harvest, as evidenced by the vibrant white stigmas.

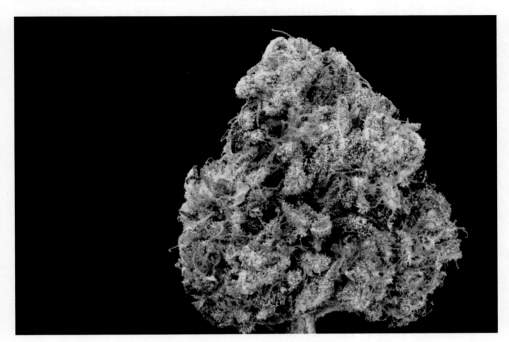

This beautiful cluster of female flowers, here from the variety 'Blackberry', is called a nug. A nug most often refers to a dried, dense, often small bud about the size of a thumb's end joint. Fresh flower clusters are almost always called buds; dried clusters are also commonly called buds. Botanically, marijuana buds are racemes. *(MF)*

Calyx, False Calyx, and Bract

Those general terms—*bud, nug, cola,* and *foxtail*—are widely accepted and consistent, but botanical terms are often confused in popular culture. Foremost is the incorrect use of the term *calyx*. Growers read or hear about swollen calyxes being a sign of maturity and an indication of readiness for harvesting. What are incorrectly called calyxes or false calyxes are correctly identified as bracts.

Bracts might seem a foreign term, but everyone has seen bracts. On poinsettias, the ubiquitous potted plant sold around Christmas, those large red "petals" are actually bracts. On bougainvilleas, the many-colored vines seen everywhere in warmer climates, bracts make up the colorful "petals" that surround a tiny, white inner flower. Cannabis bracts have the densest covering of large, stalked resin glands of any plant part. Bracts make up most of substance and weight of high-quality marijuana buds.

Colas and Foxtails

Cola, a commonly used term for female flower clusters, more often refers to an aggregate of buds that, having formed so closely together, looks like a single, very large bud. Colas form at the ends of stems and branches. Outdoors, meter-long colas can form along the main stem of large plants. *Foxtail,* another term for cola, is rarely heard these days except from those whose history with cannabis goes back to the 1960s or 1970s. At that time, foxtail most often referred to high-quality individual colas from Mexico in contrast to bagged or compressed bricks of low-quality Mexican colas.

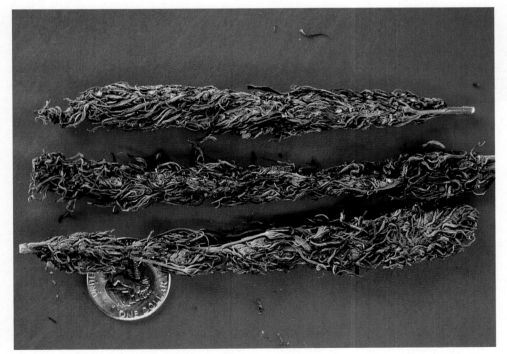

The terms cola *or* foxtail *describe a branch of flower buds that originated in Mexico. Mel Frank snapped this photo of Mexican foxtails in 1976. (MF)*

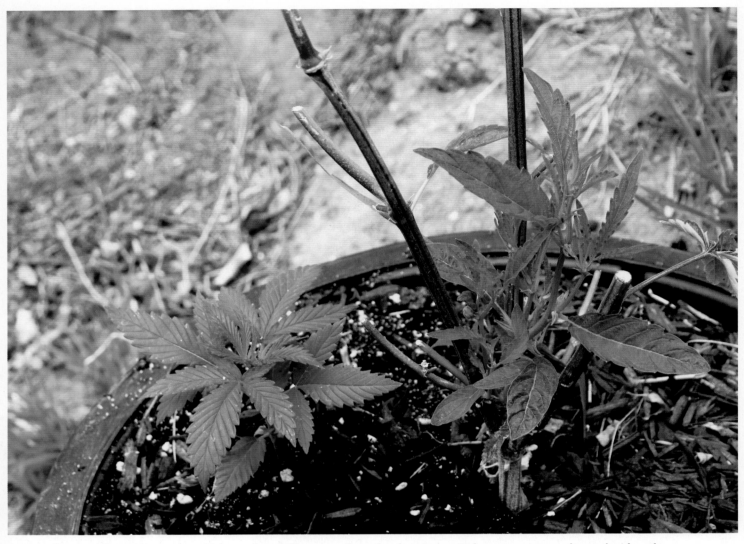

Store seeds in airtight containers along with a packet of silicon crystals to absorb moisture. Make sure to remove, dry, and replace the silicon regularly. (MF)

Rejuvenation

Rejuvenate harvested females by leaving several undeveloped lower branches with foliage on plants. Give re-vegetating females an 18/6 day/night photoperiod. Or keep the lights on 24 hours. Keep the temperature above 70°F (21.1°C) and below 80°F (26.7°C) both day and night. Cool temperatures now will slow reversion to vegetative growth. After several weeks harvested females will stop flowering and "rejuvenate"—revert to the vegetative growth stage.

Leach out old fertilizer in each container and give the harvested leafy, buddy stem stubs a dose of high-nitrogen fertilizer to promote leafy growth. The plants will show signs of reverting to vegetative growth in 4 to 6 weeks. New, green, leafy growth will sprout from branches and flower tops. Leaves will continue to grow more and more "fingers" as re-vegetation progresses.

Let the rejuvenated cannabis plants grow until they are the desired size before taking clones or inducing flowering with a 12-hour photoperiod. If second crops are allowed to grow too tall and lanky, they produce sparse buds. Rejuvenated plants can also be placed outdoors in the spring. Indoors, rejuvenated plants should be induced to flower once they have enough strong foliage.

Rejuvenating harvested cannabis plants is most often used to save the genetics of a particular variety. Rejuvenating plants is never absolute and the results are, for the most part, not pretty. Furthermore, old harvested plants have more problems with diseases and pests. Few cannabis gardeners rejuvenate plants because doing so makes inefficient use of their time and space. A completely new, healthy crop could be grown in the time it takes to rejuvenate plants.

9

HARVEST, DRYING & CURING

indoors is normally open for about 5 to 7 days, and not all flower buds are ripe at the same time. A few gardeners harvest their crops early—after 45 to 50 days of flowering, and before it reaches peak maturity. The vast majority of gardeners harvest their gardens when at peak maturity. Cannabinoid profiles, especially THC content, are highest at peak harvest.

A BOUNTIFUL HARVEST of consistent, disease- and pest-free medicinal cannabis is the reward for your financial investment and hours of work and worry about the garden. Strong, healthy, well-grown clones and seedlings yield the heaviest harvests. A well-organized harvest will cut the workload, and a basic knowledge of what is happening in the cannabis plant will help you preserve its medicinal qualities during and after harvest. Cannabinoid levels increase as plants approach peak ripeness. Proper harvest timing is essential to achieve the desired medicinal cannabinoid levels. The peak harvest window

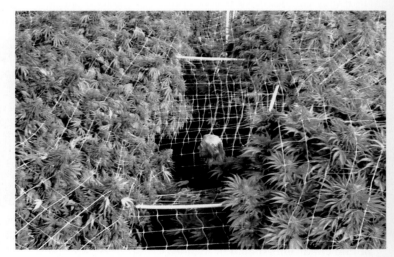

I have been fascinated with outdoor gardening for the last 15 years, since I was able to grow cannabis legally with the help of Mother Nature. Growing big plants outdoors during a long season allows them to express their genetic potential to the fullest.

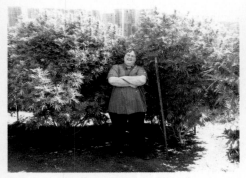

Paul Stanford, organizer of Hempstalk (www.hempstalk.org), is pictured in his medicinal cannabis garden in Portland, Oregon. He is standing in front of two female 'AK47' plants in full flower.

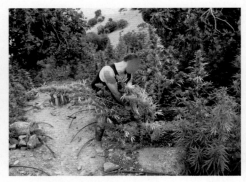

To make the harvest experience as stress-free as possible, there are a few things you should know.

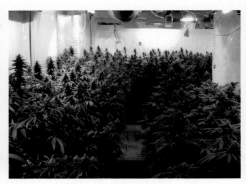

Medical gardeners are harvesting gardens like this one, full of cannabinoid-rich flower buds grown to test the varieties of DNA Genetics.

The bulk of cannabinoids, including THC, are found in resin glands that cover flowers and leaves; lesser amounts are present on stem surfaces and in interior cells of the plant. Stems and roots may smell like they contain cannabinoids, but they actually contain much lower levels of desirable cannabinoids. Male plants contain much lower quantities and levels of cannabinoids than do females, and are normally harvested before they pollinate females. Unpollinated female plants (sinsemilla) have the greatest amount of resin glands and cannabinoids, and are harvested when resin glands show peak ripeness. Leaves and flower buds are harvested, separated, manicured, dried, and cured.

Growth stops at harvest, and thereafter the THC (cannabinoid) content cannot increase. Some plant processes continue until they run out of stores. Overall cannabinoid levels are fixed, but the type changes with harvest from inactive cannabinoids to active ones or back again.

Drying removes about 75 percent of the water weight found in foliage. Drying concentrates cannabinoids in relation to overall weight. The actual cannabinoid content of resin glands will remain the same or decrease after harvest. Proper handling is the key to retaining cannabinoid potency. Prolonged periods of light, temperatures above 80°F (26.7°C), friction from fondling hands, and damp, humid conditions should be avoided because they all degrade resin glands and cannabinoids.

Washing branches of harvested flower buds in a mild solution of H_2O_2 (hydrogen peroxide) is becoming popular. We wash vegetables before consuming them, and cannabis is no different. A gentle bath of H_2O_2 removes surface bacteria, mold, dirt, dead pests and their feces, and other bad stuff. Such a bath also creates free radicles*.

*An H_2O_2 free radicle drench changes anything composed of carbon, just like using ozone in a garden room or curing room. Washing treated buds with plenty of fresh water is essential. No studies have been done to determine potential for damage to carbon chains of cannabis after an H_2O_2 bath.

Avoid excessive damage to resin glands by manicuring fresh flower buds immediately after harvest. Manicure when foliage is supple, by hand or by using a trimming machine to remove outer, less

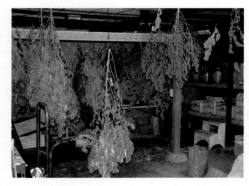

Hanging plants upside down to dry is simple, convenient, and effective. Contrary to rumor, hanging plants upside down does not drain existing cannabinoids into flower buds. Cannabinoids do not migrate to other parts of the plant after harvest.

cannabinoid-potent foliage from flower buds. Once manicured, flower buds are dried slowly to equalize moisture content, preserve cannabinoids, and shed chlorophyll. After drying, flower buds must cure to achieve full aroma and flavor. Too often beautiful buds are dried too hot and fast, and are not cured properly. Mishandling cannabis may rupture and degrade resin and terpenes. Such flower buds lose their bouquet. As resin glands degrade, cannabinoid content decreases. Poorly and quickly dried cannabis still contains various amounts of chlorophyll, starch, nitrates, etc.

Once cured, proper storage will ensure that medicinal cannabis retains all its essential qualities.

Before Harvest

Do not water for 1 or 2 days before harvest. The soil should be fairly dry, but not dry enough that plants wilt. This will speed drying time by a day or more and will not affect the quality of cannabinoids and terpenes.

The fragrance of flowering medicinal cannabis is often pungent before, during, and after harvest. If air in and around drying and manicuring rooms is stagnant, odors will linger and accumulate. To help control fragrance, keep drying and manicuring rooms well vented. If possible, allow plenty of fresh, circulating air to pass through the drying room to remove fragrances quickly. Keep temperatures below 70°F (21.1°C) to minimize aroma.

Loss of Fragrance

"Terpenes, or terpenoids, are the compounds in cannabis that give the plant its unique fragrance. THC and the other cannabinoids have no odor, so marijuana's compelling fragrance depends on which terpenes predominate. It's the combination of terpenoids and THC that endows each strain with a specific psychoactive flavor."
—Martin A. Lee, "Talking Terpenes," *High Times*

The aroma, taste, and ultimately the effects of smoked cannabis depend upon the mix of terpenes and cannabinoids. Often cannabinoids and terpenes volatize and are destroyed during flowering, harvest, and storage as a result of high temperatures and maltreatment. The absence of these compounds diminishes bouquet and taste. It can also change the overall effect of the cannabis.

Cannabis plants lose their fragrance for a combination of reasons, all of which involve destruction of terpenes or the creation of a poor environment for terpene development. During flowering, plants that are subjected to heavy weather—including wind, rain, and hot sunlight or artificial light—are often less fragrant. Outdoor plants also accumulate surface dust, bacteria, and other bad stuff. When allowed to remain on the plant, these pollutants can smell and may possibly speed cannabinoid and terpene degradation. Funny thing is that poorly ventilated indoor environments are often more polluted than the great outdoors. Such pollutants can also play a role in diminishing fragrance.

Terpenes and cannabinoids evaporate into the air in a wide range of temperatures: 246°F to 815°F (118.9°C–435°C). As temperatures climb, more and more terpenes evaporate into the air. Terpenes can be destroyed by high temperatures, humid weather, wind, rain, and fondling or rough handling. Also, terpenoids may not have a chance to develop properly on plants that grow under stressful conditions caused by climate, poor care, or attacks by pests and diseases.

Cannabis can lose its fragrance when it dries too hot and fast. Fast drying does not allow enough time for chlorophyll and other pollutants to dissipate, and they may remain in the foliage. Lingering smells and tastes of these undesirable elements can impart detectable odors and tastes when consumed.

When poorly dried, and allowed to stay too wet, as if in a compost pile, cannabis starts **anaerobic decomposition**. This process causes cannabis to smell like wet hay and, in extreme cases, to have an ammonia-like odor.

Plants can harbor powdery mildew or another disease within their tissue. Powdery mildew is impossible to detect without laboratory analysis. Such diseases weaken plants and could also play a part in the deterioration of fragrance.

Bacteria, dead microscopic pests and their feces, dust, and many other pollutants remain on the surface of cannabis foliage at harvest. These elements could also affect fragrance. Washing harvested cannabis with a dilute bath of H_2O_2 will remove and disinfect plants. Clean plants smell "fresh"; the fragrance of cannabis is all that remains.

Genetically, some plants appear to be predisposed to less aroma and to losing fragrance over time. In combination with climatic conditions, genetics could play a role in minimizing cannabis fragrance.

Negative ion generators act within a small area and have little impact on the fragrance of growing cannabis. Ozone generators introduce ozone (O_3) into an enclosed area. The O_3 converts to O_2 within a few minutes. Carbon filters remove fragrances before air is expelled outdoors*.

*A free radicle of O floating next to O_2 becomes stable when they combine to form O_2, oxygen. However this O molecule could attach to any carbon it finds and strip it away. Much of the O_3 is converted to O_2 in the air, but laws of equilibrium and diffusion also apply.

Ozone generators should be located outside of occupied cannabis drying and manicuring rooms. See chapter 16, *Air*, for more information.

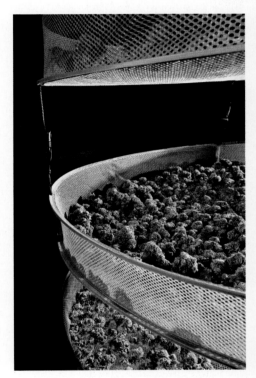

Plenty of air circulation and ventilation is necessary for manicured flower buds to dry. The buds in these net trays are turned once or twice a day by hand for even drying.

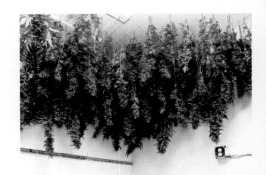

Hanging complete branches is a great way to dry flower buds of medical cannabis. These branches have just been harvested. The large leaves have been removed and the buds lightly trimmed.

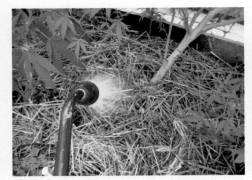

Watering is important during the flowering stage. Check soil moisture daily to avoid overwatering. Always irrigate in the morning so that the majority of water is used during the day. Soggy roots at night will slow growth substantially.

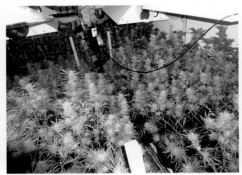

This big, healthy crop of 'Blue Dream' is ready for harvest.

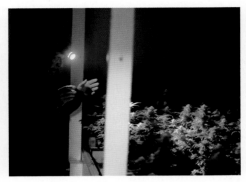

A green light or a UVB lamp makes pest trails and diseases very easy to see.

The fragrance of cannabis can also be controlled by sealing the drying and manicuring rooms. Set up a fan and carbon filter in the room to remove fragrances before venting the air out of the room. See "Fragrance" in chapter 16, *Air*, for more information.

Avoid the taste of chemical and organic fertilizers in harvested buds by leaching with plain water or a clearing solution to remove any residuals and chemicals that have built up in soil or plant foliage. Five to six days before harvesting, leach the growing medium with clean tap water or reverse osmosis water. Use a clearing solution such as Final Flush to remove any built-up nutrients in soil.

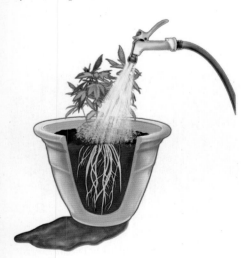

Leach soil heavily 5 to 7 days before harvest. Leaching soil will wash out any fertilizer salts that have accumulated in the soil. This allows the plant to use the balance of the nutrients in its system before harvest.

Some indoor gardeners fertilize with a liquid salt-based fertilizer until 2 or 3 days before harvest, and use a clearing solution to remove fertilizer residues. They say the practice helps plants retain weight in flower buds. But it does not make buds grow any faster, and fertilizer residues are still present in plant tissue. The tradeoff is that fertilizer adds weight at the expense of medicinal quality.

Apply the leaching solution according to directions on packaging. Always let at least 10 percent, preferably more, drain out the bottom of containers. If using a recirculating hydroponic system, change the water after the first 4 to 6 days of application. Continue to top off the reservoir with "clean" fresh water.

How to Tell When Fertilizer Could Affect Taste
1. Leaf tips and margins are burned.
2. Leaves are brittle at harvest.
3. Flower buds smell like chemicals.
4. Flower buds crackle when burning.
5. Buds taste like fertilizer.

Do not water cannabis for 1 or 2 days before harvest. The soil should be fairly dry but not dry enough that plants wilt. This will speed drying time by a day or more and will not affect the quality of cannabinoids.

Inspect plants at night with a green light or a UVB light. Powdery mildew and insect feces and trails are visible; they actually jump out at you as if you were reading an eye chart in the optometrist's chair. Carefully remove all signs of powdery mildew before it enters plant

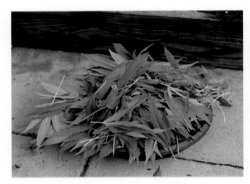

Save large leaves for making concentrates or for use in cooking.

tissue. Spray fungus with an organic fungistat before removing affected plant parts to ensure that the disease does not contaminate the rest of the crop. This method works only when there is very little mildew.

Some gardeners keep plants in 24 to 48 hours of darkness before harvesting. They say this practice causes buds to become more resinous.

Leaves
Once the large leaves are fully formed, cannabinoid potency has generally peaked out. Potency increases from the bottom of the plant upward. Large, old bottom leaves are not as cannabinoid-potent as younger smaller leaves toward the top of the plant. The most cannabinoid-potent part during much of the growth stage is found at the tips of branches in the small leaves and well-formed shoots.

Cut the entire leaf, including the leaf stem (petiole) and toss it into a bag. If left on the plant, the petiole shrivels and may attract fungus. Paper bags breathe

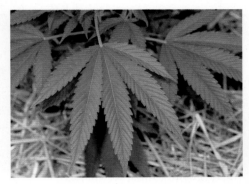

Once cut, turn plants or branches upside down, and start removing large leaves by hand. Make sure to inspect all leaves for resin!

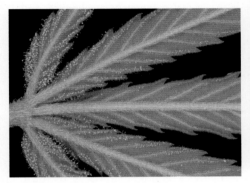

Leaves on this 'Maui' plant are developing resin as it matures. Leaves closer to flower buds and near the tops of plants tend to have more resin than those closer to the bottom of the plant. Always check leaf undersides for visible signs of resin. Start another paper bag to segregate leaves that show visible resin. These leaves are great for making hashish. (MF)

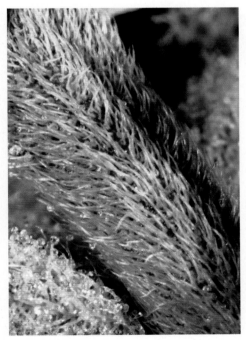

The leaf stem (petiole) has few resin glands that contain cannabinoids. This image shows many cystolith glands.

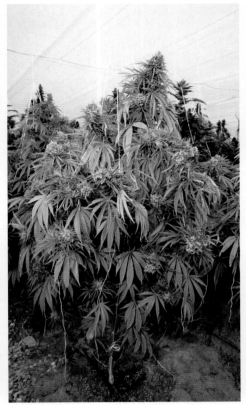

Harvest leaves if they show signs of disease or rapid yellowing that fertilizer has failed to cure. Once they start to yellow and die, their potency decreases rapidly. This is true especially with large, older "fan" leaves that turn yellow when nitrogen-rich fertilizer is withheld during flowering.

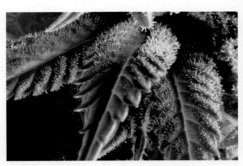

The resin on these 'Jack the Ripper' leaves is as thick as found anywhere on a flower top. It is easy to separate the resin glands from foliage into a concentrated form. Save leaf trimmings laden with visible resin to make concentrated hashish. (MF)

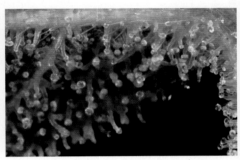

This 'Garlic' leaf is magnified 4X. Often small leaves around flower buds harbor as much resin as the flower buds themselves. These small leaves continue to develop resin until buds are ripe. These small leaves can be left with flower buds or separated to be used for a different purpose. (MF)

well and can be closed by folding over the top. Plastic bags do not breathe and often "sweat" inside, so the top of the bag must be left open.

Keep the paper bag in a closet or area with 40 to 60 percent humidity and 60°F to 70°F (15.6°C–21.1°C) temperature. Reach into the bag once or twice a day and stir leaves by hand. Leaves should be dry to the touch in 5 to 7 days. Once dry, place small resinous leaves in the freezer so resin glands will readily separate from foliage. Large leaves carry fewer cannabinoids and are most useful to make tinctures, food dishes, and drinks. See chapter 26, *Medicinal Concentrates & Tinctures*, and chapter 27, *Cooking with Medicinal Cannabis*, for more information.

Male Harvest

Harvest male cannabis plants as soon as they are identified, unless they are to be used for breeding. Males produce less and lower-quality cannabinoids, as well as taking up valuable space in the garden. Male flowers can produce pollen indoors or in light-deprivation greenhouses as early as 2 weeks after inducing flowering with the 12-hour day/night schedule. Outdoors, male pre-flowers contain pollen too. Watch out for early openers. Three to 6 weeks after initiating flowering, pollen sacks open. Plants continue producing flowers for several weeks after the first pods have begun to shed pollen. Once male flowers are clearly visible but not yet open, cannabinoid production is at peak levels. Remember, though, that cannabinoid content is low in male flowers even at peak production. After males have released their pollen, the degradation process speeds up and flowers fall.

Harvest males carefully, especially if they are close to females. Spraying males

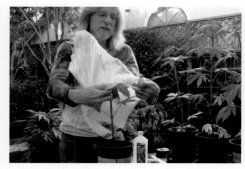

Before removing male plants from the garden, cover them with a plastic bag to help contain pollen.

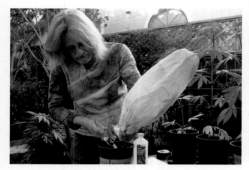

Branches full of male flowers can be stored in a glass of water for several days. Their pollen sacks will continue to open. The pollen is easy to collect once it is contained in the bag.

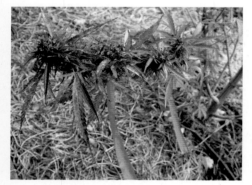

This is the last branch on a harvested outdoor female plant. A couple of plastic ties mark this branch full of flower buds that was fertilized by male pollen and left to mature after harvest.

with water will render pollen useless and help avoid accidental pollination. Cut the plant off at the base, taking care to shake it as little as possible. To help prevent accidental pollination by an unnoticed open male flower, carefully cover the male plant with a plastic bag, and tie it off at the bottom before harvesting. Or, if you can see an open male flower, spray it with water to make pollen unviable. Keep males used for breeding as far from

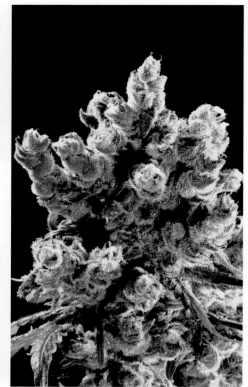

Swollen seed bracts on a ripe 'Jack Herer' female

flowering females as possible. Make sure to install fine screens for air coming into the flowering room and wet them down regularly to discourage rogue pollen. Isolate males until needed. After a month, the male often starts reverting to vegetative growth even though it retains viable sacks of pollen. Males can also be cloned and held in the vegetative stage until needed. Induce flowering about 3 weeks before viable pollen is needed. Within 3 to 5 weeks, the male will be full of viable pollen sacks.

Prolong harvest on 1 or 2 males by removing flowers with tweezers or fingernails as they appear. New flowers soon emerge after plucking old ones. Continue to remove pollen sacks until females are 2 weeks from full bloom. Picking off individual male flowers is a tedious, time-consuming process, and it is easy to miss a few.

Harvesting most of the branches and leaving only 1 or 2 pollen-bearing limbs is practical. A single male flower contains enough pollen to fertilize many

female ovules; a single branch full of male flowers is more than adequate to produce enough pollen for most home seed crops and breeding needs.

See "Making Seeds at Home" in chapter 25, *Breeding*, for complete information on harvesting.

Sinsemilla Harvest

According to cannabis expert Mel Frank, "the "peak potency window" lasts at least a week while the potency stays within a few percent of its highest. It is not critical whether to harvest today or tomorrow, but it is critical whether to harvest this week or next."

Harvest sinsemilla when the flowering cycle is coming to an end and further growth will be slow and minimal. Besides slowed growth, bracts, stigmas, and resin glands function as 3 easy-to-use indicators to help you determine when to harvest. When using commercial seeds from reputable breeders, medical gardeners also have the breeders' recommendation for weeks-to-maturation, particularly indoors.

Bracts: Especially look at the bracts, all of which should be mature and swollen except for bracts at the very tops of the buds. The topmost bracts should have begun to swell but not yet be fully swollen.

Stigmas: Most of the stigmas (a good 90 percent)—the pollen-catching "fuzzy white "hairs"—will have withered and turned rust/brown. The few remaining, still-white stigmas will have started to curl and will no longer look fresh, straight, and receptive to pollen. All cannabis plant parts except roots, seeds, and stigmas are covered with resin glands. Stigmas are devoid of resin and claims that these are potent are simply wrong. The only resin stigmas might have would come from contact with resin from broken or secreting resin glands on the bracts.

The images opposite follow different varieties of cannabis through the last few weeks of flowering. Notice how the bracts and stigmas change to indicate peak harvest time.

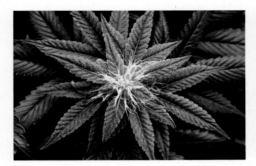

This indica variety, 'Garlic', is just starting to develop white stigmas to attract male pollen. (MF)

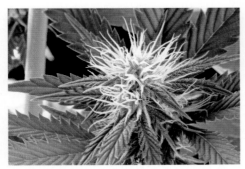

This 'Maui' bud continues to flower and develop stigmas while waiting for male pollen to land. When there is no male pollen available, growth continues. (MF)

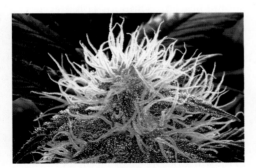

White female stigmas from this 'Skywalker' grown indoors continue to grow from seed bracts. Notice that resin is starting to become visible with the naked eye. (MF)

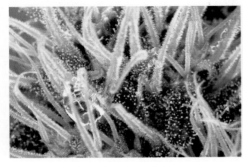

Overhead watering and sprays should be avoided during the last 2 weeks before flowering. A drop of dew water is suspended between the stigmas of this 'MK Ultra' × 'Sensi Star', but any more water would stay in between seed bracts and attract rot. (MF)

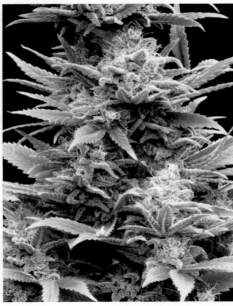

During flowering, changing the fertilizer to a high-phosphorus, high-potassium, low-nitrogen mix causes larger leaves to yellow as harvest progresses. (MF)

Stigmas tend to die back at the same rate as capitate-stalked resin glands start to weather and experience oxidation, turning amber in the process. The images on pages 105–107 show the change in stigmas as they die back. The next pictorial will run through a progressive sequence of capitate-stalked resin gland maturity through harvest.

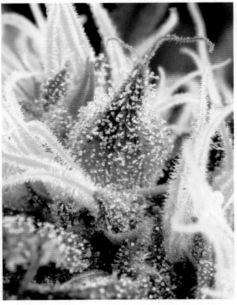

Here is a close-up of a 'Maui' bud on which pairs of white female stigmas are just starting to senesce. You can see that a few pairs of stigmas are completely dark. In this case, the stigmas have been fertilized by male pollen. (MF)

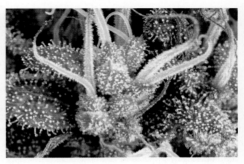

Stigmas on this 'Haze' × 'Northern Lights 5' × 'Sensi Star' cross are dying back a little at a time and will continue to convert from white to reddish-brown as flowers mature.

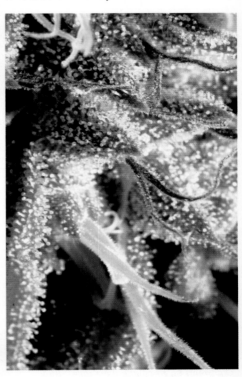

More and more stigmas on this 'OG Kush' × 'Master Kush' are dying back as harvest day nears. Look at the way the resin is continuing to pile up on the buds, small leaves, seed bracts, and foliage. (MF)

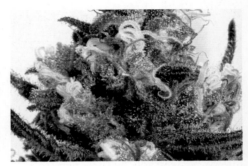

Half the stigmas on this 'Purple Heart' bud have died back and about half are healthy. This bud has so much resin that looking at resin glands could be the best indication of harvest time. (MF)

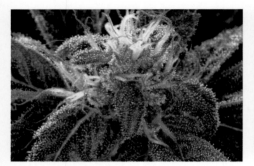

Stigmas on this 'Diesel' bud continue to die back and resin continues to populate buds. More resin is forming on small leaves now. (MF)

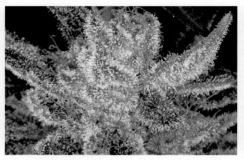

This plant bud is perfect and ready to harvest. All the resin glands are glistening in the light, and just a few resin glands have started to deteriorate.

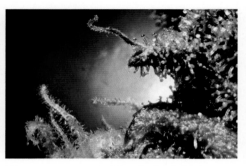

The stigma on top is dying back while the stigmas below are still healthy. This plant has a few more days until harvest.

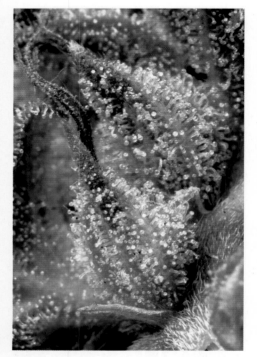

Seed bracts on this 'Jack the Ripper' bud continue to swell even though they contain no seeds. The seed bracts are packed with resin glands that still glisten in the light, although the stigmas have completely died back. (MF)

Capitate-Stalked Resin Glands

The best time to harvest is when capitate-stalked resin glands have developed a spherical head and have not yet begun to senesce. The glands start to degrade, turn amber, and fall apart; cannabinoid content diminishes and continues to digress. Check flower buds from each plant and harvest them individually as they become ready. Often the uppermost buds will be ready and harvested, while lower buds are left for another week or two to finish. Treat plants individually.

Resin glands that are bruised from being squeezed or jostled about deteriorate quickly changing color. The process is gradual, and individual resin glands change at different rates. Of course there are exceptions such as the variety 'Blueberry', which bears darker, even purplish resin glands.

On **indoor plants** a majority of the glands should be clear or translucent; fewer should be cloudy or milky, and very few, if any, should have color. Resin glands with an amber color signify oxygen has entered the gland and the degradation process is under way. Look for well-formed capitate-stalked resin glands that are fully intact and translucent.

Resin glands on outdoor plants are entirely different. More often, a good number of the visible glands will be cloudy or milky rather than clear or translucent, although after harvesting, a look inside the buds reveals predominantly clear or translucent glands. Larger bud-leaves often have yellow or amber resin glands, but glands with color should be a small minority on bracts. Having some yellow or amber glands is typical on full-sun outdoor-grown plants, where lots of sun, significant swings in temperatures, bad weather, wet or dry soil, and physical damage affect resin glands.

This section focuses on capitate-stalked resin glands. The images show the resin glands just before peak maturity through senescence.

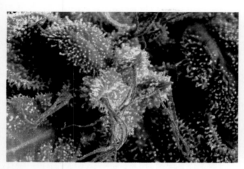

All the stigmas on this 'Haze' × 'Northern Lights 5' × 'Sensi Star' bud have turned a rich reddish brown and the resin glands are ready to harvest. This plant was grown indoors. Indoor plants tend to show resin turning amber at the same time both on seed bracts and small leaves around them. (MF)

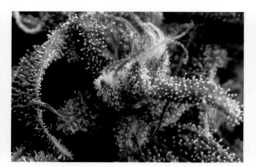

This outdoor 'Haze' × 'Northern Lights 5' × 'Sensi Star' bud ripens a little different than indoor cannabis flowers. The small leaves around the seed bracts tend to show oxidation first, which is demonstrated by the change in color from clear to amber. This is a sign of deterioration and loss of cannabinoid content. (MF)

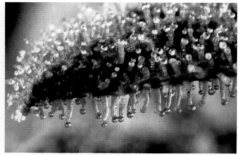

The tip of this resin-coated leaf of 'Garlic' shows a clear view of capitate-stalked resin glands. The majority of the cannabinoids, specifically THC, will be located at the base of the stalk, where the bulbous top connects. You can see that some of these resin glands have started to turn amber. (MF)

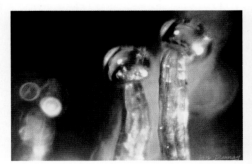

This close-up view shows beautiful resin glands at peak harvest. They are fully formed, strong, and healthy.

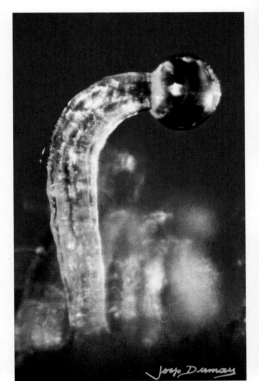

An amber color signifies oxidation and senescence of capitate-stalked resin glands. Once the inside of the bulbous top is exposed to oxygen, cannabinoids dissipate at a rapid rate.

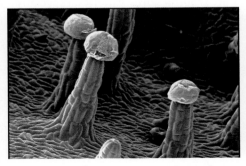

This scanning electron microscope image shows how the bulbous tops of the capitate-stalked resin glands suffer lesions from friction, wind, or rain, or start to naturally senesce—all of which will decrease cannabinoid content and potency. Such resin glands appear with an amber-colored bulb on top of a clear stalk under natural light.

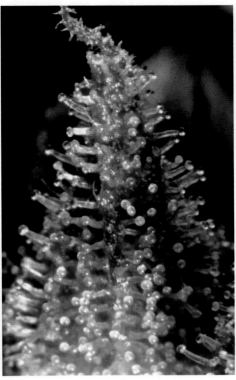

This 'Skunk #1' seed bract has some capitate-stalked resin glands that are perfectly clear and others that have started to turn amber. Time to harvest! (MF)

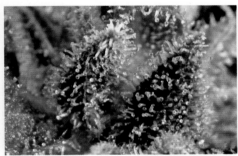

Ready to harvest! Look at the resin glands on this 'Skunk #1' bud to see that they are continuing to turn amber in color. (MF)

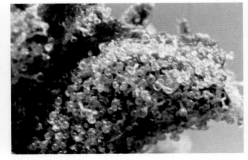

Here is the first in a three-photo sequence of the variety 'Garlic', showing resin glands on a small leaf. The first photo shows the resin glands completely clear to translucent. They cover the leaf! (MF)

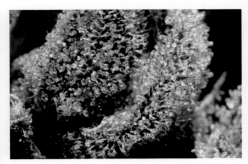

The second photo shows that some of the resin glands are starting to turn amber. Notice that the heads are the first part of the gland to turn amber. (MF)

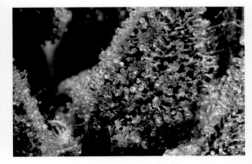

The third photo shows resin glands continuing to mature and turn amber as maturity slowly turns to senescence. (MF)

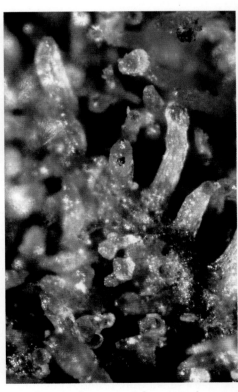

This close-up of a 'Mexican' from 1976 shows that the resin glands are well on their way to impotency. The bulbous heads have all ruptured and cannabinoids have volatized into the air. Few potent cannabinoids are left in the residue. (MF)

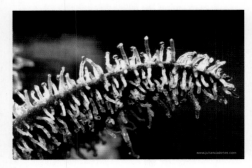

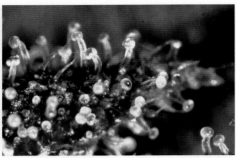

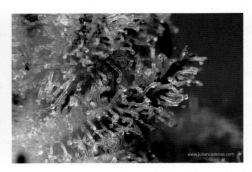

You can see that the resin gland heads are decomposing on the top of this leaf, and many resin gland heads on the bottom of the leaf have already disappeared. This plant is past peak harvest.

'Cocoa Kush' from DJ Short shows short, stocky resin glands.

Resin glands on this 'Critical Mass' flower bud have long stalks and small resin heads.

Qualities of *Indica, Sativa,* and *Ruderalis*

The difference between resin glands is striking—*indica* and *indica*-dominant resin glands tend to have a short, pyramid-like stalk with a big strong bulb on top. *Sativa* and *sativa*-dominant varieties tend to have a long, thin stalk with a large or small bulb on top. The bulbs on top of stalks are also different sizes. Large and small bulbous resin glands fall through different mesh sieves, making different grades of kief. Thin stalks tend to fall through sieves and create a "fiber" in the kief.

Flower buds harvested when the majority of resin glands have started to senesce generally deliver a more corporal or physical effect. Pure *indica*, *afghani*, and *indica*-dominant varieties harvested at this late point will possess a heavy body or tranquilizing effect. Waiting to harvest pure *sativa* and *sativa*-dominant varieties until this late stage does not take advantage of the high cannabinoid content. Such varieties are best harvested when resin glands are clear and ripe but not yet senescing.

Indica and *Indica*-Dominant Varieties

Pure *indica* varieties and *indica*-dominant crosses grown in greenhouses and indoors are harvested 6 to 9 weeks after inducing flowering with a 12/12-hour day/night photoperiod. Outdoors, *indica*-dominant plants often initiate flowering when they receive about 13 hours of daylight and 11 hours of darkness. Flowering increases as nights grow longer.

Some medical gardeners choose to harvest 6-week-old flower buds with showy resin glands that have lower cannabinoid content. Shorter flowering times make harvesting one more crop every year possible.

Sativa and *Sativa*-Dominant Varieties

Pure tropical *sativa* varieties, especially Thai and Asian varieties that were grown from native seed, take longer to bloom after turning the light to 12 hours. Seeds brought directly from the tropics can take 4 months to finish blooming under 12 hours of light. These types tend to form buds at an even rate throughout flowering, with no marked decline in growth rate.

Few indoor gardeners have the time or patience to grow pure *sativa* varieties because of their long flowering period, leggy stature, and low yield. Buds at the top of the plant often reach peak potency long before lower buds. See chapter 8,

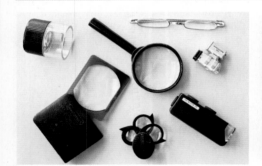

(MF)

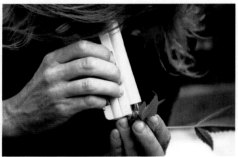

Sometimes it is easiest to remove a small piece of a bud so that you can get a complete view of it on the inside.

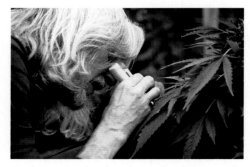

Look at resin glands right on the plant to make sure their growth is progressing properly. It is fun to watch them develop over time.

Magnifiers and Microscopes

Use a magnifying lens or mini microscope to examine capitate-stalked resin glands. Use a 10X magnifying glass, jeweler's loupe, or a 20X to 50X handheld microscope. My preference is a 45X handheld microscope with a battery-powered LED lamp. Look at resin glands without harvesting buds, or take a small, thin, resinous portion of a ripe bud and place it under the microscope at a low 30X to 50X magnification setting. If the microscope does not have a lamp, a flashlight will be necessary for an unshadowed view.

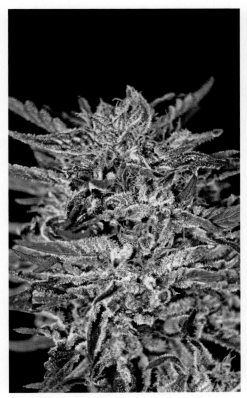

'Granddaddy Purple' is a cross between 'Purple Urkle' and 'Big Bud'; both parents are indica-dominant.

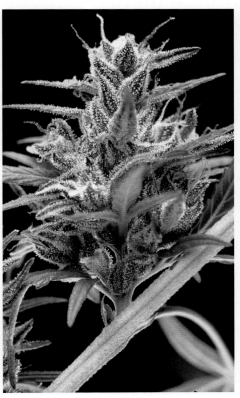

Sativa-dominant varieties like this 'Afghani #1' × 'Chiba Colombian 60' × 'African 3' from 1980 tend to ripen later and also grow differently. (MF)

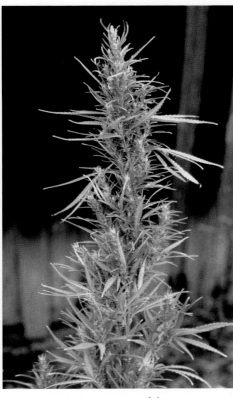

Mexican varieties are some of the most pronounced of this type of flower bud growth. (MF)

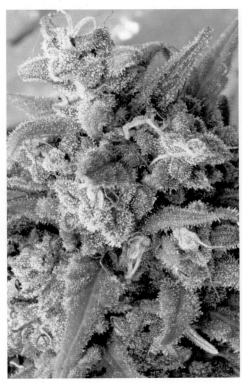

Indica- and sativa-dominant varieties tend to flower differently. Indica-dominant 'Purple Hen' flowers tend to come ripe at the same time if they receive the same amount of light. (MF)

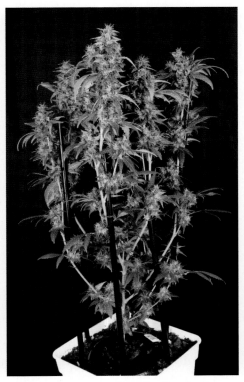

This 'Amnesia Haze' from Hy-Pro Seeds shows classic 'Haze' growth habit. Small buds grow at branch unions and tips of branches are loaded with flowers.

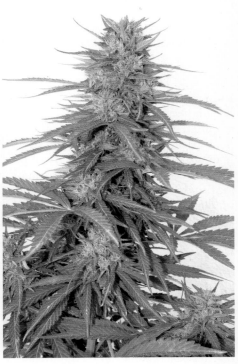

Ruderalis cross 'Chaze' takes longer to mature and produces more than most autoflowering varieties.

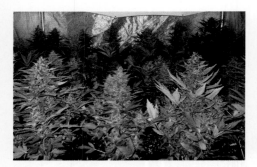

Cannabis ruderalis *is crossed with* indica *and* sativa *varieties to yield short, autoflowering plants with big buds!*

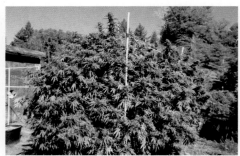

Big outdoor plants are often harvested in stages. First the outer 2-foot (61 cm) layer of flower bud–filled branches is removed. Two weeks later a second harvest is taken after smaller buds have had a chance to fatten up in the sunlight.

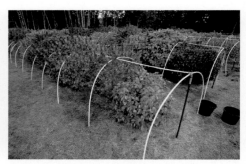

Small plants toward the front of Humboldt-locals's garden have been harvested once and will be harvested again and again. Medical cannabis gardeners growing outdoors in Northern California harvest plants twice or even 3 and 4 times. The purple plant in the second row has been harvested once and will be harvested in another week or two.

Flowering, for more information on altering the photoperiod to increase production and shorten flowering time.

Sativa-dominant crosses with *indica* varieties may not be ready for 10 weeks or more.

Ruderalis and Ruderalis-Dominant Varieties

Ruderalis crosses (autoflowering and autoflowering-feminized) varieties are daylight-neutral and ready to harvest about 70 to 80 days after germinating seed. These crosses are harvested the same as other varieties, when cannabinoid production has peaked out.

Harvest Timing

Indoors and in "light deprivation" greenhouses, sinsemilla flowers are mature from 6 to 12 weeks after the photoperiod has been changed to 12 hours to induce flowering. Seed companies list "flowering time" in their catalogs, and much information is available on the Internet about maturation dates. Outdoors, the first early harvest is ready in late spring. Fall crops are harvested from late September through November, depending on varieties grown and climate. The best time to harvest sinsemilla is when cannabinoid production has peaked but the degradation process has not yet started. Established indoor varieties are bred so the entire plant reaches peak potency at the same time. Lower flower tops that received less light are not as heavily frosted with resin as upper branches and could be slower

to mature. Varieties that ripen all at once tend to go through 4 to 5 weeks of rapid bud formation before growth levels off. The harvest is taken 1 to 3 weeks after growth slows.

Outdoor harvests depend upon weather. Fall rains and cold weather arrive late in some years, and the harvest can be taken at its peak. Plants are often harvested early in bad weather years. Harvest when there is no longer enough intense sunlight for buds to grow. At a point of diminished sunlight, resin development virtually stops. There are several reasons to harvest plants early, such as lack of light, cold rainy weather, and freezing nights.

Cold weather also influences the development of resin. Most often prolonged 40°F to 50°F (4.4°C–10°C) nights and cool days with ample sunlight will slow foliage growth and promote resin development.

Harvest large outdoor plants up to 4 times. Harvesting 2 to 4 times over the course of 2 to 6 weeks can increase harvest weight by as much as 40 percent. The top 1 to 2 feet (30.5–61 cm) is removed at the first harvest. Secondary smaller buds receive more sunlight and become heavier. The second layer of medicinal buds is then harvested. If it is a big, 10-foot-tall plant, up to 2 more harvests are possible in a good growing year. We found this technique to work best with the variety 'Mr. Nice'. An inexpensive liquid chromatogra-

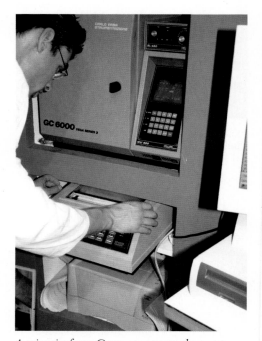

A scientist from Canna measures the exact THC content of harvested buds with a gas chromatograph. Canna provides this free service at Spannabis in Barcelona, Spain. Spannabis (www.spannabis.com) is the biggest cannabis fair in the world.

phy test can also be performed. These tests are relatively inexpensive, about $10 USD, and are fairly accurate. See chapter 2, *Measuring Cannabinoids*, for more information on liquid chromatography tests.

Laboratory analysis, though More expensive, is also available in many states and countries that sanction medical cannabis. Many countries have decriminalized small amounts of cannabis, and it can be measured legally by third-party labs.

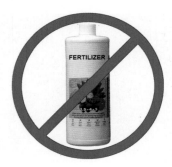
Stop fertilizing container plants before harvest.

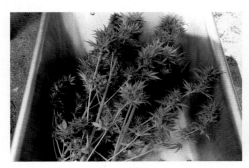
Bud-heavy branches will be covered with a dilute H_2O_2 solution to sanitize against residuals of pests and diseases.

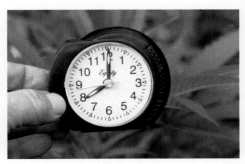
Harvest early in the day.

Harvest: Step-by-Step

Step One: Stop supplemental fertilization 5 to 7 days prior to harvest. Latent nutrient accumulation in foliage imparts a fertilizer-like taste and a "nutrient residual." Leach nutrients from the growing medium 7 to 10 days before harvest. Some gardeners continue to fertilize until 3 days before harvest if using a commercial "leaching" product that expedites the removal of built-up chemicals in the substrate.

Step Two: If sprays have been applied during the last 2 weeks (not recommended), mist plants heavily to wash off undesirable residues that may have accumulated on foliage. A 5-minute pre-bath in a dilute (5%) hydrogen peroxide (H_2O_2) solution will disinfect and wash away pest feces, bacteria, dust, etc. Remove branches from the H_2O_2 bath and gently rinse with a spray of water. The spray bath will not affect resin production. Gently jiggle buds after rinsing to shake off any standing water. To prevent fungus and bud blight, remove large leaves and wash the garden early

in the day to allow excess water to dry before nightfall. If bud mold (*Botrytis*) is visible, carefully remove infected bud an inch below damage. Remove contaminated growth from garden and destroy. Wash hands. Insert "amputated" branches in H_2O_2 bath.

Step Three: You may want to give plants 24 to 48 hours of total darkness before harvest. Some gardeners do this and say the buds are a little more resinous afterward.

Step Four: Harvest early in the morning, before direct sunlight warms the plants. This is when cannabinoid content is at its peak. Harvest entire plant or one branch at a time by cutting near the base with pruners. Jerking the root ball creates a mess and is unnecessary. All of the cannabinoids are produced in the foliage, not in the roots of the cannabis plant.

Step Five: Once formed, resin does not move and therefore cannot "drain into the foliage." Drying the entire plant by

hanging it upside down is simply convenient. When stems are left intact, drying is much slower.

Step Six: To harvest branches or entire plants:

a. Remove large leaves 1 or 2 days before actually harvesting plants. Or remove leaves upon harvest. Harvesting large leaves early starts the drying process, gets them out of the way, and makes manicuring easier and faster.

b. Harvest entire plants by cutting them off at the base before manicuring.

c. Or cut each branch into lengths of 6 to 24 inches. Manicure the freshly harvested tops, trimming away leaves with clippers or scissors. Hang the manicured branches until dry. Once dry, cut the tops from the branches, taking special care to handle tender flower buds as gently as possible.

d. Or leave larger leaves on branches to act as a protective sheath to flower buds.

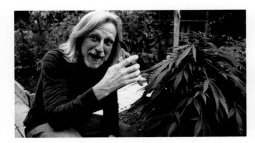
Harvest with clippers or a saw. Depending upon how buds mature, you may want to harvest the entire plant at once, or harvest individual buds as they become ripe. Indica-dominant plants are usually harvested all at once.

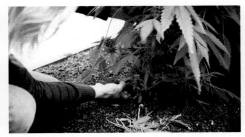
Cutting small plants at the stem is the easiest way to harvest. This plant is about 3 feet tall (about a meter) and easy to handle. I always cut it just below the soil line so that all the branches are attached to the stem.

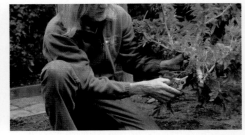
Next, trim up the bottom branches. I discard the small growth on the bottom and throw it in with the big leaves.

Tender resin glands are protected from bruises and rupture until final manicuring, but manicuring is much slower and more tedious when trimming dry foliage. Resin glands are also more apt to bruise and resin tends to fall from the dry foliage when handling.

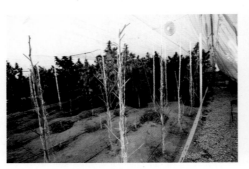

Plants can be harvested a branch or bud at a time. The main stem of the plant remains in the ground, and large leaves are left in the garden. The stem and leaves are cultivated into the soil to benefit the next crop.

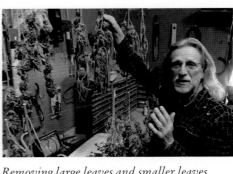

Removing large leaves and smaller leaves around buds is much easier immediately after harvest when foliage is still supple.

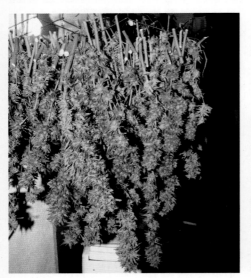

These branches full of flower buds were lightly manicured before being hung to dry on hangers in a dark, well-ventilated closet.

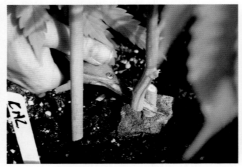

Cut smaller plants at the base to harvest.

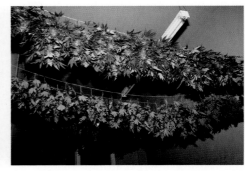

Drying bud-filled branches before manicuring causes many resin glands to be damaged.

Manicuring

Manicuring is easiest when foliage is soft and supple immediately after harvest. Keeping the trimming room at 45 to 50 percent humidity will ensure that buds stay supple longer. Trimming off leaves now will also speed drying. Waiting until foliage is dry to manicure will make manicuring buds a more tedious and time-consuming job than it already is. And removing leaves now keeps dry buds from being handled again. However, some gardeners prefer to take the extra time and energy, citing a slower and more uniform drying process.

Manicuring is easiest and most efficient with a good pair of trimming scissors that has small blades to facilitate reaching in and snipping off leaf stems and leaves around flower buds. An ergonomic pair of scissors with comfortable handles is indispensable when manicuring cannabis for hours. Small scissors are preferred because they require much less motion and energy to operate.

Manicure over a fine silkscreen (see chapter 26, *Medicinal Concentrates & Tinctures*) or a table with a smooth, slick surface. Scrape up the cannabinoid-rich resin from under the screen or on the flat surface. The resin can be consumed immediately or pressed into blocks of hashish for easy and practical storage.

Wear inexpensive rubber gloves to collect "finger resin." After trimming for a few hours, remove accumulated finger resin on gloves by putting the rubber gloves in a freezer for an hour. Cooling will make it easier to remove the accumulated resin from the gloves.

Budget enough time to harvest and manicure your crop. Properly manicuring one pound (454 gm) takes 1 person 6 to 8 hours by hand with scissors.

Trimming machines speed the manicuring process. There are many different models to choose from. Small manually powered trimmers cost less than $300 USD and work well for small harvests. Large machines that can trim 3 to 4 pounds (1.4–1.8 kg) of flower buds per hour cost $12,000 USD or more. A single machine can do the work of 6 to 10 pairs of hands with scissors. Of course, 1 or 2 people must feed the trimmer untrimmed buds, and the buds must be carted away to another room.

You can informative videos on YouTube about each of the following trimmers: Big Red Trimmer, Bonsai Buddy, Magic Trimmer, Rolling Thunder Trimmer, Samurai Power Trimmer, Trimbox, Trim Reaper, Trimpro Automatic, Tumble Trimmer, and my favorite, the Twister. However, the videos lack the close-up detail necessary to see what condition the buds are in after trimming.

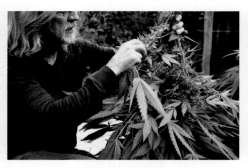

Manicuring scissors come in a couple of basic shapes. Many trimmers prefer small, compact scissors that require little hand movement. (MF)

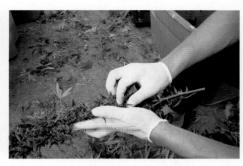

Remove large leaves and large stems upon harvest. Fresh supple leaves are easier to work with than when dry. Remove large "fan" leaves and leaf stems (petiole) to avoid possible rot. Plants with outer leaves intact take longer to dry and require much more time to manicure.

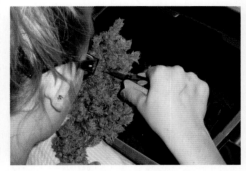

Inexpensive rubber gloves keep the resin on gloves rather than sticking to hands. The resin can be removed from gloves later to make "finger hash."

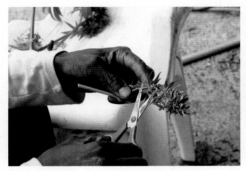

Some gardeners wet a concrete floor, or employ inexpensive swamp coolers or humidifiers. Gardeners in cold, rainy climates must ventilate adequately and possibly employ heaters. Using a dehumidifier in a large drying room is often impractical.

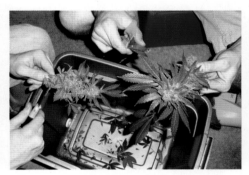

Snip off smaller, low-potency leaves around buds that show little resin, so a beautiful cannabinoid-potent flower bud remains.

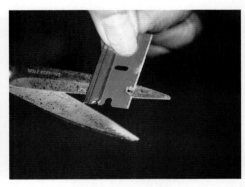

Small scissors make it easier to reach in between dense buds when manicuring.

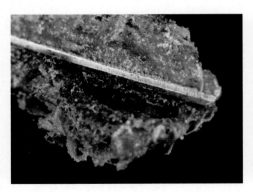

Resin can build up heavily on scissors!

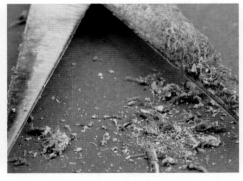

Once frozen, resin is easier to remove from scissors.

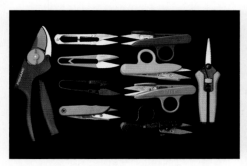

Scrape accumulated resin from scissors when it impairs blade movement. Use a small knife or razor blade to remove built-up resin from blades. Ball up small bits of scraped resin by rubbing it together between fingers. The ball of "finger hash" will grow as manicuring progresses.

Drying

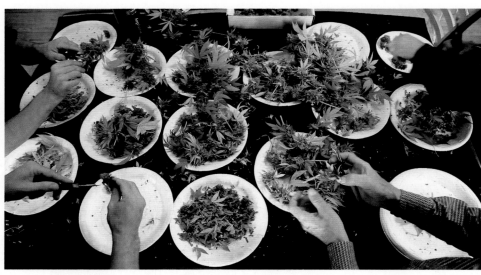

45 - 55%

Relative humidity of about 50 percent keeps leaves supple when manicuring.

After passing through the trimming machine, buds are touched up and further manicured by hand. Hand-manicuring removes rough edges. These trimmers are manicuring over smooth paper plates. Scrape up fallen resin glands on the table or under the screen.

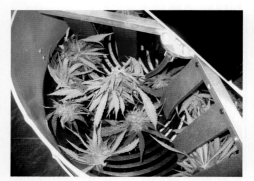

This SpinPro trimmer has a blade spinning below a steel grate. Buds are dumped on top of the grate and moved around with pliable plastic fingers.

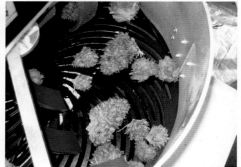

Buds are trimmed after a few spins around the grate of the SpinPro. Once trimmed, buds are removed and a new batch is dumped in.

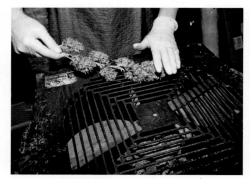

This TrimPro trimmer consists of a rotating blade below a protective steel grate. Buds are manually moved across the grate. The blade trims off any foliage that hangs below the grate.

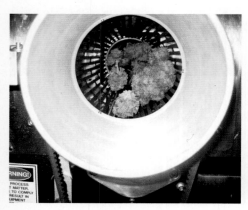

The Twister is a top-end trimmer. Buds are fed into a hopper and passed through a cylinder with a cutting deck below. Above you can see trimmed buds coming out the cylinder.

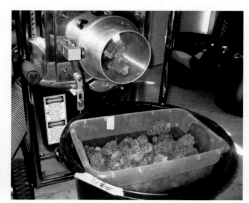

Once trimmed by the Twister, flower buds fall into a container to be further manicured by hand.

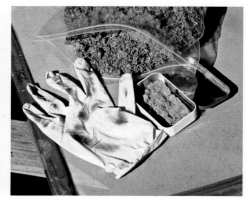

Wear tight fitting latex gloves when manicuring. Remove gloves after trimming to collect the accumulated resin.

Drying

When an entire plant or branch is harvested and hung to dry, the transport of fluids within the plant continues, but at a much slower rate. Stomata close soon after harvest, and drying is slowed since little water vapor escapes. The natural plant processes slowly come to an end as the plant dries. The outer cells are the first to dry, but fluid still moves from internal cells to supply moisture to outer cells, which are dry. When the drying and curing processes occur properly, plants dry evenly throughout. Removing leaves and large stems upon harvest speeds drying; however, moisture content within the "dried" flower buds, leaves, and stems can become uneven. If flower buds are dried too quickly, chlorophyll and other pigments, starch, and nitrates or other fertilizer salts are trapped within plant tissue, making it burn unevenly and taste unpleasantly "green."

The smell of ammonia in drying cannabis indicates a lack of air circulation, anaerobic bacteria, and an excess of nitrogen in foliage. Avoid the formation of ammonia by keeping cannabis buds and foliage well aerated during drying.

Drying facilitates storage for later use. Drying converts 75 percent or more of a freshly harvested plant into water vapor and other gases, and converts carbohydrates to simple sugars. Drying also converts chlorophyll and other pigments so that no "green" residuals remain.

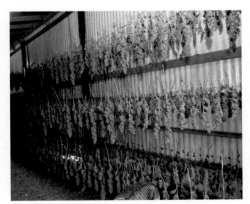

Manicuring bud–laden branches and hanging them individually allows them to dry longer. All the moisture from the stem must dry too.

During drying, starch is converted into reducing sugars*. As starch degrades, reducing sugar concentration increases and peaks out during the first few days of drying. After that, respiration is slowed, which oxidizes reducing sugar into carbon dioxide and water. The stored starch is broken down to simple sugars, which are used for food. This imparts a sweet earthy aroma and taste.

*See http://en.wikipedia.org/wiki/Reducing_sugar for complete definition of "reducing sugars."

Chlorophyll degradation is apparent as the green colors pale and fade into yellows, browns, reds, and purples. Although independent of one another, starch and chlorophyll degradation occur at about the same rate. The minty green taste of cannabis also dissipates with the degradation of chlorophyll.

When dried slowly, over 5 to 14 days, moisture evaporates evenly into the air, yielding uniformly dry flower buds with minimal cannabinoid decomposition. Slowly dried flowers retain terpenes and cannabinoids, providing medical users with full medicinal benefits. Slow, even drying—where moisture content is the same throughout stems, foliage and buds—allows enough time for pigments to degrade. After 5 to 14 days of slow drying, all the chlorophyll is gone from "dry" buds. Hanging entire plants to dry, although more laborious, allows this process to take place more slowly over time.

Circulation and ventilation fans will help control heat and humidity and keep them at proper levels. You can also use a dehumidifier to control humidity. Air conditioners are ideal to dial in temperature and humidity in warm climates, but they are environmentally expensive to operate. Large drying areas may require a heater to raise temperature and lower humidity. Do not train fans directly on drying plants; it causes them to dry unevenly.

With temperatures above 75°F (23.9°C) buds may dry too fast, and humidity can more easily fall below the ideal 50

percent level. Temperatures above 85°F (29.4°C) cause buds to dry too fast, after which they burn inconsistently and are unpleasant to consume. High temperatures also ignite fragrance. Relative humidity below 30 to 40 percent causes buds to dry too fast and retain chlorophyll, giving them a "green" taste. Quick-dried buds are easy to mistakenly dry unevenly and for too long, making

---

To find the approximate moisture content of dry buds, weigh a specific bud upon harvest, when it is wet. Weigh it again during the drying and curing process to learn how much moisture it has lost. For example, a bud that weighs 0.5 ounces (15 gm) upon harvest, will weigh 0.14 ounces (4 gm) when it has lost 75 percent of its moisture.

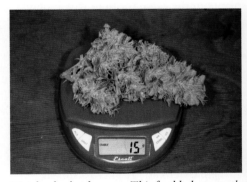

Weigh a bud at harvest. This freshly harvested bud weighs 0.5 ounces (15 gm).

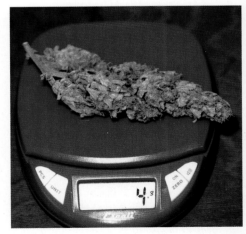

When dry, the same bud pictured above weighs 0.14 ounces (4 gm)—75 percent less.

them crispy on the outside and moist on the inside. Low humidity also causes buds to lose flavor and odor. If humidity is between 30 and 40 percent, allow for minimum air movement to slowly dry buds. Always use an accurate maximum/minimum thermometer and hygrometer to ensure that temperature and humidity are kept in the ideal range.

Suspending plants is a laborsaving way to facilitate slow, even drying. Large, moist stems can be removed and small branches hung from the ceiling to cut drying time by a few days. Use clothespins to attach branches to drying lines, or poke a paper clip through the base of branches and hang the clip from a line. Another option is to trim branches to form a hook and hang from the "hook."

Use the grow area as a drying room when not growing a garden. Do not dry plants in the same room in which plants are growing. Different climates are required for growing medicinal cannabis and for drying it. Fungus, spider mites, and other insects can also migrate from dead plants to live ones. Inspect drying buds daily for any signs of disease, spider mites, or insects. Smear Tanglefoot around the end of drying lines to form a barrier that keeps mites from migrating to live plants. Mites congregate at the barrier and are easy to smash between fingers.

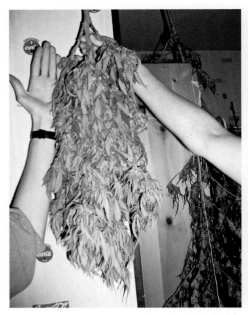

Small harvests like this 'Sensi Star' plant are manicured before hanging to dry.

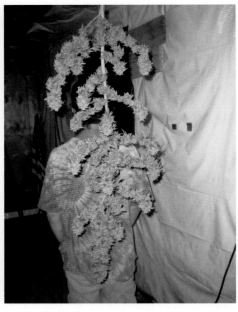

Excess foliage has been manicured from this plant. It is difficult to trim an entire plant and keep the branches intact.

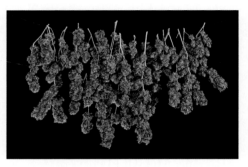

These bud-filled branches were removed and manicured individually before hanging to dry.

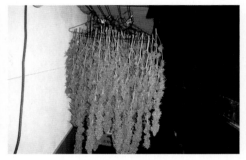

This nice crop of 'Power Plant' was manicured and hung to dry on clothes hangers in a well-ventilated closet.

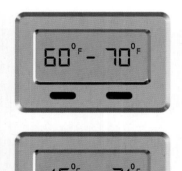

The ideal air temperature range for slow drying is between 60°F and 70°F (15.6°C–21.1°C) and humidity from 45 to 55 percent. Temperatures below 60°F (15.6°C) slow drying, and humidity often climbs quickly. Humidity above 80 percent extends drying time and heightens the threat of bud mold.

Drying Small Harvests

Small harvests can easily be dried in a closet, cabinet, or a cardboard box that is smaller than the growing area's size. If drying space is a problem, using a staggered planting schedule or planting varieties that ripen both early and late carries over to a staggered harvest that frees up drying space as buds dry.

A cardboard or wooden box makes an excellent drying space to hang small harvests. Airflow in the enclosed area is diminished, so buds and leaves must be turned daily to even out the moisture content and discourage mold. Thread a large needle with dental floss, and string the floss back and forth through the open box near the top to make drying lines. If the box is tall enough, you can install several levels of drying lines.

Lock the flaps on the box and set it in a closet or spare room. Open flaps to allow air circulation as needed. Or, cut holes near the bottom and top of the box to allow air exchange and circulation. Check daily to see how buds are drying. If buds and leaves start drying too quickly, open the box top and set the box in a cooler location.

Use a portable, foldable clothesline to make a quick and mobile drying room. Unfold clothesline, hang buds from lines, and cover with a large black bedsheet or cloth to allow for the exchange of air while maintaining darkness. Train a fan on the outside of the sheet so air circulates underneath to help dry the flower buds.

Building a small drying room is as easy as tacking some plywood together at

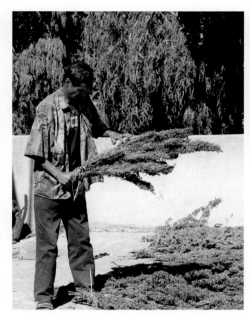

Moroccan plants are being dried in the sunlight on a warm slab. This practice degrades resin.

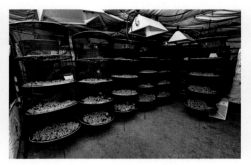

Compartmentalized net bags are inexpensive, collapsible, and easy to hang, expand into a drying rack, and store. These drying racks are perfect!

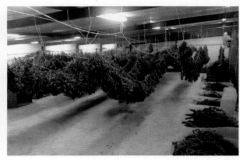

Hang manicured buds to dry for a day or so before placing on drying screens to allow the bulk of the moisture to dissipate. Once on screens, buds should be turned every day or two to ensure even drying.

right angles and hanging lines across the enclosure. Or you can tack or tape black Visqueen plastic to the ceiling and floor to make "walls."

Manicured buds can also be placed in boxes to dry. Move buds daily so new surfaces are exposed to air. Drying might be slower because the airflow is reduced. Line boxes with cardboard or paper to contain and collect resin glands that fall to the bottom. Or seal cracks with tape to contain resin glands for collection.

Drying Large Harvests
Stagger large harvests on big 10- to 15-foot-tall plants by harvesting the top 2 to 3 feet (60–90 cm) from the top of the plant. The buds located lower on the plant, now exposed to sunlight, will continue to grow and swell. Harvest again in a couple of weeks (weather permitting) by cutting the next 2 to 3 feet (61–91.4 cm) from the top branches. Most varieties can be harvested 2 to 3 times over a 4-to-6-week period.

Note: Gardeners in Northern California prefer to keep flower buds harvested last for use as personal medicine.

Drying a large harvest requires a large, dark, cool space with good airflow. Do not harvest more cannabis than avail-

able drying space can accommodate. Stagger the harvest so that there will be enough drying space. Friends in Switzerland were compelled to buy a 4-story industrial building to dry several acres of cannabis. Other surprised gardeners have to quickly erect tents and temporary buildings to serve as drying sheds. Large spaces such as bedrooms, barns, and sheds are also used.

Cut plants at the base or pull whole plants from the ground. Remove large leaves and hang the harvested plants on lines in the drying room. Cut branches from 12 to 40 inches (30.5–101.6 cm). Manicure each branch and hang on drying lines to complete the drying process.

Save space by building or buying drying racks for the buds. Make drying racks from window screen or plastic agricultural netting. Stretch the screen or netting over a wooden frame and secure with staples. Put 3- to 6-inch (7.62–15.2 cm) spacers between framed screens to allow for adequate airflow. Or build a drying box with removable screens.

Drying Time
Checklist for Proper Drying
- Temperature 60°F–70°F (15.6°C–21.1°C)
- Humidity 45–55 percent.
- Dry under minimal or no light.
- Handle buds as little as possible.
- Hang manicured buds until dry.
- Exact conditions may vary; use parameters below as a guideline.

Drying time depends upon temperature, humidity, and bud density. Most flower buds will be dry enough in 3 to 5 days before passing to the curing process, but they may take longer. It takes up to 2 weeks before all chlorophyll—the stuff that gives the "green" taste—has dissipated from foliage. Big, fat, dense flower buds can take 3 to 4 days longer to dry than smaller buds. Gently squeeze buds after they have been drying for a few days to check for moisture content. Bend stems to see if they are dry. If the stem breaks rather than folds, it is ready to cure.

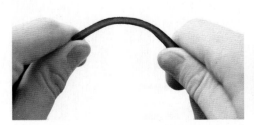

The harvest is not dry if the stem does not snap when bent.

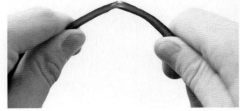

The harvest is dry or nearly dry if stems break when bent.

Check for dryness by bending a stem. The stem should snap rather than fold when bent. The bud should be dry to the touch but not brittle. The bud should burn well enough to smoke when dry.

Light—especially ultraviolet (UV) rays from natural sunlight—heat, and friction hasten biodegradation of resin glands and cannabinoids. Do not place dried cannabis in hot automobile glove compartments, and keep it away from heat vents and so forth. Friction and rough handling can bruise and rupture resin glands. Even with proper drying and curing, brutal handling of harvested cannabis will diminish cannabinoid content.

Fast Drying
Here are 6 ways to dry flower buds quickly. Remember, buds that dry quickly burn hot, are harsh to the pallet, and may taste "green" when vaporized.

One: Manicure fresh buds and remove all branches and leaves containing no visible resin. Spread evenly on tin foil or wrap in paper or enclose in an envelope.

Place the paper or envelope on a warm refrigerator, radiator, television, etc. Depending upon heat level, buds will be dry in a few hours or the next day. Buds will be a bit crispy when dry but may contain moisture deeper within. Place them in an airtight container until they sweat. Put back in the paper and dry until dehydrated enough to burn well.

Two: Cut up fresh buds and/or foliage. Place on a 12-inch (30.5 cm) square of tinfoil. Hold or place it over a 60- to 100-watt incandescent lightbulb. Stir every 15 to 30 seconds. It will be dry enough to consume in a few minutes.

Three: Place diced buds and/or foliage on a cookie sheet in an oven at 150°F (65.6°C) for 10 to 15 minutes. Check regularly and stir if needed until dry. Do not increase temperature above 200°F (93.3°C) or the cannabinoids will vaporize into the air.

Four: Place chopped buds and/or foliage on a paper plate in a microwave oven. Turn the microwave on in short, weak (50%

power) bursts of 15 to 30 seconds each. Re-cycle until dry, and stir if necessary.

Five: Dry buds in a food dehydrator for 24 to 48 hours. Food dehydrators have a series of stackable screens. Place bud and leaf on screens and stack. A fan blows temperature-controlled air gently upward to quickly dry the cannabis.

Buds and/or foliage can be cut into small pieces and place in a glass jar with an airtight lid. Place several silica gel desiccant packs (the kind that come with electronic devices and cameras) into the glass jar and seal. Moisture will migrate to the silica gel in a few hours. Remove the packets and dry using a dry heat source. Replace silica packs until cannabis is dry enough to consume. Find silica gel pack at auto parts or electronics stores.

Six: Dry buds in a food dehydrator for 24 to 48 hours. Food dehydrators include a series of stackable screens. Place bud and leaf on screens and stack. A fan blows temperature-controlled air gently upward to quickly dry the cannabis.

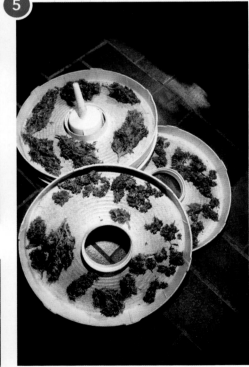

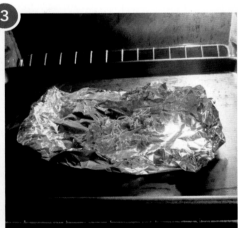

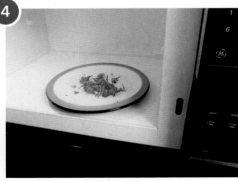

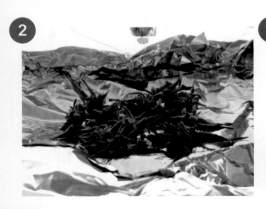

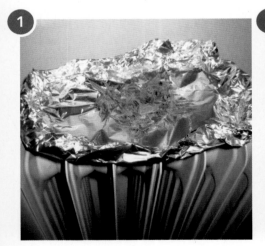

A food dryer is a good way to dry flower buds quickly. Turn its fan and heat to the lowest setting so that buds do not dry too fast and thus retain impurities.

Water "Drying": Step-by-Step

Water can be used to remove excessive chlorophyll, salts, and impurities in harvested cannabis. Cannabis that is imported from Paraguay, parts of Africa, and Mexico is often soaked in a water bath to wash out dirt, chlorophyll, and other bad stuff, but this method of curing is seldom used by home gardeners. Branches are soaked in water that is replaced daily for several days. The undesirable soluble plant matter leaches into the water and after four to seven days is almost gone. After water curing, manicured buds on branches are lightly shaken to remove water before being hung to dry.

Once completely and evenly dry, buds smoke smooth and burn evenly. Water-dried buds are about 30 percent smaller, but cannabinoids are intact and more concentrated than with air-dried buds. Lackluster color, fragrance, and overall appearance of water-cured cannabis result in low "bag appeal," a term popular at medical cannabis dispensaries. However, using this method, salts are removed even if plants were fertilized until harvest.

Note: Be very gentle when handling buds in water. Resin is not water soluble, but when branches are knocked around indiscriminately, resin glands can fall into the water. Be gentle with tender buds.

Step One: Cut branches from plants and remove large leaves including stems (petioles). Small leaves are usually left intact around buds.

Step Two: Carefully place bud-filled branches in a container of distilled or RO (reverse osmosis) water. Keep the temperature between 60°F and 70°F (15.6°C–21.1°C). It may be necessary to gently push the branches down by hand or with a weight to keep them completely submerged.

Step Three: Pour off the chlorophyll/salt–contaminated water and replace daily. Chlorophyll, salts, and contaminants are drawn out of the plant via osmosis (see chapter 20, *Water*). The water must be changed daily and replaced with fresh; old water is full of the bad stuff.

Step Four: After 4 to 7 days, remove branches from water, carefully shake off excess water, and hang to dry. Use a circulation fan to ensure that all latent water evaporates and dries from buds. Manicure small leaves while they are still soft and supple.

Step Five: Hang bud-filled manicured branches to dry (see "Drying Small Harvests" earlier in this chapter).

Dry Ice "Drying": Step-by-Step

Dry ice drying retains cannabinoids and freshness and causes very little degradation of resin glands from heat, light, and air. When vaporized or smoked, dry ice–cured cannabis has a mint-like taste because the chlorophyll does not break down. This curing method is expensive and time-consuming.

Dry ice is frozen carbon dioxide. When it warms, CO_2 converts from a frozen solid to a gas, without turning into a liquid. When moist cannabis is enclosed with dry ice, low relative humidity occurs and water molecules migrate from the cannabis to the dry ice. This causes the relative humidity of the CO_2 to increase and the moisture content of the cannabis to decrease. This process occurs below 32°F (0°C), and it preserves cannabis. Dry ice is expensive and this method is best used for drying small amounts of flower buds.

Step One: Place one ounce (28.3 gm) each of dry ice and flower buds about three-fourths dry into a 4-quart (3.8 L) container. Put dry ice on the bottom and flower buds on top.

Step Two: Make a few small 0.25-inch (6.4 mm) holes in the lid of the container for excess gas to exit. Seal the lid on the container.

Step Three: Defrost freezer. Turn freezer to coldest setting. Place the entire container in the freezer. Check every 12 to 24 hours.

Step Four: When the dry ice is gone, the buds should be completely dry. If not dry, add dry ice until cannabis is dry. Conserve dry ice by partially drying buds for a few days before enclosing with dry ice.

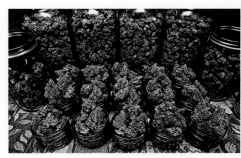

Canning jars are excellent containers to store these dry 'Black Shaman' flower buds. The rigid glass protects buds from damage. Always store jars in a cool, dark location to avoid heat and sunlight.

Curing

Curing after drying helps remove any remaining chlorophyll, other pigments, latent fertilizer salts, and so on that have accumulated in flower buds, leaves, and stems. If dried too quickly, flower buds retain more chlorophyll and have a "green" taste. When vaporized or smoked these imports are harsh on the pallet and often burn too hot. Removing chlorophyll, salts, etc., can be achieved with air, water and air, and with dry ice (CO_2).

Curing is not essential; in fact, many medical patients prefer the often minty flavor of uncured cannabis.

Even after plants, branches, or buds have dried on screens or been suspended in a drying room for five to seven days and appear to be dry, they still contain moisture inside. This moisture affects taste, fragrance, and cannabinoid content (potency). Curing will remove this excess moisture and all it contains. Curing makes buds uniformly dry and pleasant to consume, and preserves natural cannabinoids and terpenes.

Light, air, and water are all that aerobic bacteria need to start consuming chlorophyll, salts, and so forth. When the bacteria consume all the available food and oxygen dissipates, bacteria die. This action frees up carbohydrates, chlorophyll, and other contaminants. Properly dried and cured cannabis flower buds burn evenly and have a smooth, rich taste. The vibrant green color fades when chlorophyll dissipates and reddish hues become more prominent.

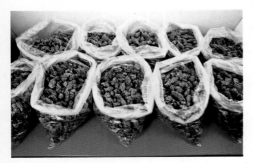

Dry cannabis flower buds are packed into turkey bags to cure.

The first week of curing affects potency in that it evenly removes moisture within the foliage so that few impurities — pigments, salts and contaminants that affect taste and fragrance — remain in the dry foliage and flowers. Curing also allows cannabis to dry so that mold does not grow when it is stored. Well-cured flower buds are soft and pliable but dry inside. Flower buds should feel like they are dry and only the dry pliable foliage is holding resin onto stems. When smoked it should have an even glow and enter the body smoothly. When vaporized, there should be no apparent "green" taste.

Air Curing: Step-by-Step

Step One: Remove flower buds from branches and place in an airtight container. Some plastic bags may impart a plastic or metallic odor. Clear and opaque turkey bags used for long-term storage are airtight. I prefer Black Magic Odor Barrier Bags because they are black, durable, and airtight. There are also bags that reflect heat and are airtight (when properly sealed) and infrared-proof, which protects them from heat.

Step Two: Write today's date on each curing container.

Step Three: Gently pack as many buds into container as possible without forcing or damaging them. Place containers in a cool, dry, dark place.

Step Four: Once enclosed in an airtight container, moisture inside buds migrates to dry portions of stems and foliage. Check in 2 to 4 hours to see if buds feel different. Gently squeeze a couple of buds to see if they feel moister now. Be careful! Resin glands bruise easily.

Step Five: Open the drying container 2 to 3 times daily for the first 7 days to release moisture. Take a whiff the instant you open the container. The fragrance should be sweet and somewhat moist. Close the container quickly. If necessary, remove buds from jar for a short time to inspect for mold and disease.

Step Six: After the first week, open containers once or twice a week for a quick whiff. Do not open too many times or the slow curing process will not work.

Step Seven: Some gardeners cure flower buds slowly for 6 months or longer. However, after 2 to 3 weeks they should be fully cured and remain fresh, firm, and pliable. Flower buds can be sealed in containers and stored.

Once cured, keep medicinal cannabis flower buds in an airtight container. Open the container periodically to let out moisture that may have condensed. Or you can keep the container sealed and store in a cool, dry, dark place. Buds should store well for 2 years or longer. However, most are consumed earlier!

Packaging and Storage

Packaging dry cannabis in an airtight or similar environment will help preserve aroma, taste, and potency. Excessive exposure to oxygen causes the cannabinoid profile and the medicinal effect to change. Dry cannabis oxidizes when exposed to the oxygen in air. Oxidation breaks down THC molecules, converting them to cannabinol (CBN).

Plastic bags are commonly used to package and store cannabis. Such containers preserve cannabis best when the bags are handled very little. Handling bruises and degrades resin glands. A rigid container (I prefer dark glass) will help protect resin glands from extra movement and abrasion.

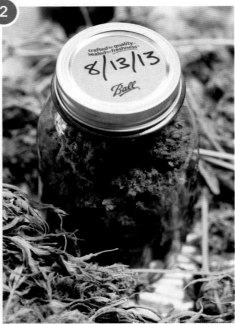

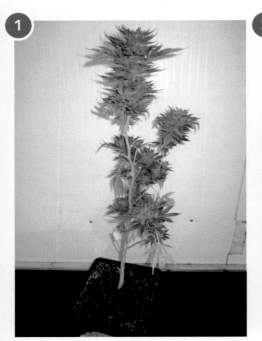

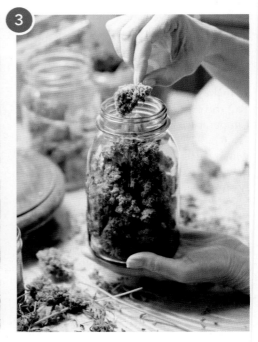

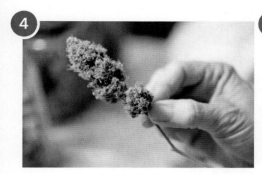

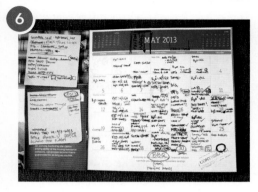

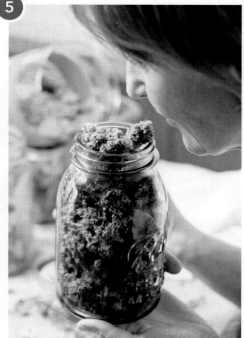

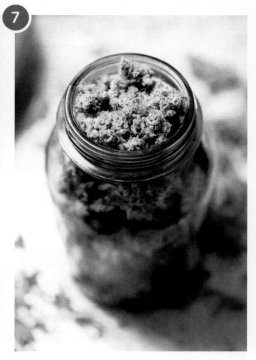

Store dry, cured medicinal cannabis in a cool, dark, dry place to preserve aroma, taste, and cannabinoid content. Cannabis quality is best preserved under these conditions. Patients store the bulk of their medicinal cannabis in a cool, dark, dry location and keep only a few days supply close at hand. The cannabis does not have time to degrade and remains potent.

Silicon packets, newspaper, or paper towels placed in the drying container will absorb excess moisture. Make sure to remove the silicon packets, paper, and so forth regularly to dry them out before returning them to the container.

Packaging cannabis for long-term storage (6 to 48 months) requires a little more effort to ensure the qualities of cannabis are retained. Cannabis can be stored for more than 2 years, but this is seldom the case. If cannabis must be stored for more than 2 years, be sure to make the preparations listed below.

Refrigeration and freezing are also means of preserving cured and dry cannabis. Although refrigeration slows decomposition, household and commercial refrigerators and freezers have high humidity levels. High humidity can cause condensation inside the sealed containers. Many refrigerators have a "low humidity" drawer, but the humidity is still quite high. Expensive "low humidity" refrigerators are available for health care and other industries. These are the refrigerators many seed purveyors use. The storage container must be well sealed to slow condensation inside. Place silicon packets in the container to absorb condensed moisture. Check stored cannabis periodically for deterioration.

Other ways to store cannabis include concentration into hashish, oil, or alcohol.

Vacuum Sealing

Vacuum seal cannabis for long-term storage. Vacuum packaging removes oxygen from the airtight storage container, which slows biodegrading of cannabis flowers to a crawl. The absence of oxygen in airtight bag makes an impossible environment for pests and diseases. Inexpensive vacuum packagers use a jar with a twist off lid. A small air suction pump is attached to a tube with a one-way valve in the top. The air is sucked out of the jar to form a vacuum seal. There are simple manual vacuums for small amounts of cannabis.

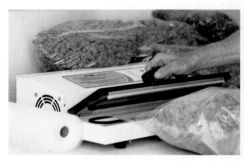

A vacuum sealer will help keep harvested cannabis from biodegrading quickly.

Food Saver and Seal-A-Meal vacuum sealer machines are very popular in North America. These vacuum sealers remove air from the plastic bag full of cured cannabis, which reduces oxidation to nil. Once the air is removed from the bag, the machine forms a hermetic seal that keeps the cannabinoid profile and flavor intact. More sophisticated vacuum packaging machines use special impermeable plastic bags. The more expensive models are able to inject CO_2 and nitrogen,* gas into the bag. Models of these sealers range in price from $50 to $2,000 USD. Inexpensive vacuum sealers are also available in the canning section of many grocery and variety stores in late summer and early autumn. Containers sealed with inexpensive vacuum sealers can lose the vacuum after

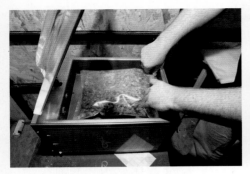

An industrial vacuum sealer removes the air inside a strong plastic bag and melts closed the open end of the bag to hermetically seal in freshness.

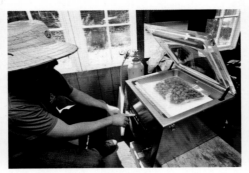

A sophisticated vacuum sealer is able to inject inert nitrogen gas into sealed bags.

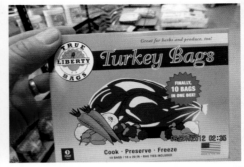

Turkey bags are the favorite storage container for many medical cannabis gardeners. True Liberty Bags makes opaque black bags to exclude light.

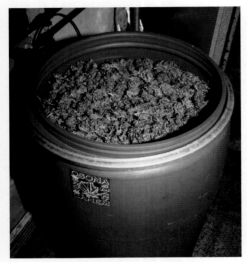

Cannabis flower buds must be perfectly dry to store in 30-gallon (113.6 L) containers. Excess moisture in such a large amount tends to attract mold and rot.

a few days. Properly vacuum-packed, medicinal cannabis flower buds will stay as fresh as the day they were sealed in the airtight container. Visit the site of my good friends at Trim Scene Solutions in Northern California (www.trimscene. com). They are experts on the subject.

*Carbon dioxide (CO_2) gas in a concentration of 35 percent, or nitrogen (N_2) gas concentrated at 98 percent will displace oxygen inside the sealed bag. In the absence of oxygen, degradation of cannabis essentially stops. Pests and diseases cannot survive without oxygen. The inert gases (CO_2 and N_2) do not alter the cannabinoid profile.

What to Do with a Moldy Crop

Moldy flower buds, whether infected with bud rot (*Botrytis cinerea*) or powdery mildew (or oidium, a catchall term for a fungal disease caused by a powdery mildew), and depending upon severity, will have a lower overall harvest weight. If mold has entered the plant's system, it will remain there after harvest. Medical patients or anybody with respiratory ailments should not vaporize or smoke moldy cannabis. For more information, see chapter 24, *Diseases & Pests*.

Medical patients or anybody with respiratory ailments should not vaporize or smoke moldy cannabis.

Stop molds and mildews before they start and spread through the entire crop. Inspect plants at night with a UVC flashlight to spot newly forming fungus. Spray with a hydrogen peroxide (H_2O_2) solution to kill fungus. If the infection is bad, spray the entire plant with hydrogen peroxide solution before harvesting. Harvest plants carefully so that any remaining spores from the fungal disease do not contaminate other plants in the garden. Pour one cup (8 oz [236.6 ml]) of 3 percent H_2O_2 into 5 gallons (19 L) of water.

Bathe harvested branches full of buds for 1 to 5 minutes in the diluted H_2O_2, then shake dry and hang in a well-aerated room until excess surface water is gone. Manicure buds while plants are fresh and supple. See "Powdery Mildew" in chapter 24, *Diseases & Pests*, for complete information on control.

Too often gardeners harvest their moldy crops and trim off mold-affected foliage. This practice spreads mold spores and does not control the disease. Drying the crop will result in lingering mold living in and on harvested flower buds, branches, and leaves. Making water- or dry-sieve hashish will not kill the disease either. Once the diseases have entered the system of the harvested foliage, they will stay even if washed off the surface of the plant.

Two ways to clean include soaking in hydrogen peroxide and passing under a UVC lamp.

Soak freshly harvested cannabis in a container filled with diluted H_2O_2 (see recipe earlier in this section). Mildews and surface molds will float to the top and can be skimmed off. Rinse bud-filled branches with a spray of fresh water, shake lightly to remove water, and then manicure and dry.

Pass harvested foliage under ultraviolet (UVC) light to kill surface molds and bacteria. About a second or two is all the UVC light a plant can withstand. Check with manufacturers for application times.

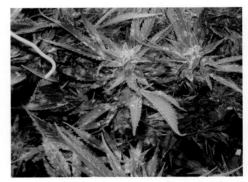

A moldy crop is a big problem. Always keep a close eye on the garden, and inspect for early signs of mold so that it does not spread.

10 GARDEN ROOMS

GARDEN ROOMS REQUIRE a secure space, consistent environment, and a regular maintenance schedule. They also increase your carbon footprint. Climate, consistency, and security are the best reasons to garden indoors. Medical cannabis can also be started in a garden room and moved into a greenhouse or outdoors. Plants get an early start with minimal environmental impact when moved outdoors.

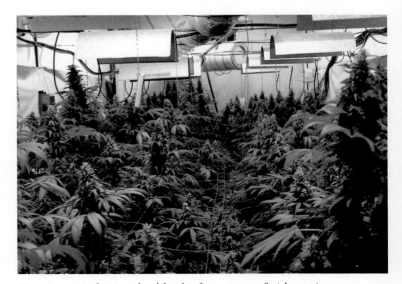

Growing an indoor garden like this from start to finish requires an investment of time, money, planning, and hard work.

To set up a garden room, you must first assess needs and desires. How much medical cannabis do you want to grow? How much time, space, and money are you able to invest to achieve this goal? Do you want to build the garden room, or do you prefer to purchase a prefabricated "grow closet?" Building a garden room takes time, skill, and a budget. The room will also need adequate electrical power, an air ventilation outlet, and a source of clean water.

Your personality traits and habits are also important to consider. Do you have a regular schedule? Do you have enough time to dedicate to this project? Do you start projects and tend to not finish them? Are you away from home several days at a time? All of these factors figure into your ability to maintain an indoor medical cannabis garden.

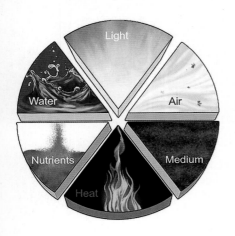

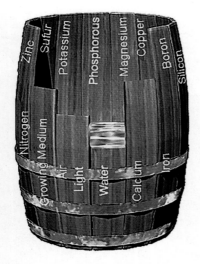

This barrel full of water illustrates that cannabis will grow only as fast as its most limiting factor. Light, air, and imbalanced soil are most often the factors that limit growth indoors.

You will have to make your own clones if a source of clones is not readily available. You will have to divide the room in two to form a clone/mother room and a flowering room. The harvest can be periodic or perpetual.

Once divided, the rooms need filters and vent fans, circulation fans, hygrometers/thermometers, and sources of water and electricity.

The size of the garden space dictates the type, wattage, and number of lamps. The most efficient lights with the highest lumens-per-watt conversion include CFLs (compact fluorescent lamps) and HIDs (high-intensity discharge lamps). CFLs are available in various lengths and wattages. See chapter 17, *Light, Lamps & Electricity*, for more information on each type of lamp.

The goal of the garden room is to supply everything that medical cannabis needs to grow well.

Air 20%
temperature
humidity
CO_2 and O_2 content

Light 20%
spectrum (color)
intensity
photoperiod (hours of light per day)

Water 20%
temperature
pH (a measure of acidity or alkalinity)
EC (electrical conductivity)
O_2 content

Nutrients 20%
composition
purity

Growing Medium 20%
air content
moisture content

Carbon Footprint
According to a study by Evan Mills, PhD*, indoor cannabis gardeners use 1 percent of all electricity in the USA,

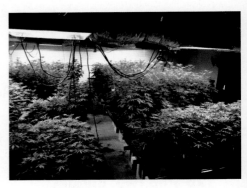

Even efficient indoor rooms like this one create a carbon footprint. Fortunately, these plants will be moved outdoors in the coming weeks.

shelling out $5 billion dollars to electric utility companies every year. This is the equivalent use of 2 million average households. Approximately 22 billion kilowatt hours are consumed. California, one of 16 states to allow cultivation of medical cannabis, is estimated to consume 3 percent of all electricity in the state. Gasoline and diesel electric generators use about 140 gallons (530 L) of fuel to produce 1 plant.

*Read the summary and full report, *Energy up in Smoke: the Carbon Footprint of Indoor Cannabis Production*, at http://evan-mills.com/energy-associates/Indoor.html.

Gardeners cultivate medical cannabis indoors to produce high-quality crops and keep their high-value produce from thieves. Keeping cannabis illegal increases the carbon footprint of gardeners. Criminalizing cannabis contributes to long driving distances, odor and noise suppression, and off-grid fossil fuel power production.

Reduce your carbon footprint by reducing your use of electricity, gas, and diesel fuel. Promote renewable energy generation. Use indoor grow-room heating, cooling, and lighting systems more efficiently. Install photovoltaic (PV) solar panels.

More efficient growing practices reduce carbon footprints, as does using lower-wattage lamps and fewer electrical and fossil fuel–using devices. Employing all the natural principles possible will help lower carbon footprints. Human caloric energy is much less expensive than fossil fuel energy, and we can make more human energy quickly, but fossil fuel energy takes a very long time to recreate. Growing medical cannabis outdoors eliminates most costs other than for a few tools, transport, water, soil amendments, and fertilizer.

Mix your own fertilizers from simple, readily available elements. When you purchase local ingredients and mix your own organic fertilizers, you are supporting local industry and farmers. You are also lowering your overall carbon footprint by decreasing transport, packaging, and sales costs.

Use online tools to qualify your carbon footprint. Enter information on electricity, gas and diesel fuel usage, vehicle fuel consumption, and renewable energy generation to measure your total carbon footprint. Take a couple of minutes to fill out the Nature Conservancy's carbon footprint calculator (www.nature.org/greenliving/carboncalculator/index.htm) to get an idea of the environmental waste you produce.

Closed (Sealed) Rooms

Closed or sealed garden rooms have most all of the qualities found in a phytotron, a scientific growth chamber, and they create a very big carbon footprint. Just like a phytotron, precise control of each factor—light, temperature, humidity, CO_2, and so forth—can be individually controlled in a closed room. The room is sealed completely so all air that enters and exits is controlled. Targeted specifically at the high-tech gardener, sealed rooms are for gardeners with advanced skills.

The room must be sealed completely so that no air enters or exits. Caulk all corners and put weatherstripping around doors. Some gardeners install a vent fan to create a very small amount of negative pressure. An air conditioner is essential to supply fresh filtered air.

A sophisticated air filter can be installed to scrub ethylene, nitrous oxides, and other contaminants such as fungi from the air in the room and precisely control fresh air exchange.

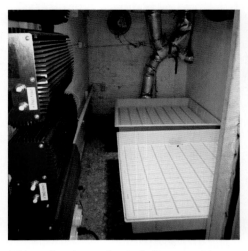

This enclosed room has its ballasts outside so the entire room can be sealed off. In fact, a fire started in this room several months before this photograph was taken. Since the room was tightly sealed, limited oxygen was available and the fire went out. After the fire, the gardener moved the source of the fire—ballasts—out of the room. Do not count on fires putting themselves out in sealed rooms, however. This gardener got lucky!

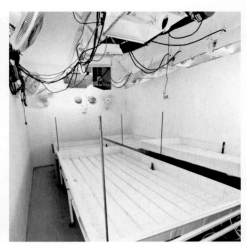

This sealed room is set up and ready for the gardener to bring in clones and start growing. The entire room is spotless and free of pathogens.

RECOMMENDED BTU REQUIREMENTS FOR A/C IN SEALED ROOMS

	Cumulative Watts		A/C Btus Moderate Temp.		A/C Btus Low Temp.	
1	1,000	600	4,000	2,400	3,300	2,000
2	2,000	1,200	8,000	4,800	6,600	4,000
3	3,000	1,800	12,000	7,200	9,900	6,000
4	4,000	2,400	16,000	9,600	13,200	8,000
5	5,000	3,000	20,000	12,000	16,500	10,000
10	10,000	6,000	40,000	24,000	33,000	20,000

A 20-pound CO_2 tank lasts two weeks in a sealed room with ten 1000-watt lamps. The room must be equipped with a big air conditioner to adequately dehumidify and cool the air. The grower must figure out how many watts the air conditioner uses, and how much it will cool the room.

Fuel Type	Btus per Unit of Fuel
shelled corn	6,300 Btus per pound
propane	91,500 Btus per gallon
natural gas	100,000 Btus per therm
kerosene	127,000 Btus per gallon
electricity	3,413 Btus per kilowatt hour

GrowBots (www.growbot.com) are able to perform robotic control, including remote iPhone video monitoring. A fully equipped 12-light grow room costs $80,000 USD and has a big carbon footprint. The initial out-of-pocket cost is more than $6,500 per installed 1000-watt lamp. It will take two perfect and heavy harvests to cover the initial cost—not including genetics, growing supplies, and electricity. Turnkey convenience is expensive in both money and carbon footprint. A small single-light homemade semi-sealed garden room costs about $1,000 USD to set up and performs nearly the same level of control.

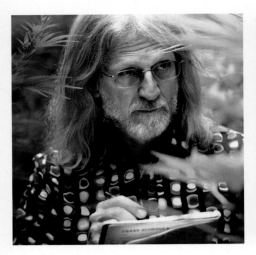
Plan the garden room on paper first.

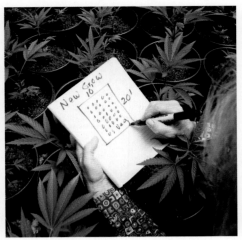
Make a rough sketch of the garden room showing lights, plants, fans, etc.

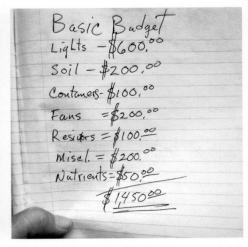
First make a rough budget to get an idea of future expenses. Next make a detailed budget that fits your needs.

Setting Up the Garden Room: Step-by-Step

Set up the garden room and make sure each step is completed before introducing plants. Construction requires space, a financial budget, and planning. A garden room under construction is a terrible environment for plants. Once the garden room is set up and totally operational, you will be ready to move in plants and start growing.

Step One: Define Needs and Desires

Needs and desires are at the basis of a garden room. The first decision is whether or not to purchase a prefabricated garden room. Start shopping by typing "garden closet," "garden tent," or "garden box" into an Internet search engine. Garden closets with flexible plastic walls are the most economical. Fixed-wall (rigid) models are more expensive. If this is your first indoor garden, consider starting with a simple soil garden rather than more expensive and often complex hydroponics.

Take an inventory of the prerequisites to cultivating a medical cannabis garden.

Needs and desires:

1. Legal medical gardener card
2. Time to dedicate to a small, medium, or large garden
3. Financial budget
4. Desired harvest
5. Available space indoors, in a greenhouse, or outdoors

How much cannabis is necessary to fulfill your patient's medical needs? Will you need 1 ounce or 6 pounds (28 gm or 2.7 kg) every month to satisfy patient needs? A properly managed room with a perpetual crop using one 600-watt flowering lamp and two 65-watt compact fluorescent lamps in a garden space of 4 × 4 × 8 feet (1.2 × 1.2 × 2.4 m) will produce from 0.25 to 0.5 pounds (113–227 gm) every month when using clones purchased at a medical dispensary. Buy clones at medical cannabis dispensaries for about $15 USD each. When properly managed, growing 16 clones to harvest 4 to 6 times every year under a 600-watt HID will yield 4 to 6 pounds (1.6–2.7 kg) of dried flower tops and about the same in leaf annually.

Setting up a small indoor garden usually takes a full weekend. Plan to dedicate about 2 hours per week to maintaining a small garden. Budget 1 hour per HID lamp per week when maintaining larger gardens. Maintenance time will fluctuate from planting to harvest. Maintenance consists of fertilizing and watering by hand or automatically, staking plants, measuring growth, cleaning up, and making sure all systems are functioning well and all plants are healthy.

Flowering Time: 60 to 70 days

Watts	Yield gm	Yield oz
200	100–200	3.5–7.0
400	200–400	7.0–14
600	300–600	10.5–21
800	400–800	14–28
1000	500–1,000	16–32

Step Two: Budget

Budget about $1,000 USD to construct a do-it-yourself indoor medical cannabis garden room. Budget $1,500+ if you purchase a prefabricated "garden closet." This is an approximate budget for a 600-watt HP sodium lamp and two 65-watt CFLs and the necessary construction and growing supplies. If you are on a super tight budget, you can purchase secondhand equipment by applying ingenuity and finding deals. Of course costs will vary depending upon prices in your area and the components you need to purchase.

Step Three: Tools

There are some tools an indoor gardener must have and a few extra tools that make indoor horticulture much more precise and cost effective. The extra tools help make the garden so efficient that they pay for themselves in a few weeks. Procure all tools before bringing plants into the room.

If the tools are on hand when needed, chances are they will be put to use.

EXPENSES FOR CONSTRUCTING A GARDEN CLOSET*

Equipment, Supplies, and Tools	Average	Economical	Used
grow lights	$300	$200	$50
ventilation fan	$100	$50	$50
circulation fan	$40	$30	$20
charcoal filter	$200	$200	$50
thermometer/ hygrometer	$30	$30	$30
white walls	$30	$20	$0
containers	$30	$0	$0
soil or soilless mix	$30	$20	$20
tools	$100	$50	$0
fertilizer	$30	$30	$30
construction supplies	$110	$50	$10
Total (in USD)	$1,000	$680	$260

*Both financial and environmental costs increase as the level of sophistication increases. For example, if electricity costs $0.15 per kWh (1000 watts for 1 hour), then 30 days × 12 hours = 360 hours × $0.15 = $54 per month for electricity.

Electricity for 2 months of flowering would cost $108.

A hygrometer is a good example. If plants show signs of slow, sickly growth due to high humidity, most gardeners will not identify the exact cause right away. They will wait and guess, wait and guess, and maybe figure it out before a fungus attacks and the plant dies. When a hygrometer is installed before plants are brought into the garden room, the horticulturist will know from the start when the humidity is too high and is causing sickly growth.

Tools

Here are a few tools you will need to set up your garden room.
I like to use both hand tools for small jobs and power tools when appropriate.

Tools Normally Needed

- saws—Japanese
- Two manual saws: one (flat) for cutting boards and one for cutting holes. (You can also use a power saw.)
- electric drill with a set of drill bits for wood, metal, and ceramic
- claw hammer
- manual screwdriver or battery-powered screwdriver
- hygrometer
- light meter
- moisture meter
- pH tester
- pliers
- pruners or scissors
- putty knife
- tape measure
- thermometer
- 400-watt lamp
- 15-watt timer
- 150-watt fan

Supplies Normally Needed

- pencil and notebook
- spray bottle
- biodegradable liquid dish soap
- indelible marking pens to mark distances and identify plants
- measuring cup and spoons
- butterfly screws
- butterfly bolts
- ceramic and wood screws
- screws and nuts for Mecalux
- Sheetrock screws
- cable ties
- wire ties
- duct tape
- Velcro to seal doors and section off rooms
- Visqueen plastic for walls
- Teflon tape to seal treads and prevent moisture leaks
- caulk
- plywood for ceiling
- several hooks to hang lamps, cords, timers, etc.
- 560 total watts of electricity
- yardstick (metrico) to measure plant growth!

Step Four: Site Selection

The location of the garden room is often an unused space in a home or outbuilding. The garden room will need irrigation water, air circulation and air exchange, grow lights, soil, and medical cannabis plants. Walls and ceilings may need to be insulated to facilitate regulating temperature. The flowering room space should be a minimum of 5 feet (1.5 m) high to allow space for containers, lights, and maximum plant growth.

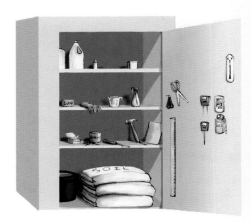

Keep tools and supplies organized in a closet.

Clone gardens using fluorescent lamps can have a low, even profile so that light is best used.

Four basic locations for a garden room include: basement, attic, ground floor, and outbuilding.

Step Five: Design the Room

Once you know how much room you need in order to grow, where you want to grow, and if you will need 1 garden room or 2, you are ready to design your garden or purchase a ready-made grow closet. I like to draw the room to scale on paper before constructing it so that I can figure out what will be needed to construct the room. In any event, constructing a garden room always takes more trips to the hardware and hydroponic stores than planned!

This prefabricated garden closet with a single growing space measures 4 × 4 feet (120 × 120 cm). The ballast for the 600-watt HPS lamp is located outside the room. The space below the growing bed serves as a storage area.

Garden Room Options
Single room for vegetative and flowering

a. Purchase clones at a dispensary, grow them for 2 to 4 weeks before flowering

b. Take clones and grow for 2 to 4 weeks after roots strike before flowering

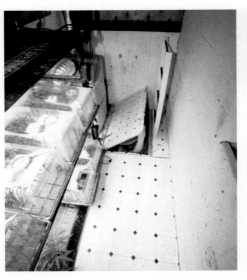

This medical cannabis gardener uses a trapdoor to access an unused part of the indoor facility. The clone room stays closed and clean.

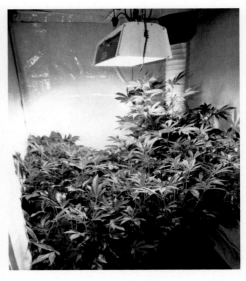

Most gardeners start out with a crop grown in a single room. After they harvest the crop, they introduce a new batch of seedlings or clones. The photoperiod is switched back to an 18/6-hour day/night photoperiod and the cycle continues.

c. Grow seedlings of autoflowering feminized plants

d. Grow seedlings, cull/separate males, flower females

e. Grow seedlings, open pollinate males and females. See chapter 25, *Breeding.*

Two rooms, one vegetative and one flowering

1. Grow clones and mother plants

    a. Grow consecutive crops of clones, harvest every 2 months

    b. Grow perpetual crops of clones, harvest 1 to 3 times weekly

2. Grow consecutive or perpetual crops of F1 hybrid feminized seedlings

3. Grow consecutive or perpetual crops of F1 hybrid regular seedlings, cull male plants

Set up 2 rooms: Productive indoor gardens consist of 2 rooms, a vegetative/mother/cloning room, about a quarter the size of a second room used for

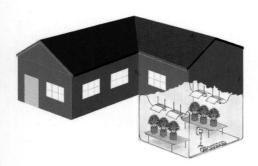

A basement is a great location for a garden room because the temperature and humidity stay relatively constant. Concrete walls backed with soil serve as insulation. Open earth or subterranean cellars with a dank moist atmosphere should be avoided. Basements are also more isolated and have less traffic.

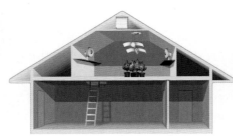

Attic garden spaces are isolated and more difficult to access. Limited access can make garden room setup and maintenance more time consuming. Heat buildup can be a problem too. If the roof is not insulated, the garden may suffer from cold in the winter and high temperatures in the summer. Unexposed roofs with attics located under trees or shade are easiest for controlling temperature and humidity. Cautious gardeners go so far as to construct a false wall and doorway or a trapdoor to enter the garden room.

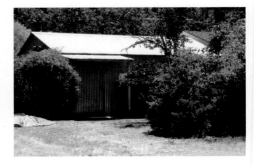

Outbuildings are less secure and should have an alarm system. Outbuildings, barns, and garages not attached to homes often lack security unless equipped with a security fence, motion-detecting floodlights, an alarm system, and possibly a guard dog. Less-secure structures are easier for thieves to break into; a garden is much easier to secure when the entry is within another building.

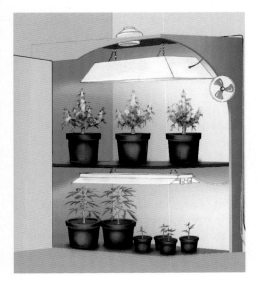

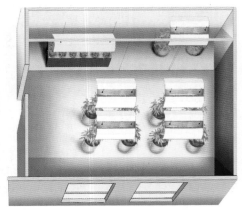

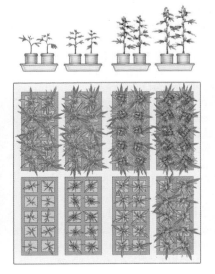

This grow closet is divided by a shelf just below the center point. The vegetative room for seedlings, clones, and mothers (shown in the photograph of the garden below) is illuminated by two 55-watt compact fluorescent bulbs. The flowering room above is illuminated by a 600-watt high pressure sodium lamp.

Clones and mothers can be grown in the same room.

In this simple sea of green layout, there are ten plants in each tray (80 total plants) illuminated by a single 1000-watt HID. Each week one tray of ten plants is harvested, and ten new plants are started.

flowering. The light is on in the vegetative room 18 to 24 hours a day, and the flowering room has a light schedule of 12 hours on and 12 hours off. Smaller vegetative plants take up less space than older flowering plants and can be huddled together. For example, a 250- or 400-watt metal halide could easily illuminate vegetative plants and clones that would fill a flowering room lit by 2 or 3 600-watt HP sodium lamps. If the metal halide in the vegetative room is turned off, fluorescent and compact fluorescent

lamps are more economical and will work well to root clones.

Consecutive harvests every 60 to 70 days: F1 hybrid seedlings or clones and mothers are grown in the vegetative room in the lower portion of the closet. Seedlings or clones advance into strong vegetative growth and are moved upstairs

to the flowering room every 60 to 70 days, after ripe buds from the previous crop are harvested. This room requires a bit more knowledge and care but is very productive. Gardeners should harvest about 7 to 14 ounces (198–396 gm) every 60 to 70 days from this garden.

Perpetual Crops: Harvesting a single flowering plant every 1 to 4 days is the most efficient way to employ artificial lighting, but it is more labor intensive. Mothers, clones, and F1 hybrid seed-

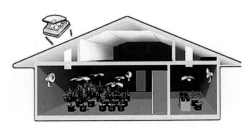

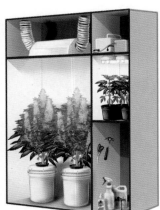

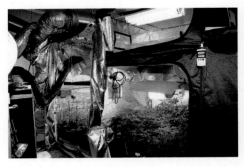

Main-floor garden rooms located in closets, cabinets, bedrooms, and spare rooms are very common. These rooms are easy to access and maintain. The atmosphere is usually easy to regulate because it is controlled along with the temperature and humidity of the home. Sometimes finding a readily accessible window or air vent is difficult.

This compact setup has 2 garden rooms: one vegetative room for growing seedlings, clones, and mothers, and a separate room for flowering. A 600-watt HPS lamp is in the flowering room and two 65-watt CFLs illuminate the vegetative room. The side-by-side orientation of the rooms allows the vegetative room to be taller and narrower and the closet a little wider. The higher profile of the flowering room allows space for a hydroponic reservoir below. It also provides space above and below for appliances and storage.

Three gardens in this photo show a continuous growth cycle. Clones are growing under fluorescent lights above a vegetative garden under CFL light below. To the left HP sodium and LED lamps illuminate the flowering garden.

lings are grown in the vegetative room. Seedlings and clones are grown into strong vegetative plants that are moved to the flowering room whenever a flowering plant is harvested. This room requires a little more organization but is about 20 percent more productive than harvesting an entire crop and replanting. Several clones are taken every day or every week. Every one to three days a plant or two is harvested. A new cutting takes the place of every plant harvested.

Step Six: Electrical Needs

A typical home has a breaker box, but older homes may have fuse boxes. Each fuse or breaker switch controls an electrical circuit in the home. In North America using 120-volt service, fuse or breaker switches are rated for 15, 20, 25, 30, or 40 amperes (amps). Breakers list the amp rating on the switch lever.

The average small 1- or 2-room garden closet will need a single 15- to 20-amp electrical circuit at 120 volts and a 10- to 15-amp circuit at 240 volts. An electrical circuit is overloaded when it is at 80

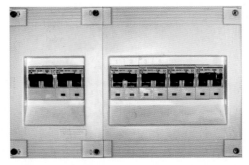

European breaker boxes control 240 volts of electricity at 50 cycles. The amp rating is printed on the end of the switch lever.

percent capacity. For example, a 120-volt 15-amp circuit is overloaded when it draws 12 amps, and a 20-amp circuit is overloaded at 16 amps.

To find out which electrical outlets are controlled by a fuse or breaker switch, remove the fuse or turn the breaker switch off. Test each and every outlet in the home to see which ones do not work. All the outlets that do not work are on the same circuit. All outlets that work are on other circuits.

When you have selected a desirable circuit, unplug everything—lights, TVs, stereos, toasters, and so forth—on that circuit. Look at the circuit's amp rating on the breaker switch. If it is rated for 20 amps, you can plug one 600-watt HID into it. A leeway of about 5 amps is there to cover any power surges and incongruence. If the circuit is rated for 20 or more amps, it may be used for a 1000-watt HID and a few other low-amp appliances. To find out how many amps are drawn by each appliance, add up the number of total watts they use, and divide by 120. If you are using 240-volt service, add the total number of watts and divide by 240.

Typical electricity consumption for small room

600-watt lamp

160-watt fluorescents

15-watt timer

200-watt fan

100-watt fan

875 total watts

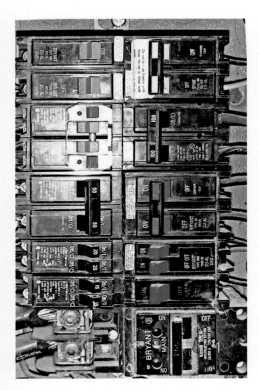

This large circuit box from a North American garden is full of breaker switches that meter 120 volts of electricity at 60 cycles to the garden room.

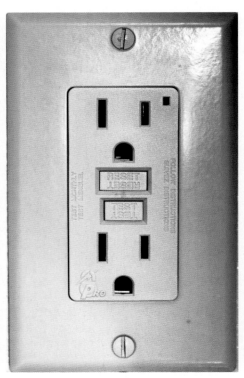

Ideally a ground fault interrupter (GFI) electrical outlet with a separate breaker switch inside will be in the garden room; if not, they are inexpensive and easy to install. A GFI outlet is essential for safety! Keep water away from outlets.

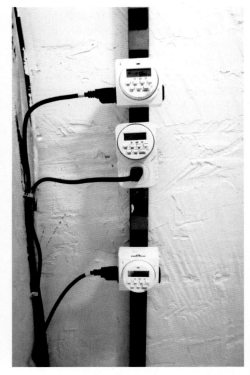

Grounded timers connected to an electrical power strip control several nutrient-solution pumps at the same time.

Volts × Amps = Watts		
Volts	Amps	Watts
120	7.3	876
120	4.7	564
120	6.5	780

Volts	Amps	Watts
240	3.65	876
240	2.35	564
240	3.25	780

Appliance Watts	Amps @120 V	Amps @240 V
100-watt lamp	0.83	0.42
250-watt lamp	2.08	1.04
400-watt lamp	3.33	1.67
600-watt lamp	5.00	2.50
1000-watt lamp	8.33	4.17
100-watt circulatory fan	0.83	0.42
150-watt vent fan	1.25	0.60
50-watt pump	0.42	0.21

IMPORTANT! Employ a certified electrician to complete any work that requires wiring or opening the fuse box!

An electrician friend recently checked the new wiring in a small medical cannabis warehouse garden. It was three-phase electric service with three hot wires. The original "uncertified electrician" had wired the garden room in a way that easily could have created fires in two places. ALWAYS employ a certified electrician when installing electrical devices!

If an extension cord must be used, make sure the wire for the extension cord is at least 16/3 (16-gauge wire with 3 strands, one of which is grounded) for 120-volt systems or it will lose voltage enroute. When using 240-volt systems, wire thickness can be smaller. Do not let the run of the electrical cord extend more than 10 feet (3 m)—the shorter the better.

Step Seven: Enclose the Garden Room

Enclose the room with white Visqueen plastic, plywood, or moisture-resistant green Sheetrock known as "sound board" in the United States. Secure plastic to walls with staples, and screw down 1 × 2-inch (2.5–5 cm) strips

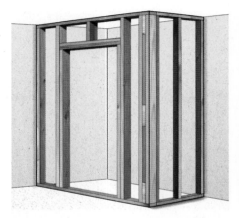

Enclose the room, if it isn't already enclosed. Remove everything that does not pertain to the garden, including furniture, drapes, rugs, and curtains that may harbor fungi and other undesirables. An enclosed room allows easy, precise control of everything and everyone that enters or exits, as well as what goes on inside.

with Sheetrock screws or duct tape. Join seams together with duct tape. Insulating the room will help contain sound and help control temperature and humidity. Cover the outside walls with Sheetrock once it is insulated. Sheetrock will further deaden the sound and make the room blend in with the rest of the rooms in the home.

Insulate windows and walls to keep room cool in summer and warm in winter. If covering a window, make it look

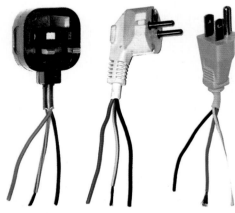

Always use 3-prong grounded plugs. If your home is not equipped with working 3-prong grounded outlets, buy a 3-prong grounded plug and outlet adapter. Ground wires are either green or brown, or brown with a green stripe. Attach the ground wire to a grounded ferrous metal object like a grounded metal pipe or heavy copper wire driven into the earth to form a ground, and screw the ground into the outlet face. NOTE: All electrical outlets and plugs require a ground wire for safety.

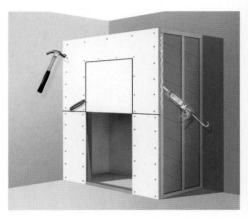

Frame in the new garden room with wood or metal studs. Cover framed garden closet with sheet rock or plastic.

aesthetically pleasing and conform to the architecture of the home. Basement windows often are insulated and painted to look like the foundation. Avoid light leaking through a crack in an uncovered window, which could annoy neighbors.

Step Eight: Divide into Two Rooms

Divide the room to make a vegetative room for seedlings, clones, and mothers on the bottom third and a flowering room on top. Install a plywood shelf to form a partition between the top and bottom of the garden closet. Or purchase a small garden closet and set it inside the larger flowering room.

Frame 1 × 2-inch (2.5 × 5 cm) boards (or Mecalux) 3 to 3.5 feet (91–107 cm) from the floor around the walls of the room. Secure 1 × 2-inch (2.5 × 5 cm) boards with screws. Cut a 3 × 4-foot (91 × 122 cm) piece of 0.75-inch (1.9 cm) plywood with a 6 × 6-inch (15 × 15 cm) piece cut from the right rear corner for the duct vent. Set the plywood on the ledge of the 1 × 2-inch (2.5 × 5 cm) boards with the vent hole toward the back wall.

Install rigid 6-inch (15 cm) ducting through the hole to connect the vegetative and flowering rooms. Use small screws to install a small inline fan in the pipe to direct air up from the vegetative room to the flowering room.

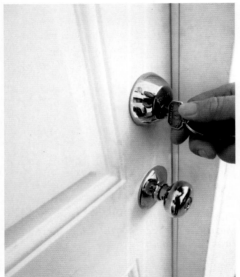

Install a door with a lock and key. Make sure to seal the perimeter of the door with plastic or carpet to prevent leaks and help control temperature, humidity, light, and sound inside the garden room. Make certain no pest-attracting light is visible from outside.

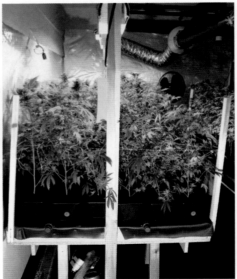

A freestanding garden is a good alternative to making holes in walls.

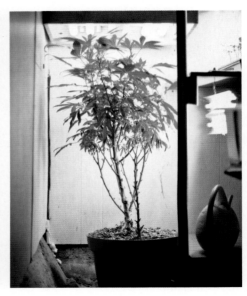

Clones root under fluorescent lamps on the right and the mother plant grows on the left.

Step Nine: Increase Light Reflectivity

Cover walls, ceiling, floor—everything—with a highly reflective material like flat white paint or Mylar. Good reflective light will increase the effective coverage of an HID lamp by more than 10 percent—all for a few dollars' worth of paint on the walls! Reflective white Visqueen plastic is another inexpensive way to "white out" a garden room, with the added benefit of protecting walls and floors from moisture.

When painting walls and ceiling white, use high-quality semigloss latex paint.

Do not use inexpensive paint; it takes longer to apply. Ask the store clerk to add a fungicide if the paint does not already contain one. For fast application, use a roller to apply paint on large flat surfaces and brush-paint corners.

Ideally, the floor should be concrete or a smooth surface that can be swept and washed down. A floor drain is also very handy. If the floor is not concrete or tile, cover with heavy plastic or impermeable painter's drop cloth to form a large tray to protect the floor from dirt and water. Fold the plastic so that at least 6 inches (15 cm) run up the wall. Attach the plastic floor covering to the walls with duct tape or staples.

Step Ten: Install a Vent Fan

Constant air circulation and a supply of fresh air are essential but often inadequate for healthy plants. A vent fan is necessary in virtually all garden rooms, and there should be at least one fresh-air vent in every garden room. Vents can be an open door, window, or duct vented to the outside. An exhaust fan vented outdoors that pulls new air through an open door usually creates an adequate exchange of air within the room. Larger rooms will need an intake fan too. If the room contains a heat or air conditioning vent, it may be opened to supply extra heat or air circulation.

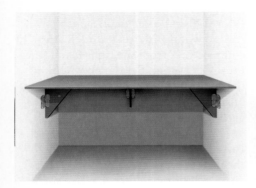

Secure shelf to upright vertical supports.

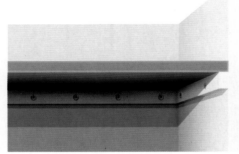

Secure partition to supporting wood around the perimeter.

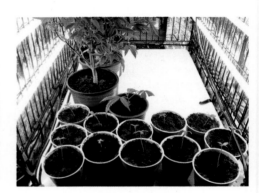

A dog carrier was modified to form a small seedling clone and mother plant room for these 'OG Kush' × 'Master Kush' feminized plants.

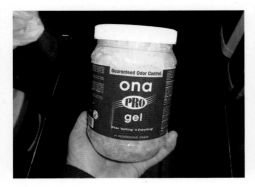

Masking agents work well for small garden rooms.

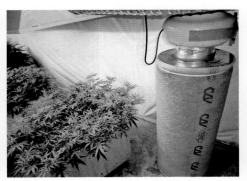

Heavy air filters can also be set on end or set on a table. The important thing is that they are able to whisk out the air and filter it through the carbon.

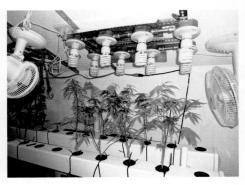

Ventilation fans can be affixed to the ceiling so that they are out of the way. A fan on the ceiling can provide ventilation to the top parts of the garden room.

One of the biggest obstacles to constructing a garden room is where and how to run the exit ducting for the ventilation fan with a minimum of work and structural change to the room. Often the vent can run out a window, chimney, or other preexisting exit. The last-choice option is to cut a hole in the ceiling or wall.

See "Setting Up the Ventilation System" in chapter 16, *Air*, for complete information on setting up a vent fan.

Step Eleven: Install an Air Filter

Most garden rooms require some sort of fragrance control to keep air fresh. A charcoal filter is often the best option.

Masking fragrance is often less expensive than purchasing a carbon filter, especially in small grow rooms. Mask lingering fragrances with a strong air freshener or a host of odor masking products. See "Fragrance" in chapter 16, *Air*, and search "air freshener reviews" on the Internet for more information.

Activated charcoal filters are the most popular and effective method to filter outgoing air. Unless made from new lightweight carbon-impregnated material, carbon filters can be quite heavy and will require stout mounting. Make sure to choose the right one for your garden area so you don't have to mount a filter that is too heavy. For example, a carbon filter rated at 200 cfm (cubic feet per minute) is more than adequate for the average closet garden room.

See www.carbonactive.ch for information on outstanding new lightweight carbon filters. The site also has a good calculator for filter and fan size in relation to room size.

Check www.canfilters.com and phatfilter.com for more on standard activated charcoal filters. Note: They are quite heavy.

For more information on air filtering and fragrance control see chapter 16, *Air*.

Step Twelve: Install Circulation Fans

Air circulation is necessary in all garden rooms, especially during flowering. Usually air circulation must be increased with circulation fans. Small clip-on oscillating fans come in very handy to circulate air in small garden rooms. They are easy to move in order to direct air where it is needed. Mount inexpensive oscillating fans to the ceiling or buy wall-mounted fans. See the fan size table in chapter 16, *Air*, to help choose the proper circulation fan(s) for your room. In general, rooms require at least one 12-inch (30.5 cm) circulation fan for every 400 watts of light. Install fans so that all leaves on plants can be seen to be slightly moving in the airflow.

When installing oscillating fans, make sure they are not set in a fixed position

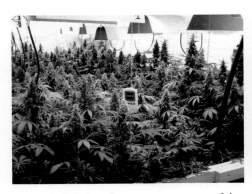

White walls help reflect up to 10 percent of the light in a room. This reflective light ensures that plants on the edges of the garden receive all possible light.

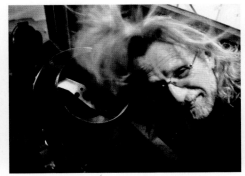

A good ventilation fan is essential!

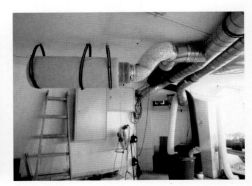

A carbon filter is essential equipment in most garden rooms in order to strip fragrances from the air before it is expelled outdoors.

and blowing too hard on tender plants, which could cause windburn and dry out the plants, especially tender seedlings and small clones. Regardless of plants' size, excessive wind will slow growth.

Step Thirteen: Install a Hygrometer/Thermometer

You can control the climate in most garden rooms with a vent fan attached to a timer or a rheostat. See sections on "Temperature" and "Humidity" in chapter 16, *Air*, for more information. Personally inspecting the meter and plants daily will help you gain experience and learn exactly how much ventilation the room needs in order to keep the temperature about 75°F (24°C) day and 65°F to 70°F (18°C–21°C) at night and the humidity below 50 percent (day/night) in the flowering room, and the vegetative room at 75°F (24°C) day and 65°F to 70°F (18°C–21°C) at night and 50 to 60 percent humidity day and night.

Environmental controllers control temperature and humidity and other garden room functions. Prices range from $80 to $1,500 USD. Quality atmospheric controllers cost a little more and are well worth the money. Check these

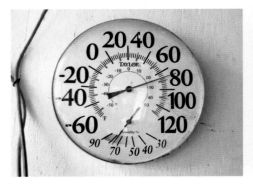

At least one thermometer is essential in every garden. Mounting 3 thermometers is a good idea, 1 near the ceiling, 1 at plant level, and 1 near the floor. This allows you to distinguish all temperature zones.

sites for more information on atmospheric controllers:

www.greenair.com

www.hydrofarm.com

www.sunlightsupply.com

Step Fourteen: Install Lights

To install a lamp in the flowering room, insert 2 hooks strong enough to support 30 pounds (13.6 kg) for each light fixture. Position the hooks in a beam or 2 × 4-inch (5 × 10 cm) board and

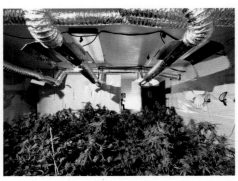

The lamps and ventilation system are suspended from recoiling hangers that are anchored to the ceiling with hooks screwed into wooden beams behind the Sheetrock. The entire system can be raised and lowered to change the distance from plants.

mount to the ceiling. Mount the HID reflective hood/bulb fixture, attaching it to the hook(s) with chain or cord. If using cord, attach the other end to a cleat mounted on the wall so that it is easy to move the fixture up and down.

Hang fixtures from an adjustable chain or cord. Attach the cord's loose end to a cleat mounted on the wall. If a ballast is attached to the fixture, its hooks should be strong enough to support 30 pounds (13.6 kg) for each lamp.

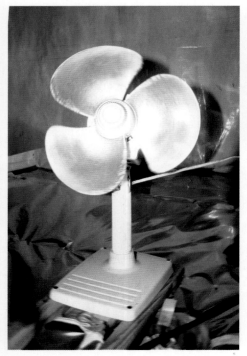

Inexpensive fans are often used in garden rooms. Removing the fan shroud lowers air friction and extends the fan's life. Be careful to not hurt yourself on a fan with no shroud.

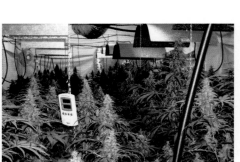

Install at least 1 maximum/minimum thermometer/hygrometer in each garden room to measure temperature and humidity. Digital models are relatively accurate and easy to use. Calibrate them against 1 or 2 other thermometer/hygrometers so they remain accurate. Place the thermometer/hygrometer equidistant between ceiling and floor, and fasten it to a wall or hang it from a string. Check the meter daily. Preferably install 3 units, 1 near the ceiling, 1 halfway up the wall, and 1 near the floor. Compare readings daily. Increase air circulation if air is stratified with different temperature readings.

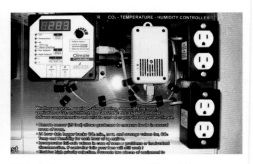

This CO₂, temperature, and humidity controller makes it easy to plug in appliances and start growing.

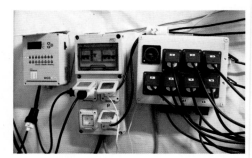

Atmospheric controllers are normally located next to timers and all the control systems for the garden room.

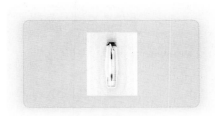

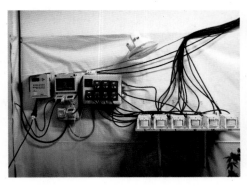

This garden room has all the electrical controls in one place, including the light timer. The lamps are on a dedicated circuit that is able to handle the load (amperage) drawn by the six lamps.

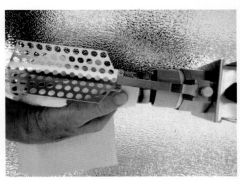

Using a paper towel, clean smudges off the bulb after screwing the bulb in place. Fingerprints attract dust that dims light. A light deflector is placed under this bulb so that the bulb and reflector can be placed closer to the canopy of the garden.

Orient the reflective hood fixture so that light shines most efficiently. Less light shines from the ends of the fixture and more from the sides, thus throwing a rectangular footprint of light below. For example, if the room is 3 × 4 feet (91.4 × 121.9 cm), orient the HID fixture so that the ends of the bulb run on the 3-foot (91.4 cm) axis and the sides along the 4-foot (121.9 cm) axis.

Setting Up the HID System: Step-by-Step

Step One: Both the lamp and ballast radiate quite a bit of heat. Take care when positioning them, so they are not so close to plants or flammable walls and ceiling that they become hazardous. If the room has limited space with a low ceiling, place a protective, nonflammable material such as sheet metal between the lamp and ceiling to protect from heat.

When hanging the lamp on the overhead chain or pulley system, make sure electrical cords are unencumbered and not too close to any heat source.

Buy and use a good electronic or analog timer to keep the photoperiod consistent. It is most effective to place the remote ballast near the ceiling to keep the room cool. Place it outside the garden room if the room is too hot.

Step Two: Insert the HID lamp plug into an electrical circuit dedicated to the garden room. A 1000-watt HID lamp will use about 9.5 amperes (amps) of electricity on a regular 120-volt house current.

Step Three: Once the proper circuit is selected, the socket and hood are mounted overhead, and the ballast is in place (but not plugged in), screw the HID bulb finger-tight into the socket. Make sure the bulb is secured in the

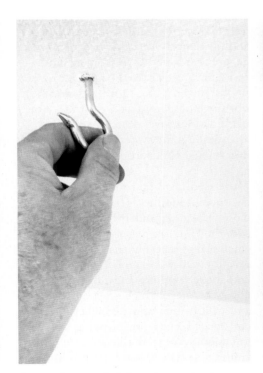

Screw a large eyebolt into the wooden beam behind the Sheetrock. Larger threads may require drilling a smaller diameter hole first.

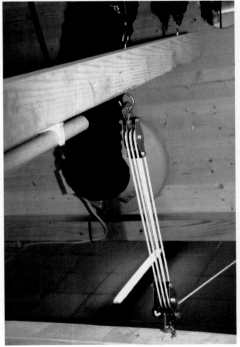

Attach the lamp to a chain or a pulley system so that it is easy to raise and lower.

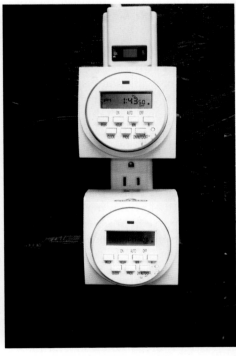

A timer is essential in every garden room. Simple inexpensive digital timers will take care of most tasks.

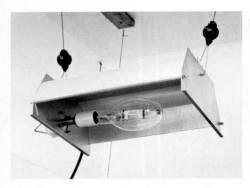

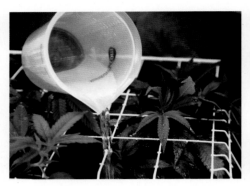

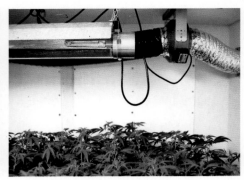

Plug the HID system into the timer and turn it on!

Small gardens are easy to water by hand using a container; for a large garden, hand-watering with a container is time consuming, tedious, and exhausting.

The lighting system is all set up and turned on. This interesting reflective hood and ventilation system support two 600-watt HP sodium bulbs.

socket, but not too tightly, and make certain there is a good, solid connection. When the bulb is secure, wipe off all smudges in order to increase brightness. Some gardeners prefer to handle HID bulbs with latex gloves to avoid leaving greasy fingerprints.

Step Four: Insert the 3-prong plug into a timer that is in the OFF position. Plug the timer into the grounded outlet, set the timer at the desired photoperiod, and turn the timer on. The ballast will hum, and the lamp will flicker as it slowly warms up, reaching full brilliance in about 5 minutes.

Step Fifteen: Water Source and Reservoir

A readily accessible source of water will reduce labor. The larger your garden becomes, the more water it will need. A 10 × 10-foot (3 × 3 m) garden could use more than 50 gallons (189.3 L) per week. Carrying water is hard, regular work. One gallon (3.8 L) of water weighs about 8 pounds (3.6 kg); 50 × 8 = 400 pounds (181.4 kg) of water a week! It is much easier to run in a hose with an on/off valve or install a hose bib in the room than to schlep water back and forth. A 3-foot (91.4 cm) watering wand attached to the hose on/off valve makes watering easier and saves cannabis branches from being broken when watering in dense foliage. Hook up the hose to a hot and cold water source so the temperature is easy to regulate.

Step Sixteen: Install a Hydroponic or Soil Garden

Move in soil-filled containers and hydroponic systems. Set up the irrigation system and make sure it is functioning properly.

Step Seventeen: Systems Check – Ready to Grow!

The room is all set up. Now is the time to test everything to make sure it operates properly before bringing in the plants. Turn on the lights, fans, and everything else. Turn it all on at the same time to make sure it will not blow

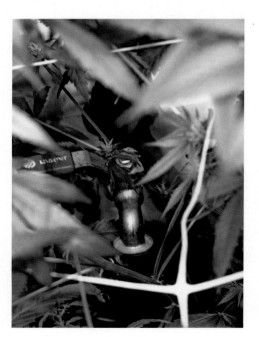

A water source in the garden room makes watering easy. But sometimes the source of water is overgrown!

a fuse or trip a breaker. Make sure the humidity and temperature are at safe levels. Set a large pan of water on the main growing beds to simulate plant transpiration. Close the doors of the garden room and let everything run for an hour or two. Open the doors and check the temperature and humidity in the room. Next turn off the fans and let the light run for 60 minutes with the doors closed. Check the temperature and humidity levels to see if the room is hotter and more humid with no ventilation, just in case the vent fan malfunctions.

Test hydroponic garden systems before adding plants. Cycle all the systems to ensure that water flows from all emitters and runs back to the nutrient tank unobstructed. Check for leaks, and clear out any blockages. Cycle the timer's on/off functions several times while you are watching the system to ensure that everything works properly.

Move seedlings and rooted clones into the room. Huddle vegetative plants closely together under the lamp. Make sure the HID lamp is not so close to small plants that it burns their leaves. Position 400-watt lamps 18 inches (45.7 cm) above seedlings and clones. Place a 600-watt lamp 24 inches (61 cm) away, and a 1000-watt lamp 30 inches (76.2 cm) away. Hang a precut string from the hood to measure the distance from lamp to plants. (Measure daily!) Move in plants and turn on the lights. The indoor medical cannabis garden is ready to grow!

11
GREENHOUSES

GROWING MEDICINAL CANNABIS in greenhouses is efficient and much less taxing on the environment and pocketbook than gardening indoors. Unheated or heated-and-cooled greenhouses extend seasons and protect plants from the elements. Containerized plants are mobile, raised beds warm early, or you can plant directly in the ground. Greenhouses can also be equipped with lights to extend vegetative growth or augment natural sunlight. Greenhouses can be blacked out to induce flowering with a 12/12 day/night schedule during the summer.

The type of structure you select depends on the size and location of your growing area, your budget, and how much time you can dedicate to your garden. Small, movable, "pop-up" greenhouses are convenient and practical. Simple cold frames and greenhouses can be assembled from common materials such as old framed windows and 2 × 4s (5.1 × 10.2 cm). Small heated-and-cooled greenhouses are a little more complex. Hoop houses are inexpensive, practical, and easy to

install. Large commercial greenhouses are best purchased from and installed by professionals. A good specialized greenhouse can be used year round in most climates. However, heating and cooling costs vary in relation to climate and seasonal weather changes.

When deciding on a garden structure, first take a look at your budget in terms of both money and time. Greenhouses

can be just as much or more work as an indoor garden. Start with a small greenhouse and learn the ins and outs of growing in your climate. Greenhouses tend to warm up quickly when the heat of the sun hits them, and cool rapidly when the sun goes down. Keeping the temperature from fluctuating too much can be difficult. It takes understanding, experience, and a little luck to master temperature management.

Growing in a greenhouse is easy once the structure is set up and covered. Plants often grow so fast that they fill the entire greenhouse!

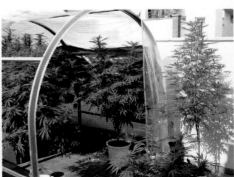

Plant in the earth or in containers when growing in a greenhouse. This gardener is experimenting with growing the same varieties in soil and in containers.

Start your greenhouse project by considering how much area you have for the footprint and how much space you will need for the desired number of plants. Think about how many plants you can grow. For example, if allowed to grow only 6 plants outdoors, they should be big plants.

Here are some great greenhouse sites to get you started:

www.vitallandscaping.com
www.become.com/greenhouses
www.charleysgreenhouse.com
www.cpjungle.com
www.doityourself.com/scat/
    basicinformation#b
www.floriangreenhouse.com
www.greenhousemegastore.com
www.hobbygreenhouse.org
www.igcusa.com
www.permies.com
www.turnergreenhouses.com

Greenhouses must have:

• full sun to partial midday shade
• proper air circulation and ventilation
• good humidity and pest control
• water-resistant electrical outlets
• a hose bib to provide water
• insulated water lines to avoid freezing, if necessary
• tables, benches, and places to hang plants (if they are not on the floor)
• a dry place to store fertilizers, potting soil, and tools

Siting the Greenhouse

Choosing a site for the greenhouse may be easy because certain factors—size of backyard, property limits, location of existing buildings and trees, and so on—may already limit location possibilities.

Greenhouses can be temporary or permanent. Permanent structures are more expensive to construct and may require a building permit.

No matter what, greenhouses should receive ample light, especially when plants are flowering. However, midday sun could create more heat and problems than simple cooling and shading are able

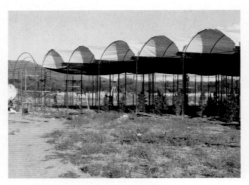

Site the greenhouse where it will receive full sun all day long. Remember, though, that the sun may need to be blocked with shade cloth to cool the greenhouse.

to control economically. In such a case, it is advisable to site the greenhouse in filtered sun or so that it is under filtered sunlight or a shadow during the hottest part of the day.

Unless square or round, site the greenhouse so that the sun passes from one end to the other rather than from one side to the other. This way plants receive the most direct light possible in relation to the path of the sun. Shadows are reduced to a minimum when the greenhouse is oriented parallel to the arc of the sun.

The site will dictate how plants are able to grow. A good site has:

• super soil
• lots of light
• good ventilation
• nutrients
• water
• flat land
• easy access—you are able to drive to it to provide the tender loving care your plants deserve

Location and exposure will depend on climate, but in general, you will want the greenhouse to receive ample sunlight yet not be exposed to strong winds. The structure should be away from any areas where falling limbs or other debris might create problems. Greenhouses in hot and tropical climates will require more shade and water. See "Sunlight and Siting the Garden" in chapter 12, *Outdoors*, which is full of pertinent information.

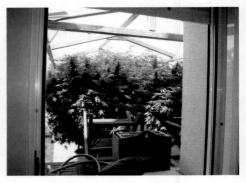

This greenhouse is located inside a large tool-shed. The walls are white, and the ceiling is clear plastic to let in sunlight. Discreet greenhouses help keep neighborhood relations pleasant.

Types of Greenhouses

The type of greenhouse you choose is governed by your climate, your budget, and your desires. The first consideration is climate. An unheated greenhouse in the mild Pacific Northwest can easily extend spring and fall growing seasons by 6 weeks each, 3 months total. Coastal California gardeners can grow all year in the same greenhouse and spend little on heating or cooling. With a little heat and proper setup, a greenhouse can produce nearly year round in Michigan and other northern climates. But be careful when planting early in the year. Plants outgrow the confines of the greenhouse and are difficult to cover before harvest if weather is rainy.

Use miniature greenhouses—cloches, plastic milk jugs, Wall O Water, and so forth—to extend the spring planting season by 2 to 6 weeks. Miniature greenhouses protect plants from cold weather and wind. They are easy to use when hardening-off cannabis transplants too. In many climates, extending the spring season could allow a gardener enough time to plant both a spring crop and a fall crop.

Cloches are individual protective coverings that keep plants warm at night. A simple cloche is a plastic milk container with its bottom cut off and its lid removed. Placed over a plant, the plastic will capture and retain heat while allowing ventilation through the open top. Make cloches out of wax paper, glass, or jars. You can also buy commercial units made of rigid, transparent plastic or

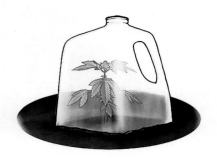

Cut the bottom from a plastic container to form a cloche. Remember to remove the lid for ventilation.

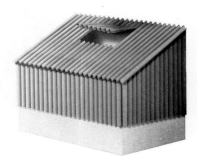

Cover greenhouses with corrugated fiberglass to exclude inquisitive passersby.

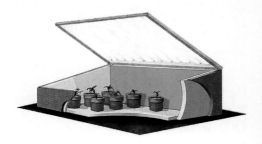

A window box greenhouse or freestanding greenhouse is a great place to start seedlings and clones. With enough light, vegetative plants do well. Most window box greenhouses are too small to accommodate large flowering plants.

heavy-duty wax paper. They are easy to use and stack well for storage.

The Wall O Water is a plant lifesaver. It is a water-filled teepee that uses the heat-emitting properties of water to shield plants from excess heat and keep them warm in the cold. It holds 3 gallons (11.4 L) of water and fits over the plant. During the day, the water absorbs the heat of the sun, moderating the temperature inside the teepee. At night, as the air temperature drops, the water releases its heat, keeping the plant comfortable. The Wall O Water does its best work in the spring when there is still a chance of freezing. As water freezes, it releases more heat into the teepee and can protect plants down to 20°F (-7°C).

Covers protect early transplants and can help produce a spring crop. The simplest option is a lightweight row cover spread over the plants and held down with stones or soil. Spun-fiber products Agronet and Reemay also have sun-

protection properties that can be used as covers in place of the sheet or blanket.

Low-profile greenhouses are perfect for crops of short plants. It is easy to set up a low-profile hoop house or greenhouse alongside a building that gets full sun. The short greenhouse or cold frame is easily darkened during full summer and lets you reap the benefits of the harvest early! (See "Light Deprivation" on page 149.)

A lean-to or attached greenhouse uses an existing structure for one or more sides. The wall of the structure provides stability and free heat if it is warmed by sunlight. Attached greenhouses are usually close to water and electricity; however, light might be lacking due to poor siting or orientation. If the wall gets too hot, it can be covered with white plastic to reflect light and cool the wall.

The freestanding greenhouse offers the most flexibility in size and location. It

can be built to take full advantage of the sun, but it does not retain heat well and can be expensive to keep warm. Numerous steps can be taken to minimize heating and cooling costs and environmental impact of maintenance. Many frame types and coverings are available in kits or raw materials. Coverings can also be easy to open for ventilation. There are also a number of good websites listed at the beginning of this chapter to help you choose the plan that works best for you.

For more information on types and prices, visit websites such as www.hoophouse.com.

Hoop houses are inexpensive, practical, and easy to build. They can be made to cover raised beds or be constructed on flat ground. They consist of a series of parallel PVC plastic or more durable steel pipes arched over two points of anchor. The arches are connected across the top with a stay to add strength to

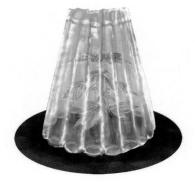

A Wall O Water will keep plants warm when temperatures approach the freezing point.

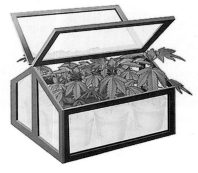

Garden stores sell many different kinds of small greenhouses.

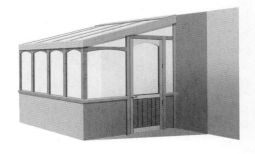

A lean-to greenhouse uses heat from the house wall to stay warm.

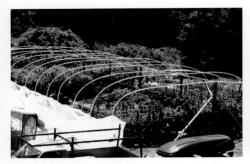

A crop of 1–2-foot-tall (30.5–61 cm) clones or seedlings planted on May 1 can be harvested in mid-July in a greenhouse that is darkened for 12 hours daily.

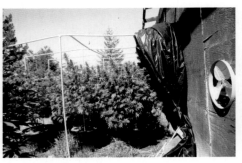

This greenhouse was built next to a sunny barn wall. The wall holds heat and protects the garden from wind.

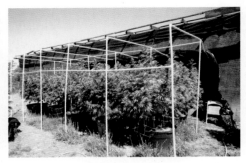

The black plastic is pulled over the PVC irrigation pipe frame of the greenhouse every afternoon to give the plants 12 hours of uninterrupted darkness to induce flowering.

the structure. A plastic skin is secured over the arches with tape or removable clamps. Ends can be closed or kept open at night for ventilation.

The outer skin can be manually removed during hot weather and replaced during cool nights. Once the plants outgrow the plastic skin it is removed. It is

replaced with a 6-inch (15.2 cm) plastic mesh that supports and trellises the plants as they grow.

Hoop greenhouses with removable plastic coverings work well when growing medium-to-large plants. The plastic is removed when weather warms and is replaced with 6-inch (15.2 cm) plastic mesh

that acts as a trellis to keep branches from breaking under the weight of buds. See chapter 11, *Greenhouses*, and chapter 13, *Case Studies*, for more information.

Hoop houses are inexpensive as well as quick and easy to set up. Plants can be moved in before or after a hoop house is set up. Once plants outgrow them,

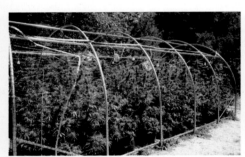

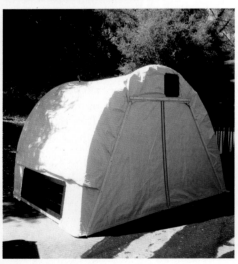

This prefabricated greenhouse comes with its own covering for blackout. The covering comes equipped with ventilation inlets and outlets.

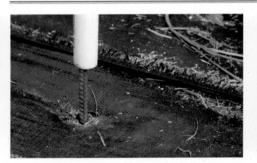

Hoop houses are easy to set up. First, weed barrier cloth is set down and secured. The greenhouse is laid out in a grid in sections measuring 10 × 8 feet (3 × 2.4 m). Two-foot-long (0.6 m) steel rebar stakes are driven through the weed barrier and halfway into the ground.

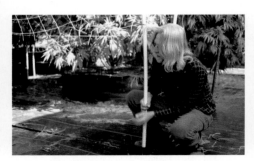

Slide a 20-foot (6.1 m) piece of schedule 40, 0.075-inch (1.9 mm) PVC irrigation pipe over 2 opposing pieces of rebar 10 feet (3 m) apart to form an arch.

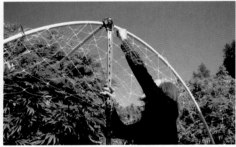

Several arches are erected and connected with individual pieces of PVC irrigation pipe secured with duct tape. A long, steel fencepost provides added stability. The hoop house is covered with plastic in the spring. When hot summertime weather arrives, the plastic is replaced with trellis netting.

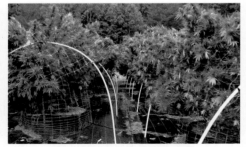

Hoop houses are inexpensive as well as quick and easy to set up. Plants can be moved in before or after a hoop house is set up. Once plants outgrow them, hoop-house structures turn into trellises to help support heavy flowering plants.

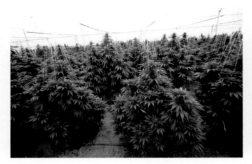

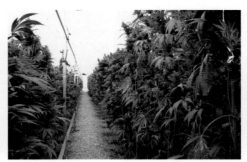

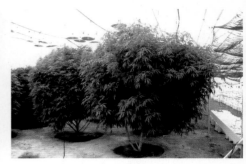

Adequate airspace is often forgotten when growing in a greenhouse. This Mexican greenhouse has plenty of extra space to let air circulate.

Always leave enough walkway space so that a wheelbarrow or small cart can pass through. Overplanting greenhouses makes maintenance difficult and cuts air circulation.

Big plants grow well in the greenhouse floor. In hard clay soils, a large planting hole filled with well-amended organic soil is as good as a large aboveground fabric container.

hoop-house structures turn into trellises to help support heavy flowering plants.

Prefabricated greenhouse kits are more expensive but come with all the parts and assembly instructions. They can be complicated to assemble. Some may offer a video to help with assembly. Often you can find small and miniature portable greenhouses at home improvement centers and on the Internet. Medical gardeners interested in larger greenhouses can see interesting automated greenhouse videos by searching for "forever flowering greenhouse" on YouTube.

Setting up a big commercial greenhouse is beyond the scope of this book. Search for "commercial greenhouse" using an Internet browser and you will find all the greenhouses you could want!

Greenhouse Construction

Both large and small greenhouses cost money, time, and space. Greenhouses with a foundation are also more permanent. Regardless of the type of greenhouse you construct, it should be on flat ground and have easy access.

This section of the chapter on greenhouses discusses different construction options, touching on main points to consider. However, providing construction instructions with diagrams is beyond the scope of this book. For more specific information, type "greenhouse plans" into an Internet browser.

Size of Greenhouse

Total area of the greenhouse is determined by the number of plants you

intend to grow and how long they will be in the ground or in pots. The longer plants grow, the more room they will need and the more problems that can occur. Induce plants to flower when they are 3 feet tall, and allow a minimum of 1 square yard (0.8 m²) for *indica*-dominant varieties and up to twice as much space for *sativa*-dominant varieties. Air circulation between plants can be a problem if plants become too big. Large plants that are planted early in the season often outgrow the greenhouse, which requires that the outside skin of the greenhouse be removed so growth is not impaired.

Ample airspace is essential in greenhouses. At least half the space in a greenhouse should be airspace. This space is necessary for air exchange, air circulation, and ventilation. Molds, mites, and insects become problems in greenhouses with inadequate airspace. As a general rule, plants should take up about 0.33 to 0.5 percent of the space in a greenhouse and air 0.5 to 0.66 percent. This ratio allows adequate air circulation.

Framing

Framing can be wood, bamboo, metal, or plastic. Framing to specific dimensions and building with premade framed panels has the advantage of quick installation and breakdown for winter storage. Build all structures using standard dimensions for framed glass, plastic panels, and sheeting to get the most from your materials and work more efficiently. For example, an 8-foot (2.4 m) greenhouse can be made with two 48-inch-wide (122 cm) fiberglass panels. Center height depends on the

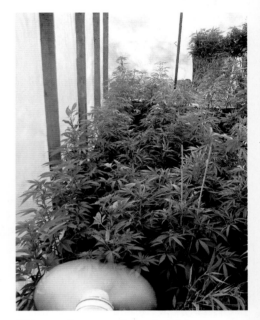

This greenhouse was framed with inexpensive lumber.

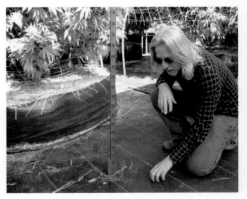

A weed barrier helps retain moisture and prevents many soil-borne insects from having easy access to the greenhouse. This medical cannabis gardener ran the weed barrier outside the greenhouse for extra protection. It also keeps mud away and makes the garden floor easy to clean.

level of the eaves. Low-growing plants can take an eave of 5 feet (1.5 m); tall plants need 10 to 14 feet (3–4.3 m).

Greenhouse **walkway space** is important for easy access. Too many gardeners are surprised when it turns into "crawling room only!" Overgrown foliage in large or small greenhouses cuts air circulation and promotes disease and pest attacks, as well as broken foliage. Room to move a wheelbarrow in a large greenhouse is especially valuable when plants grow beyond beds.

The **floor** of the greenhouse can be covered with weed barrier cloth, gravel, bricks, or concrete. Place a thermal blanket under floor covering to insulate from cold ground. A Styrofoam base in a small greenhouse keeps cold soil from cooling containers and greenhouse. You can also make raised, flat, or sunken beds in the greenhouse floor. Dirt floors can get muddy and are difficult to keep "clean." Cover muddy floors with sawdust or straw. A wood, brick, or concrete base around the bottom of the greenhouse adds stability to the structure.

Planting in the earth floor of the greenhouse allows you to use organic methods. The plants cannot be moved easily, but they grow bigger and require less maintenance than container-grown plants. Without containers, plants also retain a lower profile, but I still like raised beds. Growing in Mother Earth is always better than planting in pots when growing big plants. Most all the principles that apply to outdoor growing apply to growing in a greenhouse, too. Check out chapter 12, *Outdoors*, and chapter 18, *Soil*, for more information.

Benches

A greenhouse equipped with benches makes tending plants much easier. Water catchment systems can also be set up to recycle nutrient solution. I like a greenhouse with tables because when plants are off the floor, they stay warmer and are easier to access. Airspace below benches can serve as storage area for containers and water reservoirs.

Set up tables along the length of the greenhouse to make the best use of

space. Allow at least 3 feet (91.4 cm) between tables and greenhouse walls to accommodate plant growth and provide for comfortable access.

Metal benches are much stronger and more durable than wood but they are expensive. Frame wooden benches with enough lumber to support the center of tables. Cover wood with waterproof epoxy paint or set plastic ebb-and-flow tables on benches.

Hoop-House Construction

Mark a rectangular area 6 to 10 feet (1.8–3 m) wide and up to 50 feet (15.2 m) long where the greenhouse will be located. Purchase 20-foot lengths (6.1 m) of 0.75-inch (1.9 cm) Schedule 40 PVC pipe for every 4 to 8 feet (1.2–2.4 m) of greenhouse. Two 2-foot-long

(0.6 m) pieces of 0.5-inch (1.3 cm) rebar are necessary to anchor each end of the PVC pipe in place. Larger, stronger steel hoops can be ordered from greenhouse supply outlets.

Drive the 2-foot (61 cm) rebar 1 foot (30.5 cm) into the ground on 4- to 10-foot (1.2 to 3 m) centers to form a rectangle. Place each end of the 20-foot (6.1 m) PVC pipe over opposing 1-foot (30.5 cm) pieces of rebar to form an arch. Use duct tape or zip ties to attach a stay of 0.75-inch (1.9 mm) Schedule 40 PVC pipe across the top of the arches. Cover the hoops with a plastic skin and secure in place with duct tape or clamps. Remove plastic and replace with 6-inch (15.2 cm) plastic mesh that supports and trellises the plants as they grow beyond the confines of the hoops.

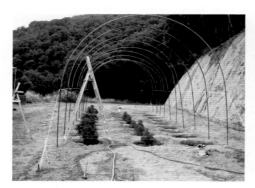

A metal hoop superstructure is constructed over small plants. Long, arced pieces are pushed into the moist earth. The superstructure is lightweight and fastened together with duct tape.

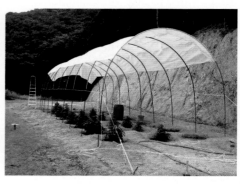

A lightweight shade cloth is stretched over the hoop house to cover the garden and provide shade during the hot days of summer.

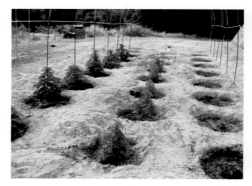

This garden was started earlier in the year in 3 different phases. The little clones are planted 2 weeks apart. Planting in sunken beds in the clay soil allows plants to stay cooler.

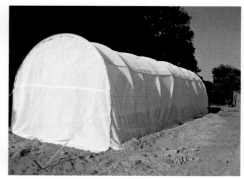

Once covered, the plants inside the hoop house cannot be seen from a distance. The shade cloth breathes so that minimal ventilation is necessary.

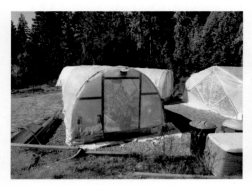

Typically a new gardener will cover a greenhouse with inexpensive plastic. A door is framed and installed, as is a vent fan. This greenhouse is covered with a light-reflecting shade cloth called Aluminet.

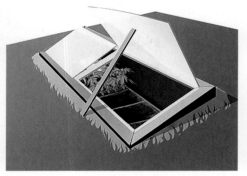

There are many interesting videos about greenhouse design, construction, heating, and so forth. Search "greenhouse construction" on YouTube for much more information.

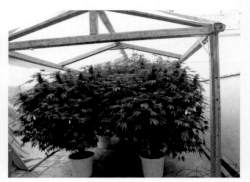

This small backyard patio greenhouse shielded plants from drizzly rain and kept plants warmer at night.

Coverings

Greenhouse coverings protect plants from the elements, but not all are created equal. Some greenhouse coverings transmit more light than others, while some hold heat and stay cool better than others. Price and durability also vary substantially. Overall, plastic and fiberglass coverings provide safe, economical alternatives to glass. The best greenhouse films are UV (ultraviolet) resistant.

Glass greenhouses are traditional. They enjoy very high light transmission, but glass is expensive, heavy, and brittle. It is not practical for most cannabis gardeners. Keep costs down and use only small glass greenhouses. Often they can be assembled from scrap windows.

Plastic Skins

Plastic designed for greenhouses is more durable than regular plastic, which tears easily when cut. Greenhouse plastic resist rips and tears. Quality greenhouse plastic is knitted instead of formed into sheets. It costs a little more than regular plastic but withstands destructive ultraviolet light from the sun. Greenhouse plastics last for 2 to 3 years before they need to be replaced. Of course, this does not take into account extreme weather such as hurricanes, tornadoes, hail, or severe icing.

An economical plastic covering is easy to control and helps to maintain heat and humidity in the greenhouse. Clear plastic is equal to glass in producing quality plants and flower buds. Plastic greenhouse film is available in clear and white that diffuses light but still allows high light transmission.

Choose the plastic that suits your needs. How long will you need it? Can you use it and then store it to use for additional seasons? How will you secure it to the greenhouse? How will you patch holes?

Rated in mils of thickness, greenhouse plastics are from 3 to 6 mils thick (1 mil = 1 thousandth of an inch [0.054 mm]). Greenhouse plastic is designed to last

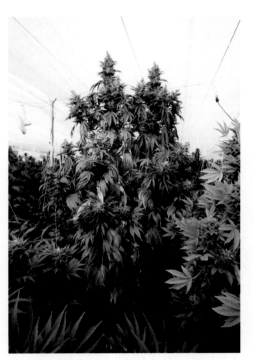

This 8-foot-tall (2.4 m) plant is growing in a large 18-foot-high (5.5 m) greenhouse. Extra airspace is needed for the transfer of carbon dioxide and oxygen.

for 2 to 5 years, depending on grade. Rigid panels are designed to last for 10 years or more.

Polycarbonate multiwall sheeting is lightweight, almost unbreakable, and available in double or triple hollow wall grades. Dual-wall construction makes this type of covering strong enough to withstand hailstorms, snow, and temperature fluctuations. Clear corrugated polycarbonate is very durable and has excellent light transmission.

Biodegradable plastic coverings are good for a month or two, maybe longer, depending upon the weather. These coverings are best used for a short time to cover individual clones or seedlings. Normally biodegradable plastic is available as plastic bags. Sheeting is expensive, and the short life renders it impractical.

Polyethylene plastic (PE) is low-cost, lightweight, provides ample light, and can withstand fall, winter, and spring weather. It does not tolerate summer UV levels. Ultraviolet-inhibited PE lasts longer, but both types lose heat more quickly than glass and other plastics. During the day, this can help keep plants cooler, but at night the heat loss requires the use of an artificial heat source. PE is available in commercial (6 mil) and utility (4 mil) grades. Most home improvement centers carry lighter-weight utility grade. Commercial grade is available via the Internet. Polyethylene plastic will last for a year or two when kept in good condition. Smaller tears can be repaired with a poly repair kit.

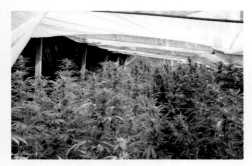

Inexpensive plastic and 2 × 4-foot (5 × 10 cm) boards and a few screws are all that is needed to construct a greenhouse. Just a little bit of work building a greenhouse will keep plants warm and dry and extend growing seasons.

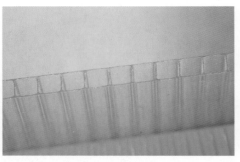

Lexan is one of the best greenhouse coverings available. The dual-wall construction traps heat between the outer panes to insulate the greenhouse. Durable Lexan lasts for years and is fairly rigid.

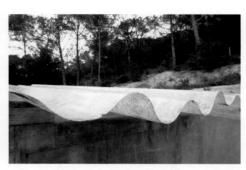

Corrugated fiberglass panels are easy to find at hardware and building supply stores.

Copolymer plastic is more durable and lasts longer than polyethylene plastic. Copolymer plastic lasts up to 3 years before becoming brittle and then breaking. Freezing and thawing will cause plastic to become brittle more quickly. More expensive copolymer plastics are more durable and equal the light transmission of glass.

Polyvinyl plastic is more durable than polyethylene or copolymer plastics. It is strong and provides structural strength when covering a greenhouse. Polyvinyl plastics will last 5 years or more when regularly maintained (cleaning it and fixing any rips or tears).

Polyvinyl chloride (PVC) is 2 to 5 times more expensive than PE but can last 5 years or longer. Polyvinylchloride is pliable and transparent or translucent, and it comes in 4- to 6-foot (1.2–1.8 m) widths that can be sealed together to provide a super wide piece. Ultraviolet-inhibited corrugated plastic panels provide another option; with their

excellent insulating properties (2.5 R insulation/3.5 mm panels, 3.0 R/5.0 mm panels), these panels can be used in cold frames, propagation houses, and greenhouses to provide excellent wind and snow protection and optimal solar heat collection.

Polycarbonate plastic is the most durable plastic. The double (twin wall) construction can last up to a decade. It maintains heat and humidity well and is the best plastic covering for year-round growing in cool and cold climates.

Lexan is one of the first dual-wall greenhouse coverings. This stuff is tough! One grade is even bulletproof! This thermoplastic lasts for years. It transmits almost as much light as glass and retains more heat. Lexan is rigid and full of thermo-storing channels. Clear panels like those in glass or Lexan may require shading during the heat of the day.

Corrugated fiberglass panels are readily available in different colors from clear to

black. Light transmission for corrugated fiberglass is fair to good, depending upon color. Poor grades will discolor, reducing light penetration, but a good grade of clear fiberglass can cost as much or more than glass. This covering transmits enough light under full sun conditions to grow a good crop of cannabis. It is lightweight, strong, and comes in 8- to 12-foot (2.4–3.7 m) panels. Fiberglass holds in heat in the winter and cool air in the summer.

Make sure to use clear or uncolored fiberglass panels. Colored panels will exclude light frequencies. For example, green panels will exclude both red and blue wavelengths, giving it its green color and denying plants their two main sources of energy.

Insulation is most efficiently used when the sun goes down. It is extremely important for greenhouses in cold climates. Throw a blanket, tarp or piece of "bubble plastic" over the top of the greenhouse to hold in heat at night.

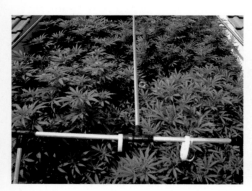

This rooftop garden is set up as a greenhouse. On rainy days and cold nights plastic is stretched over the top of the garden.

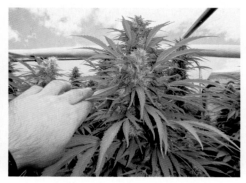

This photo from the same rooftop garden above shows how well buds grow under natural sunlight.

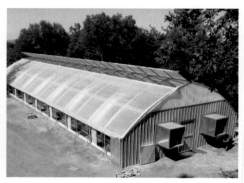

This brilliant grower cut the hillside away to site the greenhouse. It receives maximum sunlight all year and is protected from wind.

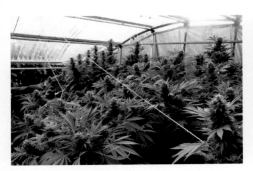

This nice little greenhouse garden was grown in France in a populated residential zone.

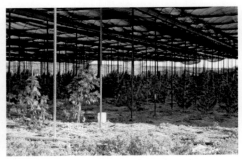

Shade cloth cuts intense heat from direct sunlight and creates a natural breezeway above plants. A covering of shade cloth cuts plants' water consumption, lowers temperatures, and reduces plants' stress levels.

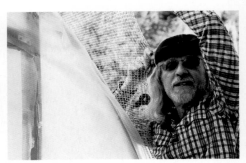

Jorge is holding up the Aluminet covering for this greenhouse. The high-tech shade cloth is lightweight and reflects intense heat from sunlight.

Larger greenhouses have automatic coverings that cover the top half of the greenhouse from inside. The space to be heated is reduced and it is more economical to heat at night.

Small greenhouses covered in plastic can be insulated inexpensively with double-wall construction. Two skins are affixed to the superstructure frame. An air pocket is formed between the skins. Nylon rope is stretched over the outer skin in several places and anchored on either end to hold it down. A small squirrel cage blower is mounted and attached to blow air in between the skins to form a 2- to 3-inch (5–7.6 cm) insulating layer of air. Light transmission is lessened, but the insulation value of the air makes it much easier to moderate the temperature inside the greenhouse. This insulation principle is most simply and easily applied to inexpensive hoop houses.

Higher R-value coverings make heating and cooling greenhouses more efficient and cost-effective. An efficient LP gas, propane, or kerosene heater will keep the greenhouse warm at night and during cold spells, but water vapor and high humidity are the by-products. Evaporative swamp coolers are the ideal way to keep greenhouses cool during hot summer temperatures, however, these coolers are less effective as temperatures and humidity rise outdoors.

Shade Coverings

Shade coverings serve to cool the greenhouse by blocking light transmission and, in turn, heat. Shade paint can be applied as a covering on the outer skin or glass of the structure. Reusable plastic shade film can cover the outside of the greenhouse or be fitted against rigid coverings inside. Roll-up shade coverings made of cloth or aluminum are flexible, removable, and reusable.

Shade paint is relatively easy to apply with a hose-end sprayer or a paint roller on a long pole. Water-based whitewash is inexpensive and easy to apply, although somewhat messy. Once applied, it can be washed off with a brush on an extended hose when sunlight intensity diminishes as the heat of summer passes. Remember, cannabis needs ample light to form big flower buds in the fall.

Colored plastic can also be used to shade plants. See "Plastic Skins" on page 143 for more information.

Shade cloth is used to cover greenhouses to help keep them cool. It is available in different opacities—from 10 to 80 percent—and 3 predominant colors:

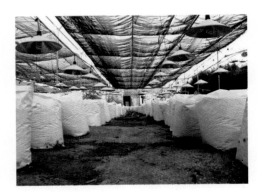

Shade cloth can be hung on part of the greenhouse to help nurture young plants. Large, well-established plants on the right receive full light.

green, black, and white. Traditionally a permeable cloth fabric, several new synthetic products, such as Aluminet, have emerged. This lightweight economical covering reflects heat and light as well as cutting light transmission.

Shade cloth can be used as the only covering for a greenhouse. It cuts light transmission, provides ventilation through the permeable cloth, and keeps pests and diseases outside.

Shade cloth, when used as a canopy with no greenhouse, creates a breezeway between plants and the cloth. The extra air circulation and ventilation provide added cooling. Used on the sides of the greenhouse, shade cloth is an excellent permeable windbreak. Shade cloth can also be affixed against walls or fences that are heated by sunlight. Attaching shade cloth to a fence can cut emitted heat by 20 to 30 degrees.

A **lath house** is built from thin, narrow strips of wood that allow filtered sun to enter the structure. In warm climates lath houses are a good place to take cuttings and harden-off plants grown indoors. Lath houses can provide 25 percent shade or more depending on the placement of the laths. Traditionally lath houses have been used to keep supplies, transplant, start seedlings, and so on.

Greenhouse construction and decision-making about greenhouse coverings are only the beginning. Growing plants in a greenhouse is often more demanding than growing plants indoors. Air temperature, humidity, light, and air

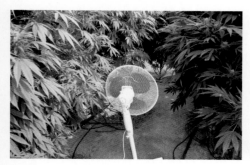

This gardener placed an oscillating fan on a stand in the middle of his greenhouse in order to increase air circulation between his flowering plants.

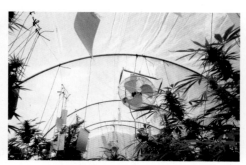

Setting up a ventilation fan was an afterthought in this greenhouse.

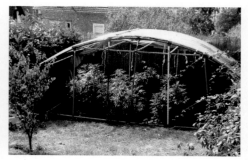

This backyard greenhouse garden in suburban Paris, France, uses the fence to hold heat and to block the neighbors' view.

quality must all be controlled in relation to a constantly changing greenhouse climate.

Climate Control

Greenhouses heat up quickly on sunny days and cool equally fast when the sun ducks behind a cloud or drops below the horizon. When the air inside the greenhouse cools, relative humidity rises, often beyond 100 percent. Water droplets condense on all surfaces—walls, ceiling, containers, and foliage. This fluctuation of heat and humidity is difficult and expensive to control. Temperature fluctuations also affect the ratio of nutrient to water that plants need and use, which makes growing in a greenhouse more demanding than growing indoors.

Air Circulation

The greenhouse must be big enough for air to circulate. A ratio of 33 percent plants to 63 percent air is ideal. Keeping air flowing inside small greenhouses is easy on a cool day, but when it heats up, air inside the greenhouse is trapped and temperatures climb beyond outdoor temperatures. Circulating greenhouse air is essential and may require large fans.

Small greenhouses can be cooled and heated relatively easily. Larger spaces are more demanding.

Condensation

Condensed water droplets that form on the inside of a greenhouse can reduce light transmission by up to 50 percent. Condensed droplets also attract fungus. Rainy and warm weather, increased plant transpiration, poor airflow and ventilation, and insufficient roof slope all contribute to condensation. Often a surface tension modifier is included in the greenhouse plastic to prevent formation of condensation droplets.

Condensation occurs because the greenhouse is warm and humid. When the temperature drops at night, hot air rises and condenses on plants and the ceiling of the greenhouse. If these drops do not run down the sides of the greenhouse, they block light transmission and are a source of problems. The little water droplets also spread disease. Not to mention how it feels to get a shower when you bump the wall of the greenhouse!

Condensation is especially bad when there are hot days and cool nights. The easiest way to ensure that condensation does not occur is to have an adequate ventilation system to remove humid air at sunset. Also, construct greenhouse ceiling/roof and sides with enough slope for gravity to carry condensed water droplets to the ground. Condensed water droplets can severely impair light transmission.

Even the best greenhouses will lose heat through radiation; conduction and convection through glass, walls, and floor (or soil); and also through vents, doors, and cracks. To counteract external variables, the internal structure of the greenhouse can be more complex than construction and siting.

Vents control temperatures in all seasons and improve growing conditions. Hand-operated roof vents will require frequent checks, or you may install automatic vents with an electric motor and thermostat that will respond to conditions around the clock. Venting is important with a cold frame, too. The high-end models have wax-filled vents

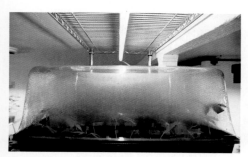

Water condenses out of the air when there is more humidity than the air can hold. Humidity condenses into moisture when humid air cools.

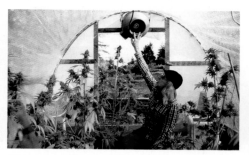

This super-efficient inline fan evacuates hot air near the ceiling of the greenhouse.

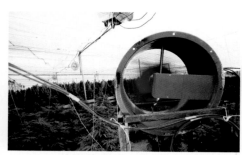

A high-rpm fan moves air across a large area.

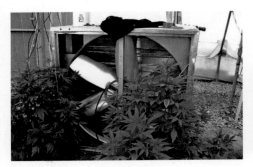

Sometimes vent fans break down!

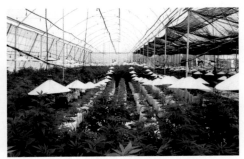

This large greenhouse has plenty of airspace inside, and hot air is vented out the top of the structure.

that operate automatically, opening when the heat rises in the frame and contracting as the temperature cools. You can find the paraffin-filled "Optivent" and many other supplies at greenhouse supply centers.

Heating systems are important to keep plants healthy during cold nights. Cannabis thrives with nighttime temps of 60°F to 65°F (15.5°C–18.3°C), but colder nights call for an additional heat source for sustained growth.

All greenhouses need ventilation, and most greenhouses need fans. Look for an extraction fan with the capacity to change the air every 1 to 5 minutes.

Cooling
Minimum-Impact Greenhouse Cooling
- Site in cool spot—shade or a natural breezeway
- Covering— insulate
- Vents—mechanical or automatic
- Shade cloth or shade covering
- Vent fans
- Humidity increase—misting
- Evaporative cooling

The eco-friendly way to cool a greenhouse is to take advantage of the microclimate. Locate it to receive shade or a breeze during the hottest part of the day and to have natural wind circulation. Greenhouses that receive full sun all day long must be covered with shade cloth or cooled artificially. This eco-friendly balance between time, money, and physical environment costs more resources

in cold and hot climates. Warm climates are the most economical location for a greenhouse.

Evaporating water increases humidity and lowers temperature in a greenhouse. Make walkways out of gravel that drains and holds water that will dissipate into the air, creating humidity. Setting up misters to increase relative humidity is very effective in dry climates, but more expensive. Remember, increasing humidity could cause cultural problems if overdone or mismanaged. Excess water sitting on leaves or clinging to the inside of the greenhouse invites cultural, disease, and pest problems.

Venting off hot air is one of the fastest and easiest ways to cool greenhouses. Since heat rises, venting hot air from the top of the greenhouse is the most efficient. If natural breezes are not enough to keep the greenhouse cool, electric fans and evaporative cooling are the next options.

Louvers on vent fans also force the hottest, most humid air out while protecting the plants from draft. Installing louvers that close when vent fans are off will help prevent entry of pests. See chapter 16, *Air,* for more information.

Lifting the sides of the greenhouse serves as ventilation but is much less efficient than venting from the top. When greenhouse sides are lifted, much warm air still stays within the upper portion of the greenhouse.

Evaporative cooling eliminates excess heat and adds humidity, reducing water

needs. Moist air circulates through the structure while warm air is expelled through roof vents or exhaust fans. Properly installed, an evaporative cooler can reduce interior temperature by as much as 30 to 40 degrees in hot, dry climates, less in wetter areas. As with fans, cooler size is determined by greenhouse size. A general guideline is to find a cooler equal to the total cubic space of the structure plus 50 percent.

Evaporative coolers are also known as swamp coolers because they introduce humid, swamplike air in order to cool homes and greenhouses. A typical greenhouse evaporative cooler consists of a big fan with large bats of straw or corrugated, concrete-impregnated pads that are fixed at the end of the greenhouse wall. Water is circulated through the pad. The large fan blows the humid air from the water-soaked pad into the greenhouse.

Air conditioners are very expensive to operate and are not practical in large greenhouses.

Misting and watering are important components of greenhouse gardening. Extended growing periods and higher sustained temperatures make adequate water essential. Again, there are methods to suit every temperament from low-tech to automatic. Most companies offer watering and misting systems by component, which can be mixed and matched to suit the grower's needs.

Automatic misting systems are a good investment for busy or forgetful growers. The timer triggers the mist or water

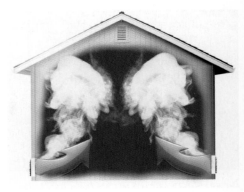

Bring fresh air into greenhouses and garden rooms from vents located near the floor, and expel stale air near the ceiling.

at preset intervals. You may want a toggle switch that allows you to rotate between manual and automatic watering. For more information on specific uses and types of watering systems, check out www.cloudtops.com. It has good information about misting systems for greenhouses. Atomize water for best results.

A lower-tech method of mist-and-watering control consists of a series of screens that tilt downward with the weight of the water shutting off the flow, and then raise to restart the cycle as the screens dry. It is fully automated by the weight of the water or lack thereof. Of course, there is also hand-watering, which is very effective and requires no mechanical intervention. Automatic systems, both high and low-tech, are alternatives to hand-watering that can be most helpful during a gardener's absence.

Heating

Heating a greenhouse with coal, gas, kerosene, electricity, or wood is expensive and often unnecessary or wasteful. Big greenhouse growers with permanent greenhouses can economically use a coal, wood, or gas boiler to supply hot water or steam through steel heating pipes run through the greenhouse. Environmentally conscious gardeners often grow in small greenhouses where steam heat is not a viable option. They heat greenhouses with the least expensive means and progressively invest resources according to the dynamics of

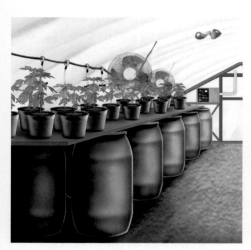

Large, black-painted drums full of water absorb heat from sunlight during the day. Heat is stored in the water, and at night it slowly dissipates into the greenhouse to warm the air.

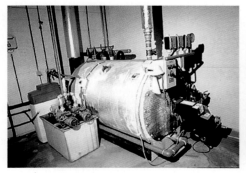

This is a photo of the original boiler that heated Sensi Seeds' main indoor growing facility. Heating a greenhouse or large indoor garden is much more economical with a fuel-fed boiler.

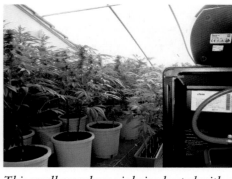

This small greenhouse is being heated with a propane gas heater.

the greenhouse. Closing all uncontrolled air leaks is the first step toward efficient, effective greenhouse heating. Next, control wall and ceiling insulation, soil heat, air temperature, and humidity.

1. Close all cracks—enclose greenhouse
2. Insulate skin—see "Coverings" on page 143.
3. Bank heat—install water barrels
4. Insulate soil—thermal blanket
5. Heat soil—manure/compost, soil heating cables/mat
6. Heat air—water and stone bank, soil bank, steam/water, gas, electricity

Thermal blankets can be placed along walls and ceiling or on the floor to hold in the heat. Such solutions are somewhat effective in cold climates with clear skies. A layer of air between two plastic skins is also somewhat efficient to hold in heat. However, the insulation value of plastic is low.

The **floor** can cool the greenhouse substantially. To keep the greenhouse warmer, cover the floor with a permeable thermal blanket and weed barrier. The floor of a small greenhouse can be covered with a layer of Styrofoam for added insulation.

Soil-heating cables with a thermostat are the most efficient use of electricity for heat when air temperatures get down to 50°F (10°C) at night and go up during the day. Place the cable on the soil at the bottom of the bed or on a bed of sand or vermiculite and cover with about 2 inches (5 cm) of sand. You will need to provide 10 to 15 watts of electric heat for every square foot (0.09 m²) of growing area. Heat cables are also useful in greenhouses for warming seedlings, clones, or flowering plants without the cost of heating the entire structure.

Heat Source	Efficiency
warm floor (insulated)	90%
warm floor (uninsulated)	80%
hot water pipes	85%
hot air heaters	60%

HEATING-FUEL EFFICIENCY

Fuel	Efficiency (%)	Unit Heat Value
electricity	95–100	3,413 Btu/kWh
natural gas	80	1,000 Btu/ft³
propane	80–91	000 Btu/gal

Check this link to learn more about the efficiency of specific fuels: http://www.ag.ndsu.edu/pubs/ageng/structu/ae1015.pdf.

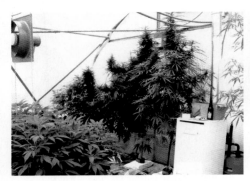
The white box is a gas heater. Notice how the plants are growing in short blocks of rockwool. This is how Nevil (Seed Bank, Holland, 1985) grew plants for breeding.

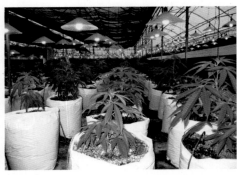
These CFLs do not throw a lot of light, but it is enough to keep these plants in the vegetative growth stage.

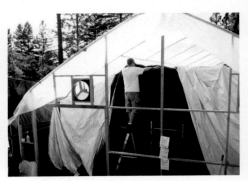
This grower covers his garden daily. He removes the shade covering after dark so that plants receive 12 hours each of light and dark. The plastic above protects the dark covering below from wind.

Heating small greenhouses can be relatively economical with an electric space heater, or be more effectively heated with thermostatically controlled forced air using ducts or plastic tubing to evenly distribute the heat. Large greenhouses may be heated with forced air or by a coal or natural hot water or steam system. But both hot water and steam heating are expensive to install. The inexpensive, low-tech-but-labor-heavy method of greenhouse warming: compost. A grower in Portland, Oregon, stacks organic matter on the sides of the greenhouse to a height of about 5 feet (1.5 m) inside and out. The compost gives off heat as it decomposes, keeping the structure warm at a very low cost.

A CO2 burner also generates heat as a by-product. Closed greenhouses often have too little CO_2 during the day for plants to be able to use light effectively. Increasing the level of CO_2 with a generator will accelerate plant growth. An infrared sensor/controller can be

attached to the CO_2 generator to control it automatically. Detailed information on CO_2 can be found in chapter 16, *Air*.

Big gas air heaters are available from horticultural supply stores. With a web browser, search for "greenhouse heater." Everything from gas to electric to kerosene heaters will pop up. Remember to keep hot air from blowing directly on plants.

Artificial Lighting

When combined with natural sunlight, artificial light is most efficiently used in most climates during non-daylight hours. Above 50° north latitude, light intensity diminishes quickly in the fall, winter, and spring. Supplemental lighting is very effective in greenhouses in these northern latitudes. Anybody who has flown into Schiphol Airport in Amsterdam at night has seen the deep orange glow emitted by HPS lamps in greenhouses.

Greenhouse growers turn the HID lights on when sunlight diminishes (30 minutes before sunset) and off when sunlight strengthens (30 minutes after sunrise). Turn on the HPS when the daylight intensity is less than 2 times the intensity of the HPS. Measure this point with a light meter. Turn off the HPS when the daylight intensity is greater than 2 times the intensity of the HPS. A simple photocell that measures light intensity can be used to turn the lights on and off automatically when light levels fall below a specified level. Supplementary lighting has greatest effect when applied to the youngest plants.

It is least expensive and most efficient to light plants when they are small. These artificial lighting principles work for flowering and vegetative growth cycles.

Exclusively HPS lamps are used because natural sunlight supplies enough light in the rest of the spectrum. Lamps with small reflective hoods and attached ballasts are used in greenhouses. The small reflective hood blocks very little natural sunlight and the attached ballast delivers electricity more efficiently to the bulb. Maintain vegetative growth in the spring with inexpensive CFL lights. Supplemental nighttime lighting is necessary to interrupt the dark period and prevent cannabis plants from flowering. The lighting can be from HPS lamps or small 60- to 75-watt equivalent CFL lamps. The small lamps are hung over plants and turned on for an hour or so in the middle of the night (dark period).

Small vegetative plants do not need as much light in the spring. This is when plants establish a big strong root system and strong vascular system. Once warm weather and long days arrive, plants really start to grow!

Light Deprivation

For many years Dutch growers, commercial growers, and other cannabis gardeners have been using "thermal blankets" in greenhouses to hold heat in at night and to black out greenhouses to simulate 12-hour nights and days that induce cannabis to flower. Darkening greenhouses to induce flowering during midsummer will allow 3 or more medicinal cannabis harvests annually in

The CFL lamps above this garden are turned on at night to interrupt the dark period. The extra hour of light in the middle of the night is enough to keep these plants from flowering.

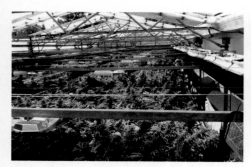

With this Forever Flowering greenhouse, a gardener is able to control the photoperiod during the entire year.

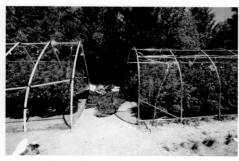

Both of these light-deprivation greenhouses are covered with black plastic every night.

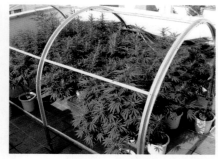

This greenhouse is blacked out by covering it with black plastic until darkness falls. The blackout plastic is removed at night.

mild climates. Cannabis plants (except *C. ruderalis*)* flower when nights are long (12 hrs) and days are short (12 hrs). To induce flowering, darken the greenhouse so that plants receive 12 hours of uninterrupted darkness every day.

*Specific medicinal varieties may react differently to the light schedules outlined in this section. See chapter 3, *Medical Cannabis Varieties*, and chapter 25, *Breeding*, for more information.

Midsummer sunlight is much more intense than sunlight in the spring and fall. Cannabis requires high levels of light to produce the biggest and heaviest medicinal flower buds. Inducing cannabis to flower under high light levels will produce a heavier harvest.

Automatic darkening greenhouses can be constructed or purchased. (Designing and constructing an automatic-darkening greenhouse is beyond the scope of this book.) Automated greenhouses have different degrees of automation. There are many greenhouse companies that offer automatic darkening greenhouses. The

most popular automated light deprivation greenhouses in the USA are from Forever Flowering (www.foreverflowering.net.) Search YouTube for videos that demonstrate how the greenhouses operate.

Imposing the day/night schedule to darken a greenhouse is not as difficult as it might appear, but it is a daily event. For example, the longest day of the year, June 21, can be 15 hours long; the greenhouse must be blacked out for 3 hours so that plants receive 12 hours of darkness.

Daily, at about the same time, the greenhouse must be blacked out. The darkening material must be removed after darkness falls, to ensure that plants are adequately ventilated during hot summer nights.

For example, if you black out a greenhouse at 7:00 a.m. and it is dark at 9:00 p.m., you can remove the cover from the greenhouse before going to bed. The ritual does not repeat until the next day/night. Make sure the cover is lightweight and the entire "job" of covering the

greenhouse is as easy as possible. I find that easy jobs are more likely to be completed regularly.

Tropical greenhouses from latitudes of 0° to 30° north and south receive from 12 to 13 hours of light/dark daily and do not need to be blacked out. In fact, to keep plants in vegetative growth, artificial light must be infused to keep plants from flowering.

In spring and fall, greenhouses do not need to be darkened to induce flowering, since darkness and daylight are close to 12 hours each. Check your latitude and the hours of light your garden receives to calculate the black-out period.

Use black opaque plastic to completely cover greenhouses. Small greenhouses are easy to cover by dragging the plastic over the superstructure of the greenhouse. Black plastic should be divided into 2 lighter-weight pieces to facilitate work when covering larger greenhouses.

Secure the bottoms of the plastic around the base of the greenhouse to prevent light from entering and wind from lifting the plastic. Use flexible elasticized bungi cords to secure the opaque covering to eyebolts along the bottom perimeter of the greenhouse. Toss ropes over the outside skin of the covered greenhouse to secure it from wind.

Store the black plastic alongside the greenhouse when not in use.

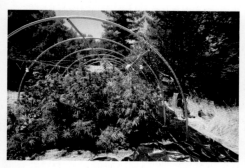

The black plastic on the right is stretched over the hoop house after plants receive 12 hours of light. The plastic is removed at night so plants are able to breathe.

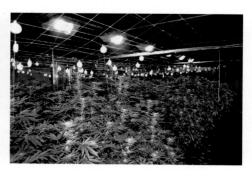

An automatic darkening system in a greenhouse at the Cannabis Castle in the Netherlands blacks out gardens to induce flowering. I shot this photo in 1986!

12
OUTDOORS

GROWING MEDICAL CANNABIS outdoors is the first option for most gardeners in states and countries where growing medical cannabis is legal or tolerated. Cannabis evolved naturally and grows best outdoors naturally. Growing medical cannabis outdoors is ecologically sound and works in concert with Mother Nature. Sunlight and air are virtually free; water and nutrients are also much less expensive in outdoor gardens. Bulk organic nutrients—composts, manures, rock powders, and so forth—are inexpensive and most often environmentally friendly. Outdoor gardening is more popular than indoor gardening in countries with progressive medical cannabis laws. More cannabis is grown outdoors than indoors, for these simple reasons: Cannabis is a strong plant that can be grown successfully almost anywhere. Virtually any sunny growing area can be coaxed into yielding a healthy crop.

Harvesting two crops, one in spring and another in the fall, is possible in temperate climates. Long nights and short spring days trigger cannabis to flower. Savvy gardeners harvest the spring crop and then plant the fall crop the next day! Harvest the fall crop when nights become long and days short. Adventurous gardeners can plant the new autoflowering feminized seeds; such stable hybrids yield 3 to 4 ounces (85–118.3 gm) 70 days after planting seeds. Autoflowering feminized plants can be harvested in the middle of summer when sunlight is most intense and resin production is at its peak.

Research local garden trends, read local garden columns, and talk to local gardeners about the best time to plant and grow medical cannabis, tomatoes, peppers, or similar vegetables, and then plan accordingly. Also inquire about common pests and diseases and when they are most prevalent. Collect publications on local growing conditions. These are often available at hydroponic stores, nurseries, and garden centers, or through your local department or ministry of agriculture.

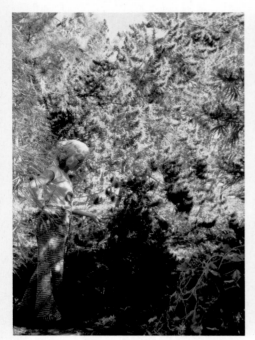

Big cannabis plants like these Colombian plants have been growing for many years. This giant plant was photographed by Mel Frank in 1977. (MF)

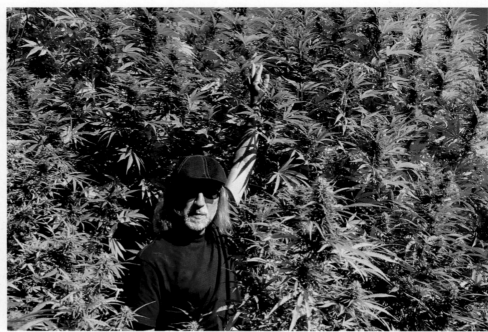

Organic soil preparation, plenty of sunlight, water, and a long growing season are all most plants need to thrive.

Security is still a concern when cultivating medical cannabis outdoors. Theft can be a problem, and so can uninformed law enforcement. Make sure to have all your paperwork in order should law enforcement knock on your door. Posting your medical recommendation at the garden is a common practice.

Much of the information that pertains specifically to outdoor cultivation is in this chapter; however, many of the subjects within this chapter are covered in great detail in other chapters of this book. References to these chapters are made in the appropriate places.

Climate

Cannabis will grow in nearly all climates. Specific varieties of cannabis grow better in some zones than others. Most varieties of cannabis need a minimum of 120 frost-free days to produce a decent harvest; gardens in such climates should be protected with plastic in the springtime. Transplanting or setting out autoflowering feminized seedlings in short-season climates is an excellent option. Gardens in short-season climates with 90 frost-free days require a greenhouse to protect plants from cold at night. Southern and warm-climate gardens suffer from excessive heat and sometimes humidity both day and night.

Outdoor gardens are dominated by climate, soil, and water supply whether in a backyard, on a balcony, in a greenhouse, or at a remote location. Microclimates are mini climates that exist within larger climates. Many maps such as the United States Department of Agriculture (USDA) Hardiness Zone map (www.usna.usda.gov/Hardzone/ushzmap.html) detail limited climatic boundaries. The USDA Hardiness Zone map divides North America into 10 zones plus an eleventh zone to represent areas that have average annual minimum temperatures above 40°F (4.4°C) and are frost-free. Look into detailed microclimate maps for your growing zone. One of the most detailed climate maps for western North America can be found in Sunset Publishing's *Western Garden Book*. The map details 26 distinct climate zones in 13 states in the western United States, as well as British Colombia and Alberta, Canada. This is the best climatic map available for the area. See information on climate zones in the western United States at www.sunset.com. Search "Sunset climate maps picture" on the Internet to learn more about climate zones.

Europe and industrialized countries have much climatic information available via the Internet. Check out charts showing rainfall, temperature, and humidity for virtually all large cities in the world and most geographic regions. Visit www.weather.com for specific information on your local weather. Temperature, rainfall, and sunlight vary widely across the globe, providing unique growing environments and countless microclimates. Look for specific information for your climate at local nurseries and in regional gardening books and magazines or through the department or ministry of agriculture (called County Extension Agents in the USA) in your area.

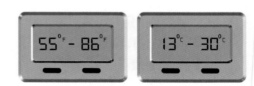

Cannabis grows best between 55°F and 86°F (13°C–30°C).

Below is a brief description of 4 distinct climate zones where cannabis grows. Reference the basic climate for your garden location in terms of the climate, light, and soil charts in this book.

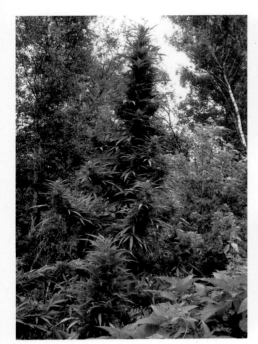

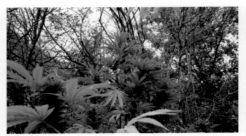

Rainy climates create a constant battle with mold and diseases. This garden in the Basque Country of Spain receives rain throughout the growing season.

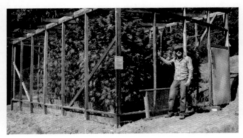

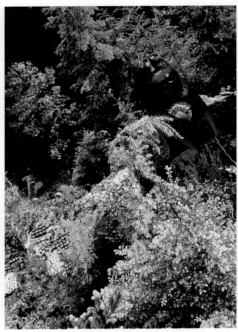

This 'Annapurna' super-autoflowering plant grows well in most outdoor climates.

Many medical cannabis gardeners post their medical data at the garden site.

Some medical cannabis gardeners are forced to grow in mountainous terrain to avoid detection. This gardener from British Colombia, Canada, has to put on a special pair of rock climbing boots to descend the last 80 feet (24.4 m) to the garden.

Fill out the brief "Garden Climate Data" form on page 154 so that you will understand the overall qualities of your climate.

Alpine Short-Season Climates

Alpine climates are particularly challenging for growing a strong, healthy medical crop. Medical gardeners in Colorado, most of Canada, and northern or alpine regions such as Switzerland are growing at elevations ranging from 4,600 feet (1,402.1 m) to 1,000 feet (304.8 m) in elevation. Most often soil is difficult to manage in alpine climates, but a little bit of light and heat works wonders!

Rainy Climates

Rainy climates can be cool and wet during winter and spring and hot and humid during other months. Annual rainfall most often exceeds 40 inches (100 liters per m³) and can top 100 inches (250 L/m³)! Winter often blows in early in these areas, bringing a chilling rain and low light levels. The more northern zones experience shorter days and wet, freezing weather earlier than the southern zones. Medical cannabis grows well in temperate maritime climates. Growing further inland often requires more protection. The temperature seldom

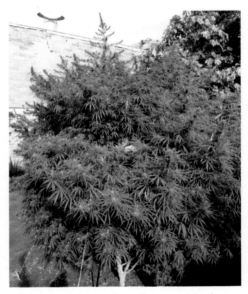

The Mediterranean Coast has an arid subtropical climate that is perfect for growing long-season sativas such as this giant 'Haze' plant.

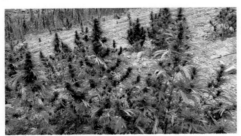

Water is the most precious commodity in a dry climate. Pounding sunlight heats soil and plants, which then must use more water. Plant in sunken beds and use mulch to conserve water.

drops below freezing in many coastal rainy climates, which contributes to larger insect populations. Some cold coastal rainforests are packed with lush but invasive foliage and fungal growth brought on by the cold, damp weather.

Arid Climates

Arid climates have little rainfall and low humidity. Wind and poor soil often accompany dry climates. Landscape flora consists of plants with small leaves that conserve water. Water is at a premium. Sunlight is intense and heat pervasive. Often cannabis needs to be planted under shade cloth to lower foliage temperatures that cause heat stress. Placing mulch around the base of plants is essential to prevent water loss. Planting in sunken beds also keeps plants cooler and attracts moisture.

Tropical and Subtropical Long-Season Climates

Tropical and subtropical climates are generally warm to hot and humid. Rainy and dry seasons vary by location. Most "selva" or jungle and tropical climates experience 10 to 30 minutes of daily

GARDEN CLIMATE DATA	YOUR TOWN NAME
number of days above 50°F (10°C)	
monthly rainfall	
monthly nighttime temperature lows	
monthly daytime temperature highs	
monthly mph/kmph wind	
monthly average humidity	
percent of sunlight monthly	
percent of cloudy days monthly	

Sunlight intensity diminishes as the angle declines in the sky. Sunlight is about 15 percent less bright from September to October when the sun is lower in the sky. The drawing shows the sun at a 75-degree angle in summer and near its lowest angle, in winter, of 28 degrees.

rainstorms. Protecting flowering females from rain with a greenhouse or shade house will help avoid bud mold and other problems. Nighttime temperatures and humidity are often high in these climates. In fact, extended nighttime temperatures above 85°F (29.4°C) will cause most plants to stop growing.

See chapter 18, *Soil*, for more information on soils in different geographic regions.

Microclimates

Each of the 4 climates (alpine short-season; arid; rainy; tropical and sub-tropical long-season) contains more localized climates or microclimates. Within these microclimates are even more micro-microclimates, all of which affect cannabis growth. For example, south-facing hillsides receive more solar heat than flat-topped or north-facing slopes. Hills and valleys also affect wind patterns as warm air rises and cold air drops.

Each and every garden has even more microclimates! For example, some places are shady and others get much more sunlight. Some growing beds are located next to a wall or fence that holds heat. Each one of these variations will influence the microclimate.

We can measure the factors that constitute microclimates and apply this knowledge in order to grow the best medical cannabis possible. Cannabis growth is governed by climatic conditions:

Collect all the information you need to garden outdoors in your climate. Precise answers to climate questions will solve most cultivation dilemmas before they arise. Take the time to learn the best times to plant and harvest in your climate—and a lot more. Use the charts in this book and find additional information on the Internet to answer questions related to your climate. A couple of hours spent on research before planting a medical cannabis garden will save you time, money, and gardening-misery.

One of the best measures of outdoor gardening variables can be found in *Sunset* magazine's climate zone maps, which take these factors into account. Agricultural hardiness zone maps devised by the US Department of Agriculture and other government agencies divide

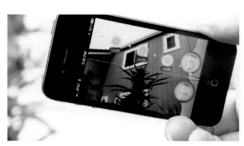

Several different "sun position" apps can be downloaded for iPhones and Android phones that will help you site your garden so that it gets the maximum amount of sunlight.

zones based strictly on winter low temperatures. *Sunset's* climate zone maps consider what every medical cannabis gardener should consider: temperature, yes, but also latitude; elevation; ocean influence; continental air influence; and mountains, hills, and valleys—all of which together form many microclimates. To grow the best garden possible in each of these climate zones, search the Internet for specific weather information about your local climate.

Sunlight and Siting the Garden

Before siting the garden, remember that all tools, irrigation equipment, soil, fertilizer, and so on must be carried to the garden. Bulk soil and amendments are easiest to move on flat ground. Make plans with this in mind when constructing backyard or terrace gardens and large gardens of any type.

Cannabis plants need 5 to 6 hours of direct sunlight, preferably during midday, at minimum levels of 4,500 foot-candles (48,437.6 lux), to flower well and produce a good crop. Lower levels of light prolong harvest and lower both quality and yield. Cannabis requires the most intense sunlight during flowering. Receiving more hours of direct sunlight during flowering promotes thick, dense flower buds. Ideally cannabis should be planted in an open, level field with no shade. But most often gardens are shaded by trees, houses, buildings, and

HOURS OF LIGHT PER DAY AT DIFFERENT LATITUDES

City	Latitude	Jan 21	Feb 21	Mar 21	Apr 21	May 21	Jun 21	Jul 21	Aug 21	Sep 21	Oct 21	Nov 21	Dec 21
Honolulu, HI	21° N	11:03	11:34	12:08	12:45	13:14	13:26	13:14	12:45	12:09	11:33	11:03	10:50
San Diego, CA	32° N	10:21	11:14	12:09	13:11	13:58	14:19	13:59	13:11	12:11	11:12	10:21	10:00
Sacramento, CA	38° N	9:56	11:01	12:11	13:26	14:26	14:52	14:28	13:27	12:12	10:59	9:55	9:28
Philadelphia, PA	40° N	9:45	10:56	12:11	13:33	14:38	15:06	14:40	13:34	12:13	10:53	9:44	9:15
Portland, OR	45° N	9:19	10:43	12:12	13:49	15:07	15:41	15:09	13:50	12:14	10:40	9:17	8:42
Seattle, WA	47° N	9:05	10:37	12:13	13:58	15:22	15:59	14:24	13:58	12:15	10:34	9:04	8:25
Calgary, CAN	51° N	8:40	10:25	12:13	14:12	15:49	16:33	15:52	14:13	12:16	10:22	8:39	7:54
Anchorage, AK	61° N	6:51	9:38	12:19	15:17	19:22	19:01	18:01	15:17	12:22	9:32	6:48	5:27

so forth, and it is not possible for them to receive full sunlight all day long.

On the summer solstice (the longest day of the year), the angle of the sun at 40.3° north latitude* is 73.2°. On the winter solstice, the shortest day of the year, the angle of the sun at the same latitude is 26.2°. As the angle of the sun climbs in the sky, sunlight intensifies and lower shadows are cast from objects over gardens. In the fall when the angle of the sun drops in the sky, intensity diminishes and objects throw a longer shadow. Measuring the path of the sun through the sky can be guesstimated by standing at planting sites and looking toward the sun. Hold your arm up and track the arc of the sun. Figure the sun will climb and drop in the sky, and guess about how much shadow it will throw. Or you could buy one of several applications such as the Sun Seeker for an iPhone or an Android phone that allows you to

type in any date and see the path of the sun. I love this application!

*The angle of the sun changes in relation to latitude. In the USA, Eureka, California; Salt Lake City, Utah; and the border between Kansas and Nebraska, are all about 40.3° north latitude.

Direct sunlight can heat foliage and cause plants to transpire excessive amounts of water in order to stay cool. Shade cloth stretched over plants will lower temperatures by blocking a percentage of the sunlight that hits foliage. A natural breezeway is also formed between the shade cloth and plants, which helps to cool them even more. If shade cloth is not an option, give plants heavier doses of magnesium and calcium. See also "drought" in the Index.

Scout garden sites in winter and try to visualize how trees will cast shadows

during summer months, and how plants will get 5 to 6 hours of midday sun. Use one of the many iPhone or Android phone apps that tell you exactly where the sun will be on specific dates. Remember that the sun takes a higher path in the late spring and summer. Six hours of direct midday sun per day is essential for acceptable growth. More is better. South-facing gardens, hillsides, and terraces receive full sun all day long.

See chapter 11, *Greenhouses*, for more information on hours of light per day for various climates.

Outdoors, hours of daylight are short in spring and increase in length during summer. Daylight hours diminish in fall and winter. The shortest day of the year falls on or near December 21, and the longest day of the year falls on or near June 21.

Check the soil drainage by digging a small hole and filling it with water.

Site the garden in the spring by standing where the plants will grow. Hold up your hand and cover the sun. Trace an imaginary line through the sky where the path of the sun will be.

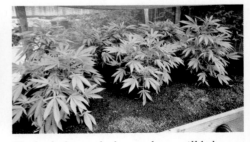

Shade cloth stretched over plants will help keep them cooler during the day and a little warmer at night.

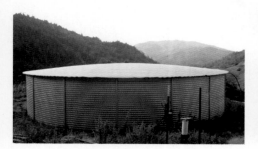
This 20,000-gallon (75,708 L) reservoir is located on top of a small hill. Water gravity flows from the reservoir to the garden.

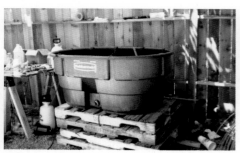
Store daily irrigation water in a large reservoir.

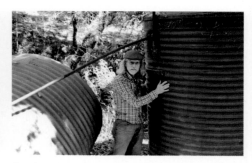
Storing water is an option for gardeners who want a constant supply of water but have only a sporadic water source.

The table on page 155 shows the number of daylight hours at different latitudes in the USA. Note that at 40° north latitude, the maximum amount of sunlight is only 15.2 hours on June 21. If plants are grown in a greenhouse, supplemental light could be applied to increase production.

Special Planting Considerations

Little research has been done on cannabis and plants that produce allelotoxic chemicals.* Some plants are immune to these toxins, and others are not. These chemicals may not affect cannabis, or all varieties of cannabis. Nonetheless, avoid planting under trees or near bushes that produce allelotoxic chemicals, including: black cherry, cottonwoods, hackberry, junipers, sassafras, sugar maples, and walnut trees. Black walnut trees are the worst.

*Allelotoxic chemicals are released by one plant that has an effect on another plant. The release of allelotoxic chemicals is a survival mechanism that allows certain plants to compete with or kill other plants. The chemicals often inhibit seed germination, root development, or nutrient uptake.

Water and Irrigation

Medical cannabis plants grown outdoors use a lot of water, especially when they grow large. Big vegetative and flowering plants may need 5 to 10 gallons (38–75 L) of water or more daily during the heat of the growing season. Adequate water can make the difference between success and failure. Water use and conservation is essential now. Backyard gardens are easy to water with a garden hose, or automated irrigation systems can be set up. Watering remote gardens is more of a challenge. Water may have to be pumped from a well, stream, irrigation ditch, or river and then stored in a reservoir. Check local regulations on using water with regard to public and private water rights.

Water quality also affects fertilizers and nutrient availability. Pay special attention to water pH and mineral content (measured in ppm or EC) of irrigation water regardless of the source—reservoir, tap, or well. Active live organic soil teaming with microbes is blessed with chemistry that rectifies high- or low-pH water, seemingly like magic. Nonorganic gardeners can use one of several commercial hydroponic fertilizer formulations to solve "hard water" problems.

Irrigate the garden during morning hours so that plants have time to use all the water necessary during the heat of the day. Do not water late in the day; unused water that sits in the ground or in containers displaces much-needed oxygen for roots. If plants are slightly overwatered, especially late in the day,

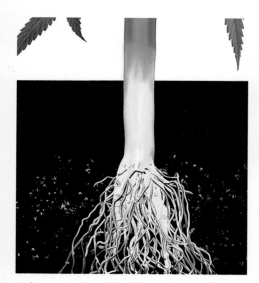
Polymers in the soil hold water longer than soil does.

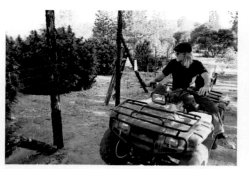
The garden needs a readily available water source. If water is not at hand, it must be hauled to the garden. Big plants can use 5 to 10 gallons (18.9–37.9 L) of water a day. Hauling water takes time and is a lot of work. One gallon (3.8 L) of water weighs 8 pounds; 100 gallons (380 L) weighs 800 pounds (360 kg)! Even carrying water by hand for short distances to water small plants is a lot of work.

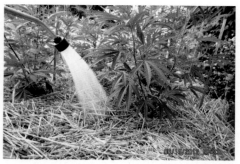
Irrigate with a hose attached to a breaker head nozzle that aerates the water. Water plants in containers daily when necessary. Small containers dry out quickly. Large containers need watering every few days. Irrigate small containers every day or two; they might require water twice daily during hot weather. A 200-gallon (757 L) container with a full-grown plant in full sun will use 5 to 10 gallons (18.9–37.9 L) of water daily.

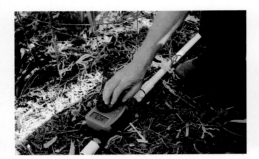

Many inexpensive battery-operated irrigation timers are available. This timer took just a few minutes to set up, and the batteries last a long time.

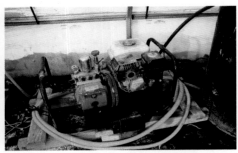

This gasoline pump is built on a small frame so that it is easy to move around.

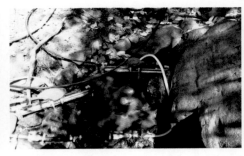

The High Lifter pump in this creek has provided three growing seasons of uninterrupted service. The pump runs quietly and is very efficient.

this oxygen depletion slows growth and could lead to root rot.

Check the garden daily, if possible, and water when soil is dry 1 inch (2.5 cm) below the surface. Irrigate containers until 10 to 20 percent of the water comes out the drainage holes. Irrigate plants in the ground until they are completely wet, but let them dry somewhat between waterings to accommodate more air (oxygen) in the soil. See "Sources of Water" in chapter 20, *Water*, for more information.

Automatic watering systems deliver a regular supply of water to plants. Consistent and fail-proof operation are two indispensable qualities for automatic irrigation systems. Type "drip irrigation" into your favorite search engine; hundreds of company sites will pop up on your screen and tell you all about drip irrigation and automated watering. See chapter 20, *Water*, for more specific information on irrigation.

Avoid nutrient buildup problems by leaching container gardens monthly with three quarts (2.8 L) of water for each dry quart (liter) of soil.

Many different types of receptacles and reservoirs can store irrigation water. Use the biggest storage unit that you can manage; plants will always need water. One good option for storing a lot of water is to dig a big hole and line it with a plastic pond liner. For all kinds of water storage devices, see www.realgoods.com.

Pumps
Regardless of the type of water pump, it will need a filter that is easy to clean. A

pre-filter before the fine filter will also cut maintenance, especially if pumping from an open water source. Remember to clean the filter periodically. Put "clean the pump filters" on your regular weekly checklist.

Pumps can be operated by hand, electric current, batteries, gasoline, gravity, and pressure from moving water. Moving water uphill requires a powerful pump. A gasoline-powered pump is necessary when lifting water more than 100 feet (30.48 m). Battery-powered pumps can lift water 10 to 15 feet (3–4.6 m) before they become inefficient. Ram pumps and the High Lifter can lift water many feet over time. Manual pumps require a lot of physical energy to operate and are impractical for moving a large volume of water uphill.

Water flow / pressure pumps
With a small flow of water under pres-

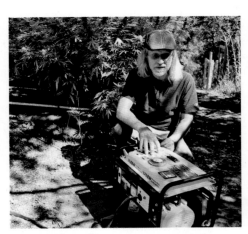

The neighbors all agreed to operate their gasoline pumps in the morning, two days a week to avoid local noise pollution. Many residents in this part of Northern California pump water from a well and store it in a large reservoir.

sure, water pressure pumps use the power of water running downhill to lift part of the water uphill. These pumps are very efficient and can run 24 hours a day to lift water up to a storage reservoir, where it is stored until used for irrigation. Here is a great website with more information on pumps: http://journeytoforever.org/at_waterpump.html.

Pumps can move water long distances and uphill. Pump size, horsepower, pipe size and length, vertical lift, and elevation above sea level all play a part in water-moving dynamics, but the specifics are beyond the scope of this book.

Always drain the pump before an expected freeze. Water frozen within it can rupture the pump. Before shopping for a pump, copy the following 9-item list. This necessary information will tell you everything you need to know to purchase the proper pump.

Before purchasing a pump, find out:
1. Vertical pipe length
2. Horizontal pipe length
3. Pipe diameter
4. Pump GPM—gallons per minute (LPM, liters per minute)
5. Elevation above sea level
6. Determine the height of the tank above water source: (net lift) = _____ ft (m)
7. Next determine the drop from the water source to the pump: (fall) = _____ ft (m). To estimate lift or fall, consult topographical maps or use a tape measure, a handheld sight level, an altimeter, or a tube and a water-pressure gauge. Remember that 1 psi = 2.3 ft.

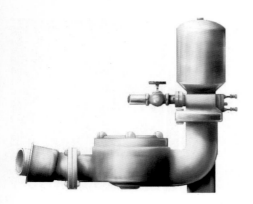

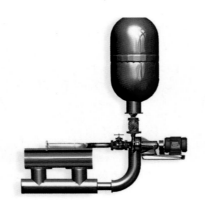

A hydraulic ram pump lifts water from a source of flowing water located above the pump. The natural force of gravity and flowing water is all the power needed. Ram pumps are rugged and dependable but noisy. For more information see www.rampumps.com.

The Bamford Hi-Ram Pump is a simple, self-powered water pump using a plastic ball, which makes the pump run much quieter than conventional ram pumps. This pump is economical and has many interesting features. www.bamford.com.au/rampump

8. Use a gallon container and a watch to measure or estimate the flow of water at the source = _____ gallons per minute (LPM).

9. Determine the amount of water required at the tank _____ gallons per day.

Make sure all of these specifications conform to your needs for water pressure and volume of water. Most often water is pumped to a reservoir located above the garden. Periodically it is dispersed as irrigation water via gravity-flow drip irrigation.

Gasoline-powered pumps are reliable and can lift much water uphill quickly, but they are noisy and polluting. You can purchase a pump already attached to the motor, or connect one yourself and mount it on a board or metal platform. For example, a 4-horsepower pump that weighs 56 pounds (25.4 kg) and pumps 6,300 gallons (23,848 L) per hour costs about $450 USD.

Noise is a major factor in starting up a small, gasoline-powered engine in the middle of a quiet rural area. An oversized muffler and small baffle will deaden most of the exhaust sound, but

will lower the efficiency and will strain the motor. You can also build a shroud around the pump or bury it in a large hole to baffle noise. I was recently in a Northern California area where neighbors agreed to run their pumps the same day of the week to minimize noise pollution.

Battery-powered pumps are an option if noise is a factor. A 1,400 gallons-per-hour (5,300 LPH) electric pump at a 9-foot (2.7 m) head pressure costs about $400 USD. Battery-powered pumps quickly lose lifting ability after 15 feet (4.6 m).

Solar energy is an outstanding way to move water. On a sunny day a 75-watt solar panel supplies enough power to a pump to move 75 gallons (284 L) of water 35 feet (10.7 m) uphill and more than 400 feet (121.9 m) away to a reservoir. Here are 3 great sites to learn more about solar power, www.realgoods.com, www.sargosis.com, and www.otherpower.com.

Set up the pump so that the intake will be able to draw in water easily. An adequate filter on the intake of the pump is essential. A hydraulic ram pump lifts water from a source of flowing water located above the pump. The natural force of gravity and flowing water is all the power needed. Ram pumps are rugged and dependable but noisy. See www.rampumps.com for more information.

The Bamford Hi-Ram Pump is a simple, self-powered water pump using a plastic ball, which makes the pump run much quieter than conventional ram pumps. This pump is economical and has many interesting features. www.bamford.com.au/rampumptial. Pump intakes can be placed in proprietary ponds and ditches, but consult laws about local water rights before using public sources of this precious resource.

Siphoning water downhill is free when the natural force of gravity is applied. With a little effort and knowledge, however, gravity-flow water will also run uphill. The principle is simple: water flowing downhill develops energy. This energy can be used to move it uphill. Water flowing down a hose that is 10 feet (3 m) long can be bent at the

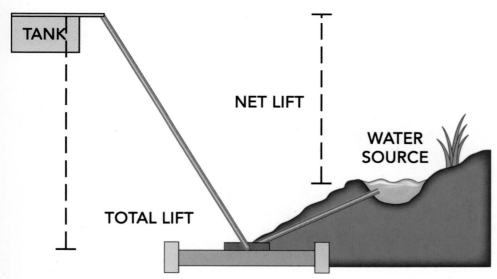

The High Lifter Water Pump is water-powered and will work with a low flow of water. The unique design uses hydraulic pressure and is self-starting and self-regulating. If inlet water stops, so does the pump; the pump starts by itself as soon as water flow begins. They are very quiet and lightweight. Investing in this pump is expensive, but it will last for many years. Check it out at http://high-lifter.com/. I love this pump!

bottom and flow uphill for at least 5 feet (1.5 m). The flow rate decreases as the elevation increases. Experiment with your flow rate and pressure to find out how high water will flow. This is the secret behind making water run uphill. For example, as long as the outlet of the pipe remains below the water surface, water will move higher than the stored water, in a pipe that runs over a hill but then continues until the outlet is below the actual elevation of the water tank or siphon pipe. Make sure to install an on/off valve to stop siphoning. The valve can be manual, or set on a timer or gallon (liter) meter.

Large-diameter hose (0.75 and 1 inch [1.9 and 2.5 cm]) is more expensive but allows for better flow rate and more volume. However, if time, flow rate, and debris blockage are less important, use less-expensive 0.5-inch (1.3 cm) diameter hose. Lightweight hose, which is normally available in green and black, will not disturb foliage.

Temperature and Humidity

Temperatures below 50°F (10°C) and above 86°F (30°C) virtually stop cannabis growth. Temperatures below 40°F (4.4°C) can cause green tissue damage in many varieties, especially when succulent or weak. Low temperatures cause stress in plants. On the other hand, plants in high alpine climates tend to produce more resin and 10 to 20 percent more cannabinoids than those in lower-elevation gardens.

Continental influences cause temperatures to drop more rapidly at night and remain high during the day. Maritime influences buffer and moderate day and nighttime temperatures. Microclimates caused by geography, artificial structures, and so on, influence temperatures too.

Nighttime temperatures are as important to plant growth as daytime temperatures. Nighttime temperatures below 55°F (12.8°C) can slow growth. Nighttime temperatures that drop more than a few degrees cause humidity to increase proportionally. Conversely, nighttime temperatures above 86°F (30°C) stop growth. Southern and tropical gardeners are often faced with this dilemma and must find ways to cool plants at night.

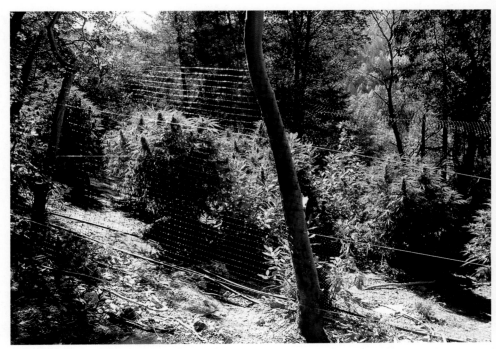

This outdoor garden in Mendocino County, California, is located in a small clearing about 500 feet (152.4 m) from a country home. These plants enjoy a 9-month growing season.

Some *indica*- and *ruderalis*-dominant varieties are able to withstand freezing temperatures but often suffer nutrient imbalances as a result. See chapter 23, *Container Culture & Hydroponics*, for more information on temperature.

The best way to control temperature outdoors is to plant in the proper place. Normally hot temperatures are common during midday in full sun. If you are planting in a hot climate, make sure plants receive filtered sunlight during the heat of the day. Or plant in natural breezeways so a breeze will cool cannabis during the heat of the day. Cold

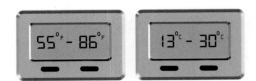

Cannabis grows best between 55°F (13°C) and 86°F (30°C).

temperatures can be avoided by planting at the proper times—well after last frost.

Temperature is difficult to control on sunny terraces and balconies. The reflection and heat-holding ability of tile, concrete, and stone make these spaces a challenge to cool. Shade cloth

shades balcony plants from scorching midday sun. And dousing soil surfaces with water also keeps direct sunlight from heating containers enough to cook roots. See chapter 19, *Containers*, for more information on keeping containers cool.

Growing in Tropical and Subtropical Humid Climates

Temperature can be an issue in tropical climates because there is a dormancy period in summer when nighttime temperatures rise beyond 86°F (30°C). Plants start growing again when nighttime temperatures fall into the seventies (20°C–29°C). For example, an Alabama gardener who plants by July 15 will still produce a leafy plant if it is watered well.

Hot wind is better when it is humid but not so good when it is arid amid high temperatures. Reduce heat stress with shade in the afternoon to block the strongest sunlight. Climates change— and there are many microclimates—so each gardener has to fine-tune his or her garden individually. Select proper plants for your climate, provide filtered light from 2:00 p.m. on, balance the humidity and watering, avoid high-EC feedings (especially nitrogen), and wish for cooler weather in September.

Cool plants by misting them with superfine atomized water. Avoid spraying plants with droplets of water during the heat of the day. Sunlight can burn foliage, leaving small spots on leaves. These spots will also stress plants.

Combat hot temperatures by irrigating with plenty of water. Mulch is essential and will cool roots and soil and cut down on water loss. Also make sure plants have optimum levels of calcium. Do not overfertilize plants in hot weather. High EC (ppm) levels of fertilizer salts and heat do not work well together. See chapter 18, *Soil*, for more information.

Humidity is almost impossible to control outdoors. Locate the garden in a breezy location or microclimate to lessen the effects of humidity. You can plant in cooler, more humid locations in a garden. Natural breezeways are under any tree or structure, between two fences, or in a gulch or canyon. Shady spots in the garden tend to be cooler and a little more humid. See chapter 16, *Air*, for more specific information about humidity.

Wind

Wind is one of the strongest forces medical cannabis plants must withstand outdoors. Sustained desiccating wind sucks moisture from plants. Wind causes plants to draw moisture from the roots and shed it through the leaves as a defense mechanism to regulate internal temperature and chemistry. Severe problems can arise if the water supply is limited for any reason.

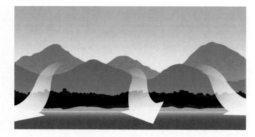

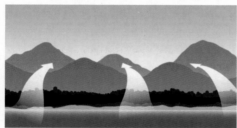

Cool air tends to sit in natural and man-made valleys, which are often a few degrees cooler than surrounding areas. Coastal breezes generally carry air from land out to sea at night. Valleys and exposed hillsides experience more wind. Coastal winds tend to flow inland during the day, creating cool zones.

Both cold and warm winds cause moisture loss, and plants dry out quickly in windy conditions. Moisture must be replaced by irrigating every day or two. Plants that are allowed to dry out completely suffer stress and are soon stunted. Stress also weakens plants and leaves them open to attack by disease and insects.

Wind patterns will affect your garden and influence where plants should be located. Pay attention to conditions and research average wind direction and

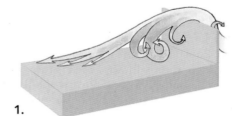
1.

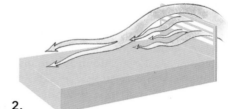
2.

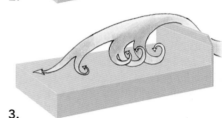
3.

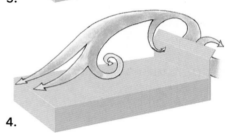
4.

1. A solid wall causes air to drop and whirl about the same distance equal to the height of the wall.

2. A louvered wall diffuses air and protects plants placed 6 to 12 feet (1.8–3.7 m) from the wall.

3. A solid wall that is angled into the wind protects plants close to the wall.

4. A solid wall that is angled away from wind protects plants up to 8 feet (2.4 m) from the wall.

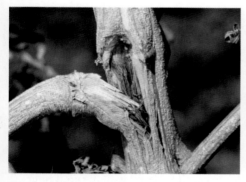

Wind coupled with rain can cause broken branches.

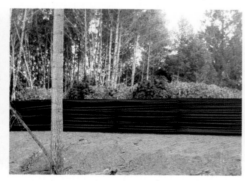

Black shade cloth protects plants from wind and lets some air through. Or protect by planting among other annuals and perennials to block heavy wind. When planting, look for areas that are protected from the wind.

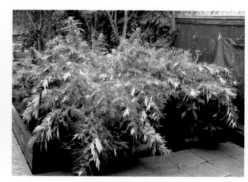

A heavy rainstorm laid this garden on its side. The 'Green Crack' plant in the back has the stoutest stems. I shook off the plants and installed a wire fence around the garden as a trellis.

force in your area. Windbreaks can help protect plants from wind, heat, and water loss. See chapter 16, *Air*, and check your local weather station via the Internet for wind patterns and local conditions over time.

On our terrace, 1.5 miles (2.4 km) from the Mediterranean Sea, the wind often blows throughout much of the day and more in the morning and evening. Plants grown in 5-gallon (18.9 L) containers on a terrace that receives full sun and constant moderate winds use about 2 gallons (7.6 L) of water daily. Indoors, the same plant would use 75 percent less water!

Wind carries pollutants, including male cannabis pollen, dust, and sand. Coastal winds carry salty seawater mixed with fine desert sand. All winds carry fine particles of earth. In Spain "kalmia" is grit mixed with saline air from the Mediterranean. These winds can destroy crops. If your climate is plagued by such abrasive winds, protect plants with windbreaks. Wash foliage with plenty of water to remove the particles after windstorms. Moderate sustained winds will dry out container- and field-grown crops within a few hours. Container crops suffer the most.

Wind also promotes degradation of trichomes on flowering plants. Light breezes cause little damage, but heavy winds cause branches and leaves to rub together and damage fragile trichomes.

Rain
Some gardeners in some climates are able to count on regular spring and summer rains for irrigation. But most growers cannot count on Mother Nature to water their gardens. Cannabis gardens in most climates must be irrigated for best results.

Given the value of medicinal cannabis and the limited cultivation possibilities, most gardens are irrigated. Rain is considered by most gardeners as something to avoid.

Rainwater is heavy and it weighs down blooming cannabis. Rainwater collects between leaves and flowers in buds and on the overall foliage. Many varieties

with weak stems and excessive foliage are unable to support the extra weight and will fall over, often one on top of another. Also, excess moisture creates a perfect environment for the growth of mold.

Avoid damage from rainstorms by staking buds adequately before rain arrives. Use 6-inch plastic or nylon netting to trellis branches in 1- to 2-foot (30.5–61 cm) layers as the plant grows. This will give support to plants in the wind and when heavy rain falls. Bud-laden branches will fall into the netting and not tend to lie over on the side.

A plastic covering over plants is more work to install but can be the best option for many backyard and terrace gardeners. Watch local weather reports and cover plants with a plastic roof before heavy rains fall.

Gardeners in rainy climates can black out greenhouses in mid-summer to induce plants to flower while sunlight is intense and before autumn rains start to fall (see "Light-Deprivation Greenhouse" in chapter 11). Inducing early flowering is also a good tactic to avoid powdery mildew, which is common in gardens after summer ends. Sunlight is also brighter when flowers are ripening.

Protect plants—organically—from desiccating heat and wind. Mix extra calcium, in the form of gypsum, into the soil mix so that plants have the optimum amount available. Fertilizing with the proper levels of calcium will help leaves become more rigid and assist them in retaining moisture. Organic growing techniques help soil retain moisture and toughen up leaves. For more information, see "drought" in the index.

Soil
Soil is divided into 3 basic categories: clay, sand, and silt. Most soils, including those found in grasslands, mountainous areas, bogs, and backyards are combinations of the 3 basic soils. Land alongside most rivers and ancient lakebeds is fertile, while nearby hillside soil is much less fertile. Fertile topsoil is often scraped away around houses during construction. Ask local gardeners and farmers for details on local soils.

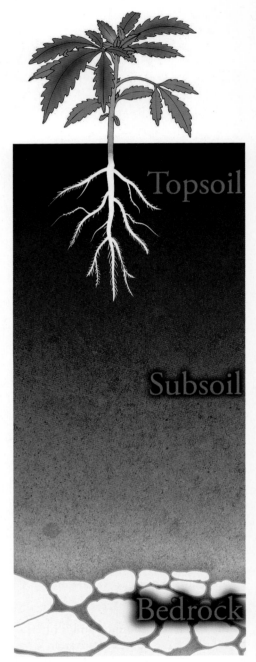

Topsoil is rich and fertile. Soil structure and fertility change with depth.

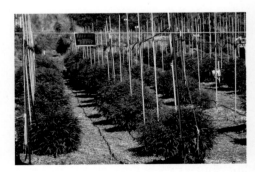

Wooden stakes support plants and provide a frame for irrigation tubing in Eddy Lepp´s garden in Northern California.

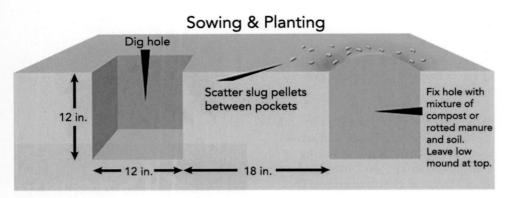

Sowing & Planting

Dig hole

12 in.

12 in.

18 in.

Scatter slug pellets between pockets

Fix hole with mixture of compost or rotted manure and soil. Leave low mound at top.

Always make sure to dig a big planting hole to give roots space to spread out.

Clay soil holds water well and provides slow, even drainage. Clay soils are slow to warm in the spring but hold warmth well into autumn when sunlight is fading. The density of clay does not allow for proper air circulation, however, and root growth is inhibited. Extremely hard and dry clay soil is often referred to as hardpan or adobe. Lime (calcium carbonate) can also form a thick layer in some desert soils and is referred to as hardpan too.

At least a month before planting, prepare clay soil by adding lots of compost and manure. Clay soils can hold water too well, which can smother roots. Adding organic matter will lighten the heavy soil, thus creating air pockets, improving drainage, and promoting root growth. The month's delay gives the manure and compost a chance to assimilate into the soil.

Sandy soil is less common and is often found near large bodies of water, in deserts, and in many inland areas. It is comprised of small, medium, and large particles and is easy to till even when wet. Plants can achieve excellent root penetration. Sandy soil feels and looks gritty.

Sandy soil is easy to work and warms quickly in the spring, but it does not hold fertilizer well, especially when overwatered, which causes the nutrients to wash out. Compost, peat moss, and coco peat help bind the large particles providing food and air circulation, but in hot climates the organic matter decomposes rapidly and is soon consumed by bacteria and other soil organisms. For

best results, keep sandy soil cool and retain moisture with mulch and additional compost. Winter season cover crops will hold moisture and prevent runoff while retaining life in the soil.

Silty soil has all the advantages of clay and sand; it holds moisture and water like clay but is quick to warm and has good drainage and a work-friendly structure like sand. It is the perfect growing medium. Most soils are a combination of sand and clay. Silty loam falls in between and feels almost greasy when rubbed in your hand, though it is less slippery than clay. The ultimate soil for growing plants is loam found in ancient river bottoms and lakebeds where sedimentary soil builds up. It is dark, fertile, and crumbly in the hand.

Forest soils vary greatly in pH and fertility. Needles and deadfall from the trees usually make the soil acidic. Most forests remaining in North America and Europe are on hillsides, since flat land is used for farming, recreation, and urban sprawl. Long-needle pines can grow in poor soils such as those found in mountainous and tropical regions. They have deep roots to look for all the elements in the soil. When a layer of humus evolves, however, short-needle conifers dominate. The roots on these trees spread out on the surface to search for nourishment and bury roots to anchor it in place.

Jungles are usually low-growing, moist, hot, and dense. Jungle soil is shallow and alive. The hot weather makes all foliage that falls to the ground decompose quickly. Often nutrients are

available to plants, but the soil does not have a chance to build density. Layers of tropical soils can be very thin. However, throughout much of Mexico, Central America, and other parts of the world volcanic eruptions have brought much rock and minerals to the surface. Mountain valleys and lowlands are full of alluvial plains packed with nutrient-rich soil.

Grasslands often have wonderful soil that recycles nutrients. Sunshine is likely to be good, but detection could be a problem in wide-open spaces. Plant in areas that are protected from wind.

Mountain soils are often very rich in minerals but lack humus. Alpine valleys hold the best alluvial-plain soil that is the product of volcanic rock erosion. Hillsides are generally less fertile, and soil must be amended to grow a good crop. Most alpine soils lack humus, and strong winds will dry out the plants. For best results, look for patches where pasture grass grows. You can help your plants deal with mountain stress by backfilling planting holes with a mix of peat moss, soil, polymer crystals, and slow-acting layers of organic fertilizer.

Bog soils are moist and spongy. Bogs are filled with vegetation and often have very rich soil. They may present a perfect place to grow individual plants. However, bogs are located in northern climates and most often present a short growing season.

Cut a square yard (0.8 m²) of moist sod from the ground, turn it over, and plant. Marsh ground supplies sufficient water on its own. Add a bit of time-release fertilizer during transplanting and another handful of "flowering" formula during a checkup in early August.

Prepare Soil
To harvest a strong healthy crop, all soils except for silt should be amended before planting. Amendments improve soil, nutrient uptake, root penetration, and soil water retention. Here we will look at how to amend and get the most from outdoor soils. Compare the descriptions of the soils above with your garden soil to learn its basic type. Then follow amendment recommendations.

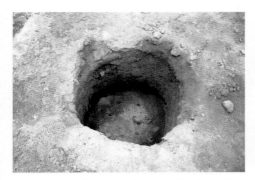

Driving a spade into soil, especially clay soil, causes a microscopic clay soil barrier (aka glazing, as in pottery) in which soil particles lay vertically and are very difficult for roots from transplanted seedlings and clones to penetrate.

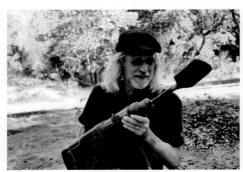

Rent an electric jackhammer and power it with a generator at your garden in the country. A jackhammer with a wide blade makes digging heavy clay and rocky soil much faster.

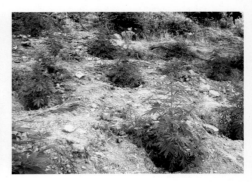

Preparing soil in an arid climate requires large holes and a lot of work! This gardener in Morocco planted in sunken beds to conserve water.

Once you have discerned the type of soil, amend it with appropriate amounts of compost, manure, coco coir, bone meal, minerals, etc. Dig as large a hole as possible for each plant. Dig holes at least 18 inches (45.7 cm) wide by 18 inches (45.7 cm) deep for each plant. Dig holes 3 to 6 feet (0.9–1.8 m) wide and 2 feet (0.6 m) deep if planting big outdoor plants. Spending a little extra time digging a big hole will pay off in fewer problems and a heavier harvest.

Adding water-absorbing polymers in the planting mix is a good defense against dry soil. The crystals expand up to 15 times when watered, making moisture available to the roots for longer periods of time. Slow-release crystals will allow an extended period between watering. This is very helpful if your patch is in a remote location that you cannot visit often.

When adding amendments, backfill in layers. For example: Fill a 2 × 3-foot (0.6 × 0.9 m) deep hole with an 8-inch (20.3 cm) layer of steamed bone meal and soil; cover this with a thin layer of topsoil blended with a rich compost-manure-straw mixture, rock phosphate, and seaweed meal. Build a mound of compost and soil about a foot above ground level. The mound will settle to about half height during the growing season. See "Organic Fertilizers" in chapter 21, *Nutrients*, for more information. See also chapter 13, Case Studies #3 and #4.

On hillsides, planting holes must be terraced and be large enough to catch runoff water. Dig extra gulleys to channel runoff to growing plants, and make a sunken "dish" around the plants to hold runoff water.

If excessive drainage is a problem, which seldom occurs if soil is properly amended, place a substance with different surface tension, such as clay soil or rocks, a foot or two below the bottom of the planting hole. The difference in surface tension will slow downward drainage. You can add many amendments including compost, peat moss, coco peat, good soil, organic nutrients, polymers, and dolomite lime—to help soil hold water—then top with a concave "bowl" of soil that will catch rain and irrigation water.

Soil Tests

Total dissolved solids (TDS) levels for soil and water are very important. Taking a soil test is the only accurate way to know the contents and profile of your soil. The soil scientist will also give recommendations to improve soil.

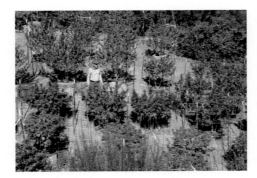

Planting on a hillside requires a small terrace. Containers are set into the hillside to form terraces in this Lake County, California, medical cannabis garden.

Well water and tap water should also be analyzed for high levels of sodium and other dissolved solids that may affect the soil. See chapter 18, *Soil*, for more information on soil tests.

Note: All of these soils and amendments are discussed in detail in chapter 18, *Soil*.

Raised Beds

Raised beds are wonderful for growing in the backyard or in greenhouses. Raised beds warm earlier in the spring and hold warmth longer in the fall. But they may heat up too much in the summer when soil enjoys direct sunlight. Cultivation and weed control are easier in a raised bed, and soil quality is easy to maintain. Build a raised bed on top of poor soils. Planting in a 6- to 8-inch (15.2–20.3 cm) raised bed eliminates the necessity of trying to dig in wet sticky clay while providing the early warmth and good drainage clay lacks. Plants can be put into the ground 2 weeks to a month early and may even produce an early spring crop. I like raised beds framed with lumber because the wooden sides serve as a base for cold frame green house construction. See chapter 11, *Greenhouses*. Find information on building and ready-made raised beds by typing "raised beds" into your favorite web browser.

Raised beds are similar to giant 200- to 500-gallon (757–1892.7 L) containers, except they are often bigger and bottomless, directly in touch with Mother Earth. Make raised beds outdoors, in a greenhouse, or in an indoor garden with

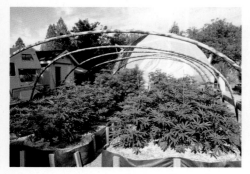

Raised beds were set up by pounding stakes into the ground and lining the "walls" with permeable fabric.

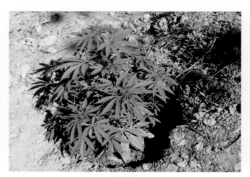

Sunken beds help hold in moisture. The beds need to be dug 6 to 12 inches (15.2–30.5 cm) deep and amended well. Sunken beds allow water to collect during rainstorms.

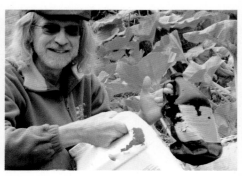

Bears and other animals can be problematic in remote gardens! Organic fertilizers left at the garden site can attract scavengers.

earthen floors. New soil can be added on top of the old. If drainage is poor, dig soil deeper and backfill with well-draining soil. Dig deep ditches to drain excess water away if necessary.

A raised bed with a large soil mass can be built up organically after several crops. To hasten organic activity within the soil, add organic seaweed, manure, and so forth, and let Mother Nature go to work. Do not overdo it! When mixing soil or adding amendments, use the best possible organic components and follow organic soil food web principles. There should be good drainage, and the soil should be as deep as possible, 12 to 24

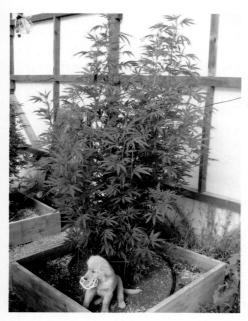

Large planter boxes make a great place for plants and puppies!

inches (30.5–61 cm). See "Organic Soil" in chapter 18, *Soil*, for more information.

A friend of mine plants on top of the compost pile. He plants 6, 12-inch-tall (30.5 cm) clones in 3 to 4 inches (7.6–10.2 cm) of good soil that is on top of a 2- to 3-foot high (61–91.4 cm) compost heap. By the time the roots penetrate into the compost, it has cooled enough and is releasing nutrients.

See also chapter 19, *Containers*; chapter 12, *Outdoors*; and chapter 13, *Case Studies*.

Sunken Beds

Sunken beds conserve moisture in hot climates. Make a sunken bed by digging down 6 to 12 inches (15.2–30.5 cm) and across 2 to 4 feet (0.6–1.2 m) or more to form a big, shallow bowl. (Do not dig deeper; subsoil in hot climates is very poor.) Dig the planting hole in the center of the sunken bed. Make sure to augment the soil with plenty of appropriate amendments. Place a heavy layer of straw, dry foliage, or rocks as mulch in the basin around each plant to conserve water. To accommodate more water and disperse it better, amplify the sunken bed a little as the plant grows.

Use low-sodium manure contains few salts. Cows are fed sodium nitrate, among other things, to make them gain and retain weight. The extra salt is passed into their manure and it will lock up nutrients, burning plants and stunting their growth. Test loads of bulk manure with a sodium (Na) meter or make sure manure is well-composted (3 to 6 months) in an open area to leach out bad salts.

Fertilizers

There are two basic approaches to outdoor fertilization: (1) adding salt-based (synthetic) fertilizers to soil, and (2) building the soil with organic nutrients and supplemental organic fertilizers. Often gardeners build organic soil, yet use salt-based fertilizers that impair or kill soil life. Smart medical cannabis gardeners grow organically.

Once soil has been prepared, it is usually amended with organic fertilizers such as manures and composts that also serve to condition the soil, improving water retention and drainage. Most often a complete range of macro- and micro-organic nutrients are also added to the soil mix. These nutrients will become available as plants mature. Supplemental fertilization may be necessary if soil nutrients become depleted. Supplemental fertilizing is easy with organic (or salt-based) fertilizers applied in a liquid or dry form as per directions. Be careful to avoid overfertilizing—your soil may already contain ample nutrients.

Growing in a container, especially a small container with less than 10 cubic feet (283.2 L) of soil, is much different than growing in living organic soil found in Mother Earth. The difference is buried in the soil biology. When cannabis is grown in a small container for 2 to 4 months, there is no time for soil biology to kick in and build the soil. When growing in containers, regular supplemental fertilizing is necessary.

Organic products such as mycorrhizal fungus and *Trichoderma* will get organic gardens off to a good start. See chapter 22, *Additives*, for more information.

When choosing organic fertilizers, remember that many of them are "alive"—some more so than others! Dry organic fertilizers can be full of dormant soil biology that springs to life and multiplies when water and air are added. See chapters 18, *Soil*, and 21, *Nutrients*, for more information on fertilizers and fertilizer mixes.

Properly mixed in a large container, organic soil can have all the nutrients necessary in an available form from transplant through harvest. The large growing container and rich organic mix are the first secrets to success. Build organic soils using natural elements such as manures, composts, peat moss and coco coir, rock powders, kelp and seaweed. Whenever possible, use the most readily available and least expensive ingredients.

Be sparing with fertilizer during the first month after transplanting. Depending upon the fertilizer, application could be as often as every watering or as seldom as every week or two. Often gardeners fertilize with a mild, soluble flowering

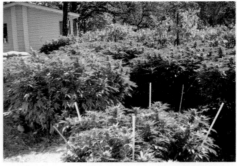

This vegetable garden was transformed into a medical cannabis garden. To facilitate maintenance, the gardener left plenty of space between plants.

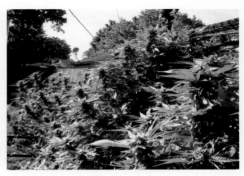

Medical cannabis plants can also supply shade. Four plants shade one wall of a home, which keeps it cooler indoors. These plants are 8 feet (2.4 m) tall!

solution for germination and seedling growth. Change to a high-nitrogen formula during the vegetative stage and back to a "super-bloom" when long nights induce flowering.

If fertilizing every few irrigations or every irrigation, you may need to dilute the food to half-strength or less until you figure out the proper dosage. Use the instructions on the fertilizer label as a guide.

If you must transport fertilizers, make sure they are in dry or powder form, lightweight, and not bulky. Avoid leaving fertilizers at remote gardens, especially those with ingredients such as molasses, blood meal, or bone meal, which attract animals—including bears. I recently visited a garden where containers had been ripped open and the fertilizer consumed by a bear.

Backyard Gardens

Backyard medical cannabis gardeners are available to give their garden the tender loving care it deserves. Paying close attention to plants' cultural needs pays off in big, healthy plants and abundant harvests at the end of each growing season.

Site the garden in the sunniest part of the yard, usually where the vegetable garden is located. Growing medical cannabis in flower and vegetable gardens allows a gardener to glean experience from past gardens.

Prepare soil in the fall. Remove rocks, debris, and weeds, and dig planting

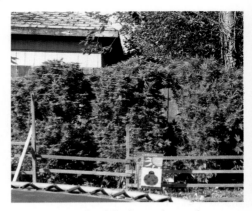

A backyard garden full of cannabis can be ornamental.

holes or garden beds. The best gardens grow in tilled soil with plenty of organic amendments. Many gardeners prefer raised beds. No-till organic gardeners leave the soil "as is" and add a heavy layer of mulch. Either way, a layer of mulch is helpful. A 4- to 6-inch (10.2–15.2 cm) layer of mulch will keep soil elements intact, as well as attract moisture. Bare soil loses some of its valuable topsoil and nutrients to erosion during winter months.

In the spring, mulched amended soil should be well-mixed and ready for planting. If soil is poor and was not amended the previous fall, dig large holes 3 feet (0.9 m) in diameter by 2 feet (0.6 m) deep, and backfill with good soil/compost, potting soil, or planting mix. Otherwise, break up the top 6 to 8 inches (15.2–20.3 cm) of soil in a 6-foot (1.8 m) radius to provide room for root penetration.

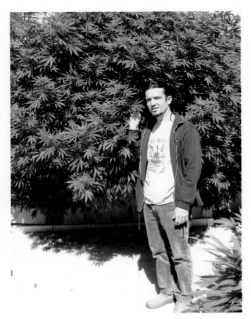

Backyard gardens are easy to grow. Wismy, editor of Yerba *magazine in Spain, stands in front of a healthy cannabis plant in one of the many backyard gardens found in Spain.*

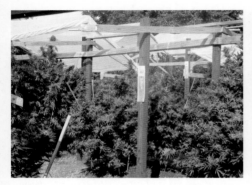
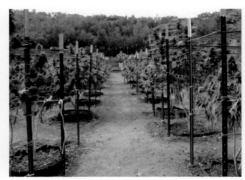
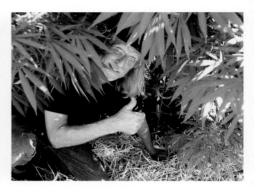

A little plastic stretched over a simple structure keeps plants much warmer at night. It also keeps plants from suffering damaging effects of wind and pounding rain.

Some medical cannabis gardeners are fortunate to have big backyards!

Mulch is essential and serves to keep soil cool and protected from temperature extremes and compaction by heavy rains.

Transplant cannabis seedlings or clones into the garden after threat of frost, and if temperatures dip below 50°F (10°C) at night, protect with a cloche, hot cap, or Wall O Water. Follow planting guidelines for setting out tomatoes.

Water and fertilize as needed. Make sure to keep up with watering during hot weather. Irrigate in the morning so that water has a chance to be used all day long. Mixing fertilizer with water is a simple and effective way to fertilize. If fertilizing with dry powders, mix them into the top few inches (cm) of soil so that they are effective.

Be on the lookout for pests and diseases, and take appropriate control measures. Flower and vegetable gardens can contract seasonal diseases and pests including powdery mildew, spider mites, and thrips that can spread to cannabis gardens. Control diseases and pests on flowers and vegetables early on so they do not spread to the cannabis garden. Follow guidelines below for planting, maintenance, and harvest.

Container Gardens

Growing in containers is the easiest option for gardeners with limited space or very bad soil. Containers can be moved into sunny and warm locations. Grow cannabis outdoors in containers that can hold from 1 to 500 gallons (3.8–1892.7 L). Small containers are easy to pick up, scoot around, or move with a caster platform. Handles on 5- to 20-gallon (18.9–75.7 L) containers make them easier to pick up and move. Large 200-gallon (757 L) containers

can be placed on a pallet and moved with a forklift–equipped tractor. Always move plants *before* watering!

Backyard gardening techniques depend upon the location and microclimate in the garden. City building rooftops, terraces, and balconies tend to be windy, as do hilltops and hillsides. The higher the garden, the more wind. Wind quickly dries plants and soil. Patio gardens are often protected from strong winds. If not, erect a wind block made from 50 percent shade cloth, lattice or another semipermeable material. Wind

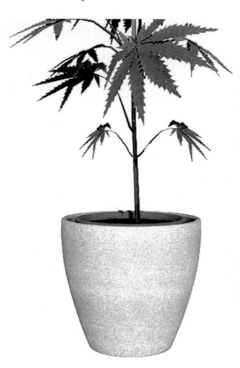

Setting the growing container inside a larger container will help protect soil from heating in the direct sunlight.

can also carry rogue male pollen or industrial hemp pollen creating problems for terrace gardeners. Plan ahead and know your neighbors. For more information, see "Rogue Pollen" in chapter 25, *Breeding*.

Small containers fit easily on a patio, balcony terrace, or rooftop. Plants need a sunny location, good genetics, good soil, water, and nutrients. Direct sunlight beaming down on containers can cook roots, however; shade containers from direct sunlight. Putting pots inside other containers can help protect roots

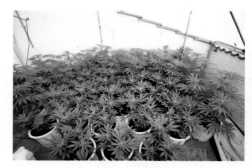

This terrace garden is flowering in the springtime.

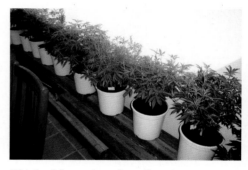

This healthy garden of 5-gallon (18.9 L) containers is being moved outdoors to flower.

from the sun. See chapter 19, *Containers*, for more information.

Daily watering and maintenance are essential during hot and windy weather. An automatic watering system is often a good idea in such gardens to ensure they receive adequate water, especially if you will be away from the garden for days at a time.

For more information, see chapter 19, *Containers*, and chapter 13, Case Study #4.

Follow guidelines below for planting, maintenance, and harvest.

Large Gardens

Large gardens require a full-time investment of time and assets. For example, a 99-plant garden full of big 10-pound (4.5 kg) plants can yield about 990 pounds (449.1 kg) of dried cannabis and almost the same amount of stems, leaves, and trim, all of which must be processed. Planting, growing, harvesting, curing, and packaging a big garden is a big job. Planning is essential to the success of large outdoor gardens. Smart gardeners lay out a week-by-week plan.

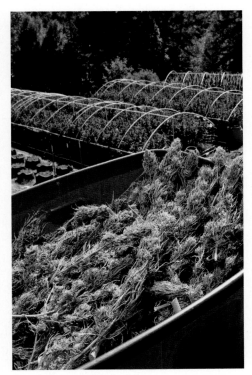
Big plants grow big buds!

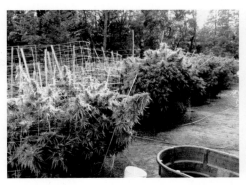
Large outdoor plants require more garden and soil preparation, water, and maintenance.

First, a perfect variety for your climate (preferably an F1 hybrid), must be grown from seeds or clones. It must be planted in January or February indoors and moved outdoors in April or May. Lights must be installed in the temporary greenhouse over the plants to keep them from blooming. Hundreds of gallons (L) of soil must be mixed and potted. In midsummer, individual plants will need up to 10 gallons (37.8 L) of water daily. This garden will need up to 1,000 gallons (3,785.4 L) of water every day! At harvest, 1 person can manicure 1 pound per day. The fastest machine can trim 3 to 4 pounds in an hour. A team of 12 people (that must be paid) with 1 trimming machine can process about 30 pounds (13.6 kg) a day; 1,000 pounds / 30 pounds (453/13.6 = 33) = 33 10-hour workdays. I have never seen an operation this efficient. Normally 1,000 pounds (453.6 kg) takes 12 workers with a trimming machine 3 months to manicure, dry, and preserve. A detailed plan with a timeline is in order!

Large gardens are a full-time job and must be cared for at all times. Roaming around in between the plants is always fun and informative. Inspecting all the plants daily is very rewarding; they teach you something every day. Remember that any problem such as trellising, diseases, and pests occurs in a big way to many plants. It is very important to avoid problems before they occur. Keen observation skills will be necessary. See chapter 13, *Case Studies*, for more information about large gardens.

Follow guidelines in this chapter for planting, maintenance, and harvest.

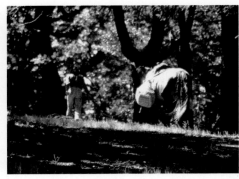
This clandestine cannabis gardener hauled her supplies in on a horse in the late 1970s. (MF)

Remote Gardens

Remote gardens are sometimes referred to as "guerrilla gardens," a term coined in the early 1970s. Remote gardens require strategy, time, and frequently, physical prowess. Unfortunately, international, national, state, and local laws can deem growing medical cannabis illegal. Clandestine guerrilla growing in remote locations is the only option for medical cannabis gardeners in such hostile areas. Location and security are the main concerns for a medical cannabis guerrilla grower. Choose a location that has limited public access. Check regulations for hunting, recreation, and insurgent movements. Consider who might be using the area, such as hunters, mushroomers, illegal marijuana growers, hikers, dirt-bikers, and Boy Scouts. Select a remote site unlikely to be used casually.

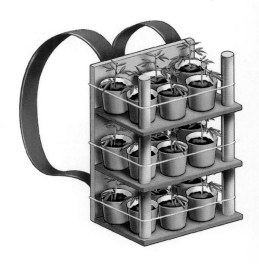
Loading clones and seedlings in a backpack in boxes is a safe convenient way to transport them to the garden site.

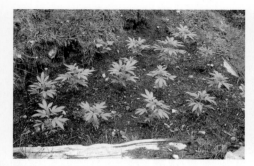
'Little Bonkers' seedlings from NGSC are planted on this fertile hillside terrace.

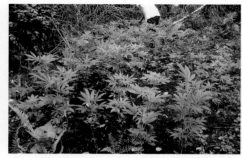
These seedlings were moved out and transplanted six weeks before the photo was taken. Clearing thick undergrowth in the British Colombia, Canada, forest was a big job.

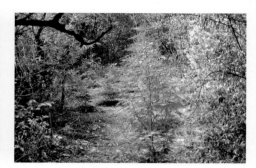
This Basque cannabis gardener turned an unused road into a remote garden patch.

Some gardeners go so far as to bury 8 × 8 × 40-foot (2.4 × 2.4 × 12.2 cm) shipping containers underground to serve as a garden area. These gardens are quite interesting. The containers are set in a trench or hole on 2- to 4-foot (0.6–1.2 m) blocks. The area underneath the container serves as ventilation ducting. Earth is filled in around and over the container; it also serves to insulate the subterranean garden.

Other clandestine gardeners have buried large, 12- to 14-foot (3.7–4.3 m) culverts (big pipes) in the ground. These were divided into top and bottom garden rooms.

Growing cannabis on federal or public land is not advised. Unfortunately, park rangers in the USA now carry lethal firearms and have the authority to arrest "suspected" gardeners. A few trigger-happy survivalists and a minority of South American organized crime factions have also moved into national forests, installing illegal immigrants with guns to grow and defend large stands of guerrilla grass. However, many times Latin immigrants band together in small groups and plant in the wild. These small groups of people have nothing to do with organized crime across borders. They want only a better life for their families. The War on Drugs has turned

gardening into a crime, and much of the world, particularly the Americas, into an unsafe place to live.

Remote gardens are often located in or near big green stands of vegetation. Cannabis is a vigorous plant and can have a large root system. A flowering female will stand out if surrounding vegetation dies back before cannabis is harvested. Stands of thorny blackberry bushes, ferns, and meadow grass are good options for planting locations.

Prepare the medical cannabis garden up to 6 months before planting. Remove green vegetation in the fall for a spring

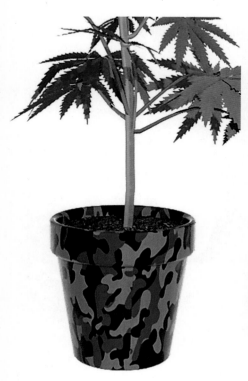
Camouflage grow bags and pots are available.

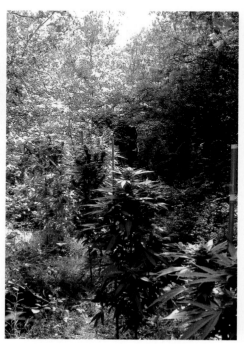
Poor soil and lack of water are two of the biggest problems remote gardens face. These plants weighed in at between 6 and 12 ounces, respectively (170.1 and 340.2 gm).

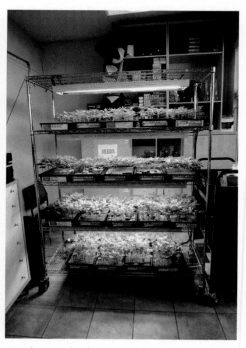
Outdoor medical cannabis gardeners can purchase clones grown indoors at dispensaries such as this one in Oaksterdam. Gardeners take the clones home and grow them indoors for a month or two before transplanting outdoors.

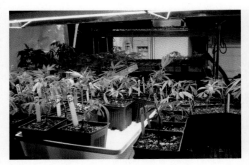

Clones growing in 4-inch (10.2 cm) containers will soon start the vegetative growth stage. When the clones are a foot (30.5 cm) tall, they will be ready to move outdoors.

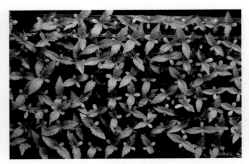

These seedlings will be transplanted into deep containers and moved outdoors in 2 months, after their sex has been determined.

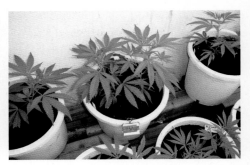

Move transplanted clones outdoors for a few hours every day to harden-off and acclimate them to the harsher outdoor climate. After about a week, they should be acclimated.

garden. Clear a few patches to allow sufficient sunshine, cut back roots of competing plants, and dig planting holes 2 to 3 feet square (61–91.4 cm³). Dig holes wider than deep so that surface roots can take hold. If possible, allow amended soil to sit for a month or longer before planting. Remote locations are hard to visit on a regular basis, so proper planning and preparation is important. If home and remote gardens are similar, you can plant an indicator crop like tomatoes as a backyard guide to your hidden plants' condition.

Ample water is an important factor for site selection. If you cannot count on rainfall, locate your garden near a water source that does not dry up in the summer; doing so will make watering easier. Water may have to be piped in from another source, including pumped uphill and stored in a reservoir. Exclusive access by boat may reduce the risk of discovery, but make sure your plants cannot be seen from the water. Many people use waterways and explore land bordering rivers.

Follow guidelines in this chapter for planting, maintenance, and harvest.

Starting Clones & Seedlings Indoors

Get a jump on the season by starting cannabis clones and seedlings under lights indoors. Move small, containerized plants into heated greenhouses to harden-off. Transplant them to a backyard or remote garden once they have become hardened-off and are more resistant to environmental stress.

Grow seedlings in tall containers (3 inches square by 6 inches tall) (7.6 × 7.6 × 15 cm), which will produce a strong, deep root system and a plant that has a better chance of surviving in tough conditions. Water seedlings and clones heavily before transplanting. A little effort preparing the planting holes will result in healthier plants and a heavier harvest.

Start seedlings and cuttings indoors and move them into a heated greenhouse in March or April or as soon as you can in your climate. A 400-watt HP sodium lamp on a timer can augment the less-intense natural light of early spring. Seedlings and clones will need at least 16 hours of artificial and natural light per day until plants are transplanted outdoors.

Transplant into a temporary greenhouse as soon as nighttime outdoor temperatures are 50°F (10°C), or earlier if the structure is heated.

Getting plants outdoors and established early in the spring allows plants to take advantage of the entire growing season. Given favorable conditions, a plant that is 3 feet (0.9 m) tall the first of May will produce about twice as much as a plant that is 3 feet (0.9 m) tall by the first of June.

Some medical gardeners keep a stream of plants moving from the indoor garden to the outdoor garden. The first crop of clones is planted in 3-gallon (11.4 L) pots in a greenhouse. Once they are hardened-off they are moved to their final location outdoors. The second crop

is moved into the greenhouse when the first crop is moved out. This process can be repeated 3 to 4 times during the season.

Transplant 1-foot-tall (30.5 cm) seedlings and clones by removing the first few sets of leaves and burying the root ball deeper, with only 8 inches (20.3cm) of foliage left above ground. Roots will grow along the belowground stem in a few weeks. Outdoors, when planted in Mother Earth, deep roots will create more self-sufficient plants. This is of particular importance in remote areas that are hard to get to, and in the mountains where rainfall may be sporadic.

Note: Outdoors in the ground only! This technique does not work the same in containers. Strong roots do not always grow off the stem and the main root ball often stays at the bottom of the pot.

Hardening-Off Plants

Seedlings and clones grown indoors are very tender. Indoors, seedlings and clones lose much of their protective waxy coating when they are pampered with the indoor climate. Hardening-off is the process of toughening-up clones and seedlings so they can be transplanted outdoors. During hardening-off the protective wax coating has a chance to grow back on foliage. Gradually hardening-off clones assures that they will suffer a minimum of stress and will continue to grow rapidly outdoors.

To harden-off seedlings and clones, set them outdoors for progressively more hours over the course of a week. Set transplants out in the shade on the first day. Gradually move them into the sun so they receive progressively more hours of sunlight every day. If temperatures are below 50°F (10°C), bring transplants in at night. Or you could set them out under a plastic greenhouse.

Transplants suffer a huge climate and temperature shock when moved outdoors. Wait to move clones and seedlings outdoors until they are fully rooted and growing well. It takes time to toughen up to the climate outdoors. Transplant seedlings and clones outdoors when nighttime temperatures are above 40°F (4.4°C). Planting under plastic will help protect tender plants from cold temperatures and winds.

A temporary cold frame greenhouse will give plants a much stronger start when temperatures are below 50°F (10°C). The superstructure of a greenhouse provides a place to hang lights if there are not enough hours of daily sunlight for early spring plantings.

Planting Time

Planting time outdoors depends upon the weather. There has been little scientific research into planting temperatures for cannabis outdoors. In general, do not transplant seedlings or clones until nighttime temperatures are above 50°F (10°C). If the garden bed is raised or heat is added to a greenhouse at night, temperatures can be lower. Hardened-off plants should be protected from cold weather, rain and wind with a small plastic greenhouse until weather warms. The plastic skin or greenhouse is removed during hot days and replaced when temperatures drop at night. Some years the crop can have full exposure in May. Other years we have to cover the greenhouse until the middle of June.

Maintenance

Backyard gardens can be watered along with vegetables, lawns, and trees. Plants need plenty of water when days get hot. Keep an eye out for cultural problems, pests, and diseases. In the USA you can telephone the local master gardeners at the County Extension Agency to ask about current pests and diseases.

THREE GARDEN PLANS

Planting Dates	Plant	Harvest
spring crop	March 15	May 15-30
fall crop	May 1	October 15-30
summer greenhouse crop	May 1	August 15-30*

*Note: Darken greenhouse every evening to black out plants so they receive 12 hours of uninterrupted darkness.
Note: Dates are the opposite by 180 days in the Southern Hemisphere.

Container gardens require regular watering—usually daily. Set up a sun-block around containers to keep soil cool. Containers left to cook in the sun suffer fried roots and stopped growth.

Large gardens need regular, daily maintenance. Routinely check plants for diseases and pests. Water the garden every day or every other day when temperatures climb. Add extra mulch around plants to conserve and attract moisture.

Remote gardens require a complete low-maintenance setup. Loosen the soil, amend it, and throw in a few handfuls of polymers to retain moisture. A thick layer of mulch, early in the year, will attract water, keep the soil cool, and prevent evaporation. Water and fertilize as needed.

Regular irrigation is the primary maintenance medical cannabis plants require outdoors. Basic information about irrigation is given under the heading "Water."

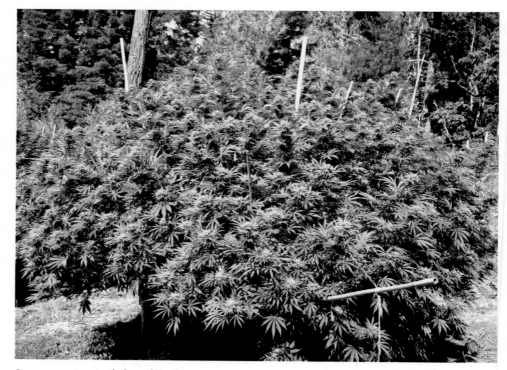

Large containerized plants like this one require water every couple of days. Always check foliage for pests and diseases while watering.

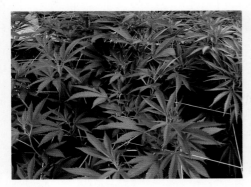

A nylon horizontal trellis is easy to stretch over the garden.

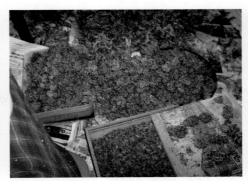

This manicured cannabis will be dried on screens.

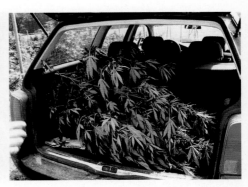

A Swiss gardener harvested a couple of plants. Transporting whole plants requires extra space, but he took them home to manicure.

Plants should also be inspected regularly for pests and diseases. Caterpillars, spider mites, thrips, and more can move into a garden unnoticed. Careful scrutiny is necessary to find and destroy pests quickly and efficiently. Pay close attention to plants every time you are in the garden. Check foliage for signs of mold, insects, caterpillars, and fertilizer excesses or deficiencies. See chapter 24, *Diseases & Pests*, for more information on identification and treatment of disease and pest attacks.

Trellis plants as needed. Always plan ahead. It is easier to build a trellis when plants are small. See "Trellises and Ties" in chapter 6, *Vegetative Growth*.

Pest prevention is crucial for all medicinal crops, especially low-maintenance gardens. It is easier to keep pests from attacking plants in the first place than to do damage control later. Build a fence to protect seedlings and small vegetative plants from deer. A low, electrified fence is in order for wild pigs and various

other rodents. See chapter 24, *Diseases & Pests*, for more information.

Water and fertilize as needed. See chapters in this book that pertain to specific outdoor needs.

Harvest

Backyard and container-garden harvests are easy because all facilities are at hand. Harvest as for indoor gardens. See chapter 9, *Harvest, Drying & Curing*, for more information.

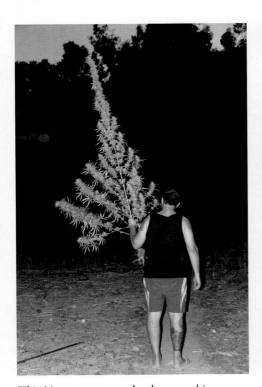

This Moroccan grower has been working all day. This is one of the many plants he harvested on a very productive day.

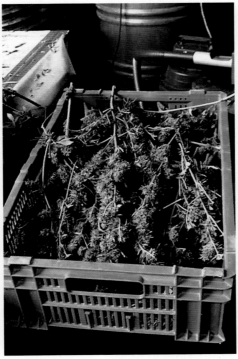

Branches full of flower buds are cut from plants and transported to the manicuring room in this lightweight plastic container.

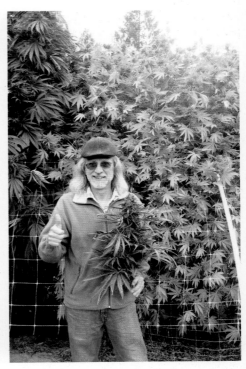

This is one of the top buds from the 'Purple Star' plant behind me. The local variety is well acclimated to the area and produces exceptionally well there. The entire plant yielded 12 pounds (5.4 kg) of dried flower buds!

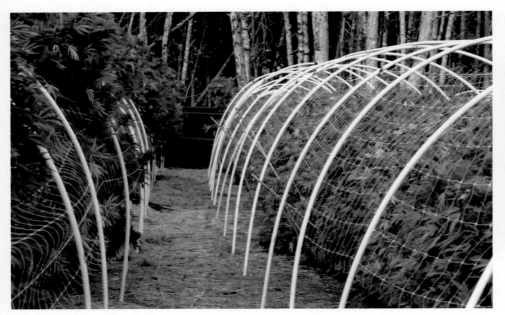

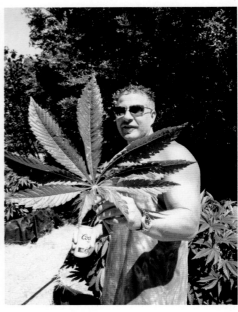

The garden on the right has been harvested once and will be harvested one more time. The garden on the left will be harvested for the first time.

Some leaves should be framed!

Large outdoor harvests require planning and hard work. Harvesting a 5- to 10-pound (2.3–4.5 kg) plant takes time, space, and physical energy. Read about harvesting large gardens in chapter 9, *Harvest, Drying & Curing.*

A trick that helps prolong harvest and increase harvest weight is to harvest the top 2 feet (60.9 cm) of large plants. Let secondary buds continue to mature in the newfound sunlight. Some varieties, such as 'Mr. Nice', can be harvested up to 4 times when grown as big plants!

Harvesting remote gardens is challenging. Harvest before cold, damp autumn weather sets in. This weather causes fungus—*Botrytis* (bud mold) and powdery mildew. Many *indica*-dominant plants can take a short, mild freeze (30°F–32°F [-1°C–0°C]). But if the temperature stays below freezing for more than a few hours, it could kill plants. Pay close attention to weather forecasts and apply the information to the microclimate where your plants are growing. Be ready to harvest quickly if weather dictates.

Accidents and thieves can force a harvest, too. Limit potential discovery by hunters, hikers, and others by harvesting at night. Find out when hikers are prone to visit the area, and plan accordingly. Some gardeners even use police scanners that pick up local police activities.

Should you encounter other hikers or unwanted people while visiting or harvesting the crop, have a believable story to explain your presence in the area. Offer nothing, explain little, and keep conversations simple. Always remember Bart Simpson's words, "I didn't do it. Nobody saw me. You can't prove a thing!"

Take a sharp pocketknife or pruners to cut plants, and a backpack to haul away the harvest. If large amounts must be harvested, it is easier to "field strip" plants before transporting. If harvesting more than one variety, put each of them in separate bags, or wrap them in newspaper before they go into the backpack.

See chapters 8 and 9 for more information on flowering and harvesting.

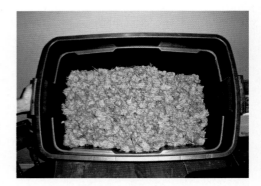

Harvested flower buds are tossed into this large bin after manicuring. They will be moved to drying racks.

Catch and save all leaves and small trim around buds. Separate into low, medium, and high grades. See chapter 9, *Harvest, Drying & Curing*, for more information on drying leaves and leaf trim around buds. Convert leaves and trim into concentrates (chapter 26, *Medicinal Concentrates & Tinctures*) or cook with it (chapter 27, *Cooking with Medicinal Cannabis*).

PART 2 ESSENTIAL MEDICAL CANNABIS HORTICULTURE

13
CASE STUDY #1
INDOOR GARDEN

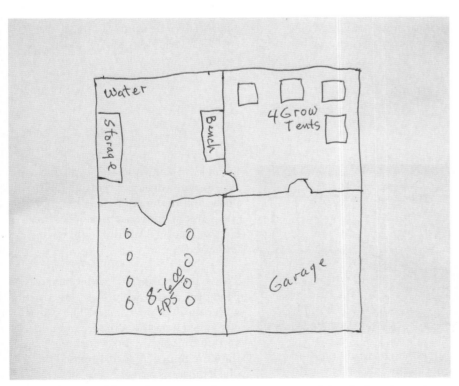

A rough drawing of the garden rooms and garage was an essential tool when the gardeners were in the initial planning stages. A detailed drawing with precise measurements was made before starting construction.

TWO GROWERS, Mitch and Tim, personify many new growers that have learned the basics of crossing and feminizing cannabis. They are crossing autoflowering feminized plants with "regular" photoperiod-reactive males and females. The regular male and female plants are grown from seed for selection and then multiplied into cuttings.

The beautiful indoor garden is in a basement with a concrete floor. The single secure point of access is through a secret door in the garage. The entry door, secured with a deadbolt lock, is hidden inside a locked storage cabinet.

A doorway to the left leads to a 10 × 10-foot (3 × 3 m) work and storage room. An immediate left turn leads through a doorway to the main flowering room. The storage room is full of soil, containers, two 55-gallon (208.2 L) reservoirs for water and nutrient solution, a potting bench, garden supplies, and a few garden tools.

Construction

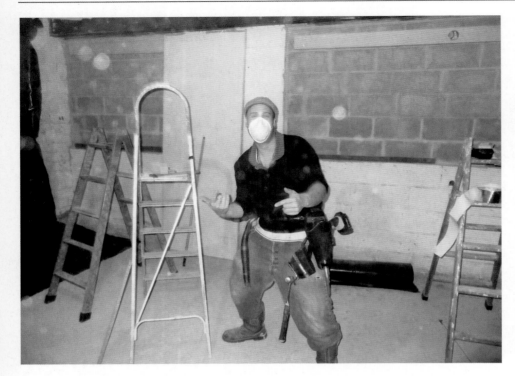

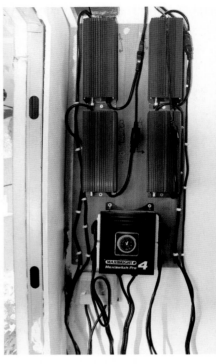

Ready and working! Tim kept all his tools at hand on a tool belt and in special pockets. A dust mask protected him from ever-present construction dust when working with Sheetrock and plaster.

In the original space, water seeped through the basement walls. To remedy this perpetual problem, the gardeners built a new inside wall of cinder blocks. They sandwiched a layer of heavy-duty water barrier material to keep the seepage behind the cinder block wall.

The floor was lined with a double-layer plastic water barrier. The barrier developed small holes after the first year and had to be replaced with a more durable product.

Four adjustable (400- to 600-watt) ballasts and a timer were mounted on a separate board for each side of the garden room. They were mounted at eye level for easy monitoring and to avoid splashes of irrigation water.

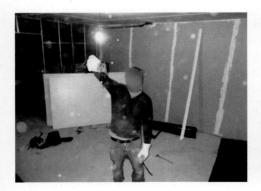

Drywall (aka Sheetrock) is color-coded green to signify it is water-resistant.

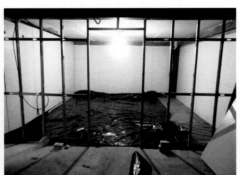

Aluminum-stud construction is easy to manage; aluminum studs weigh

much less than wood studs. Wiring can be threaded through premade holes in the aluminum studs. The big room was wired with two separate electrical circuits, each side of the room having a dedicated circuit.

The walls were covered with reflective panels filled with Styrofoam and covered with thin aluminum sheets. The panels dovetailed together and were mounted to a wood backing. Lights were hung from the aluminum beams that framed the ceiling, which was covered with Sheetrock.

Soil, Water, and Nutrients

Soil, water, and nutrients had to be sorted out before gardening could start.

Soil

Used soil was kept outdoors in 3-foot-tall (91.4 cm) plastic bins. The gardeners added an enzyme product whose manufacturer claims leaches out any built-up salts. They also include a dose of Gnat Off to kill gnats and gnat eggs before bringing the used soil back indoors. Used soil was left outdoors, exposed to the elements for a minimum of 30 days, before being reintroduced to the indoor garden room.

Water

The water for the gardens came from a well, and the composition of the well water changed throughout the year. In the late summer, more dissolved solids were in the water supply. Readings for input water EC were 610 ppm and pH 8.2. Plants would grow well for the first 3 to 5 weeks, and then nutrient problems would manifest.

The gardeners installed a reverse osmosis filter to remove salts from water and lower the pH. However, water pressure in the garden room was at 1.4 bars. The RO device required 2.4 bars of pressure to force water through the filter. They replaced the pump, after which the pressure was 2.7 bars and the RO filter worked perfectly.

Nutrients

Once a week, 2 heaping teaspoons of molasses were added to every 8 gallons (30.3 L) of irrigation water. Fertilization with molasses started 2 weeks after transplanting into 3-gallon (11.4 L) containers. Weekly fertilization with molasses continued until the end of flowering.

Epsom salts were applied once during late vegetative growth and once after 3 to 4 weeks of flowering. Varieties that needed a higher dose of nutrients received a topdressing of chicken manure. This tactic made it much easier to care for many plants with different fertilizer needs.

SOIL MIX			
Amount	Measure	Metric	Notes
7	cubic feet	200 liters	used soil
2.6	gallons	10 liters	Biobizz Premix
1.3	gallons	5 liters	perlite
1.3	gallons	5 liters	vermiculite*
1	pound	450 grams	dolomite lime
2.2	pounds	1 kilogram	worm castings
1	pound	450 grams	bat guano

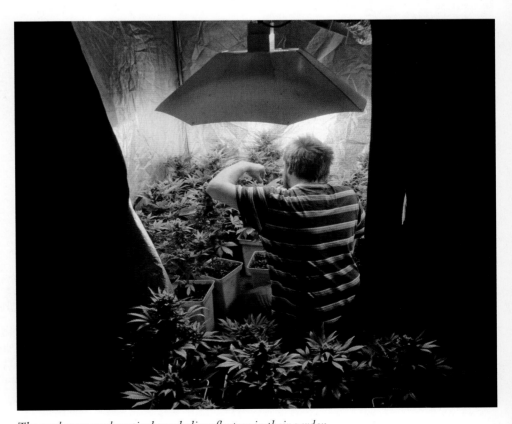

The gardeners used vertical parabolic reflectors in their garden.

Grow-Tent Rooms

The main door to the gardens opened into a room that measured 10 × 15 feet (5 × 4.6 m) and contained 4 grow tents, each 4 × 4 × 6 feet (1.2 × 1.2 × 185 m) and equipped with a 600-watt HPS lamp.

There are many different grow-tent manufacturers, and most grow tents are easy to set up and start using. Setup takes about 30 minutes, and the tents come with written setup instructions; some even have video instructions that can be found on YouTube.

The grow tents were filled with flowering crops or clones, seedlings, and mother plants. A workbench along the wall was stocked with indoor garden supplies, and tools were hung on hooks above. A big open space in the middle of the room served as a staging area to move plants, soil, and supplies in and out of the garden area.

Each 4 × 4-foot (1.2 × 1.2 m) tent yielded from 12.6 to 26 ounces per 600 watts (0.6–1.2 grams per watt). Clones were taken as needed 4 to 5 weeks beforehand, and seeds were planted 3 to 5 weeks before moving them into the flowering room.

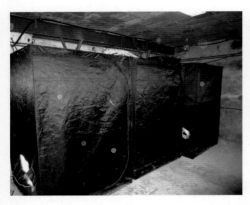

Grow tents stay a few degrees warmer when set up off the floor on pallets. Setting up individual garden rooms allowed complete control of the environment. Each tent could grow a different seeded variety of cannabis. Or cuttings or seedlings could be grown in the tent and later moved into the big flowering room. The tent could also be used as a drying room.

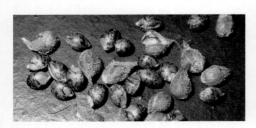

Seeds from breeding crosses were collected and planted once the grow tents were completed.

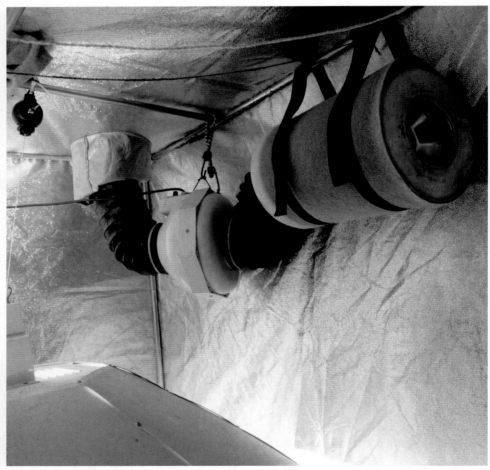

A carbon air filter with an inline 4-inch (10.2 cm) temperature-controlled, 138 cfm (270 m³/hr) fan was connected to a short run of ducting that efficiently eliminated cannabis fragrances from the grow tent. The fan also kept the air in the tent changed and the temperature perfect. The high-quality inline fan ran very quietly, day and night.

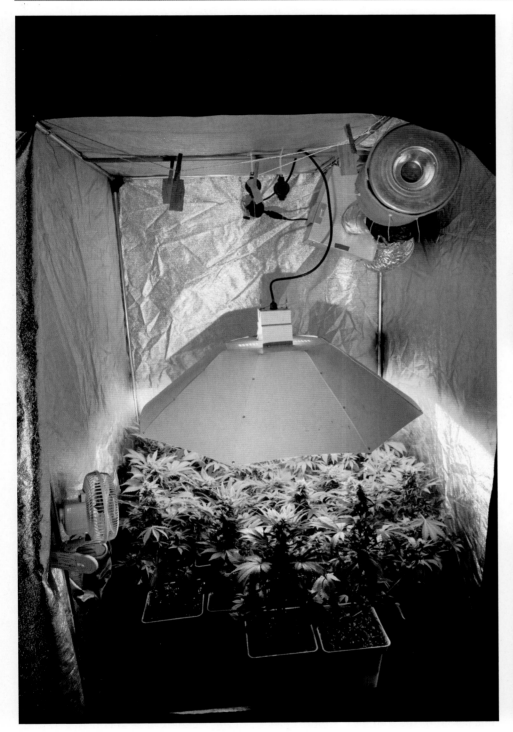

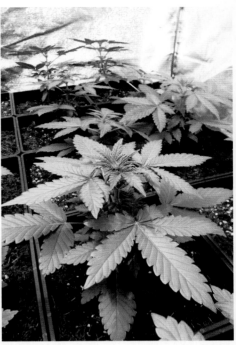

This 18-day-old autoflowering feminized seedling showed healthy foliage growth. Strong vegetative growth transforms into robust flowering, which is perfect for a sea of green garden.

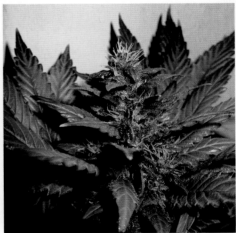

A parabolic dome reflector and 600-watt HPS lamp provided an even canopy of light to the seedlings in this grow tent. The gardeners kept temperatures lower, which allowed the lamp to be placed closer to plants.

Genetic differences in flowers became more pronounced closer to harvest. This 'Blueberry'-based automatic turns purple for harvest.

Grow-Tent Rooms (cont.)

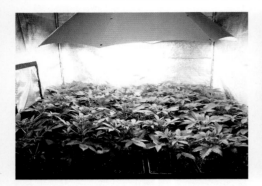

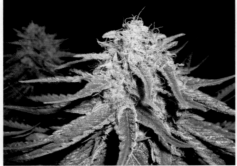

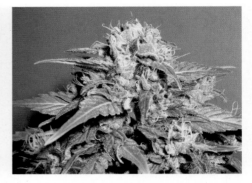

At just 21 days after breaking ground, these little autoflowering feminized seedlings were already starting to flower! The rapid growth phase starts at flowering and continues for another 2 weeks. During this growth phase, growth can quadruple.

This regular, resinous 'Panama' × 'Deep Chunk' bud was on the verge of harvest. The gardeners grew both autoflowering plants and regular females from clones in this garden. This particular plant was part of an autoflowering breeding project.

Another close-up view of the same harvest shows us the quantity of cannabinoid-rich, capitate-stalked resin glands covering the floral clusters of this autoflowering breeding parent plant.

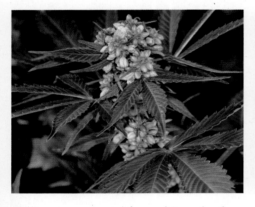

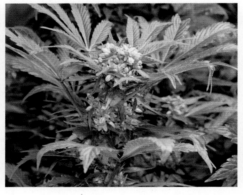

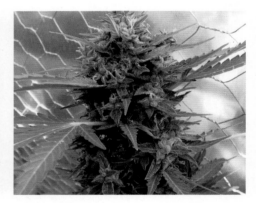

Pollen was captured from this male plant to use for breeding.

Male plants were segregated into a single grow tent.

This breeding female was recently pollinated and will produce seeds in a few weeks.

Big Rooms

The 13.8 × 19-foot (4.2 × 5.8 m) flowering room had eight 600-watt HPS lamps—4 on each side. Each lamp had a vertical parabolic reflective hood and remote ballast. The lamps were mounted overhead with 2 adjustable nylon cords that kept hoods hanging evenly. The 1 × 2-inch (2.5 × 5 cm) boards were attached to the Sheetrock and aluminum beam ceiling with screws driven into concrete anchors. Lamps were hung

from hooks screwed into the board in the ceiling.

The layout of the room was simple and easy to access with a wheelbarrow, which was essential for moving soil and supplies in and out of the garden rooms. A big open aisle in the center of the room was used as a staging area and to grow small plants.

Plants in 3-gallon (11.4 L) pots were lined up in neat rows. A few larger containers and plants were mixed with some of the 3-gallon (11.4 L) containers. The aisle in the middle allowed easy access to plants.

The autoflowering feminized plants received 18 hours of light and 6 hours of darkness during their entire lifetime, seedling through flowering. Light leaks between rooms were not a concern!

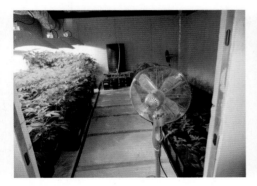

The floor fan was later replaced by wall-mounted oscillating fans. Four new fans were mounted on the walls and directed above plants. Air circulation improved dramatically, and there were no electrical cords on the floor.

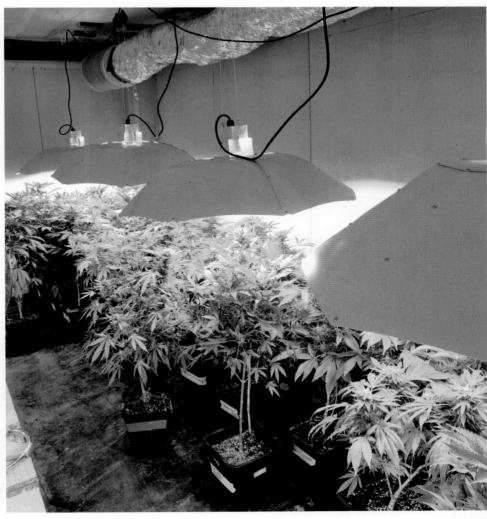

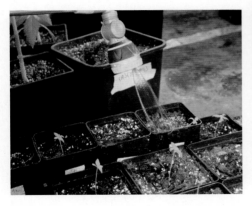

Water flow was regulated with a button on the hand-controlled watering wand attached to the hose bib.

These 3-gallon (11.4 L) containers were clearly labeled on 2 sides. The plants grew for about 2 weeks too long in the containers, in addition to suffering from an invasion of thrips. Lower growth slowed down and showed signs of nutrient deficiencies and spider mite damage, and was then removed.

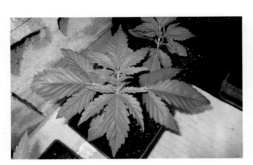

This robust F1 'Sour Boggle' × 'LPI' (autoflower) 21-day-old seedling was developing well. Note the minor lack of nitrogen at growing tips, signified by a light-green color. More nitrogen is used at growing points, causing leaf color to become lighter.

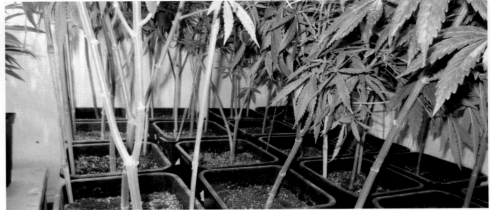

Square 3-gallon (11.4 L) containers fit closely together to get the most out of floor space. These plants stayed in vegetative growth too long. Spindly lower growth was removed to improve air circulation and facilitate maintenance.

Temperature, Humidity, and Ventilation

During the summer months, garden-room temperatures climbed a few degrees above outdoor ambient temperatures of 77°F to 86°F (25°C–30°C). Just a few degrees above the ideal 75°F (23.9°C) caused nutrient problems to manifest much more quickly than during cooler months of the year.

The gardeners purchased a small, portable air conditioner for use during hot summer days and nights. Cooling the room by a few degrees and lowering the humidity made a big difference in growth. When temperatures were around 80°F (27°C) in the indoor garden, growth was slow and weak, leaves curled under, and water and nutrient uptake were depressed.

Lowering the temperature and humidity bolstered overall plant health. Nutrient and water uptake were improved, and leaves became much stronger and were oriented toward the light. A minor change was visible within a few hours, and the garden looked much healthier a week later.

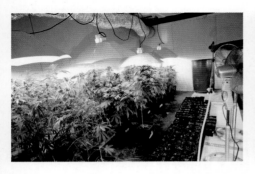

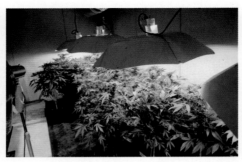

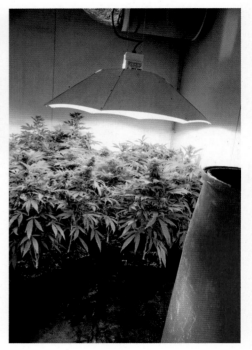

The carbon air filter at the end of the room was attached to 10-inch (25.4 cm) acoustic ducting 13-foot (4 m). Identical carbon filters were located on either side of the room.

Air was drawn through a carbon filter at each end of the room and pulled out by a 10-inch (25.4 cm) temperature-controlled inline fan that moved 1130 cfm (1980 m³/hr). The ducting continued through the wall to a short run outdoors where the flowing air was passively moved up and out by natural convection.

Small plants were easy to move into the large flowering room to take advantage of the excess light. They were placed on the floor and received just the right amount of light for the seedling growth stage.

At 5 weeks into flowering, this mixed batch of clones and seedling varieties had different nutritional needs. For example, *indica*-dominant varieties required more water and frequent fertilizing, while *sativa*-dominant varieties required more water and less-frequent fertilizing. *Sativa*-dominant varieties must be bent, and the lamp must be moved closer to *indica*-dominant varieties.

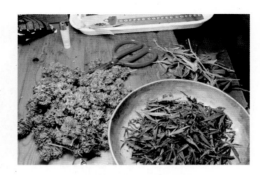

Manicuring and trimming away excess foliage is a time-consuming job!

13

CASE STUDY #2
INDOOR LED HPS LIGHTS

TONI IS A PASSIONATE and precise medical cannabis gardener. He knew nothing about cannabis until 2006 when he was diagnosed with fibromyalgia, a painful and debilitating disease. After seeking relief through prescription pills and, later, through cannabis, Toni found that consuming cannabis makes his days less painful. Cannabis also gives him an appetite and energy to enjoy life. Like so many medical cannabis patients, Toni traded a handful of prescription pills for medicinal cannabis.

As a medical patient, Toni has a passion for cannabis cultivation. He is constantly experimenting with new varieties and products, collecting information, and fine-tuning his gardens. This case study follows one of his gardens and interjects a few examples from past gardens.

Toni is an expert photographer. When it came time to write up the research from my garden visits and interviews with Toni, it was difficult to pare down the photos and detailed information about his gardens. Please see Toni's forum, "Cultivando Medicina," at www.marijuanagrowing.com for complete details on many more of his gardens, including experiments and comparisons. The Spanish-language forum is easily translated to English and other languages with the translator available on the site. His photos are incredible!

Toni is a stickler for cleanliness and order in the garden. Cleanliness and the prevention of diseases and pests are at the top of his list. He took weekly steps during the vegetative growth stage to prevent fungus, insects and mites, and their eggs.

Cleanliness + Organization = Success!

Variety Grown	Seed Company	Vegetative Days	Flowering Days
'Jack 47'	Sweet Seeds	37	67
'Black Jack'	Sweet Seeds	37	67
'Kalashnikova'	Green House Seed Company	41	57
'Lavender'	Soma Seeds	33	55
'Somango'	Soma Seeds	36	70
'Pakistan Chitral Kush'	CannaBioGen	40	63

Seeds and Seedlings

Toni avoids growing autoflowering feminized plants. He finds they require too much light (20 hours daily) and electricity for the amount of production rendered. (But increasing the hours of light increases harvest weight up to 30 percent.)

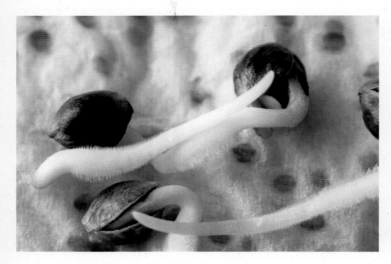

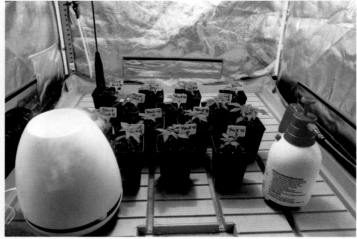

The feminized 'Black Jack' (Sweet Seeds) seeds shown here had been germinated in moist paper towels and were ready to plant. Much of this rootlet was covered with delicate feeding roots that quickly spread out into the growing medium.

Eight feminized 'Black Jack' and 8 feminized 'Jack 47' (Sweet Seeds) were germinated in 1.1-quart (1 L) containers growing under a 400-watt metal halide. This photo was taken 20 days after germination. The small plants were watered with dilute Root Juice (EC 720 mS, pH 6.2). A humidifier helped protect clones from moisture stress.

Vegetative Growth

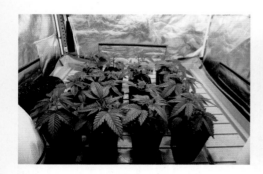

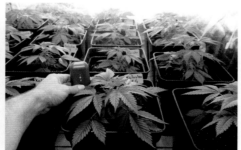

Toni applied the following fungicides in weekly rotation: tetraconazole, penconazole, and myclobutanil. He used a handheld UVC lamp (CleanLight Hobby Unit from HortiTec) to kill fungus and insects, as well as mites and their eggs. He also used a sulfur vaporizer; see "Sulfur Burners" on page 184.

A 400-watt metal halide illuminated 16 feminized 'Kalashnikova' seedlings (Green House Seed Company) grown in 1.1-quart (1 L) containers. The plants had recently been sprayed with nutrient solution having an EC of 250 mS at pH 6.0.

Sixteen feminized 'Kalashnikova' seedlings were transplanted into 3-gallon (11.4 L) containers and packed into this grow tent. A fertometer was used to measure electrical conductivity in the substrate to reveal the overall fertilizer strength.

HPS and LED Lights

A combination of light-emitting diode (LED) and high-pressure sodium (HPS) light illuminated this garden. Plants needed less light during vegetative growth. Toni used 400 watts for the first 33 to 40 days of growth. At flowering, the ballast was set to full power, and the HPS emitted the maximum amount of light.

GROWTH STAGE	ILLUMINATION	WATTS	HOURS
seedling	fluorescent	40	18
vegetative	metal halide	400	18
flowering	HPS 600+ LED 420 watts	1120	12

The LEDs were of different colors and emitted the perfect spectrum for medical cannabis growth. They were placed around the HPS lamp to augment spectrum. The entire canopy of plants grew evenly because it received the same amount and proper spectrum of light.

As a rule, HIDs were kept at 14 inches (35.6 cm) from the canopy of the garden to provide maximum intensity and even coverage. LEDs were kept about 6 inches (15.2 cm) above the tops of plants. But if the temperature climbed beyond 75°F (23.9°C) at the tips of buds, Toni raised the lights so plants would not get too hot.

LEDs must run at the correct temperature to operate properly. Beyond the narrow operating-temperature band of maximum efficiency, LED light output falls drastically and spectrums become unstable. See "Light-Emitting Diode (LED) Lamps" in chapter 17, *Light, Lamps & Electricity*.

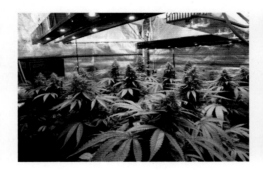

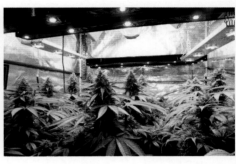

This beautiful view of the garden shows 600-watt HPS and 420-watt LED fixtures illuminating 16 flowering plants growing in 3-gallon (11.4 L) containers. The electronic ballasts made it possible to regulate the intensity of HID light emitted.

Toni used only high-quality Cree or Osram LEDs. He cited the notable difference in manufacturing process that makes these LEDs brighter and more long-lasting. LED technology is changing rapidly. Please check Toni's forum to learn up-to-date information about the lighting in his garden.

With a 600-watt HPS (Cool Tube) + 420-watts LED, light intensity/wattage could be regulated in both fixtures. Light intensity and spectrum were dialed in so that plants received intense light of the proper spectrum. Quickly evacuating the hot air allowed for placing the HID closer to the garden's canopy.

Electronic ballasts allowed Toni to increase light output when necessary. Plants needed lower light levels during vegetative growth, so light output was cut to 400 watts to save electricity without affecting growth rate.

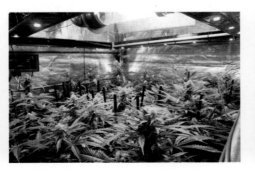

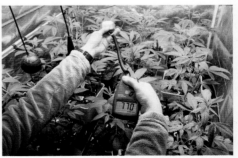

The concentrated HID and LED light penetrated 28 inches (71.1 cm) into the canopy covered in buds.

Even with the intense light provided by the 600-watt HPS (Cool Tube) and 300 watts of LEDs, all the light was used by plants. No light shined on the floor.

After changing a metal halide bulb for an HPS bulb at the initiation of flowering, light intensity was tested to ensure high light levels.

Air

AIR QUALITY

Quality	Day	Night
temperature	75°F (23.9°C)	68°F (20°C)
humidity	40%	50%
ventilation	238 cfm (405 m³/h) inline fan	195 cfm (330 m³/h) inline fan
circulation	14-inch (35 cm) oscillating fan	14-inch (35.6 cm) oscillating fan
CO_2	800-1000 ppm	not used
sulfur burner	not used	used after lights-out every 7-10 days
fragrance	activated carbon filter, ozone generator	activated carbon filter, ozone generator

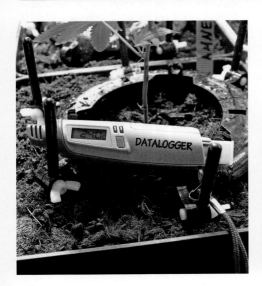

The device shown here measured temperature and humidity and logged it so Toni could download data via a USB connection. Internal memory holds 32,000 records.

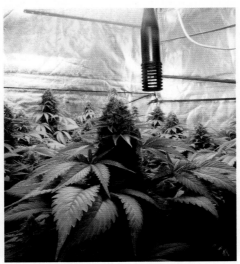

Horizontal bars in the grow tent added structure so the walls would not bow in from negative pressure created by the extractor fan. This roomful of 'Kalashnikova' flowered for 48 days under a 600-watt HPS lamp.

There were four thermometers in the room: one above, one at the plant canopy, one in the plants, and the other on the floor to measure temperature at different levels.

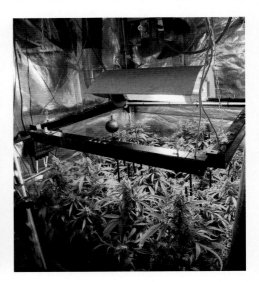

Light from a 600-watt HPS and 300-watt LEDs was optimized with a CO_2 generator and analyzer from Ecotechnics. Toni found that adding CO_2 during vegetative growth increased growth by 10 to 20 percent. At the same time, he advised that CO_2 is the last thing to add to optimize garden production.

Sulfur Burner

Toni turned on the sulfur burner as a preventive measure against diseases and pests—a weekly application during vegetative growth only. Vaporized sulfur lands on foliage, quelling diseases and pests—*Botrytis*, spider mites, and thrips. Remember that sulfur burners have a small coverage area; sulfur tends to fall close to where it was vaporized.

Sulfur sublimes (changes from a solid to a gas) between 291°F and 311°F (143.9°C–155°C). At 320°F (160°C), toxic sulfuric acid forms. This is why it is super important to use and maintain quality equipment.

Water and Fertilizer

FERTILIZER AND ADDITIVE SCHEDULE

Growth Stage	Fertilizer/Additive	Fertilizer/Additive pH	Dose in ml/L	To Start	Weekly
seedling	Root Juice		0	max EC 0.4	0
vegetative	BioGrow and	5.6	0	max EC 0.8	max EC 0.8
flowering	BioBloom	6.2	follow instructions on label	EC 0.8–1.0	increase from 200 mS each week to max of 1800 mS

This was Toni's base schedule for fertilizer and additives. He was also experimenting with other Biobizz fertilizers at the time of my visits to his garden.

Water came out of Toni's tap with 1,100 ppm of dissolved solids (salts). A reverse osmosis filter was used to purify raw water before adding fertilizer.

The substrate was Coco-Mix Biobizz. Toni added a finger-deep layer of expanded clay pellets at the bottom of each container before filling it, and he left a little extra space on top to hold water.

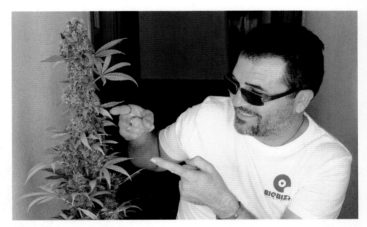

Toni with 'Mr. Bubba'!

Flowering

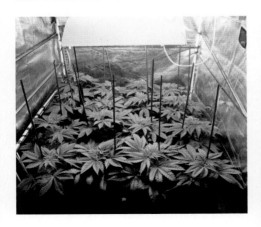

Eight feminized 'Black Jack' and 8 feminized 'Jack 47' in 3-gallon (11.4 L) containers are packed into the 48 × 48-inch square (1.2 × 1.2 m) grow tent. Toni found this the most efficient configuration for growing medicinal cannabis.

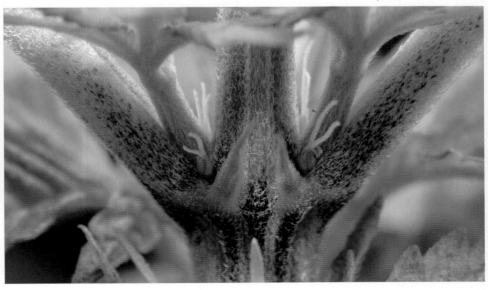

Note the white female stigmas at the seventh internode from the top of this feminized 'Kalashnikova' at 37 days of growth.

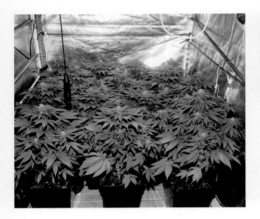

Here is the garden under a 600-watt HPS at 25 days of flowering.

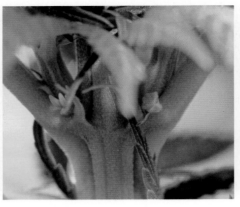

Note the male (intersex) flower on a feminized female plant after 14 days of flowering.

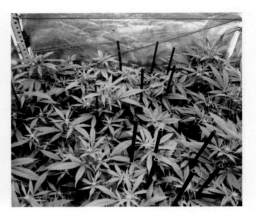

Some of the plants in this experiment were trellised using a "plant cage" with six stakes. Plants grew so densely that they covered the entire cultivation area. You could not see the floor!

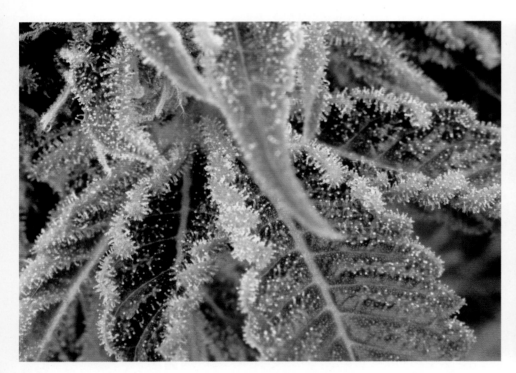

By day 43 of flowering, leaves next to this feminized 'Kalashnikova' bud were packed with resin along the edges, and formed a small spiral.

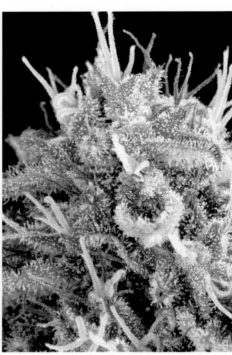

Bud of feminized 'Kalashnikova' at 49 days of flowering

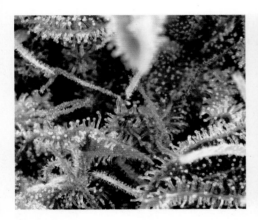

Look closely at the glandular trichomes on this feminized 'Kalashnikova' at 44 days of flowering, and you can see the first amber trichomes and a few broken resin heads.

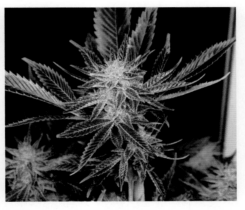

On harvest day, after 53 days of flowering, this terminal bud of a 'Lavender' female (Soma Seeds) was packed with resin.

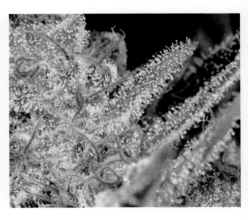

In this macro close-up of a 'Lavender' bud at 53 days of flowering, you can see that about 10 percent of the resin glands have turned amber.

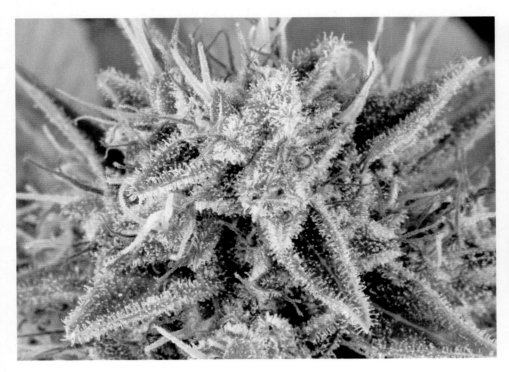

This photo of a feminized 'Kalashnikova' (phenotype) at 57 days of flowering was snapped on harvest day.

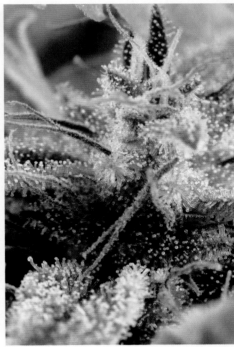

This is a different bud (phenotype) of feminized 'Kalashnikova' at 57 days of flowering at harvest. Note the subtle differences between this phenotype and the phenotype shown at left.

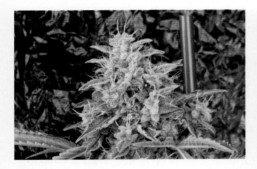

Here is a terminal bud of a 'Somango' female (Soma Seeds) at 68 days of flowering, 2 days before harvest.

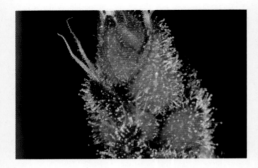

A close-up shows the tip of a bud of 'Pakistan Chitral Kush' (CannaBioGen). The blood-red color is seldom seen.

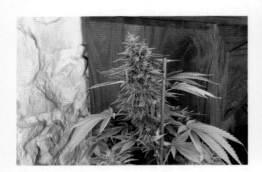

This 'Somango' in a 3-gallon (11.4 L) container was ready to harvest after 70 days of flowering. Large, older leaves exhibited chlorosis caused by washing nitrogen from the soil.

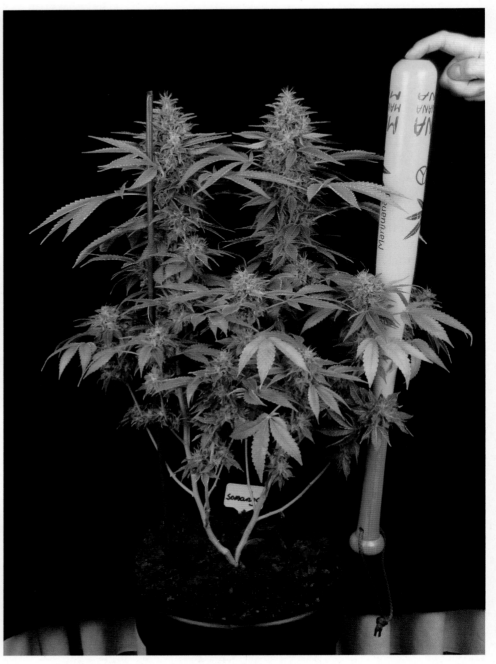

This 'Somango' was pruned to leave just 2 main branches. The result was a single plant that grew as if it were 2 individual plants.

Toni harvested 4 plants at a time in a perpetual-harvest rotation. Depending upon the variety and growth conditions, each plant weighed in at between 2 and 2.3 ounces (60–65 gm) of dried medicinal flower buds.

PART 2 ESSENTIAL MEDICAL CANNABIS HORTICULTURE

13
CASE STUDY #3
OUTDOOR BACKYARD GARDEN

AFTER A DECADE of living in Spain where I could legally grow cannabis for personal consumption, I returned to the USA. Even though I was examined by a doctor and prescribed a Medical Marijuana Identification Card from the State of California, my new home, I still felt uncomfortable with the legal system. When I left the USA years earlier, convicted "criminal medical cannabis gardeners" received long prison sentences, and their homes and assets were confiscated under civil law. It took me a few months to warm up to the new life in California.

This is a brief, three-year history of a backyard garden located in California at latitude 38° north and influenced by Pacific Ocean maritime weather. It is in Sunset Garden Climate Zone 14.

This simple history demonstrates that soil is the essential base of the garden. Sunlight, temperature, and the varieties grown are the next most important fac-

tors. Once these elements are in balance, growing outstanding medical cannabis is easy!

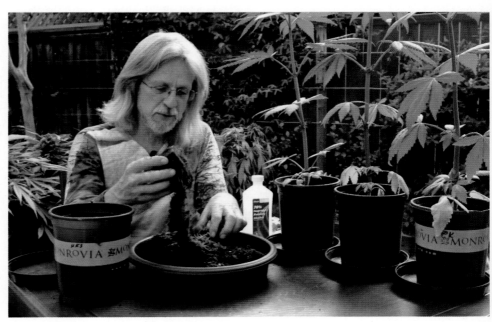
Jorge is always gardening in his backyard!

The first year, the soil was very bad: heavy clay littered with river-bottom rocks. Drainage was slow, and the soil contained little oxygen or organic matter. Water would accumulate on top of the soil after heavy rains.

I started amending the soil in February, tilling in plenty of organic matter—compost, bark dust, sand, and used indoor soil. Chicken manure was added to help break down the bark dust. Bone and kelp meal were added too, but no lime or other supplemental fertilizers.

The soil texture was transformed. Water drained readily with good retention. However, the soil still lacked the proper balance of organic life that it would take two more years to attain.

2010 Backyard Garden

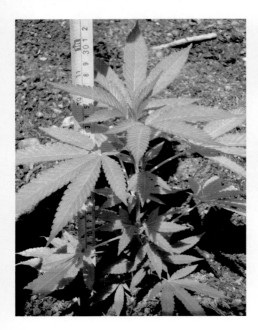

Transplanting date: July 4, 2010

My first crop maintained a low profile; I grew three each of 'Bubba Kush' and 'OG Kush'. These varieties, purchased from a local medical cannabis dispensary, were developed to be grown indoors under lights.

I transplanted the clones in rockwool cubes into 1-gallon (3.8 L) containers. I let them harden-off for more than a week, and then patriotically transplanted the 12-inch-tall (30 cm) clones on the 4th of July—Independence Day in the USA.

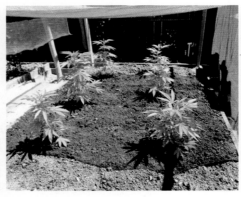

The plants, in a 6 × 10-foot (182.8 × 304.8 cm) bed raised 8 inches (20.3 cm) were covered with green 50 percent shade cloth. The shade cloth was extended over one side to help block ocean breezes.

A week after transplanting, the plants were growing slowly. July days were hot, 86°F (30°C), but the nights were cool, 45°F (7.2°C). The shade cloth over the plants kept them cooler during the day and warmer at night.

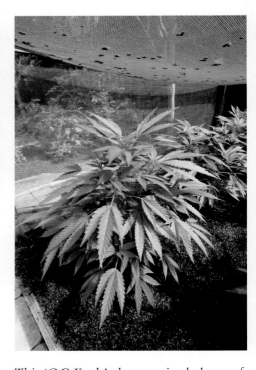

This 'OG Kush' plant received plenty of light for rapid growth.

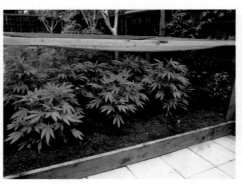

By August 4, the plants were growing well. The shade cloth cooled the soil and lowered water consumption.

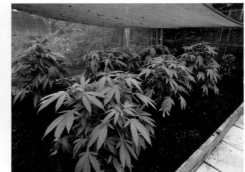

The garden is located between a two-story wall and a tall fence. Once the sun disappears behind the trees and walls, the garden receives low levels of light. Back when the sun was directly overhead, on June 21, the garden area had received almost 6 hours of direct sunlight, but by the first of October the sun was lower in the sky, and just over half the plants received 1 to 4 hours of direct sunlight; the rest received only ambient light. Plants in the foreground were also subjected to light from an adjacent window. Shade cloth helped block the nighttime light so that all parts of the plants matured at the same time.

Five pounds (2.3 kg) of bat guano was applied and cultivated into the top layer of soil on August 1. The bat guano was expensive, but it helped buds swell and also imparted a sweeter taste.

This appeared to keep the disease at bay, but it did little for the disease that had already migrated inside the plant. Bud mold progressed and was cut out when visible.

The cannabinoid-potent crop was harvested one branch at a time, on the first of October.

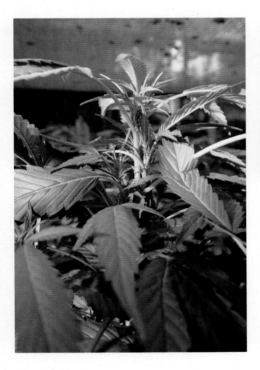

On August 10, female flowers started to grow under 13 hours and 50 minutes of sunlight! By the end of the month, flowering was in full force under 13 hours of daylight and 11 hours of darkness.

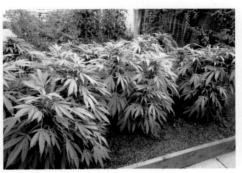

Two weeks before harvest, all foliage was green—including large leaves. A heavy dose of nitrogen (chicken manure) was necessary to combat the bark dust in the soil.

All 6 plants grew to about 3 feet (91 cm) tall, with big, thick flower buds. The first signs of powdery mildew and bud mold started in mid to late August as buds began to thicken. The mold became progressively worse until control measures were taken. Serenade Garden, a broad-spectrum preventative biofungicide, was applied as a spray at 1-week intervals until the first of September.

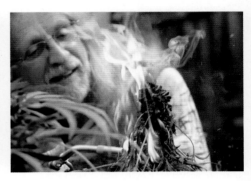

As an experiment, branches with large amounts of bud mold were left in the ground so the disease would progress.

The bud mold infected about a dozen big buds. I let them go to see how it would grow. At the end of the experiment, I decided that the best way to banish the mold from these buds was to send it up in smoke!

Caution: Do not try this at home!

2011 Backyard Garden

Transplanting date: June 14, 2011
The second year, clones were transplanted a couple of weeks earlier. The soil absorbed water and retained it much better; 12 months of biological activity had helped the soil mature. The varieties—'Chemdawg', 'Headband', and 'Blue Dream'—were more robust; they grew taller and were more resistant (but not immune) to powdery mildew and bud rot (*Botrytis cinerea*).

At planting time, dispensaries offered the best commercial cuttings available—and the easiest to acquire. Of course my research at the time was based on convenience, and I chose from stock on hand. The indoor varieties were not acclimated to the rigors of outdoors, where stems must be strong, and growth must be sturdy and fast.

The second-year garden was easier to tend because the weather was milder, and the clones were established before high temperatures arrived in late July. Water penetrated the soil better, too. I watered by hand every few days—about 10 gallons (37.9 L) per plant—using an aerating watering wand and local tap water.

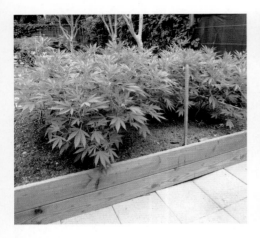

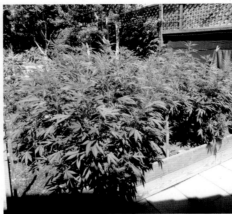

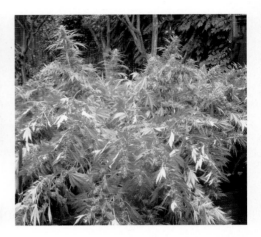

Plants were growing robustly by August 20, and female flower stigmas and bracts had just started to grow.

Branches blew in the wind, and many of them could not support the weight of newly forming flower buds. I installed a horizontal nylon trellis consisting of 6-inch squares. I fastened it to light-weight stakes set in the ground. Aside from transplanting, installing the horizontal trellis was the most work involved in this garden. It took 2 hours to press the posts into the ground, string the trellis, bend the top branches, and clean up.

On September 6, just over half the plants received 2 to 5 hours of direct sunlight; the rest received only ambient light.

A big rainstorm blew in on October 2. Here, 'Headband', a leafy variety with a narrow stem, is shown lying over in front. Strong stems, few leaves, and compact buds kept the 'Green Crack' variety standing upright in the background.

Powdery mildew once again haunted the crop but was kept at bay with applications of Serenade Garden every 10 days.

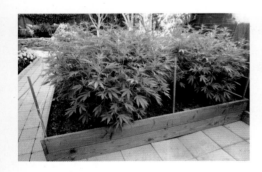

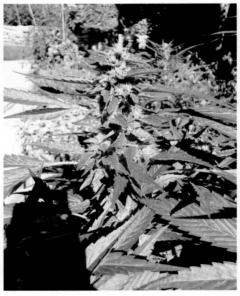

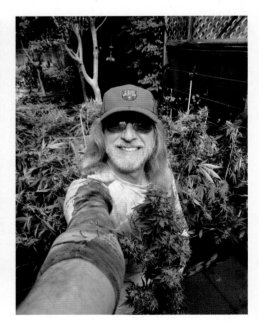

By the last day of August, more small flower buds had formed and branch tips were elongating. The extra 8 inches (20.3 cm) of sideboard added to the raised bed increased the height to 16 inches (40.6 cm). I also added compost-enriched soil to fill the void. The bed warmed sooner in spring, but it got too hot in summer until plants shaded the soil.

Buds had started to plump up by September 20. Branches of big buds would be harvested in 30 days. Lower branches were left to fatten-up a week or more before harvest.

The first bud, with a 2-ounce (56 gm) flower, was taken from 'Blue Dream' on October 4. Flower buds from different varieties ripened at different rates, extending the harvest by 2 weeks.

2012 Backyard Garden

Transplanting date: May 15, 2012

The third year, I started with good, strong clones—three 'Queen Mother × Elvira' and three 'Lamb's Bread × Mother Teresa'—from an expert indoor medical cannabis gardener. They were in 4-inch (10.2 cm) pots and were 12 to 18 inches (30.5 x 45.7 cm) tall, overgrown. The roots were in fair condition: even though a few were brown, most were strong, white, and vibrant.

I left the little clones outdoors in the shade and brought them in at night for 3 days. On May 15, I removed a few lower branches and transplanted the clones about 8 inches (20.3 cm) deep. Planting deeper gave the roots a cool, moist environment. The subterranean stems grew strong new roots in about a month.

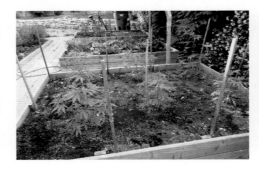

Here, in the first week of June, the established clones were growing well and needed no protection from intense sunlight. Planting earlier took advantage of less-intense sunlight and cooler temperatures. Plants had a chance to become established before warm weather set in.

On June 7, the temperature of the raised bed was about 86°F (30°C) during the heat of the day, and about 72°F (22.2°C) at a depth of 2 inches (5.1 cm). The raised bed had helped when the days were cool, before the soil warmed. After 2 days, sunlight was heating the bed to temperatures that slowed growth to a crawl.

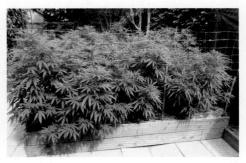

By July 12, the plants had outgrown the bed and needed support and bending. A new 4-foot (121.9 cm) wire fence with 6-inch (15.2 cm) squares around two thirds of the garden provided support to bent branches. I left the shady sides open to provide easy access to the interior of the bed. I trained branches on the perimeter through the 6-inch (15.2 cm) squares in the fence to provide stability. Bending slowed upward growth and kept plants below the fence. Bending branch tips also promoted bushier growth.

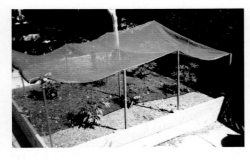

Shade cloth protected the recently transplanted clones from intense sunlight and kept soil cool the first 3 weeks after transplanting. This photo was taken on June 3, after plants were established and had started to grow.

To mount the shade cloth, I drove a few lightweight posts into the ground around the interior of the raised bed and draped 50 percent shade cloth over the tender cuttings and stapled cloth to posts. These clones were planted during a cool spell that lasted several days. (Weather reports are right much of the time!)

The shade cloth was removed a week later, but I put it back on for a few more days when the weather grew hot.

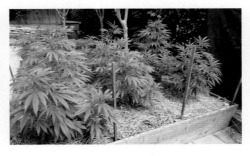

The surface of bare soil was 120°F (38.9°C) on June 21. Four inches (10.2 cm) belowground, temperatures had climbed to 86°F (30°C). A 6-inch (15.2 cm) layer of straw mulch cooled the surface to 70°F (21.1°C) and 4 inches (10.2 cm) belowground to 66°F (18.9°C). Plants began to grow 1 to 2 inches (2.5–5.1 cm) daily.

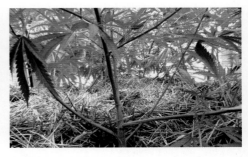

Overgrown bent plants needed thinning below to allow for air circulation and promote growth aboveground that received intense sunlight. On July 17, I cut off branches and leaves, using sharp pruning clippers to avoid wounding the plants.

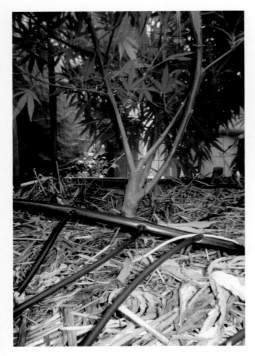

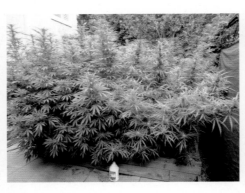

Flower-filled branches grew a foot (30.5 cm) or more between August 21 and September 5. Notice the 'Apollo 13' plant in the right foreground. Its buds were clearly much more developed than others. Note that the 'Jack's Cleaner' branches on the left were not as far along in flowering. They received light from a nearby window during the nighttime.

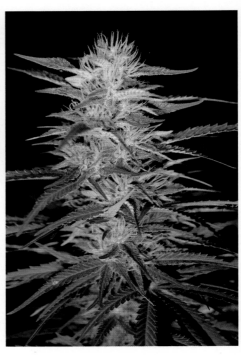

The plants used so much water that I installed a drip irrigation system to water plants daily. The drippers were unable to supply water evenly, so, as needed, I watered heavily using a wand with a breaker head that oxygenated the water. By August 24, plants were consuming even more water and were kept on the every-other-day schedule of about 40 to 60 gallons (151.4–227.1 L) in the entire 6 × 10-foot (182.9 × 304.8 cm) bed.

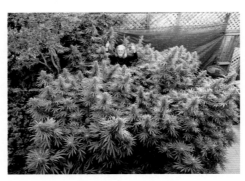

Here is a photo taken in late September from an upstairs window. The plants were from 5 to 7 feet (1.5–2.1 m) tall. Flower buds were getting so heavy that they weighed down the branches.

Here is a view of a 'Jack's Cleaner' branch of flower buds that was photographed the same day as the previous image of 'Apollo 13'. Notice that this bud was bigger and slower to mature.

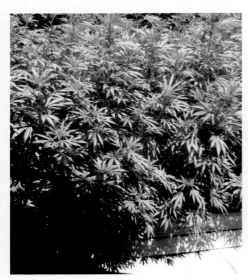

By August 21 the plants had overgrown the 6 × 10-foot (182.9 × 304.8 cm) raised bed. In this photo you can see that the top branches had started to shoot upward and small bracts and pistils had started to grow on the buds that were forming.

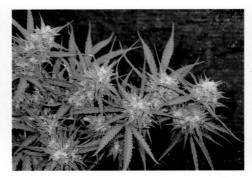

'Apollo 13' was the first to ripen, a full 2 weeks earlier than the rest of the garden. This image was taken September 27, a few weeks before harvest.

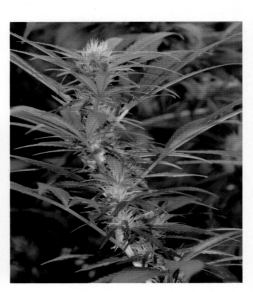

This photo is of a branch of flower buds from the same 'Jack's Cleaner' plant as above. It was taken the same day, September 27, as the previous 2 images. It was underdeveloped and smaller overall because it received light from a nearby window during nighttime hours.

13

CASE STUDY #4
OUTDOOR LARGE GARDEN

HUMBOLDTLOCAL IS A CANNABIS gardener from Garberville, California, 40.1° north latitude, about 20 miles (32.2 km) from the Pacific Ocean, tucked into a valley behind the King Range of mountains and the Lost Coast. The winters are rainy and summers are hot. Cannabis gardens require irrigation.

This garden is located on the border of the legendary Humboldt and Mendocino counties in Northern California, where Humboldtlocal grows big plants. Very big plants—10 pounds (4.5 kg) plus.

Many states that allow legal medical cannabis cultivation limit the number of plants a patient or a patient caregiver can grow. They therefore grow big plants that produce more medicine—legally.

There are no secret tricks to growing giant plants. The only requirements are simple, consistent organic garden practices and proper genetics in the seeds or clones that are acclimated to your local climate. Of course, strong knowledge of biology, horticulture, and soil and water chemistry always helps! Once the

genetics are secured, the most important factors to grow big plants are a long growing season (6 to 7 months), and plenty of light, good soil, clean water, and desire.

The big plants cost from $300 to $500 USD per plant to grow, which includes all labor, supplies, rents, and so forth. The production cost is $50 USD per pound (0.45 kg). Healthy harvests weigh in at 5 to 10+ pounds (2.3–4.5 kg) of dried flower tops and about the same volume in leaves. Post-harvest expenses

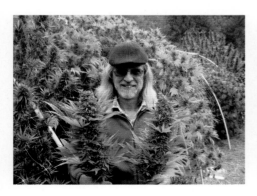
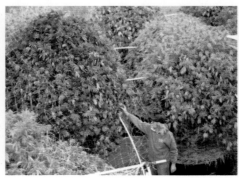
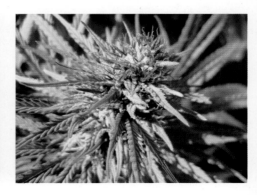

such as trimming, drying, and storing are not included in these estimates.

So much of harvesting a big crop has to do with timing and the weather. In 2010, Humboldtlocal got lucky. Seeds were started at the optimal time for the climate. Seedlings were transplanted at the right times. The weather made it easy to give them optimal conditions. Once transplanted into hoop houses, the plants took off! Plants were transplant-ed and moved to the hoop houses on April 20, 2010. (The late spring in 2011 prevented the move to hoop houses until July 1 that next year. Of course, harvest was affected.)

March

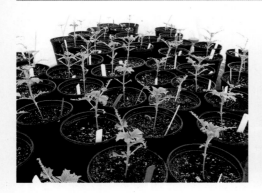

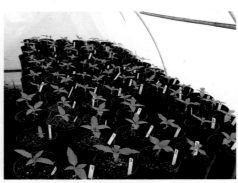

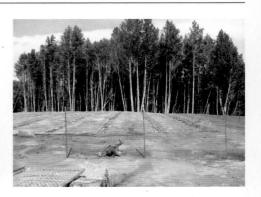

On the night of March 3, the plants were looking good in the heated greenhouse, but a sudden storm had blown in and covered the ground with snow. The little quail around the farm sought shelter from the storm by ducking into the heated greenhouse. There they found a banquet of tender young seedlings, and picked and munched the seedlings for hours before slipping out at daylight. The next day there were feathers and bird poop everywhere. The fan leaves had been pecked away but the growing tips were untouched. With no other plants ready to go, Humboldtlocal de-cided to nurse them back to health and plant them in the garden.

Planted on the first of March, these seedlings were 3 weeks old when this photo was taken. They were growing in 1-gallon (3.8 L) containers full of Hum-boldtlocal's homemade potting mix. Each plant was meticulously labeled with variety name, planting date, and transplanting date.

Nighttime temperatures dip as low as 40°F (4.4°C) in this area of California, but a small heater kept the interior of the greenhouse between 55°F and 60°F (12.8°C–15.6°C).

This is the site for the garden. It is in the best possible place located on flat land. The entire parcel receives full sun all day long. Large fir trees around the perim-eter protect the big garden from strong Pacific Ocean winds.

In 2010, tools, irrigation equipment, soil, fertilizer, and everything else had to be carried to the garden. All gardens need a readily available source of water, or it too must be hauled to the site. Plants can use 5 to 10 gallons (18.9–37.9 L) of water a day. The water source for this garden is a nearby pond.

Local varieties were planted that were developed to grow well in this climate. Smart gardeners in Northern California grow seeds and clones developed locally for their own climate.

Clones or seedlings can be started indoors or outdoors in a heated green-house in temperate climates. Small plants can be moved from indoors to a heated greenhouse when plants are a month old.

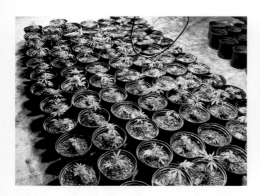

The little clones were looking better just a few days after the viscous quail attack.

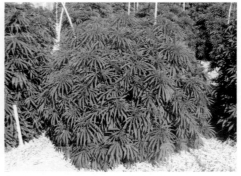

It is hard to believe that the little seed-lings that were attacked by a covey of quail could produce big healthy plants like this one just a few months later. Mother Nature works in miraculous ways.

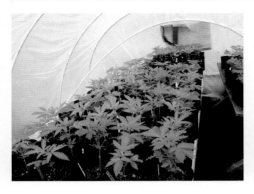

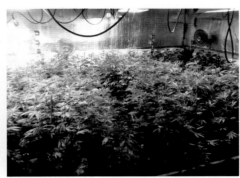

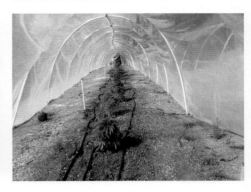

The result of the quail attack was positive! By April 15 the seedlings were 12 to 18 inches (30.5–45.7 cm) tall and had started showing male and female pre-flowers. Seedlings were bushier and demonstrated sex earlier than in other years. Empirical observations say it was

This indoor garden room was full of 'OG Kush' and 'Mr. Nice' clones. They were moved into a hoop house just days after this photo was taken. The greenhouse was wired with CFL lamps to provide just enough light to prevent flowering under fewer hours of sunlight.

This row of seedlings was planted directly in amended soil. Irrigation tubing was laid alongside plants. Next a string of lights would be installed overhead to keep plants in the vegetative growth stage.

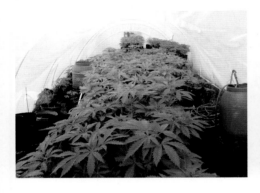

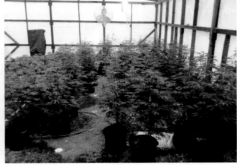

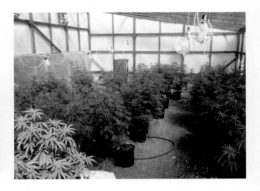

from the attack of the killer quail. Here are the same seedlings 8 days later. They had grown so quickly that the plants were shading one another. They had to be moved apart and transplanted because roots had also overgrown the 1-gallon (3.8 L) containers.

The 'OG Kush' plants were transplanted into 5-gallon (18.9 L) pots. The greenhouse protected the plants from heavy spring rains, and the supplemental light kept them in the vegetative growth stage.

By May 12, plants in the greenhouse were continuing to put on new growth. They would be transplanted into hoop houses outdoors in the next few days.

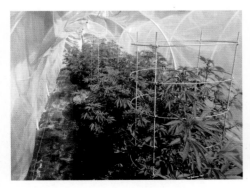

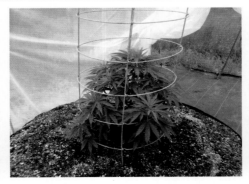

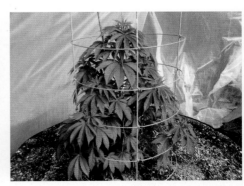

Small CFL lamps illuminated this hoop house full of 'Mr. Nice' in the springtime to keep plants in the vegetative growth stage.

Here the 'Shoe Goo' variety was also kicking into gear.

Here is the 'Burmese Kush' × 'Shoe Goo', as it was starting to get cranking.

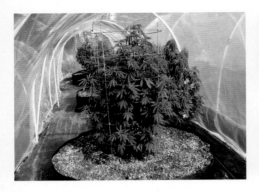

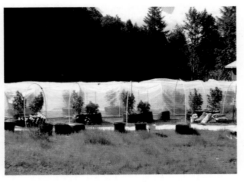

Containers were large (200–300 gallons [757.1–1,135.6 L]) and organic soil was rich in available nutrients; it drained well, and retained moisture too. The soil was covered with permeable weed barrier cloth and 300-gallon (1,135.6 L) pots were set on top. This practice contained the root ball and conserved water.

Hoop houses have access from either end. On hot days the ends can be rolled up for ventilation. Plants can usually withstand 86°F to 90°F (30°C–32.2°C) and a little more when well established. Humboldtlocal pushed his plants to higher temperatures so they would be ready for 100°F (42°C) temperatures in summer.

The ends of hoop houses can be closed in late afternoon to keep the heat inside during much of the night. Small hoop houses heat up faster and must be vented frequently.

Here are a couple of soil mixes from expert medical cannabis gardeners from the Emerald Triangle in Northern California. Both soil mixes are similar. Humboldtlocal's mix includes dolomite, oyster shells, and kelp as additional sources of calcium, magnesium, and trace elements. Nitrogen is also supplied by worm castings and chicken manure. Tom Hill's soil mix relies on Brix Mix for trace elements and does not add magnesium and calcium in the form of dolomite. Ever seeking the perfect soil mix, both gardeners change their mix slightly every year.

Humboldtlocal's Soil Mix

Makes 50 cubic feet (1,415 L) of soil

Fills 6, 300-gallon (1,135.6 L) containers
25, 1.5 cubic-foot bags (42.5 L) Sunshine Natural and Organic #4
3 cubic feet (85 L) Nutri Rich high-calcium chicken poop
1 cubic feet (28.3 L) Super Soil Earthworm Castings
4 cubic feet (113.3 L) Pahroc Perlite #4
25 pounds (11.3 kg) steamed bone meal
5 pounds (2.3 kg) kelp
5 pounds (2.3 kg) oyster shells
20 pounds (9.1 kg) dolomite lime
20 pounds (9.1 kg) gypsum

Mix well, water thoroughly; let rest for minimum of 2 to 3 weeks before using.

Tom Hill's Soil Mix

Makes 50 cubic feet (1,415 L) of soil

Fills 6, 300-gallon (1,135.6 L) containers
25, 1.5 cubic foot-bags (42.5 L) good-quality organic potting soil
4 cubic feet (113.3 L) chicken manure
4 cubic feet (113.3 L) perlite
50 pounds (22.7 kg) steamed bone meal
20 pounds (9.1 kg) gypsum

Mix well, water thoroughly; let rest for minimum of 2 to 3 weeks before using.

Add Brix Mix Powder as per package instructions a week before moving in transplants.

June

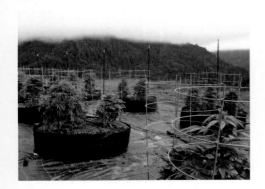

These 300-gallon (1,135.6 L) containers were planted in early May with no protection from wind and cool weather. Each container held 2 or 3 plants. Although the plants were smaller than plants in hoop houses, the extra number of plants took advantage of large containers full of great soil.

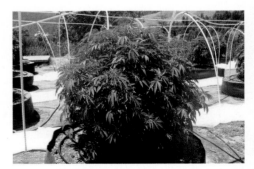

Drip irrigation tubes encircle the plant.

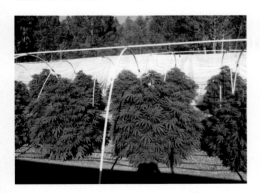

These plants were spaced on 10-to-12-foot centers—a bit close. Humboldtlocal wanted them to look like a big, continuous hedge from the air.

down the length of Humboldtlocal's hoop house. The plants grew through the trellis netting and were supported.

Hoop houses are not covered when autumn rains come because bud mold and mildew are compounded in dense foliage. Rain can always be shaken off.

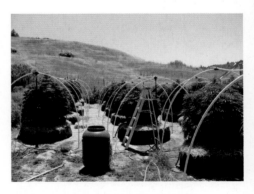

Water is essential during the entire cannabis life cycle. Humboldtlocal irrigated each plant with 20 gallons (75.7 L) every other day.

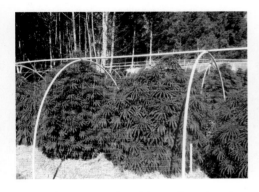

Hoop houses made with 20-foot (6 m) PVC pipe are 6 to 7 feet (182.9–213.4 cm) tall at the crown. They are designed so that plants outgrow hoops by several feet. The plastic is taken off as soon as nighttime weather warms, usually late June to early July. Two 4-foot-wide (121.9 cm) trellis nettings were run

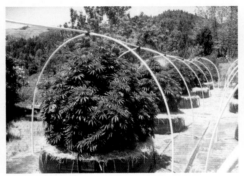

Rice straw makes good mulch and was readily available in Humboldtlocal's area. It was not full of seeds, but rodents loved it. Humboldtlocal relied on the skills and appetite of several farm cats to keep the rodent population in check. However, an occasional plant was lost to girdling of the stem.

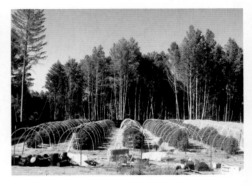

Here is the same view of the main garden a few months later. The plants stood 6 to 7 feet (182.9 213.4 cm) tall

July

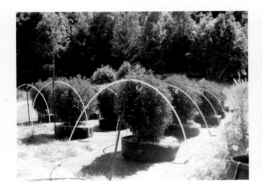

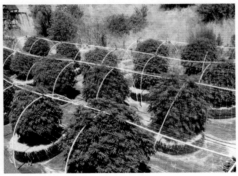

Instead of using commercial bottled fertilizers, Humboldtlocal used a "hot" soil mix and top-dressed with high-nitrogen bat guano and earthworm castings during vegetative growth. He changed to high-phosphorus bat guano during flowering. He also used a local compost tea that was rich in micronutrients, as well as earthworm castings (EWC) diluted in water as a soil drench.

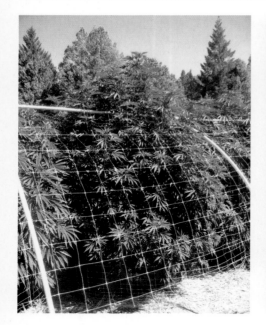

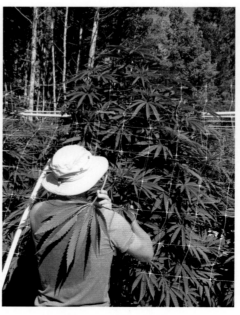

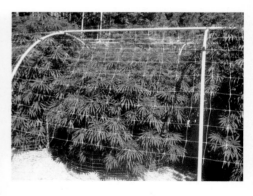

Organic gardening is the secret to huge plants and rock-hard buds.

Good genetics play a major role as well.

However, he did use a couple of organic mite and pest sprays. During this gardening year he started using Brix Mix as a foliar spray; it is known to repel and kill insects and mites.

By mid July vegetative growth was full speed ahead. This shade leaf was big enough to cover half of the gardener's back!

August

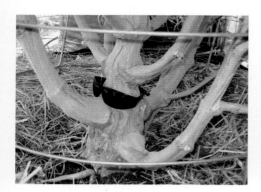

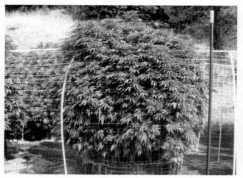

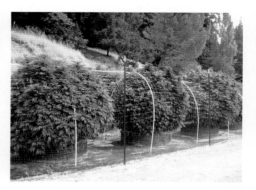

For large plants, it takes a huge stem to support branches and foliage. This stem grew so fast that it got stretch marks. Stretch marks are usually the result of infrequent watering.

Water is the key to success when growing large plants. These plants needed 20 gallons (75.7 L) or more every other day (10 gallons [37.9 L] daily) to sustain life and continue to grow.

Irrigating in the morning ensures that much of the water is used during the first part of the day. Roots do not go to bed with wet feet, and oxygen is able to speed nutrient uptake.

September

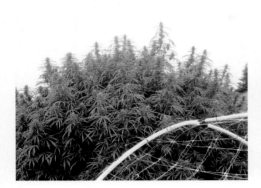

Chance of bud mold and powdery mildew increases exponentially when sprays are applied in the evening. Extra moisture is a sure breeding place for fungus.

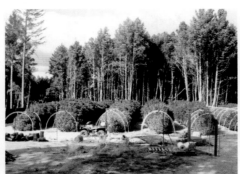

This photograph was taken on September 8, but the view itself had appeared two times in the year, in March and June. You can see that some of the plants in the foreground had been harvested once. New growth had sprouted up, and light-starved flower buds had already begun plumping up.

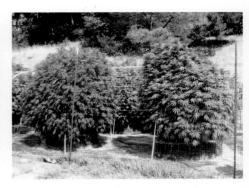

These plants will ultimately obscure the plastic netting.

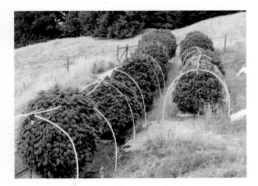

Hoop houses are able to follow the contour of the land.

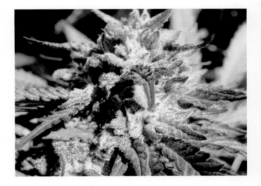

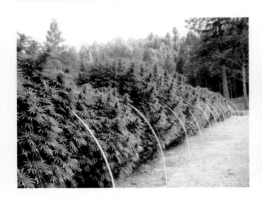

By September 8, plants had grown 2 to 3 feet (61–91.4 cm) past the first layer of trellis netting. Buds were starting to flap in the wind. Luckily, branches were tough, and no damage occurred.

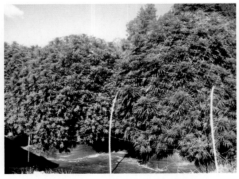

Plants had grown to more than 12 feet (365.8 cm) tall by September 20, and a second trellis netting was added to help protect bud-laden-branches from wind damage.

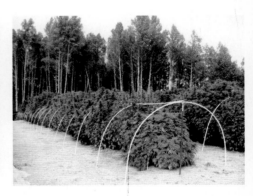

During the flowering stage, budding plants received fertilizer. Progressively more of the bloom formula was added in 2 to 3 fertigations, until the fifth or sixth week.

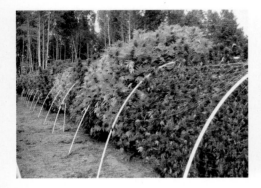

By the first of October, a 2-foot (61 cm) layer of bud-filled branches had been harvested from the purple plant in the foreground. Two weeks later, the secondary buds were fattening for harvest.

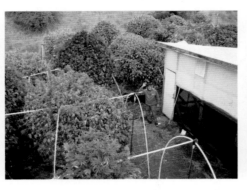

This photo provides perspective on the size of some of the plants in this garden.

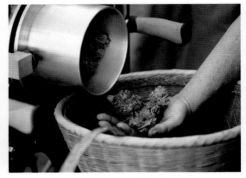

Once buds pass through the cutting deck they fall out into a receptacle. Machine-trimmed buds are taken to a table full of professional trimmers with scissors. The trimmers manicure the fresh buds to perfection.

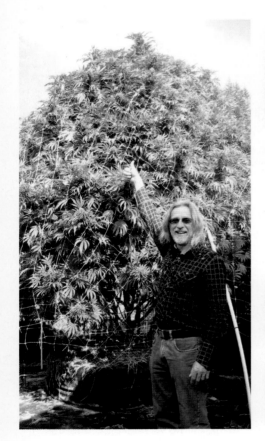

This is the photograph that was seen in more than 20 magazines and countless digital media outlets around the world. For many gardeners, Humboldtlocal and the growers in the Emerald Triangle of Northern California provide the inspiration to grow big plants beyond their wildest dreams!

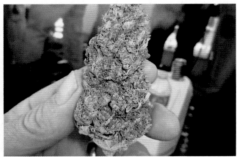

After being machine-trimmed, buds are hand-manicured to remove excess foliage before they are placed on net shelves to dry.

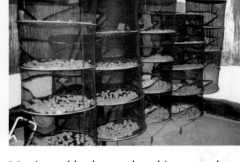

Manicured buds are placed in expandable net drying racks. One half-pound (226.8 gm) will easily fit on a tier of these 2-foot (61 cm) drying racks suspended from eyebolts in the ceiling.

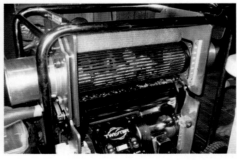

A Twister trimming machine trims most of the small leaf. Buds are prepared and dropped in the hopper. They pass through the cutting deck, where the small leaves are trimmed from compact fresh buds.

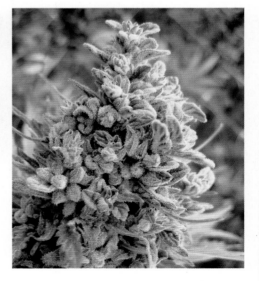

Beautiful bud!

PART 3

ADVANCED MEDICAL CANNABIS HORTICULTURE

14
PRESERVING THE SANCTUARY

THE INTERNET DOMINATES information today. We can check www.google.earth.com and see actual cannabis gardens with big plants in northern California. Amazing views of legal cannabis gardens! Security issues have changed immensely during the last few years in the United States and countries that allow or tolerate medical cultivation of the cannabis plant. As legal patients and cannabis gardeners, we do not have to worry about losing our homes in the USA to "double jeopardy" laws that prosecute gardeners as criminals, and later in civil court where we are subject to asset forfeiture laws and unsavory "criminal" vultures extorting "favors" while we cower in the shadows. We can talk freely with fellow gardeners, patients, and caregivers without fear of being labeled as so-called mafia or organized crime and subject to RICO* and other prejudicial laws. The Internet gives cannabis cultivators—medical and recreational alike—the ability to gather information yet remain anonymous in this worldwide legal turmoil. Digital

cameras and camcorders allow us to share our gardens with fellow gardeners with little or no fear of being discovered. The flood of Internet information is overwhelming to prohibitionists that criminalize sick people and work counter to the laws of Mother Nature and the cannabis plant.

*Racketeer Influenced and Corrupt Organizations [Act] (RICO) USA.

Many politicians, law-enforcement agents, and ill-informed people continue to wage war on the cannabis plant, US citizens, and citizens of many countries. They have an impressive arsenal, including draconian laws, misinformation, and high-tech surveillance gizmos. The USA Patriot Act and the Homeland Security Act of 2002 further erode personal rights of individuals. Unfortunately, the US government has done its best to export this paranoia.

"Legal" medical cannabis gardeners are obligated by local law to keep their

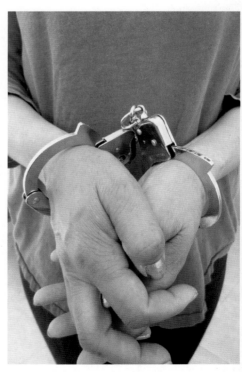

Even though medicinal cannabis is legal in many states in the USA, countless US citizens are arrested every year. Please pay attention to local laws!

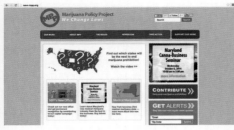

The Marijuana Policy Project (MPP) is behind many state cannabis initiatives. The MPP lobbies Congress to reduce Drug War budgets and stop deceptive anti-cannabis campaigns.

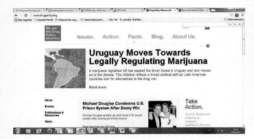

Headed by Ethan Nadelmann, the Drug Policy Alliance (www.drugpolicy.org) is an excellent website to look for current Drug War facts and political action to stop the crazy war.

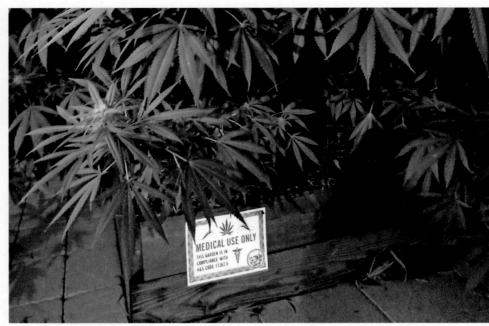

Posting a "Medical Use Only" notice that states the garden complies with state law can be used as "evidence" should problems arise.

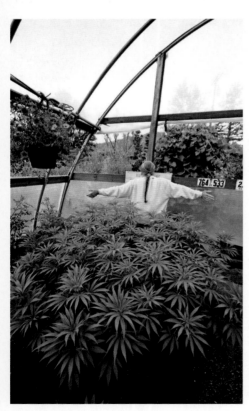

Outdoor and greenhouse gardeners are subject to climate change and Mother Nature's needs. Some years are better than others. For example, in 2011 the outdoor harvest in California was lighter overall than in 2010 because of a cold, wet spring and early autumn rains. Insightful gardeners planted more plants overall to make up for difficult growing conditions.

paperwork in order. At press time there are 18 states and the District of Colombia (19 total) in the USA with medical cannabis laws.* Around the world, laws vary immensely between countries, zones, states, provinces, and cantons. And the laws in many areas are unclear and often change from jurisdiction to jurisdiction. Cultivating cannabis for any reason is illegal under US Federal Law Statutes, and the international "Single Convention on Narcotic Drugs of 1961."** However, even the Federal Government has designated medicinal cannabis legal in a handful of cases. Confused? So is everybody else—including law enforcement and politicians. Consequently, medicinal cannabis laws are open to interpretation. Check the NORML (National Organization on the Reform of Marijuana Laws) website, www.norml.org, for updated laws and requirements for medical cannabis patient cardholders in the USA. Study news from other countries to learn how their cannabis laws are changing. For the first time in recent history, cannabis antiprohibitionists are on equal ground with prohibitionists in the world.

*Alaska, Arizona, California, Colorado, Connecticut, Delaware, Hawaii, Maine, Massachusetts, Michigan, Montana, Nevada, New Jersey, New Mexico, Oregon, Rhode Island, Vermont, Washington state, and Washington, DC.

**http://en.wikipedia.org/wiki/Single_Convention_on_Narcotic_Drugs

Even though the sunlight afforded by complete legalization can be seen among the clouds, medical cannabis gardeners in "medical" and "nonmedical" cannabis states must still be concerned with security. The retail market value of medicinal cannabis is about $15 USD per gram and $15,000 USD per kilo (2.2 pounds) at medical dispensaries. Gourmet tomatoes, a comparable legal crop, fetch up to $10 USD per pound (454 gm). On the black market a gardener can sell the crop for 10 to 50 percent or more. However, wholesale prices are much less than $15,000 USD/kg. For example, the retail price in the USA for one pound (454 gm) oscillates between $800 USD for low-quality outdoor cannabis and high-quality indoor/greenhouse cannabis that fetches from $2,500 to $3,200 USD per pound (454 gm).

The inflated value of medicinal cannabis makes gardens an easy target for criminals and law enforcement. The monetary value of cannabis has made it a hostage

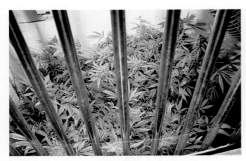

Unfortunately, medicinal cannabis has been kept behind bars for many years. During the last 15 years' progress in California, Colorado, Washington state, and other medical cannabis states, this condition is changing.

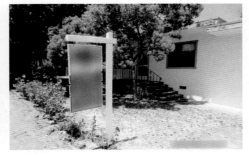

Medical cannabis gardeners in currently non-medical states in the USA often garden in rental houses.

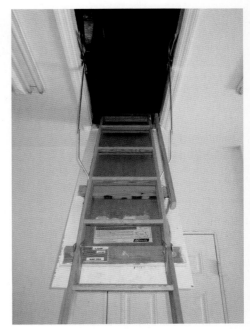

This medical cannabis garden in an attic is accessible via a pull-down stairway.

of the black market. Secret medical cannabis gardens are just like the name says: secret. I asked members on my website, www.marijuanagrowing.com, about sanctuary preservation concerns. Secrecy and maintaining a normal lifestyle—paying bills and taxes, going to little league games, and so on—topped the list. Untold quiet medical cannabis gardeners have been harvesting crop after crop for decades in Drug War–torn America and many other countries around the world. Every year cannabis-related arrests increase but actually appear to promote a disproportionate increase in cannabis cultivation. Supply increases, demand increases, and market prices drop. It is simple economics. See www.norml.org for more information.

Security—personal, family, home, and sanctuary—comes first. Thieves, both illegal and legal, can do you, your family, friends—human and animal—physical harm or worse. Thieves and government officials violate private homes and garden sanctuaries with little or no threat of legal recourse from you. In many countries, states, and provinces, law enforcement can detain you, your friends, and your family—they can even kill your pets!—all under the cloak of law.

Indoors, efficient medical cannabis gardeners in this Drug War–torn world should be able to harvest 0.4 to 0.5 grams of (dried) flower buds from heavy varieties (less for others) every month for each watt of light in the flowering room. Often, indoor medical cannabis gardeners harvest half (or less!) of the possible harvest. A half harvest is inefficient and a

misuse of assets. Even such "successful" harvests leave twice the carbon in the environment relative to harvest weight. Indoor gardeners who do not harvest this much may be inexperienced, working too hard, or lazy in regard to achievable results, and often cheating the environment. Master the basics of growing medical cannabis, and you will be rewarded with a more robust harvest. Remember, greenhouse and outdoor gardeners are subject to climate and space restrictions and should plant early and harvest often!

In the USA, individual medical cannabis gardeners who cultivate fewer than 99 total plants are seldom prosecuted under federal laws that require a 5-year minimum sentence with no parole when convicted of growing 100 to 1,000 plants.

Sanctuary Preservation

The vast majority of medical cannabis gardeners are normal people with a regular schedule, simple lifestyle, and pleasant demeanor. They keep their gardens and grounds in line with neighborhood standards. They do not have noisy, wild parties, and they get along well with neighbors.

Showing a medical garden to anyone who has no direct involvement invites problems. People like to talk and embellish. Once the word gets out, your garden may be subject to compromise and theft. Strangers can also bring diseases and pests into the garden.

Even though medical cannabis may be legal where you live, neighbors, visitors,

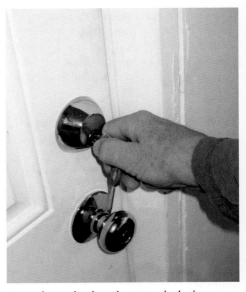

Keep the medical garden room locked to prevent unwanted visitors.

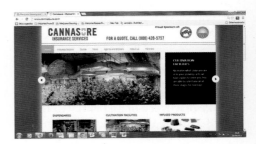

A simple search for "marijuana insurance" will net several bona fide insurance companies.

and family members may oppose it and create conflict. Indoor medical cannabis gardeners are able to attain peace of mind for themselves and loved ones by installing a secret entrance to gardens via false doors and difficult-to-find entrances through workshops, basements, and attics.

Some gardeners mount a tool pegboard or painting over the door to disguise the garden room's entryway. The locked door is controlled with a remote electric door opener.

Insurance: If you are concerned about medical cannabis crop theft and equipment theft you can buy insurance and security services. Many companies sell home security systems. Search "home security systems" on the Internet to learn about current security issues and surveillance devices. Companies such as Medical Marijuana Insurance (www.medicalmarijuana-insurance.com) will insure your medical cannabis crop. This company insures medical cannabis gardeners, processors and dispensaries against economic loss to their crop from natural and unnatural hazards. Use your favorite search engine to check for other companies that insure valuable medical cannabis.

Sanctuary Preservation Precautions

- Purchase seeds and clones at local medical cannabis dispensaries.

- Do not have seeds or gardening products sent directly to your home or garden site. Have the merchandise sent to a "safe legal" address.

- Pay for mail order merchandise with a money order.

- Have a reasonable electric bill. Pay all bills and make all garden purchases with cash.

- Do not visit illegal cannabis gardens or real criminals who lie, cheat, and steal.

- Restrict access to your garden. Keep gardens under lock and key whenever possible.

- Make discovery of and entry to the garden difficult.

- Secure the perimeter around the garden house, greenhouse, or outdoor

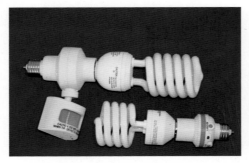

Inexpensive motion detectors are often attached to lightbulbs.

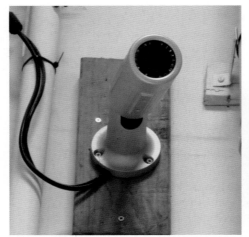

A closed-circuit security camera is simple to mount. All data can be fed directly to a computer, and it is easy to access the camera via an iPhone.

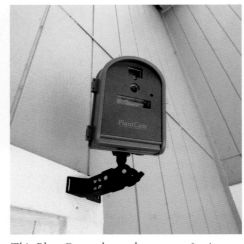

This PlantCam takes a photo every 5 minutes. It records the progress of the garden and any movement in the garden. Photos are recorded on a small camera chip.

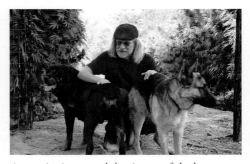

A convincing guard dog is one of the best deterrents against thieves.

garden. A sturdy fence, motion-detecting floodlights, security cameras, and possibly a guard dog will help ensure security for the sanctuary.

- Unload grow supplies a little bit at a time or from within a locked garage.

- It is a bad idea to talk on the telephone about medical cannabis in states that do not sanction it.

Sanctuary Surveillance

Motion detectors are an inexpensive ($10–$200 USD) added level of security for most all medical cannabis gardeners. A central receiver can be used to collect signals from several different wireless sensors. Motion sensors are also built into garden and industrial security floodlights. The lamps turn on when a small sensor detects motion. Other motion detectors can be used to activate alarms, security cameras, and sprinklers via a solenoid valve. Indoor gardeners use motion-detector floodlights around

the exterior of the garden area to intimidate and expose unwelcome guests. Outdoor gardeners use motion detectors and security cameras to activate lights and sprinklers to scare off destructive plant predators such as deer, rabbits, and thieves. Check www.homesecuritystore.com/ for burglar and fire alarms, security cameras, and motion detectors.

Predator trail cameras: Security cameras are affordable ($100+ USD) and easy to set up. With a security camera, you can monitor video and sound from your television or computer. Indoor gardeners set up cameras outside the building, usually trained on entry points such as doors and windows. Outdoor gardeners mount cameras to monitor activity in the garden. More expensive security camera systems can be remotely monitored via computer, iPhone, or Android telephone. Using your cell phone, you can literally watch your garden grow!

Inexpensive security cameras do not encrypt the video signal and can potentially be viewed by anyone with a similar camera that operates at the same GHz. Higher-quality models encrypt the signal and are much more secure. Medical cannabis insurance policies usually require garden-security video surveillance.

Outdoor gardeners can also use a garden camera ($80 USD) or, as deer hunters do, a trail camera ($100+ USD). Mount battery-operated weatherproof digital cameras in discreet locations in the garden and on trees along the trail. Some cameras are motion activated and others take photos at specific intervals. Download the digital images—stills or video clips—every week. Review the images to see if birds, deer, rabbits, thieves, or other perpetrators have been visiting your garden. Images have date and time codes to identify when the culprits appeared. Also use the cameras to take timed photos of your garden during the growing season. Compile all the photos sequentially to form a time-lapse video of the garden growing from beginning to end. Some cameras are equipped with a flash for nighttime photos. The flash also frightens and drives nocturnal deer and other animals away from the cannabis garden. Often, the flash is all the deer control needed. Check www.gandermountain.com, a hunting, fishing,

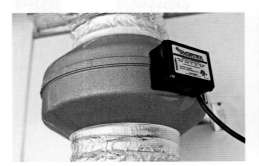

Inline fans run quietly. They efficiently move a lot of air out of the garden room.

and camping website that has a huge selection of predator trail cameras.

After having had his cannabis crop stolen, a gardener friend installed predator trail cameras around the garden and on the nearby trail. When suspected thieves found his garden again, the cameras snapped their pictures along with the date and time they visited. The gardener had plenty of time to move the plants to a safe spot. He also had photos of the thieves and was able to identify them.

Keep predator trail cameras in place all year to monitor hunters, potential thieves, and plant-predator animals. Find out where there is no human traffic, and grow there. Search YouTube for actual predator trail camera videos.

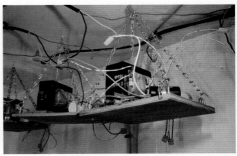

These exposed ballasts are not only a fire hazard, they vibrate and make a lot of noise.

Remember that others use trail cameras too! Trail cameras are inexpensive, and hunters often use them to find prey. Do not fall victim to these cameras. Self-portraits are not a good idea!

Sound Security

Insulate garden structures with a mass barrier like brick, thick glass, concrete, or metal to prevent sound transmission. "Sound board" is popular in North America. Absorb sound with spongy or porous open-cell foams and spun fiberglass. Stop vibrations by dampening the energy and shunting it off into a pad made of foam, cork or carpet, with rubber or spring mounts.

When making a sound barrier, use construction adhesive instead of screws

SOUND TRANSMISSION CLASS (STC) RATING*

Decibels	What You Can Hear
25	Normal speech is easy to understand.
35	Loud speech is audible but intelligible.
45	Loud speech sounds like a murmur.
45	A single layer of half-inch drywall is fixed to 6-inch (15.2 cm) lightweight concrete block wall.
60	Most sounds are inaudible.
60	A double layer of half-inch drywall covers wood on both sides of stud wall. The double wall is spaced 1 inch (2.5 cm) apart with batt insulation in between.

Sound Transmission Class (STC) Rating

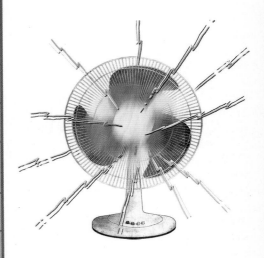

A squeaky fan is annoying and a telltale sign of a garden room.

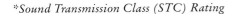

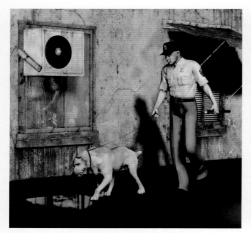

The fragrance of cannabis is concentrated in water expelled from an air conditioner. Always keep condensed water from the air conditioner inside the growing area.

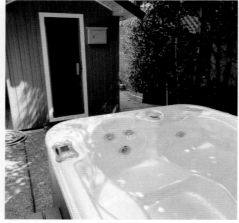

Turn off hot tubs and saunas to conserve electricity for use in the indoor medical cannabis garden.

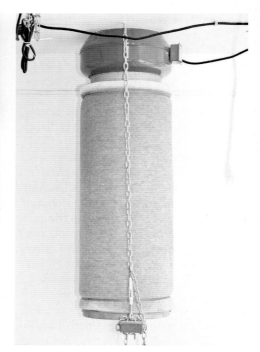

A carbon filter is essential equipment to remove unwanted fragrances in the air before evacuation.

driven into the walls. Screws touching both interior and exterior walls transmit sound to the outside wall.

Build a box or an extra room around analog ballasts to muffle noise. Remember to allow for airflow. Digital ballasts require minimal noise insulation, sometimes none at all. Place a thick pad under ballasts to absorb vibrations.

High-quality inline fans are much quieter and more efficient than squirrel-cage blowers. Install large inline fans and operate them at a low rpm to reduce noise levels.

Wrap ducting with insulation to baffle noise. Insulated ducting is also available. Fit duct outlets with a dryer hose wall outlet or something similar. The vent fan is then placed near the ceiling so it vents out hot, humid air.

Weight and thickness of a partition dictate its ability to block sound. Soundboard added to a wall drops about 5 decibels (dB) of sound. A 3-inch (7.6 cm) airspace will lower sound transmission by 6 dB. Walls insulated with dense or batt insulation cut sound well.

Use a decibel meter (see chapter 15, *Meters*) to measure the sound from your garden room.

Noise cancellation generators offer old technology to indoor gardeners. A microphone records the sound that is then analyzed by a computer. Sound waves with opposite polarity (180-degree phase at all frequencies) are generated and output through a speaker. This causes "destructive interference" and cancels most of the noise. Noise cancellation generators work best when sound can be contained in a small area such as ventilation ducting.

Light Leaks
If light escapes from vents, give ducting a 90-degree turn and paint the inside of the ducting black where it turns to eliminate unsightly light leaks. Baffle light shining out chimneys and roof vents. Check for light and air leaks. Set up the fan and go outdoors after dark to inspect for light leaks so that neighbors are not concerned or annoyed.

Fragrance
To minimize ground-level fragrances, expel carbon filtered and ozone-treated air via a roof vent or chimney. Treat air with a deodorizer or filter that traps odors before evacuating them. See "Fragrance" in chapter 16, *Air*, for a complete rundown on deodorizers and air filters. To ensure safety, Check with a qualified professional when installing a ceiling vent or when venting a chimney. See "Setting Up the Vent Fan" in chapter 16, *Air*.

Do not let air-conditioner water expelled from sealed garden rooms drain outdoors; it smells like cannabis and could draw cannabis- or catnip-loving felines, drug-sniffing dogs, and other pests.

Surround garden property with a bed of fragrant cedar shavings or chips in the flowerbeds. Few flowers have such pungent odors during the fall, and we have no examples of fragrant flowers to thoroughly mask the fragrance of flowering cannabis.

Greenhouse fans are equipped with louvers (flaps or baffles) to prevent backdrafts. During cold and hot weather, undesirable backdrafts can alter the climate in the room and usher in pests and diseases. Installing a vent fan with louvers eliminates backdrafts but may present a security risk.

Law enforcement in some jurisdictions collects information via hearsay evidence—trash, surveillance records, and so forth—to obtain a "warrant" to search the premises of medical cannabis gardeners. If law enforcement discovers a cannabis garden, they can legally continue to build the case against the gardener by using anything the gardener says. They legally collect most of the information from the gardener, friends,

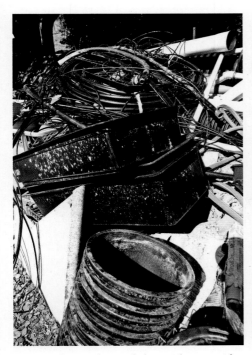

Keep garden trash out of plain sight to avoid drawing attention and to keep the garden area clean.

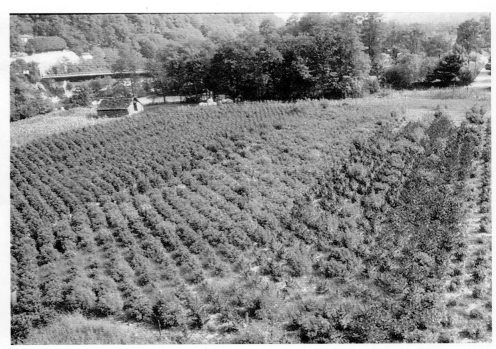

This legal cannabis garden was grown a few years ago in Ticino, Switzerland. All the paperwork was in order with local authorities to harvest a very large field of outstanding cannabis!

and family. Do not be the weakest link in the chain.

Electrical Security

Keep electrical use to a reasonable amount for your home and neighborhood. And above all, do not steal electricity. See sections on "Electrical Safety," "Electricity Consumption," "Conserve Electricity," and "Smart Meters" in chapter 17, *Lights, Lamps & Electricity.*

Internet Security

Internet traffic is so dense that it is virtually impossible to monitor or investigate all perceived crimes. Arresting medical cannabis gardeners who post photographs and text on the Internet is beyond the means of most law enforcement agencies, which are overwhelmed with budget cuts and controlling violent criminals, not to mention addressing property theft, policing traffic, and helping citizens in need.

What is true today can easily change tomorrow on the World Wide Web and iPads, iPhones, Androids, and other "smart" technology. Smart medical

cannabis gardeners can easily have several levels of security. Personal privacy and preservation of your sanctuary are of utmost importance when communicating with other cannabis sites, including those related to activism, cultivation, nostalgia, and social networking.

Simple security measures for garden photos and videos uploaded to the Internet mandate that no tattoos, photographs, license plates, addresses, buildings, or landmarks be identifiable. Medical cannabis gardeners practice these simple measures to prevent theft and other possible problems.

Cell phones may record their location and time with an internal global positioning system (GPS), even when turned off. Newer cell phones can be turned off and will not record the location on GPS. Turn off the "location services" and put the phone on "airplane mode" with Wi-Fi disabled. Some gardeners remove the battery to ensure that their device is off. When the GPS and Wi-Fi are not disabled, locations of gardens photographed and videoed with cell phones can be pinpointed. Removing the battery from your cell phone is a

simple way to avoid being tracked when traveling to secure locations.

As a precaution against automatic transmittal of data, turn off iCloud and other mobile tech services and devices when in the vicinity of the garden sanctuary.

Facebook and other traceable photos of your cannabis garden should not be posted if you are concerned about crop theft. Be careful if your employer frowns upon medical cannabis cultivation. Everybody in the world has access to your "private" Facebook information. Strangers can access it from any cell phone or computer.

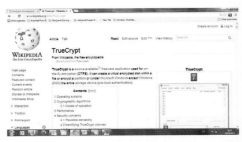

TrueCrypt is a well-known Internet encryption site. Security experts recommend carefully researching all security measures.

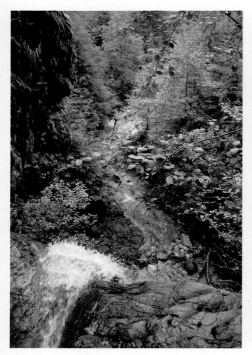

One way to help ensure that nobody finds your garden is to make the trail to the garden difficult to follow.

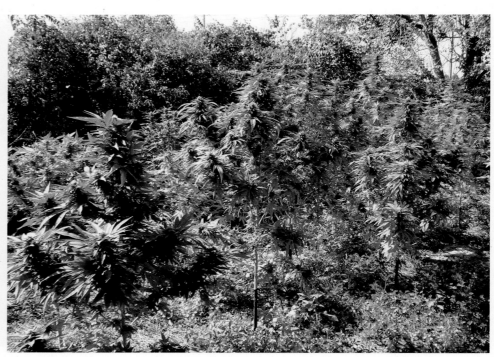

Ideally, a remote garden can be planted reasonably near the home so it can be maintained properly.

You can find many websites about online security. Type "Internet anonymity" into a search engine to find simple, easy ways to conceal your Internet identity from unsavory types.

Keep your computer secure from criminals and government snoops. Check such sites as www.pgp.com, www.pgpi. org/products/pgp/versions/freeware/ and http://en.wikipedia.org/wiki/Open-PGP#OpenPGP, and google "proxy server" for more information about Internet security.

Outdoor Security

A safe gardening location is the primary concern for medical cannabis gardeners. Make sure to have all your paperwork in order. Medical cannabis gardens are private. Doctor's patient records are private too. All records should be confidential. It is the business of the doctor and the medicinal cannabis gardener and patient; nobody else need be concerned. Check with local authorities and with www. norml.org for current status of laws.

If you should happen to come across another cannabis garden while walking in the forest or countryside, do not touch it; leave no sign you were there. Respecting other gardens is the honorable thing to do.

Gardens planted on public land risk detection by hikers, fishermen, other outdoor enthusiasts, and people surfing on Google Earth. Passersby are normally interested in their specific sports and recreation; they will not go out of their way to find your garden unless you lead them to it. Internet surfers are different. Anybody with a computer and an Internet connection can use Google Earth to spot large outdoor gardens in medical cannabis states. Greenhouses and ponds really stand out!

Remote Garden Security

In many parts of the world, gardeners are forced to cultivate remote gardens and must therefore be prepared with an array of skills to be able to plant and harvest a small garden in backcountry. Gardeners are likely to encounter curious hikers, fishermen, or hunters, any or all of whom might wonder why you are out there in remote country. Most often, these folks are just concerned citizens. A late-afternoon garden visit is a good time to "see wildlife," since most backwoods tourists are on their way home late in the afternoon.

All medical patients and gardeners should carry a cell phone to communicate with a partner or call for help when in danger. Turn off the ringer. Paranoid gardeners know that some smartphones track their geographic location and route. Some gardeners go so far as to remove the battery before going to their gardens.

Here are a few of the tactics medical cannabis gardeners in remote areas are forced to employ to ensure that they harvest their crop:

- Park vehicles discreetly, away from the trailhead that leads to your medical garden.

- Bring growing supplies such as PVC pipe, pumps, water tanks, soil, bricks of coconut fiber, and compost to the garden site and stockpile them over time. Tote a few things to the garden each visit.

- Cover shoe soles with duct tape. The style, size, and sole pattern of shoes can be determined by tracks that could ultimately lead thieves or

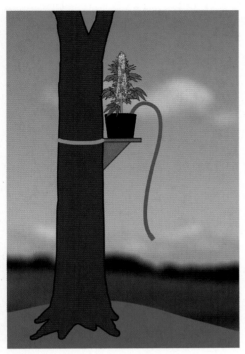

Growing cannabis up in trees is one way to avoid detection.

cops to the medical garden. Shoe-prints could be used as evidence if the medical garden is discovered by law enforcement.

- Look for motion-activated, trail cameras perched in trees, especially in open areas!

- Install a trail camera or garden camera to see who and what is frequenting the remote garden.

- Disguise plants by bending, pruning, or splitting the stem down the middle. Bending branches is the least traumatic method and has more subtle effects on hormones, liquid flow, and physical shape. See "Pruning and Bending" in chapter 6, *Vegetative Growth*. There are also camouflage sleeves available to cover pots.

- Plant cannabis among other plants of similar size and foliage. Grow in a thicket of thorny bushes or other unpleasant foliage such as poison oak, poison ivy, or stinging nettles to discourage intruders. (Stinging nettles disguise cannabis fairly well, but brushing up against them is met with a burning sensation for about 20 minutes.) Look for bushes that are dense and high enough to shelter the

medical garden from view. This deters large animals or people from wandering into the site. Protect yourself from these plants with a slick rain suit and gloves. Wash after each visit to remove irritating toxic oils and thorns. Some gardeners plant where there are a lot of mosquitos or wasps, and at least one gardener I know plants near a skunk's den. The pungent spray keeps people and animals at bay.

- Some gardeners climb 30 feet or higher up into the trees to plant on stands in the canopy or use deer and elk stands as growing platforms. Set up a pulley system to lift large containers and potting soil up to the platform. Install an irrigation hose from the base of the tree up to the planting area and arrange around the pots so you can perform weekly watering with a battery powered pump rather than climbing the tree, and be sure to use climbing belt with harness and safety lines. Do not overextend yourself. I used to climb trees for a living, and my hard-and-fast rule when I was 25 years old was to spend no more than four hours climbing per day. When you get tired, accidents happen. If you hurt yourself, you will not be able to care for your plants! Avoid making a distinguishable path to the garden by taking a different route every visit. Walk on logs and rocks and in stream beds to avoid disturbing the natural habitat. Rapid growth of native plants will erase any obvious trail. Fertilizing the trail may cause wild plants to overdose on nutrients. In late summer and early fall, most native plants in dry climates will not re-grow.

- DO NOT use booby traps, bear traps, or firearms attached to tripwires to protect your crop.

- DO NOT have anything that could be construed as a clandestine protection device or firearm near garden areas. Such things are dangerous and could be implicated in legal proceedings.

- Always locate the garden in a different area every year. Do not use the same location twice. Always clean up the garden site so there is no trace of cannabis cultivation.

Finally, search for "electronic device detector" on Google for more information about detecting electronic devices. Cannabis gardeners in Northern California used to carry police scanner radios to listen to police conducting raids for the Campaign Against Marijuana Planting (CAMP). Informed gardeners could decipher the location of the next raid. Radio scramblers and decoders are also available.

Law Enforcement

A COP is a "constable on patrol," according to the old English acronym. In theory cops are a force in the community to "serve and protect or protect and enforce" our legal rights. Many law enforcement officers do not believe in unjust laws that they are contracted to enforce; others do. However, cops are subject to the same rhetoric that many of us have endured for years as victims of the War on Drugs, and they often make uninformed legal decisions based upon misinformation.

Avoid contact and confrontations with law enforcement whenever possible. If you should happen to come into contact and speak to a police officer, be polite, direct, and busy—going somewhere. The first place most people meet a police officer is in a traffic stop. Officers are aware of what is going on around them, and they know what burned cannabis smells like. Do not smoke cannabis in the car. It is illegal in many places.

Know your legal rights. Study local, province, state, and federal laws in your

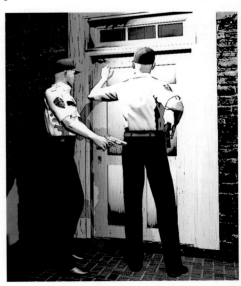

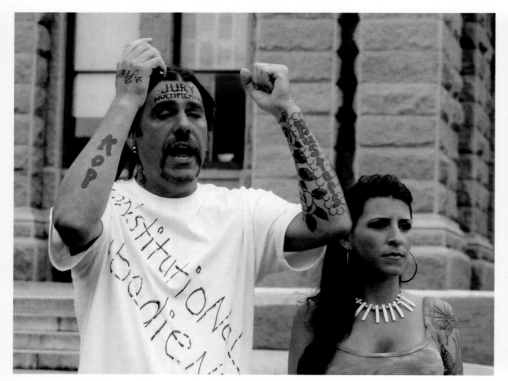

Since Barry Cooper, a retired drug cop from Texas, stopped busting citizens, he and his wife, Candi, have been endless campaigners for an end to the War on Drugs.

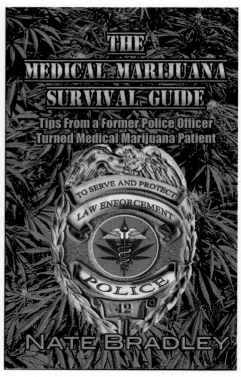

Nate Bradley is one of many ex-law enforcement officials from LEAP, Law Enforcement Against Prohibition.

jurisdiction. Be better prepared than law enforcement is!

We had no rights in Spain during the time of "El Caudillo," Francisco Franco, the last dictator in Europe (1939–1975). Paramilitary Guardia Civil could enter your home (or anywhere else) with an administrative "search warrant." Extreme repression, long prison sentences, and death orders dominated the system.

Today, with no dictator to fear, we enjoy more personal freedoms in Spain than in the majority of states in the USA!

Depending upon the country in which you live, law enforcement must first have a search warrant to use infrared or thermal imaging devices. But if they have a search warrant, such high-tech snooping is perfectly legal. If you want to take a look at what they see, rent heat-sensitive night-vision glasses from your local military supply store, or take a photo of the outside of your grow operation with infrared film. You can also add a filter to your digital camera and convert the photos with a few clicks of Photoshop to show heat signatures.

Law enforcement has sophisticated telephone bugging devices, sensitive directional microphones, infrared scopes, thermal imaging, and more. They can also subpoena telephone, Internet, and electrical company records. Intimidating police officers coerce electric company employees to break the law, violate personal rights, and give them the records of unsuspecting consumers. Tracking telephone numbers—including the location and route of a cell phone—is very easy. There has been more than one case where US law enforcement illegally acquired telephone records and illegally listened to garden store telephones. Unscrupulous law enforcement officials use telephone records to target gardeners.

Here is a real eyeful of how the Internet has spawned a slew of law enforcement seminars (www.indoorgrowtraining. com). Some of these seminars look to expand city, state, and national law enforcement budgets in the future; others are contemporary. Once you watch the video you will understand the importance of not keeping cash and scales at the garden house.

Barry Cooper was a drug cop in Texas; now he is a friend. But Barry will always be a Texan! After years of being a home-grown drug cop hero, Barry realized he was part of the problem in the War on Drugs, not part of the solution. If you want to know how a cop reacts and what is on his mind, check our Barry Cooper's video and website at www. nevergetbusted.com. It is crammed with details of legal (normally called "clandestine" and "overt") activities peace officers use every day to enforce laws.

Law Enforcement Against Prohibition (LEAP) is a wonderful group of current and former law enforcement and criminal justice officials who speak out about the failures of existing drug policies in the USA. Check out their website

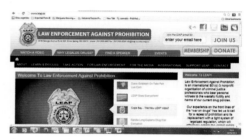

Check out the LEAP website
http://www.leap.cc/.

National Organization for the Reform of Marijuana Laws (NORML)

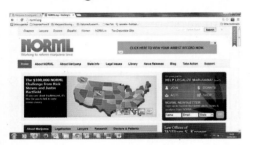

The National Organization for the Reform of Marijuana Laws is one of the many cannabis legalization organizations around the world that provide legal information.

Always keep a lawyer's card with a 24-hour contact telephone number with you!

Check out the site of the National Organization for Reform of Marijuana Laws (www.norml.org) and download your NORML Foundation Freedom Card.

THE NORML FOUNDATION FREEDOM CARD

The U.S. Constitution prohibits the government from interfering with your right to remain silent, to consult with an attorney, and to be free from unreasonable searches and seizures by law enforcement. However, it is up to you to assert these rights. This NORML Foundation Freedom Card will help you do so effectively.

If you are confronted by a police officer, remain calm. Be courteous and provide your identification. Politely refuse to answer any further questions. Ask to talk to an attorney. Do not consent to any search of your person, your property, your residence or your vehicle. Tell the officer you would like to give them this card, which is a statement of the constitutional rights you wish to invoke. Do not reach for this card until you have obtained the officer's permission to do so.

If the officer fails to honor your rights, remain calm and polite, ask for the officer's identifying information and ask him or her to note your objection in the report. Do not attempt to physically resist an unlawful arrest, search or seizure. If necessary, you may point out the violations to a judge at a later time.

(http://leap.cc/) and learn how law enforcement is changing.

Here is a brief excerpt from the LEAP website:

1. Don't leave contraband in plain view. Law enforcement can confiscate your medicine and arrest you. They have discretion.

2. Never consent to a search or talk to an officer if you want to reserve your rights.

3. Don't answer questions without your attorney present.

Like me, most of the Law Enforcement Against Prohibition members, are older and have seen and felt their fair share of good and bad. They have been enforcers of the War on Drugs and understand that the war on the cannabis plant and the people who cultivate and consume it is contrary to Mother Nature.

Informants

In many countries, including states in the USA, a cannabis gardener is considered a criminal and can suffer endless legal turmoil including a long stint in prison. In many countries, conspiracy laws and "incitement and conspiracy to grow cannabis" laws—including the RICO statutes in the USA—were enacted to break up real mafias and political uprisings. Conspiracy, incitement, and racketeering laws are used every day to incarcerate medical cannabis gardeners. Conspiracy and incitement laws are wide-ranging and a catchall way to use hearsay evidence to convict medical cannabis gardeners. They are used all over the world to enforce restrictive cannabis laws. Until the proliferation of Internet communication, these laws have silenced many publications. See "About Jorge" in the back of the book for more information.

The USA Patriot Act 2001 also curtails many personal and human rights in the USA. Ed Rosenthal's *Marijuana Grower's Handbook*, 2011, has a very good section on the USA Patriot Act and how to avoid informants and cops. Ed speaks from experience! See www.edrosenthal.com for more information.

A lawyer friend told me that the USA is an "adversarial" law community. This is

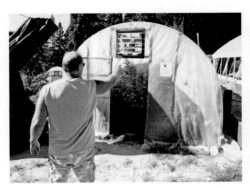

Police informants like the one above are often weak-minded "friends" or disgruntled neighbors that "get even" by squealing on your gardening activities.

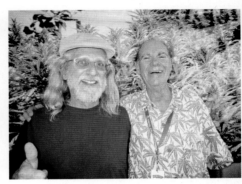

Ed Rosenthal is an expert on the court system in California in relation to cannabis prohibition laws.

why some medical cannabis gardeners always deny growing—always, even if proven otherwise. Some medical cannabis gardeners transform into helpless victims once arrested. Other proud medical cannabis gardeners have their paperwork in order and do not allow law enforcement to waste their time and tax dollars. But when arrest an un-prescribed "friend" that has seen your garden is arrested, police in the USA and other countries can legally use deception and intimidation to trick your "friend" into betraying you and your medical garden. Investigations and interrogations can last for months in many countries.

High-Tech Surveillance
Thermal Image Technology
Unfortunately we are obligated to include this page in the book. Thermal imaging technology is an issue among cannabis gardeners in some countries. Thermal image technology is an invasion of citizen household privacy and is illegal in every country with specific privacy laws. In the USA thermal images are illegal as a means to secure a search warrant, but in Canada, Holland, and other countries, authorities fly in matrix patterns over urban areas to look for alleged indoor cannabis gardens. Thermal imaging technology is the same technology that guides missiles, including smart

bombs. Nonetheless, thermal imaging technology is seldom a problem for small gardeners who use less than 2000 watts of light and have a small greenhouse or a few cannabis plants.

Relatively inexpensive (less than $1,200 USD) thermal imaging devices are now affordable for smaller police forces. Thermal imaging devices have been used legally to measure the heat signature escaping from structures. This invasive "evidence" is used with other "evidence" to secure a search warrant. According to US police sources, the devices are legal only to find heat escaping from windows, vents, and so forth. Most often, narcotics agents use the cameras illegally to secure a search warrant.

Some gardeners avoid potential thermal imaging problems by turning grow lights on during the daytime to confuse thermal imaging devices. Daytime heat and light make accurate measurement of heat coming from vents and windows impossible; thermal imaging cameras are therefore of limited use during sunlit daytime hours. Shield and insulate walls and windows against heat loss from lamps. Store ballasts in separate rooms, and channel the heat away from the garden. Gardeners further safeguard their gardens by cooling garden room air before exhausting outdoors so it

does not leave a heat trail. Air vented out underneath a structure is nice and cool before mixing with the outdoor environment.

Learn more about thermal imaging at http://en.wikipedia.org/wiki/Thermography.

Mini Helicopters
A mini helicopter called the "Smell MJ Growing" or "Sniff-O-Copter," in German, was developed in Switzerland and first used in the Netherlands in 2009. The remote-controlled drone helicopter is able to search and stay in the air for up to 8 hours. According to its manufacturer, its fragrance sensors are so accurate that the garden room location and level can be accurately pinpointed. It can fly over houses and sniff chimney and other vent exhaust.

To date, no law enforcement budgets have been able to pay for a mini helicopter to sniff around my home and others. We are pleased that law enforcement budgets do not include such frivolous items to entrap honest citizens.

In some US jurisdictions where firearms are legal, and where mini helicopters are being used to spy on residents, expert marksmen have been known to shoot the little copters out of the air.

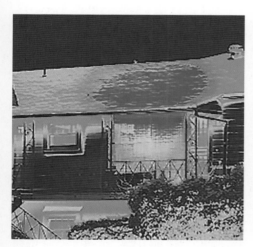

Thermal imaging technology has become less expensive and more accessible to law enforcement and citizens.

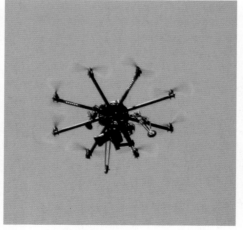

Drone helicopters are relatively inexpensive and easy to outfit with a camera that sends video to a computer.

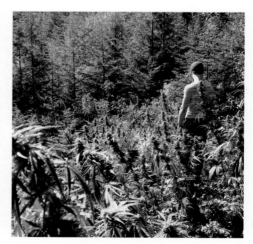

Caution! Thieves can find remote gardens!

15 METERS

THIS CHAPTER GIVES an overview of various inexpensive meters and tests available today, what they measure, and how to use the information they provide to help make medical cannabis gardens more efficient and productive. Meters allow gardeners to measure specific elements so each can be incrementally improved. Meters also help you find the weakest point in the chain of growth.

Meters and test kits measure air, water, growing mediums, electricity, light, sound, and more. They can be analog, digital, or reagent test kits. Digital and analog meters perform hundreds of tests; reagent kit tests are limited to consumables, which must be replaced.

Meter housing should be durable and waterproof, and meters should be easily calibrated (if necessary) or self-calibrating, although some more sensitive meters with a sealed housing must be periodically returned to the factory for calibration. Other important features include: automatic temperature compensation (ATC), temperature readings in degrees Fahrenheit (°F) or degrees Celsius (°C), backlit liquid crystal display (LCD), microprocessor, memory, replaceable electrode, a broad range of accurate measurement, accuracy (+/-) listing, the ability to interface with computers or cell phones, and availability in hand-held/portable or wall- or counter-mounted units with battery and instructions included. Some meters are available with remote probes at an additional cost. Some meters may have several components and wireless communication capabilities. Also note that some meters are subject to contamination and aging.

GARDEN METERS	BASIC*	ADVANCED*
anemometer	$50	$200
hygrometer	$20	$20
thermometer	$10	$30
smoke detector	$20	$20
carbon dioxide (CO_2) sensor	$200	$800
carbon monoxide (CO) detector	$20	$50
decibel (sound) meter		$50
ELECTRIC AND LIGHT METERS	**BASIC***	**ADVANCED***
electric circuit tester 3-prong plug	$5	$20
electricity monitor		$30
light meter	$40	$100
volt/amp meter		$30
SOIL, NUTRIENT-SOLUTION, AND WATER METERS	**BASIC***	**ADVANCED***
ppm meter—CF (conductivity factor), EC (electrical conductivity factor)	$50	$20
moisture meter	$20	$20
pH meter	$50	$50
TDS (total dissolved solids) meter		$50
ERGS (energy released per gram of soil) meter		$80
compost thermometer		$20
ORP (oxygen reduction potential) meter		$100
sodium (Na) meter		$80
water pressure gauge		$10
N-P-K test (reagent) kits	$20	$20
MISCELLANEOUS METERS	**BASIC***	**ADVANCED***
refractometer		$80
digital refractometer		$180
distance		$30
microscope (handheld)	$40	$40
ultraviolet light	$50	$200
Total	**$265**	**$1,075**

Approximate prices in USD

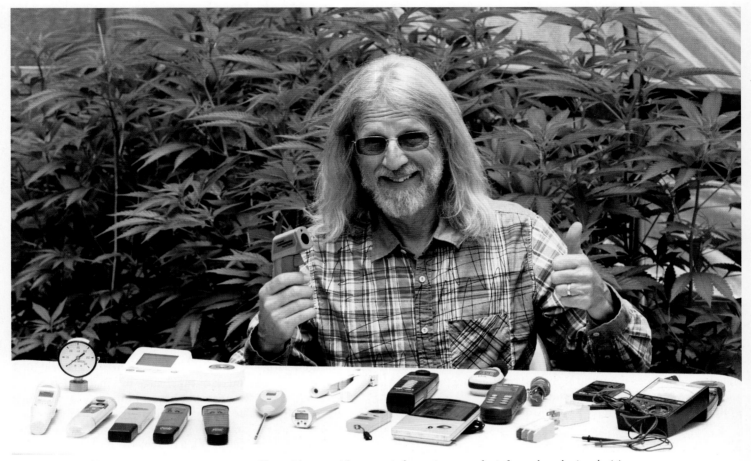

A relatively small investment in accurate meters will provide you with correct information to make informed gardening decisions.

A few meters are essential—electrical circuit testers, thermometers, and hygrometers top the list. These meters will allow you to measure air temperature and humidity (moisture) content. Thermometers can also measure the temperatures of soils and nutrient solutions. The next most essential meters include pH and electrical conductivity (EC) meters, which measure parts per million (ppm) and total dissolved solids (TDS). More expensive models of these meters will take measurements perpetually and store a record that can be uploaded to a computer, mobile telephone, or Internet site. (It is easy to set up a security camera and monitor it with an iPhone, iPad, Android telephone, or computer. The data can then be analyzed and acted upon. However, many medical cannabis gardeners prefer not to send such delicate information by telephone.)

The Garden Meters table shows recommended meters for "Basic" and "Advanced" gardens. Use this informa-

tion only as a guideline. The prices are approximate and may vary from country to country. Prices were current as of summer 2014.

To see more than 1,800 scientific videos on how to master any meter that you could possibly imagine, type "MIT Digital Lab Techniques Manual" into a web browser. Click on the YouTube link to go to the Massachusetts Institute of Technology's videos.

You can also type "video digital (name/type of) meter" into Google and see numerous videos on how to calibrate and use specific meters.

It can be difficult to find all the meters you want at one store. I had to go to the auto parts store to buy a digital laser thermometer, for example, rather than a gardening center. Find, research and order any meter you need by typing in "buy (name of meter)" into a web browser.

Air Meters

Anemometers measure air or wind speed. They are common weather station instruments. There are two classes of anemometers; one measures wind speed and the other measures wind pressure, both of which are related. Anemometers designed for one will give information about both. Handheld meters work well to measure wind outdoors in microclimates.

I use my anemometer to measure wind around my outdoor garden. Indoors, I use it to measure air speed when setting up ventilation and circulation fans. Move it around the garden and see just how bad airflow is in between plants! See chapter 16, *Air*, for more information about airflow.

Electrochemical **carbon dioxide (CO_2) sensors** measure electrical conductivity of an air sample in either an alkali solution or distilled/deionized water. These

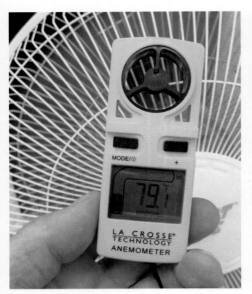
Anemometer

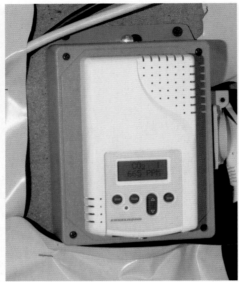
CO_2 sensor

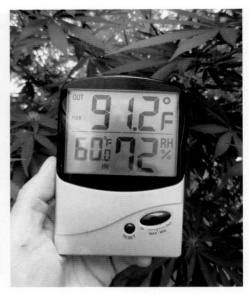
Thermometer

systems are relatively inexpensive, but they have drawbacks: limited accuracy and sensitivity to temperature and air pollutants.

Most CO_2 sensors or meters are non dispersive infrared (gas) sensors (NDIR) and chemical gas sensors. These sensors are used in the air conditioning, horticulture, building, and safety industries to monitor air quality and CO_2 levels. NDIR sensors measure infrared radiation emitted from a heated surface. Most devices can measure from 0 to 5,000 ppm CO_2. Set up sensors in the garden room or in air ducts. CO_2 sensor/controllers will turn compressed CO_2 and generators on and off at desired levels. More sophisticated CO_2 controllers can be synchronized with controllers that operate heat, ventilation, and CO_2 generators. Shop around to find sensors that are battery

or AC-powered and wall mounted with remote probes.

Disposable comparative colorimetric CO_2 test kits are fairly easy to use and inexpensive. CO_2 detector tubes are used to make spot tests. The tubes contain a chemical enclosed in a glass tube with a break-off tip. The tube is placed in a small hand pump (syringe), the tip is broken off, and a sample of air is drawn into the tube. The tube color length or intensity indicates the approximate intensity of CO_2. They test from a trace to about 7 percent (7,000 ppm). Colorimetric kits are reliable to within about 40 ppm. Tubes cost about $5 USD each and make one test.

Hygrometers measure relative humidity (RH)—moisture content in the air at a given temperature. Most hygrometers convert measurements of tempera-

ture, pressure, mass, or an electrical or mechanical change in a material as it absorbs moisture. Humidity is difficult to measure accurately. Hygrometers are available in three basic types: metal/pulp coil, hair tension, and electronic. I cannot recommend metal/pulp coil types because their accuracy is limited. Hair tension hygrometers use human or animal hair under tension that changes length as humidity changes. Hair tension hygrometers are more accurate, but still not as accurate as electronic versions.

Electronic chilled mirror dew point hygrometers give precise measurements—as accurate as ± 0.5 percent RH when clean and calibrated.

Capacitive humidity sensors are pretty accurate (± 2%) and are little affected by condensation and high temperatures over short periods.

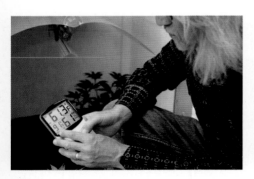
Hygrometer

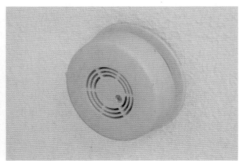
Smoke detector

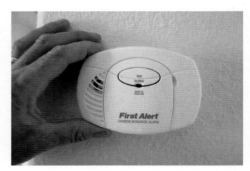
Carbon monoxide (CO) detector

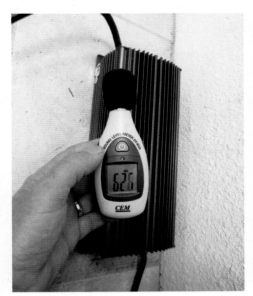

Decibel (sound) meter

LIGHT MEASUREMENT SCALES	
fc	foot-candles
Lux	lux
LM	lumens
PAR	photosynthetic active radiation
PPFD	photosynthetic photon flux density
K	Kelvin temperature
µmol m²·sec	micromol per square meter per second
µE·m²·sec	microeinsteins per square meter per second
2,000 µmol·m²·sec	intense sunlight
W/m²/nm	watts per square meter per nanometer
W/cm²	watts per square centimeter

Resistive humidity sensors measure electrical resistance relative to humidity. Meters with capacitive sensors are more sensitive than those with resistive sensors. Resistive humidity sensors usually have an accuracy rating of ± 3 percent.

Thermal conductivity humidity sensors measure absolute humidity.

A **humidistat** is a hygrometer with a control feature. See chapter 16, *Air*, for more information.

A **psychrometer** also measures relative humidity. It has 2 bulbs: 1 dry and 1 wet. Water on the wet bulb evaporates and the temperature of each bulb is measured. The difference between temperatures is logged and correlated on a chart to find the relative humidity. A psychrometer can also be used to measure dew point and make basic weather predictions.

Thermometers measure temperature. Many people prefer old reliable liquid-and-glass thermometers with a Fahrenheit scale on one side and a Celsius scale on the other. Inexpensive spring-type thermometers are not accurate enough for medical cannabis gardeners. I prefer digital thermometers that record both indoor and outdoor temperatures. They also have a maximum and minimum readout that can be reset. More

expensive thermometers record daily data and store it for downloading to a computer.

Digital laser thermometers are a lot of fun and incredibly informative to use. The thermometer projects a laser beam and records the temperature at the end of the beam. I use mine to measure leaf and stem surface temperatures, and those of water, soil, and walls—any temperature, really. See "Temperature" in chapter 16, *Air*, for more information about temperature differentials and what they mean.

Accurate temperature readings come in very handy when solving culture issues or pest and problems. Always take temperature readings at different points in the room. For more information, see "Temperature" in chapters 16, *Air*; 18, *Soil*; and 20, *Water*.

A **thermostat** measures temperature and perpetually controls heating and cooling devices such as heaters, fans, and air conditioners.

Smoke detectors detect smoke. And where there is smoke, there is usually fire. Some detectors are connected to a fire alarm. Inexpensive and readily available battery-powered smoke detectors should be placed at high points in garden rooms, where smoke will collect. Most

of these devices detect smoke by optical detection (photoelectric) or by ionization. More expensive models use both detection methods.

Automatic fire extinguishers come with a built-in smoke detector.

Mount handheld fire extinguishers by exit and entrance doors so you will know where they are when a room you are in fills with smoke.

Carbon monoxide (CO) detectors identify the presence of deadly CO gas, to prevent carbon monoxide poisoning. A product of incomplete combustion, colorless odorless CO, the "silent killer," is virtually undetectable without a CO detector. Elevated levels of CO are dangerous to humans, and low concentrations can be harmful over time. Use a CO detector to guard against high levels of CO if using a kerosene or fossil fuel CO_3 generator or internal combustion motor.

Note: It can take up to a year for CO to release from the blood. CO accumulates over time!

Decibel (sound) meters measure sound pressure level with an LED (light-emitting diode) screen readout in decibels (dB). Most meters are relatively accurate. Look for a meter with high

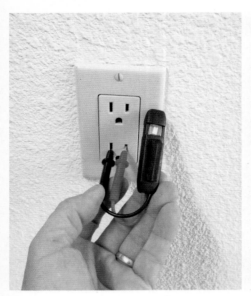

Electric circuit tester 3-prong plug

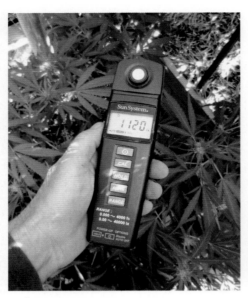

Light meter

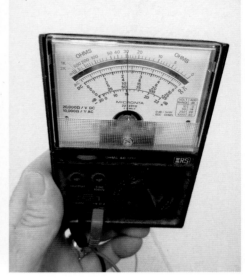

Volt/amp meter

(65 to 130 dB) and low (35 to 100 dB) measuring ranges—great for measuring noise from fans, analog ballast, pumps, and so forth. I was most amazed when I went into the backyard at night with still, quiet air that carries sound. The slightest "click" or muffled exhaust fan echoes! The 4-inch (10 cm) vent fan registers 50 dB at 10 feet away from the outlet. Ambient noise levels register 20 dB when the fan is off.

Electric and Light Meters

An **electric circuit tester 3-prong plug** shows circuit status for an individual outlet. I like the 3-light color-coded display that shows ground, neutral, and hot circuits. More-advanced plugs have a GFI (ground fault interrupt) trip button. These testers are essential for electrical safety and for solving simple electrical problems. Keep the circuit tester in your tool kit. Check all electrical circuits periodically to prevent problems before they start!

Electricity monitors measure electricity use. Inexpensive monitors plug into electrical outlets and monitor the electrical use of specific appliances. More expensive models monitor electrical use history that can be uploaded to a computer. Sophisticated meters are wireless and can monitor electricity use in the entire household or garden. There

are many different brands and levels of technology. Learn more by searching "electricity monitor" using your search engine or Amazon.com.

Light meters measure light intensity and spectrum. Inexpensive to moderately priced meters measure light in foot-candles, lux, and lumens. These scales measure light that is visible to humans—400 to 700 nm (nanometers). But not all light is created equal.

Plants do not use the entire light spectrum equally, and light sources do not generate spectrums equally. While our eyes may see only the blending of the light frequencies, plants are looking for specific wavelengths to trigger responses in the various photosystems. PAR (photosynthetically active radiation) light is the spectrum fingerprint plants need to see, and anything else, while we

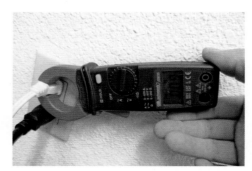

Electricity monitor

may see it as very bright, the plant does not see or use. Matching lamp spectrum to the PAR requirements of the plant is important. Having a measuring device that effectively does this for the grower is a luxury.

You can use a light meter that measures foot-candles, lux, or lumens to measure the intensity of sunlight, HP sodium, metal halide, CFL, and fluorescent light. Sunlight is generally perfect for cannabis growth, and there is little we can do to change it. Light intensity meters that measure foot-candles, lux, and lumens are accurate when measuring the intensity of lamps with known PAR ratings. Indoors, always use lamps with the highest PAR rating. For more information, see "PAR Light" in chapter 17, *Light, Lamps & Electricity*.

PAR or quantum light meters often claim to accurately measure the photons or light particles that plants need to grow. Check the technical data closely on meters before making a purchase. Meters often measure lux and then convert to PAR. High-quality sophisticated quantum meters can switch to measure "sunlight" or "electric lamps." Quantum light meters display a specific numeric PAR value in the LED screen. A PAR meter is not necessary to measure natural sunlight.*

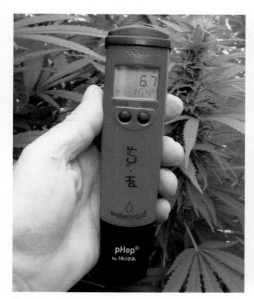

Medium-priced pH meters must be regularly calibrated and the sensor properly maintained.

A pH test kit measurement can be somewhat difficult to read but accurate nonetheless.

*Search "Electric and Light Meters" at www.marijuanagrowing.com for more information about measuring PAR light.

Volt/amp meters: This essential device tells you how many volts and amperes are flowing in an electrical line at any point and time. This meter helps you troubleshoot line amperage and voltage excesses and deficiencies. Use this meter to probe electrical outlets for deficiencies and measure voltage and ampere line drop when running electrical wires for more than 10 feet.

Soil, Nutrient-Solution, and Water Meters

pH meters measure the potential hydrogen (pH) in a substance or solution. Measurement and control of pH are essential to healthy medical cannabis gardens.

Digital meters measure electrical current between two probes and are designed to work in water and moist soil. The growing medium must be moist for an accurate reading. Digital electronic meters can make thousands of measurements with little or no additional cost per test.

Electronic pH meters are economical and convenient. Less expensive pH meters lack automatic temperature compensation but are accurate enough for casual use. Intermediately priced digital pH meters contain a glass bulb electrode that must be kept clean and moist at all times. Proper maintenance ensures accurate readings. Digital pH meters—when properly maintained and calibrated—can accurately perform hundreds of tests. More expensive models are quite accurate when properly calibrated.

These meters must be regularly calibrated to ensure their accuracy. The inexpensive probe meters are not very accurate, and the intermediately priced meters also have accuracy issues. The pH sensor must be replaced at required intervals based on age and usage.

Insert the probe(s) into the nutrient solution or soil, and the pH value will appear on a small LCD screen. Pay special attention to soil moisture when taking a pH test with an electronic meter. The meters measure the electrical current between two probes and are designed to work in moist soil. If the soil is dry, the probes do not give an accurate reading. I prefer electronic pH meters to reagent test kits and litmus paper because these meters are convenient, economical, and accurate. Once purchased, you can measure pH thousands of times with an electronic meter, while the chemical test kits are good for about a dozen tests. Perpetual pH-metering devices are also available and are most often used to monitor hydroponic nutrient solutions.

More-expensive models contain a glass bulb electrode that must be kept clean and moist at all times. Failure to maintain the tester properly could lead to inaccurate readings. An automatic temperature compensation (ATC) feature makes meters much more convenient and accurate. Keep litmus paper or a liquid dye reagent kit as a backup in case the meter malfunctions.

The pH level can also be measured with a liquid reagent kit that is similar to the N-P-K test kits discussed in this chapter. Liquid pH reagent test kits work by adding a drop or drops of pH-sensitive dye to the nutrient solution. Mix by shaking, and compare the color of the treated nutrient solution to a color chart. Such tests are a little difficult to read but quite accurate.

Do not measure pH with phenolphthalein and phenol red (aka phenolsulfonphthalein or PSP) test kits. They are frequently used in cell biology laboratories but can distinguish only between a pH of 6.8 and 8.2.

Nutrient (Ionic Salt) Meters

EC = electrical conductivity

ppm = parts per million

CF = conductivity factor

TDS = total dissolved solids

Different measurement systems all use the same base, but they interpret the information differently. Let's start with **electrical conductivity (EC)**, the most accurate and consistent scale. EC is measured in millisiemens per centimeter (mS/cm) or microsiemens per centimeter (μS/cm). One millisiemen per centimeter = 1,000 microsiemens per centimeter.* EC is the most accurate measure of total ionic salts in solution. An EC meter measures the overall volume or strength of elements (ionic salts) in water or solution.

*millimhos and micromhos are other units of measurement often used for

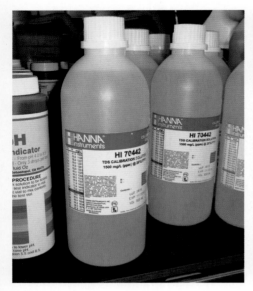

This TDS calibration solution is rated at 1,500 mg/L.

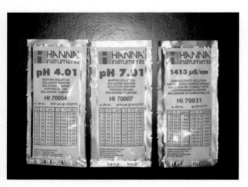

Calibration solution is available in packets.

plant recommendations. 1 millisiemens = 1 millimhos = 1,000 microsiemens = 1,000 millimhos

Parts per million (ppm) meters actually measure in EC and convert to ppm. Unfortunately, the two scales (EC and ppm) are not directly related. Each nutrient or salt gives a different electronic discharge reading. To overcome this obstacle, an arbitrary standard assumes that "a specific EC equates to a specific amount of nutrient solution." Consequently, the ppm reading is only an approximation. Also, manufacturers of nutrient testers use different standards to convert from EC to the ppm reading.

Every salt in a multielement solution has a different **conductivity factor (CF)**. Pure water will not conduct electrical current, but when elemental salts/metals

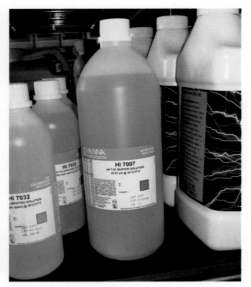

The pH 7.0 buffer solution is color-coded.

are added, electrical conductivity increases proportionately. Simple electronic meters measure this value and interpret it as **total dissolved solids (TDS)**. Nutrient solutions used to grow cannabis generally range between 500 and 2,000 ppm. If the solution concentration is too high, the internal osmotic systems can reverse and actually dehydrate the plant. In general, try to maintain a moderate value of approximately 800 to 1,200 ppm. The EC should stay below a high of 2.7.

Electrical conductivity (EC) meters measure the overall volume or strength of elements in water or solution. A digital LCD screen displays a reading of electrical current flowing between the two electrodes. Pure rainwater has an EC close to zero. Check the pH and EC of rainwater to find out if it is acidic (acid rain) before using it.

Distilled bottled water from the grocery store often registers a small amount of electrical resistance, because it is not perfectly pure. Pure water with no resistance is very difficult to obtain and is not necessary for a hydroponic nutrient solution. Electrical conductivity measurement is temperature-sensitive and must be factored into EC readings to retain accuracy. High-quality meters have automatic and manual temperature adjustments. Calibrating an EC meter is similar to calibrating a pH meter. Simply

follow manufacturer's instructions. For an accurate reading, make sure your nutrient solution and stock solution are at the same temperature.

Inexpensive meters last for about a year; expensive meters can last for many years. However, the life of most EC meters, regardless of cost, is contingent upon regular maintenance. The meter's probes must be kept moist and clean at all times. This is the most important part of keeping the meter in good repair. Read instructions on care and maintenance. Watch for corrosion buildup on the probes of your meter. When the probes are corroded, readings will not be accurate.

Digital dissolved salt meters are used to measure the overall strength of a nutrient solution. Nutrient (ionic salt) concentrations are measured by their ability to conduct electricity through a solution. Several scales are currently used to measure how much electricity is conducted by the concentration of ionic salts (nutrients) between two electrodes. A digital LCD screen displays the reading in one of the following scales: CF, DS, EC, ppm or TDS, which all measure the same thing: dissolved ionic (fertilizer) salts. Each meter has a different scale but more sophisticated meters are able to make readouts in several scales including CF, EC, ppm, and TDS. Most North American gardeners use the ppm scale to measure overall fertilizer concentration. European, Australian, and New Zealand gardeners use EC, however they still use CF in parts of Australia and New Zealand. Parts per million is not as accurate or consistent as EC to measure nutrient solution strength.

The difference between CF, EC, ppm, TDS, and DS is more complex than originally meets the eye. Different measurement systems all use the same base, millisiemens per centimeter, but they interpret the information differently.

A **dissolved solids** (DS) measurement indicates how many parts per million of dissolved solids exist in a solution. A reading of 1,800 ppm means there are 1,800 parts of nutrient in one million parts of solution, or 1,800/1,000,000.

Make sure to calibrate your meter before using it.

A total dissolved solids (TDS) meter measures solution EC and uses an approximate conversion scale to convert to ppm. The conversion is not very accurate because solutions that are composed of different elements will have different ppm values. One conversion figure becomes exceedingly inaccurate. The most accurate measure is osmotic concentration (or EC) because this is what the root systems respond to in a nutrient solution.

Parts per million meters measure the overall level of dissolved solids or fertilizer salts. Each fertilizer salt conducts different quantities of electricity. Use a calibrating solution that imitates the fertilizer in the nutrient solution to calibrate ppm or EC meters. Using such a solution ensures that the meter readings will be as accurate as possible. For example, 90 percent of ammonium nitrate dissolved in water is measured, and a mere 40 percent of magnesium is measured! Do not use sodium-based calibration solutions. They are intended for other applications than gardening. Purchase calibrating solution from the manufacturer or retailer when you buy the meter. Ask for a stable calibrating solution that mimics your fertilizer.

Calibrate EC and ppm meters regularly. A good combination ppm-EC-pH meter that compensates for temperature costs about $200 USD and is well worth the money. Its batteries last a long time, too.

Inexpensive digital dissolved salt meters last for about a year. Expensive meters can last for many years. However, the life of most EC meters, regardless of cost, is contingent upon regular maintenance. The probes must be kept moist and clean at all times, which is essential to keep the meter in good repair. Read instructions on care and maintenance. Watch for corrosion buildup on the probes, and keep them clean. When the probes are corroded, readings will not be accurate.

Check the scale each manufacturer uses to measure mS/cm with their meter. Here are the values that three major manufacturers assign:

Hanna: 1 mS/cm = 500 ppm

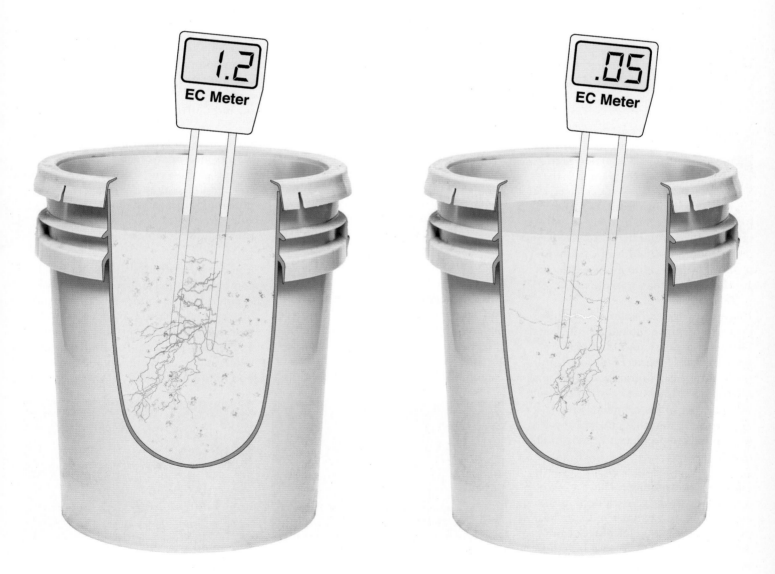

Digital DS meters measure dissolved solids (salts) by their capacity to conduct electricity through a solution.

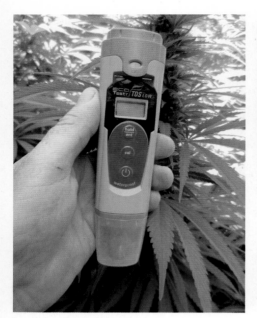

Total dissolved solids meter

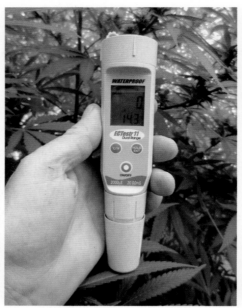

Electrical conductivity (EC) meter

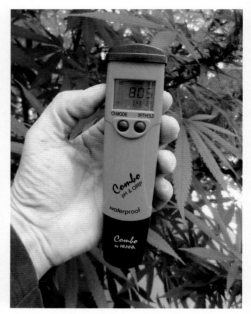

ORP (oxygen reduction potential) meter

Eutech: 1 mS/cm = 640 ppm

New Zealand Hydro: 1 mS/cm = 700 ppm

Moisture meters measure moisture levels in soil and growing mediums and should be used as a backup device to common sense. They work under the same concept as EC—with an electrical charge—and temperature, EC, and pH will all affect the reading, as will improper or nonstandardized placement, meter calibration, and media composition. Even the pros do not use these as anything other than to see trends.

Use moisture meters outdoors to test overall moisture content around plants. Dry spots are easy to find. Note how the moisture level increases deeper in the soil, especially outdoors. Outdoors, the top few inches of soil often dry out, while deeper soil is completely moist. Nonetheless, watering only the top few inches leads to problems; all irrigations should be deep.

Compost thermometers have a 2- to 3-foot-long probe to stick deep into compost piles so you can measure heat in the center. The gauge ranges from 50°F to 220°F (10°C–104.4°C) because compost piles heat up tremendously while breaking down organic matter.

Use a compost thermometer to check the level of activity in your compost. Make sure all compost has cooled to 90°F (32.2°C) before using it in the garden.

Testing at different depths will give you an idea of the biological activity that occurs at different temperatures. Once compost experiences the digestive system of bacteria, fungi, microbes, and other soil live, the entire aspect changes. See "Compost" in chapter 18, *Soil*, for more information.

ERGS (energy released per gram of soil) meters measure the available nutrient level in ERGS, mobile ions of fertility. For cannabis, the soil's conductivity (mobile ion reading) should be between 50 and 500 ERGS. Higher ERGS levels

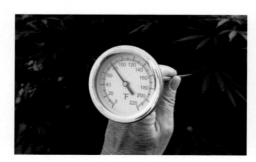

Compost thermometer

mean optimum production. This meter can also test fertilizers, soil amendments, and compost to help determine the most effective fertilization strategies.

ORP (oxygen reduction potential) meters measure oxygen reduction potential or potential available oxygen in soil and foliar sprays. Oxygen reduction potential is measured in volts or millivolts. Available oxygen is essential to roots' ability to uptake nutrients.

You can measure available oxygen and combine the ORP and pH readings to get an rH value, a more precise measure of available oxygen. Low oxygen levels indicate limited biological activity and less humus-building. Too much oxygen oxidizes organic materials and loses carbon to the atmosphere. More oxygen in

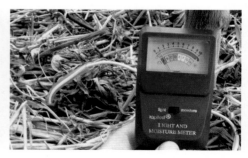

Inexpensive moisture meters are handy, and, when used properly, they take the guesswork out of watering.

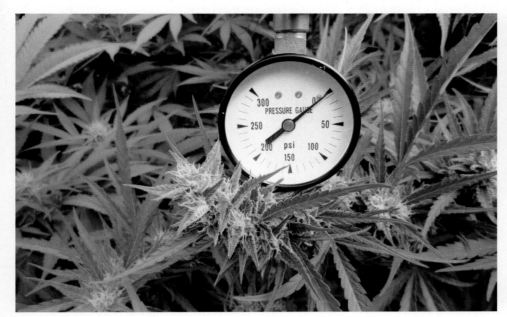

Water pressure gauge

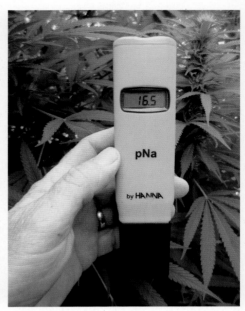

Sodium (Na) meter

foliar fertilizer and pest control sprays increases plants' absorption ability.

Handheld electronic **dissolved oxygen (DO) meters** measure dissolved oxygen in solution. Inexpensive aquarium test kits are also available but less accurate. DO meters record temperature and give oxygen levels in percentage of solution saturation. The nutrient solution in the reservoir should be a minimum of 5 ppm (5 mg/L) dissolved oxygen (DO) at 50°F (10°C), 6 ppm (6 mg/L) at 65°F (18.3°C). Very cold fresh water will hold up to 14 ppm (14 mg/L) of dissolved oxygen. Aerating the nutrient solution can inject 5 to 8 ppm (5–8 mg/L) oxygen into the water and hold it for about 24 hours.

Sodium (Na) meters measure sodium levels in growing medium, compost, and organic fertilizer. Use in conjunction with an ERGS meter. High levels of sodium reduce fertilizer effectiveness and become toxic to microorganisms. If the ERGS reading is high due to high sodium levels, corrective action will be necessary to prevent harm to soil microbes, humus formation, and, ultimately, plant growth.

Manure often contains salt that is given to livestock along with feed. If manure

is not fully leached and composted, the salt remains. Incompletely composted manures and other materials that contain toxic levels of salt are often ingredients in both bulk and bagged soil. Always test new bulk soil, compost, and manure for high sodium levels before purchasing and using.

Water pressure gauges test pressure at the water source and along the water line. Most gauges fit into the water line and read out in pressure on a dial. A pressure gauge is inexpensive and especially handy to check irrigation pressure for a pump outlet or on a hillside.

N-P-K test (reagent) kits will give you a basic idea of soil fertility for a few pennies per test. A small bit of soil and water are mixed with a reagent. The soil solution is agitated and left to settle. The liquid turns color and is then compared with the color on a chart. An exact reading of nutrients is difficult to achieve.

Miscellaneous Meters

Refractometers (aka Brix meters) measure sugar content (Brix) in cannabis leaves and stems. High Brix readings indicate adequate nutrition and fertilizer absorption. Cannabis with Brix above 12

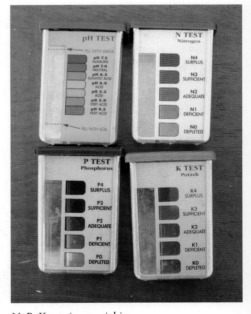

N-P-K test (reagent) kits

has a healthy immune system. Use clean pliers to squeeze sap from leaves onto the refractometer's glass plate, and then turn it toward the sun to read the Brix count in the viewer. Most meters are very accurate and measure from 0 to 30 Brix.

A **Digital refractometer** measures sugar content (Brix) of cannabis foliage. Measurements are simple and quick after calibration with deionized or distilled

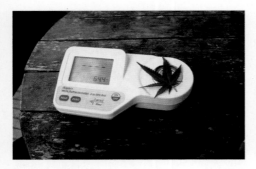
Digital refractometers make measuring sugar content in foliage easy and very precise.

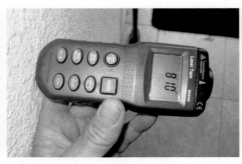
A digital laser tape measure adds precision to garden room construction.

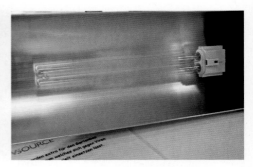
Ultraviolet (UVC) light is deadly to many diseases and pests when briefly exposed.

water. This meter measures the refractive index of the sample and converts it to percentage of Brix concentration. I like this meter because it eliminates the uncertainty associated with mechanical refractometers.

Laser tape measures are a high-tech alternative to a mechanical tape measure. These little meters are very useful in the garden. I use mine all the time to measure garden rooms and outdoor garden areas, even distance between plants. I can stand in the same place and calculate complete garden room dimensions in seconds. Just point it at a large flat object and get distance readings in feet or meters. Press two more buttons to figure square and cubic feet, both of which are very handy when setting up a garden room and calculating space.

Microscopes—30X to 50X—can be handheld, desktop, and with or without a computer interface. I like the small handheld 45X LED light microscope. It fits in my pocket, the light is bright, the battery is long-lasting, and it is easy to keep clean. Another favorite is the 30X

fold-open microscope originally used by stamp collectors. This scope is perfect to take a close look at resin glands but is not so powerful that depth of field is limited. More powerful desktop microscopes provide a closer view but are difficult to focus on all resin glands. Computer interface microscopes are relatively inexpensive and show close-up shots of resin but often lack definition.

Ultraviolet lights expose body fluids, molds, and insect excrement. Use a UVB flashlight to detect insect droppings and trails, fungus spores, and damage. UV light has been used in the hotel industry and by law enforcement for many years to detect body fluids and other residues that are not easily visible to the naked eye. Ultraviolet rays that are transmitted across a surface show a chemical signature. More sophisticated devices available to law enforcement are able to read the signature.

Spot the bad bugs and the despicable destruction in their wake. Use the UVB flashlight to snoop around the garden room, greenhouse, and outdoor garden

at night. UVB light makes slug and snail slime trails glisten and both bug exudates and bud excrement glow. It also makes powdery mildew spores take on iridescent hues and tones.

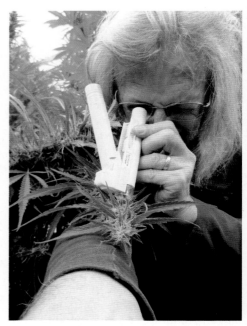
A handheld microscope simplifies garden research.

PART 3

ADVANCED MEDICAL CANNABIS HORTICULTURE

16
AIR

FRESH AIR IS ESSENTIAL to grow healthy gardens. Greenhouse and indoor gardens depend on a supply of fresh air. This precious resource often defines crop success or failure. Outdoor air is abundant and packed with the carbon dioxide (CO_2) necessary for plant life. For example, the level of CO_2 in the air is about 0.039 percent (389 ppm), but in a field of rapidly growing cannabis it could be only 250 ppm—approximately a third of normal on a very still day. Wind blows in fresh CO_2-rich air. Rain washes air and plants of dust and pollutants. The outdoor environment is often harsh and unpredictable, but there is always fresh air. CO_2-rich air is even more critical in indoor and greenhouse gardens. It must be carefully controlled to replicate the best of the outdoor atmosphere.

Air in a garden room or greenhouse must be moved either by natural currents or mechanically to simulate outdoor environments. Stale, depleted air is ventilated out and new CO_2-rich air is drawn or forced into garden rooms and greenhouses. Air must be circulated to prevent stagnant air and stratification around leaves and within the structure.

Carbon dioxide and oxygen provide basic building blocks for plant life. Oxygen (O_2) is used for respiration—burning carbohydrates and other foods to provide energy. CO_2 must be present during photosynthesis. Without it, a plant will die. CO_2 combines light energy with water to produce sugars. These sugars fuel the growth and metabolism of cannabis plants. With reduced

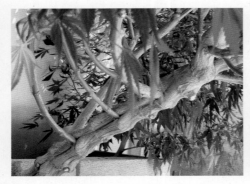

Bottom branches are pruned to allow for extra airflow under plants. Fresh air is essential to keep plenty of carbon dioxide available for plants.

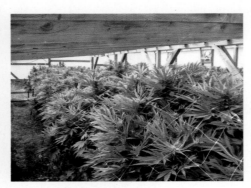

Extra airspace in this greenhouse will run out before harvest. The buds will soon touch the roof. The ventilation fans run full speed 24 hours a day.

Temperature

Temperature is a dominant factor for plant growth as well as most life processes on earth. An accurate thermometer is essential to measure temperature in *all* garden rooms. Mercury or liquid thermometers are typically more accurate than spring or dial types, but they are ecologically unsound. An inexpensive thermometer will collect basic information, but the ideal thermometer is a day/night or maximum/minimum type that measures how low the temperature drops at night and how high it reaches during the day. See chapter 15, *Meters*, for more information on thermometers.

levels of CO_2, growth slows to a crawl. Except during darkness, a plant releases more O_2 than is used and uses much more CO_2 than it releases.

Roots use air, too. Oxygen must be present along with water and nutrients for the roots to be able to absorb nutrients. Compacted, water-saturated soil has little space for the air that roots need, and nutrient uptake stalls.

Stomata

Animals regulate the amount of air inhaled and the carbon dioxide and other elements exhaled through the nostrils via the lungs. In cannabis, O_2 and CO_2 flows are regulated by stomata. The larger the plant, the more stomata it has to take in CO_2 and release O_2. The greater the volume of plants, the more fresh, CO_2-rich air they will need to grow quickly. When stomata are clogged with dirt and filmy spray residues, they do not work properly, thus restricting airflow. Keep foliage clean. To avoid clogging

stomata, spray foliage with tepid water a day or two after spraying with any pesticides, fungicides, or nutrient solutions.

Stomata function is rather complex and is controlled by many variables, including external triggers such as light; increased or decreased internal pressure based on supply and evaporative potential; and the presence or concentration of certain gases such as CO_2. For example, a 40-inch (1 m) tall plant can easily transpire a gallon (3.8 L) per day when the humidity is below 50 percent. However, the same plant will transpire about a half-pint (0.2 L) on a cool, humid day.

Molecules—O_2, CO_2, H_2O, etc.—are moved to the leaf surface in a mass flow situation known as the atmosphere. When the air is still, molecules migrate around under the energy of their own vibration—a slow process. When the atmosphere moves, molecules move more quickly. When they reach the stomata, molecules encounter their first barrier to movement, the one at the opening, and like a port on the sea with lots of ships, this slows the movement because the molecules diffuse under their own power into the stomata and out of the stomata; the opening is a two-way street. Circulation in the area moves away those molecules that have exited faster and brings new ones to the stomata faster. Once inside, they vibrate their way across the cavity to the next barrier, located at the cell membrane, and the crowding begins again. Ventilation brings new molecules in while flushing old ones out. Ventilation can also be used to distribute heat and to control humidity.

Under normal conditions, the ideal temperature range for cannabis growth is 72°F to 76°F (22.2°C–24.4°C). At night, the temperature can drop 5 to 10 degrees with little noticeable effect on growth rate. The temperature should not drop more than fifteen degrees or excessive humidity and mold might become problems. Daytime temperatures above 85°F (29.4°C) or below 55°F (12.8°C) will slow or stop growth. Maintaining the proper, constant temperature in garden rooms and greenhouses promotes strong, even, healthy growth. Make sure plants are not too close to heat sources such as ballasts, heaters, and heating vents, or they may dry out, maybe even get heat scorch. Cold intake air will also stunt plant growth.

Cannabis regulates its oxygen uptake in relation to the ambient air temperature rather than the amount of available O_2. Plants use a lot of O_2; in fact, a plant cell uses as much O_2 as a human cell. The air must contain at least 20 percent O_2 for plants to thrive.* Leaves are not able to release O_2 at night, but roots still need it to grow. A plant's respiration rate approximately doubles every twenty degrees. Oxygen use by roots increases as they warm up, which is why fresh air is important both day and night. Temperatures above 85°F (29.4°C) are not recommended even when using CO_2 enrichment. When it's too warm, photorespiration occurs faster than the plant can compensate, the system short-circuits, and O_2 takes the place of CO_2; this in turn shuts down the Calvin cycle** and thus the conversion of light to carbohydrates and energy.

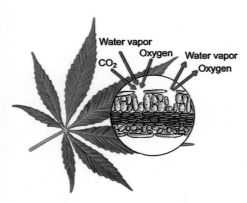

Water vapor
Oxygen
CO_2
Water vapor
Oxygen

Stomata are microscopic pores on leaf undersides that are similar to an animal's nostrils.

Stomatal function: Increased internal pressure from active roots, increased temperature, or a blockage in the exit pathway, along with suitable triggers such as a decrease in internal CO_2 levels and appropriate light triggers (usually UV light), allow for the guard cells of the stomata to become turgid and thus open (through other sometimes-complex processes involving potassium shifts and so on).

Decreased internal pressure from low temperatures, decreased water availability in the root zone, high internal levels of CO_2, lack of environmental triggers, or a faster demand at the exit pathway than can be supplied, cause a wilting or slacking in the guard cells, which partially or totally closes them. This limits the amount of water escaping the plant and provides some protection. Either case can cause an imbalance between water need and fulfillment.

Humidity is similar to the pipe in a water line. The temperature is the power to run the pump, which is the vascular system of the plant. The valve after the pump and before the end is the stoma. The other side of the valve is the container or sink—demand. As the power is increased to the pump, it pumps faster and more will flow. The larger the pipe, the more that will flow. The more open the valve the more that will flow. The larger the container at the end of the lines, the bigger the results of the system, because it can deliver more. Even though the pump may be pumping as fast as possible, the pipes have to be big enough to deliver the load. The valve has to be open enough to deliver, and the

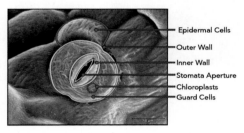

This photo of half-opened stomata, the mouthlike openings on leaf undersides, was magnified 2500 times.

container has to be big enough to handle the load. If the pump is barely moving but the pipes are huge, then there is no pressure and the water will stop flowing or reaching all the containers (the valve is closed more and more to hold pressure in the system to keep water available for the life reactions in respiration, etc.).

The opposite is true when the pump runs rapidly and the pipes are really small: not enough load is delivered and the process stops. If the pump runs wide open and the pipes are really big, then pressure drops to zero again and function stops; the same is true the other way. The overall system will deliver zero load at the extremes of these four situations. So, in a situation where water (load) was available, where the temperature (power) was normal, where the container (sink) was appropriate, and the pipes very small, the valve would be more and more open to get the load delivered.

---

*By volume, dry air contains about 78.09 percent nitrogen, 20.95 percent oxygen, 0.93 percent argon, 0.039 percent carbon dioxide (390 ppm), and trace amounts of other gases. Note the ambient level of CO_2 has increased from 350 ppm 50 years ago; as CO_2 rises, the earth gets warmer.

**The Calvin cycle [aka Calvin–Benson-Bassham (CBB) cycle, reductive pentose phosphate cycle, or C3 cycle] is a series of biochemical redox reactions that take place in the stroma of chloroplasts in photosynthetic organisms. The light-independent reactions of photosynthesis are chemical reactions that convert carbon dioxide and other compounds into glucose. Melvin Calvin, James Bassham, and Andrew Benson discovered the cycle at UC Berkeley by using the radioactive isotope carbon-14.

Photorespiration, is a process in plant metabolism by which RuBP (a sugar) has oxygen added to it by RuBisCO (an enzyme) instead of carbon dioxide during normal photosynthesis. This is the beginning step of the Calvin-Benson-Bassham cycle. This process reduces efficiency of photosynthesis in C3 plants.

Under proper conditions when the water supply is abundant, higher air temperatures step up metabolic activity and speed up growth. The warmer the air is, the more water it is able to hold. This moist air often restrains plant functions and decelerates growth rather than speeding it. Typically, as air temperature rises, humidity falls and plants use water faster; then later in the light cycle, because more water moves into the air, the air becomes more humid. When the lights go out or air temperature naturally cools, humidity levels begin to rise until saturation, at which point moisture condenses out of the air. Moving the air slows or eliminates this process. Nighttime—when the lights go out—often causes complications; problems result

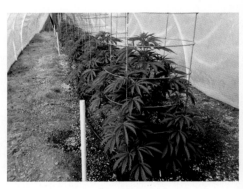

A plastic greenhouse helps regulate temperatures outdoors. Indoors, temperature regulation is accomplished in a variety of ways: air ventilation, air circulation, air conditioning, and more.

from excess humidity and moisture condensation when the temperature drops.

Heat buildup during warm weather can catch any gardener off guard and cause serious problems. Ideal garden rooms are located underground, in a basement, taking advantage of the insulating

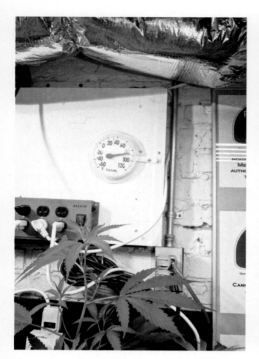

An accurate thermometer is necessary equipment for all indoor, greenhouse, and outdoor cannabis gardens.

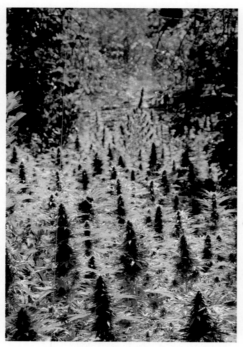

Ambient temperature regulation is essential for healthy cannabis growth regardless of whether plants are grown indoors, outdoors, or in a greenhouse.

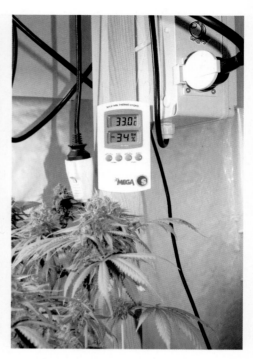

A combination thermometer/hygrometer that registers maximum and minimum readings helps keep the garden room's atmosphere constant.

qualities of Mother Earth. With the added heat of the HID and hot, humid weather outdoors, an indoor room can heat up rapidly and greenhouse temperatures can soar. More than a few gardeners in the USA have lost their crops to heat stroke during the Fourth of July weekend, which is the first big holiday of the summer, and everybody wants to get away to enjoy it. Some gardeners forget or are too paranoid to maintain good ventilation in the garden room while on vacation. Temperatures can easily climb to 100°F (37.8°C) or more in garden rooms and greenhouses that are poorly insulated and vented. The hotter the air temperature, the more ventilation and water that are necessary.

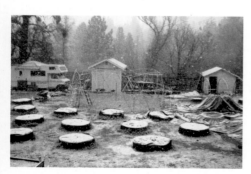

Winter weather comes early to some gardens. This gardener was able to harvest his crop a long time before the snow arrived.

The cold of winter is the other temperature extreme. Think back and remember past winter storms in your climate. Electricity often goes out in cities and surrounding areas. Water pipes freeze and heating systems fail. Some residents are driven from their homes until electricity can be restored, often days later. In such cases gardeners return to find their beautiful gardens wilted, stricken with the deepest, most disgusting green only a freeze can bring. Broken water pipes, ice everywhere! It is difficult to combat such acts of God, but if possible, always keep garden rooms and greenhouses above 50°F (10°C) and definitely above freezing, 32°F (0°C). If the temperature dips below this mark, the freeze will rupture plant cells, and foliage will die back or, at best, grow slowly. Growth slows or stops when the temperature dips below 55°F (12.8°C). Stressing plants with cold weather conditions is not recommended; it may yield a proportionately higher THC content, but it will reduce plants' overall productivity.

A **thermostat** measures temperature and controls it by turning on or off a device that regulates heating or cooling, keeping the temperature within a predetermined range. A thermostat can

be attached to an electric or combustion heater. Often indoor garden rooms can take advantage of individually thermostat-controlled electric baseboard heaters in each room.

A thermostat can be used to control cooling vent fans in all but the coldest garden rooms and greenhouses. When it gets too hot in a room, the thermostat turns on the vent fan, which evacuates hot, stale air. The vent fan remains on until the desired temperature is reached, then the thermostat turns off the fan. A thermostat-controlled vent fan offers adequate temperature and humidity control for many garden rooms and greenhouses. A refrigerated air conditioner can be installed if heat and humidity are a major problem, but such devices draw a lot of electricity. If excessive heat is a problem but humidity is not a concern, use a swamp cooler. These evaporative coolers are inexpensive to operate and keep garden rooms and greenhouses cool in arid climates.

Common thermostats include single-stage and two-stage. The single-stage thermostat controls a device that keeps temperature the same both day and night. A two-stage thermostat is

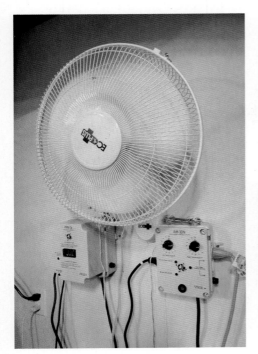

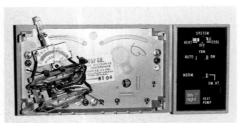

This thermostat is controlled with a mercury switch visible in the center-left of the photo.

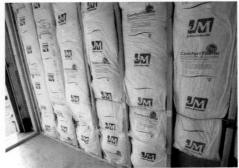

This garden room is equipped with a thermostat that controls both day and night temperatures. On the left is a CO₂ controller.

Insulated garden-room walls help immensely to keep garden-room temperature independent of outside atmospheric conditions.

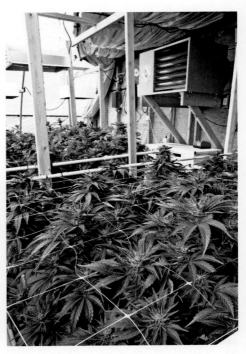

A directional air conditioner directs cool air over the entire area of this garden room.

more expensive but can be set to maintain different daytime and nighttime temperatures. This convenience can save money on heating and provides exacting control over plant growth.

Note: Sometimes a slight day/night differential in temperature, even as slight as two degrees, can bring about physiological changes in plant growth, such as intense foliage coloration or an increased production of resin and other metabolites.

Many **electronic garden room and greenhouse controllers** have been developed in the last decade. These controllers can operate and integrate every appliance in garden rooms and greenhouses. More sophisticated controllers integrate the operation of CO₂ equipment and vent and intake fans. If temperature and humidity regulation are causing cultural problems in your garden rooms and greenhouses, consider purchasing a controller.

Uninsulated garden rooms and greenhouses experience significant temperature fluctuations and require special consideration and care. Before growing in such a location, make sure it is the

only choice. If forced to use a sunbaked attic that cools at night, make sure maximum insulation is in place to help balance temperature instability. Enclose the garden room or greenhouse to control heating and cooling.

When **CO₂ is enriched** to levels of 0.7 to 0.9 percent (700–900 ppm), a temperature of 75°F to 80°F (23.9°C–26.7°C) promotes faster exchange of gases. Photosynthesis and chlorophyll synthesis are able to take place at a faster rate, causing plants to grow more rapidly. Remember, this higher temperature increases water, nutrient, and space consumption, so be prepared. Unless in a functioning sealed room, CO₂-enriched plants still need ventilation to remove stale, humid air and promote plant health.

The temperature in the garden room tends to stay the same, top to bottom, when the air is circulated with an oscillating fan or fans. In an enclosed garden room, HID lamps and ballasts keep the area warm. Placing remote ballasts near the floor on a shelf or a stand also helps break up air stratification by radiating heat upward, while protecting them from water splashes and floods. Garden

rooms in cool climates stay warm during the day when the outdoor temperature peaks, but they often cool off too much at night, when cold temperatures set in. To compensate, gardeners turn on the lamp at night to help heat the room, but leave it off during the day. Sometimes it is too cold for the lamp and ballast to maintain satisfactory room temperatures.

A **barrel filled with water** (or a nutrient reservoir) will collect heat during the day. At night, when temperatures cool, the heat banked in the water slowly radiates to warm the growing area. This passive means of heating requires only a container and space to locate it. See chapter 11, *Greenhouses*, for more information.

Garden rooms in homes are usually equipped with a **central heating and/or air conditioning** vent. The vent is usually controlled by a central thermostat that regulates the temperature of the home. By adjusting the thermostat to 72°F (22.2°C) and opening the door to the garden room, it can stay a cozy 72°F (22.2°C). However, using electric power is expensive and often wasteful. Keeping the thermostat between 60°F and 65°F (15.6°C–18.3°C), coupled with the heat

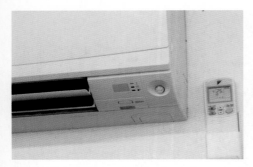

Air conditioning is expensive but often already installed in many homes.

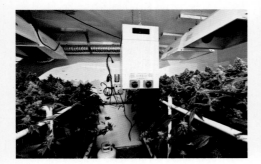

This propane heater is also a CO_2 generator.

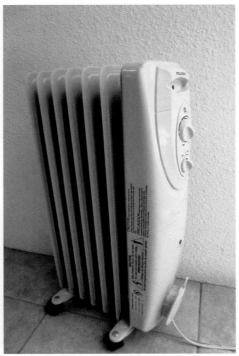

Electric oil-filled radiators are a good option for many small gardens. They can supply just enough heat during nighttime hours to maintain temperature levels and not let humidity get out of control.

from the HID system, should be enough to sustain 75°F (23.9°C) temperatures. Other supplemental heat sources such as inefficient incandescent lightbulbs and electric heaters are expensive and draw extra electricity, but they provide instant heat that is easy to regulate. Propane and natural gas heaters increase temperatures and burn oxygen from the air, creating CO_2 and water vapor as by-products. This dual advantage makes using a CO_2 generator economical and practical, especially in greenhouses. Make sure to properly vent all enclosed spaces when generating CO_2 with fossil fuels.

Kerosene heaters with an open flame generate heat and CO_2. Look for a heater that burns its fuel efficiently and completely with no telltale odor of the fuel in the room. Do not use old kerosene heaters or fuel-oil heaters if they burn fuel inefficiently. A blue flame is burning all the fuel cleanly. A red flame indicates only part of the fuel is being burned. I'm not a big fan of kerosene heaters and do not recommend using them. The room must be vented regularly to avoid build-up of toxic carbon monoxide (CO), also a by-product of combustion.

Diesel oil is a common source of indoor heat. Many furnaces use this dirty, polluting fuel. Woodstoves pollute too, but work well as a heat source. A vent fan is extremely important to exhaust polluted air and draw fresh air into a room heated by an oil furnace or a woodstove.

Propane and LP gas heaters are the most common way to heat greenhouses. Some of these heaters have an open flame, others do not. Combustion burns oxygen out of the air, which in turn increases CO_2 levels in the greenhouse.

WIND SPEED		WINDCHILL	
MPH	KMH	°F	°C
0	0	50	10
5	8	48	8.88
10	16	40	4.44
15	24.1	36	2.22
20	32.2	32	0
25	40.2	30	-1.11
30	48.2	28	-2.22

Use an **infrared heater** to raise the temperature in enclosed garden rooms and greenhouses. Infrared heat energy is directed at objects to be heated. The energy does not convert to heat until absorbed by plants, pots, soil, and so forth. Temperature is easy to control and accurate because the temperature sensor receives the same infrared energy that the plants receive. Infrared heating allows the air in enclosed gardens to be 5 to 7 degrees lower than if air is heated with fossil fuels and electricity. Temperatures also vary less from the top to the bottom of the enclosed area. And leaf surfaces stay drier and are less prone to attack by airborne diseases, allowing more plants and denser foliage in the same area.

The heating system should be designed around the greenhouse or garden room. Hang the infrared heater high enough so that infrared pattern can cover the desired width. Outdoor gardeners can suspend infrared heaters 16 feet above growing beds for nighttime heat. See manufacturer recommendations for coverage.

Outdoors, temperature is more difficult to control. Planting in a location that remains warm, especially at night, is the easiest way to keep plants warm. Remember that cool air sinks and tends to stay in the bottom of canyons or low geographic spots. Avoid windy planting locations because windchill lowers temperature in relation to the velocity of wind. If wind is a factor, erect a permeable windbreak or plant next to a building or natural wind barrier to lessen the effect.

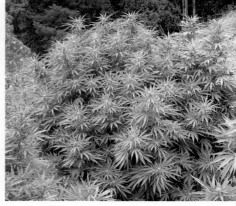

Windchill is more difficult to control outdoors.

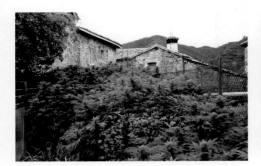

Planting next to or in between buildings protects plants from wind, which in turn helps keep them warmer.

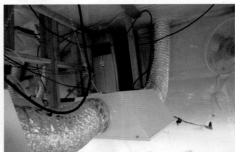

Heat generated by the HID bulb is evacuated before it affects the room's temperature and humidity.

According to popular calculations at 50°F (10°C) the windchill factor drops the temperature ten degrees when the wind is blowing at 10 mph (16.1 kmh).

Cooling the great outdoors is even more difficult than heating it. The easiest way to cool plants outdoors is to plant in partial shade. Plant in a location that is shaded during the heat of the day so that plants do not get warmer than 86°F (30°C), at which point growth virtually stops. A shade cloth can also be installed above plants. A natural breezeway occurs between the canopy of plants and the shade cloth.

Note: Cannabis will grow better outdoors in higher temperatures than it will indoors or in a greenhouse at the same temperatures. Mother Nature is the best!

Disease, insect, and spider mite existence and survival are also affected by temperature. In general, the cooler it is, the slower the insects and fungi reproduce and develop. Temperature control is effectively integrated into many control programs for diseases, pests and spider mites. Check recommendations in chapter 24, *Diseases & Pests*.

Humidity

Humidity is relative; that is, air holds different quantities of water at different temperatures. Relative humidity is the ratio between the amount of moisture in the air and the greatest amount of moisture the air could hold at the same temperature. In other words, the hotter it is, the more moisture air can hold; the cooler it is, the less moisture air can hold. When the temperature in a garden

room drops, the humidity climbs. If humidity climbs beyond 100 percent, the moisture in the air condenses into water droplets. For example, dew forms on plant surfaces outdoors when the temperature drops at night.

For example, an 800 cubic foot (10 × 10 × 8 feet) (22.7 m³) garden room will hold about 14 ounces (414 ml) of water when the temperature is 70°F (21.1°C) and relative humidity is at 100 percent. When the temperature is increased to 100°F (37.8°C), the same room will hold 56 ounces (1.7 L) of moisture at 100 percent relative humidity. That is four times more moisture! Where does this water go when the temperature drops? It condenses onto the surface of plants as well as ceilings and walls, just as dew condenses outdoors.

Relative humidity increases when the temperature drops at night. The greater the temperature variation, the greater the relative humidity variation will be.

Supplemental heat or extra ventilation is often necessary at night if temperatures fluctuate by more than 15 degrees. Seedlings and vegetative plants grow best when the relative humidity is from 60 to 70 percent. Flowering plants grow best in a relative humidity range of 40 to 60 percent.

The lower humidity range discourages most pests and diseases. As with temperature, consistent humidity promotes healthy, even growth. Relative humidity level affects the transpiration rate of plants via the stomata (see "Stomata" above). When humidity is high, water evaporates slowly. The stomata close, transpiration slows, and so does plant growth.

Water evaporates quickly into drier air, causing stomata to open, thus increasing transpiration, fluid flow, and growth. Transpiration in arid conditions will be rapid only if there is enough water available for roots to draw in. If water is inadequate, stomata will close to protect the plant from dehydration, causing growth to slow.

When relative humidity climbs beyond 70 percent, the pressure slows the movement of gas molecules from solution to the air. This results in the increase in energy or temperature in the overall system because it is not used up in evaporation. The stomata typically lodge wide open.

A 10 × 10 × 8-foot (800 cubic feet) (22.7 m³) garden room can hold:			
Water (ounces)	**Water (milliliters)**	**°F**	**°C**
4	118	32	0
7	207	50	10
14	414	70	21.1
18	532	80	26.7
28	828	90	32.2
56	165	100	37.88

The moisture-holding capacity of air approximately doubles with every 20°F (10°C) increase in temperature.

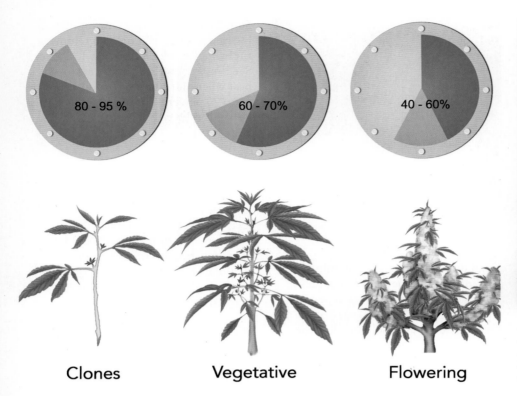

80 - 95 %   60 - 70%   40 - 60%

Clones   **Vegetative**   **Flowering**

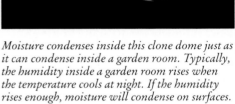

Moisture condenses inside this clone dome just as it can condense inside a garden room. Typically, the humidity inside a garden room rises when the temperature cools at night. If the humidity rises enough, moisture will condense on surfaces.

Measuring and Controlling Relative Humidity

Measure relative humidity with a **hygrometer**. By knowing the exact moisture content in the air, humidity may be adjusted to a safe 40 to 60 percent level that encourages transpiration and discourages fungus growth.

Inexpensive spring-type hygrometers are accurate within 5 to 10 percent. They are adequate for most hobby gardeners whose main concern is to keep the humidity near 50 percent. More expensive psychrometers are very accurate. Today there are many exceptionally accurate high-tech gadgets; plus they are equipped with memory! See chapter 15, *Meters*, for more information.

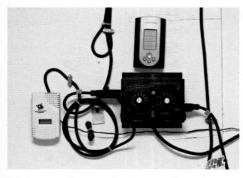

Sophisticated atmospheric controllers also control humidity with a humidistat.

A **humidistat** is attached to a vent fan, air conditioner, humidifier, or dehumidifier to regulate humidity in a garden room or greenhouse. Humidistats are inexpensive (about $20 to $100 USD) and make controlling the environment very easy. A humidistat and thermostat or a combination unit can be set up to control a vent fan and other appliances. Each can operate the fan independently. As soon as the humidity (or temperature) exceeds the acceptable range, the fan turns on to vent the humid (or hot) air outdoors.

The HID lamp and ballast radiate heat, which lowers humidity. Heat from an HID system and a vent fan on a thermostat/humidistat are all the humidity control necessary for many garden rooms. Other dry heat sources, such as hot air vented from a furnace or woodstove, dry the air and lower the humidity. But be careful; do not let piped-in, warm, dry air blow directly on foliage. It will rapidly dehydrate plants.

Increase humidity by misting the air with water or setting out a bucket of water to evaporate into the air. A humidifier is convenient and relatively inexpensive. Humidifiers evaporate water into the air to increase humidity. Just set the dial to a specific level and the humidity

changes to the desired level as soon as enough water is evaporated into the air. A humidifier is usually not necessary unless there is an extreme problem with the enclosed garden area drying out. Problems seldom occur that can be remedied by a humidifier. All too often, there is too much humidity in the air because of irrigation and transpiration.

A **dehumidifier** is more sophisticated and expensive than a humidifier and will remove moisture from an enclosed garden area by condensing it from the air. Once the water is separated from the air, it is captured in a removable container. This container should be emptied daily. For example, when the temperature drops just ten degrees, about ten ounces (~300 ml) of water from the saturated air will condense in a 10 × 10 × 8-foot (800 cubic feet) (22.7 m³) room.

A dehumidifier can be used anytime to help guard against fungus. Just set the dial at the desired percent humidity, and presto! Perfect humidity. Dehumidifiers use more electricity and are more expensive and complex than humidifiers. But to gardeners with extreme humidity problems unsolvable with a vent fan, dehumidifiers are worth the added expense. Check rental companies for large dehumidifiers if only needed for a short

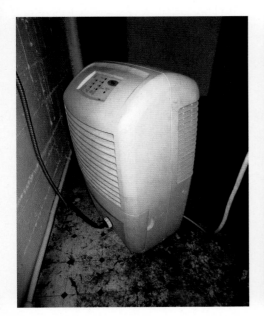

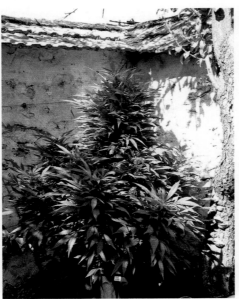

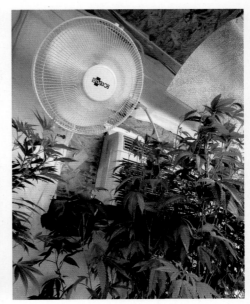

Dehumidifiers are less expensive than air conditioners. A dehumidifier is an excellent way to lower the overall humidity of a room if vent fans are unable to do the job.

Humidity tends to hang around this sheltered corner of the building in the morning and at night.

Oscillating circulation fans attached high on garden-room walls are essential to provide proper air circulation between plants.

time. Air conditioners also function as dehumidifiers but use a lot of electricity. Water collected from a dehumidifier or air conditioner has a very low electrical conductivity (EC) and can be used to water plants.

Pests and diseases can also be prevented by controlling humidity. In general, humidity above 80 percent discourages spider mites but impairs growth and promotes fungus, as well as root and stem rot. Humidity levels below 60 percent reduce the chances of fungus and rot.

Outdoors, humidity is difficult to regulate. Lowering humidity in the wide-open outdoors is virtually impossible because it is impractical to enclose. Raising humidity outdoors is possible by installing windbreaks so that plants do not dehydrate. Air around plants can also be misted, which will increase humidity. However, the best way to control humidity outdoors is to plant in a climate with the desirable humidity levels.

Change or regulate humidity outdoors by planting in a microclimate that is less humid, such as on a hillside or in a natural breezeway.

Change or regulate humidity in a greenhouse with vent fans and evaporative cooling methods, such as a swamp cooler that uses big evaporative cooling pads.

High humidity reduces the ability of the air to hold water, which slows evapotranspiration, reduces water movement in the plant, and diminishes the plant's cooling ability. High temperatures demand water-cooling; and in the light, the inside of the leaf is 10 to 20 degrees hotter than the air. As a result, high humidity is a bigger problem during the day than it is at night for plant stress.

Note: Disease spores like high humidity, and they will attack both day and night!

Air Movement
Air ventilation and circulation are essential to healthy harvests indoors and in greenhouses. Fresh air is one of the most overlooked factors contributing to a healthy garden and a bountiful harvest. Fresh air is the least expensive essential component required to produce a healthy medicinal garden. Experienced, successful gardeners understand the importance of fresh air and take the time to set up an adequate ventilation system.

Air Circulation
Plants use all CO_2 around the leaf within a few minutes. Outdoors, gentle breezes replace CO_2; in greenhouses and indoor garden rooms, air must be managed. A dead air zone forms around leaves when no new CO_2-rich air replaces the used CO_2-depleted air. CO_2-depleted air stifles stomata and virtually stops growth. If it is not *actively* moved, air around leaves and in the garden room stratifies.

Warm air stays near the ceiling, and cool air settles near the floor in enclosed areas. Air circulation breaks up these air masses, mixing them together. Avoid these would-be problems by opening a door, window, or vent and/or installing oscillating circulation fans. Air circulation also helps prevent harmful pest and fungus attacks. Omnipresent mold

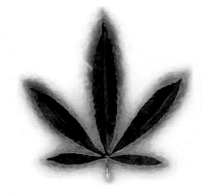

This drawing demonstrates how leaves use virtually all the surrounding CO_2 in a short time.

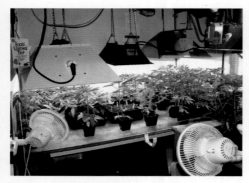

Small oscillating circulation fans move the heat generated by lamps away from the garden. Position circulation fans below and above the canopy of the garden. Do not blow heavy streams of air directly on plants or they will dry out quickly.

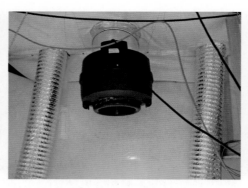

An inline fan attached directly to the ceiling removes any hot air near the ceiling.

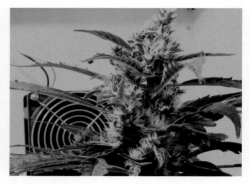

Small computer fans can be used to ventilate small garden rooms.

spores do not land and grow as readily when air is stirred by a fan. Insects and spider mites find it difficult to live in an environment that is constantly bombarded by air currents.

Improve air circulation in and around all cannabis plants by pruning out lower, spindly branches and foliage that do not receive much light.

Air Ventilation

Fresh air is easy to obtain and inexpensive to maintain—it is as simple as hooking up and placing the proper-sized exhaust fan in the most efficient location of a garden room or greenhouse. An intake vent or fan may be necessary to create a flow of fresh air in enclosed areas. Outdoors, planting in a location that receives adequate air circulation is all it takes.

A 10-foot square (0.9 m²) garden will use from 10 to 50 gallons (37.8 to 189.3 L) or more of water every week. Plants transpire most of this water into the air. Every day and night, rapidly growing plants transpire more moisture into the air. If this moisture is left in the garden room or greenhouse, humidity increases to 100 percent, which stifles stomata and causes growth to screech to a halt. It also opens the door for disease and pest attacks.

Replace moist air with fresh, dry air, and transpiration increases, stomata function properly, and growth rebounds. A vent fan that extracts air from the garden room is the perfect solution to remove this humid, stale air. Fresh air flows in through an intake vent or with the help of an intake fan.

Ventilation is as important as water, light, heat, and nutrients. In many cases, fresh air is even more important. Greenhouses use large ventilation fans. Garden rooms are very similar to greenhouses and should follow their example. Most garden rooms have an easy-to-use opening such as a window in which to mount a fan, but security or room location may render it unusable. If no vent opening is available, one will have to be created.

All garden rooms require ventilation. The ventilation system could be as simple as an open door or window that supplies and circulates fresh air throughout the room. But open doors and windows can be inconvenient and problematic. Most gardeners elect to install a vent fan instead. Some gardeners need to install an entire ventilation system, including ductwork and several fans.

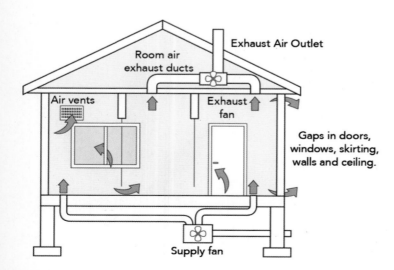

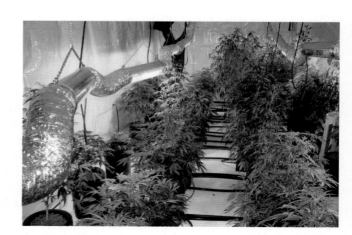

Connecting light reflectors to a ventilation system removes hot air generated by lamps. Oftentimes, lamps generate the majority of heat in a garden room.

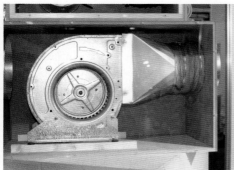

This squirrel cage blower has been set inside a box to dampen the noise it generates.

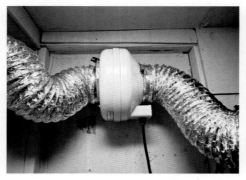

This inline fan is placed in the middle of ducting to speed air movement.

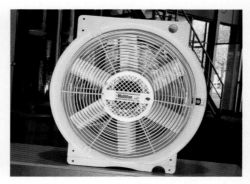

Propeller fans are very efficient and move a lot of air, but they are noisy when running at higher speeds.

Squirrel cage blowers are efficient at moving air, but they are very loud. Blowers with a balanced, well-oiled wheel run most quietly. Felt or rubber grommets below each foot of the fan will reduce noise caused by vibrations. Run motor at a low rpm (revolutions per minute) to lessen noise.

Inline fans are designed to fit into a duct pipe. The propellers are mounted to increase the airflow quickly, effortlessly, and as quietly as possible. Inline fans are available in quiet, high-quality models that run with little friction.

Propeller or muffin fans with large fan blades expel air through a large opening, and are most efficient and quiet when operated at low revolutions per minute (rpm). A slow-moving propeller fan on the ceiling of a garden room will quietly and efficiently move the air.

A vent fan *pulls* air out of a room four times more efficiently than a fan is able to push it out. Do not set up a circulation fan in the room and expect it to vent the area by pushing air out a distant vent. The circulation fan must be very large to adequately increase air pressure and push enough air out a vent to create an exchange of air. A vent fan that pulls air out of the garden, on the other hand, is able to change the pressure and exchange the air quickly and efficiently.

A vent fan *pulls* air out of a room 4 times more efficiently than a fan is able to *push* it out.

Vent fans are rated by the amount of air they can move, measured in cubic feet per minute (cfm) or cubic meters per hour (m³/h). The fan should be able to replace the air volume (length × width × height = total volume in cubic feet or meters) of a large garden room in less than five minutes, and in a small garden room in less than one minute. Once evacuated, new air is immediately drawn

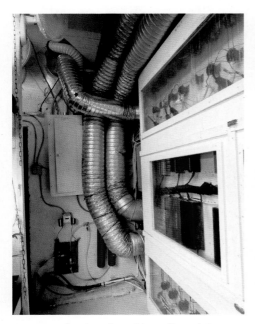

Run vent ducting alongside walls and the ceiling so they are out of the way. Keep the vent ducting as straight as possible so air flows freely.

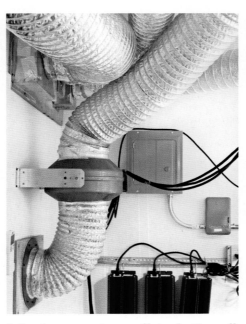

Inline fans move air very efficiently. Here, all four ventilation ducts are connected to inline fans.

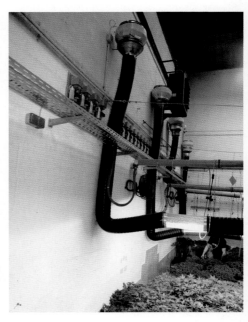

Inline fans can be placed at the end of ducting, where they are most efficient, or they can be placed in the middle of a run of ducting to pull and push air.

in through an intake vent or via an intake fan. An intake fan might be necessary to bring an adequate volume of fresh air into the room quickly. Covering the intake vent with fine mesh silkscreen will help exclude pests. (see "Filtering Intake Air" below). Some rooms have so many little cracks for air to drift in that they do not need an intake vent.

Ducting

Ducting should be as big as possible so that air can be moved passively whenever possible. Hot air rises. Adept gardeners locate air exit vents in the hottest peak of garden rooms or greenhouses for passive, silent air venting. The larger the diameter of the exhaust ducts, the more air that can travel through them. By installing a big, slow-moving vent fan in this vent, hot stale air is quietly and efficiently evacuated. A fan running at 50 rpm is quieter than one running at 200 rpm. Smart gardeners install 12-inch (30.5 cm) or larger ducting and inline fans whenever possible. Most often, the vent fan is attached to ducting that directs air out of enclosed garden areas.

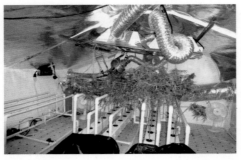

Airflow is impaired proportionately to the number and angle of turns ducting takes.

Flexible ducting is easier to use than rigid ducting. Insulated ducting will lessen noise. Run ducting the shortest possible distance, and keep curves to a minimum. When turned at more than a 30° angle, much of the air that enters a duct whirls into turbulence, restricting flow. Keep the ducting straight and short.

Intake Air

Some garden rooms and small greenhouses have enough fresh air coming in via cracks and holes, but most enclosed

areas require fresh air to be ushered in with the help of an intake vent or fan.* An intake vent allows air to passively flow into an enclosed area. An intake fan blows fresh air into the garden room or greenhouse. The ratio of 1:4 (100 cfm [m³/h] incoming and 400 cfm [m³/h] outgoing) should give the room a little negative pressure.

An intake fan blows fresh air into the room. The ratio of 1:4 (100 cfm [m³/h] incoming and 400 cfm [m³/h] outgoing) should give the room a little negative pressure.

Indoor garden rooms can often take full advantage of the preexisting household heating, ventilation, and air conditioning (HVAC) system. The HVAC system often contains an adequate filtering system to keep air clean and fresh smelling.

Delivering fresh air to plants ensures that they will have adequate CO_2 to continue rapid growth. One of the best ways to deliver air directly to plants is to pipe it in via flexible ducting. Ingenious

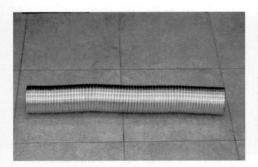

Straight ducting (with no bend) is the most efficient for air transmission.

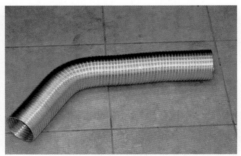

A 45° curve cuts up to 40 percent of air transmission.

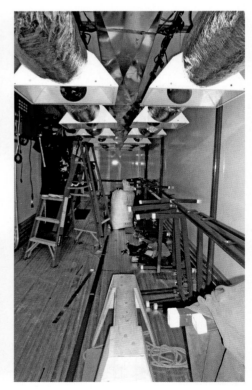

Ducting can also be insulated, which lowers noise levels. Prefabricated, insulated, flexible ducting is readily available.

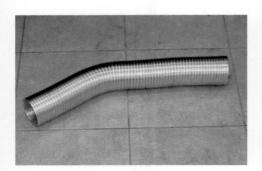

A 30° curve cuts up to 20 percent of air transmission.

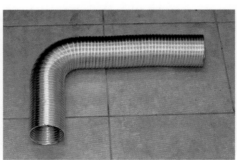

A 90° curve cuts up to 60 percent of air transmission.

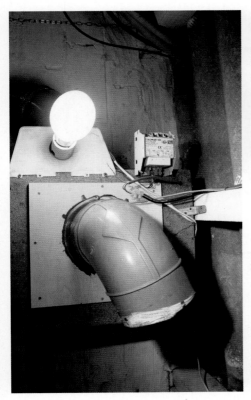

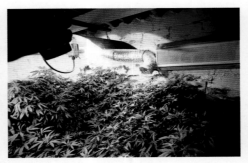

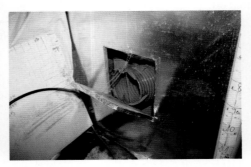

Cool intake air is being delivered into this garden via flexible ducting. You can see where plants directly receiving cold intake air do not grow as well as plants on either side.

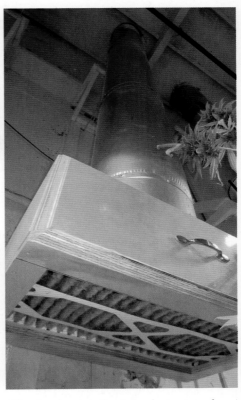

Intake air in this garden room is heated and directed downward upon entry.

This intake air vent near the floor can be sealed off at night to help hold heat in the room.

Filter intake air before introducing it to the garden room or greenhouse.

gardeners cut holes in the intake ducting to direct air where it is needed. The air is dispersed evenly throughout the room. Fresh air for each plant is essential for fast, consistent growth. Sealed rooms get all their air via the air conditioner exchange.

Always make sure fresh air is neither too hot nor too cold. Keep the temperature differential less than 10 degrees for intake air. And bring in cooler air to cause fewer problems in an overheated garden room. For example, one friend who lives in a hot, arid climate brings fresh air in from the crawl space under the house, where the air is a few degrees cooler than ambient air.

Filtering Intake Air

Covering intake air vents with a filter will help exclude pests and diseases from the garden area. Often a nylon stocking stretched over the intake vent is all that is needed. Some gardeners go so far as to put a superfine mesh screen over intake vents. Just remember, fine mesh screens

will restrict airflow and put extra pressure on the intake fan, causing it extra wear and a shorter life.

CO₂ Enrichment

Cost versus benefit: CO_2 provides the biggest bang for the buck at a saturation point of 700 to 900 ppm.

The most common ways to introduce CO_2 into garden rooms and greenhouses include:

1. Combustion: burning fossil (hydrocarbon) fuels such as propane, butane, natural (LP) gas, and kerosene. Alcohols—ethyl, ethanol, methyl, isopropyl, and so forth—are too expensive to consider using for this purpose.
2. Compressed (bottled) CO_2
3. Chemical reaction
   a. Excellofizz
   b. Co2 Boost
   c. Dry ice
   d. Fermentation
   e. Decomposition of organic matter

Carbon dioxide (CO_2) is a colorless, odorless, nonflammable gas that surrounds us all the time. Atmospheric CO_2 content has increased rapidly in the last 60 years, from about 300 ppm to 380 ppm—more than 25 percent, as a conservative estimate. Today the air we breathe contains about 0.038 percent (380 ppm) CO_2. Rapid-growing cannabis can use the available CO_2 in an enclosed garden room or greenhouse within a few hours. Photosynthesis and growth virtually stop when the CO_2 level falls below 0.02 percent (200 ppm).

Carbon dioxide enrichment has been used in commercial greenhouses for more than 40 years. Adding more CO_2 to air in garden rooms and greenhouses stimulates growth by as much as 30 percent. Cannabis can use more CO_2 than the 0.38 percent (380 ppm) that naturally occurs in the air. By increasing the amount of CO_2 to 0.7 to 0.9 percent (700–900 ppm)—the optimum range widely agreed upon by professionals—plants can grow up to 30 percent faster,

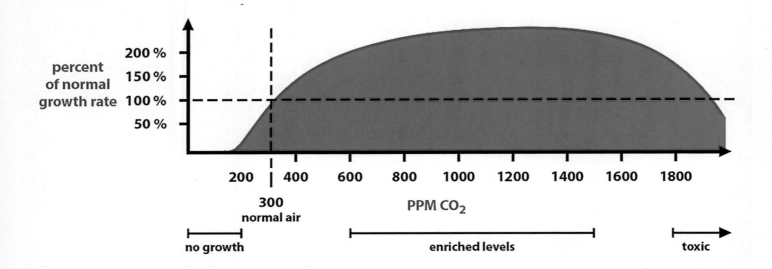

providing that light, water, and nutrients are not limiting. Carbon dioxide enrichment has little or no effect on plants grown under standard T12 fluorescent lights. However, brighter T8 and T5 lamps supply enough light for the plants to process the extra available CO_2.

Caution! Carbon dioxide can make people woozy when it rises above 4000 ppm and can become toxic at higher levels. When CO_2 rises to such high levels, it displaces oxygen, causing a lack of O_2. In fact, high levels of CO_2 (5000+ ppm) can be used for insect and spider mite control.

Carbon dioxide enrichment does not make plants produce more potent cannabinoids; it causes more foliage to grow in less time. CO_2 provides more energy for their production and the basic building blocks from which they are made. And while the volume does increase in the entire plant, the concentration per dried weight unit remains the same.

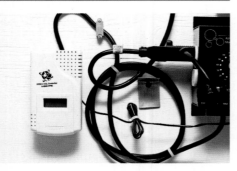

A CO_2 monitor makes it easier to keep the carbon dioxide level in the room precise.

Carbon dioxide-enriched cannabis demands a higher level of maintenance than normal plants. CO_2-enriched plants use nutrients, water, and space faster than unenriched plants. A higher temperature, from 75°F to 80°F (23.9°C to 26.7°C), will help stimulate more rapid metabolism within the super-enriched plants. When temperatures climb beyond 85°F (29.4°C), CO_2 enrichment becomes ineffective; and at 90°F (32.2°C) growth stops.

Carbon dioxide-enriched plants use more water. Water rises from plant roots and is released into the air by the same stomata the plant uses to absorb CO_2 during transpiration. Carbon dioxide enrichment affects transpiration by causing the plants' stomata to partially close. This slows down the loss of water vapor into the air. Foliage on CO_2-enriched plants is measurably thicker, more turgid, and slower to wilt than leaves on unenriched plants.

CO_2 at Night

Plants do not use CO_2 at night or during a dark period. There is no extra O_2 and this ratio should remain constant all the time. CO_2 from outside the plant is used exclusively in the photosystem; without light, it is no longer used. Using CO_2 at night wastes money and natural resources, and is harmful to plants.

Carbon dioxide affects plant morphology. In an enriched growing environment, stems and branches grow faster, and the cells of these plant parts are more densely packed. Flower stems carry more weight without bending. Because of the increased rate of branching, cannabis has more flower initiation (budding) sites. Plants are more likely to set flowers early if CO_2 enrichment is used.

With CO_2-enriched air, plants that do not have the support of the other critical elements for life will not benefit at all, and the CO_2 will be wasted. Plants can be limited by just one of the critical factors. For example, the CO_2-enriched plants will use water and nutrients much faster, and if they are not appropriately supplied, the plants will not grow. They might even be stunted.

To be most effective, the CO_2 level must be maintained at 700 to 900 ppm everywhere in the room. To accomplish this, the garden room or greenhouse must be completely enclosed. Cracks in and around the walls should be sealed off to prevent CO_2-rich air from escaping. Enclosing the room makes it easier to control the CO_2 content of the air within. The room must also have a vent fan with flaps or a baffle. The vent fan will remove the stale air that will be replaced with CO_2-enriched air. The flaps or baffle will help contain the CO_2 in the enclosed garden room or greenhouse. Venting requirements will change with each type of CO_2-enrichment system and are discussed on the next page.

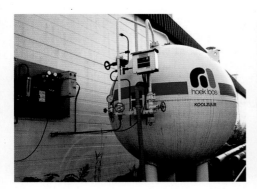

A big tank of CO_2 can be placed outside large grow rooms.

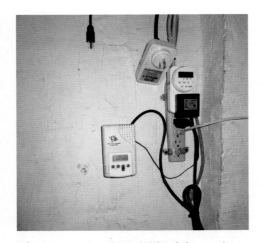

Set this CO_2 monitor and controller to manage two different rooms and provide a log 24 hours a day.

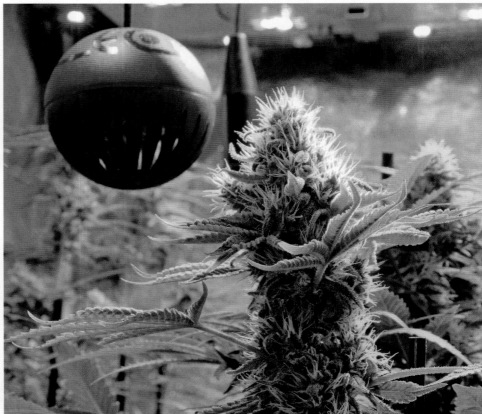

The big ball on the left is one of the many new solid state CO_2 sensors available to cannabis gardeners. The Evolution NDIR CO_2 Sensor works with a controller to regulate carbon dioxide in a room full of MK Ultra plants laden with flower buds.

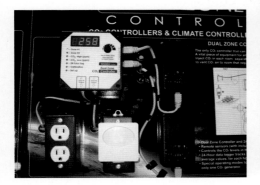

This inexpensive ($300 USD) CO_2 monitor and controller is easy to mount and use.

Measuring and monitoring CO_2 levels in the air is expensive. Monitoring CO_2 levels in greenhouses or garden rooms with six or more lights is economically feasible and helps keep the levels consistent.

Note: Anytime you vent any gas that replaces oxygen in a sealed environment that you might work in, you should definitely know and monitor the level of that gas and oxygen as well.

See chapter 15, *Meters*, for more information.

Stay Safe! Store bottled propane and other explosive gases outdoors.

The easiest way to calculate CO_2 use in a garden room or greenhouse is to search "CO_2 grow room calculator" in www.google.com. You will find several pages of calculators that give CO_2 needed and flow-rate calculations for emitters and generators they sell.

At a concentration of approximately 2000 ppm, carbon dioxide becomes detrimental to plant growth: the stomatal guard cells become confused and quit functioning. Plants need a concentration of about 20 percent oxygen; adding CO_2 displaces O_2, and at a certain point these levels will begin to affect respiration in the plant.

Effects of Altitude and CO_2 Enrichment

A CO_2 monitor/regulator must be calibrated for altitude to provide the proper level of the gas. Air is much denser at sea level than it is at, say, 3,000 feet (915 m). Conversely, air is thinner at higher elevations, so if CO_2 is added, it must be added in proportion to the available air. Too much CO_2 will cause problems.

In fact, when using a CO_2 generator at higher altitudes, incomplete combustion occurs, the result of which is the release of ethylene gas. At night in a sealed or semi-sealed room, both the plants and the CO_2 generator (pilot light) are using oxygen, so more O_2 is depleted, exacerbating the problem. In such situations, bottled CO_2 with a calibrated monitor/regulator used in conjunction with a little nighttime ventilation will keep the environment copacetic. Or use a CO_2 generator that is kept outside the garden room and duct the gas into the sealed area. Make sure to place a CO_2 monitor/regulator inside the garden room.

If you are using CO_2 and plants' growth rate does not increase, check to make sure the entire garden room is running properly. Verify that plants have the proper light and nutrient levels, as well as the correct temperature and humidity, and that grow medium moisture and pH levels are appropriate. Make sure roots receive enough oxygen both day and night.

CO_2 Emitter Systems

Compressed CO_2 systems store the gas in a tank (cylinder) and meter it out into the garden room over time. Compressed CO_2 systems are ideal for sealed rooms. They cost about $0.50 USD per pound (453.6 gm) of compressed gas and are virtually risk-free—producing no toxic gases, heat, or water vapor. Carbon dioxide is metered out of a cylinder of compressed gas using a regulator, flow meter, solenoid valve, and short-range timer. There are two types of compressed CO_2 systems: continuous flow and short-range dispersal. Metal cylinders hold CO_2 gas under 1000 to 2200 psi (68.9–137.0 BAR), depending upon temperature.

In North America, cylinders are available in four sizes: 10, 20, 35, and

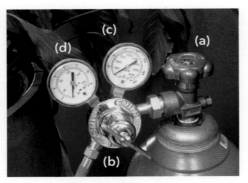

This CO_2 emitter has an (a) on/off valve, (b) solenoid valve, (c) regulator, and (d) flow meter.

50 pounds (4.5, 9, 15.9, and 22.7 kg). Tanks must be inspected annually and registered with a nationwide safety agency. The 20-pound (9 kg) tank is the most common and easiest to handle. Purchasing a complete CO_2-emitter system at a hydroponic store is the best value for most small gardeners. Purchasing component parts—regulator, a flow meter, and a solenoid valve— is also an option. For more information, see *Marijuana Horticulture: The Indoor/ Outdoor Medical Grower's Bible.* Most hydroponic, beverage, and welding supply stores rent, sell, exchange, and refill tanks. The latter two often require an identification card. If you purchase

a lighter and stronger aluminum tank, make sure to request an aluminum tank exchange. The tank you buy is not necessarily the one you keep.

Make sure CO_2 tanks have a protective collar on top to shield the valve. If the valve is knocked off by an accidental fall, there is enough pressure to send the top (regulator, flow meter, valve, etc.) straight through a parked car! Distribute CO_2 from the tank to the garden room by using a tube or fan. Suspend lightweight perforated plastic tubing from the ceiling to disperse the CO_2. The tubing carries CO_2 from the supply tank to the center of the garden room. The main supply line is attached to several smaller tubes that extend throughout the garden. CO_2 is heavier and cooler than air and cascades onto the plants below.

To make sure CO_2 is evenly dispersed from the tubing, submerge the lightweight plastic tubing in water and punch the emission holes under water while the CO_2 is being piped into the line. This way you know the proper diameter holes to punch and where to punch them to create the ideal CO_2 flow over the garden.

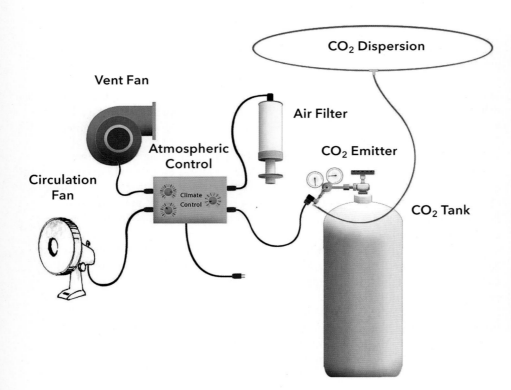

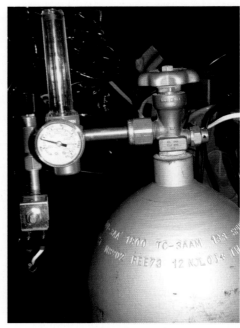

This CO_2 emitter system combines the regulator and flow meter into a single unit.

TANK SIZE	TYPE	WEIGHT FULL
10 lb (4.5 kg)	aluminum	25 lb (11.3 kg)
10 lb (4.5 kg)	steel	35 lb (15.9 kg)
20 lb (9 kg)	aluminum	50 lb (22.7 kg)
20 lb (9 kg)	steel	70 lb (31.8 kg)
35 lb (15.9 kg)	aluminum	75 lb (34 kg)
50 lb (22.7 kg)	ateel	170 lb (77.1 kg)

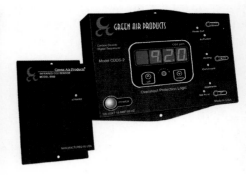

CO_2 controllers are a wise investment. They keep CO_2 at the proper level in the indoor (and greenhouse) atmosphere.

Overhead fans help evenly distribute CO_2 throughout the room. The CO_2 is released directly below the fan, into its airflow. This evenly mixes the added CO_2 throughout the air and keeps it recirculating across the plants.

CO₂ Generator Systems

CO_2 production is dictated by the rate at which the fuel is burned. For example, one pound of fossil fuel yields about 3 pounds (1.36 kg) of CO_2 gas, 1.5 pounds (0.68 kg) of water vapor, and 22,000 BTUs of heat. Amounts vary relative to fuels being burned.

CO_2 generators use a pilot light with a flow meter and a burner with an open flame to burn oxygen from the air. When used in an enclosed area, excess CO_2 is generated. CO_2 generators burn fossil (hydrocarbon) fuels, including natural (LP) gas, butane, and propane gas. CO_2, heat, and water vapor are by-products of the combustion process. The inside of the generator is similar to a gas-stove burner with a pilot light enclosed in a protective housing. The generator must have a cover over the open flame. You can operate the generator manually or synchronize it with a timer to operate with other garden room equipment such as ventilation fans that expel air at intervals so that less fuel is burned.

Even though CO_2 is heavier than air, when generated via combustion it is hotter and less dense, and therefore rises in a garden room. Good air circulation promotes even distribution of CO_2. CO_2 generators can burn fossil fuels such as kerosene, propane, or natural gas. Low grades of kerosene can have sulfur content as high as one tenth of one percent (0.001%)—enough to cause sulfur dioxide pollution. Use only high-quality "1-K" kerosene even though it is more expensive. Maintenance costs for kerosene generators are high because they use electrodes, pumps, and fuel filters. Propane and natural gas burners are the best choice for most applications.

When filling a new propane (cylinder) tank, first empty it of the inert gas, which is used to protect it from rust. Never completely fill a propane tank. Propane expands and contracts with temperature change and could release flammable gas from the pressure vent if too full.

Note: In the USA, as of April 1, 2002, all new cylinders must be equipped with an overfill prevention device (OPD). It is illegal to refill old tanks that do not have this new valve. Check with your local propane dealer for current regulations on refilling tanks.

Hobby CO_2 generators are generally priced from $250 to $500 USD, depending on size. The initial cost of a generator is slightly higher than a CO_2 emitter system that uses small, compressed-gas cylinders. CO_2 generators are about three times less expensive to operate than bottled CO_2 emitters. One gallon (3.8 L) of propane, which costs about $3 to $5 USD, contains 36 cubic feet (1019.4 L) of gas and over 100 cubic feet (2831.7 L) of CO_2 (every cubic foot [28.3 L] of propane gas produces three cubic feet [85 L] of CO_2). For example, if a garden used one gallon (3.8 L) of propane every day, the cost would be $90 to $150 USD per month. In contrast, bottled CO_2 for the same room would cost more than $250 USD per month.

One pound (0.5 kg) of fuel produces 1.5 pounds (0.7 kg) of water and 21,800 BTUs of heat. For garden rooms less than 500 cubic feet (14.2 m³), this makes CO_2 generators very difficult to use. Even for larger garden rooms, the added heat and humidity must be carefully monitored and controlled so as to not affect plants. Gardeners in warm climates do not use generators,

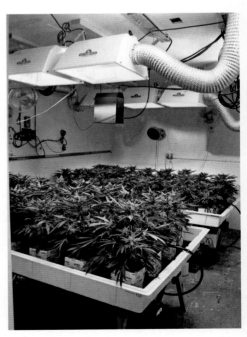

A CO_2 generator from Green Air supplies extra carbon dioxide to this fast-growing garden.

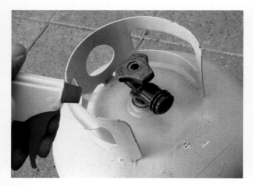

Check for gas leaks by spraying tank fittings with soapy water. Leaky valves and connections are easy to spot when they form bubbles.

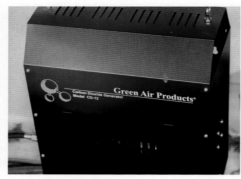

Hobby CO_2 generator.

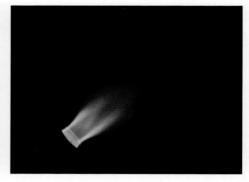

The blue flame from this torch is burning clean. A red flame signifies inefficient combustion.

because they produce too much heat and humidity.

If fuel does not burn completely or cleanly, CO_2 generators can release toxic gases—including carbon monoxide—into the garden room. Nitrous oxide, also a by-product of burning propane, can grow to toxic levels—not a laughing matter! Well-made CO_2 generators have a pilot and timer. If leaks or problems are detected, the pilot and timer will turn off automatically.

A CO_2 monitor is necessary if you are sensitive to high levels of the gas. Digital alarm units or color-change plates (used in aircraft) are an economical alternative. Carbon monoxide is a deadly gas and can be detected with a carbon monoxide detector/alarm available at most hardware and building supply stores. See "Carbon Monoxide Monitors" in chapter 15, *Meters*, for more information.

Check homemade generators frequently, including kerosene, propane, and natural (LP) gas heaters. Propane and natural gas produce a blue flame when burning efficiently. A yellow or red flame indicates unburned gas (which creates carbon monoxide) and needs more oxygen to burn cleanly.

Oxygen is also burned. As oxygen becomes deficient in a room, the oxygen and fuel mixture changes. The flame burns too rich and turns yellow. This is why fresh air is essential.

Leaks in a system can be detected by applying a solution of equal parts water and concentrated dish soap to all connections that are under pressure. If bubbles appear, gas is leaking. Never use a leaky system.

1 pound (453.5 gm) of CO_2 displaces 8.7 cubic feet (0.2 cm³) of CO_2.

0.3 pounds (136.1 gm) of fuel produces 1 pound (453.5 gm) of CO_2.

Divide the total amount of CO_2 needed by 8.7 and multiply by 0.33 to determine the amount of fuel needed. In our example, we found we need 1 cubic foot (28.3 L) of CO_2 for an 800 cubic foot (22.7 m³) garden room.

You could either do the math or enter your raw data into a CO_2 calculator such as the one available on Greentrees Hydroponics.net (www.hydroponics. net/learn/co2_calculator.asp), which does all the calculations for you.

It is best to use a CO_2 emitter in a closed (sealed) garden room so that heat build-up is not an issue.

Turn off CO_2 generators at night, since plants do not use CO_2 at night. (See "CO_2 at Night" on page 240.) They create excess heat and humidity in the garden room, and they need oxygen to operate. At night, roots need the extra oxygen in the room for continued growth.

Other Ways to Make CO_2

You can generate CO_2 using such methods as dry ice or other chemical reactions, fermentation, and burning ethyl or methyl alcohol in a kerosene lamp.

The Excellofizz puck (check out www. fearlessgardener.com) releases CO_2 into the atmosphere. It is simple to use; just add a few ounces of water and a puck or two to cause a chemical reaction that will disperse enough CO_2 to augment the air in a 10-foot-square (0.9 m²) room to about 1000 ppm all day. Excellofizz also releases a eucalyptus fragrance to help mask odors. Make sure to keep the fizz contained so that it does not splatter on plants and damage them.

Decomposing organic materials like woodchips, hay, leaves, and manures release large amounts of CO_2. The company named Co2 Boost (www.co2boost.com) has a proprietary product that decomposes to make CO_2. I have received numerous good reports about their method of generating CO_2.

Although you can capture CO_2 from this decomposition and direct it to a garden room, it is most often impractical for indoor gardeners. Piping indoors the CO_2 and fumes from a compost pile is complicated, expensive, and more work than it is worth. Greenhouse gardeners can actually compost in the greenhouse, but it could also complicate matters with undesirable diseases and pests.

Norwegians are studying charcoal burners as a source of CO_2. When refined, the system will combine the advantages of generators and compressed gas. Charcoal is much less expensive than bottled CO_2 and is less risky than generators in terms of toxic by-products. Others are studying the use of new technology to extract or filter CO_2 from the air.

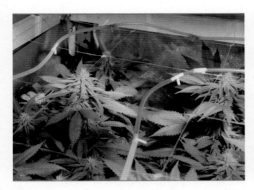

The plastic tubing and emitters hooked up to a Co2 Boost system deliver carbon dioxide directly to individual plants.

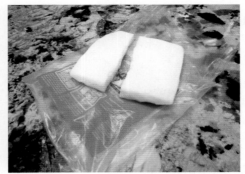

This 5-pound (2,268 gm) chunk of dry ice lasted 3 days in my home freezer.

Fermentation

Combine water, sugar, and yeast to produce CO_2 via fermentation. The yeast eats the sugar and releases CO_2 and alcohol as by-products. Mix one cup (23.7 cl) of sugar, a packet of brewer's yeast, and three quarts (283.9 cl) of warm water in a gallon (3.8 L) jug to make CO_2. You will have to experiment a little with the water temperature to get it right. Yeast dies in hot water and does not activate in cold water.

Once the yeast is activated, CO_2 is released into the air in bursts. Punch a small hole in the cap of the jug, and place it in a warm spot (80°F to 95°F [26.7°C to 35°C]) in your garden room. A fermentation lock (available for under $10 USD at beer-brewing stores) prevents contaminants from entering the jug, and they bubble CO_2 through water so the rate of production can be observed. The hitch is that you must change the concoction up to three times a day. Pour out half the solution, and then add 1.5 quarts (1.4 L) of water and another cup (23.7 cl) of sugar. As long as the yeast continues to grow and bubble, the mixture can last indefinitely. When the yeast starts to die, add another packet. Several jugs scattered around the garden room have a significant impact on CO_2 levels.

Fermentation releases no heat, toxic gases, or water, and it uses no electricity. But it stinks. It is unlikely that a gardener could tolerate the stench of a large-scale fermentation process. And with this method, CO_2 production is difficult to measure and keep uniform.

Dry Ice

Two pounds (907.2 gm) of dry ice will raise the CO_2 level in a 10 × 10-foot (3 m²) garden room to about 2000 ppm for a 24-hour period. Dry ice is expensive, $3 to $4 USD per pound (453.6 gm). One chagrined gardener remarked, "I can't believe that stuff melts so fast!"

Dry ice is carbon dioxide that has been chilled and compressed. As it melts, it changes state (sublimes) from solid to gas. Gaseous CO_2 can be mixed into the air with fans that circulate it among the plants. Dry ice works best in small-scale gardens. It is readily available at supermarkets. Because CO_2 has no liquid stage and emits no toxic gases as it melts, the transformation from solid to gas is clean and tidy. It's also easy to approximate the amount of CO_2 being released.

One pound (453.6 gm) of dry ice is equal to a pound (454 gm) of liquid CO_2. Determining the thawing period for a particular size of dry ice will allow you to estimate how much CO_2 is released during a particular period. To prolong the thawing process, put dry ice in an insulating container such as a foam ice cooler and cut holes in its top and sides to release the CO_2. The size and number of holes allow you to control the rate at which the block melts and releases CO_2. The melting can be slowed through insulation, but it cannot be stopped.

Because it is extremely cold, dry ice can cause tissue damage or burn the skin by freezing (frostbite) after prolonged contact. Dry ice sublimates at -109.3°F (-78.5°C) at atmospheric pressure. This makes the solid dangerous to handle without protection. While generally nontoxic, the outgassing from dry ice can cause asphyxiation due to displacement of oxygen in confined locations.

Baking Soda & Vinegar

Mixing vinegar and baking soda to produce CO_2 eliminates excess heat and water-vapor production, and requires only household items. Create a system that drips vinegar (acetic acid) into a bed of baking soda.

The main disadvantage of this system is the erratic level of CO_2 produced. It takes a considerable amount of time for the CO_2 to build to a level where it helps plants, and once it reaches an optimum level, it can continue to rise until it reaches levels detrimental to plants, especially in small, enclosed gardens. If you have time to experiment, it is possible to set up a drip system operated by a solenoid valve and a short-term timer. With such a system, CO_2 could be released periodically in small increments and coordinated with ventilation schedules.

Caution! Some recipes replace vinegar with muriatic (hydrochloric) acid. Use vinegar—DO NOT USE HYDROCHLORIC ACID! It off-gases Cl_2, chlorine gas, which will kill everything! Hydrochloric acid is extremely dangerous. It can burn flesh, eyes, and the respiratory system; it can even burn through concrete.

Fragrance

A good exhaust fan, vented outdoors, is the first step in cannabis fragrance control and the easiest way to keep garden rooms and greenhouses from smelling of fresh cannabis. The exhaust fan simply carries away fragrances, dispersing them into outside air so that odors and other pollutants do not build up in the enclosed space. Seedlings, cuttings, and vegetative cannabis odors are much less pronounced than when flowering. Fragrance continues to build as flowering progresses. Often, minimal fragrance control is necessary until the last four to six weeks of flowering.

If strong fragrance in your indoor garden is not controlled by expelling air, follow the progression-control list on page 246.

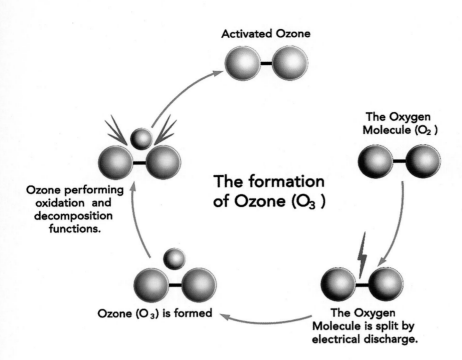

The formation of Ozone (O₃)

Activated Ozone

The Oxygen Molecule (O₂)

Ozone performing oxidation and decomposition functions.

Ozone (O₃) is formed

The Oxygen Molecule is split by electrical discharge.

This diagram shows how ozone (O₃) sheds a molecule to become oxygen (O₂).

A good air filter will keep the area in and around the garden room smelling fresh and clean.

1. Air conditioner
2. Negative ion generator (deionizer)
3. Deodorizing liquid, gel, puck, or spray
4. Ozone generator—keep it out of the garden and drying rooms!
5. Activated charcoal filter

Most gardeners skip the first four steps and move directly to efficient charcoal filters.

Air Conditioners

Classic air conditioners are mechanisms that extract heat and dehumidify air in an area. Humid air is condensed within the device into water, which is collected in a receptacle, removed, or directed down a drain. Much of the fragrance of growing cannabis is trapped within the condensed water vapor. Other air conditioners dehumidify the air without cooling it. Regardless of the air conditioner used, keep runoff (condensed moisture) inside the garden room so that fragrant water does not escape outdoors.

Air conditioners can contain only a portion of the fragrance, but it is often enough to minimize escaping odors.

Deodorizers

Kill odors by changing their structure at the molecular level. Products such as Odor Killer, Ona, VaporTek, Ozium, etc. are made from essential oils that kill odors by creating a neutral atmosphere at the atomic level. Such products are usually available in gel and spray form. Many gardeners prefer to use gel over the long term and spray for emergencies.

Deodorizers can be set out in the garden room, around the house, and near doorways. Several companies offer products that affix to a wall or other surface. One ingenious gardener I interviewed stuck one such deodorizing puck to the inside of the front door, just below the mail slot, to keep the house fresh. Other products are designed to be attached to the ventilation ductwork system.

Often these products are used not only to alter the odor of cannabis, but also to alter the somewhat unpleasant odor produced by an ozone generator. Other companies offer aerosol spray cans with a dispenser that periodically meters out a burst of spray.

Negative Ion Generators

Negative ion generators are small and somewhat efficient in controlling odors, smoke, airborne pollen, mold, dust, and static electricity. They pump negative ions into the atmosphere. Negative ions are attracted to positive ions containing odors and other airborne pollutants. Negative ions attach to positive ions, and odor becomes neutralized. The particles fall to the floor and create a fine covering of dust on the ground, plants, walls, and objects in the room.

These devices work fairly well for small garden rooms with minimal odor problems. They plug into a regular 115-volt current and use very little electricity. Check the generator's filter every few days, and make sure to keep it clean.

Ozone Generators

The presence of natural ozone in the atmosphere after a rainstorm gives the air a clean fresh fragrance. Man-made ozone has many applications including food and water sterilization and the removal of odors from the air at the molecular level. Some gardeners even use high levels of ozone to exterminate garden-room pests. See chapter 24, *Diseases & Pests*, for more information.

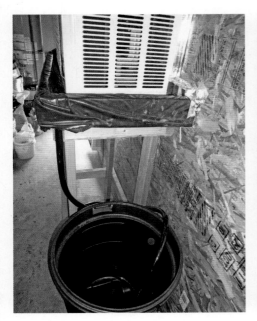

Collect the water from air conditioners inside so that the smell does not linger outdoors.

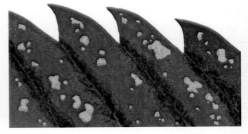

Deodorizers work for short periods in enclosed areas. Some deodorizers are adequate for small garden rooms.

Give ozone enough time to mix with smelly air to neutralize fragrances. Excess ozone exiting a building has an unpleasant and distinct odor. For this reason and safety concerns, many gardeners use a carbon filter to further scrub the air.

Ozone generators are rated by the number of cubic feet (m^3) they are able to treat. (To figure cubic feet or meters, multiply the length × width × height of the room). Do not set up the ozone generator in the garden room and let it treat all the air in the room. It can diminish or remove the fragrance of flower buds. Set up an ozone generator in a spare closet, or build an ozone exchange chamber and route fragrant garden-room air through the closet for ozone treatment before being evacuated outdoors. Or set up the ozone generator in ventilation ductwork to treat air before it exits. Once generated, ozone has a life of about 30 minutes. It takes a minute or two for O_3 molecules to combine with oxygen to neutralize odors.

Ozone generators do not enjoy the popularity they had 10 to 15 years ago. For best results, keep the ozone generator in another room or isolated from the growing plants. Ozone can cause chlorotic spots on leaves. Mottled spots at first appear to be magnesium (Mg) deficiency, and then increase in size and turn dark. Most often, the symptoms are found on foliage near the generator. Leaves wither and drop, and overall plant growth slows to a crawl.

Ozone generators neutralize odors by converting oxygen (O_2) into ozone (O_3) by exposing the smelly air to ultraviolet (UV) light. Ozone is a neutral molecule that is bipolar: it has both an internal positive and negative charge that cancel each other out to become a neutral molecule. Ozone reacts with positively charged fragrance cations that are present in the air, neutralizing the odor. Once the extra molecule is shed, O_3 is converted back into O_2. The chemistry takes a minute or longer to occur, so treated air must be held in a chamber to be converted effectively.

Watch for important features such as "self-cleaning" (or easy to clean), and

easy, safe bulb replacement. When UV light encounters moisture in the air, nitric acid is produced as a by-product. This white, powdery nitric acid collects around the lamps at connection points. This is an unpleasant, very corrosive acid that will severely burn skin and eyes. Before purchasing and using an ozone generator, verify that it has proper safety features such as a switch that turns off the lamp for maintenance, making it possible to work without looking at the retina-searing UV rays. Legal exposure to ozone for humans is about 0.1 ppm for a maximum of eight hours. Most garden-room ozone generators produce about 0.05 ppm at timed intervals. See chapter 24, *Diseases and Pests*, for plant symptoms of ozone damage.

Caution! UV light is very dangerous. In a flash, intense UV light can burn your skin and the retinas in your eyes beyond repair. Never, under any circumstances,

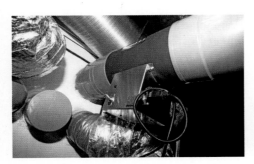

Ozone generators that fit in exhaust ducts ensure that no ozone will remain in the garden area.

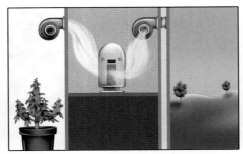

This drawing demonstrates how to use an ozone generator so that it will not affect the fragrance of cannabis. Tainted garden-room air is ushered into another room to be treated with ozone before being expelled outdoors.

Ozone damages foliage. Always keep ozone generators outside of garden rooms, greenhouses, and drying rooms.

look at the UV lamp in an ozone generator. Sneaking a peek can cost you your eyesight! Ozone is also capable of burning your lungs and other internal body tissue. At low levels, there is no damage, but at higher levels, danger is imminent. Never use too much ozone!

Ozone disrupts and changes various chemical compounds and can entirely remove fragrance from cannabis. The free radicals involved in ozone generation will take any organic compound they can find!

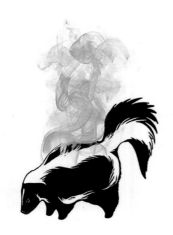

'Skunk #1' is a well-known variety of cannabis that smells like a skunk. Avoid problems with the neighbors by abating this odor before it leaves the garden area.

Air Filters

Air filters used by indoor medical cannabis gardeners fall into two basic categories: particulate air filters and activated carbon air filters. Particulate air filters are made from fibrous materials that are designed to remove solid particles such as dust, mold, bacteria, and pollen from the air. These volatile organic compound (VOC) particles measure from 10 to 100 nanometers (nm).

Particulate air filters found in home heating and air conditioning systems do not remove fine pollutants from the air. These filters are designed to remove some of the larger particles of dust and pollution but fail to remove fragrances.

Activated carbon filters remove fragrances (airborne molecular contaminants) by absorption. Activated carbon is the most common active ingredient in air filters used by medical cannabis gardeners. Fragrance must be filtered out at the molecular level. Passing garden-room air at a constant rate and pressure through an activated carbon filter will remove pollutants at the molecular level.

High-efficiency particulate air (HEPA) filters have been used since the 1950s in the medical, automotive, and aeronautic industries. These expensive filters are used by a few medical cannabis gardeners to remove extremely small particles including bacteria from garden-room air. **Buyer Beware!** HEPA-type, HEPA-like, HEPA-style, etc., filters DO NOT meet HEPA standards and are inferior to a true HEPA filter. The HEPA standard ensures quality.

Activated Carbon Filters

Activated carbon (aka activated charcoal and activated coal) filters are the choice of most gardeners to remove unwanted cannabis fragrance from garden room and greenhouse air before venting it outdoors. Activated carbon is contained in a perforated, flow-through metal canister or made into a carbon filter.

Look for filters that contain plenty of the proper activated carbon to clean garden air. Make your selection based on the filter's efficiency in relation to the weight and absorption ability of the activated carbon. Some filters are so heavy that they are mounted upright in the garden rather than hung from the ceiling, where the warm, fragrant air collects.

Use duct tape to seal all joints when setting up the air filter. Accidental leaks may cause unfiltered air or an inefficient exhaust system.

Always follow the manufacturer's filter and fan specifications. Filters are designed to work with specific fans. Most manufacturers include instructions to help set up the air filter for maximum efficiency. To calculate the proper filter and fan for a room, use CarbonActive's online calculator, www.carbonactive.ch/calculator/.

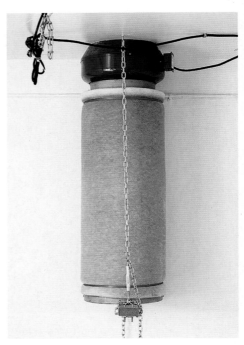

This efficient activated carbon filter is connected to ducting that runs straight up through the roof.

Many medical marijuana gardeners make their own activated carbon filters. Check the Marijuana Growing Forum (www.marijuanagrowing.com) for more information.

Activated carbon consists of at least 90 percent carbon and has an extremely porous structure. For example, a single gram of activated carbon has more than 500 m² in surface area! Sources of raw carbon include wood, peat, coal, or coconut shells. First they are processed similarly to charcoal, and then they are "activated."

Charcoal is activated chemically or with steam and pressure. The activation process opens millions of minute pores. These extra passageways increase charcoal's ability to adsorb odor and pollution molecules. Extra surface area is also charged with positive ions that attract negative ions—odors and pollutants.

A charcoal filter needs:

- Relative humidity below 70 percent
- Enough time for charcoal to absorb fragrances
- A pre-filter, regularly changed to keep clean—dust blocks pores of carbon!

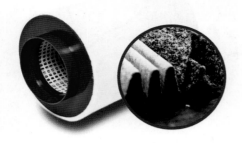

Multilayer fleece mats are sealed airtight in the base and cover, which are made from recycled plastic, preventing any accidental intake of (unfiltered) air.

(cfm)	(m³/h)
0.588	1
59	100
147	250
294	500
589	1,000

cfm = Cubic feet per minute
m³/h = Meters cubed divided by hours

Activated Carbon Basics

Activated charcoal adsorbs odors but also absorbs moisture. At 65 to 70 percent relative humidity, charcoal absorbs moisture and starts to clog. At 80 percent or higher humidity, adsorption drops tremendously, even though carbon never completely stops working. Once activated charcoal is saturated with moisture (humidity), it will shed moisture back into the air as ambient humidity levels drop, and the filter will start to extract pollutants once again. But some moisture will still be trapped deep within the internal pores of the activated charcoal, which reduces efficiency and life expectancy.

Note: An ultrasonic water atomizer will produce lime and other salts. Retain lime with a pre-filter. Use only salt-free water for humidification.

Air must move slowly through charcoal filters to extract odors. The fan should let just enough air through the filter so the odors have enough dwell time to be

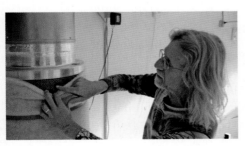

Both passive intake air and air brought in by a fan require a filter to minimize airborne pollutants in enclosed gardens. Install an intake air filter or fine screen to remove large particles such as dust and other pollutants from intake air.

absorbed by the carbon filter. Check with filter manufacturers or retailers about venting specifications. To ensure success, always buy a bigger filter than the fan's maximum output. Employing a smaller fan will cause air pressure to drop, and the contact time between fragrant air and charcoal will increase. The capacity of the fan should be 20 percent lower than the capability of the filter so the activated carbon has enough time and capacity to neutralize the air continuously. Lowering fan capacity more than 30 percent does not make carbon more effective, and it restricts airflow. The overall lifespan of charcoal also increases when properly maintained.

Use a pre-filter to remove fine dust and pollutants (100 nm or larger) and thus avoid damaging the carbon. A pre-filter is typically fitted around the superstructure of the carbon filter to remove larger particles so they do not clog the activated carbon. Use the pre-filter designed specifically for the charcoal filter.

Caution! Microparticles such as concrete dust and smoke pass through the pre-filter to the carbon. Tobacco smoke reduces the life of activated carbon.

Caution! DO NOT wash pre-filters with water. Clean them with a vacuum or a jet of high-pressure air. Water destroys the structure of pre-filters. Remove and clean pre-filters outside the room to prevent intake of microdust that could damage activated carbon. Replace pre-filters when dirty and difficult to clean thoroughly.

Use CarbonActive's calculator (www. carbonactive.ch/calculator/) to determine which pre-filter, carbon filter, and extraction fan are best for your airspace.

Types of Activated Charcoal

Activated carbon's ability to adsorb fragrances is a function of the carbon's hardness, regardless of its crushed or pelletized form. Harder carbon is less dusty and more expensive than semihard or soft carbon/charcoal.

Some gardeners prefer to spend the extra money on activated carbon made from coconut fiber. Coco carbon is very hard, with little dust and the highest charge of ions.

A volume of activated carbon is necessary to remove fragrances from the air of a garden room. Different forms of activated carbon react differently to filtering air. Granular activated carbon (GAC) is designed to absorb all gases and fragrances. This is the best activated carbon filter to use.

Activated Carbon Classifications

granular activated carbon (GAC)—absorption of all gases

powdered activated carbon (PAC)—water purification

extruded activated carbon (EAC)—gas phase applications

beaded activated carbon (BAC)—water filtration

impregnated carbon—water purification and chemical absorption

polymer coated carbon—human blood purification

Crushed or Particle Carbon

Particle carbon is highly active and heavily charged with ions. This type of carbon is the most efficient air-cleaning system. Particle carbon is used in lightweight, low-pressure systems that stir up no dust. Production is consistent, with less than 5 percent variation in batches.

Irregular granular and crushed activated charcoal disperses air, forcing it to travel farther through the filter. Its irregular surfaces give more contact between air and carbon, providing more filtering area, which in turn absorbs more pollutants.

CarbonActive filters have tiny particles of activated carbon (0.4–0.8 mm). Since these particles are much smaller than pellets, the odor-neutralizing surface is 10,000 times larger so that the effect is amplified enormously. Special fleece mats ensure an optimal arrangement of the activated carbon particles.

Granular Crushed Carbon
Granular crushed carbon is actively charged with ions. It is mostly used to purify water. MESH 4 to 12 filters are specifically for filtering water.

Carbon Pellets
Carbon pellets activate slowly and, by volume, contain fewer charged ions. Their low evaporative ability makes them perfect to clean paints and gases such as benzene and methanol.

Activated carbon pellets are smooth and cylindrical in form. The surface provides a short, direct path for air to flow through and out the filter, effectively lowering the filtering ability for minute odor molecules. Pelletized activated carbon is less expensive than other forms of activated carbon, with density per volume of 50 to 60 g/cc.

Extending the Life of Carbon Filters
Carbon filters typically last about a year when properly maintained. Active life depends upon maintenance, climatic conditions, and the total volume of pollutants that are filtered. The quality of carbon is directly proportionate to its ionic charge and filtering ability.

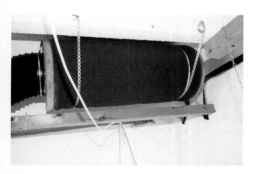

This pre-filter is filthy! Its ends are the original color (white), but the filter itself is very dirty where it is drawing in air.

Many other factors affect the longevity of activated carbon. Plants have 2,500 different molecules, and each plant is unique. Controlling fragrance is relative to the microclimate— indoors, outdoors, greenhouse, and location— Canada, Switzerland, Argentina, and so on. Many other factors influence the air, including CO_2, pre-filter maintenance, and even the fan being used. Changing the pre-filter is critical because this is where dust, dirt, heat, and humidity form a perfect environment for bacteria and insects to reside.

Caution! Clean the pre-filter monthly with a vacuum or jet of compressed air. Remove the pre-filter from the garden room to clean. Change pre-filter at least once every 12 months to avoid disease and pest problems.

Store activated carbon and filters at room temperature in a dry, airtight place.

Reactivating and Reusing Carbon
Spent, clogged carbon can be reactivated with chemicals or by exposure to very high temperatures 1,472°F (800°C) under controlled conditions. It is not recommended unless done by a professional. Furthermore, repacking carbon requires precision packing. When the carbon loses its filtering ability, it is much easier to purchase newly activated charcoal.

Dispose of used carbon along with normal household garbage. Or it can be broadcast in the garden to help sweeten the soil.

The following sites offer more technical information and setup instructions for activated charcoal filters:
CarbonActive, www.carbonactive.ch— an expert Swiss site, dense with information

Can-Filters, www.canfilters.com

Organic Air Filters, www.organicairfilter.com

Phresh Filters, www.phreshfilter.com

Phat Filters, http:// http://phatfilter. com.au/

Rhino Filters www.rhinofilter.com

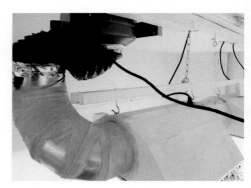

You do not need a wind velocity meter to know that this vent fan is not working efficiently!

The Ventilation System
Construct a ventilation system that brings in cool air to the bottom of the room and expels hot air from the top of the room.

Locate the vent in the ceiling or near the ceiling, where hot air naturally accumulates. Carefully cut a hole in the wall or ceiling in the exact place you want it.

Filter incoming air to prevent insects, spider mites, diseases, and pollen from entering the room. Filter outgoing air to neutralize unwanted fragrances (and to avoid bothering your neighbors). Filtering incoming air requires a nylon stocking or a similar fine mesh stretched over incoming air sources.

The following sites offer exhaust fan calculators:
Ask the Builder, www.askthebuilder. com/B98_Sizing_an_Exhaust_Fan_. shtml

ACF Greenhouses, www.littlegreen house.com/fan-calc.shtml

Setting Up the Ventilation System: Step-by-Step
Note: Set up intake vents near the floor in a corner of the room. Install exhaust fan(s) in the opposing corner near the ceiling so that air is drawn through the enclosed area.

Step One: Figure the total volume of the garden room. Length × width × height = total volume. For example, a garden room that is 10 × 10 × 8 feet (21.5 m³)

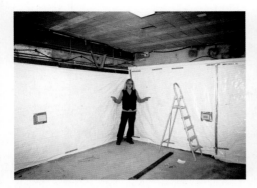

Measure the dimensions of the room: length, width, and height.

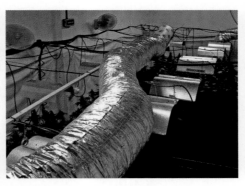

Stretch flexible ducting so it is as smooth and straight as possible inside. Irregular interior surfaces cause air turbulence and seriously diminish airflow.

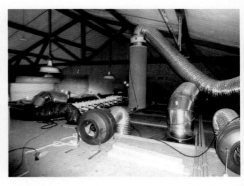

Install vent fans in the attic, ceiling, or high in the garden room or greenhouse, where they are most efficient.

has a total volume of 800 cubic feet (10 × 10 × 8 feet = 800 cubic feet or 21.5 m³). A room measuring 4 × 5 × 2 meters has a total volume of 1,400 cubic feet (40 m³).

Step Two: Use a vent fan that will remove the total volume of air in the enclosed garden in less than five minutes for large rooms and one minute for small rooms. Warm garden rooms need more frequent ventilation. Figure one complete air change for the maximum temperature the enclosed garden will need to operate.

Divide the volume of the growing area by the number of minutes required to get one full air change:

A 640-cubic foot (18 m²) room / 4 air changes = 160 cfm (18 L2/hr) fan (640/4 = 160).

A 640-cubic foot (18 m²) room / 1 air change = 640 cfm (18 L2/hr) fan (640/1 = 640).

Step Three: Place the fan high on a wall or near the ceiling of the garden room so it vents off hot, humid air.

Buy a fan that can easily be mounted on the wall or inline in a duct pipe. Quality inline fans move much air and make very little noise. It's worth spending the extra money on an inline fan. Small, enclosed areas can use a fan that can be attached to flexible 4-inch (10.2 cm) dryer ducting. Many stores sell special ducting to connect high-speed squirrel cage blowers with the 4 inch (10.2 cm) ducting.

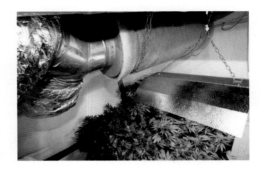

Step Four: If possible, use an existing window, chimney, or sewer vent to expel garden-room air. The last and most-involved option is to cut a hole in the ceiling or wall.

To place a fan in a window, cut a 0.5 to 0.75-inch (1.3–1.9 cm) piece of plywood to fit the windowsill. Cover window with a lightproof, dark-colored paint or similar covering. Mount the fan near the top of the plywood so it vents air out of the garden room. Secure the plywood and fan in the windowsill with sheet rock screws. Open the window from the bottom.

Make a lightproof vent using 4-inch (10.2 cm) flexible dryer ducting. Vent the hose outdoors, and attach a small squirrel cage fan to the other end of the ducting. Make sure there is an airtight connection between the fan and hose by using a large hose clamp or duct tape to fix the connection.

Use rigid ducting instead of flexible ducting, if possible. Air flows more freely and quietly in larger ducting. Choose

between 4-, 6-, 8-, 10-, and 12-inch (10.2, 15.2, 20.3, 25.4, 30.5 cm) ducting.

Vent air up the chimney where fragrances are seldom a problem. First, clean the chimney of excess ash and creosote by tying a chain to a rope and lowering the chain down the inside, banging and knocking all debris to the bottom. There should be a door at the bottom of the chimney to remove the debris. If cleaning the chimney yourself is inconvenient, hire a chimney-sweep service. Tap ducting into an existing hole in the chimney.

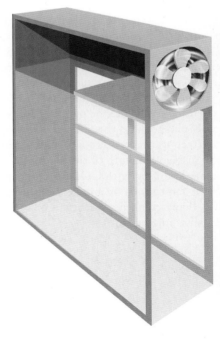

This window allows air to vent but does not allow light to escape.

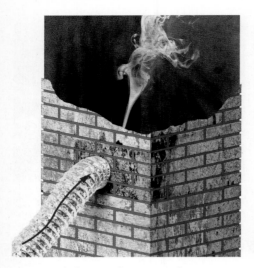

An unused chimney draws vented air up and outside.

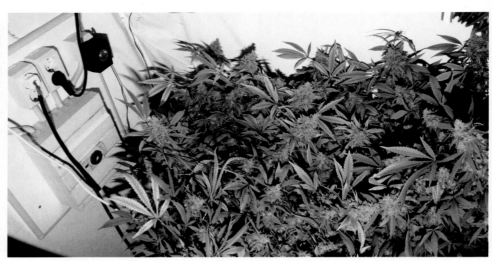

This little garden has all the electrical connections on a board. The CO_2 monitor is mounted on another wall.

Cut a hole in the ceiling and vent air into the attic. Often a hole can be cut in the ceiling and covered with a vent, then a fan is placed behind the vent.

If cutting into a ceiling with a crawl space, make sure you have a method to evacuate the garden-room air from the crawl space. Install louvers below the rafters on the outside wall of the house.

Step Five: Attach the fan to a thermostat/humidistat or other temperature/humidity monitor/control device to vent hot, humid air outside. Set the temperature on 75°F (23.9°C), and the humidity on 55 percent in flowering rooms and 60 to 65 percent in vegetative rooms. Most control devices have wiring instructions. More sophisticated controllers have built-in electrical outlets, and the peripherals are simply plugged into the outlets.
Or attach the vent fan to a timer and run it for a specific length of time. This is the method used with CO_2 enrichment. Set the fan to turn on and vent out used, CO_2-depleted air just before new CO_2-rich air is injected.

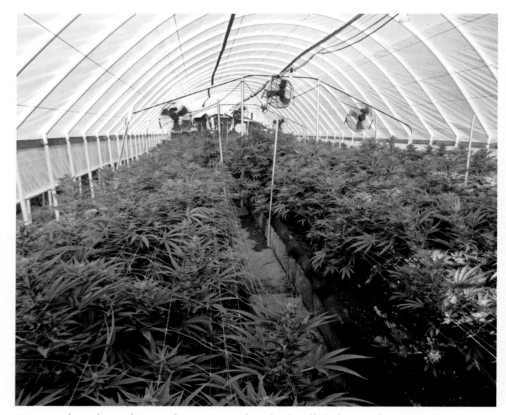

Rip-stop plastic keeps this greenhouse intact when the sheriff's helicopter hovers overhead.

PART 3

ADVANCED MEDICAL CANNABIS HORTICULTURE

17

LIGHT, LAMPS & ELECTRICITY

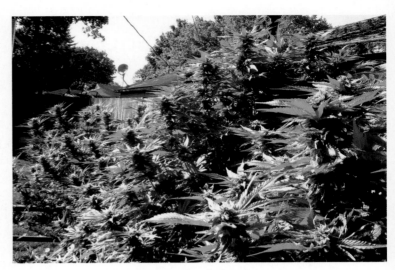

Cannabis grows best under natural sunlight, where it can express its true genetic potential.

LIGHT IS ESSENTIAL for cannabis to grow strong, healthy medicine. All plants grow and evolve under Mother Nature's sunlight and care. Plants are accustomed to natural sunlight and have adapted to her spectrum, intensity, and photoperiod. Light is comprised of separate wavelengths or bands of colors. Each color in the spectrum used by plants sends them separate signals, promoting a different type of growth.

Sunlight contains 4 percent ultraviolet radiation, 52 percent infrared (heat) radiation, and 44 percent visible light. Midday during the bright summer growing season, light intensity can top 8640 foot-candles (93,000 lux), but cannabis plants use about half the energy found in natural sunlight. Sunlight energy arrives from the heavens as electromagnetic radiation. It is both wave and particle in nature. The smallest divisible particles of light are called photons. The brightness of light is equivalent to the number of photons absorbed per unit of time. Each photon contains a fixed amount of energy. The energy in each photon dictates how much it will vibrate. The wavelength is the distance moved by a photon during one vibration. Wavelengths are measured in nanometers.*

*One nanometer (nm) = one billionth (10^9) of a meter. Light is measured in wavelengths; the wavelengths are measured in nanometers.

Electromagnetic radiation spans a broad range of wavelengths. Gamma rays with a wavelength of 10^5 nm are at the far blue end of the spectrum and radio waves with a wavelength of 10^{12} nm are at the far-red end. Red light has a longer wavelength. The photons vibrate slower and contain less energy. Photons in the far blue ultraviolet (UV) visible spectrum have shorter wavelengths and contain more energy. The human eye sees only "visible light" (wavelengths between 380 and 750 nm) a small part of the entire spectrum. Visible light wavelengths (light spectrum) appear to people as all the colors of the rainbow. Visible light is measured in foot-candles (fc) and lux (lx). Lumens are the measure of visible light emitted by a light source.

Lumens measure "luminous flux," the total number of packets (quanta) of light produced by a light source. Luminous flux is the quantity of light emitted. Use the lux measurement to know how many lumens to give the entire area for complete illumination.

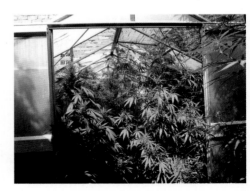

Greenhouse coverings block some sunlight, but there is still plenty of light to grow very big plants.

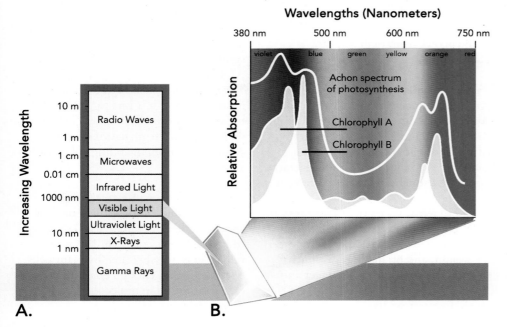

Wavelengths (Nanometers)

This graph shows visible light spectrum and includes the active photosynthesis, chlorophyll a and chlorophyll b spectrums. Note that visible light is a small part of the spectrum.

Unlike lumens, lux measures the area over which the light (luminous flux) spreads. For example, if 1000 lumens were concentrated in one square meter, the illuminated square meter would have 1000 lux. If the same 1000 lumens spread over 10 square meters, a measurement of 100 lux is registered on the 4 square meters.

Plants "see" other parts of the light spectrum than humans see. They respond to wavelengths similar to those that humans need to see, but they use different portions of the spectrum. Peak needs to occur in the blue portion (430 nm) and red portion (662 nm) of the spectrum, where chlorophyll* absorption is at the highest levels. Light used by plants is measured in PAR (photosynthetically active radiation), PPF (photosynthetic photon flux) (μmol/s).

Chlorophyll is the most important light-absorbing pigment in cannabis, but it does not absorb green light. Green light is reflected, which is why we see the color green. Other pigments include carotenoids (a group of yellow, red, and orange pigments) that absorb light energy. Other pigments (e.g. zeaxanthin [red] and phycoerythrin [red]) absorb different wavelengths. Each color of light activates different plant functions. For example, positive tropism, the plant's ability to orient leaves toward light, is controlled by spectrum.

*Phototropism is the movement of a plant part (foliage) toward a source of illumination. Positive tropism means the foliage moves toward the light source. Negative tropism means the plant part moves away from the light. Positive tropism is greatest in the blue end of the spectrum, at about 450 nanometers. At this optimum level, plants lean toward the light, spreading their leaves out horizontally to absorb the maximum amount of illumination possible.

PAR watts are a measure of light energy (radiant flux) used by plants to produce food and grow. PAR watts are the measure of the actual amount of specific photons a plant needs to grow. Light energy is radiated and assimilated in photons. Photosynthesis is necessary for plants to grow, and is activated by the assimilation of photons.

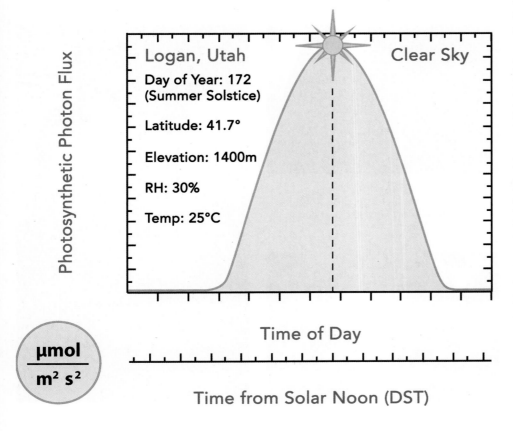

This graph shows the maximum amount of light available during June 21, the longest day of the year, at Logan, Utah, which is located at 41.7° north latitude. Note how the intensity of the sun increases and decreases dramatically before and after 1:45 pm (13:45).

Ultraviolet (UVA, UVB, UVC) Light

UVA is the most common UV light. It has little energy and is least harmful of all UV light. Used in glow-in-the-dark black lights, UVA light is also used in phototherapy and in tanning booths.

Black-light fluorescent lamps emit ultraviolet rays through a dark filter and glass bulb, but they are not appropriate to grow cannabis. According to some sources, ultraviolet light is supposed to promote more resin formation on flower buds. However, all known experiments that add artificial UV light in a controlled environment have proven that it does not make any difference.

UVB is a very damaging form of UV light. It packs enough energy to destroy live tissues but not enough energy to be absorbed completely into the atmosphere. Destructive UVB can cause skin cancer. Be careful when outdoors, especially in areas with damaged ozone layers in the atmosphere that let more UVB light pass through. These are high-risk areas for skin cancer.

UVC light is absorbed almost completely, and within a kilometer of the atmosphere. The UVC photons crash into oxygen atoms, and the result is ozone. In nature, UVC is transformed into ozone and later oxygen so quickly that it is difficult to capture. UVC light works well as a germicidal water purifier and bacteria-killer in food. It also works well to kill bacteria, mold, and pests on plant leaf surfaces.

UVC light (100–280 nm) carries too much electromagnetic radiation, or energy (the hyper atoms are moving too fast), for plants to process; the energy is sufficient to force electrons away from atoms and rupture fragile chemical bonds.

UVC light is used in short, limited, regular applications to kill mold spores in growing and harvested cannabis. UV radiation is absorbed by oxygen in the forms O_2 and O_3 (ozone). The ozone layer of our atmosphere protects life on the planet from high levels of UV radiation.

UVA (315–380 nm) and UVB (380–315 nm) light help new branch growth and have a similar effect as blue light. Ultraviolet (UVA and UVB) light emitted by natural sunlight and plasma lamps has been proven to increase overall vegetative growth in cannabis by up to 30 percent.

In experiments, vegetative plants grown under plasma lamps that emit UVA and UVB light grew up to 30 percent more dry weight, and branching was much more profuse. Cells were stronger and the outer layer of cells was tougher, which discourages attacks from diseases and pests.

I have personally seen plants grown at 1000-foot (300 m) and 4600-foot (1400 m) elevation. The plants at 1000 feet (300 m) produced more and bigger flow- er buds. The plants at 4600 feet (1400 m) were smaller, with thicker, stronger stems and smaller buds heavy with resin. Afterward, both crops were compared. The plants grown at high elevation had more resin, but it is unclear if that was because of more UVB light. There are many different explanations for heavier resin production, including cold weather and wind.

Random photons of infrared light (750–1000 nm) on the other end of the spectrum do not contain enough energy to promote plant growth. Infrared radiation is not absorbed by plant cells, because it lacks enough energy to excite electrons found in molecules and is therefore converted to heat.

Gardeners who use infrared heaters do not have to worry about light affecting plant growth. Infrared radiation is absorbed by water and by carbon dioxide in the atmosphere.

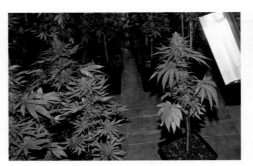

UVC light is being used to kill fungus, bacteria, pests, and their eggs. The lamp must be moved over plants so that it does not damage foliage.

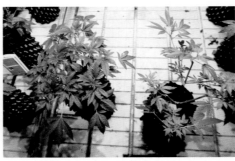

The plant on the left was grown with an LEP (light-emitting plasma) lamp, and the one on the right grew under an MH (metal halide) lamp.

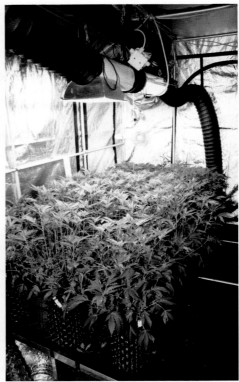

This LEP lamp produces UVA and UVB light, as well as a complete spectrum used by plants.

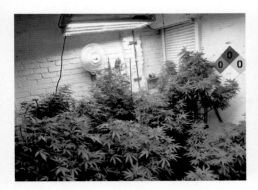

T5 fluorescent lamps supply enough light to keep this roomful of mother plants healthy.

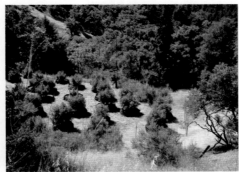

This outdoor medical cannabis garden receives direct sunlight for about 9 hours each day, all season long.

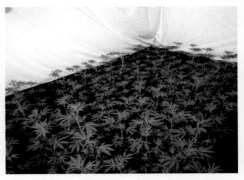

Tie a 12- to 36-inch-long string to the HID reflector. Use the string to measure the distance between the bulb and the plant canopy.

Blue photons carry more energy and are worth more PAR watts than lower-energy red photons. It takes from 8 to 10 photons to bind 1 CO_2 molecule.

PAR watts in photons-per-second became the standard to measure horticultural lamp spectrum output. This measurement is called photosynthetic photon flux (PPF), and is expressed in micromoles-per-second (μmol/s). Today PPF is the accepted lighting and greenhouse industry standard.

Outdoors, plants receive natural sunlight—100 percent PAR/PPF. Greenhouse and shade cloth coverings limit the amount of PPF. Look for the "light transmission" factor in greenhouse and shade cloth coverings to figure the amount of PAR/PPF light available to plants.

Most artificial lights deliver only a part of the necessary light spectrum that cannabis needs to grow. A higher PAR/PPF rating guarantees that more photons will be available for healthy plant growth. Under artificial lights indoors, medicinal cannabis must receive enough intense PAR/PPF light to grow well. Gardeners report that medical cannabis grown under intense lamps with high PAR/PPF ratings is healthier and stronger, with fewer disease, pest, or cultural problems.

Light Intensity

Sunlight on a hot summer day when the sun is at the highest angle in the sky produces light levels of more than 93,000 lux—all the PAR light you could possibly need!

ILLUMINANCE (LUX)	EXAMPLE
93,000	Brightest sunlight at midday
20,000	Shade illuminated by a clear blue sky at midday
10,000–25,000	Overcast day at midday
<200	Super dark storm clouds at midday
400	Sunrise and sunset on a clear day
40	Overcast sky at sunset or sunrise

Outdoors, little can be done to change the PAR rating except to plant the garden in a sunny location, and to shade the plants as needed. Greenhouses can be illuminated with HID light, but outdoors we are compelled to work with Mother Nature during cloud-covered days. We can use greenhouse coverings and shade cloth to cool plants and decrease intense light.

Indoors, artificial lightbulbs and tubes must supply intense light for medicinal cannabis to grow well. The lamp must have the proper spectrum and have a high PAR rating.

Indoors, generating intense light is expensive and requires knowledge to employ a bulb with the proper spectrum. Intensity is the magnitude of light energy per unit of area. It is greatest near the bulb and diminishes rapidly as it moves away from the source. High-wattage HID (high-intensity discharge) bulbs supply the most intense light efficiently, followed by T5 and T8 fluorescent, and CFL and plasma lamps. But remember

that T5 and T8 bulbs can be placed four times closer to plants, which makes them much more efficient than HID bulbs, according to the Inverse Square Law (see below).

For example, plants that are 2 feet (61 cm) from a lamp receive one-quarter the amount of light received by plants 1 foot away (30.5 cm). An HID that emits 100,000 lumens produces a paltry 25,000 lumens at 2 feet (61 cm) away. A 1000-watt HID that emits 100,000 initial lumens yields 11,111 lumens at 3 feet (91.4 cm) away. Couple this meager sum with a poorly designed reflective hood that has lost its shine, and the garden suffers.

For plant growth, the brilliance of a lamp has a limited effect when it does not produce the proper spectrum. For example, the efficient 600-watt HP sodium lamps have the highest lumens per watt (lm/W) conversion, but a color rendering index (CRI) of 24 and spectrum of 2000 K to 3000 K. Even though these lamps produce more light per watt, plants can use only parts of it!

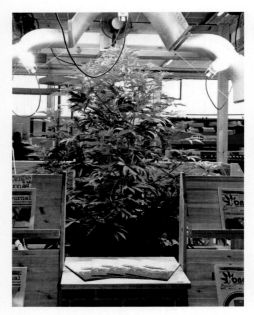

Three 600-watt HID lamps cannot supply the same amount of light as natural sunlight.

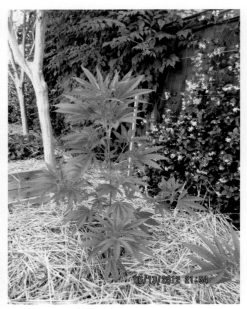

Leaves reach for the light. Strong, well-illuminated plants orient foliage to catch the maximum amount of light possible.

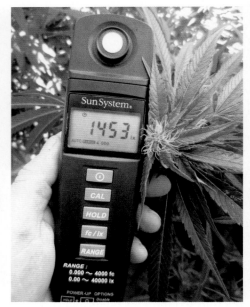

A basic light meter is an essential tool in the garden. Indoors, a light meter will help save time and electricity, as well as increase production.

LAMP	WATTS	INITIAL LUMENS	MEAN LUMENS
MH	1000	100,000	80,000
SMH	1000	115,000	92,000
HPS	1000	140,000	112,000
HPS	600	90,000	72,000

Watts per square foot (W/ft²) (W/m²) measures how many watts are available from a light source in an area. But the lumens per watt (lm/W), wattage, spectrum, mounting height of the lamp, and reflective hood are not considered.

Lumens *emitted* are only part of the equation. Lumens *received* by the plant are much more important. Lumens received are measured in watts per square foot or in foot-candles (fc). One foot-candle equals the amount of light that falls on 1 square foot of surface located 1 foot away from 1 candle.

Measuring Light

As explained earlier in this chapter, plants use the PAR portion of the light spectrum to grow. Artificial lights that produce the highest PAR rating with a high-intensity are the logical choice to grow medicinal cannabis. To find out which lightbulbs supply the most usable light for photosynthesis, reference their color rendering index (CRI) and the Kelvin (K) temperature ratings. The CRI indicates how close the lamp's spectrum is to natural sunlight. The color temperature (spectrum) of the bulb is expressed in kelvins. Kelvin is an absolute measurement of temperature that indicates the exact color spectrum a bulb emits. Lightbulbs with a Kelvin temperature from 3000 to 6500 will grow medicinal cannabis. These two figures, coupled with lamp intensity expressed in lumens, can approximate a PAR rating for lamps that do not have one.

The **color rendering index** (CRI) is a scale used to measure the ability of a light source to reproduce the colors of various objects faithfully in comparison to an ideal or natural light source, which means how true to life these colors appear in the visible spectrum when they are being illuminated with anything other than natural light.

The **color corrected temperature** (CCT) of a bulb is the peak Kelvin temperature at which the colors in a bulb are stable. We can classify bulbs by their CCT rating, which tells us the overall color of the light emitted. It does not tell us the spectrum (concentration of the combination of colors emitted).

Light is commonly measured in foot-candles or lux, two scales that measure light visible to humans, but do not measure photosynthetic response to light in PAR or PPF. Lumens are a measurement of light emitted from the sun or artificial light. Light meters that measure in PAR or PPF are very expensive and seldom used by medical cannabis gardeners. Foot-candle and lux meters can also be used to achieve an approximate measure of light available to plants. The foot-candle and lux readings are still valuable, because they record the amount of intense (PAR/PPF) light spread over a specific area.

Using an inexpensive light meter to calculate lumens, foot-candles, or lux is a way to estimate the amount of light plants receive. But it does not measure how much light is available to plants.

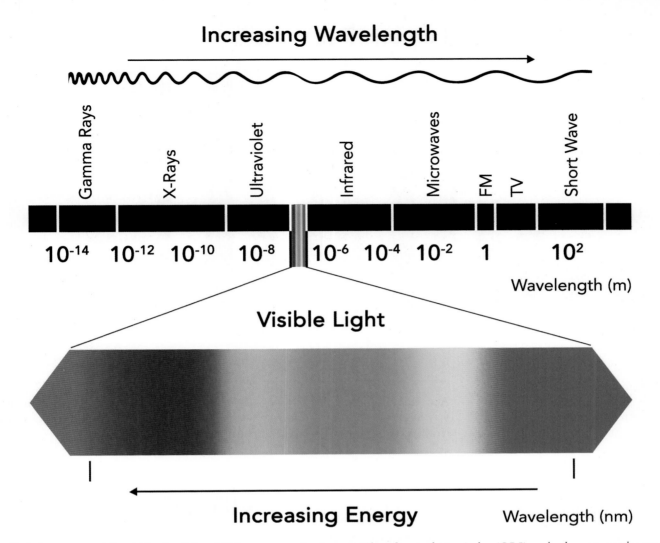

Increasing Wavelength

Gamma Rays · X-Rays · Ultraviolet · Infrared · Microwaves · FM · TV · Short Wave

10^{-14} 10^{-12} 10^{-10} 10^{-8} 10^{-6} 10^{-4} 10^{-2} 1 10^{2}

Wavelength (m)

Visible Light

Increasing Energy

Wavelength (nm)

The visible light spectrum falls within the 400 and 700 nanometer (nm) range. The color rendering index (CRI) and color-corrected temperature (CCT) of an artificial light source does not take into account the photosynthetically active radiation (PAR) or photosynthetic photon flux (PPF).

The Inverse Square Law

The relationship between light emitted from a point source (bulb) and distance is defined by the inverse square law. This law affirms that the intensity of light changes in inverse proportion to the square of the distance. Light diminishes rapidly.

$I = L/D^2$
Intensity = light output/distance²

For example:
Distance Intensity = light output/distance²

Feet	Centimeters	Lumens	Lumens/Distance²
1	30	100000	100000/1
2	60	25000	100000/2
3	90	11111	100000/3
4	120	6250	100000/4

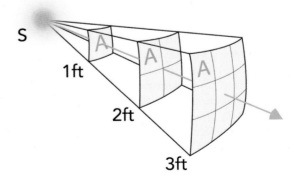

Lumens Per Watt

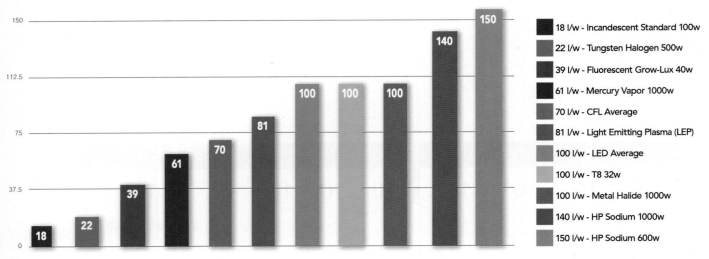

Lumens-per-watt (lm/W) output of lamps

Once you know the PAR rating of a lamp, using a foot-candle or lux meter will measure light intensity at the foliage. The foot-candle or lux light meter measures the overall intensity of visible light over a garden. Use the most efficient lamp with the highest PAR or PPF (μmol/s) rating for the application: seedling/clone, vegetative, and flowering. Outdoors and in greenhouses, plants that do not receive enough intense light grow slowly. Lack of light during flowering keeps flower buds from filling out and putting on weight.

Light meter readings vary a lot as a result of orientation. To get the most accurate readings, orient the meter at a 90-degree angle from the garden canopy when taking measurements. Avoid pointing the light sensor directly at a bulb unless measuring directly below bulb.

*Light can be measured in many different scales: foot-candles, lumens, lumens/cm², lumens/ft², lumens/m², lux, phot, nox, candlepower, meter candle, nit, stilb, lambert, foot-lambert, millilambert, candela/m², candela/cm², candela/ft², and candela/in², watts, microeinsteins, millimoles, joules, photons, radiant flux, luminous flux, PAR, PPF, etc. To figure out conversions to different scales for measuring light, OnlineConversion.com will do the math for you: www.onlineconversion.com/light.htm.

According to lighting expert Theo Tekstra from Gavita-Holland, "Micromoles is the way to express photons." Micromoles measure the number of photons per second, or irradiation of photons per second per meter. Micromole = μMol

Kelvin Scale

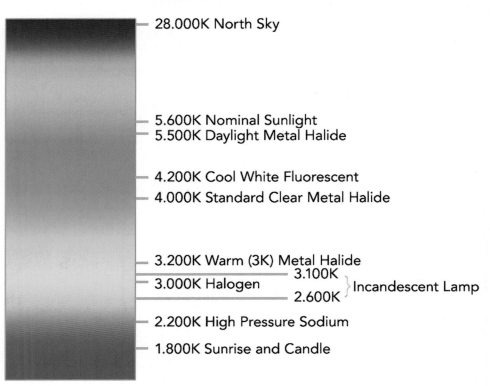

28.000K North Sky

5.600K Nominal Sunlight
5.500K Daylight Metal Halide

4.200K Cool White Fluorescent
4.000K Standard Clear Metal Halide

3.200K Warm (3K) Metal Halide
3.100K
3.000K Halogen
2.600K } Incandescent Lamp

2.200K High Pressure Sodium

1.800K Sunrise and Candle

The Kelvin temperature scale is commonly used to measure the "color" of light. Notice the difference in spectrum between metal halide and HP sodium HID lights.

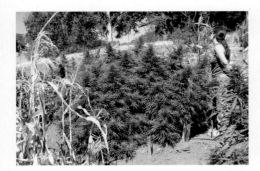
Outdoors under natural conditions cannabis flowers in the autumn, when nights are long and days are short.

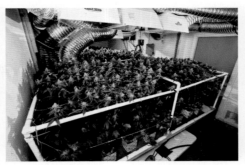
This indoor garden is flowering under 12 hours of darkness and 12 hours of HID light.

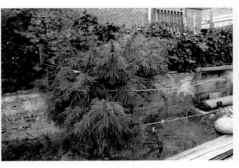
Half of this 'Haze' plant received light from a streetlamp, causing it to remain in the vegetative growth stage. The other half of the plant received total darkness at night and flowered. This example is proof that floral signals are generated in the leaf and transported to the nearest buds upstream.

To get an idea of how well a medical cannabis plant will grow under a specific greenhouse covering or lightbulb, three things must be known: (1) PAR, (2) intensity, and (3) hours of darkness.

Photoperiod

The photoperiod is the relationship between the duration of the light period and dark period. In nature, cannabis normally flowers in the fall, when nights grow long and days short.

In general, cannabis is a short-day plant that will flower when it receives short 12-hour days and 12-hour nights. (*C. ruderalis*, however, is a long-day plant.) Most varieties of cannabis will stay in the vegetative growth stage as long as an 18- to 24-hour light and a 6- to 0hour dark photoperiod are maintained. However, there are exceptions. Eighteen hours of light per day will give cannabis all the light it needs to sustain vegetative growth. Cannabis can efficiently process 16 to 18 hours of light per day, after which it reaches a point of diminishing returns and the electricity is wasted. (See chapter 25, *Breeding*.)

Flowering is most efficiently induced in most varieties of cannabis with 12 hours of uninterrupted darkness in a 24-hour photoperiod. When plants are at least 2 months old—after they have developed male and female sexual characteristics—altering the photoperiod to an even 12 hours, day and night, will induce visible signs of flowering in 1 to 3 weeks. Older plants tend to show signs of flowering sooner. Varieties originating in the tropics generally mature later, and more hours of darkness shorten flowering time. The

12-hour photoperiod represents the classic equinox and is the standard daylight-to-dark relationship for flowering in cannabis.

Some gardeners experiment with gradually decreasing daylight hours while increasing hours of darkness. They do this to simulate the natural photoperiod outdoors. This practice prolongs flowering and does not increase yields. Genetically unstable varieties could express intersex (hermaphroditic) tendencies if the photoperiod bounces up and down several times. If you plan to give plants a photoperiod of 13/11 day/night, stick to it. Do not decide you want to change the photoperiod to 15/9. Such variation will stress plants and could cause intersexuality.

Tropical gardeners that get 12 to 13 hours of light and at least 11 to 12 hours of darkness year round can grow plants with artificial light the first month or two of life and set them outdoors to induce flowering with the long nights. Such gardens can flower for two or three months, harvested and replanted year round. Other gardens in latitudes further north with good weather could grow autoflowering feminized plants during the long summer days to avoid having to cover greenhouses to induce flowering.

The photoperiod signals plants to start flowering; it can also signal them to remain in (or revert to) vegetative growth. Cannabis must have 12 hours of uninterrupted total darkness to flower properly. Dim light during the dark period in the pre-flowering and flowering stages prevents cannabis from blooming.

When the 12-hour dark period is interrupted by light, plants get confused. The light signals plants, "It's daytime; start vegetative growth." Given this signal of light, plants start vegetative growth, and flowering is retarded or stopped.

Cannabis will not stop flowering if the lights are turned on for a few minutes once or twice during the 2-month-long flowering cycle. If a light is turned on for 5 to 30 minutes—long enough to disrupt the dark period—on 3 to 5 consecutive nights, plants will start to revert to vegetative growth.

Less than one half of one foot-candle of light will prevent cannabis from flowering. That is a little more light than is reflected by a full moon on a clear night. Well-bred indica-dominant plants will revert within three days. Sativa-dominant plants take four to five days to revert to vegetative growth. Once they start to revegetate, it can take from four to six additional weeks to induce flowering again!

There are other photoperiods possible. For example, you can give plants 12 hours of HID light and the remaining 6 hours of incandescent light for a total of 18 hours to save on electric bills. But other light regimens that do not allow for 11 to 12 hours of darkness in 24 hours are going against Mother Nature. If sales people promise higher yields, watch out for disproportionate use of electricity. There are also some screwy photoperiod regimens that

A relationship exists between photoperiod response and genetics. Little scientific information is available about which specific varieties of cannabis are affected by photoperiod.

Sativa-dominant varieties that originated in the tropics respond to long days better than *indica*-dominant varieties, even though both are short-day plants. On the equator, days and nights are almost the same length year round. Plants tend to bloom when they are chronologically ready, after completing the vegetative growth stage. For example, the pure *sativa* variety 'Haze' flowers slowly for 3 months or longer, even when given a 12-hour photoperiod.

Give 'Haze' varieties more darkness and less light hours to speed harvest time and make flower buds fill in faster. Start with the 12/12 photoperiod and change to a 14 dark/10 light photoperiod after the first month. Play around a little with the photoperiod on pure *sativas* to dial it in for specific varieties.

You can start 'Haze' on a 12/12 day/night schedule, but it still must go through the seedling and vegetative stages before spending 3 months or longer flowering. Plants grow more slowly in 12-hour days than when given 18 hours of light, and inducing flowering takes longer.

Indica-dominant varieties that originated in northern latitudes tend to flower sooner and respond more quickly to a 12-hour photoperiod. Many *indica* varieties will flower under a 14/10 or 13/11 day/night photoperiod. Again, the hours of light necessary to induce flowering in an *indica*-dominant plant is contingent upon the genetics in the variety. More hours of light during flowering can cause some varieties to produce bigger plants, but flowering time is usually longer and some gardeners have reported looser, leafier flower buds as a result.

Some gardeners have achieved higher yields by inducing flowering via the 12-hour photoperiod, then changing to 13 to 14 hours of light after 2 to 4 weeks. This practice works best with early-flowering *indica*-dominant varieties, but flowering might be prolonged. I spoke with gardeners who increase light by 1 hour 2 to 3 weeks after flowering is induced. They say the yield increases about 10 percent. Flowering takes about a week longer, however, and different varieties respond differently.

Horticulturists in the "green industry" state that once the bud is competent (after the juvenile stage) and will respond to flowering signals, it is determined (changed to a floral bud), which means it is going to flower. High stress by light levels, photoperiod, temperature, etc., can delay or cause abortion and maybe a shift back to adult vegetative growth. However, it is common practice that photo controls are dropped about a third to half of the time to harvest in most green industry production. They typically add or subtract an hour or two of light a day, just like cannabis growers. Nevertheless, this stress (longer days) could also be the trigger to shock plants out of the flowering stage.

Ruderalis-dominant varieties are autoflowering. *Cannabis sativa* and *C. indica* varieties are crossed with *C. ruderalis*. Some of the offspring contain the autoflowering genes. Autoflowering plants are often feminized. The seeds are planted indoors and grown indoors, outdoors, or in greenhouses. These varieties flower under 24 hours of light after about three weeks of growth. *C. ruderalis* crosses will flower under any light regimen. However, when growing indoors many gardeners report that a light regimen of 20 hours light and 4 hours dark will spur the most growth.

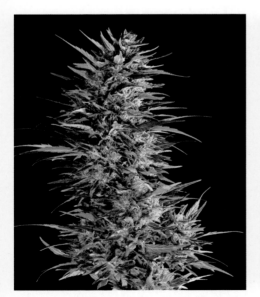

'Super Silver Haze' is a sativa-*dominant variety.*

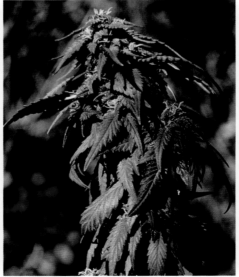

In 1978 this budding 'Kush' landrace variety represented a growing number of wild plants that were brought to the USA by cannabis breeders like Mel Frank. (MF)

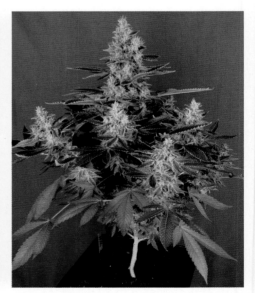

This autoflowering feminized 'NYC Diesel' from Soma Seeds is in full bloom and ready for harvest.

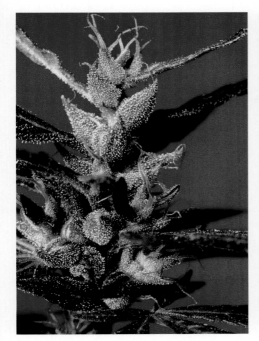

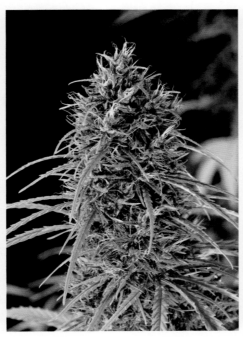

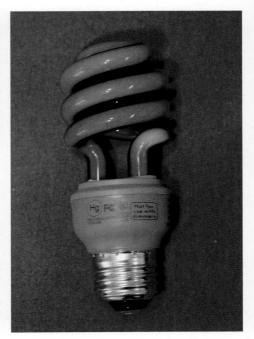

This lightweight flower has few seed bracts. The pure sativa from Colombia was pollinated and will produce seed. (MF)

This early-flowering 'Swazi' landrace came from the Kingdom of Swaziland.

Indoor gardeners use a green light to illuminate rooms at night so they can attend to plants. Plants process virtually no green light, therefore it has little or no affect on flowering.

should not be followed! To learn more about photoperiod regimens, check out www.marijuanagrowing.com.

Some gardeners give plants 36 hours of total darkness just before inducing flowering with the 12/12 photoperiod. This heavy dose of darkness sends plants an unmistakable signal that causes a hormonal change to stimulate flowering. Gardeners using this technique report that plants normally show signs of flowering, such as stigma formation, sooner than normal.

Indoor and Greenhouse Garden Lamps

Medical cannabis can be grown indoors using exclusively artificial light sources such as fluorescent, compact fluorescent (CFL), light-emitting diode (LED), high-intensity discharge (HID), and light-emitting plasma (LEP) lamps. Each of the lamps has its strengths and weaknesses. The fluorescent, CFL, LED, and LEP produce less heat than HID lamps, but HIDs produce more lumens per watt (lm/W). Many of the lamps are available in a growing range of spectrums conducive to plant growth.

All lamps used for indoor growing require ballasts or some sort of extra circuitry to regulate line electricity before reaching the bulb. Old-fashioned heavy magnetic (analog) ballasts are losing popularity to ever-improving electronic ballasts and circuitry.

There are many different bulbs and ballasts, and there are many different setups for gardens. New manufactures have entered the market and most of the old-reliable manufacturers offer more products than ever before. Next we will discuss different lighting systems and all the pertinent gardening details. Find all

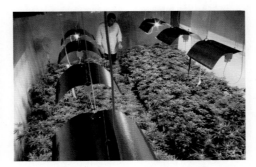

This beautiful indoor medical cannabis garden from Resin Seeds is full of CBD-rich 'Cannatonic' plants, and is illuminated with eight 600-watt HP sodium lamps.

the lamps in this chapter at local hydroponic stores and via Internet vendors.

High-Intensity Discharge (HID) Lighting Systems

Medical cannabis gardeners are compelled to employ high-intensity discharge (HID) lamps indoors in lieu of natural sunlight when they are unable to garden outdoors or in a greenhouse. Many medical gardeners start cuttings and seedlings indoors under lights before moving them into a greenhouse or outdoors. To date, some HID lamps outperform other lamps in their combined lumens-per-watt efficiency, spectral balance, and brilliance.

The HID lamp family contains mercury vapor, metal halide (MH), high-pressure (HP) sodium, and conversion bulbs (MH to HPS and HPS to MH). Metal halide, HPS, and conversion lamps have a spectrum similar to actual sunshine and can be used to grow cannabis.

Popular HID wattages range from 150 to 1100. Smaller 150- to 250-watt bulbs are popular for small gardens measuring up to three feet square. Brighter 400- to 1100-watt lamps are favored for larger gardens. The 400- and 600-watt bulbs

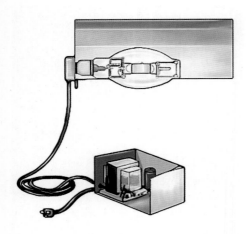

This simple cutaway drawing of a metal halide reveals the transformer and capacitor in a protective metal box. The bulb and hood are attached to the ballast with 14/3-wire and a mogul socket.

are most popular among European gardeners. North American gardeners favor 600- and 1000-watt bulbs. Super efficient 1100-watt metal halides were introduced in 2000.

The brightest bulbs measured in lumens per watt are the metal halide and HP sodium bulbs. Originally developed in the 1960s, metal halides and HP sodium bulbs were characterized by one main technical limitation—the larger the bulb, the higher the lumens-per-watt conversion. For example, watt for watt, a 1000-watt HP sodium produces about 12 percent more light than a 400-watt HPS and about 25 percent more light than a 150-watt HPS. Scientists overcame this barrier when they developed the 600-watt HP sodium. Watt for watt, a 600-watt HPS produces 7 percent more light than the 1000-watt HPS. The "pulse start" metal halides are also brighter and much more efficient than their predecessors.

An HID light "system" consists of a ballast (transformer, capacitor, and starter) attached to an HID bulb and reflector. High-intensity discharge lamps produce light by passing electricity through ionized gas enclosed in a clear ceramic arc tube under very high pressure. The combination of chemicals sealed in the arc tube determines the color spectrum produced. The mix of chemicals in the

arc tube allows metal halide lamps to yield the broadest and most diverse spectrum of light. The spectrum of HP sodium lamps is limited because of the narrower band of chemicals used to dose the arc tube. The arc tube is contained within a larger glass bulb. Most of the ultraviolet rays produced in the arc tube are filtered by the outer bulb. Some bulbs have a phosphor coating inside. This coating makes them produce a little different spectrum and fewer lumens. The outer bulb functions as a protective jacket that contains the arc tube and starting mechanism, keeping them in a constant environment, as well as absorbing ultraviolet radiation. Protective glasses that filter out ultraviolet rays are a good idea if you spend much time in the garden room.

Caution: To avoid serious damage to your eyes, *never* look at the arc tube if the outer bulb breaks. Turn off the lamp immediately.

An HID lamp requires a seasoning period of 100 hours of operation for all of its components to stabilize. If a power surge occurs and the lamp goes out or is turned off, it will take 5 to 15 minutes for the gases inside the arc tube to cool before restarting. Lamps

last longer when started only once a day. Always use a timer to turn lamps on and off.

Typically, metal halides operate most efficiently in a vertical ±15degree position. When operated in positions other than ±15 degrees of vertical, lamp wattage, lumen output, and bulb life decrease; the arc bends, creating non-uniform heating of the arc tube wall, resulting in less-efficient operation and shorter life. There are special lamps made to operate in the horizontal or any other position other than ±15 degrees.

HID lamps may produce a stroboscopic (flashing) effect, making the light appear bright, then dim, bright, dim, etc. This flashing is the result of the arc being extinguished 120 times every second. Illumination usually remains constant, but it may pulsate a little. This is normal and nothing to worry about.

The number of HID lamp manufacturers has grown during the last few decades. Today HID bulbs are often made in China by unknown manufacturers. For example, go to http://www.alibaba.com/ and search for HID lights. HID bulbs made in different countries have diverse quality standards and laws or rules that

Theo from Gavita Holland is getting a close-up view of an HID. He wears special protective lenses to avoid burning his eyes from the intense light.

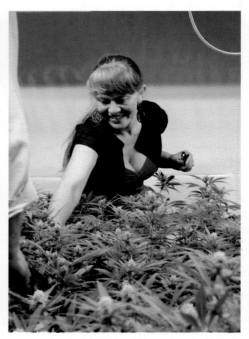

HID lamps can transform a simple indoor room into a Garden of Eden. All that is needed is a little light, cannabis, and desire!

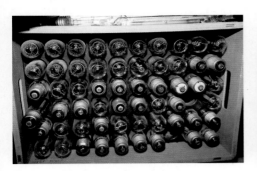

Most HID bulbs have changed shape to a tubular design because of advances in materials and technology.

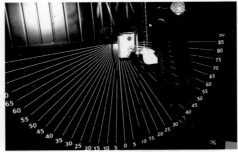

At the Gavita-Holland testing facility, bulb luminescence is measured every 5 degrees. The bulb is secured in a mogul socket against a wall when measurements are taken.

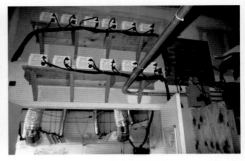

These reliable heat-producing analog ballasts are high up on shelves outside the garden room.

are not always enforced. Substandard products result. General Electric, Iwasaki, Lumenarc, Osram/Sylvania, Philips, and Venture (SunMaster) continue to manufacture good-quality HID bulbs. Go to their websites and check the official statistics for each bulb.

Certain brands of bulbs may have better attributes than others. Indoor cannabis gardeners usually come to this conclusion because they purchase two different brands of bulbs and have better luck using one brand over the other. However, many manufacturers buy and use the same components, often manufactured by competitors.

The best way to ensure that bulbs emit adequate light all the time is to check the light output with a light meter. Pulse-start metal halides operate in the same way as traditional metal halide bulbs, but their construction is slightly different. Traditional bulbs have an electrode at each end of the arc tube and an additional striker electrode close to one of the main electrodes. When the bulb starts, a short arc is formed between the striker electrode and the main electrode. This creates ionized gas that fills the tube and provides a path for an arc between the two main electrodes. A temperature-sensitive bimetallic strip acts as a switch and removes the striker electrode from the circuit when the light has fully lit. Pulse-start metal halides do not have a striker electrode; instead, their ballast contains an igniter circuit that provides a spike or pulse of electricity (1 kilovolt [kV] to 5 kV on a cold strike and up to 30 kV on a hot restrike) to start the arc.

HID Ballasts

A ballast wired in between the lamp and the electrical power supply is necessary for HID lamps to regulate specific starting requirements and line voltage. Purchase the high-intensity discharge system—ballast, lamp, reflector, and electrical cords and plugs at the same time to ensure that they all function properly and are designed to work together. Always buy the proper ballast for HID bulbs. A good rule of thumb is that ballasts can be used only with bulbs they were designed for.

A ballast converts and regulates electricity. Ballasts can be either the old-style magnetic (analog or inductive) type or the newer electronic (digital) type. Inefficient conversion and regulation of electricity will result in lost power in the form of heat. Heat is an excellent measure of efficiency. Digital ballasts "leak" about 2.5 British thermal units per hour (Btu/h). Analog ballasts lose about 3.5 Btu/h. The difference is small, but it adds up over time. More electricity goes to the bulb and less heat is generated in the room.

After all the hype of lower electric bills when using electronic ballasts, our www.marijuanagrowing.com forum member JustThisGuy converted 16 analog ballasts to 16 digital ballasts. With analog ballasts the electric bill was $1,100 USD per month, and with digital ballasts it was $1,000 USD, a savings of about 9 percent. See chapter 15, *Meters*, for more information on measuring electricity use.

Analog (Magnetic) Ballasts

Analog or magnetic ballasts have been around for decades. They are available in wattages from 150 to 1100. Magnetic ballasts contain an inductor that consists of copper wire wound around an iron core (a series of metal plates stuck together by resin). This serves to regulate the current and voltage delivered to the lamp. A capacitor and (sometimes) a starter for lamps are mounted on a separate board. The ballast is wired in between the lamp and the electrical power supply. Magnetic ballasts weigh in at 30 pounds (13.6 kg) for a 400-watt and up to 60 pounds (27.2 kg) for a 1000-watt HPS.

Analog ballast kits contain a transformer core, capacitor (HPS and some metal halides), starter, containing box, and (sometimes) wire. You can purchase components separately from an electrical supply store, but doing so is often more work than it's worth. If unfamiliar with electrical component assembly and reading wiring diagrams, purchase the assembled ballast in a package containing the lamp and reflective hood from one of the many HID retailers. Do not buy used parts from a junkyard or try to use a ballast if you are unsure of its capacity. Just because a bulb fits a socket attached to a ballast, does not mean that they will work efficiently together.

Analog ballasts generate noise and about 3.5 Btu/h of heat. As they age, the resin between plates in the core hardens and metal plates start to vibrate. Ballasts operate at 90°F to 150°F (32.2°C–65.6°C). Touch a "strike anywhere" kitchen match to the side to check if it is too hot. If the match lights, the ballast

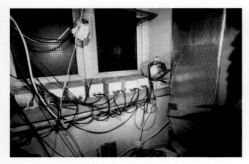

Analog ballasts are lined up on the shelf and attached to HID lamps many feet (meters) away. Much electricity is being lost during transmission from the ballast. Lamps are not as bright when they receive less electricity.

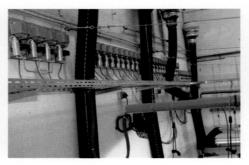

This gardener prefers to use reliable analog ballasts.

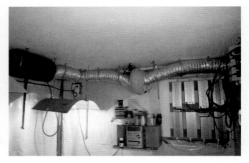

Electronic ballasts create little heat and make little noise when operating. Placing electronic ballasts close to lamps inside a garden room reduces electrical transmission loss in lines.

is too hot and should be taken into the shop for assessment. Heat is the number one ballast destroyer.

Many types of ballasts are manufactured with a protective metal box. This outer shell safely contains the core, capacitor (starter), and wiring. Dampen noise by building another box around it. Make sure there is plenty of air circulation. If the ballast runs too hot, it will be less efficient, run more noisily, burn out prematurely, and maybe even start a fire.

Electronic Ballasts

Electronic ballasts use a high-frequency oscillator circuit to provide a high-frequency current to drive the lamp. Electronic ballasts operate about 10 percent more efficiently than magnetic ballasts and consume a little less electricity to produce the same output. A microprocessor (CPU) that fine-tunes the electrical supply to the lamp can be found in some electronic ballasts, including those supplied by Lumatek.

High-frequency operation requires special "high-frequency" bulbs. Do not use a high-frequency lamp in analog or 50/60 cycle (hertz) ballast. And do not use a low-frequency bulb with a high-frequency electronic ballast. Operating requirements of each system are different, and interchanging bulbs or ballasts from digital to analog or vice versa will result in premature equipment failure.

The electrical *input* frequency, measured in hertz (Hz), to the ballast is 50 or 60 Hz. When the electricity leaves

the ballast to go to the lamp, *output* frequency increases up to 4000 Hz. The high operating hertz virtually eliminates the stroboscopic effect and output does not fluctuate with input voltage. High operating frequencies prevent acoustic resonance and optimize lamp life. The result of the stable power supply is a brighter lamp.

HID lamps designed for digital ballasts also have stronger metals inside the bulb due to the higher operating frequencies and demands of a digital system. This is why it is so important to make sure ballasts and bulbs are designed to be used together.

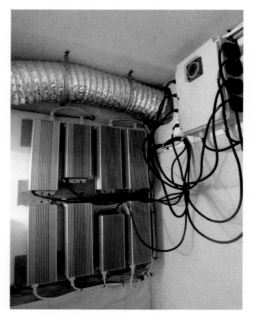

Eight electronic ballasts are mounted on the wall next to an eight-light timer. Everything is easy to monitor. Note how all the electrical components are located high in the room to avoid water problems.

Electronic ballasts are lightweight and run cool, generating about 2.5 Btu/h. They are designed to operate in environments less than 104°F (40°C).

Solid-state electronic ballasts have no moving parts and make little noise. Manufacturers often cover components in resin (a process called "potting") to protect them from water, humidity, and other damage. This is very important in a garden environment. Mount ballasts on a small pad or rubber feet to subdue any noise caused by vibration.

Available in 150- to 1150-watt models, many electronic ballasts are able to modulate in-between wattages. For example, a 1000-watt ballast could work at different settings: 600, 750, 1000, or 1150 watts.

The wattage on some electronic ballasts can be changed. For example, a 1000-watt electronic ballast could run at wattages from 600 to 1150. Dial settings are adjusted to change the wattage of the lamp. Underdriving lamps works well but is less efficient electrically.

Multiple power outputs from ballasts enable use for different bulbs. Electronic ballasts can be adjusted to operate at different wattages. The "soft dim" switch requires 60 seconds for each increase or decrease in wattage. For example:

1000-watt: 600, 660, 750, 825, 1000, 1150

600-watt: 300, 400, 600, 660

400-watt: 250, 275, 400, 440

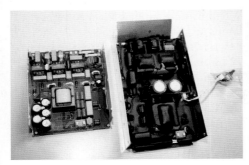

Two electronic ballasts: the one on the left is normal, and the one on the right is coated with protective resin so that parts do not move and are moisture resistant.

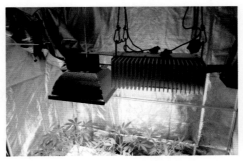

Aluminum fins quickly and evenly dissipate heat generated by this LEP lamp. Aluminum dissipates heat faster than steel. Enclosed ballasts with fins cool fastest, and run at the most consistent operating temperatures. Set ballasts so cooling fins are oriented vertically; heat is dissipated more quickly, and LEP lamps will stay cooler.

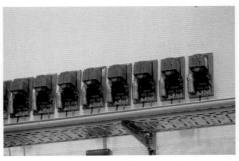

These ballasts are located up high in the garden room and do not use a protective housing.

Electronic ballasts can drive a wide range of electronic lamps (EL) and increase their output by 10 to 15 percent, but increasing output overdrives the bulb and shortens its life.

The world of indoor plant lighting is changing all the time. Keep up with new developments in plant lighting at www.marijuanagrowing.com.

Ballast Features

Avoid purchasing ballasts with enclosed fans or timers. They run too hot, and the extra appliances tend to break or cause problems.

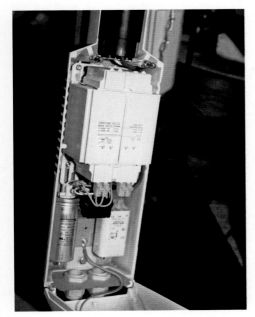

This attached, enclosed ballast from Gavita uses aluminum housing with ribs to quickly dissipate heat.

Ballasts can be attached to the light fixture or remote. The remote ballast offers the most versatility and is often the best choice for small HID gardens. A remote ballast is easy to move. Help control heat by placing a remote ballast on or near the floor to radiate heat in a cool portion of the garden room, or move the ballast outside the garden to cool the room. Do not place the ballast directly on a damp floor or any floor that might get wet and conduct electricity. Attached ballasts are fixed to the hood; they require more overhead space, are very heavy, and tend to create more heat around the lamp.

Attached ballasts have the benefit of using less electricity and creating a lower electronic profile around the garden. The electric cord between the ballast and the lamp consumes electricity, lowering lamp efficiency. It works like an antenna and emits a radio frequency signal that is very easy to pick up from afar. Thousands of luminaries can be operated in the same area.

A **handle** will make ballasts easier to move. A small 400-watt analog metal halide ballast weighs about 30 pounds (about 14 kg), and a large 1000-watt HP sodium ballast tips the scales at about 55 pounds (about 25 kg). This small, heavy box is very awkward to move without a handle.

Air vents allow a ballast to run cooler. The vents should protect the ballast's internal parts and prevent water from splashing in.

Ballasts with a switch allow gardeners to use the same ballast with two different sets of lights. This wonderful invention is perfect for running two flowering garden rooms. The lights go on for 12 hours in one garden room while they are off in a second room. When the lights turn off in the first room, the same ballasts hooked to another set of lights in the second room are turned on. There must be a 10- to 15-minute pause between initiation of lights in each room.

There are also ballasts to run both metal halide and HP sodium systems. These dual-purpose ballasts are not as efficient as dedicated ballasts. They often over-

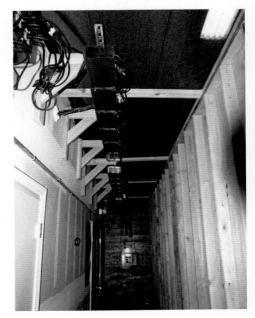

Keep remote ballasts up and out of the way to avoid risk of electrical shock or accidents involving moisture.

drive the metal halide bulb, causing it to burn out prematurely after accelerated lumen output loss. If you have a limited budget and can only afford one ballast, it is more economical to use conversion bulbs to change spectrum. (See "Conversion Bulbs" on page 272).

Most magnetic ballasts sold by HID stores are "single tap," and are set up for 120 volt household current in North America or 240 volts in Europe and other countries. Some "multi-tap" or "quad-tap" ballasts are ready for 120 or 240 volt service. North American ballasts run at 60 cycles per minute, while European counterpart runs at 50 cycles per minute.

European greenhouse HID lighting systems operate at 400 volts. Hobby lights were developed from professional lights that operate at 230 watts.

There is no difference in the electricity consumed by using either 120 or 240 volt systems. The 120 volt system draws about 9.6 amperes, and an HID on a 240-volt current draws about 4.3 amperes. Both use the same amount of electricity. Work out the details yourself using Ohm's Law.

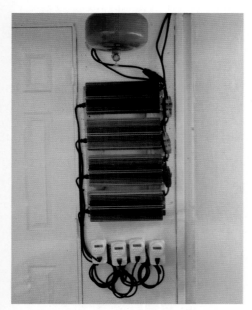

Ballast safety is super important. This set of electronic ballasts has a heat-sensitive fire extinguisher mounted above. If the ballasts catch fire or get too hot, the fire extinguisher is designed to trigger. Note that I have not seen one of these extinguishers that was UL (Underwriters Laboratories), CSA (Canadians Standards Association), or EMC (electromagnetic compatibility), approved.

Ballast Safety

The ballast has a lot of electricity flowing through it. Do not touch the ballast when operating. Do not place the ballast directly on a damp floor or any floor that might get wet and conduct electricity.

Always place the ballast up off the floor, and protect it from possible moisture. The ballast should be suspended in the air or on a shelf attached to the wall. It does not have to be very high off the ground, just far enough to keep it dry.

Place the ballast on a soft foam pad to absorb vibrations and lower decibel sound output on analog ballasts. Loose components inside the ballast can be tightened to further deaden noise caused by vibrations. Train a fan on ballasts to cool them. Cooler ballasts are more efficient, and bulbs burn brighter. Always check with a qualified source such as a hydroponic store to ensure that the ballast is designed for a specific lamp. Do not try to mix and match ballasts and lamps.

Some industrial ballasts are sealed in fiberglass or similar material to make them weatherproof. These ballasts are not recommended for use indoors. They were designed for outdoor use where heat buildup is not a problem. Indoors, the weather-protection of the sealed unit is unnecessary and creates excessive heat and inefficient operation.

Purchase only quality ballasts that come with a guarantee. Read the fine print, and do not be tricked by misleading sales phrases such as "all components UL (or CSA, EMC, etc.) approved." Each of the components could be UL, CSA, or EMC approved, but when the components are used together to operate a lamp, they are not UL, CSA, or EMC approved. Often components are approved, but not approved for the specific application.

To keep ballasts clean wipe them down with a damp cloth. Look for heat damage such as melted and burned wires. Take ballast to dealer immediately if signs of heat or malfunction occur. Often ballasts are sealed, and opening the ballast or breaking the seal will void the warranty.

When using a single ballast to light 2 lamps at 12-hour intervals, let it cool down before restarting. Run the lamp 12 hours then let the ballast cool for 15 minutes before restarting to operate the second 12-hour stint of light. Letting the ballast cool will help avoid burnout.

HID Bulbs
Ulbricht Sphere
An **integrating sphere** (aka Ulbricht sphere) is a hollow spherical cavity. The inside is covered with a diffuse reflective white paint. Its purpose is to uniformly diffuse or scatter light so that it is distributed equally to all points inside the sphere.

Measuring light in an Ulbricht sphere is the standard in photometry and radiometry. It measures light produced by a source where total (light) power can be acquired in a single measurement. The number of new HID bulbs that appear on the market today is mind-boggling. Osram Sylvania, General Electric, Gavita, Philips, SunMaster, Fulham, and Venture are a few of the manufacturers that make and continue to develop new HID bulbs.

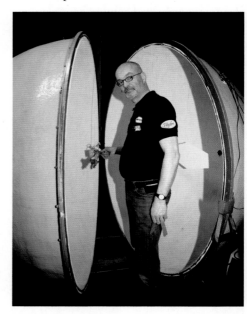

Theo from Gavita Holland demonstrates their Ulbricht sphere for measuring light. He also uses a digital power analyzer to measure the output of lights. It measures the input of the ballast and the actual output to the lamp, including power, frequency, and wave form.

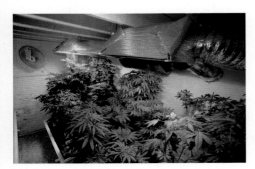

It is easy to see the difference in spectrum between the clear metal halide light in the foreground and the orange HP sodium light in the background.

Two blown tubular bulbs, an elliptical bulb dimpled in the middle, and two tubular bulbs represent some of the most common shapes of HID bulbs.

Not all HID bulbs are created equal. In fact, there are brighter brands that supply up to 15 percent more light than the closest competitor. The Philips Master GreenPower Plus TD EL 1000-watt lamp is the brightest lamp and emits more μmol than any other bulb. This exceptional HPS tubular lamp is secured at both ends, which allows a straight shot for the electricity to flow. Coupled with a bit longer arc tube, the free-flowing electricity makes the bulb generate more than 2000 μmol of light! Note that other bulbs, such as the Gavita Enhanced HPS 1000-watt, generate only 1750 μmols of light—12.5 percent less light.

Notable new bulbs have a high PAR rating and pulse-start metal halides.

High-intensity discharge bulbs are identified by wattage and by the size and shape of the outer envelope or bulb. They are further rated by voltage, ballasting requirements, lumen output, spectrum, etc.

Overall, HID bulbs are designed to be tough and durable, and new bulbs are tougher than used ones. Nonetheless, once the bulb has been used a few hours,

the arc tube blackens and internal parts become somewhat brittle. After a bulb has been used several hundred hours, a solid bump will substantially shorten its life and lessen its luminescence.

HID Bulb Maintenance

Always keep the bulb clean. Wait for it to cool before wiping it off with a liquid glass cleaner and clean cloth, every 2 to 4 weeks. Dirt and fingerprints will lower lumen output substantially. Bulbs get covered with insect spray and salty water-vapor residues. This dirt dulls lamp brilliance just as clouds dull natural sunlight. Hands off bulbs! Touching bulbs leaves them with your hand's oily residue. Baked-on residue weakens the bulb. Most gardeners clean bulbs with Windex or rubbing alcohol, and use a clean cloth to remove filth and grime; Hortilux Lighting advises cleaning bulbs with a clean cloth only.

Never remove a warm lamp. Heat expands the metal mogul base within the socket. A hot bulb is more difficult to remove, and it must be forced. Special electrical grease is available to lubricate sockets (Vaseline works too). Lightly smear a dash of the lubricant around the mogul socket base to facilitate bulb insertion and extraction.

The outer arc tube contains practically all the ultraviolet light produced by HIDs. If an HID should happen to break when inserting or removing it, unplug the ballast immediately and avoid contact with metal parts, to prevent electrical shock.

Pulse-start metal halide lighting manufacturers are required by the Energy Independence and Security Act of 2007 to meet certain efficiency standards. Effective January 1, 2009, standards require pulse-start metal halide lighting with a minimum ballast efficiency of 88 percent. Find ballast efficiency by dividing the lamp wattage by the operating wattage.

Lumen output diminishes over time. As the bulb loses brilliance, it generates less heat and can be moved closer to the garden. This is not an excuse to use old bulbs; it is always better to use newer bulbs. However, it is a way to get a few

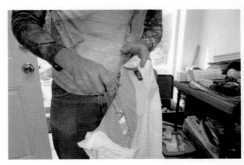

Place used HID bulbs in a plastic bag and dispose of them in a dump designated for hazardous materials.

more months out of an otherwise worthless bulb.

Write down the day, month, and year you start using a bulb so you can better calculate when to replace it for best results. Replace metal halides after 12 months of operation and HP sodium bulbs after 18 months. Many gardeners replace them sooner. Always keep a spare bulb (in its original box) available to replace old bulbs. You can go blind staring at a dim bulb trying to decide when to replace it.

You may prefer to change bulbs according to manufacturer´s recommendations. Some companies recommend as often as once every 8 months, others at 12 months. You are best to measure the light output; when it has diminished 10 to 20 percent, change bulbs.

Bulb Disposal

All fluorescent, compact fluorescent, plasma, HID, and any bulbs that may contain mercury or some other heavy metal that should not escape into the environment. Take spent bulbs to the proper hazardous materials disposal site in your area. Do not toss bulbs into the trash.

1. Place the bulb in a dry container, and then dispose of it at certified toxic waste dump facility such as a HAZMAT disposal site in the USA. Most countries have specific agencies that dispose of toxic waste.

2. Lamps contain materials that are harmful to the skin. Avoid contact, and use protective clothing.

3. Do not place the bulb in a fire.

Mercury Vapor Lamps

The mercury vapor lamp is the oldest and best-known member of the HID family. The HID principle was first used with the mercury vapor lamp around the turn of the 20th century, but it was not until the mid-1930s that the mercury vapor lamp was really employed commercially. Today they are too inefficient to consider as a light source for medical cannabis cultivation.

Mercury vapor lamps produce only 60 lumens per watt—and a poor light spectrum for plant growth. Lamps are available in sizes from 40 to 1000 watts. Bulbs have fair lumen maintenance and a relatively long life. Most wattages last up to 3 years at 18 hours of daily operation.

Bulbs usually require separate ballasts. There are a few low-wattage bulbs with self-contained ballasts. Uninformed gardeners occasionally try to scrounge mercury vapor ballasts from junkyards, and use them in place of the proper halide or HP sodium ballast. Trying to modify these ballasts for use with other HIDs will cause problems.

Metal Halide Bulbs and Ballasts

Metal Halide Bulbs

The metal halide HID lamp is still one of the most efficient sources of artificial white light available to gardeners today. Grow plants from seed through harvest with metal halide lamps. They come in wattages from 50 to 1100, and 1500 watts. They may be either clear or phosphor-coated, and all require a spe-

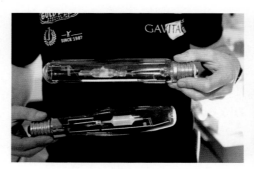

Two metal halide bulbs from different manufacturers have arc tubes of different shapes.

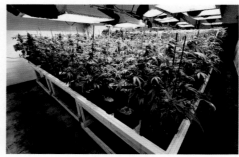

Metal halide lamps can produce a spectrum very similar to natural sunlight.

cial ballast. The smaller 175- or 250-watt halides are very popular for closet garden rooms. The 400-, 600-, 1000- and 1100-watt bulbs are most popular with indoor gardeners. The 1500-watt halide is avoided due to its relatively short 2000- to 3000-hour life and its incredible heat output. American gardeners generally prefer the larger 1000-watt lamps, and Europeans seem to almost exclusively favor 400- and 600-watt lamps.

Caution! Do not mix and match ballasts and bulbs! Ballasts are designed to be used with specific bulbs. Using bulbs with improper ballasts will shorten the life of both components and could cause excessive heat or catch fire!

More and more new metal halide lamps are being developed and marketed every year. New technology and materials have opened the door to new lighting products. The intention of this book is to show the basics of light and electricity, and how cannabis interacts with light rather than to keep up with all the new lighting developments. For more current

information on new lamps, ballasts, and reflective hoods, see www.marijuanagrowing.com.

Clear halides are most commonly used by indoor gardeners. Clear super metal halides supply the bright lumens for plant growth. Clear halides work well for seedling, vegetative, and flower growth. Phosphor-coated 1000-watt halides give off a more diffused light (and produce less light) but they emit less ultraviolet light than the clear halides. They produce the same initial lumens and about 4000 fewer lumens than the standard halide, and have a slightly different color spectrum. Phosphor-coated halides have more yellow, but less blue and ultraviolet light. Phosphor-coated bulbs were popular among gardeners in the 1990s.

The 1000-watt super clear halides are the most popular metal halides used to grow cannabis in North America. Compare energy distribution charts and lumen output of all lamps to decide which lamp offers the most light for your garden. Typically, a home gardener starts with one super metal halide.

Universal metal halide bulbs designed to operate in any position, vertical or horizontal, supply up to 10 percent less light and often have a shorter life.

Base Up (BU) and Base Down (BD) metal halide lamps must be vertical to operate properly. Horizontal (H) lamps must orient the arc tube horizontally to burn brightest.

Metal halide lamps are available in a variety of spectrums.

LAMP	KELVIN TEMPERATURE
AgroSun	3250
Multivapor	3800
Sunmaster Warm Deluxe	315 PAR
Sunmaster Natural Deluxe	315 PAR
Sunmaster Cool Deluxe	315 PAR
SolarMax	7200
MultiMetal	4200

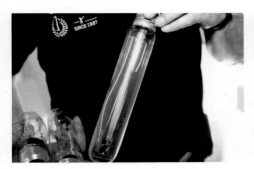

High-pressure sodium bulbs have a long arc tube that extends almost the length of the bulb.

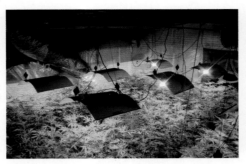

Plants tend to stretch between internodes under the limited light spectrum emitted by HP sodium lamps.

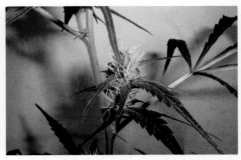

The distinctive yellow-orange-tinged glow emitted by HP sodium lamps unmistakable.

AgroSun and Sunmaster Warm Deluxe emit low (3000 Kelvin) color temperatures. The enhanced orange-red component promotes flowering, stem elongation, and germination while a rich blue content assures healthy vegetative growth. Visit www.growlights.com for more information.

The average life of a halide is about 12,000 hours, almost 2 years of daily operation at 18 hours per day. Many will last even longer. The lamp reaches the end of its life when it fails to start or come up to full brilliance. Electrode deterioration is greatest during start-up. Do not wait until the bulb is burned out before changing it. An old bulb is inefficient and costly. Bulbs lose at least 5 percent of their brilliance every year. Replace bulbs every 12 months or 5000 hours.

Metal Halide Ballasts

Read "About Ballasts." Different ballasts are required for each type of lamp. Use a magnetic ballast to operate metal halide bulbs designed for use with them. An electronic ballast is made specifically for electronic high-frequency bulbs. Ballasts must be specific to certain lamps because their starting and operating requirements are unique. Electronic ballasts are more efficient and produce less heat than analog or magnetic ballasts.

High-Pressure Sodium Bulbs and Ballasts

Approximately 60 percent of HP sodium light is infrared or heat. All lamp power and light will be converted to heat as bulbs degrade over time.

HP Sodium Bulbs

The high-pressure sodium (HPS) lamp is the most efficient source of artificial light available to medical cannabis gardeners today. HPS lamps come in wattages from 50 to 1000 watts. All require a special ballast. The smaller 175- or 400-watt HP sodium systems are very popular for closet garden rooms. The 400-, 600-, and 1000-watt bulbs are most popular with indoor and greenhouse gardeners.

HP sodium lamps emit a yellow-orange glow that could be compared to that of the harvest sun. Cannabis's light needs change when blooming; it no longer needs to produce so many vegetative cells. Vegetative growth slows and eventually stops during flowering. The plant's energy is focused on flower production so it can complete its annual life cycle. Light from the red end of the spectrum stimulates floral hormones within the plant, promoting flower production. In general, American gardeners use 1000- and 600-watt HP sodiums most often, while European gardeners use 400- and 600-watt HPS lamps.

Discount building stores often carry a good selection including 250- and 400-watt lamps. All HPS lamps will grow cannabis. Even though HPS lamps are brighter and will grow cannabis, the spectrum contains little blue and more yellow/orange. Lack of color balance makes plants stretch between internodes and experience more cultural and plague problems. But when grown properly, the lack of the proper spectrum does not necessarily diminish overall harvest.

Gardeners with small rooms often retain the 1000-watt halide and add a 1000-watt HP sodium during flowering, when plants need more light to produce tight, dense buds. Adding an HPS lamp doubles available light and increases the red end of the spectrum. This 1:1 ratio (1 MH:1 HPS) is a popular combination in flowering rooms.

The average life of an HPS lamp is about 24,000 hours, with about 5 years of daily operation at 12 hours per day. Many last even longer. The lamp reaches the end of its life when it fails to start or come up to full brilliance. Electrode deterioration is

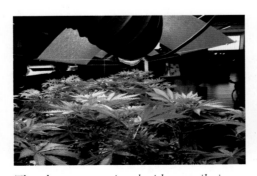

These lamps are equipped with a ventilation system that allows the bulb to be placed closer to the plants without burning them.

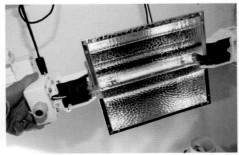

The Gavita double-ended bulb is my current favorite HID because it is more efficient than any other on the market today.

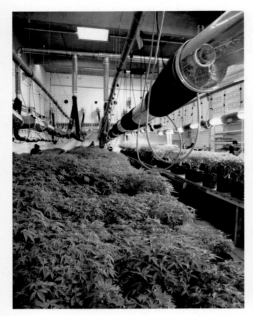

The bulbs in this mother room are attached to a ventilation system that removes heat generated by the bulbs.

Conversion bulbs are most commonly purchased for single-light gardens.

has unique needs, including operating voltages during startup and operation that do not correspond to similar wattages of other HID lamps. Magnetic HPS ballasts contain a heavy transformer that is larger than that of a metal halide, a capacitor, and an igniter or starter. Electronic ballasts are much lighter in weight and more compact, and they consume less power than analog ballasts. They also require a specific bulb that is designed for high-frequency output electronic ballasts. Purchase complete HPS systems from a reputable source.

Self-contained units that have an integrated solid-state electronic ballast, a lamp, and a reflector in a single enclosed unit produce very little EMI (electromagnetic interference, aka radio frequency [RF] interference). Large greenhouses can use up to 10,000 lamps with no RF interference.

greatest during startup. Do not wait until the bulb is burned out before changing it. An old bulb is inefficient and costly. Bulbs lose at least 5 percent of their brilliance every year. Replace bulbs every 24 months or 9000 hours.

Double-ended 1000-watt HPS bulbs
from Philips are the best grow lamp currently available. These bulbs are more efficient, and their arc tube is a little bit longer. Electricity flows from one end of the arc tube and out the other. This makes them inherently more efficient than bulbs that require electricity to travel farther. The new bulbs produce about 15 percent more light than single-ended bulbs. Since the bulb is attached at both ends, the arc tube is always mounted parallel to the reflector for maximum efficiency and reflection.

The **600-watt high-pressure sodium lamp** produces 90,000 initial lumens. HPS lamps are available in wattages from 35 to 1000. The Philips GreenPower 400v, 600-watt EL (electronic lamp) has the highest PAR light output rating and more than 95 percent light maintenance.

The 430-watt Son Agro by Philips was designed to augment natural sunlight in greenhouses. The bulb produces a little more blue light, about 6 percent, in the spectrum. Adding a touch more blue

light helps prevent most plants from becoming leggy.

High-pressure sodium lamps are manufactured by: GE (Lucalox), Sylvania (Lumalux), Westinghouse (Ceramalux), Philips (Son Agro), Iwasaki (Eye), and Venture (high-pressure sodium). Many more HPS bulbs are manufactured by others in China. Check out different Chinese manufacturers and their manufacturing standards. Chinese products are not necessarily bad; in fact, several of the above companies manufacture bulbs or components in China.

End of Life
HP sodiums have the longest life and best lumen maintenance of all HIDs. Over time the sodium bleeds out through the arc tube. The sodium-to-mercury ratio changes and the voltage in arc rises. The lamp warms up and goes out. The sequence is repeated, signaling the end of the lamp's life, which is about 24,000 hours—five years at 12 hours daily use.

Dispose of bulbs in an approved hazardous waste facility.

HP Sodium Ballasts
Read "About Ballasts." A special ballast is specifically required for each wattage of HP sodium lamp. Each wattage lamp

Conversion Bulbs
Conversion, or retrofit, bulbs increase lighting options on a budget. One type of conversion bulb allows you to utilize a metal halide (or mercury vapor) system with a bulb that emits a light spectrum similar to that of a HP sodium bulb. The bulb looks like a cross between a metal halide and an HP sodium. While the outer bulb looks like a metal halide, the inner arc tube is similar to that of an HP sodium. A small igniter is located at the base of the bulb. Other conversion bulbs retrofit HP sodium systems to convert them into virtual metal halide systems.

Conversion bulbs are manufactured in 150, 215, 360, 400, 880, 940, and 1000 watts. You do not need an adapter or any additional equipment. Simply screw the bulb into a compatible ballast of comparable wattage. Conversion bulbs operate at a lower wattage and are not as bright as HP sodium bulbs. Although conversion bulbs have less blue, they are up to 25 percent brighter than metal halide systems and their lumens-per-watt conversion is better than that of super metal halides. The 940-watt conversion bulb has a lumens-per-watt rating of 138. Similar to the HP sodium lamp, the conversion bulb has a life expectancy of up to 24,000 hours. Unlike most high-pressure sodium lamps which flicker on and off near the end of their lives, conversion

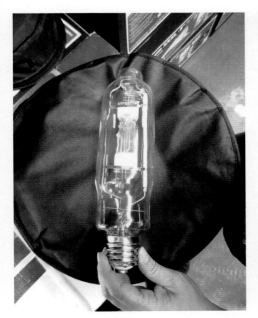

HP sodium to metal halide conversion bulb

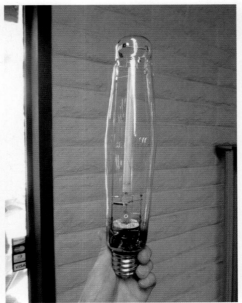

Metal halide to HP sodium conversion bulb

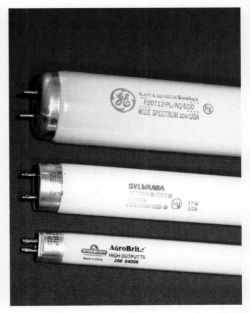

Three popular fluorescent bulbs include T12 (top), T8 (middle), and T5 (bottom). All three require different two-pin fixtures and ballasts.

bulbs go off and remain off at the end of their lives.

Although conversion bulbs are not inexpensive, they are certainly less expensive than an entire HP sodium system. For gardeners who own a metal halide system, or who deem metal halide the most appropriate investment for their lighting needs, conversion bulbs offer a welcome alternative for bright light. In the United States, CEW Lighting distributes Iwasaki lights. Look for their Sunlux Super Ace and Sunlux Ultra Ace lamps. Venture, Iwasaki, and Sunlight Supply manufacture bulbs for conversion in the opposite direction—from high-pressure sodium to metal halide. Venture's White-Lux and Iwasaki's White Ace are metal halide lamps which will operate in an HP sodium system. The 250-, 400-, and 1000-watt conversion bulbs can be used in compatible HPS systems with no alterations or additional equipment. If you own a high-pressure sodium system but need the added blue light that metal halide bulbs produce, these conversion bulbs will suit your needs.

Many gardeners have great success using conversion bulbs. If you have a metal halide system but want the extra red and yellow light of an HP sodium lamp to promote flowering, simply buy a conversion bulb. Instead of invest-ing in both a metal halide and an HP sodium system, you can rely on a metal halide system and use conversion bulbs when necessary, or vice versa.

HP Sodium to Metal Halide

Several companies make HPS to MH conversion bulbs, including the Sunlux Super Ace and Ultra Ace (Iwasaki) and Retrolux (Philips). The bulb emits an HP sodium spectrum with a metal halide system. These bulbs make it possible to use a metal halide ballast and get the same spectrum as an HP sodium lamp. Lumens-per-watt efficiency is traded for the convenience of using these bulbs. A 1000-watt HP sodium bulb produces 140,000 initial lumens. A MH to HPS conversion bulb produces 130,000 initial lumens. If you only want one lamp, a conversion bulb is a fair choice.

Metal Halide to HP Sodium

Metal halide to high-pressure sodium bulbs are manufactured by several companies, including the White Ace (Iwasaki) and White Lux (Venture). They have an MH spectrum and are used in an HPS system. The bulb converts from HPS to MH and produces 110,000 initial metal halide lumens.

Fluorescent Lamps, Ballasts, and Fixtures
Fluorescent Bulbs

Fluorescent bulbs (tubes) come in a wide variety of lengths, from 6 inches to 8 feet (15.2–243.8 cm). Two- and 4-foot (60–121.9 cm) tubes are easy to handle, readily available, and the most popular. Circular (T9) and U-shaped bulbs (B = bent) are also available.

Fluorescent bulbs are available in at least 7 different diameters. T2 bulbs are the smallest and T4, T5, T8, T9, T12, and T17 (Power Twist) are each progressively larger in diameter. Many medical gardeners still use inexpensive reliable T12 lamps grow cuttings, seedlings and small vegetative plants. They supply cool, diffused light in the proper color

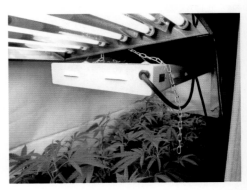

Thin, high-output (HO) T5 fluorescent bulbs are the brightest fluorescents and are very efficient.

LAMP	USA	LIFE HOURS	WATTS	KELVIN TEMP.	LUMENS
Warm White	T12	24000	40	2700	2200
Neutral White	T12	24000	40	3500	2200
Cool White	T12	24000	40	4100	2200
Full Spectrum	T12	24000	40	5000	2200
Agrosun T12	T12	24000	40	5850	2450
AgroBrite T12	T12	24000	40	6400	2200
Spectralux T8 HO	T8 HO	20000	54	6500	2700
Ecolux T8 HO	T8 HO	20000	54	6500	2700
Spectralux T5 HO	T5 HO	20000	54	3000 and 5000	5000
Spectralux T5 VHO	T5 VHO	20000	54	3000 and 6500	5000
GE Starcoat T5 HO	T5 HO	20000	54	3000 and 6500	5000
Philips T5 Alto HO	T5 Alto HO	20000	54	3000	5000
GE Starcoat T5 HO	T5 HO	20000	54	Warm	5000

USA	Inches	Millimeters
T2	0.25	7
T4	0.5	12
T5	0.625	15.875
T8	1	25.4
T9	1.125	28.575
T12	1.5	38.1
T17	2.125	53.97

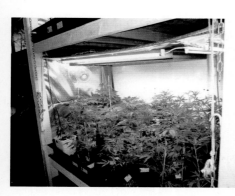

Big clones receive plenty of light for rapid growth under this bank of T5 bulbs.

spectrum to promote root growth. Other more brilliant fluorescents include T5 high output (HO), VHO and T8 HO, lamps. They are being used in gardens from seed through harvest.

HO = high output
VHO = very high output
XHO = extra high output

The average lumen output of a 4-foot (121.9 cm) 40-watt T12 is 2800 lumens per watt. A 32 watt T8 bulb yields 100 lumens per watt and supplies 100 average lumens. A 54 watt T5 throws 5000 average lumens, 92 lumens per watt.

Fluorescents produce much less light than HIDs and must be very close (2 to 4 inches [510 cm]) to the plants for best results. The light emission is strongest near the center of the tube, and somewhat less at the ends.

Fluorescent lamps are available in a variety of spectrums, from 2700 to 6500 K, including Warm White, Neutral White, Cool White, Full Spectrum, Daylight, and so forth, as listed at left.

Fluorescent lighting manufacturers include GE, Osram/Sylvania, and Philips.

The three main fluorescent tubes used by gardeners include T12, T8, and T5. The T12 and T8 bulbs were developed in the 1930s. The T12s met with immediate success; T8s became popular in the late 1980s. Today, T5 and T8 bulbs are more efficient than ever and often used to grow cannabis from clone or seedling through harvest.

Designed in the 1990s, T5 bulbs are the brightest of the fluorescent lamps. The full-spectrum, high-intensity, fluorescent T5 tubes come in high output (HO, 54 W), very high output (VHO, 95 W), and extra high output (XHO, 115 W). The intensely bright new spectrum is designed specifically for plant growth. The VHO and XHO lamps produce more heat and are more difficult and expensive to manufacturer than lower-output bulbs.

The T5 tubes are smaller and will fit in narrow spaces. The size makes for more accurate control of light direction with a reflective hood. Tubes are also rated as high efficiency (HE) and high output (HO), but the latter has lower efficiency.

High-output lamps are driven at a higher current and are brighter. The ends on the connecting pins are unique so they

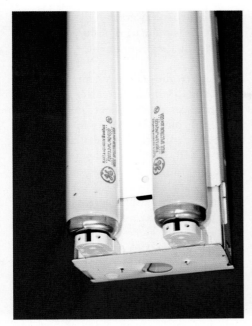

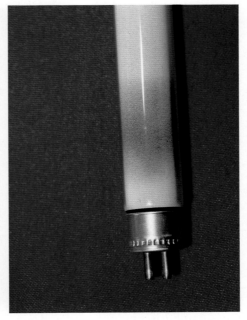

This T12 fixture with bulbs is the basic setup that can be purchased at most hardware stores. Such fixtures are commonly used when rooting clones or growing seedlings.

As a fluorescent bulb nears the end of its life, the ends become darker and the tube emits less overall light.

cannot be used in the wrong fixture. High-output bulbs are labeled HO, or VHO for very high output. The T5 lamps render peak light output at 95°F (35°C). The T8 and the T12 lamps provide peak light output at a 77°F (25°C). The bulbs run most efficiently and last longest when operated within the proper temperature range.

A fluorescent lamp consists of a glass tube coated on the inside with light-emitting phosphors and filled with a low-pressure mercury vapor. An electric current is passed through the tube, exciting the mercury vapor and causing it to emit UV light. This UV light causes the coating of the tube to fluoresce, giving off visible light. The mix of phosphorescent chemicals in the coating and the gases contained within determines the spectrum of colors emitted by the lamp. The quality of the phosphors and manufacturing process are essential to a lamp that will maintain true brilliance for a long time.

Old-fashioned T12 and T8 lamps are inefficient halophosphate tubes that do not render colors well. Today triphosphor and multi-phosphor tubes dominate the marketplace, because they are much more efficient and retain their properties well over time. A simple test with a light meter showed that inexpensive brand-new VHOs produced 30 percent less lumens than the phosphor and multiphosphor tubes.

Be very cautious when purchasing inexpensive lamps that use phosphorous from China rather than quality phosphorus (tri-phosphorous) from Japan and a few other places. Phosphorous from China generally does not hold the lumen or blue of the 6.5 K lamps. Lumen degradation occurs rapidly. Controlled studies found that inexpensive lamps start with very high lumens but can drop off by over 30 percent in a few months. Check bulbs regularly to ensure they are up to full brilliance.

Using fluorescents along with HIDs is awkward and problematic. When using them in conjunction with HIDs, fluorescents must be very close to plants to provide enough intense light for plant growth. Fixtures may also shade plants from HID light and generally get in the way.

End of Life

Fluorescents blacken with age, losing intensity. Replace bulbs when they reach 70 to 90 percent of their stated service life listed on the package or label. A flickering light is about to burn out and should be replaced. Life expectancy is around 9000 hours (15 months at 18 hours' daily operation).

The end-of-life failure mode for fluorescent lamps varies depending on their ballasts and on how the lamps are used. A lamp that turns pink with black burns on the ends of the tube lacks mercury.

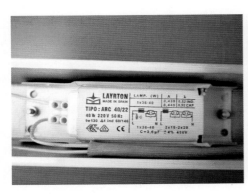

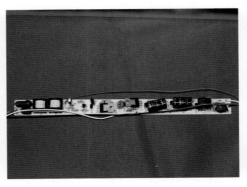

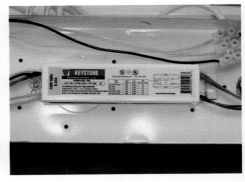

This analog fluorescent lamp ballast is efficient and provides perfect service for years.

The components of electronic fluorescent ballasts can be configured into many different shapes. In this case they conform to the restraints of a long, thin fixture.

This electronic ballast is smaller and more lightweight than its analog counterpart.

A main reason that a lamp flickers is as a result of poor electrical connections.

Change the starter on older fluorescent fixtures. The starter is the little round tube that sticks into the fixture at one end of the bulb. Starters are inexpensive and have about the same life as a bulb. A new bulb will last a short time with an old starter that is on its last leg.

Fluorescent Ballasts

Each fluorescent lamp requires a specific ballast to regulate electricity before reaching the bulb. Fluorescents require an appropriate fixture containing a small ballast to regulate electricity and household electrical current. The tube type should always match the markings on the light fixture. Ballasts are rated for the size of lamp and power frequency. Ballasts can also include a capacitor to correct the power factor. The fixture is usually integrated into the reflective hood. The ballast is located far enough away from fluorescent tubes that plants can actually touch them without being burned.

Many of the T12 and T8 fixtures use old-fashioned magnetic ballasts. Newer T5, T8 and T12 fluorescents use electronic ballasts. Gardeners prefer slimmer T8 and T5 bulbs with electronic ballasts because they run cooler, electricity cycles faster, and lights do not flicker. Fluorescent light fixtures cannot be connected to dimmer switches intended for incandescent lamps.

Self-starting "rapid start" ballasts eliminate voltage spike when they are properly grounded. There are "instant start," "rapid start," "quick start," "semi-resonate start," and "programmed start" ballasts. The old-fashioned semi-resonate start lamps are the slowest to ignite; some of them even require a separate starter. All of the others strike and start lamps much faster. Programmed start ballasts are found in premium fixtures. Fixtures and lamps do take 5 to 10 minutes to warm up.

One of the main problems with fluorescent lighting is ballast incompatibility with the bulb. Some manufacturers use ballasts and lamps because they are the least expensive, not because they are designed for specific applications. Another example comes from gardeners: running a T8 tube with a ballast for a T12 will reduce lamp life and can increase energy consumption.

Analog Ballasts

Analog (magnetic) ballasts are simple, consisting of a copper wire winding on a laminated magnetic core. They are heavy and radiate almost all heat produced by the system. Analog ballasts consume about 10 percent of the system's electricity. A wiring diagram is usually glued on the ballast. Simple wiring is also provided.

These ballasts will normally last 10 to 12 years. The end of the magnetic ballast's life is usually accompanied by smoke and a miserable chemical odor. When the ballast burns out, remove it and buy a new one to replace it. Be very careful if the ballast has brown slime or sludge on or around it. This sludge could contain carcinogenic PCBs. If the ballast contains the sludge, dispose of it in an approved location for hazardous waste.

Electronic Ballasts

Electronic ballasts run much cooler, consume little electricity, and are lightweight. They are normally located within the lamp fixture. Electronic ballasts are very quiet, with no annoying hum. Electronic ballasts use transistors to alter incoming electricity into high-frequency alternating current (AC), and regulate the current flow in the lamp simultaneously. Efficacy of a fluorescent lamp rises by almost 10 percent at a frequency of 10 kHz, compared to efficacy at normal power frequency. Electronic ballasts are also called digital ballasts because they are controlled by a microcontroller or similar hardware. The electronic controller dims lights and maintain constant light levels—no flickering.

Electronic ballasts typically work in rapid start or instant start mode. Low-cost ballasts start slowly. More expensive ballasts use programmed start, which ignites the lamps quickly.

At the end of life, electronic ballasts simply stop. No drama. One of the most common causes of lamp failure is due to a lower voltage capacitor and other parts that cost less are installed. The stress causes premature failure. Always purchase quality equipment.

Most electronics failures happen early in life and diminish thereafter. High temperatures shorten electronic ballast life. Typically for every 50 degrees the temperature rises, the ballast life is cut in half. Keep the temperature range within the operating boundaries, normally at about 77°F (25°C) in most countries. Dispose of electronic ballasts in an approved hazardous waste dump.

Fluorescent Fixtures

A "shop light" fixture/reflector that holds two 40-watt T12 fluorescent tubes and ballast available at hardware stores is perfect for growing cuttings and seedlings until they are about six inches (about 15 cm) tall. A more substantial fixture will be necessary for higher

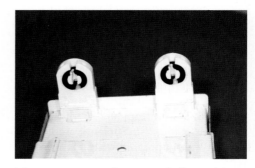

The most common fluorescent bulbs used for gardening are connected to sockets with bi-pin connectors. The bi-pins of T5 and T8 fixtures are much smaller than bi-pins of T12 fluorescent fixtures. If purchasing new tubes, make sure the bulb fits the fixture. The fixture may contain one, two, or more tubes.

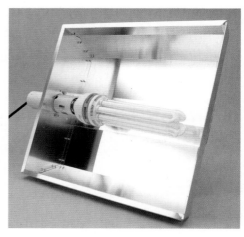

This CFL fixture is similar to a reflective hood for an HID bulb.

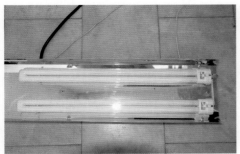

This CFL fixture holds two 55-watt bulbs. The design of the U-shaped bulbs makes reflecting light efficient.

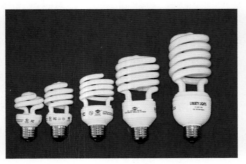

Many CFLs are designed to provide light in homes and offices. Most of these lamps are too small to be used for anything but growing clones and seedlings.

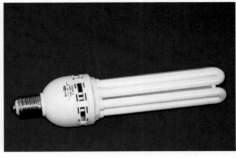

Large CFL lamps tend to throw light back through glass, losing efficiency. The 95-watt bulb is most efficient and can be placed close to plants because it runs relatively cool.

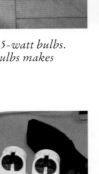

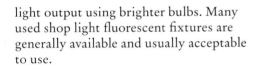

The T12 fixture on the left is larger than the T5 fixture on the right. (MF)

light output using brighter bulbs. Many used shop light fluorescent fixtures are generally available and usually acceptable to use.

If your fluorescent fixture does not work, first unplug the electricity. Next check all electrical connections to make sure they are secure. If you see any signs of burning or heat, take the fixture to the nearest electric store and ask for advice. Make sure they test each component and tell you why it should be replaced. It might be less expensive to buy another fixture.

Fluorescent Bulb Disposal
The US Environmental Protection Agency (EPA) and other similar agencies around the world classify fluorescent lamps as hazardous waste because bulbs contain mercury and ballasts contain other unpleasant stuff. They must be taken to a qualified facility for recycling or safe disposal of toxic waste.

Compact Fluorescent Lamps (CFL)
Most consumers know compact fluorescent lamps (CFL) as the new energy-efficient replacement for household incandescent lightbulbs, the ones that Thomas Edison invented. The characteristic helical spiral was developed in the mid-1970s for low wattage CFLs. By the 1980s CFLs with electronic ballasts were available. Other configurations—horseshoe, round and flat (butterfly) were later developed. For example, readily available 65-watt floodlights are configured flat so that light emitted is either direct or easily reflected. Larger wattages, 65+, can be used to grow medicinal cannabis from seed through flowering. Some of the smaller wattages fit into household incandescent lightbulb sockets. Larger 95-, 125-, 150-, and 200-watt bulbs require a larger mogul socket. Common wattages used for growing cannabis include 55, 60, 65, 85, 95, 120, 125, 150, and 200. Regardless of wattage, CFLs must warm up for about 5 minutes so the chemicals become stable before they come to full brightness.

CFL	WATTS	K TEMP.
Warm White	13	2700
Cool White	13	4100
Daylight	13	6400
GE	13	6500
Sylvania	14	3000
Bright Effects	15	2644

Compact fluorescent lamps are available in many spectrums, including Daylight, Cool White, and Warm White. Compact fluorescent lamps are perfect for gardeners with a limited budget and a small space. They run cooler than HIDs and require minimal ventilation. When CFLs were first introduced, wattages were too small, and bulbs did not emit enough light to grow cannabis. The new CFLs provide enough light to grow cannabis from seed to harvest. Beware of manufacturer and reseller websites making outrageous claims about CFL performance. Add up the actual lumens and watts to verify claims.

CFL lamps that work well for gardening are available in two basic styles and shapes:

1. Bulb shaped like a long "U" with a two- or four-pin fixture (these lamps are designated "1U"). The 20-inch (50.8 cm) long "1U" 55-watt, dual-pin-base bulbs are common in Europe. Normally, two 55-watt lamps are placed in a horizontal reflective hood.

2. The short lamps consist of several U-shaped tubes (designated 4U, 5U, 6U, etc., for the number of U-shaped tubes) that measure approximately 8 to 12 inches (20–30 cm) not including the 2- to 4-inch (5–10 cm) attached ballast and threaded base.

Short U-shaped bulbs are most efficient when vertically oriented. When mounted horizontally under a reflective hood, much light is reflected back and forth between the bulb's outer envelope and the hood, which markedly lowers efficiency. Heat also builds up from the ballast. Both conditions lessen efficiency.

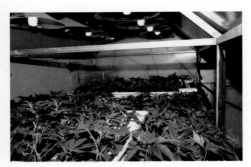

This clone garden is illuminated exclusively with small, spiral-shaped energy-saving compact fluorescents lamps.

Two Types of CFL Sockets:

The first type of CFL socket is a bi-pin tube that is designed for conventional ballasts. A bi-pin tube contains an integrated starter that averts the need for external heating pins but causes incompatibility with electronic ballasts.

The second type of CFL socket is a quad-pin tube designed for electronic ballasts or conventional ballasts with an external starter.

CFLs emit light from a mix of phosphors inside the bulb, each emitting one band of color. Modern phosphor designs balance the emitted light color, energy efficiency, and cost. Every extra phosphor added to the coating mix decreases efficiency and increases cost. Good-quality consumer CFLs use 3 or 4 phosphors to achieve a white light with a color rendering index (CRI) of about 80. Running a compact fluorescent lamp base-up will result in hotter electronics and a shorter bulb life. Standard CFLs do not respond well to dimming. They are either on or off.

Normally, CFL bulbs have a life of 10,000 to 20,000 hours (18 to 36 months at 18 hours per day). Lamps with attached ballast burn out 3 to 6 times faster than the ballast.

CFL Ballasts

The most important technical advance has been the replacement of analog (electromagnetic) ballasts with electronic ballasts—starting is much faster and flickering is almost gone. CFLs that flicker when they start have magnetic ballasts.

Integrated CFL lamps combine a bulb, electronic ballast, and a household light-bulb threaded connection or bayonet fitting into a single unit. When the lamp's life is over, the lamp and the attached ballast are both thrown away, which means you are throwing away a perfectly good ballast. My preference is to use the long CFLs that are not attached to ballasts.

Nonintegrated CFLs have remote electronic ballasts permanently installed in the light fixture and are not part of the bulb. The bulb is changed at its end of life. Nonintegrated, CFL fixture-mounted ballasts are larger and last longer in comparison to the integrated ones.

The normal life of a CFL ballast is 50,000 to 60,000 hours (7 to 9 years at 18 hours per day). The end of ballast life is signaled when it stops. When the ballast burns out, remove and replace it. Dispose of the ballast in a hazardous waste dump.

End of Life

The lifetime of any lamp depends on operating voltage, manufacturing defects, exposure to voltage spikes, mechanical shock, frequency of cycling on and off, lamp orientation, and ambient operating temperature, among other

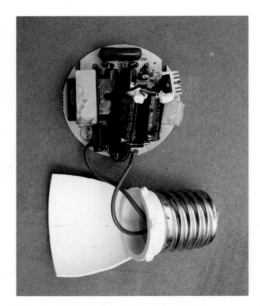

The attached encased ballast for this large CFL lamp has been broken away from the base. The integrated ballast is thrown out along with the burned out bulb.

factors. The life of a CFL is significantly shorter if it is frequently turned on and off. In the case of a 5-minute on/off cycle the lifespan of a CFL can be cut in half. Leave them on for hours. At the end of life, CFLs produce 70 to 80 percent of original light output. Replace lamps when they are at 80 to 90 percent brilliance, after 12 months of operation.

CFL Bulb and Ballast Disposal

New CFLs contain half as much mercury as old bulbs. Compact fluorescent bulbs, old or new, must be disposed of properly. Place them in a sealed plastic bag and dispose the same way you should dispose of batteries, oil-based paint, and motor oil: at your local household hazardous waste (HHW) collection site or other authorized disposal site for hazardous materials.

When buying replacement bulbs, look for deals on CFLs at Home Depot and similar discount stores, or check the Internet. For example, www.lightsite.net is an outstanding site that also has a retail store locator. Philips is producing some of the higher wattage compact fluorescent lamps. Their PL-H compact fluorescent lamp is a 4U bulb available in 60, 85, and 120 watts with Kelvin ratings from 3000 to 4100.

Plasma Lamps

Plasma lamps fall into two categories: (1) internal or light-emitting plasma (LEP) lamps, which use radio waves to energize sulfur or metal halides in a bulb, and (2) external or induction lamps, which use fluorescent induction, including a tube filled with fluorescent phosphors.

The light-emitting plasma lamp is the original and most widely used form of (internal) induction lamp. Radio frequency is used to excite gases inside a small ceramic envelope and produce a very bright light. The small lamps are about the size of a small camera storage chip.

The external inductor (plasma) lamps consist of round or rectangular tubes similar in diameter to T12 fluorescent tubes. The electromagnetic induction (plasma) lights are efficient and deliver 81 lumens per watt.

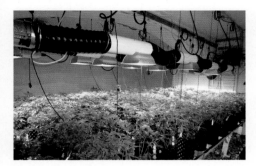

Plasma lamps produce UVA and UVB light. They have a radio frequency generator rather than a ballast.

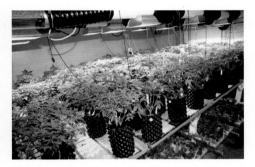

The Gavita-Holland Pro 300 (watt) LEP lamp and fixture is the only commercially available luminaire developed for indoor gardeners. With a CRI of 94, the 5600 K color temperature (spectrum) is like natural sunlight. The lamp runs cool—so cool you can put your hand on the protective glass without burning it. Not possible with an HID fixture!

Light-Emitting Plasma (LEP) Lamps

Today's light-emitting plasma (LEP) grow lights are much different than the plasma lamps popular in the 1980s. Invented by Nikola Tesla in the 1890s, the first promising plasma lamps were sulfur lamps developed by Fusion Lighting. The lamps had technical difficulties, and they were too bright and had a poor spectrum for plant growth. Today several companies are overcoming the technical problems and making the spectrum conducive to plant growth. Several high-efficiency plasma (HEP) lamps have been introduced to the market; these lamps, including models from Ceravision and Luxim, achieve 140 lumens per watt. Commercially available LEP lamps come in wattages from 40 to 300. Plasma International also manufactures a 730-watt microwave-driven sulfur plasma lamp. Gavita-Holland is the only known horticultural lighting company applying plasma lamp technology in the garden.

The plasma lamp family generates light by exciting plasma inside a bulb using radio frequency (RF) power. The small lamp is less than an inch (2.5 cm) square, and is embedded in a ceramic resonator. An RF driver, solid-state amplifier, and microcontroller are in a fully sealed lamp without electrodes and filaments.

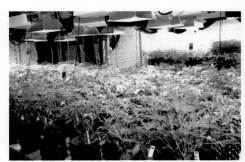

A combination of plasma (5500 K) and high-pressure sodium (2100 K) lamps in a ratio of 1:4 provides the best spectrum for rapid growth. Plasma light combined with HPS light produces more branches, increases dry matter weight up to 30 percent, and improves overall plant structure. Stronger plants are more resistant to disease and pest attacks. The extra plasma light may also promote earlier and more prolific development of resin glands. Some gardeners report that resin glands tend to develop a few days earlier and continue to form at a more rapid rate when plasma lighting is used.

Lamps use a noble gas or a mixture of these gases and metal halides, sodium, mercury, or sulfur.

The plasma lamp does not have a ballast, but rather an RF generator (aka magnetron) and semiconductors that fulfill the equivalent function. It has more than 90 percent conversion efficiency, and the solid-state driver eliminates failure. And there is no noise.

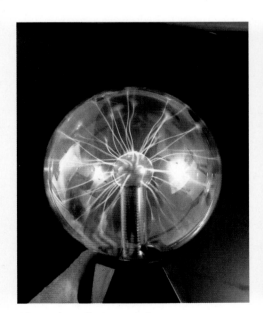

Plasma lamp from a novelty store

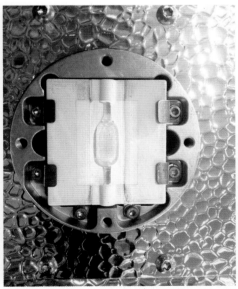

LEP bulbs are small and very bright.

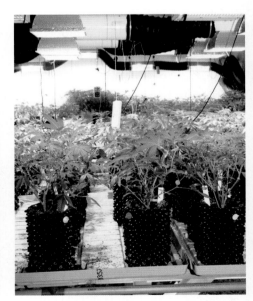

Light-emitting plasma lamps are the only light source for these mother plants. LEP lamps also emit UVA and UVB light. Natural sunlight emits UV light; HID bulbs do not. Among other things, this light is responsible for making plant cells more resilient.

LAMP	460-WATT HPS	280-WATT LEP	BENEFIT
bulb lumens	50,000	23,000	none
fixture efficiency	65%	85%	directional source
fixture lumens	32,500	19,465	directional source
light-loss factor	75%	80%	low lumen degradation
mean lumens	24,375	15,572	low lumen degradation
application efficiency	48%	82%	optical control

Light-emitting plasma is the only high-intensity light source that can be dimmed down to 20 percent of light output, with both analog and digital controls. Dimming even increases longevity of the lamp. The cost is about $1000 USD for a 300-watt LEP lamp.

Solid-state LEP lamps use electricity to energize metal halides, and argon rather than sulfur. These lamps have no electrodes and no associated failures. Overall, plasma lamps have a long life—up to 50,000 hours (7.7 years at 18 hours per day)—and are rated for 70 percent lumen maintenance. LEP-lamp efficacy ranges from 115 to 150 lumens per watt.

The directional nature of the light source means that no light is lost, trapped between the light and the reflector, and allows for the light to be spread evenly over the grow area with no overspill. The annual energy and maintenance costs are up to 45 percent less than for MH bulbs.

A solid-state electronic ballast with no moving parts is located in a sealed housing with a Gore-Tex ventilation plug. A square light pattern reflector with a UVC glass filter directs light at the garden. The Gavita lamp will last 30,000 hours (4.5 years at 18 hours per day).

Low levels of UVB light pass through a shield and UVC light is filtered out. UVB light is produced by natural sunlight and is essential for healthy plant growth. The overall light spectrum contains more blue light too. See "UV Light" on page 256.

Do not try to air-cool plasma lamps. When artificially cooled, the bulb is unable to reach full operating temperature and does not come to full brilliance or spectrum.

Magnetic Induction Lamps

Magnetic induction lamps are similar to fluorescent lamps, but the electromagnets are wrapped around a section of the lamp tube. High-frequency energy emitted by an induction coil produces a very strong magnetic field and excites the mercury atoms inside the glass tube. The mercury atoms emit UV light that

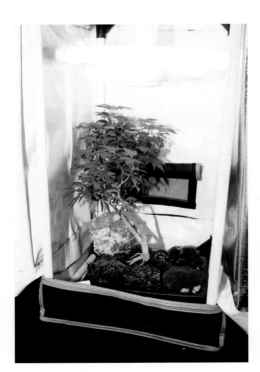

Magnetic induction lamps are considered plasma lamps, but they look more like circular T9 fluorescent fixtures.

is down-converted to visible light by the phosphor coating on the inside of the tube. The lamps contain no electrodes, and failures caused by filament erosion, vibration, or seal breach are impossible. With no electrodes to degrade, the lamps are very efficient and enjoy a longer life.

Round or rectangular 300-watt magnetic induction bulbs have a daylight color temperature of 5000 K and produce 24,500 lumens, 81 lumens per watt, and have a life of 100,000 hours. A 300-watt induction lamp system costs about $300 USD. They come with attached or remote ballast. The 300-watt induction lamp is touted to be a replacement for 600-watt HID lamps. Small, 80-watt circular induction lamps with remote ballasts produce 6000 lumens of light with a color temperature (spectrum) of 5000 K. They have a life of 100,000 hours.

Magnetic induction lamps generate little heat, and ballasts have a life of 40,000 hours or longer.

Different color temperatures are possible by changing the composition of the phosphorous inside induction lamps. Plasma spectrums contain relatively little red light. At least one company has developed a bispectrum grow light to produce one half of the bulb at 2700 K and the other half at the other end of the spectrum.

Light-Emitting Diode (LED) Lamps
About LEDs
Light-emitting diode lamps are everywhere. You see them in stoplights,

LAMP	WATTS	LUMENS	KELVIN COLOR TEMPERATURE	HOURS OF LIFE
induction	300	24,500	5000	100,000
induction	80	6000	5000	100,000

flashlights, Christmas tree lighting, household lighting, and more. The technology has come a long way since it was developed in the early 1960s, when LEDs were found in appliances and generated a faint 0.001 lumens per watt. New LED technology is advancing rapidly and they are becoming much brighter and more electrically efficient. Light-emitting diode lamps are available across the visible spectrum, and from ultraviolet through infrared. Gardeners are successfully using LEDs to cultivate medical cannabis.

Light-emitting diode lamps can be used for pre-grow and propagation in horticulture, as well as some experiments with interlighting indoors and in greenhouses. At press time, LEDs are not an economically viable replacement for HID lamps in greenhouses or indoors. However, the horticultural industry

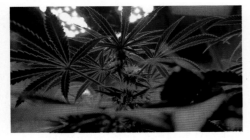

Purple LED light reflects off cannabis foliage, causing plants to look purple.

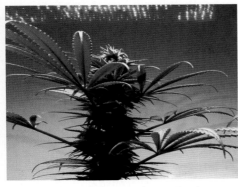

You can see the different color LEDs that make up the color spectrum.

has a very big interest in LEDs, and I suggest watching for bona fide advances in fast-changing LED technology.

There are so many new and different LED types and so much sales information about them, that it is difficult to understand which specific LEDs work best as a light source to grow medical cannabis.

Light-emitting diode lamps use solid-state semiconductor energy to produce light. The technology is similar to that found in computer circuitry. LEDs do not use filaments found in incandescent and tungsten halogen bulbs, or gas used in HID, fluorescent, and compact fluorescent bulbs. LEDs generate less heat, and are rated for regular household current—120 V and 240 V. LEDs work in both 120 V and 240 V, 50 to 60 cycle electrical service. For this reason, LED fixtures often come with no plug.

Light output from LEDs continues to increase with improved materials and technological advances while maintaining the efficiency and reliability of solid state. Solid-state components are difficult to damage with external shock.

LED lamps are a promising replacement for HPS lamps because of their high-efficiency (up to 54 percent), very long life (they still produce at least 70 percent of their original output after 50,000 hours), small size, and low operating voltage.

Outdated LEDs that produce less than 1 watt are not as bright as new 1-, 2-, and 3-watt LEDs. Also, some LEDs of the same wattage are brighter than others. See "Brilliance" on page 284.

Rather than a ballast, a series of resistors or current-regulated power supplies is necessary to deliver precise voltage and current for LEDs to operate most effi-

ciently. The power supply can be decreased to dim lights. Some LEDs have a dimming range of 20 to 100 percent. The necessary hardware is hardwired and soldered into a small (circuit board) fixture that is connected to a power supply. When purchasing a fixture, individual clusters of LEDs that can be replaced within fixtures are the most practical and economical.

Other types of lights are constant voltage—that is, they require a certain voltage to work, and they are usually fairly tolerant of slight variations in working voltage. For example, a normal incandescent bulb designed for European 230 volts of alternating current (VAC) will work fine from about 40 VAC to 270 VAC. LEDs are constant-current devices and require that voltage be controlled to maintain an exact current flow through the LED. Unlike other light sources, LEDs are nonlinear devices, which means that a small increase in voltage causes a large increase in current flow through the LED. This means LEDs have to be driven by special power supplies known as constant-current power supplies. They adjust their output voltage to maintain the current through the LEDs at a constant, preset level.

LEDs are often connected in series or string. LEDs are also unique; if they fail there is about an 80 percent chance that they will still conduct electricity (aka "slag down") rather than "blow" like an incandescent bulb and no longer conduct electricity. This causes the voltage to the remaining LEDs to increase. The current can increase to the point of causing more LEDs to fail, or even cause a chain reaction that can destroy all the LEDs in the string. A constant-current power supply will detect the increase in current and lower its output voltage to compensate—and protect the remaining LEDs.

Another option is to use a less expensive constant-voltage power supply; the output is constantly adjusted to provide an exact voltage no matter what load it is driving. These are usually 24 volts of direct current (VDC), 36 VDC, or 48 VDC. If this type of power supply is used, the circuit boards on which the LEDs are mounted need to have a small current-regulator chip mounted

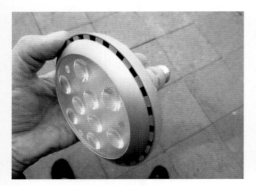

This floodlight has multiple LEDs inside, and screws into a household light socket.

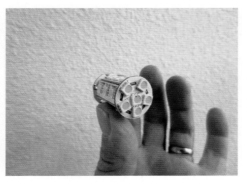

Weird-looking LEDs that resemble a bundle of chips emit more heat than light.

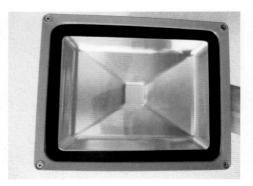

This small, yellow, 30-watt LED emitter produces 2700 lumens and a lot of heat.

on them. Some manufacturers do not use the regulator chips; instead they use resistors to adjust the voltage (and therefore the current flow) through the LEDs. This is not recommended because the voltage requirements of the LEDs vary depending on age and temperature, and can lead to all the LEDs receiving too high a voltage and then failing.

When you turn on an LED, electrons recombine with electron holes in the LED and release photons (light energy) in the process of electroluminescence. Peak performance depends on operating temperature. To date, the most efficient LED is 1 watt. Larger wattages run hotter and are less efficient, producing fewer lumens per watt. For example, a 3-watt LED produces only 35 percent more lumens than a 1-watt LED. The extra electrical energy is converted to heat rather than light.

If ambient temperatures in the operating environment climb too high, LEDs overheat and "droop," producing sub-

stantially less light. Similar to solid-state computer chips, LEDs fail sooner when overheated over time.

LEDs are driven in milliamperes (mA). Some LEDs are driven at lower mA to increase efficiency. The science and data behind all the circuitry is more complex than can be explained within the scope of this book. The best way for medical cannabis gardeners to discern the brilliance of an LED or a fixture full of LEDs is to measure light output with a light meter.

Overall, most indoor gardeners can decipher LED output with the following equation: amperes × voltage = watts

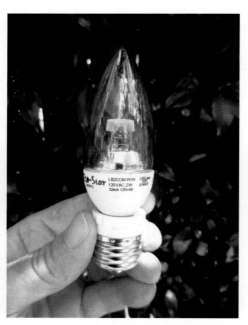

A 2-watt LED is bright, but the bulb needs a reflector.

(Ohm's Law). Otherwise, light output can become quite complicated and confusing. For example, a 3-watt LED that runs at 350 mA yields 1-watt of light.

Small LEDs heat up quickly and lose efficiency; that is, light energy is converted to heat beyond a specific operating temperature. The operating temperature is a function of electric current (mA) input.

The optimal temperature for each color of LED ensures an accurate rendering of color spectrum. At maximum temperature or too high of a temperature the LED will fail. That is, if too much current is run through the little LEDs they get too hot, become inefficient (light energy is transformed into heat), and they fail (burn out).

Humidity is detrimental to circuits. LED circuitry is exposed and must be protected from humidity to avoid corrosion. The LEDs must be enclosed to isolate them from exterior humidity.

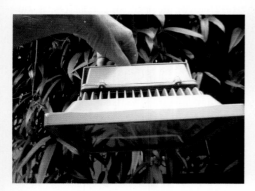

This 30-watt LED fixture uses standard heat-dissipation technology to stay cool. Excessive heat quickly lowers lumen output and efficiency.

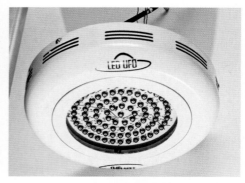

The LED UFO was one of the first LED grow lights available commercially.

LED Manufacture and Binning

Producing LEDs requires growing a thin layer of crystal on a substrate (supporting layer) of synthetic sapphire or silicon carbide. The process must be very tightly controlled across a range of factors; in fact, much of the steady increase in LED efficiency/brightness comes from improved quality control in manufacturing, rather than advances in technology. Other efficiency increases have come from modifying the structure of the LED layer to help photons that get created but then are trapped within the structure of the LED layer. This happens because the materials in LEDs have a very high refractive index, which causes any photons that strike the surface of the LED chip at much of an angle to be reflected back into the chip and lost.

After the wafer is coated, it is cut into thousands of tiny chips. It is difficult to control the manufacturing process, so each of these tiny chips will have slightly different properties. That is, the voltage requirement, wavelength, and brightness will all be slightly different for each chip! The distribution of the brightness, wavelength, and voltage qualities of the chips from each batch follows a standard bell curve.

These chips are then individually tested by machine and sorted into "bins" according to their properties. Understanding "binning," (and that all LEDs are not created equal) is super important, especially if you plan to build your own light fixture. For example, the brightness of the same make and model of LED can vary up to 100 percent, depending on the bin designation, and the voltage required can also vary by up to 50 percent. This means that the LEDs from best voltage/brightness bin put out twice the light for two thirds the power of LEDs from the worst bin. All quality LED manufacturers have the bin codes listed on their website.

LEDs are constantly improving in brightness and efficiency, but unlike the ever-increasing speeds of computer CPUs, these improvements will slow and eventually stop. This is because unlike computer CPUs, which can essentially get faster forever, LEDs will eventually reach very close to 100 percent efficiency; experts believe they will reach a maximum of about 90 percent. To achieve this percentage, chips must be individually tested by machine and sorted into bins according to their properties.

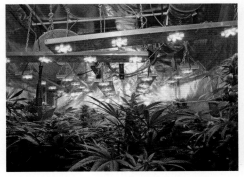

All high-quality LEDs in these EVO LED 70 fixtures are made by Cree. Each 70 cm fixture contains four groups of LEDs. Each group of 9 LEDs provides 15 watts, for a total of 60 watts.

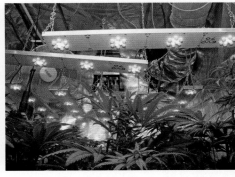

This photo was taken a few minutes after the previous one. Toni (see chapter 13, Case Study #2), the photographer, changed the light setting on his camera to show a different spectrum of light.

Cost

An inexpensive 30- to 50-watt LED fixture with emitter costs $0.65 to $0.70 USD per watt. HIDs cost less than $0.50 USD per watt. A 90-watt LED grow light costs about $300 USD when purchased at a garden store or from a specialty retailer. However, three 30-watt LED floodlight fixtures cost $66 USD when purchased at a discount retailer. Remember, all LEDs are not created equal.

LEDs have historically been more expensive than most other light sources due to complex manufacturing process, high rejection rate, the cost of both the material in the LED chip and the substrate the chip was based on—expensive synthetic sapphire. Improved manufacturing processes has reduced the reject rate, thin film technology has reduced the amount of material required to make the emitter, and many LEDs are now being made on low-cost SiC (silicon carbide) substrates. The efficiency and consequent brightness of the LEDs has also improved dramatically. Top-quality LEDs can now achieve over 50 percent efficiency. Now fewer LEDs are required to achieve the same brightness in a light, further lowering their cost.

There is a huge variation in the cost and quality of LEDs. High-quality, high-brightness LEDs from top manufacturers such as Cree, Osram, and Philips can cost 10 or 20 times as much as low-quality Chinese LEDs, and there is a large market in counterfeit LEDs.

LEDs and Heat

All electrical devices create heat, and LEDs are no exception. One of the difficulties of creating the first high-power light-emitting diode was to keep the chip from melting! All the energy consumed by an LED is converted into either light or heat. The more efficient the LED, the greater the amount of light produced and the smaller the amount of heat. For example, a high-quality blue or white LED that consumes roughly 2.4 watts, and converts 50 percent of its input into light, produces about 1.2 watts of heat. That may not sound like much heat. But the LED is concentrated into a super thin chip (1 mm × 1 mm). If the chip were 30 mm × 30 mm it would generate over 1000 watts of heat! A low-quality LED that converts only 20 percent of the electricity to light generates about 1.92 watts of heat.

The heat must be removed or the chip will overheat and fail. The cooler the LED stays, the more efficiently it will operate (produce more light) and the longer it will last. The emitter (LED chip) on high-end LEDs is mounted on a base made of a special heat-conductive ceramic. Less expensive LEDs use a small piece of metal known as a "slug."

Next the LED is soldered to a special circuit board that is designed to transfer heat. The metal core printed circuit board (MCPCB) is made from a layer of aluminum covered with a thin layer of a material that conducts heat well but does not conduct electricity. This is the dielectric layer. The higher the thermal conductivity (measured in watts per kelvin [W/K]), the better. Inexpensive boards have a conductivity of about 0.5 W/K, better quality boards have a rating of 1 W/K, and the highest quality boards have a rating of 2.2 W/K. A bit of copper is placed on top of the dielectric layer to conduct electricity and provide solder pads for mounting the LEDs and a protective layer. These circuit boards are often mounted to a heat sink that could have a cooling fan.

Some lights have the LEDs mounted on conventional plastic circuit boards to save money. These plastic boards do no conduct heat well and will cause the LEDs to overheat and fail very quickly.

LED Power Ratings

Much confusion surrounds LED power ratings. LEDs are rated in watts. However, this rating is *not* the actual power consumption of LEDs in watts. The wattage rating of LEDs (1, 3, 5, 10 watts, etc.) is actually a *class* or *family* rating, and bears no real relationship to the actual power consumed by the LED.

1-watt LEDs operate at 350 mA
3-watt LEDs operate at 700 mA
5-watt LEDs operate at 1000 mA
10-watt LEDs operate at 1500 mA

Note: Larger LEDs require higher ,voltages and are less efficient.

The "wattage classes" were set to standardize power supplies, and so that LEDs from different manufacturers could be combined within the same fixture. The standards were intended for white and blue LEDs only. The name of each rating (class) was fairly accurate—a 3-watt LED did consume about 3 watts. But the efficiency of LEDs has increased dramatically, and the voltage required to drive the LED to 700 mA has dropped. Today the average 3-watt white or blue LED consumes about 2.4 watts. Different colors of LEDs of the same class

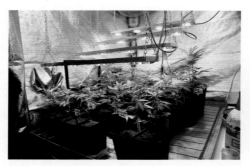

Keep LEDs as close as possible to plants, because light diminishes to the square of the distance. Regardless of the benefits of LEDs— many point sources and dialed-in light frequencies—light is light, and all natural laws remain in force.

consume different amounts of power, because different colors use different materials and require different voltages.

Wattage is calculated by Ohm's Law. The formula is:
watts = volts × amperes (W = V × A)

Here is a breakdown of the actual power drawn by 3-watt-class LEDs of several different colors.

Red/hyper red—2.4 volts, actual wattage at 700 mA is 2.4 volts × 0.7 watts = 1.68 watts
Blue/royal blue/white—3.4 volts, actual wattage at 700 mA is 3.4 volts × 0.7 watts = 2.38 watts

Brilliance

When LEDs are "ganged," or grouped together, they can produce enough light to grow medical cannabis. An LED fixture must be 12 inches (30.5 cm) or less from plants to be an effective light source for cannabis cultivation.

Depending upon manufacturer, modern LEDs produce from 40 to 70 lumens per watt (lm/W). New and experimental LEDs produce more than 200 lm/W. As of 2014, Cree Incorporated markets an LED that produces 152 lm/W. But, you will see below that lumens per watt are just part of the story.

The brightness of LEDs is rated in two different ways, depending on their wavelengths. LEDs between 640 nm and 460 nm are rated in lumens. LEDs with wavelengths longer than 640 nm or shorter than 460 nm are rated by

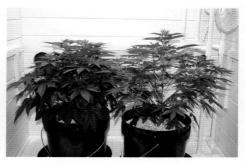

LEDs can be configured in many different color combinations. This photo shows less-intense purple light, causing lower leaves to display green.

their radiant power (radiant flux) in mW (milliwatts).

Lumens are not a good measurement system for measuring the output of LEDs. It is not a linear system, meaning that it does not measure all wavelengths/colors equally. It was developed as a measurement for visible light and measures apparent brightness—how bright a light appears to the human eye. Lumens were developed to rate white light sources rather than to measure monochromatic LED light sources. Furthermore, human eye response to light is extremely uneven. Colors in the center of the visible spectrum such as green appear much brighter than an equally bright light or red or blue.

Lumens can be used only to compare (LED) light sources with the exact same wavelength. This explains why some LEDs with wavelengths of 660 nm hyper, near the extremes of human vision, are often rated as "dominant wavelength 640 nm."

Spectrum

Note: The spectrum of each LED may also dictate brilliance and light output.

LEDs are monochromatic, unlike common CFLs, fluorescents, etc. LEDs produce a single color over a narrow range of wavelengths. White LEDs are actually blue, or sometimes ultraviolet. Some LEDs have a phosphor coating (aka downshift phosphor), which absorbs the blue light and re-emits it at longer wavelengths. The phosphor coating contains a mix of different phosphors,

MOST LED GROW LIGHTS CONSIST OF LEDS WITH THE FOLLOWING WAVELENGTHS:	
hyper red	660 nm
red	630 nm
blue	470 nm
royal blue	450 nm

THEY MAY ALSO INCLUDE SOME OF THE FOLLOWING:	
far red	740 nm
orange (amber)	617 nm
yellow	590 nm
green	530 nm
UV (technically near UV)	390 nm

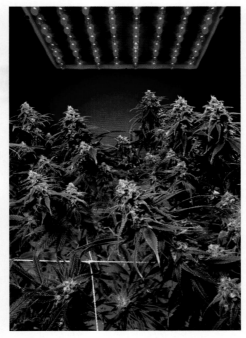

LEDs can be arranged in rows, clusters, and circles. Note the combination of red and blue light in this LED fixture.

each of which emits a different color, which combine to create white light. The proper mix of colors causes different temperatures, and that creates white light. More red and less blue creates a warmer white. More blue and less red yields a cooler white.

Note: The human eye perceives cooler whites as brighter than warmer whites. This is why they have higher lumen ratings even though they may not actually produce more photons.

White light is categorized by its color temperature. This is the temperature of a "black body" (an object that does not reflect any light) that has been heated until the light it gives off matches the hue of the white light source. The color temperature of the white light is equal to the temperature in kelvins of the surface of the glowing black body.

LED grow lights take advantage of the availability of LEDs of different wavelengths to make lamps that only create light at the wavelengths the plant can use most efficiently. In other words, the wavelengths match the plants' photosynthetic absorption peaks.

LED technology allows manufacturers to literally dial in the spectrum of fixtures to produce incredibly high PAR ratings. This point alone makes them more efficient per watt.

LED Bulbs and Tubes
A vast array of retrofit LEDs can be packed into a larger bulb that fits in a household incandescent screw fitting. Such bulbs cost from $15 to $30 USD and are generally not bright enough to grow plants well. They are rated in replacement terms for an incandescent bulb. For example, a 15.5-watt LED bulb replaces a 75-watt incandescent.

LED tubes are shaped like regular T12, T8, and T5 fluorescent bulbs, but the

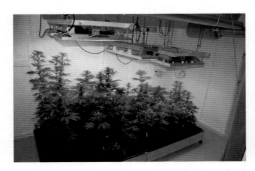

LEDs emit the characteristic purple glow that turns all the photographs purple!

tubes are filled with LEDs. More than 200 LEDs will fit in a 4-foot (121.9 cm) T12 tube. But not all LEDs are created equal. LED tubes are filled with little LEDs. An energy-efficient 22-watt 4-foot T8 LED tube produces 1248 lumens. They do not fit in existing T8 fluorescent fixtures. The flicker-free tubes have a lifetime of more than 50,000 hours.

T8 red tubes are 660 nm and contain 288 LED bulbs. Spectrums can also be split into blue and white with a 50/50 split between LEDs of 420 nm/5500 K that contain 144 red and 144 white LEDs. Some fixtures allow LED tubes to be mixed with T8 fluorescent tubes to improve spectrum. The tubes run cool and can be placed within inches of plants.

LED Fixtures
Usually, different LEDs are combined in a fixture to achieve a specific light spectrum. A series of individual LEDs can be mounted and hardwired into a single fixture that is square, rectangular, or circular. Or the fixture can contain long T12 and T8 glass tubes loaded with LEDs.

The most practical fixtures allow individual clusters of LEDs packed in a bulb to be easily replaced. Such fixtures also make upgrading to LEDs inexpensive.

LED vs. HID Lamps
We can easily compare LED and HID wattage, lumen output, and lm/W output. But comparing milliwatts per square meter (mW/m²) and PAR watts are the true measures of the light plants need for photosynthesis. Comparing PAR watts makes the best comparison. However, LEDs have several qualities

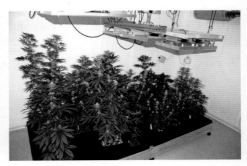

Plants show their natural green color when the LEDs are turned off.

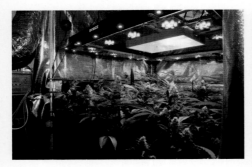

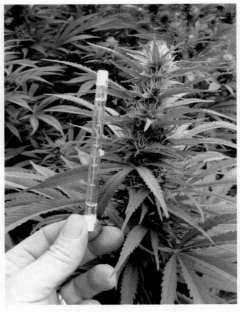

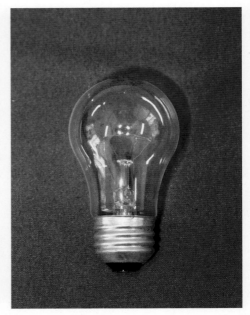

Combining HP sodium lamps with LEDs makes a winning combination for flowering.

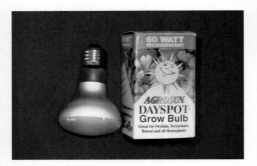

Incandescent "grow lights" are inefficient and inadequate to grow medicinal cannabis. These lamps direct heat and light with an interior reflector.

Tungsten halogen (aka quartz iodine) lamps are incandescent lamps with a little bit of a halogen, (often iodine or bromine) added to the envelope. Tungsten halogen lamps retain clarity and are operated at very high temperatures. These lamps are inefficient in terms of lumens-per-watt conversion, and produce too much heat to be practical garden lights.

Incandescent lamps are inefficient. They produce light by heating a filament wire with electricity until it glows and produces light. The filament is enclosed in a glass bulb filled with inert gas. This antiquated, inefficient technology was popularized by Thomas Edison.

that HIDs don't have. LEDs produce very little heat and can be placed closer to the canopy of the garden, which inherently provides plants with more bright light.* LED light is also able to be focused and directed through a lens, which intensifies the light. This factor can be compared when we look at overall fixture brilliance only.

There are also a few spectrum details that must be addressed. LED fixtures can contain a few to hundreds of LEDs. The LEDs can be of many different spectrums. Fixtures are manufactured to include LEDs of different spectrums to provide the highest ratings for plant growth. However, I have had a difficult time finding accurate brilliance tests for LED fixtures.

*See the "Inverse Square Law" on page 259, earlier in this chapter.

End of Life
LEDs have a life from 25,000 to 50,000 hours, and sometimes longer. They fail by dimming over time. LEDs are so new to gardeners that there is no specific information about when to replace them.

Many LEDs with a range of spectrums are packed together in fixtures. A single LED that fails or is not as bright as others may not affect the overall output of the fixture enough to warrant replacing. Overall, I can recommend replacing a fixture when it yields 85 to 95 percent light output.

Do not worry about tossing out hazardous substances when disposing of LEDs.

They contain no mercury to pollute the environment. LEDs and fixtures can be recycled.

Other Lamps
Several other lamps deserve a short mention, primarily so that they will not be used. Cannabis grows poorly under these lamps. These lamps produce more heat than light, and in a spectrum that is not compatible with plant growth.

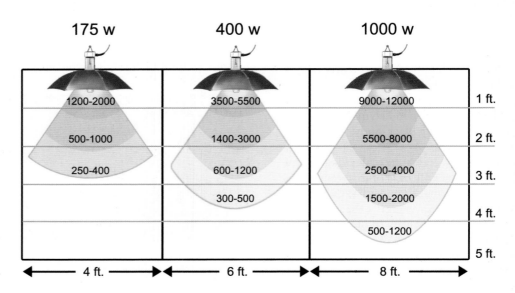

Getting the Most Artificial Light

A 175-watt HID yields enough light to effectively grow a 2 × 2-foot (61 × 61 cm) garden. Notice how fast light intensity diminishes more than a foot from the bulb.

A 250-watt HID will illuminate up to a 3 × 3-foot (91.4 × 91.4 cm) area. Keep the bulb from 12 to 18 inches (30.5–45.7 cm) above plants.

A 400-watt HID delivers plenty of light to effectively illuminate a 4 × 4-foot (1.2 × 1.2 m) area. Hang the lamp from 12 to 24 inches (30–61 cm) above the canopy of the garden.

A 600-watt HP delivers enough light to effectively illuminate a 4 × 4-foot (120 × 120 cm) area. Hang the lamp from 18 to 24 inches (30.5–60 cm) above plants.

A 1000-watt HID delivers enough light to effectively illuminate a 6 × 6-foot (1.8 × 1.8 m) area. Some reflective hoods are designed to throw light over a rectangular area. Large 1000-watt HIDs can burn foliage if located closer than 24 inches (61 cm) from plants. Move HIDs closer to plants when using a light mover.

Lamp Spacing

Light intensity almost doubles every 6 inches (15.2 cm) closer an HID is to the canopy of a garden. When PAR light intensity is low, plants stretch for it. Low light intensity is often caused by the lamp being too far away from plants. Dim light causes sparse foliage and spindly branches that are prone to disease and pest attacks.

1000 watt: lm/W = 140

1 foot (30.5 cm) away 140,000 lumens

2 feet (61 cm) away 35,000 lumens

3 feet (91.4 cm) away 15,555 lumens

4 feet (121.9 cm) away 9999 lumens

1000-watt HP sodium @ 4 feet = 10,000 lumens

4 × 4 = 16 square feet, 1000 watts/16 square feet = 62.5 watts per square foot

$1000 \ W/m^2 = 100 \ W/cm^2$

600 watt: lm/W = 150

1 foot (30.5 cm) away 90,000 lumens

2 feet (61 cm) away 22,500 lumens

3 feet (91.4 cm) away 9,999 lumens

4 feet (121.9 cm) away 6428 lumens

600-watt HP sodium @ 3 feet = 10,000 lumens

3 × 3 = 9 square feet, 600 watts/9 square feet = 66 watts per square foot

$600 \ W/m^2 = 6 \ w/cm^2$

400 watt: lm/W = 125

1 foot (30.5 cm) away 50,000 lumens

2 feet (61 cm) away 12,500 lumens

3 feet (91.4 cm) away 5555 lumens

4 feet (121.9 cm) away 3571 lumens

400-watt HP sodium @ 2.25 feet = 10,000 lumens

2.25 × 2.25 = 5 square feet, 400 watts/5 square feet = 80 watts per square foot

$400 \ W/m^2 = 4 \ w/cm^2$

400 watt: lm/W = 100

1 foot (30.5 cm) away 40,000 lumens

2 feet (61 cm) away 10,000 lumens

3 feet (91.4 cm) away 4444 lumens

4 feet (121.9 cm) away 2857 lumens

400-watt metal halide @ 2 feet = 10,000 lumens

2 × 2 = 4 square feet, 400 watts/4 = 100 watts per square feet

$400 \ W/m^2 = 4 \ w/cm^2$

Increase yield by giving gardening area uniform light distribution. Uneven light distribution causes strong branch tips to grow toward the intense light. Foliage in dimly lit areas is shaded when light distribution is uneven.

Reflective hoods ultimately dictate lamp placement—distance between lamps and above the plants. Nearly all stationary lamps have bright (hot) spots that plants grow toward.

Gardeners prefer high wattage lamps—400, 600, 1000, or 1100 watts—because they produce more lumens per watt and their PAR rating is higher than lower-wattage bulbs. Plants receive more light when the lamp is closer to the plants. Even though 400-watt lamps produce fewer lumens per watt than a 1000-watt bulb, when properly set up they actually deliver more usable light to plants. The 600-watt bulb has the highest lumens-per-watt conversion (150 lm/W), and can be placed closer to the canopy of the garden than the 1000- or 1100-watt bulbs—without burning foliage.

For example, the lumens-per-watt conversion is lower with 400-watt bulbs than with 1000-watt bulbs, but hanging five 400-watt lamps over the same area that two 1000-watt lamps cover provides more even distribution of light, and minimizes shading. The lamps burn cooler and can be placed closer to plants. The 400-watt lamps also emit light from 5 points, where the higher wattage bulbs emit from 2. Overall, bright light coverage is increased with the 400-watt lamps even though their lumens-per-watt conversion is lower.

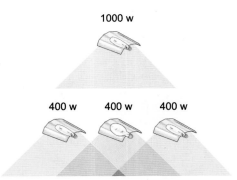

Three 400-watt bulbs (1200 watts) effectively cover up to 40 percent more growing area than one 1000-watt lamp. The lower-wattage bulbs are placed closer to plants, which increases light intensity.

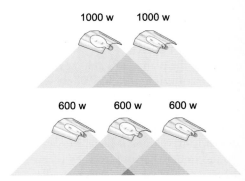

Three 600-watt bulbs (1800 watts) deliver more intense light to a garden than two 1000-watt lamps (2000 watts). Three points of light provided by the 600-watt bulbs distribute light better than when the light is generated by two lamps. The 600-watt lamps can also be placed closer to the garden canopy.

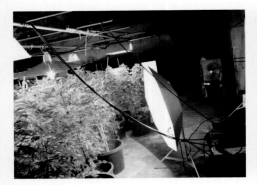

Side lighting in this room helps plants fill out all the way around. Most often, however, side lighting is much less efficient than overhead lighting.

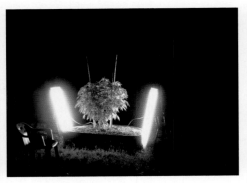

Two banks of fluorescent light illuminate this plant at night. The extra light keeps the plant from flowering in the spring. Such side lighting is impractical for most gardeners.

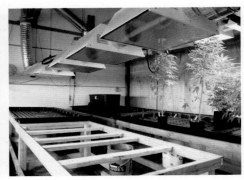

This table has wheels on the bottom and can be moved back and forth. There are three tables with wheels in this room. Tables are moved back and forth to create a walkway between them. Having only one walkway increases growing area and production.

Three 600-watt lamps that produce 270,000 lumens from three point sources, instead of two 1000-watt HPS lamps yielding 280,000 lumens from two points, decrease total light output by 10,000 lumens but increase the number of sources of light. Lamps can be placed closer to plants, increasing efficiency even more.

Side Lighting

Lighting from the side is generally not as efficient as lighting from above. Vertically oriented lamps without reflectors are efficient but require plants to be oriented around the bulb. To promote growth, light must penetrate the dense foliage of a garden. The lamps are mounted where light intensity is marginal––along the walls—to provide sidelight.

Compact fluorescent lamps are not a good choice for side lighting when using HID lamps. (See "Compact Fluorescent Lamps" on page 277.

Rotating Plants

Rotating the plants will help ensure even distribution of light. When possible, rotate plants every few days by moving them one-quarter to one-half turn. Rotating promotes even growth and fully-developed foliage. Move plants around under the lamp so they receive the most possible light. Move smaller plants toward the center, and taller plants toward the outside of the garden. Set small plants on a stand to even out the garden profile.

The longer that plants are in the flowering growth stage, the more light they need. During the first 3 to 4 weeks of flowering, plants process a little less light than during the last 3 to 4 weeks. Plants flowering during the last 3 to 4 weeks are placed directly under the bulb, where light is the brightest. Plants that have just entered the flowering room can stay on the perimeter until the more mature plants are moved out. This simple technique can easily increase harvests by 5 to 10 percent.

Add a shallow shelf around the perimeter of the garden to use light that is consumed by the walls. This sidelight is often very bright and very much wasted. Use brackets to put up a 4- to 6-inch-wide shelf around the perimeter of the garden. The shelf can be built on a slight angle and lined with plastic to form a runoff canal. Arrange small plants in 6-inch pots along the shelf. Rotate them so they develop evenly. These plants can

either flower on the short shelf or when moved under the light.

Installing rolling beds in greenhouses and garden rooms will remove all but one walkway from the garden. Greenhouse gardeners learned this space-saving technique long ago. Gardens with elevated beds often waste light on walkways. To make use of more gardening area, place two 2 inch (5 cm) pipes or wooden dowels below the gardening bed. The pipe allows the beds to be rolled back and forth, so only one walkway is open at a time. This simple technique usually increases gardening space by up to 25 percent.

Growing a perpetual crop and flowering only a portion of the garden allows for more plants in a smaller area and a higher overall yield. See chapter 4, *Cannabis Life Cycle*, for more information on "Perpetual Crops."

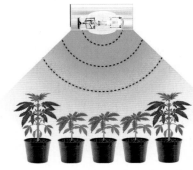

Containers on wheels rotate easily. Make sure wheels are large enough to support the weight of moisture-laden substrates.

Light intensity is brightest directly under the bulb. Arrange plants under lamps so they receive the same intensity of light. Plants can also be put up on a support to move them closer to the bulb and more intense light.

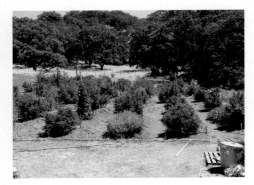

Outdoors, big plants that receive full sunlight all day long must be spaced much further apart, on 12-foot (3.7 m) centers to ensure adequate room for growth.

Plant Spacing

Outdoors and in greenhouses, medical cannabis gardeners must allow for rapid, robust growth. This requires extra space between plants. Greenhouse crops can be easily controlled with light-deprivation techniques. Outdoor plants that receive full sun and are able to grow for several months reach heights of more than 12 feet (3.7 m) and are 12 feet (3.7 m) in diameter. Proper planning requires that such seedlings and clones be planted on a minimum of 12-foot (3.7 m) centers to allow for adequate growth and ventilation. See chapter 12, *Outdoors,* and chapter 13, *Case Studies,* for more information.

When light shines on a garden, the leaves near the top of plants get more intense light than the leaves at the bottom. The top leaves create shade, making less light energy available to lower leaves. If the lower leaves do not receive enough light, they will yellow and die.

Six-foot-tall (1.8 m) plants take longer to grow and have higher overall yields than shorter 4-foot-tall (1.2 m) plants, but the yield of primo tops will be about the same. Due to lack of light, the taller plants have large flowers on the top 3 to 4 feet (91.4–121.9 cm) and spindly buds nearer the bottom. Tall plants tend to develop heavy flower tops whose weight the stem cannot support. These plants need to be tied up. Short plants better support the weight of the tops and have much more flower weight than leaf weight.

At least 99 two-week-old seedlings or clones can be huddled directly under a single 400-watt HID. The young plants will need more space as they grow. If crowded too closely together, plants sense the shortage of space and do not grow to their maximum potential.

Leaves from one plant shade another plant's foliage and slow the overall plant growth. It is very important to space young plants just far enough apart so their leaves do not touch or touch very little. This will keep shading to a minimum and growth to a maximum. Check and alter the spacing every few days. Eight to 16 mature females that are 3 to 4 months old will completely fill the space under one 1000-watt HID.

Plants can absorb light only if it falls on their leaves. Plants must be spaced so their leaves do not overlap too much. Yield increases very little when plants are crowded. Plants also stretch for light, which makes less efficient use of intense light. The most productive number of plants per square foot or square meter is often a matter of experimenting to find the magic number for your garden. In general, each 40-inch square (1 m²) space will hold from 16 to 32 plants.

Reflective Hoods

Some reflective hoods reflect more light and more evenly than others do. A reflector that distributes light evenly—with no hot spots—can be placed closer to plants without burning them. These hoods are most efficient because the lamp is closer and the light more intense.

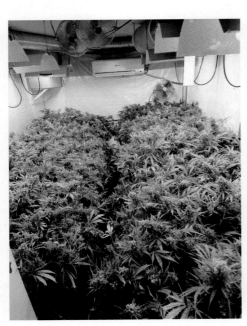

This garden is well maintained and fast-growing. Top leaves may shade bottom leaves now, but the buds receive intense light and will be harvested in about a week.

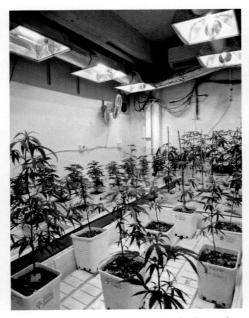

Plants in this garden are spaced a little too far apart to take advantage of all the light in the room.

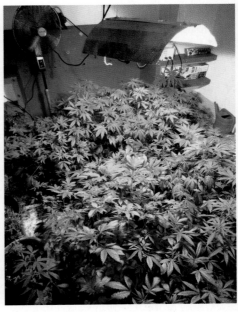

The large bed below the metal halide lamp is crowded with rooting clones.

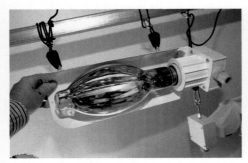

This bulb from Gavita has a reflector built in. The internal reflector is very efficient because it is close to the bulb and always in the same position.

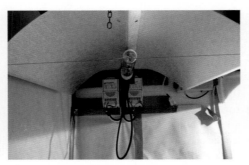

The Adjust-A-Wing is adjustable for different coverage patterns. It dissipates heat quickly and is incredibly efficient.

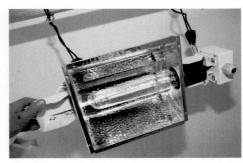

The Gavita Pro 1000-watt Double Ended lamp is attached at both ends, which allows electricity to flow in only one direction in the bulb.

The farther the lamp is from the garden, the less light plants receive.

When used in conjunction with reflective walls, the proper reflective hood over the lamp can double the gardening area. Gardeners who use the most efficient reflective hoods can harvest up to twice as much as those who don't.

Reflective hoods are made from steel sheet metal, aluminum, or even stainless steel. The steel is either cold-rolled or pre-galvanized before a reflective coating is applied. Pre-galvanized steel is more rust resistant than cold-rolled steel. This metal can be polished, textured, or painted, with white being the most common paint color. Hood manufacturers apply white paint in a powder-coating process.

Notes: There are different shades of white, and some whites are whiter than others. Flat white is the most reflective color and diffuses light most effectively. Glossy white paint is easy to clean but tends to create hot spots of light. Also, sheet metal hoods are less expensive than the same size aluminum hood, because of reduced materials expense.

Seedlings, cuttings, and plants in the vegetative growth stage need less light than flowering plants because their growth requirements are different. For the first few weeks of life, seedlings and clones can easily survive beneath fluorescent lights. Vegetative growth requires a little more light, easily supplied by metal halide or compact fluorescent lamps.

Pebble and hammer-tone surfaces offer good light diffusion and more surface area to reflect light. Hot spots are common among highly polished surfaces. Mirror-like hoods also scratch easily and create uneven lighting.

Premium reflective hood manufacturers use a special process developed in Germany that puts a mirror-like reflective surface on aluminum so that it does not oxidize. The slightest bit of oxidation cuts reflectivity.

The bulb should also fit firm and straight in the reflector, at perfect parallel angle to the reflective hood. When the bulb does not stay parallel to the reflector, the light pattern below is out of whack and inconsistent.

Reflective hoods become dirty and may be scratched when cleaned, resulting in a loss of up to 5 percent of their reflective ability every year. If they are dirty and not regularly cleaned, reflective loss increases. Changing the reflective hood every year will ensure that the reflector provides the maximum amount of reflection over time. More than 65 percent of the light is reflected by the reflector.

Clean reflectors with a mild detergent and water. Use a soft dry cloth to avoid scratching. Do not touch the reflective part of reflector hoods.

Do not use sulfur vaporizers when garden lamps are on, and do not use sulfur vaporizers and misters close to luminaires. Sulfur and calcium deposits will damage lamps' reflective surfaces and decrease the efficiency of reflectors.

Air-cooling high-frequency lamps causes them to run below peak operating temperature, which also lowers their efficiency and changes the color spectrum somewhat.

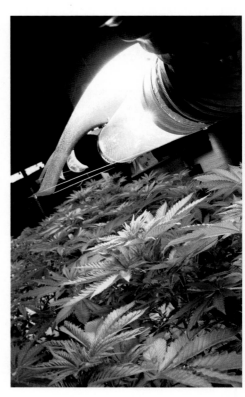

Air-cooled reflective hoods allow lamps to be placed much closer to plants without fear of heat damage. Light is much more intense when close to plants, and therefore provides greater value.

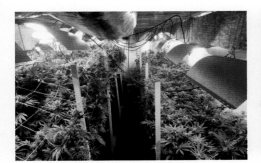

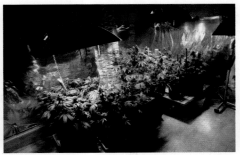

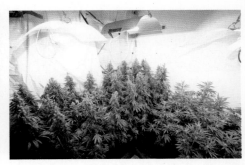

Horizontal reflectors are the most reflective.

A 1000-watt reflector with a hot spot must be placed 36 inches (91.4 cm) above the garden. A 600-watt lamp with a reflector that distributes light evenly can be placed 18 inches (45.7 cm) above the garden. When placed closer, the 600-watt lamp shines as much light on the garden as the 1000-watt bulb!

The Adjust-A-Wing was the first adjustable reflector available. This reflector has been improved over the years and is one of the most popular available.

Horizontal Reflective Hoods

Horizontal reflectors are most efficient for HID systems, and are the best value for gardeners. A horizontal lamp yields up to 40 percent more light than a lamp burning in a vertical position. Light is emitted from the arc tube. When the arc tube is horizontal, half of this light is directed downward to the plants, so only half of the light needs to be reflected.

Horizontal reflective hoods are available in many shapes and sizes. The closer the reflective hood is to the arc tube, the less distance light must travel before being reflected. Less distance traveled means more light reflected. Horizontal reflectors are inherently more efficient than vertical lamps/reflectors, because half of the light is direct and only half of the light must be reflected.

Horizontal reflective hoods tend to have a hot spot directly under the bulb. To dissipate this hot spot of light and lower

the heat it creates, some manufacturers install a light deflector below the bulb. The deflector diffuses the light and heat directly under the bulb. When there is no hot spot, reflective hoods with deflectors can be placed closer to plants.

Horizontally mounted HP sodium lamps use a small reflective hood for greenhouse culture. The hood is mounted a few inches over the horizontal HP sodium bulb. All light is reflected down toward plants, and the small hood creates minimum shadow.

Adjustable Horizontal Reflective Hoods

An adjustable reflector allows light to overlap in the middle and less light to shine on the wall on its other side.

Vertical Reflective Hoods

Reflectors with vertical lamps are less efficient than horizontal ones. Like horizontal bulbs, vertically mounted bulbs emit light from the sides of the arc

tube. This light must strike the side of the hood before it is reflected downward to plants. Reflected light is always less intense than original light. Light travels farther before being reflected in parabolic or cone reflective hoods. Direct light is more intense and more efficient.

Parabolic dome reflectors offer the best value for vertical reflectors. They reflect light relatively evenly, though they throw less overall light than horizontal reflectors. Large parabolic dome hoods distribute light evenly and reflect enough light to sustain vegetative growth. The light spreads out under the hood and is reflected downward to plants. Popular parabolic hoods are inexpensive to manufacture, and provide a good light value for the money. Four-foot parabolic hoods are usually manufactured in nine parts. The smaller size facilitates shipping and handling. The customer assembles the hood with small screws and nuts.

MAXIMUM LIGHT REQUIREMENTS FOR PLANTS

Growth Stage	Foot-Candles	Lux	Hours of Light
seedling	375	4000	16-24
clone	375	4000	18-24
vegetative	2500	27,000	18
flowering	10,000	107,500	12

These guidelines will give plants all the light they need to form dense buds. Less light will often cause looser, less-compact buds to form.

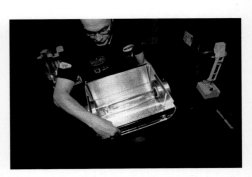

This HortiStar reflector has adjustable sides to adjust light pattern when the luminaire is next to a wall. It also has a replaceable reflector that snaps into place inside the hood.

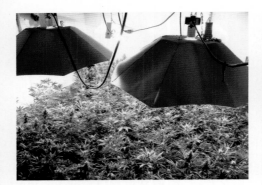
Vertical parabolic reflectors throw a wide, even pattern of light but are not as efficient as horizontal reflectors.

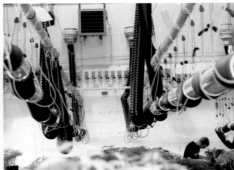
A heat vent outlet around the bulb helps dissipate heat into the atmosphere. Excessive heat around the bulb causes premature burnout.

Reflective-Hood Light Distribution

Reflective hoods are designed to throw light over a specific area. Mounting height affects the effective light coverage and intensity.

The light reflected and the overall light emitted using specific reflective hoods are scientifically measured with a 108-degree arc divided into 5-degree increments from the center of the bulb's base. Light measurements are taken along the arc and plotted on a graph to show the light output of specific luminaires.

Lightweight reflective hoods with open ends dissipate heat quickly. Extra air flows directly through the hood and around the bulb in open-end fixtures to cool the bulb and the fixture. Aluminum dissipates heat more quickly than steel. Train a fan on reflective hoods to speed heat loss.

Artificial light fades as it travels from its source (the bulb). The closer you put the reflector to the bulb, the more intense the light it reflects. Enclosed hoods with a glass shield covering the bulb operate at higher temperatures. The glass shield is a barrier between plants and the hot bulb. Enclosed hoods must have enough vents; otherwise, heat buildup in the fixture causes bulbs to burn out prematurely. Many of these enclosed fixtures have a special vent fan to evacuate hot air.

Air-Cooled Lamp Fixtures

Several air-cooled lights are available. Some use a reflective hood with a protective glass face and two squirrel cage blowers to move air through the sealed reflective-hood cavity. The air is forced to travel around corners, which requires a higher velocity of airflow. Other air-cooled reflectors have no airflow turns, so the air is evacuated quickly and efficiently.

Air-cooled reflective hoods are not recommended for use with electronic ballasts and corresponding HID bulbs. Air-cooled reflectors lower the operating temperature of bulbs, which changes the lamp spectrum and lowers efficiency.

Air-cooled fixtures are inexpensive to operate and easy to set up.

Water-Cooled Lamp Fixtures

Water-cooled lamp fixtures are expensive and impractical for environmentally conscious medical gardeners. I have never seen one being used in a garden room, even though they run cooler and can be moved closer to plants. The water and outer jacket account for a 10 percent lumen loss. On an average day, a 1000-watt bulb uses about 100 gallons of water to keep cool, if the water runs to waste. To recirculate the water requires a big reservoir. The water in the reservoir that serves a recirculating cooling system must also be cooled. Reservoir coolers can easily cost $1000 USD.

No Reflective Hood

Lamps burn cooler and emit only direct light with no reflective hood. Bulbs are hung vertically in between plants. Circular gardens use no reflective hoods so that no light is reflected and plants receive only direct light.

Reflectors are responsible for about 66 percent of all light plants receive from specific luminaries. For example, Gavita rates their lamps as 96 percent efficient, and their figures are based on 33 percent direct light from the bulb and 66 percent reflected light.

Measure the light output from reflective fixtures when the room is being set up. Make sure each square inch (cm²) receives adequate light.

You can make your own light tests; all you need is a light meter and a room with no ambient light. Hang a lamp 3 feet (91.4 cm) from the floor. Make sure the bulb and arc tube are parallel to the floor. Mark a grid on the floor, putting dots every 12 inches (30.5 cm). Mark 12-inch (30.5 cm) increments on the walls, starting from the floor. Center the grid under the bulb. Position the bulb parallel and exactly 3 feet from the floor.

Hortilux Medium 600 HPS

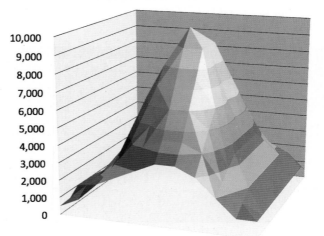

This light study was a simple matter of taking measurements and entering them into an Excel spreadsheet, then clicking the graph button.

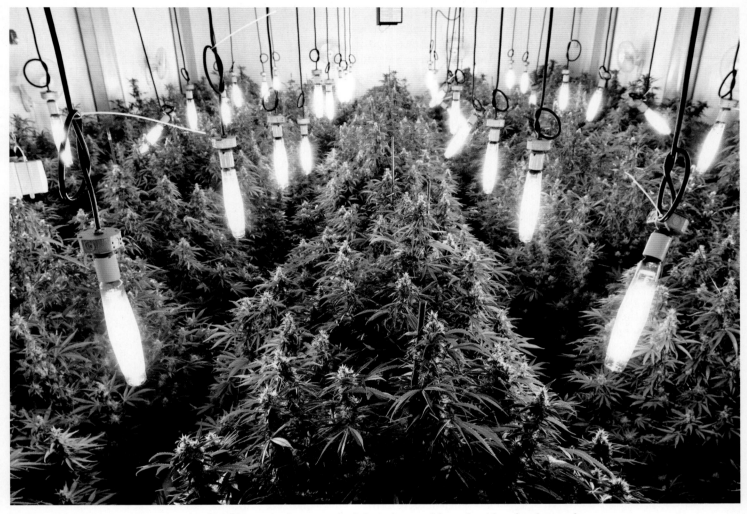

HID lamps having no reflector can be placed between plants. Bright light is dispersed from the sides of each arc tube.

Warm up the lamp for 15 minutes before taking measurements.

Take foot-candle or lux readings every 12 inches (30.5 cm) and post the results to a spreadsheet program such as Microsoft Excel. Spreadsheet graph programs have a graph button that converts the spreadsheet tabulations into several different kinds of graphs.

You will learn that all bulbs and reflective hoods are not created equal!

Check out International Light Technology's "Light Measurement Handbook" available free on the Internet. The 64-page technical book answers endless light questions. Download the book in a few minutes—drawings, graphs, charts, and all—at www.Intl-Light.com/handbook.

Reflective Light

Reflective walls increase light in the gardening area. Less-intense light on the perimeter of gardens is wasted unless it is reflected back onto foliage. Up to 95 percent of this light can be reflected back toward plants. For example, if 500 foot-candles of light is escaping from the edge of the garden and it is reflected at the rate of 95 percent, then 475 foot-candles will be available on the edge of the garden.

Reflective walls should be 6 to 12 inches (15.2–30.5 cm) or less from the plants for optimum reflection. Ideally, take walls to the plants. The easiest way to install mobile walls is to hang the lamp near the corner of a room. Use the two corner walls to reflect light. Move the two outside walls close to plants to reflect light. Make the mobile walls from lightweight plywood, Styrofoam, or white Visqueen plastic.

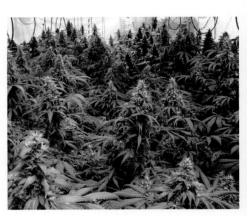

White Visqueen walls are easy to install and easy to keep clean. They add about 10 percent more light around the perimeter of the garden.

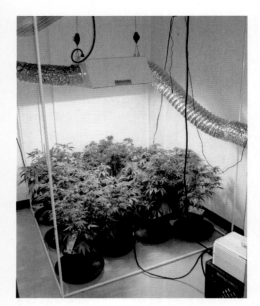

Reflective walls on two sides of the garden reflect light back to plants. The light escaping out the two open sides is wasted.

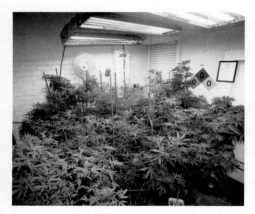

You can see the difference white walls make in this mother room.

Using white Visqueen plastic to "white out" a room is quick and causes no damage to the room. Visqueen plastic is inexpensive, removable, and reusable. It can be used to fabricate walls and to partition rooms. Waterproof Visqueen also protects the walls and floor from water damage. Lightweight Visqueen is easy to cut with scissors or a knife, and can be stapled, nailed, or taped.

To make the white walls opaque, hang black Visqueen on the outside. The dead airspace between the two layers of Visqueen also increases insulation. The only disadvantages of white Visqueen plastic are that it is not as reflective as flat white paint, it may get brittle after a few years

of use under an HID lamp, and it can be difficult to find at retail outlets. Using flat white paint is one of the simplest, least expensive, and most efficient ways to create reflective walls.

While easy to clean, semigloss white is not quite as reflective as flat white. Regardless of the type of white used, a nontoxic, fungus-inhibiting agent should be added when the paint is mixed. A gallon (3.8 L) of good flat white paint costs less than $25 USD. One or two gallons should be enough to "white out" the average garden room. Use a primer coat to prevent bleed-through of dark colors or stains or if walls are rough and unpainted. Install vent fans before painting. Fumes are unpleasant and can cause health problems. Painting is labor-intensive and messy, but it's worth the trouble.

Reflective Surfaces
Aluminum foil is one of the worst possible reflective surfaces and no more than 55 percent reflective. The foil tends to crinkle up and reflects light in many directions—actually wasting light. It also creates hot spots and reflects more ultraviolet rays than other surfaces.

C3 Anti-detection film is a specialized type of Mylar that exhibits the same properties as the 2-mil-thick (0.002 inches) Mylar, but in addition to reflecting approximately 92 to 97 percent of the light, it is also 90 percent infrared proof and virtually invisible to infrared scanning and thermal imaging.

Emergency thin polyester (camping) blankets are constructed of a single layer of polyester film that is covered with a layer of vapor-deposited aluminum. These blankets are not very effective at reflecting light because they are so thin and permeated with countless tiny holes. They can also create hot spots when wrinkled or not attached flush to the wall.

Flat white paint is a great option for large grow rooms or for people who are interested in a low-maintenance wall. Flat white paint has the ability to reflect between 75 and 85 percent of the light, and it does not create hot spots. Glossy white is easier to clean but contains light-inhibiting varnish. Semigloss paint

MATERIAL	PERCENT REFLECTED
aluminum foil	70-75
black	<10
C3 Anti-detection film emergency blanket	92-97
flat white paint	75-85
Foylon	94-95
Mylar	90-95
Styrofoam	7580
rubberized white paint	7580
Visqueen (white)	7580
white paint (flat)	85-93
white paint (semi-gloss)	75-80
yellow paint (flat)	70-80

provides a more reflective surface and is easy to clean. Adding a fungicide is recommended when painting. Paint that has lead pigment—banned in the USA in 1978—is toxic and not to be used.

Paint concrete walls with elastomeric paint to provide a tough and thick coating that also waterproofs most surfaces, including stucco, masonry, concrete with cracks, and concrete blocks. Some elastomeric paints are compatible with wood.

Foylon is a reflective material that reflects light and heat in an evenly dispersed pattern. It is durable, and it reflects about 95 percent of the light that hits it. The material is plied with ripstop fiber and is thick enough to act as an insulator. It is also heat and flame resistant. For more information on Foylon, see www.greenair.com.

Foylon is a more durable version of Mylar, made of spun polyester fabric and reinforced with foil laminate. Foylon is resistant to most solutions, won't tear or fade, and can be wiped or washed clean. More expensive and more durable than Mylar, Foylon reflects about 85 percent of heat energy and requires good ventilation. Attach Foylon to walls with Velcro, so that it can be easily removed for cleaning.

Mirrors also reflect light, but much less than Mylar. Light must first pass through the glass in the mirror before it hits the "silver" or metal amalgam. Light is lost when it is reflected back through the same glass.

Mylar, a thin (1–2-mil [0.001–0.002 in.]) mirror-surface sheeting in a roll format, provides a very reflective surface—up to 95 percent. Unlike light-absorbing paint, reflective Mylar reflects almost all light. To install reflective Mylar, simply tape or tack it to the wall. To prevent rips or tears, place a piece of tape over the spot where the staple, nail or tack will be inserted. Although expensive, Mylar is preferred by many gardeners. The trick is to position it flat against the wall. When loosely affixed to surfaces, light is poorly reflected. To increase its effectiveness, keep reflective Mylar clean.

Polystyrene foam (Styrofoam) sheeting is reflective and serves to insulate too. Light reflected from Styrofoam is diffuse, with no hot spots. Purchase rigid foam sheets to use as freestanding walls, or else tape, glue, or nail sheets to walls.

Rubberized roofing paint reflects up to 90 percent of the light that hits it. It

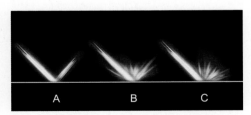

A. Specular: Mylar and mirror give the best strength of light, but it is concentrated. About 90 percent of the light is transferred.

B. Diffuse: Equivalent to a non-shiny (matte) surface

C. Spread: Flat white surface that is diffuse with reasonable spread

is mildew resistant, high viscosity, and rubberized to form a rubberlike blanket that expands and contracts. It adheres to most surfaces, wood and metal alike. Rubberized paints are available at most hardware stores.

Visqueen plastic, in both white and white/black, is easy to clean and is perfect to use as walls or to cover walls of garden rooms. Attach white Visqueen to existing walls with screws, tape, or glue, or hang white/black plastic from ceiling to form garden-room walls. The black side does not allow light to penetrate. The white side is 75 to 90 percent reflective. Always use heavy, 6-mil Visqueen.

Increase light without adding more watts of light

Use several 400- or 600-watt lamps instead of one or two 1000s.

Manually rotate plants on a regular basis.

Add a shelf around perimeter of garden.

Install rolling beds.

Grow a perpetual crop.

Use a light mover.

Move small plants closer to the light.

Movable reflective walls are easy to remove for maintenance, and they give maximum reflection. Insulated greenhouse mobile blankets also make great garden room partitions.

Light Movers

A light mover is a device that moves lamps back and forth or in circles across the ceiling of a garden room. The linear or circular path distributes light evenly. Use a light mover to get lights up to 12 inches (30 cm) from plants. The closer a lamp is to plants without burning them, the more light plants receive.

Uniform light distribution makes cannabis grow evenly, but it is not a substitute for more lumens from an additional lamp. It is a more efficient way to use each HID, especially 1000-watt lamps.

Slower-moving light movers are usually more reliable. Some fast-moving light movers can cause lightweight reflectors to wobble or list. Some light movers spin at a fairly rapid rate. I'm not sure if this makes a difference or not.

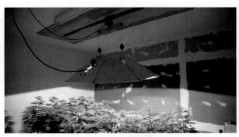

This light mover shuttles the lamp back and forth over the garden, providing more even light coverage from more angles. The moving lamp can be placed closer to the garden because it generates less heat in one place when moving.

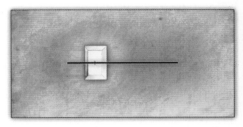

This drawing shows the overall light coverage when using a light mover. Note that the plants receive very intense light under the bulb for short periods of time.

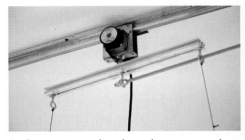

Light movers can be adjusted to run on a short or long track.

Gardeners report that light movers make it possible to use fewer lamps to get the same yield. And at the same time, I have never seen a light mover in a garden in Europe. Light movers increase intense light coverage by 25 to 35 percent. According to some gardeners, 3 lamps mounted on motorized light mover(s) will do the job of 4 lamps.

Motorized light movers keep an even garden profile. If the 1000-watt HID is on a 15- or 20-amp circuit, you can easily add a light mover that draws one more amp to the circuit, with no risk of overload.

Benefits of a light mover:

Bulbs can be placed closer to the canopy of the garden

Increases bright light to more plants

Delivers light from different angles, providing even lighting

Increases intense light coverage by 25 percent or more

Light is closer to plants

Economical use of light

Watch out for the following:

Stretched or leggy plants

Weak or yellowing plants

Foliage burned directly under the bulb

Uneven lighting

Light mover binding or getting hung up

Electricity and Safety

Before you touch anything electrical, always unplug from the electrical outlet. Work backward when installing electrical components or doing wiring. Start at the bulb, and work toward the outlet. Always plug in the power cord last!

Purchase a current ABC fire extinguisher rated to put out wood, paper, grease, oil, and electrical fires. Some fire extinguishers are smoke-activated. Place them over heat sources such as ballasts. Place regular fire extinguishers alongside the exit door. You can see it every time you enter and exit, and if there is a fire in a room, the tendency is to go out the door! Make sure the ABC fire extinguisher is UL, CSA, or EMC approved.

Study the overload table on page 298 see the definitions for *ampere, breaker switch, circuit, conductor, fuse, ground,*

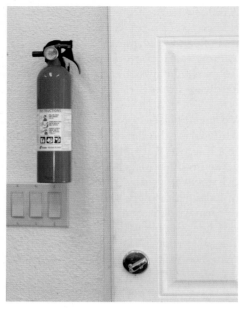

Mount fire extinguishers next to the door. If there is a fire, you will head for the door, and the fire extinguisher will be there. Always mount an up-to-date fire extinguisher that is able to put out wood, grease, and electrical fires. Such devices are filled with a dry powder and are commonly known as ABC extinguishers: A = wood, B = oil base, C = electric.

GFI (ground fault interrupter) outlet, hertz, short circuit, volts, and *watts* in the following glossary. You will need to understand these terms to gain full use of the information in this chapter.

Keep electrical service about 4 feet (about 120 cm) above the floor, and keep all water and liquids on or near the floor. Electricity and water do not mix!

To learn more about electrical safety, check out the Occupational Safety and Health Administration's website: www.osha.gov/Publications/electrical_safety.html

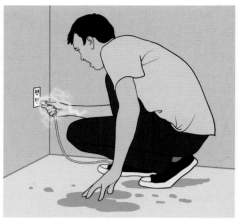

You will be working with water under and around the HID system. Water conducts electricity about as well as the human body does. A simple rule of thumb is to keep all things electrical at eye level in the room, and keep all things wet or watery below the waist.

Ampere (amp) is the measure of electricity in motion. Electricity can be looked at in absolute terms of measurement, just as water can. A gallon is an absolute measure of a portion of water; a coulomb is an absolute measure of a portion of electricity. Water in motion is measured in gallons per second, liters per minute, etc. Electricity in motion is measured in coulombs per second. When an electrical current flows at one coulomb per second, we say it has one ampere.

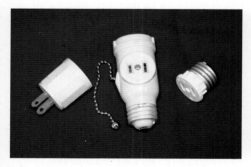

This light mover shuttles the lamp back and forth over the garden, providing more even light coverage from more angles. The moving lamp can be placed closer to the garden because it generates less heat in one place when moving.

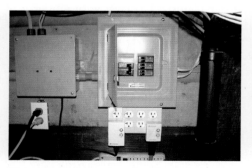

This subpanel contains 8 breaker switches. The 2 main switches on the left turn the panel on and off.

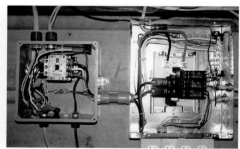

This set of subpanels shows all the wiring and connections to fuses and most outlets.

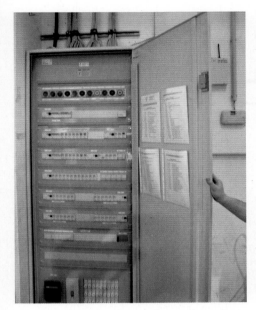

This is the most impressive electrical panel I have ever seen. All the switches and timers are contained in one big box. The four papers taped to the door show the location of each electrical circuit.

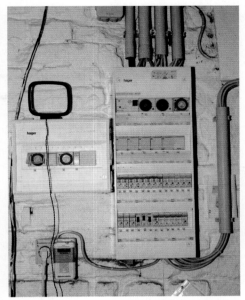

This European electrical panel contains many breaker switches and timers. Everything electric in a large garden room can be monitored in one place.

Never replace fuses with pennies or aluminum foil! They will not melt and interrupt the circuit when overloaded; doing so is an easy way to start a fire. Fuses are virtually obsolete.

A **fuse box** is an electrical circuit box containing circuits interrupted by fuses.

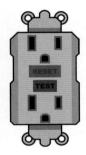

GFI: Ground fault interrupter outlets are required anywhere water is used in a home or business. Install GFI outlets in *all* garden rooms to provide an instant, safe, electrical shutoff when necessary.

Ground means to connect electricity to the ground or earth for safety. If a circuit is properly grounded and the electricity travels somewhere it is not directed, it will go via the ground wire into the ground (earth) and be rendered harmless. Electricity will travel the path of least resistance. This path must be along the ground wire.

Breaker box is an electrical circuit box that has on/off switches rather than single application fuses. The main breaker box is called a "service panel."

Sub-breaker box (aka a subpanel) is attached and located just off the main service panel. The subpanel controls specific circuits. The power to the sub-breaker box must be shut off at the service panel.

Breaker switch is an on/off safety switch that will turn the electricity off when the circuit is overloaded. Look for

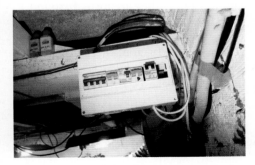

This European sub-breaker panel was wired in to add extra fuse protection in the garden room.

breaker switches in the breaker panel or breaker box. Breaker switches are rated for different amperes—10, 12, 20, 25, 30, 40, etc.

Circuit is the circular path that electricity travels. If this path is interrupted, the power will go off. If this circuit is given a chance to do so, it will travel a circular route through your body!

New circuits: Powering any more than 4 to 6 lamps usually requires adding new incoming circuits, or else the use of present circuits will be severely limited, possibly prone to fire. Employ a certified electrician to install more than 3000 or 4000 watts of indoor garden light.

Conductor is something that is able to carry electricity easily. Copper, steel, water, and the human body are good electrical conductors.

DC (direct current) is a continuous electrical current that only flows in one direction. Batteries run on DC current.

Fuse is an electrical safety device consisting of a fusible metal that melts and interrupts the circuit when overloaded.

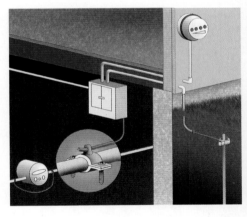

All electrical outlets, fuses, and connections must be grounded. Inspect electrical connections for signs of heat-blackened wires, melted connections, and smelly wiring.

The ground is formed by a wire (usually green, brown, or bare copper) that runs parallel to the circuit and is attached to a metal ground stake. Metal water or sewer pipes also serve as excellent conductors for the ground. Water pipes conduct electricity well and are all in good contact with the ground. The entire system—pipes, copper wire, and metal ground stake—conducts any misplaced electricity safely into the ground.

The ground wire is the third wire with the big round prong. The ground runs through the ballast all the way to the reflective hood. High-intensity discharge systems must have a ground that runs a continual path from the socket through the ballast to the main fuse box, then to the house or circuit ground.

Heat: Use a laser thermometer to inspect electrical connections for signs of heat damage; institute repairs immediately.

Ohm's Power Law

volts × amperes = watts

115 volts × 9 amperes = 1035 watts

240 volts × 4 amperes = 960 watts

An HID lamp that draws about 9.2 amperes × 120 volts = 1104 watts.

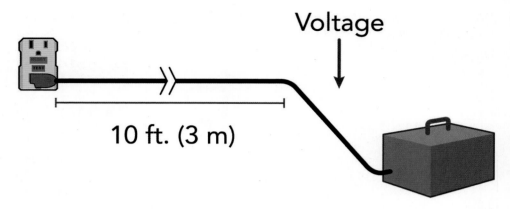

Voltage

10 ft. (3 m)

Electricity diminishes as it travels through a copper wire. The maximum distance electricity should travel from outlet to the ballast of a high-intensity discharge, light-emitting plasma, or compact fluorescent lamp is about 10 feet (about 3 m). After this distance, the voltage drops due to resistance in the wire. The problem is compounded by using wire that is too small to carry the electrical load.

Amp Rating	Amps Available	Amps to Overload
15	13	14
20	16	17
25	20	21
30	24	25
40	32	33

Wire size is important! See "Electrical Wiring and Circuits."

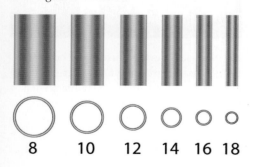

8	10	12	14	16	18

Watts measure the amount of electricity flowing in a wire. When amperes (units of electricity per second) are multiplied by volts (pressure), we get watts. 1000 watts = 1 kilowatt.

Watt-hours measure the amount of watts that are used during an hour. One watt-hour is equal to one watt used for one hour. A kilowatt-hour (kWh) is 1000 watt-hours. A 1000-watt HID will use roughly one kilowatt per hour, and the ballast will use about 100 watts. Electrical bills are charged out in kWh.

Electrical Wiring and Circuits

Electrical wire comes in many thicknesses (gauges) indicated by number. Higher numbers indicate smaller wire, and lower numbers indicate larger wire. Most household circuits are connected with 14-gauge wire in the USA and Canada. Wire thickness is important for two reasons—amperage and voltage drop. Amperage is the amount of amperes a wire is able to carry safely.

Electricity flowing through wire creates heat. The more amperes flowing, the more heat created. Heat is wasted power. Avoid wasting power by using the proper thickness of well-insulated wire (14-gauge for 120 volt and 18-gauge for 240 volt applications) with a grounded wire connection.

Using wire that is too small forces too much power (amperes) through the wire, which causes voltage drop. Voltage (pressure) is lost in the wire. For example, by forcing an 18-gauge wire to carry 9.2 amperes at 120 volts, it would not only heat up, maybe even switching off breakers, but the voltage at the outlet would be 120 volts, while the voltage 10 feet away could be as low as 108. This is a loss of 12 volts that you are paying for. The ballast and lamp run less efficiently with fewer volts. The further the electricity travels, the more heat that is generated, and the more voltage drops.

A lamp designed to work at 120 volts that only receives 108 volts (90 percent of the power intended for operation), would produce only 70 percent of the normal light. Use at least 14-gauge wire for any extension cords, and if the cord is to carry power over 60 feet (18.3 m), use 12-gauge wire.

When wiring an outlet or socket:

The hot wire attaches to the brass or gold screw.

The common wire attaches to the aluminum or silver screw.

The ground wire always attaches to the ground prong.

Caution! Keep the wires from crossing and forming a short circuit.

Plugs and outlets must have a solid connection. If they are jostled around and the electricity is allowed to jump, electricity is lost in the form of heat; the prongs will burn, and a fire could result. Periodically check plugs and outlets to ensure they have a solid connection.

If installing a new circuit or breaker box, hire an electrician and purchase *Wiring Simplified* by H. P. Richter and W. C. Schwan. It costs about $15 USD and is available at most hardware stores in the USA. Installing a new circuit in a breaker box is very easy but could turn into a shocking experience. Before trying

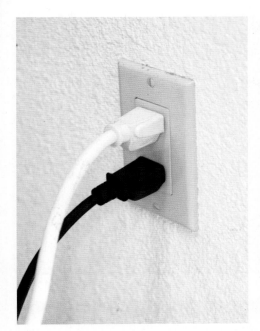

Three-prong electrical outlets with a ground are essential in all garden rooms.

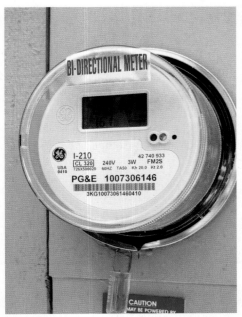

Solar panels on a home or building collect and transform solar energy into electricity. A bidirectional meter is needed when more electricity is produced than is being used. The excess generated electricity is sent (sold) back to the public electric grid.

anything of this scope, read about it and discuss it with several professionals.

A circuit with a 20-amp fuse, powering the following items:

1400-watt toaster oven

100-watt incandescent lightbulb

+ 20-watt radio

1520 total watts

1520 total watts ÷ 120 volts = 12.6 amps in use

OR

1520 total watts ÷ 240 volts = 6.3 amps in use

The above example shows that 12.6 amps are being drawn when everything is on. By adding 9.2 amps, drawn by the HID to the circuit, we get 21.8 amps, an overloaded circuit!

There are three solutions:

1. Remove one or all of the high ampere-drawing appliances, and plug them into another circuit.

2. Find another circuit that has few or no amps drawn by other appliances.

3. Install a new circuit. A 240-volt circuit will make more amps available per circuit.

Electricity Consumption

The average electric bill for a small apartment that uses about 200 kWh per month is $40 to $70 USD. A large house with a hot tub and many electrical appliances can use 2000 kWh at a cost of $200 to 400 USD per month.

Most gardeners in the USA can safely use one 1000-watt lamp per room to grow medicinal cannabis. The tables on page 300 will give you an idea of the efficiency of each type of lamp, its "cost per watt," and its "value per watt."

Electrical records are considered to be in the public domain in some jurisdictions;

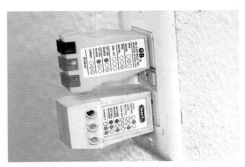

Inexpensive circuit testers are easy to use and ensure that all circuits function properly.

anybody—including disgruntled friends, thieves, and law enforcement—can access them with the touch of a computer keyboard. In some communities, judges are easily pressured or bullied by law enforcement into issuing search warrants.

There are many legitimate reasons for unqualified "suspicious" electricity consumption that are not investigated. Armed searches based upon electrical records are a recipe for failure and for law enforcement budget shortfalls.

Conserve Electricity

Lower the carbon footprint of indoor and greenhouse gardens. Avoid using diesel generators. Use energy-efficient appliances, refrigerators, water heaters, and so on. Monitor and minimize electrical consumption. To avoid electricity draw, unplug appliances when they are not in use.

Use alternative energy sources such as solar and wind energy, or any non-fossil fuel, to decrease your carbon footprint. Alternative energy sources are often more expensive at startup, but they pay for themselves many times over in the long run. Check into rebates and tax credits offered by local, state, and national governments.

To limit electrical consumption, move into a home with a basement, all-electric heat, and a woodstove. HID lamps installed in a basement garden also generate heat. Disperse excess heat with a vent fan attached to a thermostat/humidistat. Turn off the electric heat, and use the woodstove as needed.

Set the water heater for 130°F (54.4°C) instead of 170°F (76.7°C). This easy

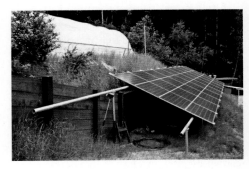

Solar panels convert sunlight into electricity. The best website for solar information is www.sargosis.com. Contact my friend Pete (contact@sargosis.com) before installing solar.

LAMP	COST PER WATT IN USD	LM/W	VALUE PER WATT IN USD
metal halide (MH)	$0.5	100	$200.00
high-pressure sodium (HPS)	$0.5	140	$280.00
T5 compact fluorescent lamp (CFL)	$0.5	100	$200.00
T12 fluorescent	$0.27	22	$81.48
light-emitting plasma (LEP)	$3	82	$27.33
light-emitting diode (LED)	$0.7	90	$128.57

COST OF ELECTRICITY (IN USD)

Cost per	12-hour days		18-hour days		24-hour days	
kWh	Day	Month	Day	Month	Day	Month
$0.10	$1.20	$36.00	$1.80	$32.40	$2.40	$72.00
$0.15	$1.80	$54.00	$2.70	$48.60	$3.60	$108.00
$0.20	$2.40	$72.00	$3.60	$64.80	$4.80	$144.00

procedure saves about 25 kWh per month. But do not turn the water heater any lower than 130°F (54.4°C). Harmful bacteria can grow below this safe point. An alternative would be to install an "on demand" water heater.

Human electric meter readers are disappearing, falling victim to smart meters. Human meter readers often use high-tech telescopes to read the meter dials that store the readings in an integrated digital entry device. The information is then dumped into the larger computer at the central office. Evidence of the DEA sending instructions to electric companies in the past exists, but it is uncommon.

Electric companies often replace meters that show a major change in electricity consumption. The first step is to change the meter. It is upgraded to a smart meter where the technology exists.

Smart Meters

Smart electric meters record electricity consumption in intervals of an hour or less and send this information back to the central office at regular intervals. Electricity consumption is therefore constantly monitored. Electric companies are replacing old analog meters with more efficient digital smart meters that do not require an employee to physically read electric meters. Utility customers can monitor electricity use via the company's website from a computer or a handheld electronic device. However, smart meters have been under increasing scrutiny by those who cite a high degree of inaccuracy, invasion of privacy, and extraordinary electromagnetic activity. Some communities have taken measures to ban smart meters altogether.

Timers and Controllers

A timer is essential to turn lights on and off at the proper times. This inexpensive

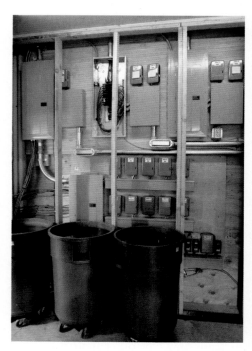

All the timers in this complex of four large garden rooms are centrally located and easy to monitor and maintain.

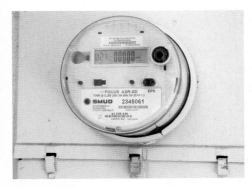

Smart meters allow electric companies to perpetually monitor electric consumption from a central office.

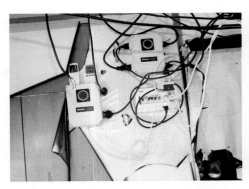

A subpanel with breaker switches controls this set of heavy-duty light timers. The timers were designed for use with high-wattage lights.

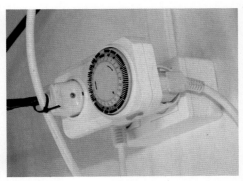

Small timers are designed for use with one lamp or to control fans and pumps. The timers are easy to plug in and set. Make sure to use a timer with a two-pole contact switch. The inrush of electrical current is not compatible with inexpensive timers.

investment can also turn other appliances on and off at regular intervals. Using a timer ensures that your garden will receive a controlled light period of the same duration every day. Purchase a heavy-duty grounded timer with an adequate amperage and tungsten rating to meet your needs. Some timers have a different amperage rating for the switch; it is often lower than that of the timer. Use a timer with a two-pole contact switch. The sudden rush of electrical current is not compatible with household timers. Timers that control more than one lamp are more expensive, because they have to be able to switch a very high current. Many prewired timers are available at stores that sell HID lights.

If running more than 2000 or 3000 watts, attach the lamps to a relay, and control the relay with a timer. The advantage of a relay is that it offers a path for more electricity without having to change the timer. There are numerous

sophisticated timers on the market that will solve every timer need you have.

Digital controllers can turn lights on and off and control fans, air conditioners, irrigation cycles, and more. Many cannabis gardeners prefer to use a controller to keep the environment in the room stable. For example, the humidity rises when the lights go out. The vent fan must be activated to evacuate the humid air; using a controller assures consistent timing.

Electric Generators

Diesel and gasoline generators are noisy, messy, and expensive to operate. More importantly, they are extremely polluting to the environment.

Gardeners in Northern California and Oregon have related many stories of diesel generators, all of which lacked glamour and reeked of petroleum and noise. Imagine a big heavy fuel truck

arriving to your rural home on a gravel or dirt road. The truck spills and splashes gas or diesel fuel on the road, leaving a "footprint." The diesel pollution can seep into groundwater.

Check out the Livingston Survey, which claims that indoor cannabis gardeners account for 1 percent of electrical use in the USA, $5 billion every year. See "Cannabis Carbon Footprint" in chapter 10, *Garden Rooms*.

Medical gardeners who use gas and diesel generators might not be carefully considering environmental impact. These generators can supply all the electricity necessary for an indoor garden to grow "off the power grid," but carbon footprint, reliability, and noise are serious considerations.

Auxiliary generators are essential when a power-outage emergency arises for a few days. A couple of small generators

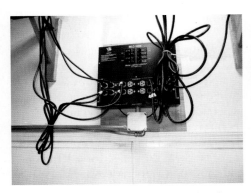

An effective light timer is set up with breaker switches, and can control up to 16 lamps. Timers like this make setting up a big indoor garden much easier.

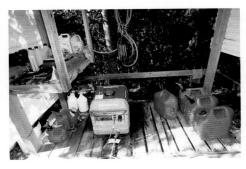

This 3000-watt Honda generator supplies enough electricity to operate lights placed over outdoor plants so they do not flower early in the spring. It also supplies enough power to operate fans in a greenhouse.

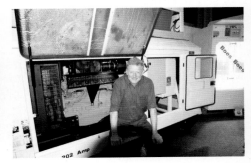

Big generators can supply enough electricity to run 20 to 30 lights easily. However, they must be supplied with diesel or gasoline fuel.

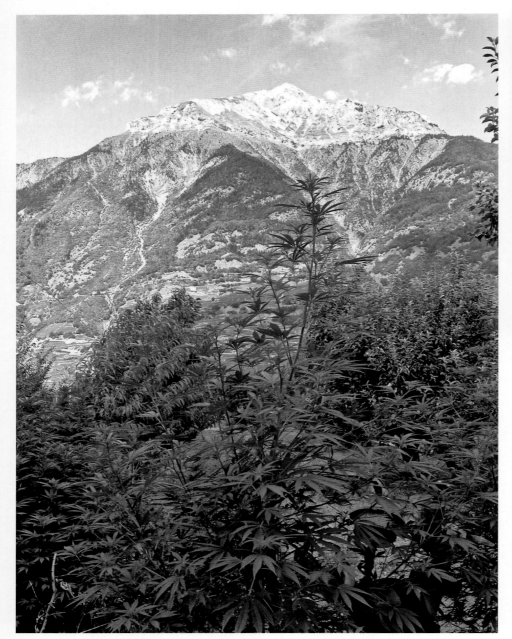

Gas and diesel generators are not necessary to grow cannabis in pristine environments.

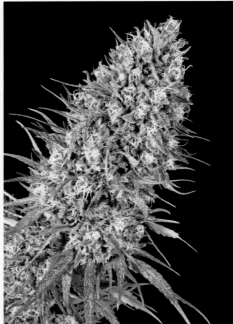

This beautiful 'Cripple Creek' bud photographed by DoobieDuck is in perfect light.

periods. Generators also guzzle a lot of gas. Diesel motors are more economical to run, but noisy, and the toxic fumes reek. Always make sure gasoline- or diesel-powered generators are vented properly. Their exhaust produces carbon monoxide, which is toxic to plants and fatal to humans.

Diesel generators for truck and train car refrigerators are fairly easy to acquire and last for years. Once set up, a "Big Bertha" generator can run many lights. Big gasoline generator motors can be converted to propane, which is a cleaner-burning fossil fuel.

Generators are usually moved to a belowground location covered by a building. With a good exhaust system and baffling around the motor, the sound is soon dissipated. Muffling the exhaust and expelling the fumes is a little more complex. The exhaust must be able to escape freely into the atmosphere. The generator will need fuel, and must be monitored regularly. Maintaining a generator that runs 12 hours per day is a lot of work. If the generator is left alone and shuts down prematurely, plants stop growing.

can save an indoor crop. If the lights go out for a few hours, no problem; but if they go out for 3 to 4 days, plants suffer. A generator that will supply enough electricity for a skeleton crew of lights will keep harvest dates on track.

Buy the generator new. Larger generators should be water-cooled and fully automated. Start it up and check its noise output before purchasing. Always buy a generator that is big enough to do the job. A little extra cushion will be

necessary to allow for power surges. If the generator fails, the crop could fail. Allow at least 1300 watts per 1000-watt lamp to be run by the generator. The ballast consumes a few watts, as does the wire. A 5500-watt Honda generator will run four 1000-watt lamps.

Honda generators are among the most common generators found in garden rooms because they are reasonably priced, dependable, and quiet. But they are not designed to work for long

18 SOIL

SOILS ARE DIFFERENT—very different—from one another. The average organic mineral soil is made up of 45 percent mineral particles; 5 percent living and dead organisms such as bacteria, protozoa, microbes, fungi, and earthworms; and 50 percent air and water. Three major factors contribute to cannabis roots' ability to grow in a soil: texture, pH, and nutrient content (organic and mineral).

Most gardeners look at soil in two basic ways. The first is to see it as a living, organic substance that must be nurtured in order for cannabis roots to extract the necessary nutrients quickly, efficiently, and in maximum amounts. There are large volumes of soil in outdoor gardens and in large containers placed in greenhouses or indoors, and for such volumes, we can apply complete organic principles. The second way to look at soil is as a growing medium that holds chemical elements, salt-based fertilizers (nutrients), air, and water. Indoors and often in greenhouses this is the way many gardeners approach growing.

Dirt, Soil, and Soilless Mix
Dirt is found under your fingernails. Soil is mineral-based and best employed to grow cannabis in fields, planting beds, and very large containers. Soilless mixes are best for growing cannabis in small containers—indoors, outdoors and in greenhouses. The dynamics of small containers are not the same as in large containers, planting beds, or Mother Earth.

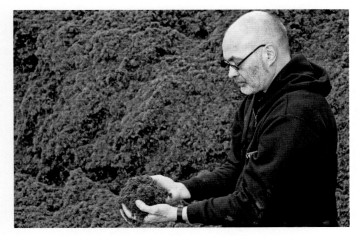

Many soils and soilless mixes used by cannabis gardeners are peat-based and are mixed with other elements.

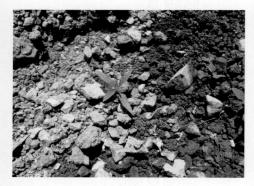

Rocky, clayey soil is packed with nutrients, but its texture restricts air and moisture content.

Soil texture is governed by the size and physical makeup of the mineral particles. Proper soil texture is required for adequate root penetration, water and oxygen retention, and drainage as well as many other complex chemical processes.

"Soil texture" is a descriptive tool used to express mineral particle sizes and grains in sediment, and is divided into three main groups, clay, loam, and sand. Most soils are a mix of three basic soil particle sizes: clay, silt, and sand (described below).

Soil pH is a measure of the acid-to-alkaline balance. Soil life and mineral (nutrient) availability and uptake by roots are affected by soil pH levels. Every full-point change in the 0 to14 pH scale denotes a *tenfold* increase or decrease. Nutrient uptake is best within a pH range of 6.0 to 6.5. Keeping the soil and water pH-balanced and within the proper range is essential to a strong, healthy cannabis crop.

Soil varies from location to location on the earth and often varies from one place to another in your own backyard.

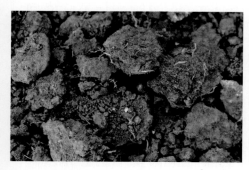

Heavy clay soil is easy to spot. It clumps up readily, is difficult to work, and drains poorly.

Soil Tests

Soil tests are remarkably inexpensive ($20–$200 USD) and save medical cannabis gardeners much time and money wasted on fertilizers. Such tests also save the environment from excessive fertilizer pollution, including nitrates and phosphates, accumulation in the soil, and runoff in the watershed. Excess fertilizer salts wash out into the water system where they cause countless environmental and health problems. For example, home gardeners use at least ten times more fertilizer per square yard (m²) than big agribusiness farms. For every $10 USD spent on fertilizer by home gardeners, $9 USD is wasted! I recently spoke to an outdoor medical cannabis gardener who spends $3,000 USD on fertilizer annually. By applying the above information we see that 10 percent ($300 USD) worth of fertilizer is actually used and 90 percent ($2,700 USD worth of fertilizer) is washed into the soil and groundwater. The gardener could easily save $2,700 USD by investing $20 to $200 USD in soil tests and the following recommendations.

Familiarize yourself with 2 basic types of soil analysis: base cation saturation ratio (BCSR) and sufficiency level of available nutrients (SLAN).

Base cation saturation ratio is commonly used by organic farmers and market gardeners in many countries. The results of BCSR testing provide the actual amounts of nutrients in soil. The goal of BCSR testing is to achieve a balanced ratio of nutrients. The methodology uses Mehlich 3 extraction with different testing parameters. The BCSR soil-testing method is supported by the National Sustainable Agriculture Information Service (ATTRA).

Standard soil tests provide information for some or all of the following:
• calcium
• magnesium
• potassium
• sodium
• phosphorus
• sulfur
• chlorine
• minor elements
• trace elements

Get a BCSR soil analysis ($110–$150 USD) from Earthfort, http://earthfort.com/lab services.html.

Also known as Index (UK) system, SLAN is used by the majority of universities, farmers, and big agribusinesses worldwide. The results of this type of test provide plant-available nutrient levels in a well-known range, ensuring neither a deficiency nor an excess. The methodology uses ammonium acetate extraction.

Standard SLAN soil tests provide some or all of all of the following and many include recommendations to improve soil nutrient content.
• pH
• ECe (dS/m)
• NO_3-N (ppm)
• NH4-N (ppm)
• PO_4-P (ppm)
• potassium (ppm)
• magnesium (ppm)
• calcium (ppm)
• sodium (ppm)
• SO_4-S (ppm)
• zinc (ppm)
• manganese (ppm)
• iron (ppm)
• copper (ppm)
• boron (ppm)

An optimum range for each reading and amendment and fertilizer recommendations are also included in many soil tests. For a little more money many labs include an easy-to-read graph.

SLAN Soil Test Labs
• Logan Labs, LLC: Least expensive soil tests I have found. Basic test $20 USD. www.loganlabs.com
• A&L Western Laboratories, Inc.: Excellent service at a reasonable price. www.al labs west.com
• Spectrum Analytic, Inc.: This lab does everything and also shows a sample soil test. www.spectrumana-lytic.com

Regardless of the type of test you choose, BCSR or SLAN, follow soil collection and submission guidelines to the letter. Gardeners living in a state

Graphical Soil Analysis Report

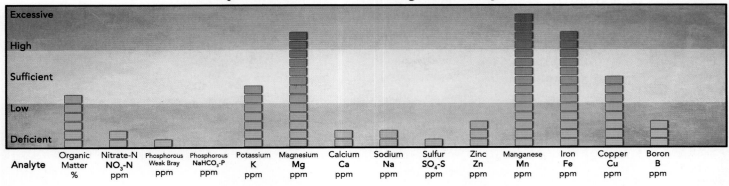

| Analyte | Organic Matter % | Nitrate-N NO₃-N ppm | Phosphorous Weak Bray ppm | Phosphorous NaHCO₃-P ppm | Potassium K ppm | Magnesium Mg ppm | Calcium Ca ppm | Sodium Na ppm | Sulfur SO₄-S ppm | Zinc Zn ppm | Manganese Mn ppm | Iron Fe ppm | Copper Cu ppm | Boron B ppm |

Graphical Plant Analysis Report

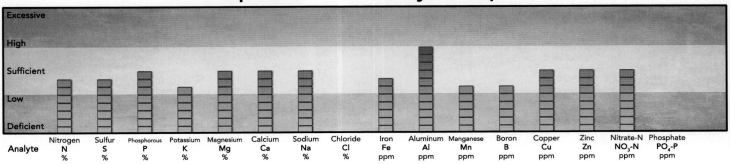

| Analyte | Nitrogen N % | Sulfur S % | Phosphorous P % | Potassium K % | Magnesium Mg % | Calcium Ca % | Sodium Na % | Chloride Cl % | Iron Fe ppm | Aluminum Al ppm | Manganese Mn ppm | Boron B ppm | Copper Cu ppm | Zinc Zn ppm | Nitrate-N NO₃-N ppm | Phosphate PO₄-P ppm |

http://www.al-labs-west.com/files/Graphical%20Plant%20Analysis%20Report.pdf

or country that sanctions medicinal cannabis can send tests to local labs and request recommendations for cannabis. Medical gardeners who do not live in such a state can send their soil samples to any soil test lab but are advised not to mention the target crop.

Excellent sites to learn more about soil:

- **Soil and Health Library** provides free e-books, mainly about holistic agriculture, holistic health, and self-sufficient homestead living. http://soilandhealth.org

- **Soilminerals.com** provides complete information on garden soil minerals, nutrients, trace minerals, fertilizers and amendments for all gardens, farms, lawns, orchards and greenhouses. www.soilminerals.com

- **University of Idaho, College of Agriculture** offers a short course in soil and plant diagnostics. www.webpages.uidaho.edu/~b-mahler/s44603.pdf

- **Acres USA** is North America's oldest magazine covering commercial-scale organic and sustainable farming. www.acresusa.com

- **National Sustainable Agriculture Information Service (ATTRA)** manages projects that promote self-reliance and sustainable lifestyles that include sustainable and renewable energy, energy conservation, resource-efficient housing, sustainable community development, and sustainable agriculture. www.attra.ncat.org

- **Jorge Cervantes Presents Marijuana Growing.** Check our site, which includes a forum for updates and current discussion! www.marijuanagrowing.com

- **Google** William A. Albrecht, PhD, a famous agronomist who pointed out the direct relationship between soil fertility and human health. www.google.com

Plant Tissue Analysis

Analyzing plant tissue for nutrient accumulation and utilization is common among professional farmers and greenhouse growers. The tests cost less than $40 USD and help growers fine-tune fertilizer application. A small investment in periodic plant tissue analysis will lower fertilizer bills and increase yields, often substantially. Legal medicinal cannabis gardeners are also able to request plant tissue analysis from agricultural laboratories within states and countries that sanction medical cannabis.

Soil tests measure nutrient levels that are potentially available for uptake by roots.

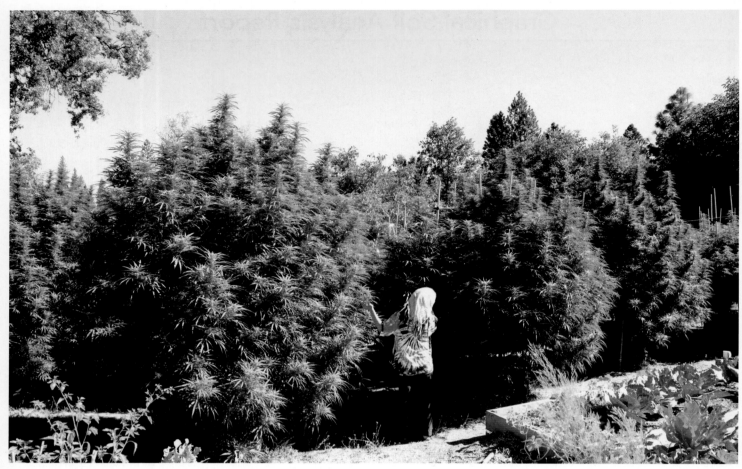

A soil test and the proper organic amendments before planting saved this gardener hundreds of dollars in fertilizer.

The test is normally performed before planting, and it does not measure the actual concentration of nutrients inside of plants. For example, nitrogen is often deficient in plants even though it may be readily available in the soil. A tissue analysis, on the other hand, will provide current data to make timely decisions.

Plant tissue analysis also helps ensure plants are not overfertilized. High concentrations of nitrogen, in particular, may affect human health because excess nitrates can convert to nitrites while being digested in the gut. Nitrates may react with other compounds to form nitrosamines that may be carcinogenic.

Fine-tuning fertilization programs, including micronutrient levels, is much easier when accurate information from analysis of plant tissue is available. Micronutrients are required in minute amounts, and an overdose could easily stunt a crop or significantly diminish yields. Soil gardeners are able to test soil, which gives them an idea of which nutrients may be lacking. They can use subsequent plant tissue analysis to concentrate on determining amounts of specific elements and how those elements are utilized by plants.

Hydroponic gardeners, who do not have soil tests at their disposal, find plant tissue analysis especially useful.

Plant tissue analysis often takes 1 to 2 weeks when a specimen is sent to a laboratory. When crops are grown for 10 to 12 weeks total, this might be 10 percent of the plant's life. But, nitrogen tests* can be completed on the spot with a handheld meter in the garden, and results are available immediately.

*A chlorophyll concentration meter measures chlorophyll content index (CCI) in foliage and the nitrogen content is extrapolated from this data. One molecule of chlorophyll contains four nitrogen atoms.

Texture and Types of Soil

To feel its texture, pick up a handful of moist outdoor soil and rub it between your fingers. Heavy clay soil will feel slick and greasy. Sandy soil feels grainy and rough. Silty soil will feel soft and spongy and be dark in color.

Pick up a handful of moist potting soil and gently squeeze it to feel the texture. The soil should barely stay together and have a sponge effect when you slowly open your hand to release the pressure. Potting soils that do not fulfill these requirements should be thrown out or amended.

The cation exchange capacity (CEC) of a growing medium is its capacity to hold cations that are available for uptake by the roots. The CEC is the number of cation charges held in 3.5 ounces (100 gm or 100 cc) of soil and is measured in milliequivalents (mEq) or centimoles/kg on a scale from 0 to 100. A CEC of zero means the substrate holds no available cations for roots. A CEC of 100 means the medium always holds cations available for uptake by roots. Growing mediums that carry a negative electrical charge are the best.

Cation exchange capacity is a calculated value that estimates the ability of a soil to attract, hold, and exchange cation elements; CEC values are reported in milliequivalents per 100 grams of soil (mEq/100 gm). Soil-sample testing laboratories report a value for the CEC. Use the CEC numeric value on your report and then compare the number to the graph below to find your soil type.

High-CEC soils hold more nutrients and water. But soils with high levels of clay (and high CEC readings) allow little room for oxygen and can slow root growth and nutrient uptake. If acidic, high-CEC soils also require more lime to buffer and lower pH.

Nutrients take more time to leach out of high-CEC soils.

Low-CEC soils hold nutrients poorly, which requires more frequent irrigation and lower volumes. These soils have a low capacity to retain cations. Add humus-based amendments to acidify and balance low-CEC soils.

Nutrients must be dissolved in (water) solution in order to be absorbed by roots. When dissolved, they are in a form called "ions." This means that they have electrical charges. An electrical charge is either positive (+) or negative (-). For example, table salt, sodium chloride (NaCl), becomes 2 ions when dissolved: sodium (Na+) and chloride (Cl-). The sodium ion with a positive (+) charge is called a "cation," and the chloride ion with a negative (-) charge is called an "anion." In chemistry, opposites attract and likes repel one another. In ionic form, nutrients are attracted to opposite charges—positive attracts negative and vice versa.

Soil chemistry can become very complex, and it is beyond the scope of this book to dig deeply into the subject. For

more information on the subject, check www.marijuanagrowing.com.

Use this table to estimate the CEC of your soil:

SOIL	MIN.	MAX.
	CEC	CEC
sand	1	4
sandy loam	5	8
silt loam	8	20
clay loam	20	40
clay	40	80

CEC of popular growing mediums measured in mEq/100 grams
- compost   90
- Sunshine Mix   90
- peat moss   80
- garden soil   70
- expanded clay   20
- vermiculite   20
- perlite   00
- rockwool   00

This list shows different growing mediums' ability to hold positive charges that are ready for root uptake. Note the zero CEC of perlite and rockwool. Roots must be constantly bathed in nutrients. Other mediums do not provide a constant flow of nutrients and the CEC regulates the ability to hold a positive charge to make nutrients available for root uptake.

Clay soil consists of very small, flat mineral particles that have a strong negative ionic charge. In fact, the negative electrical charge often ties up calcium, magnesium, potassium, and sodium in clay soil. Minute mineral particles pack tightly together, especially when wet, causing very slow drainage. Roots penetrate clay soil slowly, and damage from waterlogging is more common. Clay soil has little or no space for oxygen, the lack of which slows nutrient uptake. Clay soil can be very difficult to

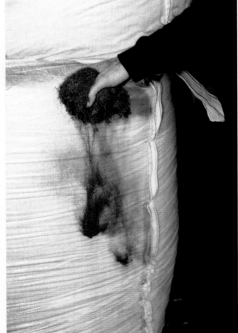

This soilless mix is super dry but light and powdery. It holds a lot of water and air at the same time.

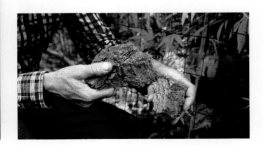

This handful of soil has everything necessary for strong plant growth.

This is very heavy clay soil. It is great for making pottery but horrible as garden soil.

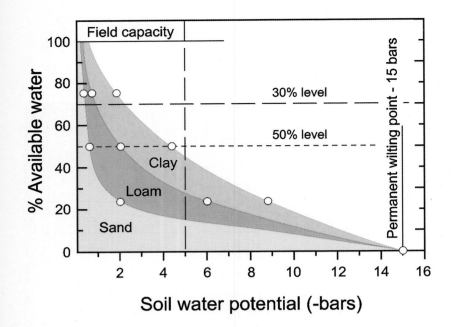

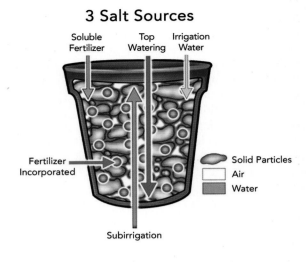

3 Salt Sources

Soluble Fertilizer

Top Watering

Irrigation Water

Fertilizer Incorporated

Solid Particles

Air

Water

Subirrigation

This cutaway drawing shows how roots penetrate the soil. Note: There must be enough air trapped in the soil to allow biological activity and absorption of nutrients.

till; it is often extremely heavy when wet and is known to clump up.

Amend clay soil with compost, manure, gypsum, etc. (See Organic Soil Amendments later in this chapter for a complete list.) Incorporating compost, manure, or other organic amendments in the fall is one of the best ways to improve clayey and poor-quality soils. Raised beds are also an excellent option to combat clay soil. Till clay soil when it is damp and workable, and add manure, compost, or both.

Sandy soil boasts the largest particles that permit good aeration and drainage. Drainage can be too fast if particles

are too big. The texture of sandy soil is somewhat gritty depending upon the size of its mineral particles. Sandy soil is easy to cultivate and warms quickly in the spring, but low water-retention rates mean that frequent watering is necessary. Amend sandy soil with compost and organic matter to help it retain water more evenly.

Silty soil is very fertile. It is composed of fine organic particles and minerals such as quartz. Silty soil is granular, like sandy soil, but it has more nutrients and offers better drainage. When silty soil is dry it has a smoother texture and looks like dark sand. This type of soil can hold more moisture and can at times become

compacted. It offers better drainage and is much easier to work with when moist.

Soils are seldom all clay, all sand, or all silt. They are a combination of different types. This table demonstrates the different percentages of soil combinations.

NAME OR TYPE OF SOIL	PARTICLE DIAMETER LIMITS
	USDA Classification
clay	Less than 0.002 mm
silt	0.002–0.05 mm
very fine sand	0.05–0.1 mm
fine sand	0.1–0.25 mm
medium sand	0.25–0.5 mm
coarse sand	0.5–1 mm
very coarse sand	1–2 mm

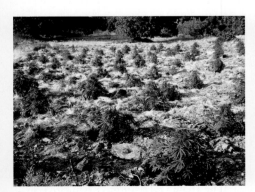

The hard, clayey, rocky soil above is packed with nutrients but restricts root growth and water drainage. Plants shown here are in sunken beds to conserve moisture.

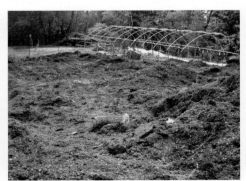

Beautiful peat-rich soil is ideal for planting. This greenhouse and the field in the foreground produce nice, big gardens of medicinal cannabis.

Other Soils

Loam soil is made up of sand, silt, and clay. Loam is considered by many to be the perfect soil. Its texture is often gritty, yet it retains plenty of air and water and drains well because of its different-sized particles. Depending upon its makeup, loam can range from heavy (clay) to light (sandy).

Peat (bog) soil is formed by the accumulation of dead and decayed organic matter. Found in rainy, marshy areas, the decomposition of organic matter in peat soil is blocked by soil acidity. Few nutrients are present even though peat soil is rich in organic matter. Peat soils are prone to waterlogging, so for best results, they must be mixed with other soils and compost before cannabis is planted.

Chalky soil is very alkaline in nature and is often packed with rocks. It is prone to dryness, and in summer chalky soil consumes much water and fertilizer. This soil also locks up iron and magnesium due to its high pH activity.

Alkali soils are packed with sodium carbonate, which is detrimental to cannabis growth. The farmland around my hometown is plagued with alkali soil. Many other regions in the world also suffer from alkali soil; the pH hovers around 8.5 and higher. Alkali salt is so abundant in many places that it appears as white powder that cakes up on the surface of soil. Alkali soils also significantly slow water absorption.

To "purge" alkali salt from soil, farmers cultivate with a tractor or tracked vehicle

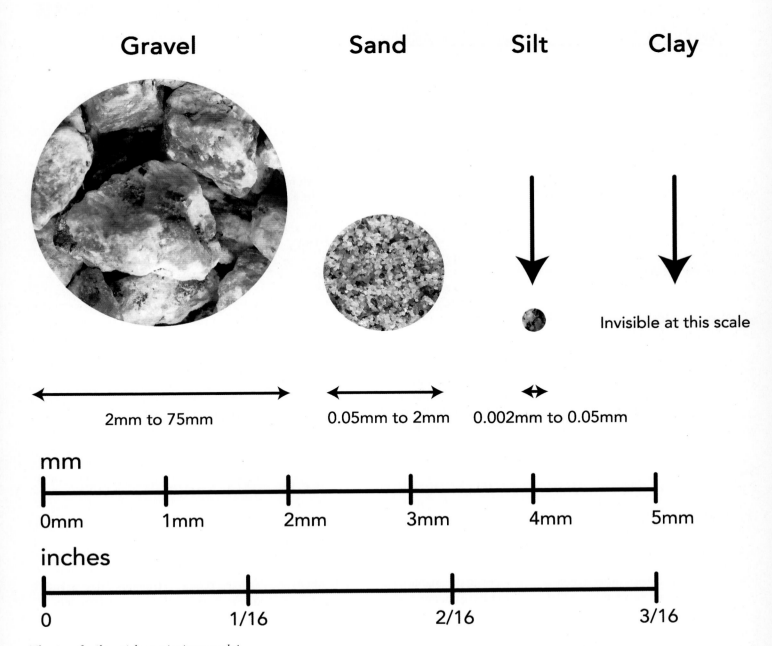

The size of soil particles varies immensely!

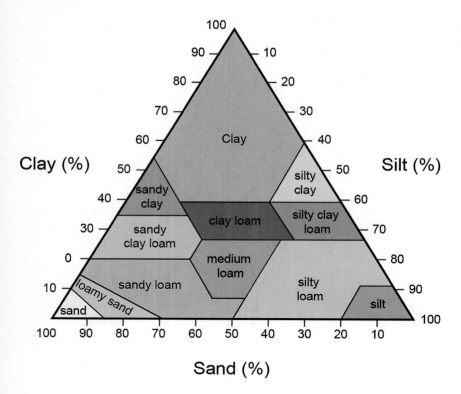

This soil pyramid demonstrates the diversity of most soils.

A simple pH chart shows the range in which most nutrients are available in soil.

equipped with 30- to 36-inch (76–91 cm) "ripping bars." Tilled fields are flood-irrigated with a foot (30.5 cm) or more of water to drive the alkali salts deep into the soil, beyond the depth of most roots. The salts rise to the surface over time, and the process is repeated every few years as needed.

Outdoor cannabis gardeners plagued with alkali soil should grow in large containers and amend alkali soils with acidic elements, including peat moss. Use as little alkali soil in the container as possible, and before planting, leach alkali soil heavily with water to wash out unwanted salts.

Soil pH
Potential hydrogen (pH) is a scale from 0 to 14 that measures the concentration of either hydrogen (H) ions or hydroxide (OH) ions. Zero is the most acidic, 7 is neutral (also known as *base*), and 14 most alkaline. Every full-point change in the logarithmic pH scale signifies a *tenfold* increase or decrease in acidity or alkalinity. For example, soil or water with a pH of 5.0 is 10 times more acidic than soil or water with a pH of 6.0. Water with a

pH of 5.0 is 100 times more acidic than water with a pH of 7.0. With a tenfold difference between each full point on the pH scale, accurate measurement and control is essential to ensure nutrient availability.

Cannabis grows best in soil with a pH from 6.5 to 7.0. Within this range cannabis can properly absorb and process all necessary available nutrients most efficiently. If the pH is too low (acidic), acid salts chemically bind nutrients (or, more correctly stated, the ion form changes in valence, or charge). The plant then only takes up a certain charged ion such as phosphate, the plant-available form (H_2PO_4-) converts to the unavailable form $HPO_4$2- on pH rise and achieves equilibrium at pH 7.2, and the roots are unable to absorb the nutrients. An alkaline soil with a high pH causes nutrients to become unavailable. Excess unused nutrients in soil also cause toxic salt buildup that limits water intake by roots. It can also make some elements available at toxic levels when pH drops below 5.4!

The pH of soil mixes is very important because it dictates the ability of specific

pH-sensitive bacteria. But I have experimented and irrigated well-managed organic soil with 8.0 pH water and higher. Once the rich organic soil absorbs the water, the soil life buffers the pH and it reverts back to 6.5 after a few minutes!

Hydroponic nutrient solutions perform best in a lower pH range than for soil. The **ideal pH range for hydroponics is from 5.8 to 6.8.** Some gardeners run the pH at lower levels and report no problems with nutrient uptake.

Measuring Soil pH
Measure pH with a litmus paper, a liquid pH reagent test kit, or electronic pH meter, all of which are available at most nurseries. When testing pH, take 2 or 3 samples and follow—to the letter—instructions supplied by the manufacturer. Soil test kits measure soil pH and primary nutrient content by mixing soil with a chemical reagent solution and comparing the color of the solution to a chart. Novice gardeners often have a difficult time achieving accurate measurements. Comparing the color of the soil/chemical mix to the color of the chart is often confusing. If you use one

of these kits, make sure to buy one with good, easy-to-understand instructions, and ask the sales clerk for exact recommendations on using it.

If using litmus paper, collect samples that demonstrate an average of the soil. Place the samples in clean jars, and then moisten the soil samples with distilled water that has a pH of 7.0. Place 2 pieces of the litmus paper in the muddy water. After 10 seconds, remove 1 strip of litmus paper. Wait a minute before removing the other one. Both pieces of litmus paper should register the same color. The litmus paper container should have a pH-color chart on the side. Match the color of the litmus paper with the colors on the chart to get a pH reading. Litmus paper will accurately measure the acidity of the substance to within a point or less. The pH readings will not be accurate if altered by water with a high or low pH, and the litmus paper could give a false reading if the fertilizer contains a color-tracing agent.

Liquid pH reagent test kits work by adding liquid drops of pH-sensitive dye to the nutrient solution. Mix by shaking and compare the color of the treated nutrient solution with a color chart. Such tests are a little difficult to read, but quite accurate.

Do not use phenolphthalein and phenol red test kits; they are not precise enough to measure and render an accurate pH value.

Adjusting Soil pH

For an accurate pH test with an electronic pH meter:

1. Clean the probes of the meter before and after each test, and wipe away any corrosion.

2. Water soil with distilled or neutral pH water before testing.

3. Pack the soil around the probes.

Lime amendments will raise pH and lower acidity, but too much lime can

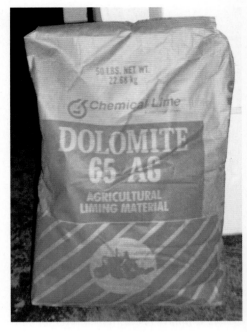

When planting, add 1 cup of fine dolomite lime to each cubic foot (1 ounce per gallon [30 ml per 4 L]) of planting medium to stabilize the pH and provide calcium and magnesium.

burn roots and make nutrients unavailable. If you need more than 1 full point of pH adjustment, check with local farmers, nurseries, or agricultural agencies for recommendations on lime application.

Lime application differs based on soil type. Some guidelines are:

• 35 pounds/300 square yards (16 kg/251 m²) very sandy soil

• 50 pounds/300 square yards (23 kg/251 m²) sandy soil

• 70 pounds 300 square yards (32 kg/251 m²) loam

• 80 pounds/ 300 square yards (36 kg/251 m²) heavy clay soil

*Rule of thumb: add 1 to 2 pounds (0.5–0.9 kg) of dolomite lime to each cubic foot (0.03 cm³) of soil.

Lowering alkaline levels is somewhat easier than raising the acid level. If your soil is too alkaline, 1.2 ounces (34 gm) of finely ground rock sulfur per square yard (90 cm²)* of sandy soil will reduce soil pH by 1 point. Other types of soil will need 3.6 ounces (100 gm) per square yard (90 cm²).

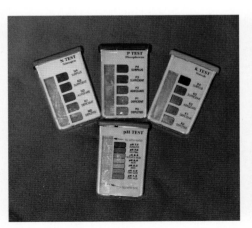

Litmus paper is relatively expensive and is fairly accurate.

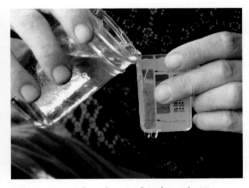

Mix water with a chemical in liquid pH reagent test kits.

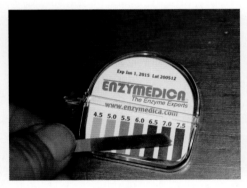

This simple N-P-K and pH reagent soil test kit is inexpensive and easy to use.

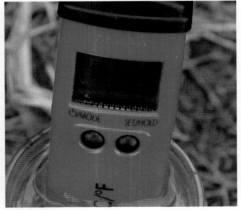

Electronic pH meters are economical and convenient. Also, remember to check the pH of irrigation water. See chapter 15, Meters, for complete information on electronic pH meters.

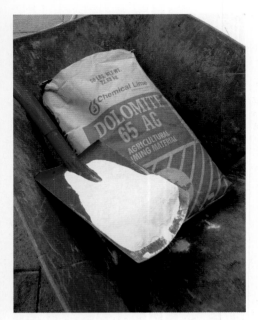

Dolomite lime is an essential additive for most garden soils and soilless mixes.

*1 cubic yard = 27 cubic feet
(1 m³ = 106 cm³) (1 cubic yard = 105 cm³)

Well-decomposed sawdust, composted leaves, and peat moss also help to acidify soil and lower pH.

Raising Soil pH

The most common way to raise pH both outdoors and indoors is to incorporate lime into the soil (see descriptions below of different kinds of lime). Other materials that raise soil pH include pulverized eggshells, clam and oyster shells, and wood ashes, all of which have a high pH. Both eggshells and oyster shells decompose extremely slowly and are not recommended. Wood ashes, with a pH of 9.0 to 11.0, are easy to overapply. They are also soluble and wash from soil quickly. Wood ashes from fireplaces are often adulterated with contaminants that are not plant-friendly.*

*Cannabis is a well-known accumulator plant that takes in heavy metals and sequesters toxins in vacuoles, which are impermeable. The heavy metals remain toxic. Cannabis was planted around Chernobyl, the toxic nuclear site in Russia, to absorb toxic radioactive heavy metals.

Agricultural Lime (aka Aglime, agricultural limestone, or garden lime) is made from pulverized limestone or chalk. Calcium carbonate is the active component, but it may also include calcium oxide, magnesium oxide, and magnesium carbonate. Aglime raises pH and ads calcium and possibly magnesium and trace nutrients. Aglime is usually available in larger particle sizes and takes much longer than finer grades to affect soil pH.

Calcitic lime is calcium, $CaCO_3$. Lime is calcium, calcium carbonate. Calcitic lime is just calcium, $CaCO_3$. Dolomite lime, on the other hand, is calcium and magnesium, $CaMg(CO_3)2$. If soil needs magnesium, apply dolomite lime. But many soils contain an adequate level to an abundance of magnesium but insufficient calcium and therefore require calcitic lime. Granular and coarse lime reacts slowly in soil. Apply lime to soil in the fall so that it has time to react. If applied in the spring it will not change pH for several months

Dolomite lime (calcium magnesium carbonate, $CaMg(CO_3)2$) stabilizes pH and adds calcium and magnesium. As long as it is thoroughly mixed into the soil, it is difficult to overapply. Dolomite has a neutral pH around 7.0, and does not raise the pH beyond 7.4, the upper range for carbonates. It stabilizes the pH safely. Compensate for acidic soil by mixing dolomite with soil before planting. It will buffer the pH, keeping it stable when applying mild acidic fertilizers. Dolomite does not prevent toxic-salt accumulation caused by impure water and fertilizer buildup. A proper fertilizer regimen and regular leaching helps wash away toxic salts. When purchasing, look for dolomite flour (powder), the finest fast-acting dustlike grade available. Coarse dolomite could take a year or more before it affects soil pH. Mix

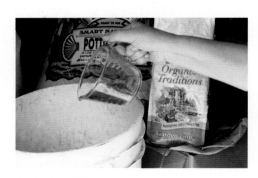

Agricultural lime

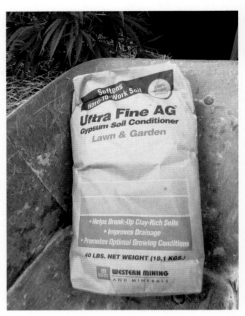

Gypsum is rich in calcium and works wonders in cannabis gardens.

dolomite flour thoroughly with the growing medium before planting. Improperly mixed, dolomite will stratify, forming a cake on soil surface or a subterranean layer that burns roots and repels water. Lime is sold as a grade of fineness with a sieve size of 10 to 100. When using different grades, the amounts are also adjusted, since 3000 pounds of course lime may equal 1000 pounds of a fine grade.

Hydrated or slaked lime (calcium hydroxide, $Ca(OH)2$) contains mainly calcium and might contain magnesium. It is improperly referred to as hydrated lime and is actually hydroxide of lime. As the word hydrated implies, this lime is water-soluble. Hydrated lime is more caustic (quickly burns skin) than quicklime and is usually made by adding water to burnt lime, forming a hydrate. It absorbs water readily from the air, and as a result becomes increasingly difficult to handle. Fast-acting hydrated lime alters pH quickly, but the results last about 2 weeks and it is caustic enough to burn skin. If you decide to use it, be very careful. Mix it thoroughly with warm water, and for fast results apply small amounts with each watering. At most, use a mix of 0.25 cup (6 cl) hydrated lime and 0.75 cup (18 cl) dolomite lime. Any larger quantity will toxify soil and stunt or kill plants.

Hydrated lime is immediately available, whereas the slower acting dolomite buffers the pH over the long term. My favorite use of hydrated lime is for a garden room fungicide. Sprinkle it on the floor and around the room. It also is used as a fungistat, killing fungus on contact.

Quicklime (calcium oxide, CaO) is made by burning rock limestone in kilns. This highly caustic lime should never be used in the garden. Quicklime reacts with water, yielding slaked (calcium hydroxide) lime. Organic certification agencies prohibit the use of quicklime. Although fast-acting, the effect is short lived and it does not have the buffering abilities of dolomite lime.

Gypsum (calcium sulfate, $CaSO_4 \cdot 2(H_2O)$ is the "magic ingredient" in many soil mixes. It is an amendment, conditioner, and fertilizer. Gypsum lowers the pH of sodium-rich soils and lowers the level of exchangeable sodium. It can also raise soil pH, albeit slowly. Here is a great link about gypsum: www.usagypsum.com/agricultural gypsum.aspx. See chapter 12, *Outdoors*, and chapter 13, *Case Studies*, for more information.

Do not mix fast-acting hydrated lime and fertilizer. At best, acidic fertilizers will cancel the effects of lime. For example, urine is slightly acidic. When it is dispersed into a toilet that was recently cleaned with bleach, which is very alkaline, it results in an unpleasant odor and neutralizing reaction. The same is true with fertilizers.

To raise pH 1 point, add 3 cups (65 cl) of fine dolomite or agricultural lime to 1 cubic foot (30 L) of soil. An alternate fast-acting mix would be to add 2.5 cups (590 cl) of dolomite and 0.5 cup (12 cl) of hydrated lime to one cubic foot (28.3 L) of soil.

Guidelines to raise soil pH from 5.5 to 6.5 in different types of soil:

Soil Type	kg/m²	lb/yd²
clay	0.9	1.67
sand	0.7	1.29
silt	0.8	1.47
organic	1.1	2.03
peat	1.7	3.13

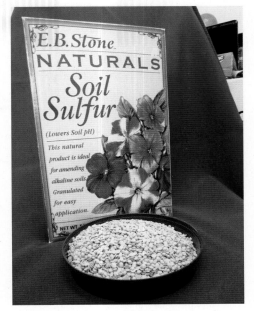

Sulfur is used to lower soil pH.

Lowering Soil pH

Soils with a pH above 7.0 are generally considered alkaline and must be lowered to accommodate robust cannabis growth. Use sulfur in the form of iron sulfate or magnesium sulfate to lower pH. Sulfur is readily available at nurseries or garden centers in geographic areas with high-pH soil. Do not confuse "elemental sulfur" (iron sulfate and magnesium sulfate) with sulfur used as a "plant nutrient." Aluminum sulfate is often recommended because it lowers pH instantly as it dissolves in the soil. Cannabis can tolerate very little aluminum. *Do not* use aluminum sulfate. Other acids in liquid, crystal, and powder form can be used to lower pH, but they kill soil life in organic soil and are not advised. See chapter 23, *Container Culture & Hydroponics*, and chapter 20, *Water*, for more information.

Needing to lower pH is not as common as needing to raise it. Fertilizers, including manures, coconut coir, peat, and many organic amendments, are naturally acidic and lower the pH of the growing medium. In fact, adding too much manure to soil actually acidifies the soil so much that nutrients become locked out. Commercial potting soils and soilless mixes are generally acidic and their pH seldom needs to be lowered.

Slower ways to lower pH include adding cottonseed meal, pine needles, shredded leaves, sawdust, or peat moss. All have advantages and disadvantages. Cottonseed meal also adds nitrogen to soil. Pine needles take a long time to break down. Unless well-rotted, sawdust consumes nitrogen in the soil, and peat moss (pH 3) is nutrient-poor and expensive.

Soil Temperature
Heating Soil
The biological processes for nutrient transformation and availability are controlled by soil temperature and moisture. Raising the soil temperature speeds the chemical process and can hasten nutrient uptake. Ideally, the soil temperature should range from 65°F to 70°F (18°C–21°C) for the most chemical activity. However, microorganisms living in the soil are very active within

POUNDS OF ELEMENTAL SULFUR NEEDED TO LOWER THE PH OF A LOAM SOIL TO A DEPTH OF SIX INCHES						
Current pH		Desired pH				
lb per 100 ft²	kg per 9.3 m²	6.5	6	5.5	5	4.5
8	3.62	3	4	5.5	7	8
7.5	3.4	4	3.5	4.5	6	7
7	3.17	1	2	3.5	5	6
6.5	2.94		1	2.5	4	4.5
6	2.72			1	2.5	3.5

For sandy soils, reduce amount by 0.33; for clay soils, increase amount by 0.5.

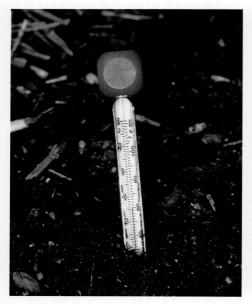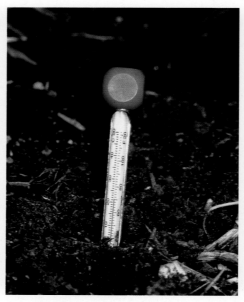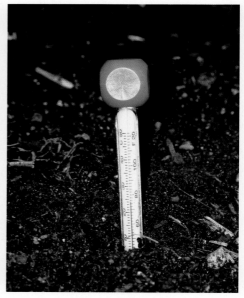

Each image of the thermometer was taken in sequence, an hour apart. Note how the temperature of the soil climbs from 60°F (15.5°C) to 75°F (24°C) in just 2 hours. High soil temperatures stifle growth.

a temperature range of 80.6°F to 89.6°F (27°C –32°C).

Raised beds and containers that are 6 inches (15.2 cm) or more above ground level are affected by ambient air temperature and thus stay warmer. With raised beds, gardeners can plant 4 to 6 weeks earlier and can grow 4 to 6 weeks later in most climates. See chapter 12, *Outdoors*, for more information.

Direct sunlight shining on raised beds and containers heats outside margins quickly. Shade your garden beds and pots to avoid overheating them. Ambient temperatures above 92°F (33.3°C) cause excessive vapor pressure within the roots, which can cause damage. At high temperatures roots send stress signals to shut down much chemistry in leaves before damage can occur.

Soil temperatures that climb above 75°F (24°C) dehydrate roots, and at higher temperatures the roots literally cook! It is relatively easy to heat the soil in a pot. If the artificial light or any heat source is too close to small pots, it can easily heat up the outside layer of soil where the majority of the feeder roots are located. Once destroyed, roots take at least 2 weeks to grow back. When growing a cannabis crop that takes 8 weeks to flower, 2 weeks accounts for a quarter of

the flowering cycle. Even the color of the container, such as black or white, will change the rate at which the growing medium warms.

Use soil-heating cables or a heating pad to warm soil in containers. Fasten heating cables to a board or table and set a heat-conducting pad on top of the cables to distribute heat evenly. Set cuttings and seedlings in shallow flats or growing trays on top of the heat-conducting pad. The added heat speeds root growth of clones and seedlings when soil temperature is below 65°F (18°C). Carefully monitor soil heat so that it does not climb beyond 70°F (21°C). To control heat more precisely, it may be necessary to attach heating cables and pads to a timer that turns them on and off at 15- to 30-minute intervals.

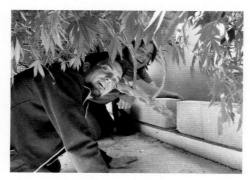

Bricks and a white stone wall supply additional heat to this large cannabis plant.

Soil heating cables cost less than soil heating pads but must be mounted on a board, whereas the pads are ready to use. Most commercial nurseries carry cables, and hydroponic stores carry heating pads.

Cooling Soil

Unless measures are taken, soil in containers heats to the ambient level of garden rooms and greenhouses, especially when there is little deviation between day and nighttime temperatures. To cool soil naturally, set containers on cold concrete or earthen floors. They will stay nearly as cold as the concrete or earth, which is usually cooler than the ambient temperature. Keep garden room temperatures below 75°F (24°C) to help keep containers cool. Irrigating containers with cool water will also help cool the soil.

Outdoors and in greenhouses, soil in containers that receive direct sunlight warms rapidly to dangerous levels that cook roots. Set containers inside other containers to insulate soil from blazing sunshine. Or insulate containers with Styrofoam or a similar material.

Cold soil, below 50°F (10°C), slows water and nutrient uptake and stifles growth. Gardeners often overwater when the soil is too cold, which further

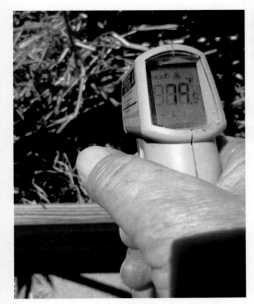

A 6-inch (15 cm) layer of straw mulch on top of the soil cooled the soil surface from 120°F to 79°F (49°C–26°C).

slows growth and can waterlog roots. Damage to roots often goes unnoticed. Even if realized immediately, however, plants could take 2 or more weeks to recover. Root temperatures below 40°F (4°C) make water expand, which causes cell damage and stifles growth.

Increase soil temperature by moving pots up off the floor a few inches. Set them on an insulating board or piece of Styrofoam. Use soil heating cables or pads if necessary.

Soil Amendments

Soil amendments increase the soil's air-, water-, and nutrient-retaining abilities. Amendments with a high CEC rating hold nutrients and water well and release them as needed. Soil amendments fall into 2 categories: mineral and organic.

Mineral amendments are near neutral on the pH scale (7.0) and contain few, if any, available nutrients. Mineral amendments decompose through weathering and erosion. They have the advantage of creating no bacterial activity to alter nutrient content and pH of the growing medium. Dry mineral amendments are also very lightweight and much easier to move in and out of awkward spaces.

Perlite works especially well for aerating the soil. This is a good medium to increase drainage during vegetative and flowering growth. Perlite has a low CEC rating, and it does not promote fertilizer-salt buildup. See chapter 23, *Container Culture & Hydroponics,* for more information on perlite.

Expanded clay pellets (calcined clay, hadite, Hydroclay, and similar fired clay products) expedite drainage and hold air within the growing medium. See chapter 23, *Container Culture & Hydroponics,* for more information on expanded clay.

Sand is heavy and has a low CEC rating. Use no more than 10 percent as a soil amendment because it tends to wash into pockets. Sand will also accumulate on soil surface. See chapter 23, *Container Culture & Hydroponics,* for more information on sand.

Vermiculite is a good soil amendment to hold moisture, but if used in large quantities it can be very expensive. It is rich in potassium (K) and magnesium (Mg). It has a high CEC rating and holds water, nutrients, and air within its fiber, and it gives body to fast-draining soils. Alone, fine vermiculite holds too much water for cuttings but works well when mixed with a fast-draining medium. See chapter 23,

Container Culture & Hydroponics, for more information on vermiculite.

Organic Soil Amendments

Organic soil amendments overall have a high CEC rating. They contain carbon, and they break down through bacterial activity, slowly yielding humus as an end product. Humus is a soft, spongy material that binds minute soil particles together, improving the soil texture and increasing nutrient uptake.

New, actively composting organic soil amendments require nitrogen to carry on bacterial decomposition. Organic amendments are not always well composted and often contain high, even toxic, levels of salts. Check bulk amendments/fertilizers/soils with a sodium (Na) meter to ensure that they contain less than 50 ppm of sodium.

Amendments must contain at least 1.5 percent nitrogen or they will "rob" nitrogen from the soil. When using organic amendments, make sure they are thoroughly composted (at least 1 year) and releasing nitrogen rather than pilfering it from the soil. A dark, rich color is a good sign of fertility.

At a reputable nursery, purchase quality organic amendments that are OMRI-approved* (or approved by a similar third-party organic-certifying agency). Look carefully at the descriptive text on the bag to see if the contents are sterilized and guaranteed to contain no harmful insects, larvae, eggs, and fungi or bad microorganisms. Contaminated soil causes many problems that are easily averted by using a clean mix.

*Organic Materials Review Institute (OMRI) is the premier independent

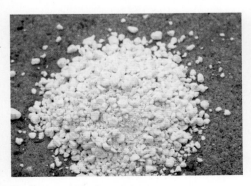

Perlite

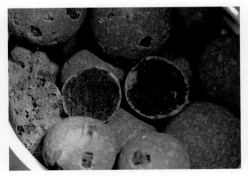

Expanded clay pellets

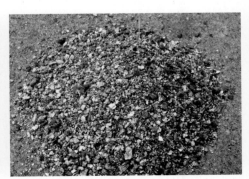

Vermiculite is available in fine, medium, and coarse grades.

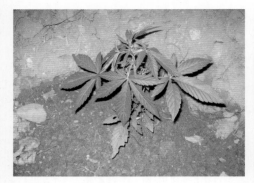

A little organic soil amendment can help immensely. Just make sure the planting holes are big enough so that heavy clay soil does not restrict root growth.

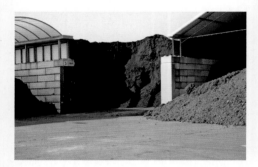

Mountains of peat-based soil—seen here at the Gold Label facility in the Netherlands—are awaiting processing into top-quality grow medium mix.

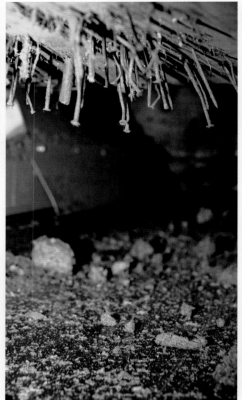

A big, powerful magnet removes an incredible amount of ferrous metals from soil before processing. Check your soil for ferrous metals by rolling a magnet around in it for a few minutes. You may be surprised.

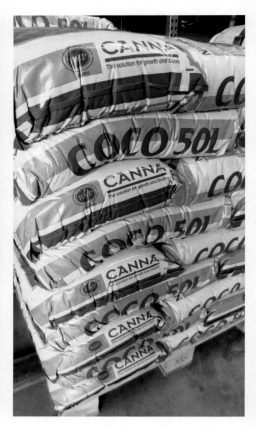

Coco coir was popularized in the cannabis cultivation industry by Canna, a Dutch company that continues to lead the industry.

agency that provides organic certification for growers, manufacturers and suppliers in North America. Check for a similar agency in your country. www.omri.org.

Buyer beware! Batches of commercially available soil and amendments are not always mixed consistently. Weather—heat, cold, rain—diseases, and pests can also alter the content of bulk and bagged potting soils that are exposed to such elements. Often when a company has a big demand for their products, they do not have enough bulk materials to mix the soil and therefore include second-class materials that are not completely composted or that contain high levels of salts.

Organic amendments break down after a year or less of use, losing much of their volume and becoming compacted. They also become contaminated. If reusing amended soil, see "Recycling Potting Soil," on page 320, for guidelines.

Bark chips, bark dust, and wood fiber are acidic and may use available nitrogen in the soil to decompose. Mycorrhizal fungi, *Trichoderma*, and many other decomposers break down bark chips. In general, cannabis prefers bacterial activity rather than fungal activity in the soil. There is virtually no CEC in the bark chips until after the breakdown into organic acids and such. Bark chips work well to impart antiseptic activity and increase airspace.

Coconut fiber is an excellent soil amendment because it holds so much water and air at the same time. Add to soil and soil mixes in garden soil or in organic mineral soil container mixes. Many gardeners prefer inexpensive coco that has been pressed into bricks because they are easy to store and transport. See chapter 23, *Container Culture & Hydroponics*, for more information on coco.

Compost and leaf mold have a medium to high CEC and are usually rich in

organic nutrients and beneficial organisms that speed nutrient uptake. When not allowed to heat to 160°F (71°C), compost can be full of harmful pests and diseases. A single cutworm in a container can kill a defenseless plant before migrating to another pot. Be extremely careful when using outdoor compost indoors.

Well-composted organic matter amends texture and supplies nutrients. Leaf mold, garden compost (at least 1 year old), and many types of thoroughly composted manure usually contain enough nitrogen for their decomposition needs and release nitrogen rather than using it.

Mushroom compost is an inexpensive soil amendment with a high CEC, and it is full of nutrients. Mushroom compost is sterilized chemically to provide a clean medium for mushroom growth. After serving its purpose as a mushroom growing medium, it is discarded. On average, mushroom compost contains low levels of nitrogen (N), potassium (P), potash (K), calcium (Ca), magnesium (Mg), and iron (Fe).

By law, mushroom compost is required to sit fallow for 2 years or more to allow all the harmful sterilants to leach out. After lying fallow for several years, mushroom compost is very fertile and contains many beneficial microorganisms. Check your local nursery or extension service for a good source of mushroom compost. Some of the most abundant harvests I have seen were grown in mushroom compost.

Manure: Barnyard manure, a great fertilizer for outdoor gardens, often contains toxic levels of salt and copious quantities of weed seeds and fungus spores that disrupt an indoor garden. If using manure, purchase it in bags that guarantee its contents. There are many kinds of manure: cow, horse, rabbit, and chicken, to name a few. When mixing manures as amendments do not add more than 10 to 15 percent to avoid salt buildup and overfertilization. Manures purchased in bulk should be checked with a sodium (Na) meter to ensure they do not contain excessive amounts (more than 50 ppm). The nutrient content of manures varies depending upon the animal's diet and the decomposition factors.

NOTE: Green or fresh manures require composting for a minimum amount of time, based on the animal source, and can range up to five years with chicken manure. Ammonium levels will be very high until composting occurs.

See "Manure" in chapter 21, *Nutrients*, for more information on manures and other additives.

Peat is one of the most common soil amendments both in container (soilless and soil) gardens and outdoor soil gardens. Although bulky, large bags and compressed bails of peat are available virtually everywhere at a fair price. See chapter 23, *Container Culture & Hydroponics*, for more information on peat.

Soil Mixes

Outdoor soil mixes that incorporate garden soil, compost, manure, coco peat, and rock powders, grow some of the biggest and best cannabis plants in the world. Outdoor soil mixes should be mixed a few months early and left in the hole to blend and mature. Remember, outdoor organic soil mixes are full of life!

The following recipes were given to me by a good friend who is a wise lifelong gardener. Here are his complete organic fertilizers (COF) and soil mixes for growing medicinal cannabis organically indoors, outdoors, and in containers within greenhouses. Make sure to mix the components thoroughly before applying.

Organic Soil Mix
All measurements are by volume
- 1/3 best organic garden soil
- 1/3 coco coir hydrated with a strong commercial fertilizer solution such as Canna Terra Vega
- 1/3 well-rotted, sifted organic compost

To each 5 gallons (19 L) of mix add 1 cup (237 ml) of COF.

Complete Organic Fertilizer (COF) Mix
- 1 quart (1 L) high-calcium aglime
- 0.5 quart (0.5 L) gypsum
- 1 quart (1 L) soft rock phosphate
- 0.33 cup (78 ml) potassium sulfate
- 3 quarts (3 L) canola seed meal
- 2 teaspoons (10 ml) borax or a smaller quantity of Solubor (1 gm actual boron)
- 1 teaspoon (5 ml) zinc sulfate
- 1 teaspoon (5 ml) manganese sulfate
- 2 teaspoons (10 ml) iron sulfate
- 0.5 teaspoon (2.5 ml) copper sulfate
- 1 quart (1 L) kelp meal

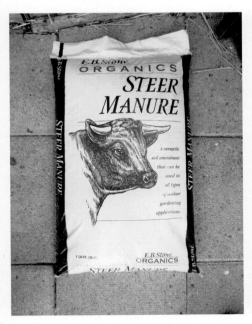

Steer manure contains low levels of nutrients and is an excellent soil amendment.

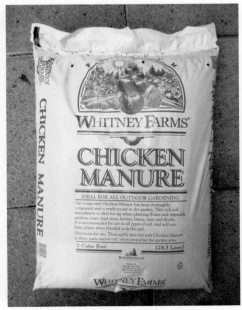

Well-composted chicken manure is a favorite organic fertilizer and soil amendment.

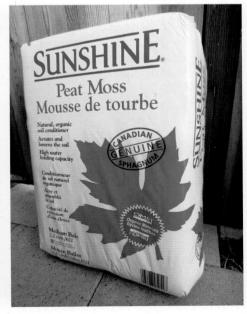

Peat is the base of many commercial soils and soilless mixes.

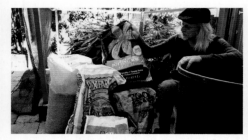

Mixing soil is best done outdoors or in an open area.

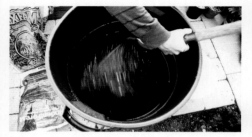

Blend soil in a large container.

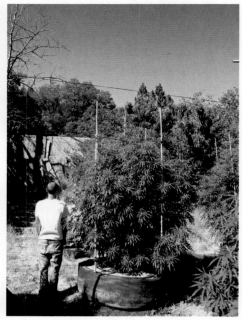

This healthy plant is the product of a good soil mix in a large container.

In indoor gardens and greenhouses, outdoor soil mixes often create problems. Soil dug up in the backyard and used to fill containers usually drains poorly and retains too much water and not enough air. Problems are compounded when this soil is mixed with garden compost that is full of harmful microorganisms and pests. The end results are low yields and possible crop failure.

Avoid soil-mix problems by purchasing all the components in sealed plastic bags. Use garden soil or compost only if they are top quality and devoid of harmful pests and diseases. Use only the richest, darkest garden soil with a good texture. Amend the soil to improve water and nutrient retention and drainage.

Solarize garden soil by setting it out in the sun in a plastic bag or a shallow 6-inch-deep (15 cm) bed and then covering it with plastic. Turn the bag occasionally to heat it up on all sides. Make sure the entire bag receives full sun and heats up to at least 160°F (71°C) for a minimum of 2 hours, or 120°F (49°C) for 3 to 4 weeks.

Lime: Do not use dolomite lime! Use only high-calcium lime and avoid magnesium. Fineness of grind is essential. Use 100-mesh screened lime.

Soft rock phosphate (SRP) is also essential. It is by far the best form that is acceptable to organics. The source of SRP is Nutri-Tech Solutions, www.nutri-tech.com.au.

Boron: Borax is 10 percent boron. At 2 teaspoons at a time, 1 kilogram of Borax from the supermarket might last months. Solubor supplies 20 percent boron, but if used, you need to calculate how much of it is needed to deliver 1 gram of actual boron.

Zinc sulfate is deliquescent; it absorbs moisture from the air and turns into a sloppy mess. Avoid such problems by storing it in an airtight container.

Measuring: There are 2 "dangerous" elements in this mix: boron and copper. These must be measured very accurately.

Tom Hill Mix

This mix was given to me by Tom Hill, a Northern California medical cannabis gardener. The mix is for 50 cubic feet

(1,416 L) and will fill six, 300-gallon (1,136 L) containers.

25 bags, 1.5 cu ft each (42.5 L) of quality organic potting soil
4 cu ft (113.3 L) chicken manure
4 cu ft (113.3 L) perlite
50 lb (22.7 kg) steamed bone meal
20 lb (9 kg) gypsum

See "Brix Mix" in chapter 21, *Nutrients.*

There are many more soil mixes listed on our website forum. Check out www.marijuanagrowing.com.

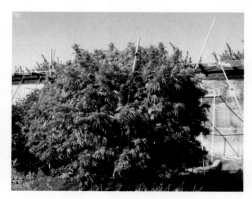

Tom is an excellent gardener, and you can see that his soil mix grows big, strong, healthy plants!

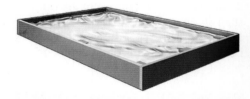

Solarizing soil will kill most all the undesirables.

Steam sterilization is the fastest sterilization method and is the method most commonly used by greenhouse professionals. It requires a strong source of steam that will completely permeate the medium, and the growing medium must be completely enclosed. Steam the medium so that it heats to at least 140°F (60°C) for at least 2 hours.

You can also sterilize soil by laying it out on a Pyrex plate and baking it at 160°F (71°C) for 10 minutes or microwaving it for 2 minutes at the highest setting. It is much easier to purchase quality potting soil at a nursery.

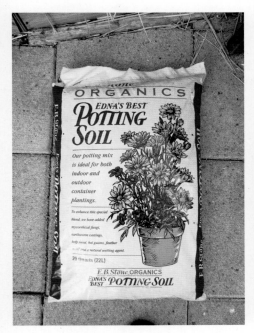

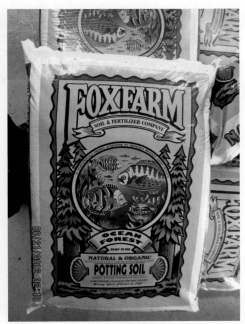

Organic potting soil is available from many different suppliers, with significant variation in quality.

Regardless of the brand of potting soil, always check its pH and sodium level.

amendments in this chapter and "Fertilizers" in chapter 21, *Nutrients*.

Blend soil components when dry to evenly disperse them into the mix. Add a light spray of water to dampen dust. To give an example of how long to mix soil, a spoonful of fritted trace elements in a cubic yard (m²) of soil requires at least 5 minutes of mixing by hand.

Caution! Fritted micronutrients are on glass particles. These are high in potassium and can overload the ratio. Sensitive cannabis varieties are easy to burn.

Here are two good soil mixes from Vic High, an expert medical cannabis gardener.

Vic High Mix #1
- 1 bail (3.8 cu ft [107 L]) Sunshine #2 or Pro-Mix or similar product
- 0.5 gallon (2 L) steamed bone meal – P
- 3.8 quarts (3.6 L) blood meal – N
- 1.3 cups (31 cl) Epsom salts – Mg
- 3.5 cups (83 cl) dolomite lime – Ca & Mg + buffering
- 1 tablespoon (17.8 ml) fritted trace elements
- 1 cubic foot (28.3 L) chicken manure – N + trace elements

Mix thoroughly, moisten, and let sit 1 to 2 weeks before use.

Vic High Mix #2
- 1 bail (3.8 cu ft [107 L]) Sunshine #2 or Pro-Mix or similar product
- 8 cups (1.9 L) bone meal
- 4 cups (1 L) blood meal
- 1.3 cups (31 cl) Epsom salts – Mg
- 3.5 cups (83 cl) dolomite lime – Ca & Mg + buffering
- 1 teaspoon (0.5 cl) fritted trace elements
- 4 cups (1 L) kelp meal
- 20 lb (9 kg) pure worm castings

Mix thoroughly, moisten, and let sit 1 to 2 weeks before use.

In regard to the above-listed ingredients, blood and bone meal are inexpensive sources of nitrogen and phosphorus. Kelp meal contains more than *60 available* (trace) elements. Worm castings

Potting Soil

Well-formulated, high-quality potting soil stored in a sealed bag frequently has the proper texture, a stable pH, and a small supply of nutrients. Often these soils are fortified with trace elements and also contain low levels of macro- and secondary nutrients. The proper porous texture allows good root penetration, water retention, and drainage. Agricultural lime or dolomite lime keeps pH stable. Many potting soils are formulated with a wetting agent to evenly retain adequate water and air. Avoid using potting soils for longer than 4 months, because their properties tend to degrade.

Since soil is heavy, transportation costs tend to keep it somewhat localized. Ask your nursery person for help in selecting a quality potting soil for fast-growing cannabis or annual flowers or vegetables.

Avoid potting soils with more than 10 percent tree bark or wood fiber. Potting soils in the eastern USA, for example, often contain high levels of wood fiber. Such soils with hold water well but their pH can fluctuate substantially. The size and shape of bark varies, and its decomposition by carbon and microbes is uneven. Furthermore, wood fiber re-

quires nitrogen to decompose, which depletes the nitrogen intended for plants. Such soils also promote an environment that is conducive to perennial "woody" plant growth rather than herbaceous annual (cannabis) plant growth.

Buyer Beware! Potting soil that has been stored outdoors is subject to direct sunlight and moisture. Any life in the organic soil could easily be compromised. Holes or tears in the plastic let moisture and adulterants enter the bag of "sterile" potting soil.

Upon purchase, always check potting soils—bagged or in bulk—with a pH meter and a sodium (Na) meter to ensure that the pH is within a safe range to grow cannabis, and that it does not contain excessive sodium (more than 50 ppm).

Read the nutrient description on the label—carefully—before purchasing.

Mixing Potting Soils

Mixing custom potting soil saves you money, and it allows you to use specific amendments and fertilizers to reduce complications and their subsequent workload. See discussion of specific

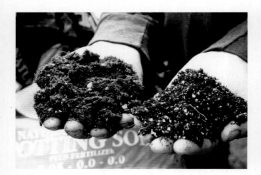

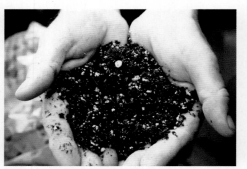

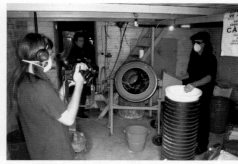

The difference between these potting soils is striking. The one on the right, with more perlite, drains best.

This soil mix is high in perlite and dark, rich elements. It will drain well and hold plenty of nutrients and water for plants.

Rent a commercial cement mixer to mix large quantities of soil.

are also a great source of micronutrients. Bat guano is expensive; use sparingly as a top dressing during the first week of flowering.

Use a layer of sand on top of soil to quell fungus gnat growth. Or use fungus gnat predators (*Hypoaspis miles*); once established they control fungus gnats, thrips, and mites.

Caution! Do not use cheap or discounted low-quality potting soil. These soils can be full of weed seeds, pests, and diseases. In addition, they hold water unevenly and drain poorly. The latest trend in "cheap" potting soils is to use composted garbage in the mix. Ultimately, saving a few pennies on soil will cost many headaches, might result in lower yields, and can even cause crop failure. Most potting soils supply transplanted seedlings and clones with enough nutrients for the first 2 to 4 weeks of growth. After that, supplemental fertilization is necessary to retain rapid, robust growth.

Adding 0.5 cup (11.8 cl) per cubic foot (28.3 L) of fine-grade dolomite lime to buffer and stabilize the pH is a good garden practice.

Trace elements in fortified soil and soilless mixes can wash out and should be replenished with chelated elements the instant deficiency signs occur. Organic gardeners often add their own blends of trace elements in mixes that contain seaweed (including kelp), guanos, and manures. However, be extremely careful *not* to overapply.

Recycling Potting Soil

At right is a recipe from Vic High for recycling soil used indoors and in greenhouses. Recycling potting soil may cause problems, the most common of which are pests and diseases, growing-medium compaction, and poor drainage. Recycling indoor and outdoor potting soil to use outdoors is much less problematic. The soil must be hot composted or sterilized with heat or steam to kill undesirable diseases and pests. Nutrients must be replenished too. New amendments often have to be added to increase water retention and to avoid compaction and undesirable CEC levels in most soils, but not necessarily in clay-based mineral soils. Carefully monitor and balance pH in peat-based soils.

Simply screening out roots or reusing the soil "as is" practically guarantees problems with pests and diseases. Even reusing half or a third of the old soil and adding new amendments can be problematic. For best results, the soil must be hot composted. Peat-based soils decom-

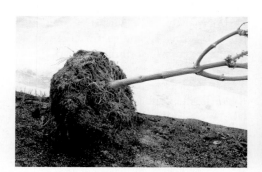

Even when planted in Mother Earth, the bulk of roots are located around the stem. Roots spread out quite a bit, but they are not usually as dense as with plants grown in containers.

pose and become more acidic. Fertilizer salt buildup is also a problem if the soil is not leached well enough with water.

Caution! Residual nitrogen that is hot composted will usually convert to the toxic nitrite form and kill the plants.

Organic soils rich in soil life can easily be mixed together and hot composted for 3 to 4 months. Once composted, mix the following into every 50 gallons (190 L) of soil.

- 2.5 cups (59 cl) dolomite
- 0.5 cup (11.8 cl) Epsom salts
- 2.1 quarts (2 L) bone meal
- 3.8 quarts (1 L) blood meal
- 3.8 quarts (1 L) kelp meal
- 1 teaspoon (0.5 cl) fritted trace elements
- Enough perlite to regain original drainage qualities

Outdoors: Used indoor soil makes excellent outdoor potting soil when broken up and mixed with compost. Let

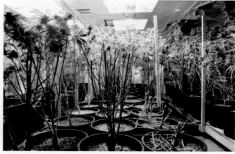

Soil from these indoor plants will be moved outdoors, and their stems will be ground up to be mixed into the outdoor garden soil.

the soil compost outdoors for at least three months before using. Do not reuse depleted soil "as is" in outdoor pots. The same problems that occur indoors when reusing soil also happen outdoors.

Dry soil is lighter and easier to transport than wet soil. Cut stems off at or below the soil line before moving dry, used soil out to incorporate in the outdoor garden. If mixed into a vegetable or flower garden, simply remove used soil from containers and till it into the top few inches of garden soil. Drench soil with dilute dark food coloring so white perlite is not unsightly. White perlite in an outdoor garden could call unwanted attention to an indoor garden.

Propagation Cubes and Pellets

Rockwool root cubes, peat pellets, and Oasis blocks are preformed containers that make it easy to root cuttings, start seedlings, and then transplant them. Root cubes and peat pots also help encourage strong root systems. Peat pots are small, compressed peat moss containers that have an outer wall of expandable plastic netting. When

watered, a peat pellet pops up into a seedling pot.

Place a seed or cutting in a moist peat pot or root cube. If the little container does not have a planting hole, make one with a chopstick, large nail, or something similar. Set the seed or clone stem in the hole. Crimp the top over the seed or around the stem to ensure constant contact with the medium. In 1 to 3 weeks, roots grow and show through the side of the cube. Cut the nylon mesh from peat pots before it becomes entangled with roots. To transplant, set the peat pot or root cube in a predrilled hole in a rockwool block or into a larger pot. Clones and seedlings suffer little or no transplant shock when properly transplanted.

Check moisture levels in peat pots and root cubes daily. Keep them evenly moist but not drenched. Root cubes and peat pots do not contain any nutrients. Seedlings do not require nutrients for the first week or two. Feed seedlings after the first week, and feed clones as soon as they are rooted.

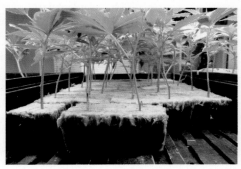

For many professional clone makers, Rockwool is the preferred growing medium in which to root cuttings.

Coarse sharp sand, fine vermiculite, and perlite work well to root cuttings. Sand and perlite are fast draining, which helps prevent damping-off. Vermiculite holds water longer and makes cloning easier. A good mix is one third of each: sand, fine perlite, and fine vermiculite. Premade seed starter mixes sold under such brand names as Sunshine Mix and Terra-Lite are the easiest and most economical mediums in which to root clones and start seedlings. Soilless mix also allows for complete control of critical nutrient and root-stimulating hormone additives, which are essential to asexual propagation.

Used, Indoor Soil Disposal

Disposing of used growing medium can be inconvenient for indoor gardeners. Soilless mixes and soils often contain perlite, which is unsightly in outdoor gardens. Dead roots must also be ground up in order to avoid other soil problems.

Dry soil is lighter and easier to work with and transport. Press and rub dry soil through a 0.25- to 0.5-inch screen to remove roots, stems, and foliage Screened soil is easier to handle, contain, and transport. Some city gardeners actually place used soil in a trash compacter to reduce size and make it more manageable. Please do not dispose of used soil in the trash. Dump it where it will benefit other plants. Always separate transport bags from soil before disposal. Reuse the bags.

Used indoor growing mediums make excellent outdoor amendments when

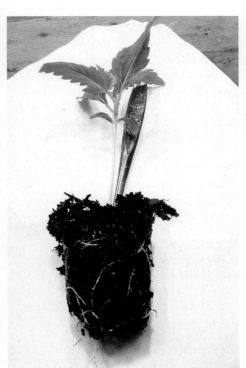

This little seedling was grown in a rooting flat along with 50 others. A spoon was used to lift it out of the container for transplanting.

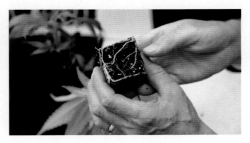

This clone is well rooted and prime for transplanting into soil or soilless mix. Roots will spread out and grow as soon as they come in contact with the new growing medium.

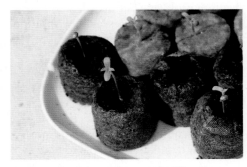

Rockwool cubes, or plugs, and Jiffy pellets are the two most popular rooting cubes for medicinal cannabis clones.

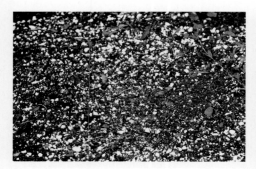

Used indoor soil can be unsightly in outdoor gardens.

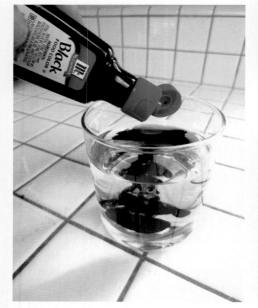

When discarding indoor mixes in backyard gardens, some gardeners add diluted food coloring to cover the white of perlite.

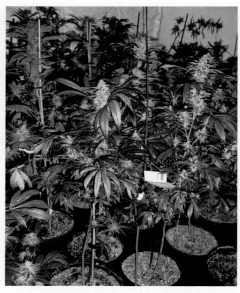

This sickly garden is a result of grow-medium stress.

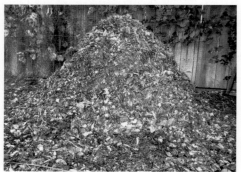

This compost pile is big enough to hold in heat and will decompose faster than a smaller pile.

mixed with compost and garden soil. Do not reuse the depleted indoor soil in outdoor pots. Many of the same problems that occur indoors will happen in outdoor pots.

Grow-Medium Problems
Visible Signs of Grow-Medium Stress
- dry, crispy, brittle leaves
- patchy or inconsistent leaf color
- yellow leaf edges that worsen
- crispy, burnt leaf edges
- chlorosis—yellowing between veins while veins remain green
- irregular blotches on leaves
- purple stems and leaf stems
- leaf edges curl up or down
- leaf tip curls down

- soft, pliable leaves
- branch tips stop growing
- leggy growth

Many maladies are caused by grow-medium problems but manifest as nutrient deficiencies or excesses. The solution is found within the growing medium.

When water is abundant in the growing medium, roots easily absorb it. Roots use more energy to absorb more water as it becomes scarce. Finally, the point comes when the substrate retains more moisture than plants are able to take in.

Well-rotted manure usually holds moisture well and is less prone to have viable weed seeds and pests.

Build compost piles high, and turn them regularly. Good compost recipes include the addition of organic trace elements, enzymes, and the primary nutrients (N-P-K). The organic matter should be ground up and in the form of shredded leaves and grass. Do not incorporate woody branches that could take years to decompose.

Before using compost indoors, pour it through 0.25-inch (0.64 cm) mesh hardware cloth (screen) to break up the humus. Place a heavy-duty framed screen over a large garbage can or a wheelbarrow to catch the sifted compost. Return earthworms found on the screen to the medium, and kill any cutworms you find. Make sure all composts are well rotted and have cooled before mixing with indoor and greenhouse soils. For more information about composting, see *Let It Rot! Third Edition*, by Stu Campbell (Storey Publishing, 1998).

Some gardeners mix up to 30 percent perlite into organic potting soil that contains lots of worm castings. Heavy worm castings compact soil and leave little space for air to surround roots. Adding perlite or similar amendments aerates the soil and improves drainage.

Organic Soil and the Soil Food Web

Serious, conscientious medical cannabis gardeners grow 100 percent organically. Cannabis gardeners can use 100 percent chemical fertilizers with outstanding yields, but the overall health benefits of the plant may suffer. Use either 100 percent organic fertilizers or (less desirable) salt-based chemical fertilizers. Do not mix the two! Chemical fertilizers kill soil life. It is that simple.

The soil food web is the population of organisms living all or part of their lives in the soil. The soil food web is a complex living system in the soil, and it interacts with the environment, plants, and animals.

The soil food web is very complex and beyond the scope of this book to fully explain. For a basic description of the soil food web and to learn how you can work with it to achieve bountiful harvests, use a web browser to search for

"Dr. Elaine Ingham." She is the world authority on the soil food web. Also, pick up a copy of *Teaming with Microbes*, by Jeff Lowenfels and Wayne Lewis, for more information on the soil food web.

A properly functioning soil food web retains nutrients in the soil. Nutrients are bound and do not leach or volatize easily. Remember, nitrogen volatizes readily if not bound up; there has to be a continuous replacement source to feed the microbes or they will dip into the nutrient pools. A soil that is too active will outcompete the plants for available nutrients.

Nutrients are available in the proper forms and rates for plants to take up. Oxygen, water, and nutrients can easily move into and through well-structured soil. Roots can easily penetrate noncompacted soil. Disease-causing organisms are suppressed via competition with beneficial organisms. Plant surfaces, both above- and belowground, are protected from disease-causing organisms by beneficial organisms. Plant-growth-promoting hormones and chemicals are produced to stimulate larger, more productive root systems. Toxic compounds are decomposed by soil life when properly managed.

The following descriptions are basic overviews of different soil organisms in the soil food web. There are millions of species involved in the soil food web, and, as you might expect, we do not have space to describe all of them here.

Bacteria
Single-celled bacteria are so small that 250,000 to 500,000 of the little single-celled organisms could fit within the period to a sentence. Bacteria are one of the main decomposers of fresh, green, organic garden matter. Different bacteria eat different organic matter. They travel short distances and promote medicinal cannabis health. Once food and nutrients are inside bacteria, they are "locked up" until bacteria are consumed by predators. There are two groups of bacteria: aerobic and anaerobic.

Anaerobic bacteria do not need oxygen to survive. In general, anaerobic bacteria are to be avoided and not promoted. By-products of some anaerobic organic decomposition include hydrogen sulfide and butyric acid, both of which smell like vomit and ammonia with the fragrance of vinegar. If you know these odors, you know the smell of anaerobic decomposition. But other anaerobic organic decomposition does not cause unpleasant odors, and such decomposition has a sweet, earthy fragrance. Conditions that promote anaerobic bacteria include compacted soil with little pore space and standing water.

Aerobic bacteria need air to live, and are the ones we want in the garden overall. Bacteria recycle three basic elements: carbon, nitrogen, and sulfur. Sulfur-oxidizing bacteria make water-soluble sulfates available to plants. The correct bacteria convert inert atmospheric nitrogen into "fixed" nitrogen—ammonium, nitrate, or nitrite ions.

Bacterial slime (biofilm—DNA, proteins, and sugars) also buffers the rhizosphere so the pH remains reasonably constant. Bacteria are attached to particles of soil, and they lock up nutrients that stay in the soil and are not leached away. The nutrients stay in the same place in the soil and are not washed out. When other organisms eat the bacteria, nitrogen is released in their poop, right next to the rhizosphere where it is readily available.

Archaea
Similar to bacteria, archaea were discovered in the early 1970s. But single-celled archaea survive in both high- and low-temperature environments, and many produce methane. They are decomposers that break down and recycle organic and inorganic materials.

Fungi
Classified as lower plants, fungi produce no chlorophyll and do not need light to live. The majority of soil fungi are virtually invisible without being magnified by a microscope. Much larger than bacteria, fungi have many cells and can stretch threadlike growth (hyphae) many feet. They can transport nutrients along their length. Once inside the soil, fungus nutrients are "locked in," and remain in the soil. Fungi also produce an enzyme that dissolves the woody compounds lignin, cellulose, and many others.

Fungi are the number one decomposers and decayers. Some fungi can decompose organic matter and move it from the soil surface down to the root zone in nutrient form. Fungi move nutrients, most notably phosphorus and sulfur, making them available to the plant. Other fungi move these nutrients horizontally in the soil to where they are needed. Some fungi trap destructive root-penetrating nematodes, absorbing nematode nutrients as nourishment. Fungi act as living banks for organic nutrients. Fungi are super fragile and do not grow well in compacted soil or when broken up by double digging and rototilling. Chemicals and salt-based fertilizers also destroy fungi.

Cannabis and the class of fungi, Mycorrhizal, form a complex relationship in the root zone, or rhizosphere. Two basic categories of mycorrhizal fungi include ectomycorrhizal and endomycorrhizal. Ectomycorrhizal fungi grow close to the root surface and are most common around conifers and hardwood trees. Organic cannabis gardeners are most interested in endomycorrhizal fungi that penetrate both roots and soil. The mycorrhizae react with nutrients outside roots and facilitate nutrient absorption and transport.

Specific types or species of mycorrhizal fungi form relationships with specific species of plants and make phosphorus, copper, calcium, iron magnesium, and zinc available. Nutrients are released for roots to take in when fungi die and decay. The key is to employ only the specific species of mycorrhizal that form the proper relationship. For more information see "Mycorrhizal Fungi" in chapter 22, *Additives*.

Endophyte fungi live in plant tissue all or most of their life. Excluding edible mushrooms and baker's and brewer's yeast and lichens, many are pathogenic to cannabis, including gray mold (*Botrytis cinerea*) and *Fusarium*. See "Gray Mold" and "*Fusarium*" in chapter 24, *Diseases & Pests*, for more information.

Algae
Algae are single-celled threadlike organisms, including seaweed and kelp. There are several kinds of algae, among them

blue-green, green, red, and brown. They can inhabit saltwater, fresh water, and terrestrial environments, including soil. Algae need sunlight in order to grow and produce their own food.

Algae participate in creating soil by forming carbonic acids during their metabolism. They also form partnerships with other organisms, including fungi. Blue-green algae fix nitrogen using the nitrogenase enzyme. Overall, algae's role in the garden is small, since algae grow at soil surface level and just below, and their growth is limited by sunlight penetration. Excess algae in soil will attract soil pests, including fungus gnats.

Slime Molds
Slime molds are slimy, amoeba-like organisms found in leaves, lawn thatch, manure, and other organic matter. Spores germinate in soil and ingest bacteria, fungi spores, and protozoa. The nutrients are thus "locked up" in the soil and prevented from leaching. Slime molds are eaten by larger predators, which digest them and then release nutrients into the soil. Slime molds surround their food and digest it internally. They are also food for larvae, worms, and beetles. Slime molds cycle nutrients and help bind soil particles together.

Protozoa
Protozoa are organisms with a nucleus within a single cell. In most cases, protozoa cannot make their own food; they survive by eating thousands of bacteria—and occasionally fungi and other protozoa.

Most of the 60,000 different kinds of protozoa are soil dwellers, but all of them need water for life, reproduction, and mobility. They travel in the thin layer of water enveloping soil particles. When this dries up they go into dormancy.

Protozoa and bacteria live in symbiotic relationships, yet at the same time, protozoa control bacteria populations. When they eat all the readily available bacteria, the big protozoa start consuming nematodes and smaller protozoa until the population becomes balanced once again. Wastes generated by protozoa are brimming with mineralized nutrients, including nitrogen compounds. Once

the waste is in the soil, nitrogen-fixing bacteria, if present, convert ammonium (nitrogen) into the readily available nitrate form of nitrogen.

According to Jeff Lowenfels, coauthor of *Teaming with Microbes*, "As much as 80 percent of the nitrogen a plant needs comes from the wastes produced by bacteria- and fungi-eating protozoa."

Nematodes
Nematodes are nonsegmented, thread-like, blind roundworms. Nematode waste is high in mineralizing nutrients liberated after consuming bacteria and fungi. There are more than 20,000 species of nematodes. Even though you can find 40 to 50 nematodes in a single teaspoon of good garden soil, most gardeners only know about the bad, root-eating nematodes. For more information on them, see "Nematodes" in chapter 24, *Diseases & Pests*.

Bacterivore nematodes live on bacteria. Their waste is loaded with mineralized nutrients. Predator nematodes eat algae, arthropods, fungi, other nematodes, protozoa, and even slugs! Wiggling and crawling through the soil, nematodes aerate and cultivate as they go. Soil structure and porous texture are essential for nematode well-being.

Arthropods
Beetles, flies, mites, mosquitoes, spiders, and springtails are all arthropods. About three-fourths of all living things are arthropods. These little critters have jointed legs and segmented bodies connected by a lightweight exterior skeleton (exoskeleton). Exterior skeletons are much stronger and give arthropods superhuman strength.

Arthropods aerate soil, shred organic material, and prey on other members of the soil food web, including bacteria, fungi, and other arthropods. Arthropods also promote fungal and bacterial activity in soil. Most live on or near the soil surface, but others burrow down into the soil, aerating it and leaving mineralized nutrient excrement in their path.

Unfortunately, most gardeners classify arthropods into three groups: bad bugs,

bad insects, and others! Of course most cannabis gardeners are familiar with a few bad ones—spider mites and thrips, to name a couple, but there are millions more, and many of them live in and are strategic to healthy soil and to medical marijuana. For example, mites (not bad spider mites) and springtails together are accountable for recycling as much as 30 percent of the forest floor in temperate climates. They want to work in your garden soil too!

We have dedicated a large part of the "Diseases & Pests" chapter to arthropods that are detrimental to plants. Just remember that not all bugs are bad!

You can find more than 300,000 mites in a square yard of good organic garden soil. Depending on species, mites prey on members of the soil food web—nematodes, algae, fungi, decaying foliage, and other arthropods. They are also prey to other mites and arthropods.

Ants mix organic materials found on the soil surface, shredding them and toting them deep into their dens.

This is just the tip of the iceberg. We do not have enough space to discuss the rest of the arthropods, including beetles, spiders, centipedes, millipedes, earwigs, grasshoppers, crickets, lice, flies, bees, wasps, sow bugs, pill bugs, and a few million more, but you should have the idea of just how important they are for a healthy soil food web.

Earthworms
Earthworms are tube-shaped, segmented worms that range from 1 inch to 3 feet in length. Earthworms are easy to identify and are an indicator of healthy organic garden soil. Most gardeners are familiar with the night crawler (*Lumbricus terrestris*) that originated in Europe. And many gardeners know the common "red wiggler" compost worm (*Eisenia fetida*), which is native to the USA, but there are 7,000 more earthworm species, some of which are found in garden soil. Good organic garden soil has 10 to 50 earthworms per square foot. Each worm can move up to a pound of soil every year. A night crawler can move 6 times its body weight. That's more efficient than rototilling, and it's free! Earth-

worms till the soil, making better access for air, fungi, and other soil life while enhancing microbial life and improving water-holding ability.

Earthworms shred organic matter, aerate soil, aggregate soil particles, and move microorganisms and organic matter in the soil. They normally live in the top 6 inches of soil, but some species can burrow down 10 feet or more. Garden earthworms primarily eat bacteria but may also consume fungi, nematodes, and protozoa in addition to all the organic material they take in.

Once through the worm's mouth, food is mixed with saliva, and powerful muscles start breaking it down before grinding it in the gizzard. Bits of sand help grind the mix before entering the intestines. Bacteria in the intestines then start to digest it. These bacteria produce nutrients that are absorbed into the worm's bloodstream. Unused materials are eliminated in the form of vermicastings, also known as "worm castings."

Vermicastings have 50 percent more organic matter than the same soil not digested and expelled by worms. Chemical bonds that make nutrients unavailable are liberated by this positive-charged worm poop. Nutrients now have the ability to attach to soil particles and become available to roots.

Gastropods
Gastropods—slugs and snails—as well as some 40,000 other species form this group. Slugs and snails not only eat your plants, they also consume algae, fungi, and rotting organic matter. Many slugs can even digest cellulose. They shred their food to help decompose and decay organic material and organisms. They spend less than 15 percent of their life aboveground.

Reptiles, mammals, and birds
Squirrels, mice, rabbits, chipmunks, moles, voles, gophers, snakes, salamanders, lizards, and birds may be annoying and even destructive in the garden, but they do have positive value. They move soil by burrowing, scratching, and simply moving their bodies, and in the process they move organic matter from one place to the other in the garden. They also

defecate in the garden, adding available nutrient-rich nutrients. Birds in the garden demonstrate that worms, larvae, insects, and bugs are also in the garden. Bird poop (guano) is chock-full of nutrients and microorganisms. Bird feet transport protozoa that drop off as birds move about.

However, once moles and gophers have "moved enough soil," you may want to escort them out of your garden. And once mice, rabbits, voles, and birds have eaten enough desirable plants, it is time for them to go too. See chapter 24, *Diseases & Pests*, for information on removing unwanted reptiles, mammals, and birds from your garden.

Salt-Based Fertilizers
Salt-based (chemical) fertilizers have the ability to destroy soil life; over applied, repeated applications continue to kill soil life—bacteria, fungi, insects, etc.—which weakens plants. If the first salt-based fertilizer application to organic garden soil does not kill all soil life, subsequent applications will finish it off. Outdoors, this scenario also prompts undesirable weeds to dominate the bleak environment.

Salt-based fertilizers are big business. Fertilizer manufacturers rely on low manufacturing costs and exponential profit margins. This "formula" allows for extravagant advertising budgets that are used to influence consumer purchasing.

Diseases and pests attack artificially supported plants. Harsh fungicides and pesticides are used to kill diseases and pests, which are secondhand problems caused by lack of soil life. Water and nutrients then leach from the soil at a faster rate, and more fertilizer is subsequently required. This downward cycle is repeated every time another fertilizer salt or killing substance is applied.

Garden and soil-life diversity is the key to healthy soil. Infuse, attract, and grow diverse soil friends and workers—bacteria, fungi, protozoa, arthropods, and beneficial nematodes. Bring life and teeming vitality back to your garden soil and grow healthy, organic, medicinal cannabis.

Rototilling Soil Kills Soil Life and Destroys Structure
Rototillers can do more work than people, but does this work need to be done? Ask the average farmer, gardener, or nurseryperson, and he or she will tell you that, yes, tilling is the way we have always done it. Tilling helps the soil; it breaks up clods and dead roots, and tills in and kills weeds. Uniformly tilled soil looks great, and most gardeners have a wonderful feeling of accomplishment after the garden or field is tilled.

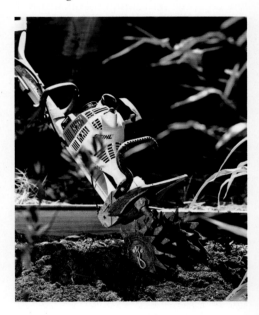

Ask well-informed organic gardeners if they till the soil, and you will receive a firm no. They understand that unnecessary tilling disrupts and kills soil life; it destroys the soil's structure and water-holding ability. Instead of tilling, they add compost, organic teas, and fertilizers to promote soil life so that bacteria, fungi, protozoa, arthropods, and earthworms do all the work. These little creatures make nutrients available to roots, increase plant vitality, and help soil retain water and nutrients. Organic gardeners also selectively use natural fungicides or pesticides, some of which may kill soil life.

Mulch
Mulch is a protective cover placed on the soil to retain moisture, reduce erosion, provide nutrients, and suppress weed growth. Mulch keeps the surface of the soil from forming a hard, cakey layer, and it promotes a lively layer of roots and soil life below the surface.

Avoid using mulch in spring when soil is cool. Mulch insulates soil. It slows warming and prevents moisture evaporation. When mulches mat down, they form a barrier that blocks the flow of air and water between soil and atmosphere. Keep an eye on mulches because they may wick water from the soil surface and dry it out.

Apply mulch after soil has warmed in early to mid summer. Soil temperatures will stay on target, and warmth will hold well into autumn. Mulch also slows evaporation, but do not forget that mulch can absorb rainfall and prevent it from penetrating soil. Irrigate mulched plants heavily so that water penetrates into the soil below.

Spread mulch by hand around plants. Keep mulch at least 6 inches or more away from stems to discourage diseases and pests. Finely chopped mulch is often more effective, but it decomposes faster than coarser mulch. A thick 6-to-12-inch (15–30 cm) layer of straw, hay, or grass mulch around a big plant in full sun will substantially reduce water consumption. Keep adding mulch as it decomposes.

Indoors, apply mulch such as expanded clay pellets or a piece of plastic that is cut to fit over containers.

Outdoors, almost anything can be used for mulch—rocks, sticks, newspaper, plastic, straw, hay, and more.

Composted mulch normally smells like freshly cut wood or sweet compost. Stay away from mulches that smell of ammonia, rot, sulfur, or vinegar, all of which signify anaerobic conditions.

Slugs, snails, mice, and other pests are attracted to mulch. Keep mulch 6 inches (15 cm) or more away from stems to discourage rodents from chewing stems. Place a plastic cuff around the base of plants to further discourage rodent damage. Use appropriate control measures for diseases and pests (see chapter 24, *Diseases & Pests*).

Cover crops protect soil in the off-season. These living mulches are tilled into the soil in the spring, adding nitrogen, organic matter, and other nutrients.

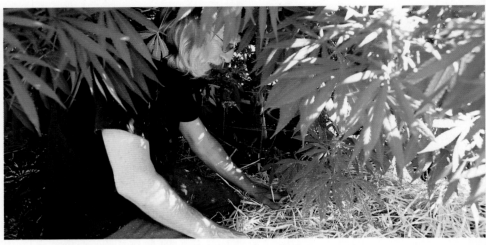

Indoors, outdoors, or in a greenhouse, mulch is often the least expensive way to conserve water, protect the soil, and reduce maintenance. Thumbs up for mulch!

The roots of some cover crops such as alfalfa and clover fix nitrogen in the soil, providing they are cut and tilled before flower set.

Straw and alfalfa hay are my favorite mulches. Straw, available at farm and garden stores in compressed bails, is best used during warm weather to keep moisture from evaporating and to promote soil life. Avoid sources of hay and straw that could have been sprayed with growth regulators or herbicides that accumulate in foliage. Such straw also tends to have less available nitrogen, so the nitrogen pool in the soil is robbed for the decomposition process. Alfalfa hay is more expensive than straw, but it is heavy in nitrogen and adds it to the soil instead of robbing it from the soil. Alfalfa hay will biodegrade faster than straw.

High-carbon mulches such as straw, woodchips, and tree bark stay on the surface and are decomposed mainly by fungi, UV rays from sunlight, and weather. High-carbon mulches form a barrier that can deflect irrigation water. They can also wick water from the ground, but this is not common. If sticks are poked into the ground, they will wick water up toward dry wood. Mulch made from wood can contain or feed termites!

Shredded cardboard and newspaper make a good base to pile organic mulch on. To hold paper in place, wet it as you put it down.

Compost used as mulch should be well rotted and void of weed seeds and heat.

Grass clippings are a high-nitrogen source that helps compost cook. My preference is to avoid adding grass that has been treated with herbicides such as Weed & Feed.

Leaves and leaf mold (composted leaves) tend to compact when they lay flat before adequate composting. Leaf mold is one of my favorite compost materials, especially when it comes from healthy hardwood trees.

Plastic bags, Visqueen, and plastic sheeting work well as mulch. I like to use biodegradable plastic, and have found that dark-colored plastic is less obtrusive than light-colored plastic.

A plastic mulch will shade weeds, prevent moisture loss, and raise the temperature of the soil by 5 to 15 degrees Fahrenheit (3–8 degrees Celsius) on a sunny day. As plants grow, their leaves will shade the plastic and stop the warming effects. A lake, pond, or small creek will also moderate air temperature, keeping it warmer in winter and cooler in summer. Do not use organic mulches in the spring; during that time of year they will cool the soil.

Rocks and gravel are great mulches. Rocks hold heat and retain it overnight. Rock mulches also extend growing seasons.

19 CONTAINERS

CONTAINER SIZE, SHAPE, construction material, color, and drainage outlets affect the maintenance schedule and ultimately the overall health of cannabis plants.

Containers come in all shapes and sizes and can be constructed of almost anything: plastic, wood, metal, clay, fiber, and more. Cannabis will grow in any clean container that has not been used for petroleum products or deadly chemicals. Fiber and wood containers breathe better than plastic or metal pots. Heavy clay pots are brittle and absorb moisture from the soil inside them, causing the soil to dry out quickly. Metal pots are also impractical for garden rooms because they oxidize (rust) and can bleed off harmful elements and compounds. Wood, although somewhat expensive, is great to construct large raised beds and planters on wheels. Plastic and fiber containers are inexpensive and durable; these offer the best values to indoor gardeners.

Growing in containers allows gardeners to control the water and nutrient regimen of individual plants. Movable potted plants can be turned every few days to let plants receive even lighting for even growth. Huddle small, containerized plants tightly together within the brightest area under the HID lamp. Move containerized plants further apart as they grow. Set small plants on blocks to move them closer to the HID. Weak, problematic, or diseased potted plants can easily be dipped in medicinal solution, quarantined, or culled from the garden.

Containers must be:
1. clean,
2. have adequate drainage holes, and be
3. big enough to accommodate plant growth.

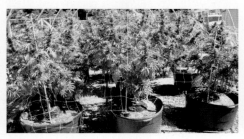

Big containers give roots plenty of room to grow and expand.

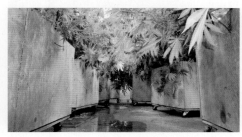

Containers on casters are easy to move, and they stay warmer since they are up off the floor.

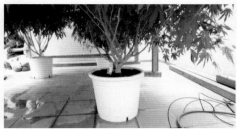

Growing big plants in 5-gallon (19 L) containers is possible but more difficult. Roots use water and nutrients quickly and must therefore be replenished quickly.

Types of Containers

Containers used to cultivate cannabis fall into three basic categories: bags, cans, and beds. Bags consist of containers with a flexible shape such as plastic grow bags and burlap or fiber bags. Cans are a group of containers with rigid sides: plastic pots, large planter boxes, and clay pots. Beds may or may not have rigid sides; the main distinction is that they have no bottom and thus drain freely.

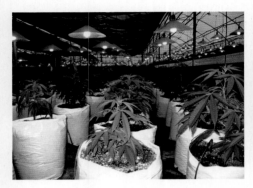

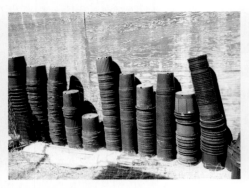

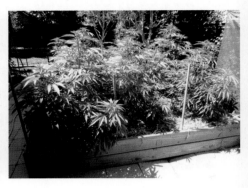

Plastic grow bags are a favorite container among cannabis gardeners. Inexpensive, long-lasting grow bags take up little storage space and are lightweight. A box of 100, 3-gallon (11 L) bags weighs less than 5 pounds (2.3 kg) and measures less than a foot square (30 cm²). One hundred 3-gallon (11 L) grow bags can be stored inside two 3-gallon (11 L) bags. Imagine storing 100 rigid pots in the same space!

Rigid plastic pots are the most commonly used containers in garden rooms. They are the standard container for nursery stock and are readily available. Most often they are black with smooth sides and large drainage holes. Black containers absorb heat and reflect very little, causing the root zone to heat rapidly. When allowed to get too hot, roots cook and rot. Once cooked, roots may take a month or more to recover.

Outdoor garden beds should be at least 6 inches (15 cm) tall to take advantage of a warmer atmosphere aboveground. They can be higher, but little benefit is reaped from extra heat. See chapter 12, *Outdoors,* for more information on raised beds.

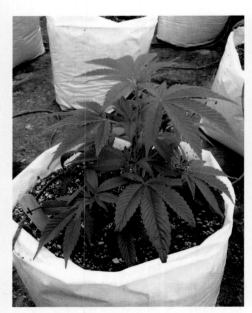

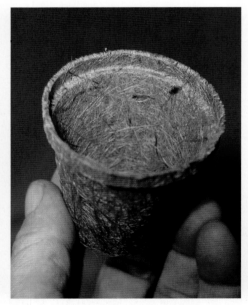

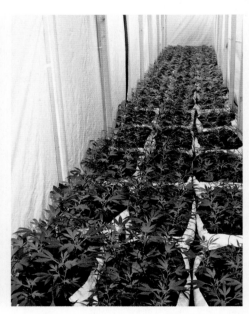

White containers reflect heat and stay cooler, but if placed in full sun they still get hot enough to cook roots. White containers must be thick or painted a dark color on the inside so that roots receive no light, since light is detrimental to their growth. See "Container Problems" in this chapter.

Rigid fiber and paper-pulp pots are popular with gardeners who move their plants outdoors. Removing the container's bottom eases transplanting into soil. Pot bottoms habitually rot out, but painting the inside of the fiber container with latex paint will keep the bottom from rotting for several crops.

The potting soil sack can be used as a container. The moist soil inside the bag expands and contracts. Keeping soil evenly moist will lessen the chance of burned root tips that grow down the side of bags. Always remember to make adequate *drainage* holes in bags!

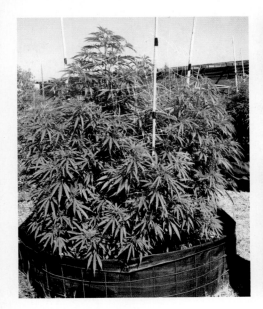

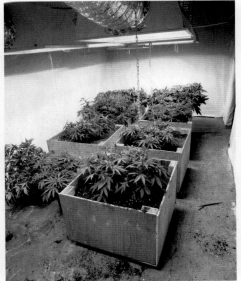

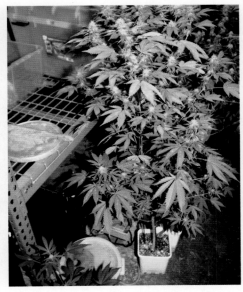

Big plants can grow in small containers but will require several irrigations daily and are likely to have problems.

Permeable-fabric grow bags are easy to make with many different types of material. Commercial brands such as Smart Pots, GeoPots, and so forth are gaining in popularity. Grow bags, whether plastic or fabric, are easy to wash and reuse. Empty out the soilless mix and submerge bags in a big container of soapy water overnight. Stir them around with a stick, wash by hand, and hang to dry. Once dry, the bags are ready to reuse. I like fiber pots the best because the air in the sides keeps the roots pruned. For more information, see "Root-Pruning Containers" in this chapter.

Large planter boxes are wonderful. Planters should be as big as possible but still allow easy access to plants. Roots will have more room to grow and less container surface for them to run into and grow down. Set large planter boxes and pots on blocks or casters to allow air circulation underneath. The soil in planter boxes stays warmer and the plants are more easily maintained.

Garden beds are my favorite! Garden beds can be raised with rigid sides or not, but they must be completely open on the bottom and drain directly into Mother Earth. Garden beds can easily be installed on the floor of a greenhouse and outdoors. In fact, I have seen garden beds in basement and outbuilding garden rooms. Please take note, however: the soil below basement garden beds is often poor-quality subsoil that drains poorly.

Container Shape and Size

Popular container shapes include rectangular, square, and cylindrical. Square and rectangular containers can butt up to one another, providing more overall growing medium in gardens. Cylindrical containers are readily available and inexpensive but lack the versatility of square pots.

Containers are wider than deep or deeper than wide. Cannabis gardeners growing indoors and in greenhouses prefer containers that are wider than deep because they are more stable and surface roots are able to spread out farther. This is true regardless of container size, small or large. Deep containers tip over more easily but promote (seedling) taproot and deep root growth. They are favored to grow small plants that will be transplanted outdoors.

The volume of a container definitely dictates the irrigation and feeding schedule. In most cases container size helps determine the size of a plant. Cannabis is an annual; it grows very fast and requires a lot of root space for sustained, vigorous development. Containers should allow space for a strong root system but be just big enough to contain the root system before harvest. If the container is too small, roots are confined and both water and nutrient uptake are limited, which in turn slows growth. But if the container is too big, it requires too much expensive growing medium and becomes heavy and awkward to move.

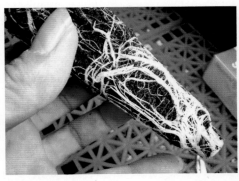

Deep containers are ideal to grow seedlings and clones that will be planted outdoors.

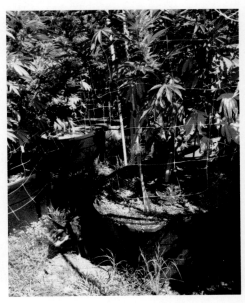

Plants grown in large containers require less-frequent irrigation and are much easier to maintain.

SELECTING CONTAINERS

Plant Age	Container Size	Metric Equivalent
0–3 weeks	root cube	root cube
2–6 weeks	4-inch pot	10 cm pot
6–8 weeks	2-gallon pot	7.5 L pot
2–3 months	3-gallon pot	11 L pot
3–8 months	5-gallon pot	19 L pot
6–18 months	10-gallon pot	38 L pot

Allow 1 to 1.5 gallons (3.8–5.7 L) of soil or soilless mix for each month that a given plant will spend in its container. A 2- to 3-gallon (7.5–11 L) pot supports a plant for up to 3 months. A 3- to 6-gallon container is good for 3 to 4 months of rapid plant growth.

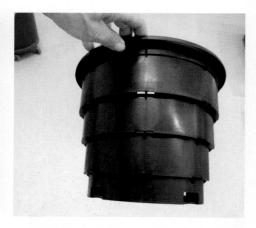

This root-pruning container diverts root growth with different obstacles on the wall. Note that it also has air holes to air prune roots that are encircling the inside of the container.

Small Containers

Three-gallon (11 L) containers are ideal for 2- to 3-foot-tall (60–90 cm) plants. Larger pots are usually unnecessary because plants grow no longer than a week or two in the vegetative stage and 6 to 10 weeks flowering. Smaller 3-gallon (11 L) pots are easy to move and handle. Roots also grow less during flowering. By the time a plant is pot-bound, it is ready to harvest. I used to recommend up to a 5-gallon (19 L) container for plants that are harvested after 90 total days of life. I now believe this is a waste. While the smaller containers require daily watering, they produce harvests comparable to those of 5-gallon (19 L) containers.

Large Containers

Mother (stock) plants usually grow larger, longer, and require 5- to 50-gallon (19–190 L) containers when grown in soil. However, mother plants grow quite well in 5- or 10-gallon (19–38 L) hydroponic containers for a year or longer. If you plan to keep a mother plant for more than a few months, grow it hydroponically in its own container for best results.

Root Pruning

Root-Pruning Containers

Root-pruning containers work on a simple principle. Roots tend to grow around and down the inside of containers having a smooth wall. Root-pruning containers place obstacles in the path of roots to divert them and stop or change the direction of root growth.

Air Root-Pruning Containers

Unpruned roots encircle the inside of

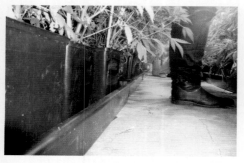

Small containers are great for small plants. They are lightweight and easy to handle. Roots soon outgrow small containers; these clones are ready to transplant.

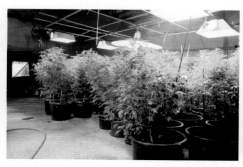

Large containers outdoors sit on top of the ground, forming a barrier to pests that enter through the soil—such as termites, a problem insect in many gardens.

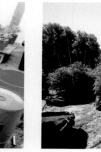

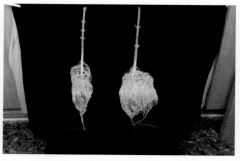

Square containers fit closely together providing more growing medium per square foot (m2).

Large containers allow space for root growth as well as biological activity. They are the next best thing to growing in Mother Earth, even indoors.

The roots on the left were grown in a smooth-sided 3-gallon (11 L) container. The root mass on the right was grown in the 3-gallon (11 L) root-pruning container above.

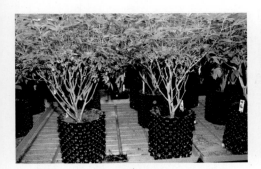
Uneven surfaces allow for more root growth, and a series of holes permits air to prune roots.

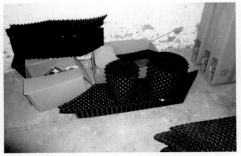
These air-pruning containers require little storage space and are easy to assemble.

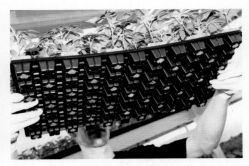
Roots on these clones grow through drainage holes. Once they hit the air, growth stops. Roots are thus "air pruned."

containers, forming thick masses that are sensitive to temperature changes and will dry out easily. Roots that become dry for long or that cook in hot temperatures will die. Dead roots soon rot, leaving plants vulnerable to diseases, pests, and nutrient deficiencies.

When roots grow to the end of a container with permeable sides and are exposed to air, the root tips stop growing. More feeder roots form along the main stem of the root. Air naturally prunes the tips of roots, and the roots form a dense mass inside the container. Gardeners can make their own permeable air-pruning containers from many different materials, or such containers can be purchased from retail or wholesale outlets.

Clone and seedling roots are easy to air prune. Holes in air-pruning flats are shaped like a cone with a hole at the bottom. Roots are directed down the container and out the hole in its bottom. The tips of the roots dry out once they come into contact with air, thus pruning them. Use these containers if you must hold clones for a week or longer than you desire.

Chemical Root Pruning

Chemical root pruning controls root growth inside containers. Commercial nurseries have been using chemical root pruning for many years with outstanding results. Uncle Ben, a charter member of the defunct site www.overgrow.com tuned us in to chemical root pruning, and we thank him!

Uncle Ben used a product called SePRO Griffin's Spin-Out that consists of copper hydroxide suspended in water-soluble paint as a carrier. To use, simply brush-paint container insides with two coats of the product. Roots grow to within a fraction of an inch of the copper hydroxide, and then stop. Roots will not touch the copper compound. The result is essentially the same as is achieved with air pruning. Plants having a dense root system dispersed evenly throughout the root ball are easier to maintain, and they grow bigger in smaller containers.

Note: Medical cannabis gardeners avoid using copper compounds to prune roots, citing root burn problems. In elemental form copper is easy to overapply, and it

quickly becomes toxic to plants. Copper sulfate (0.3 %) is less toxic than copper hydroxide. Both compounds are insoluble in water and ions do not translocate to roots.

Physical Root Pruning

Physically pruning roots may be necessary to give new life to potbound plants outdoors or in greenhouses. Removing roots will not make plants grow faster; in fact, it will slow growth for about two weeks. Once new roots start to grow, however, growth rebounds. About midsummer, root pruning can help plants that must stay in the same size container. Root pruning will keep plants manageable and much easier to maintain. Physical root pruning is the last option; try air pruning and chemical root pruning first.

Drainage and Leaching

All containers need some form of drainage. Drainage holes allow excess water and nutrient solution to flow freely out the bottom of a container. Drainage holes should let water drain easily but not be so big that growing medium washes out. Containers should have at least two

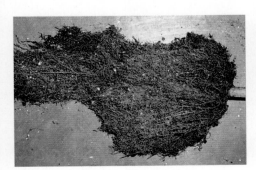
This dense mass of roots is the result of chemical root pruning. The same result can be achieved by using air-pruning containers.

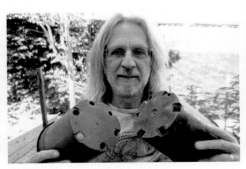
Drainage holes are essential in all containers. I prefer the container on the right with larger holes that run slightly up the sides to the one on the left with smaller holes on the bottom only.

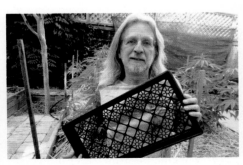
This nursery tray is used to hold small containers. It provides extra space below so that containers drain and do not sit in water.

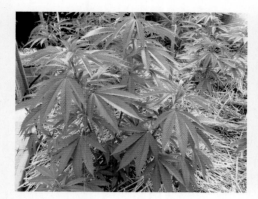

Feeder roots grow near the soil surface, just under the mulch. I like to add mulch to outdoor, indoor, and greenhouse containers.

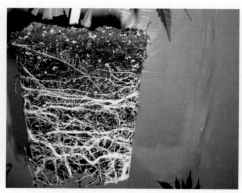

This rootbound plant appears healthy aboveground but will stop growing as soon as roots suffer heat or moisture stress.

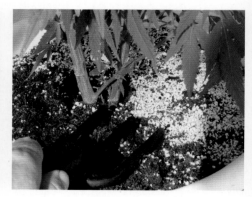

Lightly cultivate the soil surface so water penetrates evenly. Be careful to avoid disturbing the roots.

half-inch (1.2 cm) holes per square foot (929 cm²) of bottom. Most pots have twice this amount. To slow drainage and keep soil from washing out of the large holes, add a 1-inch (2.5 cm) layer of gravel in the bottom of the pot.

Surface tension created by the varying sizes of soil and rock particles, and a lot of other interesting science, causes water to be retained at the bottom of the container. Line pots with newspaper if drainage is too fast or if soil washes out of drainage holes, but be wary of overly slowing the drainage.

Put trays under containers to catch excess water. Do not let water stand in saucers for more than 20 minutes or waterlogged roots will die and rot. Set containers up on blocks so water drains into saucers or trays and roots do not sit in water. Nursery trays used for rooting cuttings and growing seedlings must have good drainage throughout the entire bottom. Once clones and seedlings are in place in the tray, the tray should always drain freely with no standing water in the bottom.

Container Problems

Do not place containers in direct heat. If soil temperature in pots climbs beyond 75°F (24°C), it can damage roots. Shade pots that are in direct sun with a piece of plastic or cardboard to keep the soil temperature of below 75°F (24°C).

A 1 to 2-inch (2.5–5 cm) layer of hydroclay mulch on the soil surface keeps the soil surface moist. Roots are able to grow along the surface, and the soil does not need to be cultivated. The hydroclay mulch also decreases evaporation and helps keep irrigation water from damaging roots or splashing out of containers.

Roots soon hit the sides of containers, grow in circles, and later grow down and mat up around the bottom. The unnatural environment inside the container often causes a thick layer of roots to grow alongside the container walls and bottom. This portion of the root zone is the most vulnerable to moisture and heat stress and is the most exposed to it. Often inexperienced or lazy gardeners set such plants in a saucer to contain irrigation water. The submerged roots soon die and rot, compounding the problems.

Avoid such problems by transplanting plants before they become rootbound, or by using root-pruning containers.

When soil dries in a pot, it becomes smaller, contracting and separating from the inside of the container wall. This condition is worst in smooth plastic pots. When this crack develops, frail root hairs located in the gap quickly die when they are exposed to air whistling down this crevice. Water also runs straight down this crack and onto the floor. You may think the pot was watered, but the root ball remains dry. Avoid such killer cracks by cultivating the soil surface and running your finger around the inside lip of the pots. Lightly cultivate the surface of the soil every few days and maintain evenly moist soil to

help keep root hairs on the soil perimeter from drying out. A layer of mulch will also help avoid the gap between soil and container.

White containers reflect light and keep soil cooler. Always use thick, white containers so light does not penetrate and subsequently slow root growth. If roots around the outside of the root ball start turning green, you know they are receiving direct light. Remedy the problem by painting the inside of the container with a nontoxic latex paint.

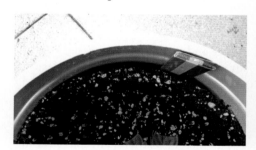

Soil shrinks when dry; it causes a gap to form alongside the container's inside wall.

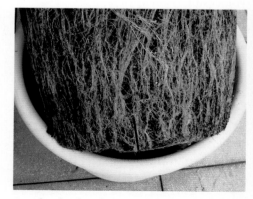

Low levels of sunlight through container walls cause unhealthy green roots. Paint containers black inside to cut light transmission.

20 WATER

WATER IS A PART of humans and all living things. Water moves the fluids that support life in plants and animals. Water (H_2O) exists in liquid, gaseous, and solid states. When pure, water is tasteless and odorless. Reflected light often gives it a blue appearance, especially when concentrated in glaciers. Many substances, including fertilizer salts, readily dissolve in water, which is known as the universal solvent. Most sources of water are rarely pure. The impurities in water are "invisible" once dissolved and part of the solution.

Determine basic water quality by measuring its alkalinity, pH, and total dissolved solids (TDS). Alkalinity, the capacity to neutralize or buffer an acid solution, affects pH, the acid-to-alkaline balance of water. Two minerals or dissolved solids, calcium (Ca) and magnesium (Mg), buffer pH so that the addition of acidic mineral salts or fertilizers does not affect the pH a great deal. Pure and nearly pure water that contains few or no dissolved minerals is considered soft because it has little or no buffering ability. The pH of soft water (see below) can experience extreme fluctuations when acidic fertilizer salts are added.

Hard Water

Hard water contains significant quantities of dissolved minerals. Calcium (Ca) and magnesium (Mg) concentrations are most often used as an indicator as to how "hard" the water is. When heated, the carbonates (formed by reaction of CO_2 with bases) in hard water precipitate (settle) out, forming scale on plumbing pipes, showerheads, and so on. Soaps do not lather well in hard water because it reacts to form calcium or magnesium salts, which are insoluble. Water containing 100 to 150 milligrams of calcium carbonate ($CaCO_3$) per liter (mg/l) is acceptable to grow cannabis. Nonetheless, water can have 400 ppm sodium and it will still be soft, but about 60 to 120 ppm Ca makes it hard (depending on whose scale is used).*

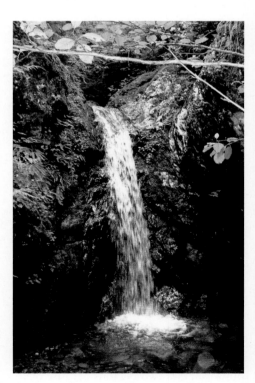

A mountain stream in Vancouver, BC, is an excellent source of fresh, clean water. But most water sources available to gardeners are far from pristine.

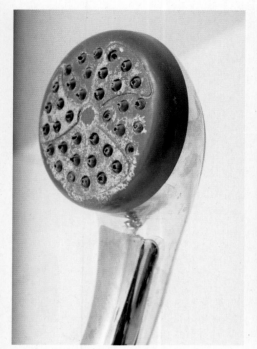

Salt has started to accumulate on this shower-head. The buildup is from the dissolved solids (salts) in the water supply. The same salts also deposit in soil and containers.

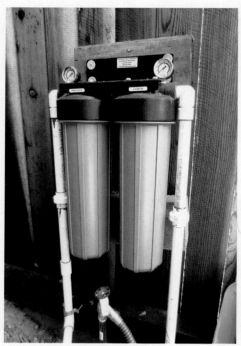

This simple filter removes particles and chlorine from the water supply.

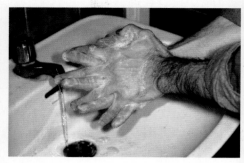

Soft water makes soap lather.

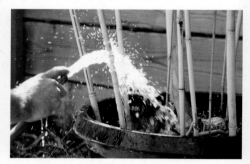

Watering heavily and filling containers completely so that 20 percent of the irrigation water drains out will help wash away built-up fertilizer salts in the growing medium.

*For much more information on hard water, search "hard water" on the www.marijuanagrowing.com forum.

Soft Water

Softened water is often treated with sodium, which binds to the calcium and magnesium ions, removing their ability to form scale or interfere with detergents. In Spain, we have hard water; we put sodium (granular salt) in the dishwasher so spots (scale) will not form on dishes. You can taste the sodium in softened water. Water softeners are used to lengthen the life of plumbing pipes, pumps, and so on, and to increase the effectiveness of soaps. Soft water contains less than 50 milligrams of calcium per liter (50 ppm) and should be supplemented with calcium and magnesium. Sodium in excess of 50 ppm is detrimental to cannabis growth.**

**The sodium ions exchange places with a chemical the sodium is attached to, pulling out all multivalent ions (Ca^2-, Mg^2-) with a similar number of monovalent charges (Na-): every Ca that binds releases two Na ions because of the charge difference, a two-for-one deal (in ppm, 100 ppm Ca removed buys 200 ppm Na in return).

A better alternative is often potassium, but it is a little more expensive. Both potassium and sodium exist as the resin used in water softeners and both are monovalent ions—potassium (K-) and sodium (Na). Potassium is a better option for cannabis and humans. Sodium is economical and widely available, but potassium is more effective.

The metric system facilitates the measurement of "dry residue per liter." Measure the dry residue per liter by pouring a liter of water on a tray and allowing it to evaporate. The residue of dissolved solids that remains after all the water evaporates is the "dry residue per liter." The residue is measured in grams. Try this at home to find out the extent of impurities in your water. Fertilizers have a difficult time penetrating root tissue when they must compete with resident dissolved solids, especially sodium. Water that is loaded with high levels of dissolved solids (salts in solution) is possible to manage but requires different tactics. Highly saline water that contains sodium will block the uptake of potassium, calcium, and magnesium. Salt-laden water will always

cause problems. If water contains 300 ppm or less dissolved solids, allow at least 25 percent of the irrigation water to drain out of the bottom of containers with each watering. *If raw water contains more than 300 ppm of dissolved solids, use a reverse-osmosis device to purify water.* Add nutrients to pure water as a way to avoid many nutrient problems.

If raw water contains more than 300 ppm of dissolved solids or more than 50 ppm sodium (Na), use a reverse-osmosis device to purify water before using it in the garden.

Built-up dissolved fertilizer salts often become toxic in container gardens. Excessive salts inhibit seed germination, burn the root hairs and tips or edges of leaves, and stunt plants. Leach excess salt buildup from growing mediums by applying 3 gallons of water per gallon of medium and repeat leaching using a mild pH-corrected fertilizer solution. Leach the growing medium every 2 to 4 weeks to avoid toxic buildup. Hard water and well water in dry climates are often alkaline, and usually contain notable amounts of calcium and magnesium. Cannabis uses large quantities of both nutrients, but too much calcium and magnesium can build up in soil. In general, water that tastes good to people also tastes good to cannabis.

Minerals dissolve into groundwater from rock and sediment. Water sources in low-rainfall or desert regions contain relatively high levels of dissolved mineral salts. For example, Southern Spain and Italy, southwestern USA, and much of Mexico all have high levels of dissolved mineral salts in their groundwater. More than 85 percent of the gardens in the USA have hard water. Many rivers and streams in Alaska, the Great Lakes region, and Tennessee have moderately hard water. Hard and very hard water flows in almost every state in America. Streams in Arizona, Kansas, New Mexico, and Southern California have the hardest water, with dissolved minerals more than 1,000 ppm.

Soft water flows in many parts of Hawaii, New England, the Pacific Northwest, and the South Atlantic and Gulf states. To get an idea of how hard the water is in different parts of the USA, visit www.qualitywatertreatment.com/city_water_guide.htm.

If your water is soft: pH continues to drift up in soft water and purified water with few dissolved mineral solids (less than 60 ppm) due to little or no buffering capacity. Remedy this problem by stabilizing the pH and adding soluble calcium and magnesium, sold at hydroponic stores under the name "Cal-Mag."

If your water is hard: Treat it with the best option: reverse osmosis (RO).

If water is acidic or alkaline: If EC is low, acidity or alkalinity are weak and will not cause problems. If acidity or alkalinity are driven by multivalent ions, they will directly add an H proton or OH (compounds that do not change things by association). For example, an organic acid is weak and requires less added hydroxide to neutralize, versus phosphoric acid, which requires more hydroxide to neutralize.

Other conditions could exist, including the concentration and strength (molality) of an acid/base solution. Remove problem-causing salts with an RO filter. Or invest in a sophisticated injector system to monitor and adjust pH. Many injectors, in particular those by Anderson, have multiple injector inputs that can inject solutions in sequence from different sources to adjust pH as well as inject specific nutrients.

Sources of Water

Air conditioner water: Water condensed from an air conditioner or dehumidifier is very clean—virtually no dissolved solids. But the water does trap cannabis fragrance. Most A/C units generate 2 to 3 gallons (7.6–11.4 liters) of water a day. Empty containers on a daily basis!

Rainwater: You can harvest 600 gallons of rainwater from 1 inch of rain that falls on a 1,000 sq ft (93 m²) roof. Although slightly acidic in urban areas, rainwater is free of chlorine and pollutants or salts that normally occur in groundwater.

Clean rainwater is an excellent choice for irrigation. Collect runoff by placing a barrel under a downspout. Mix

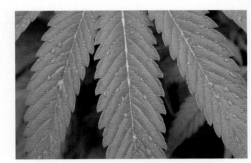

Plants love rainwater for good reason: it is the best water Mother Nature has to offer.

the rainwater with tap water to dilute dissolved solids. Roofs and terraces can accumulate trash, which will pollute the otherwise clean rainwater. Covering your catch-barrel will prevent evaporation and keep out trash. To make sure it is not too acidic (acid rain) and harmful to plants, take pH and parts per million (ppm) readings from collected rainwater before using.

Rivers and streams: Usually, these water resources are publicly controlled. Alpine watersheds supply "mineralized" water—water with elements and nutrients that plants need to produce food and grow.

Tap water: Household water often contains chlorine and other dissolved minerals. Check two or three times a year with your local water bureau to find out what is in your water. Also check the pH regularly. See discussion above about water sources.

Clean your tap water by filling barrels and setting them 2 to 3 feet (61–91.4 cm) above the ground. Add ammonium

ppm	mg/L	µg/L
100	100	1,000
200	200	2,000
300	300	3,000
400	400	4,000
500	500	5,000

HARD/SOFT WATER INDEX	mg/L	gpg
soft	0-60	0-35
moderately hard	61-210	3.5-7
hard	121-180	7-10.5
very hard	>181	>180
mg/L = milligrams per liter		
gpg = grains per US gallon		

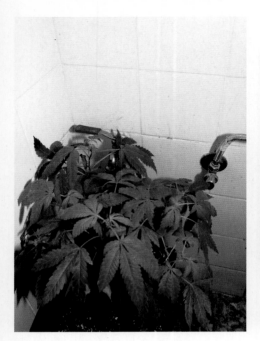

Piping water into the garden facilitates irrigation.

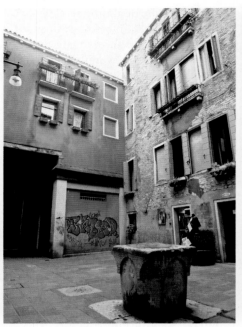

This well in Venice, Italy, has been closed because the water is brackish (salty). Test well water to ensure that it contains no harmful elements.

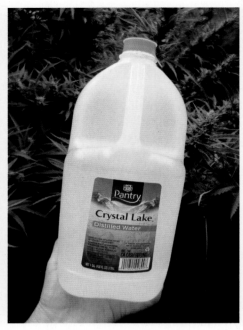

Distilled water is expensive and is best used in small amounts such as for watering cuttings and seedlings.

sulfate to settle out the sodium, then siphon water from the top of the barrel, refilling after each watering to allow the chlorine to evaporate. Chlorine, like sodium, is beneficial in small amounts. It is essential to the use of oxygen during photosynthesis and is necessary for root and leaf cell division. But too much chlorine causes leaf tips and margins to burn and leaves to turn a bronze color. Chlorine (which evaporates) and chloramine (which must be filtered to remove) are added to household water systems to kill bacteria, parasites, and other organisms. But both oxidize iron, manganese, and hydrogen sulfide, making them easier to filter out. Empty the barrel periodically, and scrub out residues and sediments. See "Chlorine (Chloride)" in chapter 21, *Nutrients*, for more information.

Well water: Ground water is pumped from a well. Have your well water analyzed at least once a year because mineral content often changes with the seasons and over time. Do not assume that the mineral content will be the same as that of your neighbors' well water. Most often well water is hard, with high levels of calcium and magnesium.

Purified Water

Bottled water enjoys minimal regulation in most countries. The US federal government for example, requires that bottled water be at least the same quality as tap water, but some studies show it is of lower quality. Frequently sold as "mineral water" for $1 to $4 USD per gallon, bottled water may contain more dissolved solids than tap water. If you are using bottled water, read labels carefully to ensure that it contains less than 150 ppm (15 mg/L) dissolved solids (aka minerals).

Carbon filters are effective at removing chlorine, chloramines, sediment, and volatile organic compounds (paints, petroleum solvents, and hazardous wastes) from water. But they do not remove dissolved mineral salts from water. Use carbon filters as a pre-filter to reverse osmosis (RO) filters.

Deionized (aka demineralized) water has had its mineral ions removed. A water deionizer moves water through special ion exchange resins, complex sodium salts. These resins bind to the mineral dissolved solids (salts), filtering them out of the "pure" water. Deionized

water is similar in purity to distilled water. Deionization does not specifically remove viruses or bacteria.

Distilled water has many of its impurities eliminated via distillation, a process that boils water. The resulting vapor is captured and condensed into clean water. Purchasing distilled water is very expensive: $0.75 to $1 USD per gallon. But home distillation systems can cut prices to $0.25 USD per gallon. Distilled water is available at most grocery stores and home improvement centers. Gardeners often use distilled water for cuttings.

Electrodialysis-filtered water is most economical to use in large- and medium-scale installations when desalinating brackish water and seawater. Smaller systems are also available. This process is most efficient when removing ionic components with a low molecular weight.

Water microfiltration systems remove suspended solids down to 0.1 micrometers in size. Use microfiltration as a pre-filter to RO filters to extend the life of RO filters.

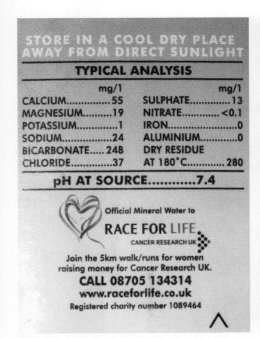

European bottled water has the guaranteed analysis printed on the label, but in the USA, no specific analysis is available on the label. The dissolved solids in this bottled water are measured in milligrams per liter (mg/L).

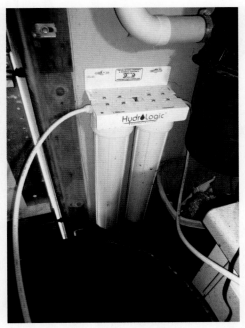

This reverse osmosis machine transforms water with a high ppm or EC into "clean" water with less than 10 ppm.

Other processes such as ultrafiltration and ultraviolet oxidation, also remove salts and pollutants from water. Check www.wikipedia.org for more information.

Reverse Osmosis (RO) Water

Reverse-osmosis machines are used to separate dissolved solids from water. These machines move the solvent (water) through the semipermeable membrane. The process is accomplished by applying pressure to the "tainted" water to force only "pure" water through the membrane. The water is not totally (EC of zero), but most of the dissolved solids are removed. The efficiency of reverse osmosis depends on the type of membrane, the pressure differential on both sides of the membrane, and the chemical composition of the dissolved solids in the tainted water. Unfortunately, common tap water often contains high levels of sodium (Na), calcium (Ca), alkaline salts, sulfur (S), chlorine (Cl) and other minerals. The pH could also be out of the acceptable 6.5 to 7 range.

Sulfur is easily smelled and tasted in water. Saline water is a little more difficult to detect. Water in coastal areas is generally full of salt that washes inland from the ocean or sea. Dry regions that have less than 20-inches (50.8 cm) annual rainfall also suffer from alkaline soil and water that is often loaded with alkaline salts.

pH

The pH scale, from 0 to 14, measures acid-to-alkaline balance. Zero is the most acidic, 7.0 is neutral or base, and 14.0 is most alkaline. Base is 7.0 or above. Just like the algorithmic earthquake Richter scale, every full point change in the pH scale signifies a tenfold increase or decrease in acidity or alkalinity. For example, soil or water with a pH of 5.0 is ten times more acidic than water or soil with a pH of 6.0. Water with a pH of 5.0 is 100 times more acidic than water with a pH of 6.0, and 1,000 times more acidic than water with a pH of 7.0. With a tenfold difference between each point on the scale, accurate measurement and control is essential to a strong, healthy garden.

Nutrients are available in a plant-soluble form within a limited pH range. The range of solubility is different for each nutrient. Cannabis grows best in soil within a pH of 6.5 to 7.0. Within this range cannabis can properly absorb and most efficiently process available nutrients. If pH is too low or high, mineral salts settle out into a solid (precipitate) from the nutrient solution. If the pH of the nutrient solution is too low, acidic salts chemically bind nutrients, which the roots are then unable to absorb. An alkaline nutrient solution with a high pH causes nutrients to become unavailable. Toxic salt buildup that limits water intake by roots also becomes a problem. Hydroponic solutions perform best in a pH range a little lower than for soil. The ideal pH range for hydroponics is from 5.8 to 6.8. Some gardeners run the pH at lower levels and report no problems with nutrient uptake.

The pH of the growing medium affects the nutrient-solution range and should be kept at a similar pH level as the nutrient solution. For example, most store-bought potting soils are slightly acidic, and rockwool hydroponic mediums are often alkaline. For more information on how pH affects plant growth see "pH" in chapters 18, *Soil*, and 23, *Container Culture and Hydroponics*, and "Cultural Problems" in chapter 21, *Nutrients*.

After repeated irrigation, water or nutrient solution with a pH that is too high or low will change the pH of the growing medium. Raw water with adequate levels of calcium and magnesium and a pH above 6.0 will help keep nutrient solutions from becoming too acidic. Climatic conditions can also affect irrigation water pH. For example, the pH can become more acidic in late autumn, when leaves fall and decompose. Large municipalities carefully monitor

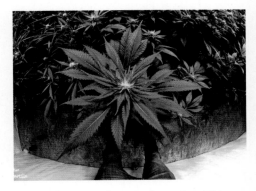

Strong plants stand out in the garden. This plant is at capacity for fertilizer, and a wide-angle camera lens helps with perspective!

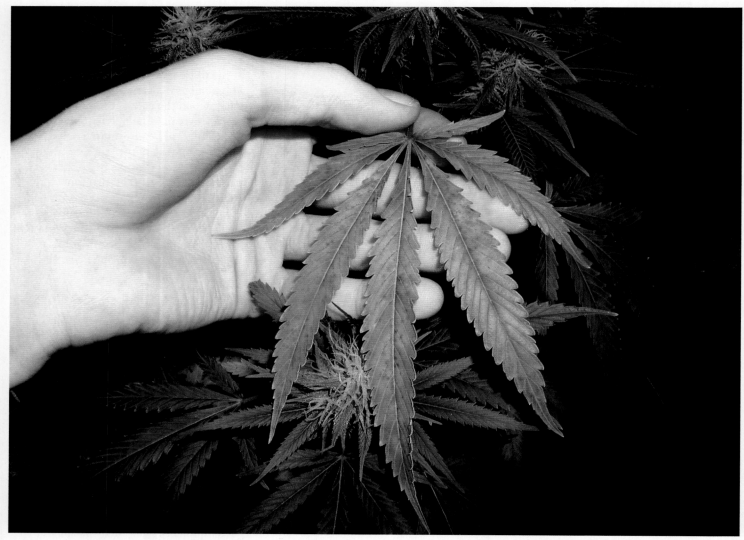

Problems with pH fluctuation or pH imbalance cause nutrients to become unavailable to plants. This leaf shows symptoms of a high pH.

and correct water supply pH, and there are few water-quality problems.

Add nutrients to water to create a nutrient solution before measuring pH because nutrients are acidic and will affect the outcome. Once nutrients are mixed in solution, wait a few minutes so that the solution can stabilize before measuring. I like to measure the pH of the original water to get an idea of how much the nutrients acidify the solution. If the pH of water is too low, add soluble potassium bicarbonate to neutralize it. Find potassium bicarbonate, also an organic fungicide, at pharmacies and hydroponic centers. However, water that is high in bicarbonate (HCO_3) makes it hard to keep the pH down, and it is difficult to avoid scale (mineral buildup) on equipment.

Once tested, the pH should be within the acceptable range for soil or hydroponics (see chart on page 340). Continue to fine-tune the pH level by adding small amounts of chemicals.

Phosphoric acid is the most popular substance used to lower pH. Potassium hydroxide is popular to raise pH. Both of these chemicals are relatively safe, although they can cause burns and should never come in contact with eyes. Most hydroponic supply stores sell easy-to-use pH adjusters that are diluted to a reasonably safe level.

Concentrated pH adjusters can cause large pH changes and can make adjusting the pH very frustrating. The pH will "bounce" up and down when adjusted with a concentrated product when added

in very small amounts. Not only does the pH overshoot the desired mark, the availability is virtually destroyed. If using such concentrates, dilute the chemical with a larger volume of water before adding it to the nutrient-solution reservoir.

Altering Nutrient-Solution pH

I like to use pH Up and pH Down from the hydroponic store rather than less-reliable citric acid, baking soda, or vinegar. Avoid using potassium hydroxide and sodium hydroxide, commonly used in hydroponic gardens, because they are caustic and require special handling.

Hydroponic gardeners use phosphoric and nitric acid to lower pH. Calcium nitrate can also be used but is less common. Such acids can be used to lower pH but must be added more often.

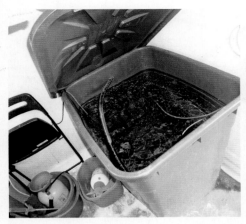

Keep the nutrient reservoir aerated to ensure maximum uptake from plants.

Measure the pH of water and nutrient solutions with litmus paper or an electronic pH tester. Both are available at most nurseries, home improvement centers, and hydroponic stores. Comparing the color of the soil/chemical mix to the color of the chart can be confusing. If you use one of these kits, make sure to buy one with good, easy-to-read color codes. Follow instructions supplied by the manufacturer.

Electronic pH testers are economical and convenient. Less-expensive pH meters are accurate enough for casual use. More-expensive models are very accurate. I prefer electronic pH meters to reagent test kits and litmus paper because pH meters are convenient, economical, and accurate. Once purchased, you can measure pH thousands of times with an electronic meter, while the chemical test kits are good for about a dozen tests. Perpetual pH-metering devices are also available and are most often used to monitor hydroponic nutrient solutions.

For an accurate pH test with an electronic pH meter:

1. Clean the probes of the meter after each test and wipe away any corrosion.

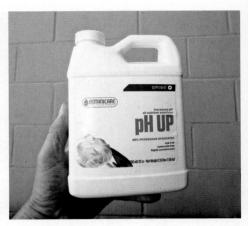

pH Up raises the pH of water or a nutrient solution.

2. Pack the soil around the probes.

3. Water soil with distilled or pH-neutral water before testing.

4. Use a dilution test of one part growing medium to one part distilled water. Stir, allow to sit, and then drain away liquid into a separate cup, using a filter for the medium, and then measure the water.

Raising Nutrient-Solution pH
Ammonium carbonate $(NH_4)_2CO_3$, aka "bakers' ammonia," is nitrogen in

Test the pH regularly, at least once a week, to ensure that it stays within the acceptable range for either soil or hydroponics. Water evaporates from hydroponic nutrient-solution tanks and transpires from foliage, using more water than nutrients. Both cause a concentration of nutrients, acidifying the nutrient solution and lowering the pH. The pH and electrical conductivity (EC) of water supplies in municipalities and cities can also change throughout the year.

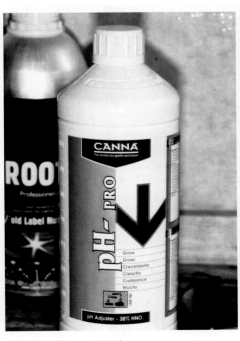

pH down lowers pH of water or a nutrient solution.

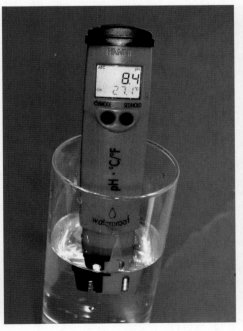
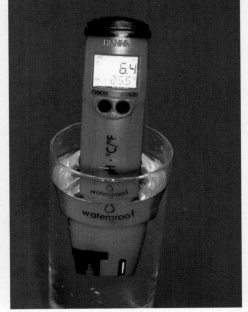

Add nutrients to the water first, and then check the pH. For example, the pH of the image on the left started out at 8.4, which is very high. Once the (acidic) nutrients were added, the pH dropped after an hour in solution. The gardener had to use pH down to drop the pH one more point to 6.4.

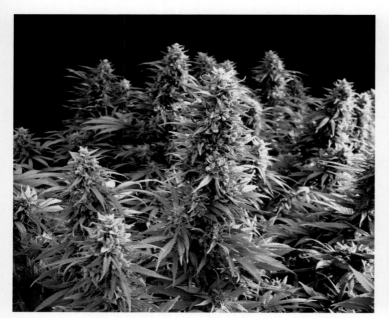

This beautiful crop of 'Jolly Bud' grown by DoobieDuck has no trouble with nutrient or water uptake.

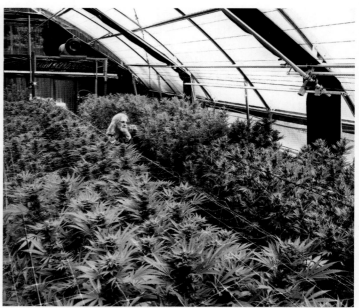

The water for this greenhouse in Santa Cruz, California, is treated with reverse osmosis to control pH and EC/ppm.

HOW pH AFFECTS PLANT NUTRIENT UPTAKE

EXPERIMENTAL AVAILABILITY OF NUTRIENTS

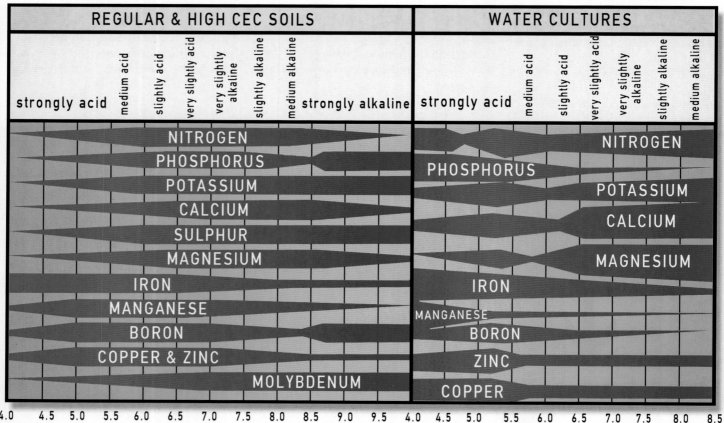

pH OF SATURATED SOIL
(pH below 5.5 cuts primary nutrients)

pH OF NUTRIENT WATER OR SATURATED SOILLESS MEDIUM
(pH above 5.5 cuts phosphorus & manganese)

the form of ammonia, but it is not a good choice to alter pH. When crushed it is used as smelling salts, and yes, it smells bad!

Calcium hydroxide ($Ca(OH)_2$, aka hydrated lime, builder's lime, or pickling lime) is an inorganic compound. Use only in small amounts because it is soluble and very fast-acting.

Potassium bicarbonate ($KHCO_3$) works well to neutralize or buffer pH. It is a common ingredient in club soda and is used as a source of CO_2 in baking and in dry chemical fire extinguishers, among other things. Potassium bicarbonate also works as an organic surface fungicide for powdery mildew. Be careful, concentrations above 0.5 percent can have toxic effects on plants.

Potassium carbonate (K_2CO_3) is a common ingredient in pH up solutions and it works well to raise pH in nutrient solutions. It is used as a leavening when baking gingerbread and as a buffering agent in wine production. It is also used for fire suppression.

Potassium (potash) silicate (K_2SiO_3) will raise pH quickly and add potassium to the nutrient solution and growing medium. It can be used as a foliar mist. Potassium silicate is also used to make welding rods and as an anticorrosive agent.

Potassium hydroxide (NOH, aka caustic potash) is relatively safe and very popular to raise pH. Potassium hydroxide is also mixed with potassium carbonate to buffer pH when using soft water. This inorganic compound is a strong base with many industrial uses, including cleaning chemicals, the manufacture of biodiesel and batteries.

Sodium bicarbonate ($NaHCO_3$, aka baking soda, bread soda, cooking soda, and bicarbonate of soda) will raise pH. It is also used as a stomach antacid. **Note:** See "Ammonium carbonate."

Sodium carbonate (Na_2CO_3) is a commonly used salt in water softeners. Do not use sodium carbonate to alter pH. It is detrimental to plant growth.

Sodium hydroxide (NaOH, aka lye and caustic soda) is very corrosive. It is commonly used as drain cleaner. Do not use sodium hydroxide to alter pH.

Safety Precautions

Dilute pH adjusters so they are safer and more forgiving, and dosages are easier to control.

Carbonates and hydroxides are bases.

Read labels completely and follow instructions.

Keep out of the reach of children.

Keep an ample supply of fresh water to dilute accidental spills.

Wear a mask, rubber gloves, long sleeves, and other protective clothing.

Do not inhale toxic fumes.

Store pH-adjusting agents in an airtight container to guard against spills and accidental activation with moisture. For example, when potassium hydroxide absorbs humidity, it turns into corrosive sludge.

Lowering Nutrient-Solution pH

Why does nutrient-solution pH constantly drop?

It depends on many things, from the medium to the air driven into it or exposed to it. The plant is also giving off protons (H+ ions) that add to the pH pool and lower the pH. This could almost be another chapter in this book!

The most common reason pH fluctuates is because native water is soft and has no buffering agents to stabilize pH.

Acids are used to lower pH. Most fertilizers are acidic and naturally lower pH. Acids that are not diluted in water are dangerous—they undergo chemical change so readily that they can react with skin and cause burns.

Use extreme caution when handling acids. The higher the concentration, the more corrosive they are. Acids can eat metals and burn your skin!

Hydroponic gardeners use **phosphoric and nitric acid** to lower pH. **Calcium nitrate** can also be used but it is less

common. Such acids can lower pH but must be added more often.

Ammonium monopotassium phosphate (KH_2PO_4, aka potassium dihydrogen phosphate, KDP, or monobasic potassium phosphate, MKP) is most effective to raise pH from 5.5 to 7.0. It also buffers pH well when within this range. The buffering ability diminishes below pH 5.5. It is a source of phosphorus and potassium. Gardeners can use ammonium monopotassium phosphate to minimize the escape of ammonia from nutrient solutions and growing mediums. It is also used as a fertilizer, food additive (in Gatorade, for example), and fungicide. The soluble salt can also be used as a fertilizer.

Ammonium nitrate (NH_4NO_3) is a high-nitrogen fertilizer, and can also be used in explosives.

Ammonium sulfate is often recommended to lower pH because it is difficult to overapply; however, cannabis can tolerate very little ammonium. Avoid using ammonium sulfate.

Calcium nitrate $Ca(NO_3)_2$ is also known as nitromagnesite, Norwegian saltpeter, Norgessalpeter, or nitrate of lime. It is an inorganic compound used in concrete.

Citric acid is unstable because plants break it down, and it tends to drift up after a few hours unless well buffered. Citric acid can be obtained from lemons and limes but is most often made from other sources. Citric acid should be used in emergencies only. It can also cause bacteria to grow, lowering dissolved oxygen in the nutrient solution and competing with roots.

Hydrochloric acid, a solution of hydrogen chloride (HCl), lowers pH quickly and efficiently. It is water-soluble. But it is a highly corrosive mineral acid that is used in cleaning supplies, PVC plastic, swimming pool maintenance, and many other products. Not recommended!

Muriatic acid (concentrated hydrochloric acid). Cannabis can tolerate low levels (<100 ppm) of chloride, which is derived from hydrochloric acid. Muriatic acid is produced from hydrochloric acid and common salt, sodium chloride (NaCl).

Nitric acid (HNO_3), a major component in fertilizers, lowers pH and does not precipitate when pH is high. It is a highly corrosive, strong, and toxic acid. Use at high dilutions and low concentrations. A concentration of 86 percent or more is called fuming nitric acid and reacts violently (often creating explosions) with many nonmetallic compounds.

Phosphoric acid* (H_3PO_4, aka ortho-phosphoric acid or phosphoric (V) acid) is one of the most popular chemicals used to lower pH in hydroponic gardens. Hydroponic stores sell it in dilute mixes that are ready to use and relatively safe. Phosphoric acid changes pH relatively quickly. Avoid using when pH is high and there is an abundance of phosphorus available to plants. Excess phosphorus tends to precipitate. Change to nitric acid in such situations.

*Phosphoric acid is also used to "convert rust" to black ferric phosphate; in gel form it is called naval jelly. Food grade phosphoric acid is used to acidify foods and beverages.

Potassium nitrate (KNO_3, aka saltpeter or saltpetre) is a food preservative and an important ingredient in gunpowder.

Magnesium nitrate [$Mg(NO_3)_2$] has 10.5 percent nitrogen and 9.4 percent magnesium.

Sodium hydroxide (NaOH) Do not use!

Sodium nitrate ($NaNO_3$, aka Peru saltpeter or Chile saltpeter) is used in fertilizer as a source of nitrate, food preservatives, and explosives.

Sulfur (S) is insoluble and unavailable to plants. Till elemental sulfur into soil, and oxygen turns sulfur into SO_4, which is readily available for uptake by roots. Most efficient oxidation takes place to convert sulfur to SO_4 in warm weather in lightly moistened, well-aerated soil. Cold temperatures and water-saturated soil slow the conversion. Elemental sulfur works well when applied a few weeks before the growing season. Take care when adding large quantities of elemental sulfur because it can quickly acidify soil.

Ammonium sulfate is an acid-forming material; K-Mag fertilizer, **potassium sulfate**, and **calcium sulfate** are neutral materials and have no effect on soil pH.

Active soil bacteria convert sulfur to sulfuric acid, lowering soil pH. The process is slow and soil temperature must be above 55°F (12.8°C). Do not flood soil (which creates anaerobic conditions) or else sulfur will convert to hydrogen sulfide that will kill roots (and smell like rotten eggs).

Ferrous sulfate also decreases soil pH, but it costs more than sulfur, and eight times more of it is needed in comparison to elemental sulfur.

Aluminum sulfate is expensive, and there are reports of aluminum toxicity when too much is applied. It changes soil pH instantly once mixed with soil.

Ammonium sulfate and **sulfur-coated urea** fertilizers have little effect on pH. For example, ammonium sulfate fertilizer 21-0-0 at 10 pounds per 1,000 square feet (92.9 m²) can change soil pH from 7.5 to 7.4.

Iron sulfate is soluble but 6 times more of it is necessary than elemental sulfur to change pH. It reacts in 3 to 4 weeks—faster than elemental sulfur—but can damage roots.

Magnesium sulfate ($MgSO_4$) contains magnesium, sulfur, and oxygen. Soluble **Epsom salts** ($MgSO_4 \cdot 7H_2O$) work well to correct magnesium deficiencies in soil and cannabis plants.

Sulfuric acid (H_2SO_4) is sold as swimming pool and car battery acid at most grocery stores, by the quart or liter. Mix 1 cup with a gallon of distilled water and get a gallon of pH down for about $1 USD. It also adds sulfur to the mix. Battery acid is 40 percent sulfuric acid. Do not use toxic battery acid from a battery; it is contaminated with lead!

Vinegar is the product of ethanol fermentation, resulting in acetic acid.

The pH of table vinegar ranges from 2.4 to 3.4. The pH climbs when diluted. Typically, acetic acid ranges from 4 to 8 percent concentration for table vinegar. Vinegar used for pickling can be as high as 18 percent. Cannabis breaks vinegar down, causing pH to climb. Vinegar also causes excess bacterial growth that uses soil oxygen and acidifies soils.

How Fluids Move within Cannabis

Water is essential to plant life. It provides a medium to transport nutrients necessary for plant life and make them available for absorption by the roots. Water quality is important for this process to work at maximum potential. With this in mind, the first question a medical cannabis gardener needs to ask about water is, "What's in the water, and how does it affect growing cannabis?"

Everything in water can affect how plant roots absorb it.

Microscopic root hairs in the rhizosphere (root zone) absorb water and nutrients in the presence of oxygen and carry them up the stem to the leaves. This flow of water from the soil through the plant is called the transpiration stream. A fraction of the water is processed and used in photosynthesis. Excess water evaporates into the air, carrying waste products along with it via the stomata in the leaves. This process is called transpiration. Some of the water also returns manufactured sugars and starches to the roots.

Roots support the plant, absorb nutrients, and provide the initial pathway into the plant's vascular system. A close-up look at a root reveals the xylem and phloem core—vascular tissue enveloped

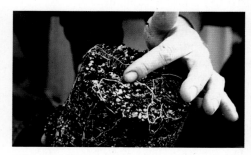
White, healthy roots absorb water and nutrients at a fast rate when grown properly.

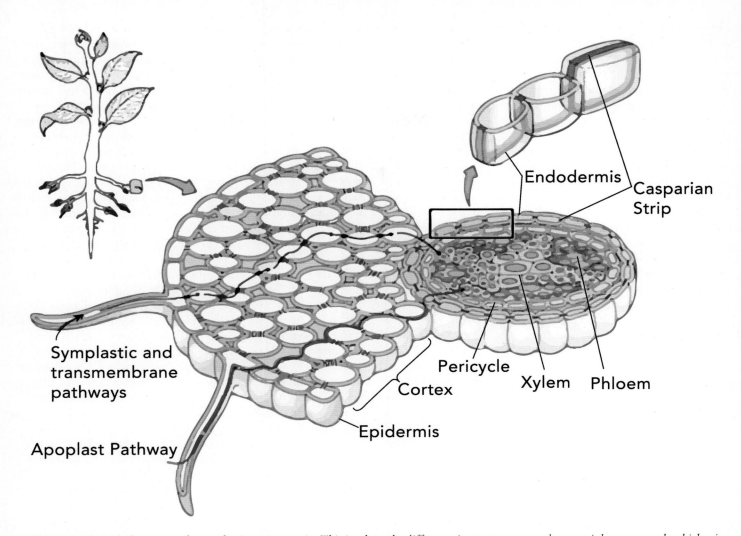

Labels in figure:
Endodermis
Casparian Strip
Pericycle
Xylem
Phloem
Cortex
Epidermis
Symplastic and transmembrane pathways
Apoplast Pathway

Everything goes through the same pathway, the Casparian strip. This is where the difference in a water root and terrestrial root occurs by thickening.

by a cortex tissue, or the layer between internal vascular and external epidermal tissue. The microscopic root hairs are located on the epidermal tissue cells. These root hair follicles are extremely delicate and must remain moist. Roots and root hairs must also be protected from abrasions, extreme temperature fluctuations, and harsh chemical concentrations. Plant health and well-being is contingent upon strong, healthy roots.

A majority of nutrient absorption begins at the root hairs, and the flow continues throughout the plant via the vascular system. Absorption is sustained by diffusion, in which water and nutrient ions are uniformly distributed throughout the plant. The intercellular spaces—apoplasts and connecting protoplasm, called symplast—are the pathways that allow the water and nutrient ions and

molecules to pass through the epidermis and the cortex to the xylem and phloem's vascular bundles. The xylem channels the solution through the plant while phloem tissues distribute the food manufactured by the plant. Once nutrients are transferred to the plant cells, each cell accumulates the nutrients it requires to perform its specific function.

The solution that is transported through the vascular bundles or veins of a plant has many functions. This solution delivers nutrients and carries away waste products. It provides pressure to help keep the plant structurally sound. The solution also cools the plant by evaporating water via the leaves' stomata.

Osmosis
Water and molecules or atoms smaller than a water molecule can move through

the semipermeable membrane. All other stuff enters through various ports and gates and controlled entry and transport. Water is given almost free reign, which is why a plant can recover from wilt so quickly when dry, but it takes three days for nitrogen to reach the right place in the plant. But flow can go the other way, too; it is all based on the principle of equilibrium, that a solution will achieve an equal concentration or disbursement of the ions dissolved in it. The solution is separated, the potential still exists, and water molecules are what move to dilute the more concentrated areas when the ions cannot move because of a barrier, in this case a semipermeable barrier through which only water molecules can pass. So water moves into the plant by a difference in the potential between the area of higher concentration (plant tissue) from a lower concentration (soil solution). If the potential is higher outside the plant tissue, such as overfertilization, water will move backward, governed by the laws of equilibrium again, from the plant into the soil, and thus burns are caused on the upper tissues.

The roots draw the water up the plant by osmosis, the process by which fluids are drawn through a semipermeable membrane and mix with each other until the fluids are equally concentrated on both sides of the membrane. Semipermeable membranes located in the root hairs allow specific nutrients that are dissolved in the water to enter the plant while the other nutrients and impurities are excluded. Since salts and sugars are concentrated in the roots, the electrical conductivity (EC) inside the roots is (almost) always higher than that outside the roots.

Here is a simplistic view of how osmosis works: It depends on the relative concentrations of each individual nutrient on each side of the (root) membrane; it does not depend on the total dissolved solids (TDS) or EC of the solution. For nutrients to be drawn in by the roots via osmosis, the strength of the individual elements must be greater than that of the roots.*

*Osmosis does depend on solution EC on either side of the root. However, the ions are allowed into the cell that may have a root hair by a larger pore structure of the membrane and is pulled in by the flow of water molecules from the soil solution into the plant. They may even be able to continue this pathway to the core, but will be switched over at the Casparian strip. In reality, for elements to enter apoplastically, they have to be smaller not stronger.

But, the transport of water (instead of nutrients) across the semipermeable membrane depends on EC. For example, if EC is greater outside the roots than inside, plants dehydrate as water is drawn out of the roots. In other words, salty water with a high EC can dehydrate plants.

Irrigation

Having a readily accessible water source is convenient, and it saves time and labor. For example, a 4 × 4-foot indoor garden of 16 healthy plants in 3-gallon (11.4 L) pots needs 10 to 25 gallons (37.9–94.6 L) of water per week. Large outdoor plants in big containers can use 5 to 10 gallons of water daily. Water weighs 8 pounds per gallon (1 kg/L). That's a lot of containers to fill, lift, and spill. Carrying water in containers from the bathroom sink to the garden is okay when plants are small, but when they are large, it is a big, sloppy, regular job.

Running a hose into the garden saves labor and mess. A lightweight half-inch (12.7 mm) hose is easy to handle and is less likely to damage plants than a hose having a larger diameter. If the water source has hot and cold water running out of the same tap, and it is equipped with threads, attach a hose and irrigate with tepid water. Use a dishwasher coupling or similar coupling if the faucet has no threads. The hose should have an on/off valve at the outlet, so water flow can be controlled. A rigid water wand prevents breaking branches while watering in tight quarters. Buy a water wand at the nursery or construct one from plastic PVC pipe. Do not leave water under pressure in the hose for more than a few minutes. Garden hoses are designed to transport water, not hold it under pressure, which may cause hoses to rupture.

Irrigation guidelines:

1. Water plants in containers when they are half-full of water; weigh pots to tell the difference.

2. Water soil gardens when the soil is dry one-half inch (1.3 cm) below the surface.

3. Water containers with a mild nutrient solution and let 10 to 20 percent drain off at each watering.

4. Do not let soil dry out to the point that plants wilt.

5. Do not let roots sit in water, such as a saucer, for more than 20 minutes at a time or roots will drown.

Large plants use more water than small plants, and small containers

differentially permeable membrane

water molecule

sucrose molecule

This simple drawing shows the basic principle of osmosis on a molecular level. When the concentration of "salts" is greater on one side of a barrier such as a cell wall in a plant, the salts migrate to the other side to equalize the pressure.

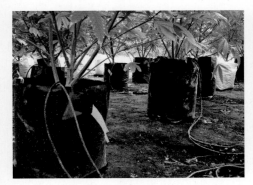

This drip system in a greenhouse uses two feeder hoses for each large container to ensure that the entire soil mass receives adequate irrigation.

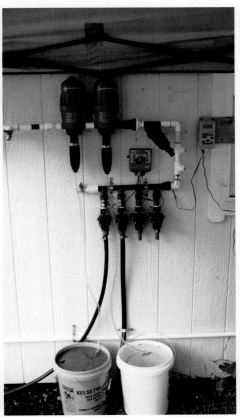

The fertilizer-injection irrigation setup above keeps fertilizer applied at a consistent rate and controls the pH.

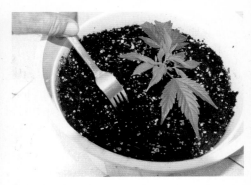

Lightly cultivating the soil surface breaks up the hard crust that often forms, allowing irrigation water to penetrate evenly.

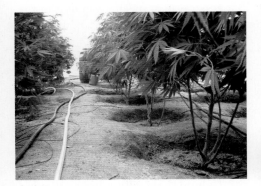

Plant in the earth outdoors or in a greenhouse.

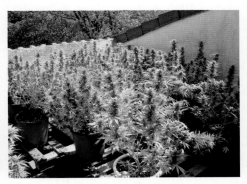

This outdoor garden is protected from wind by white walls that also reflect light. The pallets under pots allow for better drainage and keep soil up off the cold concrete floor, which keeps them warmer.

must be watered more often than large containers. But many more variables than plant or container size dictate a plant's water consumption. The health, age, variety, and size of the plant, and its container size, soil texture, as well as temperature, humidity, ventilation, and the intensity of wind and light all contribute to water needs. Change any one of these variables, and the water consumption will change. Good ventilation is essential to promote a free flow of fluids, transpiration, and rapid growth. The healthier a plant is, the faster it grows and the more water it needs.

In general, *sativa* varieties have a more extensive root system and use more water than *indica* varieties.

Small plants with a small root system in small containers of soil must be watered frequently—as soon as the soil surface dries out. If exposed to wind, small plants will dry out very quickly.

Irrigate soil and soilless mixes when they are dry one-half inch below the surface. As long as drainage is good, it is difficult to overwater fast-growing cannabis. Four-week-old clones flowering in 2- to 3-gallon (7.6 to 11.4 L) containers need to be irrigated once or twice daily. In fact, most gardeners prefer smaller containers because they are easier to control.

Flowering cannabis uses high levels of water to carry on rapid floral formation. Withholding water stunts flower formation. Plants exposed to wind dry out much faster than that are sheltered.

Mulch on top of soil surface conserves water and prevents a crust from forming. But mulch could also be difficult for irrigation water to penetrate. Always make sure water penetrates mulch evenly when irrigating.

Outdoor, terrace, and patio plants will use up to three or four times more water

than normal on a hot, windy day. Keeping up with watering is difficult and time-consuming. Use an automated watering system or a windbreak to lessen wind's impact on plants. Mulch will also lessen evaporation from the soil. Use plenty of water, and allow up to 10 percent runoff during each watering. The runoff will prevent fertilizer from building up in the soil. Water early in the day, so excess water will evaporate from the soil surface and the leaves. Letting foliage and soil remain wet overnight invites fungal attacks.

If planting in the earth outdoors, competing plants, especially established trees and bushes, suck up irrigation, depriving annual cannabis plants. For example, in my backyard, the oak trees on the other side of my fence suck up so much water that I must give the cannabis plants 3 to 4 times as much irrigation water as the same varieties in raised beds that have no competition from trees.

Sometimes the soil surface down as far as 6 inches (15.2 cm) is moist, but below the wet mark, soil may be bone dry. But the opposite may be true too. Fine topsoil and compost on the soil surface dry rapidly during windy days with a lot of sun and the soil below could remain super wet.

Moisture meters take most of the guesswork out of irrigating cannabis. They can be purchased for less than $30 USD and are well worth the money. Moisture meters measure exactly how much water the soil contains at any level or point. Often the soil will not hold water evenly, and thus it develops dry pockets. Checking the soil moisture with a finger provides an educated guess but disturbs the root system. A moisture meter will give an exact moisture reading without disturbing the roots.

Use a moisture meter outdoors to test the growing medium moisture at different depths. For example, if you continue to water plants and the water accumulates below the soil surface, oxygen could be squeezed out of the soil. However, the soil structure plays a major role. Porosity and the mix of appropriate size (large and small pore space) and any blocking actions in the mineral soil can change the equation. Water moves initially through the soil in all pore spaces while gravity pulls it through, and it is picked up by surrounding small pores through capillary action. It vacates the large pores under gravity and occupies the smaller. If the pores are all small, the amount of time to drain can increase; if the pores change size suddenly then the flow can be blocked such as the famed Texas clay pan; and if the amount of clay in the mineral soil is high, it can be smoothed during a preparation known as glazing, which stops the flow of water. But either way or mechanism, it is not

50 Percent Watering Rule

*Weigh a container after watering to get the "full" weight. Weigh the container after several days when it weighs "half" as much to find the 50 percent full weight. Water plants in containers when they are 50 percent full by weight. For example, a plant in a 3-gallon (11.4 L) container weighs 2.2 pounds (1 kg) when fully watered and 1.1 pounds (499 gm) when 50 percent full. It is time to water when the container weighs 1.1 pounds (499 gm).

One of the biggest issues with soils that dry down is that all the salts that are in solution adhere to the growing medium particles when the water disappears. As soon as water is reapplied, no matter at what EC, all of these salts, as well as any associated with the soil particles, immediately go into solution. For example, if the medium has an EC of 4.0 when dry, and very clean RO water is applied, the water will, for a short time until equilibrium is obtained, have an EC of 4.0, causing salt burn. If the EC is at 2.0 and the medium dries and watering is done at 1.6, then the EC jumps to 3.6, immediately causing issues. The solution to the problem is to run water into the container several times, which allows the medium to rehydrate and wash out the salts, then reapply fertility at normal values. Of course, this must all occur within the 20-minute time period.

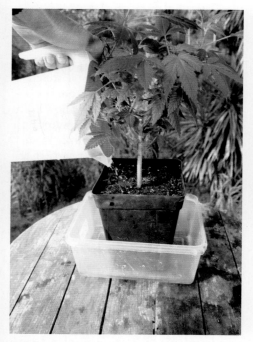

Fill the container to capacity with water.

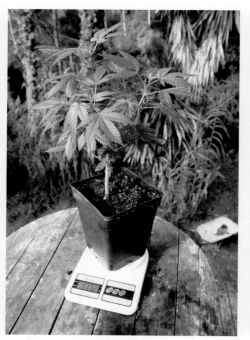

Weigh container to learn how much water it contains. When it weighs half as much as when drenched with water, it is time to irrigate.

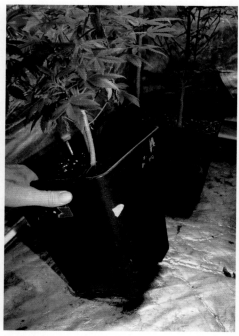

Tip the container to check if it is heavily laden with water. Irrigate the light container.

because the water is heavy, it is because the water accumulates for a given reason, indicating blocked or restricted passage.

Cultivate the soil surface to allow water to penetrate evenly and guard against dry soil pockets. Such cultivation also keeps water from running down the crack between the inside of the pot and the soil and then out the drain holes. Using Smart Pots or similar container will also solve this problem. See chapter 19, *Containers*, for more information. Gently break up and cultivate the top half-inch (1.3 cm) of the soil with your fingers, a salad fork, or a lightweight cultivator. Be careful not to disturb the tiny surface roots. After you develop some skill at knowing when the plants need water, you can check to see how heavy they are simply by tipping them.

Outdoor gardens may need deeper cultivation to aerate soil, but cultivate with care! If soil compacts around plants, insert a garden fork in the soil and wiggle it a little before removing. This will break up the soil and allow air to penetrate. Do not disturb soil much or it will break many roots.

Keep containers lined up in rows when growing and watering. It is much easier to keep track of watered and fertilized pots when they are lined up.

Overwatering
Cannabis does not like soggy soil. Soil kept too wet drowns roots, squeezing out the oxygen. This causes slow growth and possible fungal attack. Poor drainage is most often the cause of soggy soil. It is compounded by poor ventilation and high humidity.

Applying more water to the medium than it can hold against gravity for more than 20 minutes causes overwatering. Overwatering occurs when *more* water is applied to the growing medium after it has already been saturated for 20 minutes or more, or before the plant needs watering. After 20 minutes roots suffer from lack of oxygen and die.

Overwatering is a common problem, especially with small plants that have

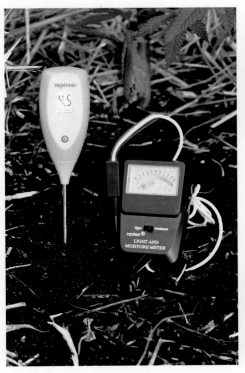

Inexpensive moisture meters help take the guesswork out of irrigation.

little volume in containers. Too much water drowns the roots by cutting off their supply of oxygen. Again, the most important thing to remember is to never let soil be saturated for more than 20 minutes.

If you have symptoms of overwatering, use a moisture meter. Pay attention to the levels of moisture in containers an in outdoor garden soil. Often dry soil pockets develop amidst moist soil. Sometimes, parts of the soil are overwatered and other soil pockets remain bone-dry. Lightly cultivating the soil surface, allowing even water penetration, and using a moisture meter will help overcome this problem. Indoors and in greenhouses, one of the main causes of overwatering is poor air ventilation. Plants need to transpire water into the air. If there is nowhere for this humid air to go, gallons of water are locked in the air of the enclosed area. Well-ventilated air carries this moist air away, replacing it with fresh, dry air. If you are using trays to catch runoff water, use a turkey baster, large syringe, or sponge to draw the excess water from the tray so that plants do not sit in stagnant water.

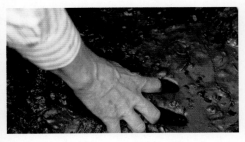

Heavy clay soil does not drain well and stays soggy for a long time. Soil or soilless mixes that drain well are essential to rapid cannabis growth.

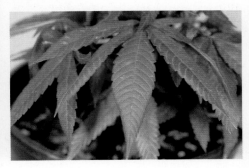

One sure sign of overwatering is when leaves curl under on the edges.

Signs of overwatering include:
1. Leaves curled down and yellowed
2. Waterlogged and soggy soil
3. Fungal growth
4. Slow growth

Symptoms of overwatering are often subtle, and inexperienced gardeners may not see any blatant symptoms for a long time.

Overwatering at the end of June, followed by a cold snap in my friend Nomaad's garden, retarded plant growth by two weeks. Plants had to be harvested later and produced about 20 percent less. If not overwatered, the plants would not have had spotty growth and would have flowered earlier. Pay attention to water temperature, too. If large outdoor pots are too wet at night, conditions are perfect for fungus growth to develop. Irrigate early in the morning so plants have enough time to absorb the water during the day.

Underwatering
Underwatering is less of a problem indoors and in backyards, but fairly common if small (1- to 2-gal) pots are used and the gardener does not realize the

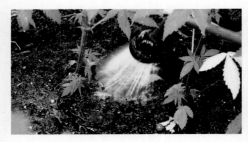

A water wand with a breaker mixes air with irrigation water just before applying.

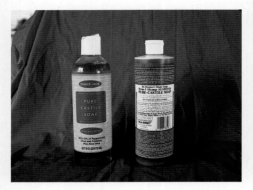

Add a few drops of biodegradable liquid dish soap concentrate to the irrigation water. The detergent helps water penetrate the soil more thoroughly.

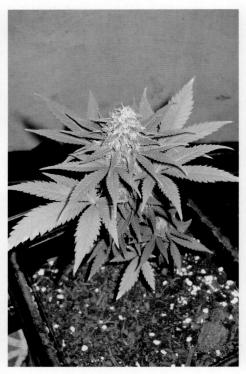

Underwatering causes plants to become stunted and take up water and nutrients at erratic rates. This little plant could have grown much better had the soil surface been cultivated so water could penetrate evenly.

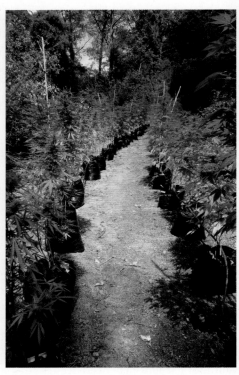

Set up a drip irrigation line to water rows of plants.

water needs of rapid-growing cannabis. Small containers dry out quickly and may require daily watering. If forgotten, water-starved plants become stunted. Once the tender root hairs dry out, they die. Most gardeners panic when they see their prize cannabis plants wilting in bone-dry soil. Dry soil, even in pockets, makes root hairs dry up and die. It seems to take forever for the roots to generate new root hairs and resume rapid growth.

Add a few drops (one drop per pint [47.3 ml]) of a biodegradable, concentrated liquid soap like Castille or Ivory to the water. It will act as a wetting agent by helping water penetrate the soil more efficiently, and it will guard against dry soil pockets. Apply about one quarter to one half as much water/fertilizer as the plant is expected to need, and then wait 10 to 15 minutes for it to totally soak in. Apply more water/fertilizer until the soil is evenly moist. Avoid letting runoff water sit in trays for more than 20 minutes after initial watering. Remove excess water with a large turkey baster.

Another way to thoroughly wet pots, especially ones that have fully dried, is to soak the containers in water. This is easy to do with small pots. Simply fill a 5-gallon (18.9 L) bucket with 3 gallons (11.4 L) of water. Submerge the smaller pot inside the larger pot, for a minute or longer, until the growing medium is completely saturated. Wetting plants thoroughly ensures against dry soil pockets. Do not submerge pot for more than 20 minutes or it will kill roots.

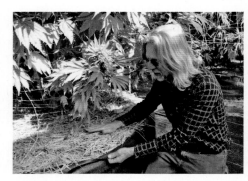

Whether in containers or planted directly in the ground, mulch plants (here with straw) to conserve moisture and protect soil surface.

PART **3** ADVANCED MEDICAL CANNABIS HORTICULTURE

21
NUTRIENTS

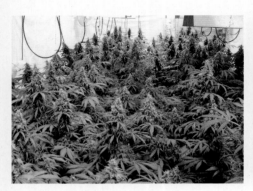

Healthy cannabis plants produce high yields.

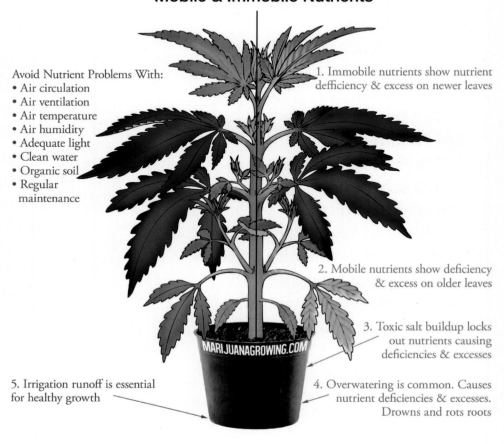

Healthy cannabis organically grown by DoobieDuck attracts birds and other wildlife.

MOST ANY NUTRIENT formula (fertilizer), regardless of its contents, will grow cannabis. But what quality will the cannabis be, and what are the residual health concerns? With the proper nutrient formula and growing conditions, medical cannabis can reach its genetic growth potential.

Nutrients

Cannabis needs the non-mineral nutrients carbon, hydrogen, and oxygen to manufacture food and grow. Carbon (CO_2) in the air is fixed via photosynthesis. Hydrogen atoms that are building blocks come almost totally from water. Oxygen from the atmosphere is used in respiration and plant processes. The rest of the elements (called mineral nutrients), are absorbed from the growing medium and nutrient solution. Supplemental nutrients supplied in the form of a fertilizer help medicinal cannabis to reach its maximum potential.

Nutrients must be *available* to roots in order to be absorbed. Nutrients occur in many chemical combinations and forms (called compounds) that are comprised of two or more nutrients' ions joined together via positive (anion) and negative (cation) attractions.* The compounds release nutrients for uptake by roots under specific conditions. The proper nutrient formula delivered at the proper pH and EC concentration makes nutrients available for uptake.

*An anion is an ion with a negative charge because it has more electrons than protons. A cation is an ion with a positive charge because it has more protons than electrons.

Well-managed life—microbes, bacteria, fungi, etc.—in organic soil interacts with naturally occurring nutrients to make them available for uptake by roots. Properly mixed and alimented soils with high fertility require very little supplemental fertilizer. For example, during the flowering stage, outdoor gardeners in Humboldt County, California, add just 2 handfuls of bat guano to grow 10-pound (4.5 kg) plants in living organic soil.

Nutrients are grouped into 3 categories: macronutrients or primary nutrients, secondary nutrients*, and micronutrients or trace elements.** Each nutrient in the above categories can be further classified as either mobile or immobile. Solving nutrient-deficiency problems is much easier when you know which nutrients are mobile or immobile.

*Some confusion exists on what the secondary nutrients are, but they are generally considered macronutrients as well as secondary macronutrients, and are measured the same way as a percentage of the overall mix.

**Trace elements are micronutrients measured in ppm.

Mobile nutrients are able to move (translocate) from one part of the plant to another as needed. When a nutrient shortage occurs, mobile nutrients travel to the area to solve the deficiency. For example, nitrogen accumulated in older leaves translocates to younger leaves to solve a deficiency. Mobile nutrients show deficiency symptoms on *older*, lower

Mobile & Immobile Nutrients

Avoid Nutrient Problems With:
• Air circulation
• Air ventilation
• Air temperature
• Air humidity
• Adequate light
• Clean water
• Organic soil
• Regular maintenance

1. Immobile nutrients show nutrient deficiency & excess on newer leaves

2. Mobile nutrients show deficiency & excess on older leaves

3. Toxic salt buildup locks out nutrients causing deficiencies & excesses

4. Overwatering is common. Causes nutrient deficiencies & excesses. Drowns and rots roots

5. Irrigation runoff is essential for healthy growth

MARIJUANAGROWING.COM

leaves first. Nitrogen will show a deficiency on older leaves because it is a part of essential enzyme structure and has to be replaced as these enzymes are denatured and disposed of. Mobile nutrients include nitrogen (N), phosphorus (P), potassium (K), and magnesium (Mg).

Immobile nutrients either stay at their destination or move very little once assimilated and transported. Immobile nutrients include calcium (Ca), boron (B), chlorine (Cl), cobalt (Co), copper (Cu), iron (Fe), manganese (Mn), molybdenum (Mo), silicon (Si), sulfur (S) and zinc (Zn). Deficiencies of immobile nutrients show symptoms first in younger leaves. These nutrients do not translocate to new growing areas as needed. They remain deposited in their original place in older leaves.

Other elements—Barium (Ba), Cadmium (Cd), Chromium (Cr), Lithium (Li), Palladium (Pd), and Vanadium (V)—may be necessary for plant growth and health. These elements should be available in low concentrations.

Leaching Growing Mediums

To leach* soil or substrate, add enough water (it takes a lot!) to the medium to wash out excess fertilizer (nutrient) salts. For a container that holds 1 gallon (3.8 L) of water, add enough water to make sure it is full—until water drips out the bottom. Then apply 1 additional gallon of water (3.8 L,) and allow 1 gallon (3.8 L) to drain out the bottom of the container. Do this a total of 7 times. Once a total of 7 gallons (26.5 L) of water has been added and drained, the process is almost complete.

Add 1 more gallon (3.8 L) of water that includes the correct ratio and concentration of fertilizer. **The entire process must be completed within 20 minutes or the excess of water will drown the roots.**

The process can be done 2 or 20 times, as long as it is completed within 20 minutes. I repeat: the container must *drain completely* within 20 minutes. "Drain completely" means drain to a point at which the water is held against gravity within 20 minutes. This practice is *not* overwatering.

Toxic Nutrient Conditions

Too often gardeners give their medical cannabis gardens too much tender loving care. This care and enthusiasm is kindled by countless nutrient and additive advertisements. As a consequence, medical cannabis gardeners frequently overapply fertilizers and additives, creating toxic soil conditions. Often the solution to this problem is to leach the built-up nutrients out of the growing medium with copious quantities of water. This will wash away excess nutrients that have built up in the soil and created toxic conditions. An overabundance of nutrients (fertilizer salts) in the growing medium disrupts the medium's chemical balance. This imbalance causes some nutrients to become unavailable for uptake by roots and other nutrients to be oversupplied.

Leaching the substrate works well for most nutrient problems, but it does not solve all nutrient problems. For more information please see specific nutrients.

*Water is used to leach fertilizer salts from a growing medium. Just before harvest, plants and soil are flushed to remove excess nutrients in plant tissue.

Note: See chapter 9, *Harvest, Drying & Curing,* for more info about leaching the substrate and flushing nutrients out of medical cannabis plants before harvest. See chapter 23, *Container Culture & Hydroponics,* for more information on leaching hydroponic mediums and water-based hydroponics.

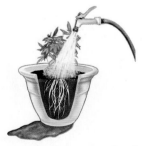

Leach substrates to wash away nutrient buildup.

In order to measure nutrients in solution, you will need an accurate, calibrated EC (electrical conductivity) meter and an accurate, calibrated pH meter.

NUTRIENT	MOBILITY
nitrogen (N)	mobile
phosphorus (P)	mobile
Potassium (K)	mobile
calcium (Ca)	immobile
magnesium (Mg)	mobile
sulfur (S)	semimobile
zinc (Zn)	immobile
iron (Fe)	semimobile
manganese (Mn)	immobile
boron (B)	very immobile
copper (Cu)	semimobile
molybdenum (Mo)	mobile
chlorine (Cl)	immobile
cobalt (Co)	immobile
nickel (Ni)	mobile
selenium (Se)	semimobile
silicon (Si)	immobile
sodium (Na)	mobile / immobile

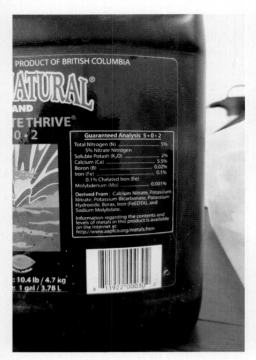

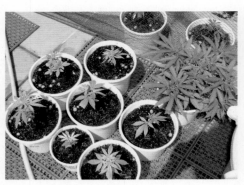

These seedlings are suffering from nitrogen deficiency.

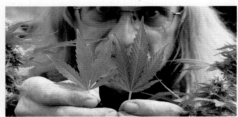

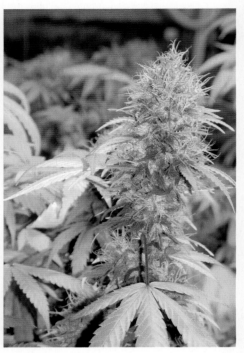

Fertilizer contents are listed on the container. Read them carefully to ensure that your plants are receiving a balanced nutrient formula.

The pale leaf on the left is nitrogen deficient; the leaf on the right is healthy.

The nitrogen level is low in flowering fertilizer formulas, causing older leaves to yellow.

Macronutrients

Macronutrients are the elements that the plants use most and must be present at all times for growth to grow well. Most fertilizers usually show nitrogen (N), potassium (P), phosphorous (K) as (N-P-K) percentages in big numbers on the front of the package. They are always listed in the same N-P-K order. These nutrients must always be in an available (soluble) form to supply cannabis with the building blocks for rapid growth. Nitrogen is the nutrient most often found deficient.

Nitrogen (N)—mobile (essential)

About: High levels of nitrogen are needed during vegetative growth, but lower levels are needed during seedling, clone, and flowering growth stages. Reducing nitrogen levels causes earlier flowering and increased abscisic acid (hormone) levels.

Nitrogen regulates the cannabis plant's ability to make proteins essential for new protoplasm in the cells, and many other functions. It is mainly responsible for leaf and stem growth, as well as overall size and vigor. Nitrogen is most active in young buds, shoots, and leaves. Cannabis absorbs nitrogen mainly in the form of ammonium (NH_4+), which is assimilated very quickly into mainly amino acids, and nitrate (NO_3-)—the nitrate form of nitrogen—is assimilated more slowly into most everything else. Small organic molecules also supply nitrogen. Be careful when using ammonium; too much can burn plants. Hydroponic fertilizers use slower-acting nitrate and mix it with ammonium. The proper balance keeps the rhizosphere pH more stable, and high ammonium levels influence taste of harvest.

Deficiency: Nitrogen is the most common cannabis nutrient deficiency in greenhouses, indoors, and outdoors. Low levels of nitrogen deficiency often go unnoticed. Deficiencies progress as follows:

First there is a lightening and slight yellow coloration to older mature leaves followed by leaf death or drop. Leaves lose luster, turning slightly pale. Stunting can also be seen when there has been

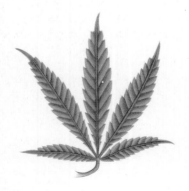

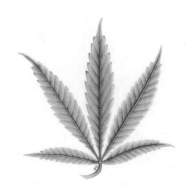

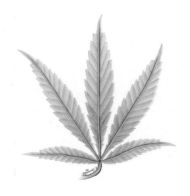

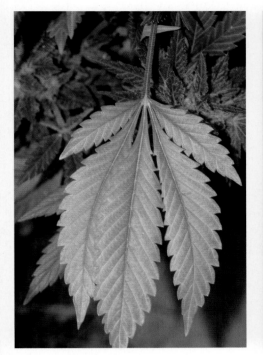

Nitrogen-deficient leaf

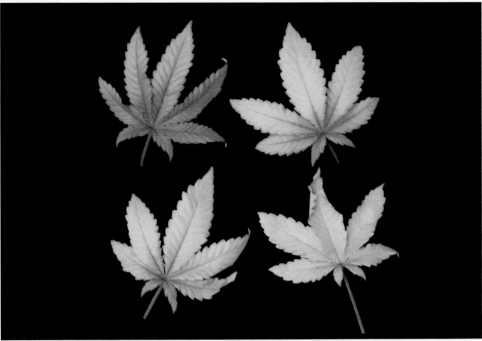

This photo of 'Pakistani' leaves shows the progression of nitrogen deficiency (clockwise from top left). (MF)

a slight deficiency for a time. Acute deficiency will result in decreased flowering.

Leaf margins may discolor. Leaves continue to yellow and may curl, develop brownish spots, and, as deficiency progresses, start to drop. Growth slows on shorter plants with smaller leaves and narrower stems. Yellowing of leaves progresses upward on plants. Signs of premature flowering appear on sickly plants. Yield is substantially diminished.

Cause: Nitrogen is highly soluble and easily washed out of growing mediums. It must be replaced regularly, especially during vegetative growth. Decaying organic matter and soil life may consume available nitrogen in soil and deplete it faster than roots can take it up.

Nitrogen is used quickly during rapid growth, and mild deficiency could occur; even if it is available, roots may not be able to supply nitrogen fast enough. Nutrient levels inside plants catch up when growth slows. The cause could also be inadequate nitrogen in the fertilization schedule or when using a growing medium with a low CEC (cation exchange capacity) that was

not designed for use with the nutrient formula. Diseases such as *Fusarium* and *Pythium* can cut fluid flow and the supply of nitrogen, but they have specific symptoms apart from nitrogen depletion.

Confused with: Potassium deficiency. Reddish stems and leaf undersides caused by potassium deficiency can be misinterpreted in cannabis varieties that naturally have reddish-purple stems and petioles.

Solution: Leach growing medium with a slightly more concentrated nutrient solution. Fertilize with the proper soluble high-nitrogen fertilizer that has the proper ratio of ammonium (NH_4+) and nitrate (NO_3-)—the nitrate for the growing medium. Organic sources of soluble high-nitrogen fertilizers include

blood meal, seabird guano, fish emulsion, compost teas, and more. Check and correct pH in the root zone. Leaves should green up in 3 to 5 days. Severely affected leaves may not recover and should be removed. For faster results in foliage, foliar feed with a soluble, dilute, high-nitrogen fertilizer. Soil application is also necessary when foliar feeding, because foliar applications do not translocate. Even though nitrogen is mobile when plants are foliar fed, it stays in the leaves.

Excess: First, older bottom leaves turn lush, dark green, and supple. As the overdose advances, leaves in the middle and top of the plant are affected. The weak foliage is susceptible to temperature and humidity stress, diseases, and pest attacks. Stems weaken and fold

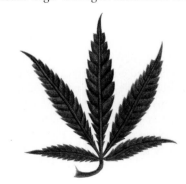

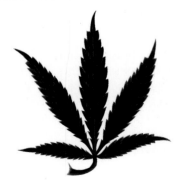

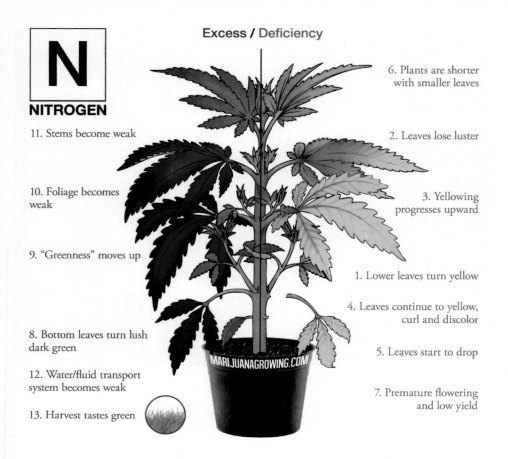

NITROGEN

Excess / Deficiency

11. Stems become weak

10. Foliage becomes weak

9. "Greenness" moves up

8. Bottom leaves turn lush dark green

12. Water/fluid transport system becomes weak

13. Harvest tastes green

MARIJUANAGROWING.COM

6. Plants are shorter with smaller leaves

2. Leaves lose luster

3. Yellowing progresses upward

1. Lower leaves turn yellow

4. Leaves continue to yellow, curl and discolor

5. Leaves start to drop

7. Premature flowering and low yield

---

if stress is allowed to progress. As the excess progresses, the water transport system becomes restricted and foliage turns brownish-copper. Leaves become thickened and brittle, excess NH_4 causes Ca deficiency. Excess levels of nitrogen in harvested plants cause the dried cannabis to taste "green" and burn poorly when smoked.

Cause: Nitrogen overdose is seldom a problem unless soil is loaded with the nutrient or too much was applied via the fertilizer mix.

Confused with: Excess nitrogen is not usually confused with anything unless salt burn becomes an issue. Some have related it to viral infections.

Solution: Leach growing medium with a dilute fertilizer solution. Severe problems require heavy leaching to carry away all the toxic elements. Leach as per "Leaching Growing Mediums" on page 351. Add a dilute complete fertilizer. Cut back on nitrogen dose if plants remain excessively green. Results should appear in 3 to 5 days, possibly earlier in hydroponic gardens.

Do not withhold nitrogen in subsequent fertilizing after leaching or when flowering. The nitrogen in the mix must be reduced but not removed. The main issue for cannabis cultivation is when the level of NH_4 is too high. When too much N is applied, especially as NH_4, it is moved to the vacuole of the cell and converts to nitrite or nitrosamines or both—cancer-causing products. Some "experts" say the ratio of nitrogen needs to be 1:1 but the experts I believe find that a more reduced ratio of 1:4 is much better and safer. This provides a balance so that the ratio of nitrogen does not deviate and turn into NH_4 quickly.

Phosphorus (P)—mobile (essential)

About: Phosphorus is indispensable for photosynthesis. It is the energy source for plants transferring energy generated in PS and during respiration, from the release of stored energy in carbohydrates. Phosphorus—one of the components of DNA, many being enzymes and proteins—is associated with overall vigor, resin, and seed production. Phosphorus is extremely important to the health of young plants. More than two thirds of

the phosphorus absorbed during the cannabis life cycle is taken in during the first quarter of life. The highest concentrations of phosphorus are found in roots' growing tips, growing shoots, and vascular tissue.

Deficiency: Lack of phosphorus is relatively uncommon and often misdiagnosed. The deficiency is first noticed when the petioles begin to take on a purple hue. Do not confuse with purpling of the main stem, which is indicative of an overall nutrient deficiency. Leaves take on a bluish green hue. Vertical growth slows, as well as lateral development. Dark copper-colored or purple-to-blackish dead blotches start to show on deformed lower leaves after a couple of weeks of deficiency. Dark necrotic spots develop on leaf stems (petioles) as leaves curl downward and drop. Severely affected leaves develop a dark bronze or metallic purple color as leaves continue to curl, contort, wither, and drop. Flowering is often delayed, buds are much smaller, seed yield is poor, and plants become more vulnerable to fungal and insect attack.

There is a big difference between petioles and stems when purpling occurs. On petioles this is a clear sign of phosphorus deficiency; on stems this is an overall deficiency indicating underfeeding. This underfeeding can come from many reasons, including lack of nutrients, but also poor water relations, high humidity, anything that slows transport, and overdosing microbes in the root zone as well as soil temp being too high or low, and overwatering. Purpling petioles or stems are NOT associated with a nitrogen deficiency, except where it was part of an overall problem including phosphorus.

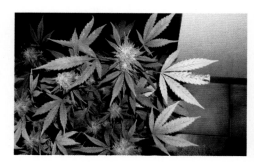

Phosphorus deficiency

Cause: When a phosphorus deficiency does occur, the pH has usually drifted up too high, beyond 7.0, which makes the macronutrient unavailable for uptake because it becomes unavailable as it changes ion form. Cold temperatures [below 50°F (10°C)] impair phosphorus uptake. Deficiencies are aggravated by clay and soggy soils. Other causes include acidic growing medium, an excess of iron and zinc, or soil that has become fixated (chemically bound) with phosphates. However, adequate zinc is necessary for proper utilization of phosphorus.

Confused with: Zinc deficiency, cold temperatures

Solution: Naturally occurring phosphate compounds accessible for uptake by roots are seldom available. Phosphorus is bound in organic compounds and is released via decomposition affected by soil life. Bat guano is a readily available source of phosphorus. Steamed bone meal, barnyard manure, and compost are the next-best sources. Thoroughly mix in the organic nutrients into living soil. Always use finely ground organic components that break down and become available quickly. Prevent deficiencies by mixing a complete organic fertilizer that contains phosphorus into the growing medium before planting. Outdoors, mix fine, steamed bone meal and pulverized rock phosphate into soil the year before planting.

Use phosphoric acid to lower the pH to within a range of 5.5 to 6.2 in hydroponic units, and lower the EC too. Correct the pH (6.0–7.0 for clay soils and 5.5–6.5 for potting soils) to facilitate phosphorus availability. If the soil is too acidic and an excess of iron and zinc exists, phosphorous becomes unavailable.

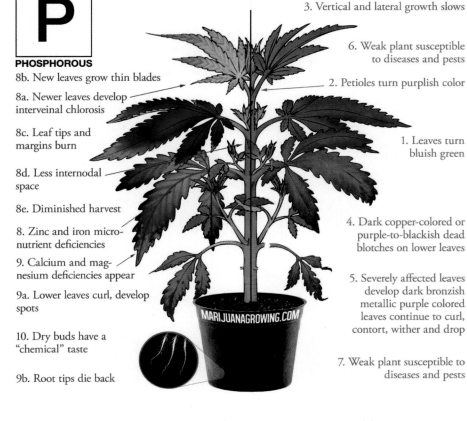

Excess / Deficiency

P

PHOSPHOROUS

8b. New leaves grow thin blades

8a. Newer leaves develop interveinal chlorosis

8c. Leaf tips and margins burn

8d. Less internodal space

8e. Diminished harvest

8. Zinc and iron micro-nutrient deficiencies

9. Calcium and magnesium deficiencies appear

9a. Lower leaves curl, develop spots

10. Dry buds have a "chemical" taste

9b. Root tips die back

3. Vertical and lateral growth slows

6. Weak plant susceptible to diseases and pests

2. Petioles turn purplish color

1. Leaves turn bluish green

4. Dark copper-colored or purple-to-blackish dead blotches on lower leaves

5. Severely affected leaves develop dark bronzish metallic purple colored leaves continue to curl, contort, wither and drop

7. Weak plant susceptible to diseases and pests

MARIJUANAGROWING.COM

Cannabis absorbs inorganic phosphates in ionic form only. Check with your local hydroponic store for appropriate phosphorous-rich, properly formulated nutrient mixtures. Use soluble forms of phosphorus when soil temperatures are below 50°F (10°C).

Excess: Relatively common, especially during flowering. In fact, an excess of phosphorus is promoted to thicken flower buds and add weight to final harvest. Excess is usually caused by adding too much high-phosphorus fertilizer in an available form. Toxic signs of phosphorus may take several weeks to surface, especially if excesses are buffered by a stable pH. Symptoms manifest in the form of micronutrient deficiencies in zinc, which is the most common, and iron. Also, as phosphorus availability increases, calcium and magnesium availability drops. If signs of zinc and iron deficiencies are present, phosphorus could also be lacking.

Excess chemical-based phosphorus in cannabis buds during flowering causes a "chemical" taste when smoked.

Cause: Many cannabis varieties can tolerate high levels of phosphorus. Available phosphorus builds to toxic levels if heavily applied and not leached from soil.

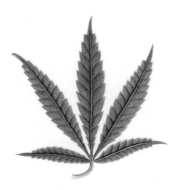

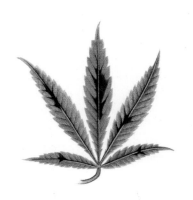

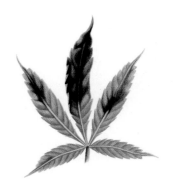

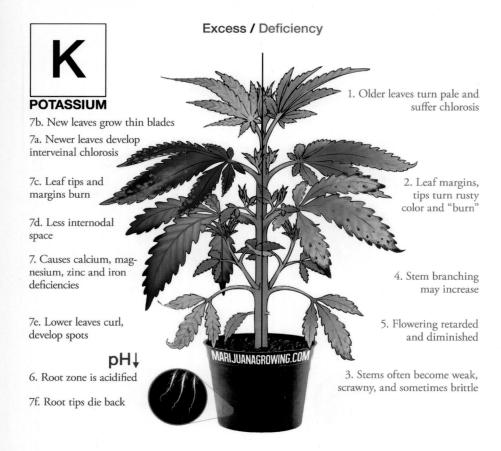

K

POTASSIUM

7b. New leaves grow thin blades

7a. Newer leaves develop interveinal chlorosis

7c. Leaf tips and margins burn

7d. Less internodal space

7. Causes calcium, magnesium, zinc and iron deficiencies

7e. Lower leaves curl, develop spots

pH↓

6. Root zone is acidified

7f. Root tips die back

1. Older leaves turn pale and suffer chlorosis

2. Leaf margins, tips turn rusty color and "burn"

4. Stem branching may increase

5. Flowering retarded and diminished

3. Stems often become weak, scrawny, and sometimes brittle

MARIJUANAGROWING.COM

Confused with: A deficiency of zinc, iron, magnesium, or calcium

Solution: Raise the pH. Phosphorus does not leach very well so leaching the growing medium has little effect. It just changes form and can combine with calcium to form insoluble compounds.

Potassium (K)—mobile (essential)
About: Potassium helps combine sugars, starches, and carbohydrates, and is essential to their production and movement. Potassium is vital to growth by cell division. It increases the chlorophyll in the foliage and helps to regulate stomata openings so plants make better use of light and air. It is necessary to make proteins that augment oil content and improve flavor in cannabis plants. It also encourages strong root growth and is associated with disease resistance and water intake. The potash form of potassium oxide is (K_2O). Soils with a high level of potassium increase a plant's resistance to bacteria and mold.

Deficiency: Potassium deficiencies are common in indoor gardens, less common in greenhouses, and somewhat common outdoors. Potassium deficiency causes the internal temperature of foliage to climb; beyond 104°F (40°C), it causes protein in cells to burn and degrade. To cool down leaves, evaporate moisture. Evaporation is normally highest on leaf edges, and that's where the burning takes place. Up to 70 percent of a plant's energy is "burned" to keep cool.

Potassium in excess also moves to these far areas, pores at the ends of the veins, and accumulates, causing this burn that is often confused with general salt burn but is not. The chlorosis must be seen first and a dulling in the cuticle layer of the leaf, all on older leaves.

Plants with a minor potassium deficiency appear healthy; leaves are a little too green and have a dull tone. Stems thin and branching may increase. Young leaf fringes and tips discolor turning a rusty brown, dehydrating and curling up. Progressively greater numbers of older leaves (first tips and margins, followed by whole leaves) develop rust-colored blotches, turn dark, and die. Stems often become weak, scrawny, and sometimes brittle. Deficient plants become very susceptible to disease and pest attacks. Flowering is retarded and greatly diminished.

Cause: Potassium is usually present but fixed or bound in humus-rich and clay soils, often locked in by toxic fertilizer (salt) buildup. Excess sodium in the water source that has built up in soil, calcium magnesium and phosphorus and cold weather impair uptake of potassium.

Confused with: Endema (an abnormal accumulation of fluids) or spots caused by bacteria or fungi. Absorption of magnesium, manganese, and sometimes zinc and iron is also slowed. Burned leaf margins are also caused by low humidity and overall fertilizer (salt) burn.

Solution: Leach the toxic salt out of the soil by leaching heavily with clean water.

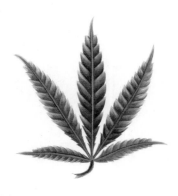

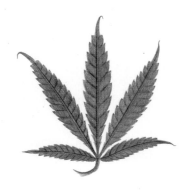

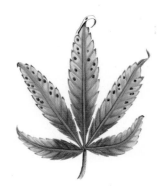

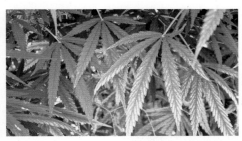

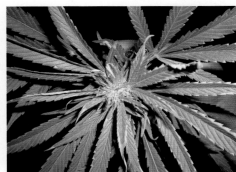

Potassium deficiency

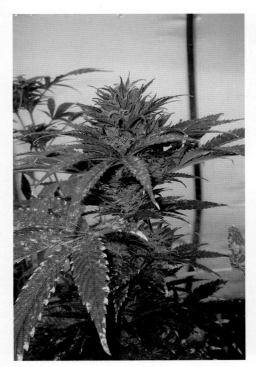

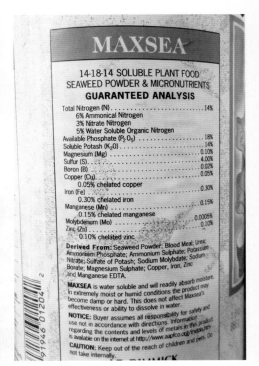

The burned leaf fringes on this 'Dynamite' clone have classic signs of potassium deficiency.

Severe potassium deficiency

This soluble plant food lists its ingredients in percentages and explains where they were derived from.

Apply a well-balanced N-P-K fertilizer with high potassium content. Organic gardeners add fast-acting potassium in the form of liquid kelp or potash. Potassium is absorbed quickly and deficiency symptoms should disappear in a few days. Add slow-acting granite dust and greensand to outdoor planting holes.

Excess: Occasionally, too much potassium is a problem, but it is difficult to diagnose because it is mixed with the deficiency symptoms of other nutrients. Excess potassium acidifies the root zone, slows the absorption of calcium, magnesium, and sometimes zinc and iron. Look for signs of toxic potassium buildup when symptoms of calcium, magnesium, zinc, and iron deficiencies appear.

Cause: Potassium has built up in soil, and too much is now available to roots.

Confused with: Calcium, magnesium, and sometimes zinc and iron deficiencies or general salt burn. However, coco coir gives off large amounts of potassium, which is readily absorbed and locks out calcium and magnesium; the result is calcium and magnesium deficiency symptoms but with tip and later marginal

leaf burn from potassium accumulating at these points. True salt burn comes not from too many ions in the tissue but from a reversal of the osmotic gradient, pulling water out of the plants not moving it into the plant. The fix in coco is to increase the EC, not back it up and leach.

Solution: Leach the growing medium of affected plants with a very mild and complete fertilizer solution. Severe problems require that more water be leached through the growing medium. Leach with a minimum of three times the volume of water for the volume of the growing medium.

Secondary Nutrients

The secondary nutrients—calcium, magnesium, and sulfur—are often grouped with the macronutrients (nitrogen, phosphorus, and potassium) because plants use secondary nutrients in large amounts. Rapid-growing cannabis is able to process more of these nutrients than most general-purpose fertilizers are able to supply. A properly balanced organic or ionic salt hydroponic fertilizer supplies all necessary macro and micro (trace)

elements in the proper formulations for maximum results.

Calcium and magnesium are dissolved in all water sources, usually in large amounts. Lower levels of sulfur are also present in most water supplies. Always take into account the amount of preexisting calcium and magnesium 'nutrients' already available in the water supply when fertilizing, especially in hydroponic formulas. Excessive calcium causes "hard water," a condition that limits nutrient uptake.

If growing in an acidic potting soil or soilless mix, correct the pH of the growing medium to 5.8 with agricultural lime. Calcium is already incorporated into the peat part of the mix. The proper rate of all lime tends to be three to five kilograms per 35 ft³ (3–5 kg per 1 m³).

With a pH below 6.0, incorporating one cup of fine (flour) dolomite lime per gallon of growing medium ensures adequate supplies of calcium and magnesium. Forms of sulfur are found as compounds in most fertilizers.

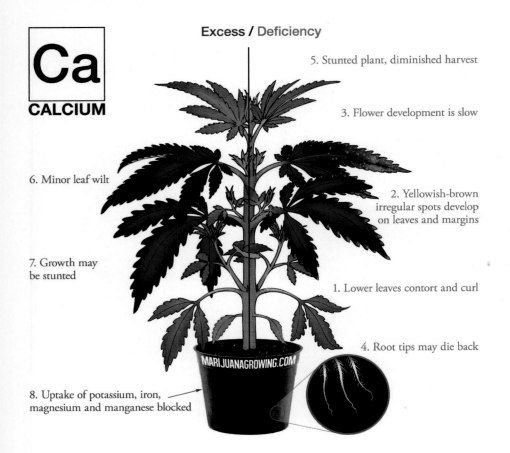

Excess / Deficiency

5. Stunted plant, diminished harvest

3. Flower development is slow

2. Yellowish-brown irregular spots develop on leaves and margins

6. Minor leaf wilt

7. Growth may be stunted

1. Lower leaves contort and curl

4. Root tips may die back

8. Uptake of potassium, iron, magnesium and manganese blocked

MARIJUANAGROWING.COM

Ca
CALCIUM

Calcium (Ca)—immobile (essential)

About: Calcium is fundamental to cell manufacturing and growth. Calcium is necessary to preserve membrane permeability and cell integrity, which ensure proper flow of nitrogen and sugars. Calcium stimulates enzymes that help build strong cell and root walls. Cannabis must have some calcium at the growing tip of each root. Since calcium has little mobility within the plant, it must be available in the root zone for uptake in order to avoid shortages. Tap water "hardness" is determined by the amount of dissolved calcium and magnesium salts. High levels of calcium help protect plant tissue from pest and disease attacks. But hard water scale contains a considerable amount of calcium carbonate, $CaCO_3$, which is almost insoluble in water.

Deficiency: Calcium is most often deficient in hydroponic gardens, but this deficiency is rather uncommon in greenhouses and indoors. Calcium is abundant in virtually all soils but occasionally lacking outdoors in cool wet climates and acidic soil. Calcium is sometimes deficient in soilless rooting mediums.

Early deficiency causes lower leaves to contort and curl. As the deficiency progresses, symptoms appear relatively quickly, first in lower leaves that develop yellowish-brown irregular spots with a dark brown border that enlarges over time. Often spots are at or near the edge of leaves. Older affected leaves develop yellowish hazy zones and spots around larger necrotic irregular spots. Flower bud development is inhibited, and root tips often die back. The plants are stunted and harvest is diminished.

Cause: An imbalanced fertilizer with unavailable calcium causes a deficiency. Calcium can be bound or fixed in (acidic) soil and unavailable for uptake. Excess ammonium, magnesium, potassium, and sodium in the root zone impair calcium uptake. Often, calcium is available in solution and growing medium but unavailable within the plant due to a transport problem (within the plant) caused by environmental conditions. Humidity that is too high or too low impairs transpiration. An EC that is too high, or improper irrigation that causes internal movement of water, will affect calcium uptake and is demonstrated in

lower leaves. Excess phosphorus could also be the cause.

Confused with: Root disease, excess nitrogen (ammonium), magnesium, potassium and sodium or deficiencies of iron, potassium and zinc

Solution: Leach soil and soilless mix with plain or low-EC water to wash out any built-up fertilizer salts that impair calcium uptake. Avert deficiencies in the soil and in most soilless mixes by adding fine dolomite lime (Ca and Mg) or gypsum (calcium sulfate hydrate $[CaSO_4 \cdot 2(H_2O)]$) to the planting mix. Acidic soils often contain low levels of calcium.

Use properly formulated soluble-hydroponic fertilizer that contains adequate available calcium, preferably calcium nitrate. Dissolve one-half teaspoon (2.5 cc) of hydrated lime per gallon of water. Water the deficient plants with calcium-dosed water as long as new deficiency symptoms persist. Remember, damaged tissue will not go away. Or use a complete hydroponic nutrient that contains adequate available calcium. Keep the pH of the growing medium stable. Reverse osmosis filtered water must have calcium added.

Excess: Leaves wilt, but very little. Excessive amounts of soluble calcium applied early in life can stunt growth. Too much calcium blocks potassium, iron, magnesium, and manganese uptake. If growing hydroponically, an excess of calcium will combine with sulfur in the solution, which causes the nutrient solution to suspend in the water and to aggregate into clumps, which then causes the water to become cloudy (flocculate). Once calcium and sulfur combine, they form a residue [gypsum $CaSO_4 \cdot 2(H_2O)$] that settles to the bottom of the reservoir.

Cause: Too much available calcium in water or nutrient solution

Confused with: Deficiency of potassium, magnesium, manganese, or iron

Solution: Change nutrient solution, attempt to wash excess from soil with heavy leaching.

Magnesium (Mg)–mobile (essential)

About: Cannabis uses a lot of magnesium. It is the central atom in every chlorophyll molecule, and it is essential to the absorption of light energy and photosynthesis. It aids in the utilization of nutrients. Magnesium helps enzymes make carbohydrates and sugars that are later transformed into flowers. It also neutralizes the soil acids and toxic compounds produced by the plant.

Deficiency: Deficiencies are common indoors and occasionally outdoors, especially in acidic soils. No deficiency symptoms are visible during the first 3 to 4 weeks. In the fourth to sixth week of growth, the first signs of deficiency appear. Interveinal yellowing and irregular rust-brown spots appear on older and middle-aged leaves and younger leaves remain healthy. Size of rust-brown spots between green veins increases and migrates to lower and finally newer leaves as the deficiency progresses. The entire plant looks sick. Rusty-brown spots appear on the leaf margins, tips, and between the veins. Leaves start dying and dropping, possibly curling before falling off. A minor deficiency will cause few problems with growth. However, minor deficiencies can quickly escalate during flowering and cause a diminished harvest as flowering progresses.

Cause: Magnesium is bound in the soil if there is an excess of potassium, ammonia (nitrogen), and calcium (carbonate). Most often, magnesium is in the soil but unavailable to the plant because the root environment is too acidic, wet and cold. Clay soils rich in calcium also tend to be magnesium poor. Small root systems are

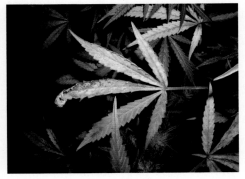

A magnesium deficiency is easy to correct with applications of Epsom salts.

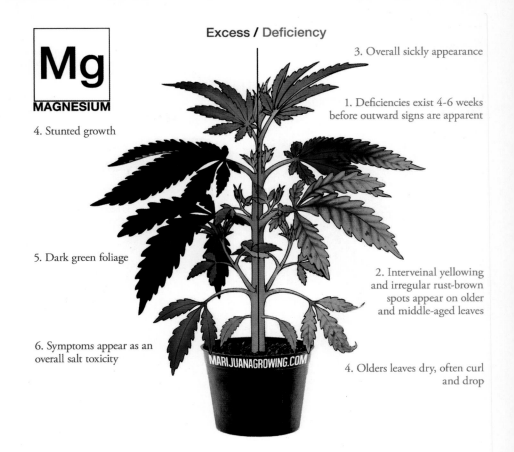

Mg
MAGNESIUM

Excess / Deficiency

4. Stunted growth

5. Dark green foliage

6. Symptoms appear as an overall salt toxicity

3. Overall sickly appearance

1. Deficiencies exist 4-6 weeks before outward signs are apparent

2. Interveinal yellowing and irregular rust-brown spots appear on older and middle-aged leaves

4. Olders leaves dry, often curl and drop

MARIJUANAGROWING.COM

also unable to take in enough magnesium to supply heavy demand. A high EC slows water evaporation and diminishes magnesium availability.

Confused with: An excess of potassium, ammoniacal nitrogen, and calcium carbonate

Spray with a 2 percent solution of Epsom salts every 4 to 5 days.

Solution: Add superfine dolomite lime to acidic potting soils before planting; it will stabilize the pH and add magnesium and calcium to the growing medium. Add 2 teaspoons (10 cc) of Epsom salts (magnesium sulfate) per gallon (3.8 L) of water with each watering to correct magnesium deficiencies if no dolomite was added when planting. Or dilute Kieserite (magnesium sulfate monohydrate, $MgSO_4 \cdot H_2O$) in water. For fast results spray the foliage with a 2 percent solution of Epsom salts every 4 to 5 days. If the deficiency progresses to the top of the plant, it will turn green there first. In 4 to 6 days, the green-up will start moving down the plant, turning lower leaves progressively greener. Continue a regular watering schedule with Epsom salts until the symptoms totally disappear. Use Epsom salts designed specifically for plants rather than the supermarket type. Another option is to apply Kieserite, found packaged as Ca-Mg fertilizer/supplement. Composted cow and turkey manure is also rich in magnesium.

Control room and root-zone temperatures, humidity, pH, and EC of the nutrient solution. Keep root zone and nutrient solution at 70°F to 75°F (21.1°C–23.9°C). Keep ambient air temperature at 75°F (21.1°C) day and 65°F (18.3°C) night. Use a complete fertilizer with an adequate amount of magnesium. Keep the soil pH above 6.5, the hydroponic pH above 5.5, and reduce high EC for a week. Reduce EC by leaching with plain water.

Excess: Excess magnesium is rare and does not appear quickly. Extra magnesium in the soil is in itself generally not harmful, but it inhibits calcium uptake. Symptoms appear as an overall salt toxicity accompanied by stunted growth and dark-green foliage.

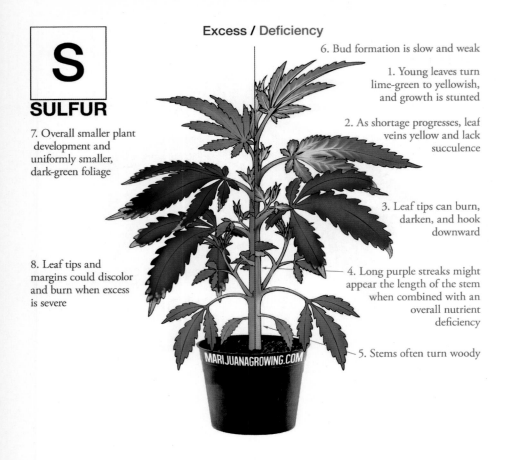

S

SULFUR

Excess / Deficiency

7. Overall smaller plant development and uniformly smaller, dark-green foliage

8. Leaf tips and margins could discolor and burn when excess is severe

6. Bud formation is slow and weak

1. Young leaves turn lime-green to yellowish, and growth is stunted

2. As shortage progresses, leaf veins yellow and lack succulence

3. Leaf tips can burn, darken, and hook downward

4. Long purple streaks might appear the length of the stem when combined with an overall nutrient deficiency

5. Stems often turn woody

MARIJUANAGROWING.COM

Cause: Magnesium toxicity is rare and difficult to discern with the naked eye. If extremely toxic, the magnesium develops a conflict with other fertilizer ions, usually calcium, especially in hydroponic nutrient solutions. Toxic buildup of magnesium is uncommon in soil that is able to grow cannabis.

Confused with: Calcium deficiency

Solution: Leach soil heavily to wash out excess.

Sulfur (S)—semimobile (essential)

About: Sulfur is an essential building block of many proteins, hormones, and vitamins, including vitamin B_1. Sulfur is also an indispensable element in many plant cells and seeds. The sulfate form of sulfur buffers the water pH. Virtually all groundwater and river or lake water contains sulfate. Sulfate is involved in protein synthesis and is part of cysteine (an amino acid) and thiamine, which are building blocks of proteins. Sulfur is essential in the formation of oils and flavors, as well as for respiration and the synthesis and breakdown of fatty acids.

Deficiency: Sulfur is not commonly deficient; many fertilizers contain some form of it. Excess sulfur is somewhat common when the EC is high. Young leaves turn lime-green to yellowish, and growth is stunted. As shortage progresses, leaf veins yellow and lack succulence. Leaf tips can burn, darken, and hook downward. Roots also elongate and stems often turn woody. Acute deficiency is usually caused by a rising pH resulting in a loss of phosphorus, which in turn causes more and more leaves to turn yellow and leaf stems to turn purple. Long purple streaks might appear the length of the stem when combined with an overall nutrient deficiency. Buds may have difficulty forming, often remaining leafy and fluffy, with reduced potency. Bud formation is slow and weak. Plants could have shorter overall life.

Mauk from Canna in the Netherlands, who has conducted detailed scientific experiments with nutrients, says, "We have repeatedly noticed that the symptoms were most obvious in the older leaves. Sulfur deficiency resembles a nitrogen deficiency. Acute sulfur deficiency causes elongated stems that become woody at the base."

Cause: Sulfur deficiency occurs indoors when the pH is too high (above 6.0) or when there is excessive calcium present and available. Hydroponic fertilizers separate sulfur from calcium in an "A" container and a "B" container. If combined in a concentrated form, sulfur and calcium will form crude, insoluble gypsum (hydrated calcium sulfate) and settle as residue to the bottom of the tank.

Confused with: Nitrogen, magnesium, iron deficiencies

Solution: Fertilize with a hydroponic fertilizer that contains sulfur. Balance the pH to 5.5 in hydroponics and above 6.0 in soil gardens. Add inorganic sulfur to a fertilizer that contains magnesium sulfate (Epsom salts). Organic sources of sulfur include mushroom composts and most animal manures. (To avoid burning the roots, make sure to apply only well-rotted manures.) Avoid elemental (pure) sulfur in favor of sulfur compounds such as magnesium sulfate. The nutrients combined with sulfur mix better in water.

Excess: Seldom seen or a problem except in coco mediums that are already rich in sulfur. Excess sulfur symptoms include

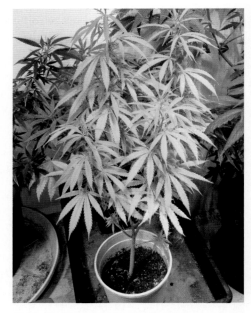

Sulfur is abundant in most fertilizers; when deficient it is usually mixed with other nutrients. Low sulfur levels cause buds to be fluffy and less potent.

overall smaller plant development and uniformly smaller, dark-green foliage. Leaf tips and margins could discolor and burn when excess is severe.

Cause: An excess of sulfur in the soil causes no problems if the EC is relatively low. At a high EC, plants tend to take up more available sulfur, which blocks uptake of other nutrients.

Confused with: Potassium and manganese deficiencies

Solution: Leach the growing medium of affected plants with a very mild and complete fertilizer. Check the pH of the drainage solution. Correct the input pH to 6.0. Severe problems require more water to be leached through the growing medium. Leach a minimum of 3 times the volume of water for the volume of the growing medium. Lower the overall fertilizer concentration (EC) of nutrient solution.

Micronutrients

Micronutrients, also called trace elements or trace nutrients, are essential to cannabis growth and must be present in minute amounts. They function mainly as catalysts to the plant's process and utilization of other elements.

Organic fertilizers such as marine algae or kelp (liquid or meal), humic acid, manures, and composts often contain all necessary micronutrients.

To ensure that a complete range of trace elements is available, use ionic salt fertilizers (designed for hydroponics) that supply all necessary micronutrients in proper proportions. High-quality hydroponic fertilizers use food-grade ingredients that are completely soluble and leave no residues.

Due to labeling requirements, many fertilizer companies do not list trace elements that are actually contained in their products. Before adding chelated trace elements, check with manufacturers to see if it is a "complete" fertilizer with all necessary nutrients.

Chelated micronutrients are available in powdered and liquid form. Add and thoroughly mix micronutrients into the growing medium before planting. Micronutrients are often impregnated in commercial potting soils and soilless mixes. Check the ingredients on the bag to ensure that the trace elements were added to the mix. Trace elements are necessary in minute amounts but can easily reach toxic levels. Follow manu-

facturer's instructions when applying micronutrients; they are easy to overapply.

Zinc, iron, and manganese are the three most common micronutrients found deficient. Often deficiencies of all three occur concurrently, especially when the soil or water pH is above 6.5. Deficiencies are most common in arid climates—such as Spain, the southwestern United States, and Australia—with alkaline soil and water. All three have the same initial symptom of deficiency: interveinal chlorosis of young leaves. It is often difficult to distinguish which element—zinc, iron, or manganese—is deficient, and all three could be deficient. This is why treating the problem should include adding a chelated dose of all three nutrients. Remember that chelation technology is expensive and really only required when mediums are alkaline.

Read your fertilizer's ingredients—chelated iron might read something like "iron EDTA."

Boron (B)–very immobile
About: Boron is still somewhat of a biochemical mystery. We know that boron helps with calcium uptake and numerous plant functions and is critical for photosynthate transfer. Scientists

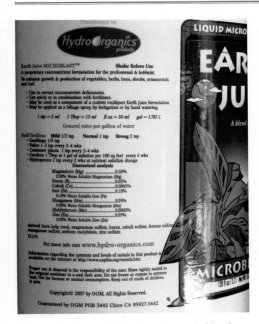

Chelated water-soluble iron is available along with a host of other micronutrients in an organic form.

Chelates

A **chelate** (Greek for *claw*) is an organic molecule that forms a clawlike bond with free electrically charged metal particles, combining nutrients in an atomic ring that is released easily for plants to absorb only at the root surface. Plants do not take up a chelate directly. First, the metal is converted in an ionic form at the root surface. There, ions are released and absorbed by the plant, where it is re-chelated and moves through the plant. This property keeps metal ions such as zinc, iron, and manganese soluble in water, and the chelated metal's reactions with other materials is suppressed. Roots take in the metals in a stable, soluble form that is used immediately.

Natural chelates such as humic acid and citric acid can be added to organic soil

mixes. Roots and bacteria also secrete natural chelates (exudates) in order to promote the uptake of iron and other metallic elements. Man-made chelates are designed for use in different situations. Chelators may move back to the growing medium to pick up another metal, but supporting evidence for this is marginal.

DTPA is most effective in a pH < 6.5. EDDHA is effective up to a pH < 8.0. EDTA chelate is slow to cause leaf burn.

Chelates decompose rapidly in low levels of ultraviolet (UV) light, including light produced by HID bulbs and sunlight. Keep chelates out of the light to protect them from rapid decomposition.

This information was condensed from Canna Products, www.canna.com.

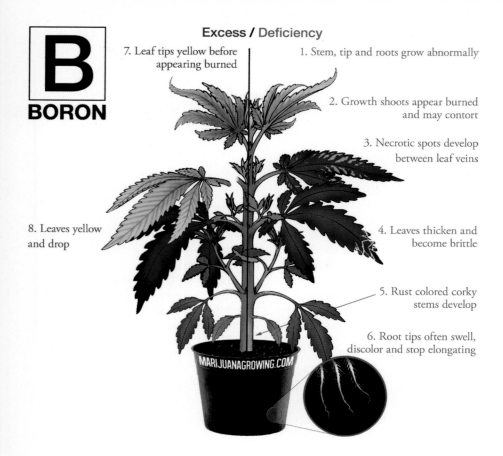

B BORON

Excess / Deficiency

7. Leaf tips yellow before appearing burned

8. Leaves yellow and drop

1. Stem, tip and roots grow abnormally

2. Growth shoots appear burned and may contort

3. Necrotic spots develop between leaf veins

4. Leaves thicken and become brittle

5. Rust colored corky stems develop

6. Root tips often swell, discolor and stop elongating

MARIJUANAGROWING.COM

---

have collected evidence to suggest that boron helps with synthesis, a base for the formation of nucleic acid (RNA uracil) formation. Strong evidence also supports boron's role in cell division, differentiation, maturation, and respiration as well as a link to pollen germination.

Deficiency: Cannabis uses minute amounts of boron, and deficiencies seldom occur indoors. Usually boron causes no problems, but it must be available during the entire life of a plant. Stem tip and root tip grow abnormally if it is deficient. Root tips often swell, discolor, and stop elongating. Growing shoots look burned, which may be confused with a burn from being too close to the light. First, leaves thicken and become brittle, and then top shoots contort or turn dark (or both), which is later followed by progressively lower-growing shoots. When severe, growing tips die, and leaf margins discolor and die back in places. Necrotic spots develop between leaf veins. Root steles (insides) often become mushy—perfect hosts for rot and disease. Deficient leaves become thick, distorted, and wilted, with

chlorotic and necrotic spotting. Rust-colored cork tissue forms on stems, and growing tips have a witch's broom appearance. Boron deficiency often brings about calcium deficiency.

Cause: Not present in extremely poor soil or lacking in fertilizer

Confused with: Calcium deficiency and light burn (See photos of each to distinguish.)

Solution: Give boron-deficient plants one teaspoon (5 cc) of boric acid or borax soap per gallon (3.8 L) of water. You can apply this solution as a soil drench to be taken up by the roots, or apply hydroponic micronutrients containing boron. Hydroponic gardeners should keep boron dosage below 20 parts per million (ppm), because boron quickly becomes toxic if it is concentrated in the solution.

Excess: Excesses are rare but can be deadly. Older leaves are affected first and symptoms are similar to salt burn. Leaf tips yellow first, and as the toxic conditions progress, leaf margins become

necrotic toward the center of the leaf. After the leaves yellow, they fall off. Be careful when adding trace elements to soil and hydroponic nutrient formulations. Avoid using excessive amounts of boric-acid-based insecticides.

Cause: Overfertilization

Confused with: Leaf spot fungus, light burn

Solution: Difficult to correct an oversupply of boron before crop is mature

Chlorine (Chloride) (Cl)—immobile (essential)

About: Chlorine (chloride) is required in the molecule that holds the water molecule, allowing and triggering the breakdown and release of hydrogen and oxygen for photosynthesis to occur. It is necessary for root and leaf cell division. It also increases osmotic pressure in the cells, which opens and closes the stomata to regulate moisture flow within the plant tissue. Chlorine is found in many municipal water systems. Cannabis tolerates low levels of chlorine and is almost never deficient in gardens that grow cannabis. Excess chlorine is somewhat common indoors. Chlorine tends to acidify soil after repeated applications.

Deficiency: Chlorine deficiency is rare. A solution concentration of less than 140 ppm is usually safe for cannabis, but some varieties may show sensitivity when new and young foliage turns pale green and wilts. Excessive chlorine causes leaf tips and margins to burn and causes the leaves to turn a bronze color. The roots develop thick tips and become stunted.

Note: Both severe deficiency and excess of chloride have the same symptoms: bronze-colored leaves.

Cause: Not available in water or soil

Confused with: Chlorine excess

Solution: Add chlorinated water

Excess: Young leaves develop burned leaf tips and margins. Young seedlings and clones are the most susceptible to damage. Later, the symptoms progress throughout the plant. Characteristic yellowish-bronze leaves are smaller and slower to develop. Most grow well with chlorine levels up to 140 ppm, but some varieties develop leaf tip and margin burn when concentrations top 20 ppm.

Note: Both severe deficiency and excess of chlorine have the same symptoms: bronze-colored leaves.

Cause: Too much chlorine in the home or municipal water system

Confused with: An excess of iron evidenced by bronze-colored leaves

Solution: Let heavily chlorinated water sit out overnight, stirring occasionally, or aerate it with a pump. Chlorine will volatize and disappear into the atmosphere in 24 to 48 hours. Place an air pump or a water pump and fountain in the chlorine-rich water to speed volatization of chlorine. Use this water to mix the nutrient solution or to irrigate the garden. If chlorine noticeably alters water pH, adjust it with a commercial pH UP product. Correct soil excesses by adding fine dolomite or agricultural lime.

Water treated with chlorine dioxide can be dealt with in this fashion, but water systems that use chloramine cannot, as it does not volatize; reverse osmosis is required, or a chemical purifier could be used, but the latter is not necessarily recommended.

Simple water filters do not clean dissolved solids from water. Such filters remove only debris emulsified (suspended) in water, releasing dissolved solids from their chemical bond isomer complex. A reverse osmosis machine uses small polymer, semipermeable membranes that allow pure water to pass through yet filter out dissolved solids. Reverse osmosis machines are the easiest and most efficient means to clean raw water.

Cobalt (Co)—immobile (beneficial)

About: Cobalt is necessary for nitrogen fixation, although the need for cobalt in plants was only recently established. It is essential for growth of the bacteria *Rhizobium* involved in legume nodule formation and fixing atmospheric

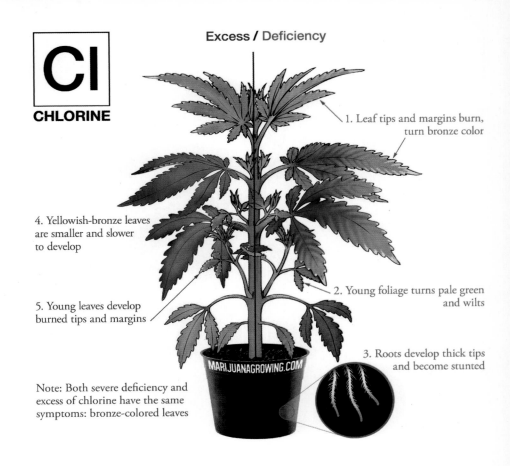

Excess / Deficiency

CI
CHLORINE

1. Leaf tips and margins burn, turn bronze color

4. Yellowish-bronze leaves are smaller and slower to develop

5. Young leaves develop burned tips and margins

2. Young foliage turns pale green and wilts

3. Roots develop thick tips and become stunted

MARIJUANAGROWING.COM

Note: Both severe deficiency and excess of chlorine have the same symptoms: bronze-colored leaves

nitrogen into amino acids and proteins. Cobalt, found in vitamin B_{12}, is synthesized by *Rhizobium* to promote nitrogen fixation.

Cobalt slows ethylene synthesis. Ethylene, a hormone, inhibits new shoot development. More new shoot development is possible when ethylene is inhibited. It is still not clear as to other direct influences cobalt might have on cannabis growth.

Deficiency: Nothing is known yet of symptoms, etc. Possible symptoms might include decreased production of Vitamin B_{12} and less nitrogen fixation

Copper (Cu)—semimobile (essential)

About: Copper is a component of numerous enzymes and proteins. Necessary in minute amounts, copper helps with carbohydrate metabolism, nitrogen fixation, and the process of oxygen reduction. It also helps with the making of proteins and sugars. Copper is also used as a fungicide.

Deficiency: Copper is used in minute amounts by cannabis. Deficiencies are uncommon indoors or outdoors. Young leaves and growing shoots slowly wilt, twisting and turning under in the process. Leaf tips and margins develop necrosis and turn dark-green to copper-gray. Occasionally, an entire copper-deficient plant wilts, drooping even when adequately watered. Growth is slow and the yield decreases. A small deficiency can cause new shoots to die back. Flowers are retarded and fail to mature properly.

Cause: Lack of copper in fertilizer and growing medium. Copper is concentrated in roots.

Confused/mixed with: possible boron deficiency or a pathogen attack (insect, virus, etc.)

Solution: Apply a copper-based fungicide such as copper sulfate. To avoid burning foliage, do not apply if the temperature is above 75°F (23.9°C). Apply a complete hydroponic nutrient that contains chelated copper. Or apply chelated trace

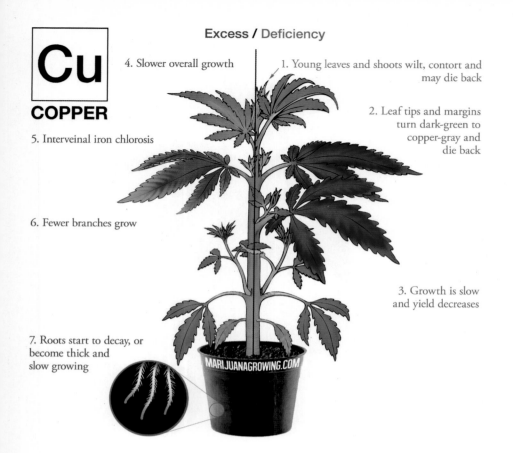

Cu

COPPER

4. Slower overall growth

1. Young leaves and shoots wilt, contort and may die back

2. Leaf tips and margins turn dark-green to copper-gray and die back

5. Interveinal iron chlorosis

6. Fewer branches grow

3. Growth is slow and yield decreases

7. Roots start to decay, or become thick and slow growing

MARIJUANAGROWING.COM

elements containing copper. Be careful not to overapply.

Excess: Excess copper is somewhat common indoors but seldom seen outdoors. Copper, although essential, is extremely toxic to the plant even in minor excess. Toxic levels slow the overall plant growth. As the toxic level climbs, symptoms include interveinal iron chlorosis (deficiency) and stunted growth. Fewer branches grow, and roots start to decay, or become thick and slow growing. Toxic conditions accelerate quickly in acidic soils. Hydroponic gardeners must carefully monitor their solution to avoid copper excess.

Cause: Too much copper in fertilizer, copper built up in soil to toxic levels, or residue accumulated on foliage or in soil from copper-based fungicides

Confused with: Iron deficiency demonstrated by interveinal chlorosis

Solution: Leach the soil or the growing medium to help expel excess copper. Do not use copper-based fungicides or foliar sprays.

Iron (Fe)—semimobile (essential)

About: Iron is fundamental to the enzyme systems and to transport electrons during photosynthesis, respiration, and chlorophyll production. Iron permits plants to use the energy provided by sugar. A catalyst for chlorophyll production, iron is necessary for nitrate and sulfate reduction and assimilation. Iron colors the earth from brown to red, according to concentration. Most soils contain plenty of iron in different forms. But cannabis often has a difficult time absorbing it under many conditions. Soil pH is a major factor dictating absorption of iron. Acidic soils normally contain adequate *available* iron for cannabis growth.

Deficiency: Iron deficiencies are most common when pH is above 6.5 and uncommon when the pH is below 6.5 in soil and 6.0 in hydroponic gardens. Symptoms may appear during rapid growth or stressful times and may disappear by themselves. Mild iron deficiencies have little effect on harvest. Young leaves are unable to draw immobile iron from older leaves, even though it is present in the soil. The first deficiency symptoms

appear on young leaves and shoots as veins remain mostly green and areas in between turn yellow. Interveinal chlorosis starts at the opposite end of the leaf tip: the apex of the leaves attached by the petiole. As the deficiency progresses more and larger leaves demonstrate interveinal chlorosis. Large leaves may yellow completely. In acute cases, leaves may develop necrosis and drop. Medium to severe iron deficiencies inhibit growth and diminish harvest. Do not confuse with magnesium deficiency where interveinal chlorosis shows on *older* leaves first.

Cause: Imbalanced pH, especially above 6.5 in soil and 6.0 in hydroponics. Manganese, zinc, and copper inhibit iron uptake. Overwatering, poor drainage, cold growing medium, and damaged or rotten roots will all lower iron uptake. Nutrient solution exposed to light causes algae growth. Algae break down chelates and robs iron from roots. Sterilizing the nutrient solution with UV light causes iron to precipitate.

Confused with: Magnesium deficiency; nitrogen deficiency; and early stages of copper, manganese, and zinc deficiencies. In contrast to magnesium, iron deficiency appears first in younger leaves because of iron's relative immobility. Iron readily oxidizes to the Fe^{3+} ion and precipitates out in the tissues of the plant, including the phloem.

Solution: Lower the soil pH to 6.5 or less; rockwool and hydroponic substrates require about 5.6 to 5.8. Avoid fertilizers that contain excessive amounts of phosphorus, manganese, zinc, and copper, which inhibit iron uptake. High levels of phosphorus compete

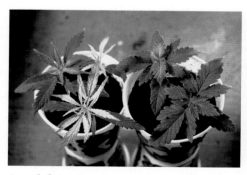

Iron deficiencies are somewhat common. The sativa *plants on the left are deficient in iron; the* afghani *plants on the right are not. (MF)*

with the uptake of iron. Improve the drainage; excessively wet soil holds little oxygen to spur iron uptake. Increase root zone temperature. Foliar feed for guaranteed results with dilute EDDTA 0.2 teaspoons per quart (0.1 gm/L) or EDTA at half a teaspoon per quart (0.5 gm/L). Apply 5 to 10 times the recommended dose of chelated iron in liquid form to root zone. Chelates are decomposed by light and must be thoroughly mixed with the growing medium to be effective. Leaves should green up in 4 or 5 days. Complete and balanced nutrient formulas contain iron, and deficiencies are seldom a problem. Organic sources of iron, as well as chelates, include cow, horse, and chicken manure. (To avoid burning cannabis plants, use only well-rotted manures.) Remember that foliar application of chelated iron is only a temporary fix.

Caution: If iron deficiency is pronounced, add only chelated iron to remedy the problem. Iron often reacts with other nutrients, causing them to become unavailable.

Excess: Excess of iron is extremely rare except in flooded soils. High levels of iron do not damage cannabis but can interfere with phosphorus uptake. An excess of iron causes leaves to turn bronze, accompanied by small, dark-brown leaf spots. Iron excess can also promote phosphorus deficiencies.

Cause: Flooded outdoor soils where iron accumulates

Confused with: Phosphorus deficiency

Solution: Leach plants heavily. Avoid deficiencies by using a high-quality hydroponic fertilizer that contains chelated micronutrients.

Manganese (Mn)—immobile (essential)
About: Manganese is engaged in the oxidation-reduction process associated with photosynthetic electron transport. This element activates many enzymes and plays a fundamental part in the chloroplast membrane system. Manganese assists nitrogen utilization along with iron in chlorophyll production.

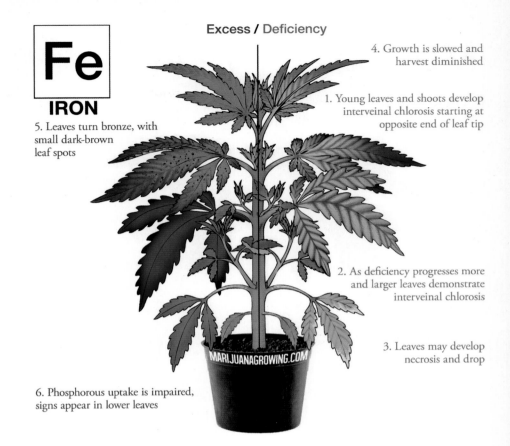

Excess / Deficiency

Fe
IRON

4. Growth is slowed and harvest diminished

1. Young leaves and shoots develop interveinal chlorosis starting at opposite end of leaf tip

5. Leaves turn bronze, with small dark-brown leaf spots

2. As deficiency progresses more and larger leaves demonstrate interveinal chlorosis

3. Leaves may develop necrosis and drop

MARIJUANAGROWING.COM

6. Phosphorous uptake is impaired, signs appear in lower leaves

Deficiency: Manganese deficiency is relatively uncommon indoors and relatively uncommon outdoors. Young leaves show symptoms first, becoming yellow between veins (interveinal chlorosis) while veins remain green. Symptoms spread from younger to older leaves as the deficiency progresses. Necrotic (dead) spots develop on severely affected leaves, which become pale and fall off; overall plant growth is stunted, and maturation may be prolonged. A telltale sign of manganese deficiency is where margins remain dark green surrounding interveinal chlorosis.

Cause: A high pH (above 6.5) or an excess of iron causes manganese deficiency. Lack of manganese in the soil or fertilize.

Confused with: Severe manganese deficiency looks similar to magnesium deficiency.

Solution: Lower the pH, leach the soil, and add a complete, chelated micronutrient formula.

Excess: Problems with manganese excess are somewhat common. Young and newer growth develops chlorotic, dark orange to dark rusty-brown mottling on the leaves. Tissue damage shows on young leaves before progressing to older leaves. Growth is slower, and overall vigor is lost.

Cause: Toxicity is compounded by low humidity. The additional transpiration causes more manganese to be drawn into the foliage. A low pH (5.0–5.5) can cause toxic intake of manganese, which in turn restricts intake of iron and zinc.

Confused with: Excess of iron and zinc
Solution: Raise pH to 6.5.

Molybdenum (Mb)—mobile (essential)
About: Molybdenum is part of two major enzyme systems that convert nitrate to ammonium. This essential element is used by cannabis in very small quantities. It is most active in roots and seeds.

Deficiency: Molybdenum deficiencies and excesses are rare, though occasional deficiencies occur in cold weather. First, the older and middle-aged leaves yellow; some leaves develop interveinal chlorosis

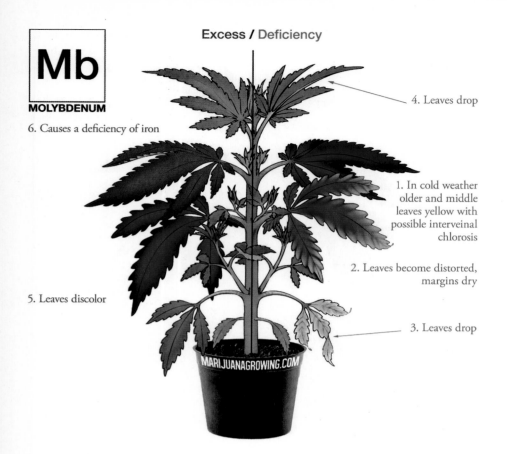

Excess / Deficiency

Mb

MOLYBDENUM

6. Causes a deficiency of iron

5. Leaves discolor

4. Leaves drop

1. In cold weather older and middle leaves yellow with possible interveinal chlorosis

2. Leaves become distorted, margins dry

3. Leaves drop

MARIJUANAGROWING.COM

and discolor around leaf edges. Leaves continue to yellow and develop cupped or rolled-up margins as the deficiency progresses. Leaves become distorted and twisted, dry along the edges die, and then drop. Overall growth is stunted. Deficiencies are worst in acidic soils. Molybdenum deficiency promotes nitrogen shortage.

Cause: Not present in fertilizer, growing medium, or water

Confused with: Nitrogen deficiency
Solution: Water with chelated micronutrients that contain molybdenum. Be careful not to overapply.

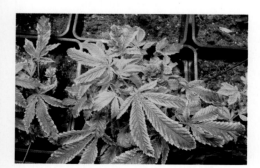

Molybdenum deficiency

Excess: Excess molybdenum is uncommon in cannabis gardens; it is difficult to detect and has little effect on cannabis. Leaves discolor. An excess of molybdenum causes a deficiency of copper and iron.

Cause: Too much in soil or fertilizer

Confused with: Copper and iron deficiency

Solution: No correction needed

Nickel (Ni)—mobile (beneficial)
About: Nickel was first demonstrated as an essential plant nutrient in 2004. Cannabis requires nickel in trace amounts. It is normally not listed on fertilizer labels because nickel is available in soil. Nickel is essential for activation of the enzyme urease, which helps metabolize (urea) nitrogen. It is also required for absorption of iron. Nickel also has a function in bacteria, and it may play a role with interaction between plants and bacteria. At a pH less than 6.7 nickel is moderately available, but at a pH less than 6.5 nickel compounds are very soluble.

Deficiency: A lack of nickel causes toxic levels of (urea) nitrogen to accumulate, causing dead lesions to form on foliage. Excessive application of zinc, copper, or magnesium could cause a deficiency. But cannabis requires so little nickel that I have never seen a case where it is deficient. Plants grown without additional nickel will gradually reach a deficient level at about the time they mature and begin reproductive growth. If nickel is deficient, plants may fail to produce viable seeds.

Cause: Excessive zinc, copper, manganese, iron, calcium, or magnesium in soil or by root-knot nematode damage

Confused with: Nitrogen (urea), zinc, copper, or magnesium excess

Solution: Apply copper, zinc and magnesium in trace amounts to fertilizers so that they do not build up to toxic levels. Nickel-deficient soils have not been identified.

Excess: A nickel overload is virtually never a problem unless gross quantities are available in soil. Cannabis as an accumulator plant can absorb a lot of nickel.

Cause: Overdose can be caused by too much nickel in soil or by soil fertilized with sewage sludge or packed with heavy metals from industrial pollution.

Confused with: Does not apply

Solution: Grow in soil that is not full of industrial waste or sewage sludge packed with heavy metals.

Selenium (Se)—semimobile (beneficial)
About: Not yet classified as an essential nutrient for plants, selenium's role as a beneficial element for plants is still being discovered. Some plants are able to accumulate large amounts of selenium, from 100 to 10,000 mg Se kg-1 dry weight. However, little work has been done regarding cannabis as a selenium accumulator plant. Selenium can be absorbed by roots in an inorganic source or via organic compounds. Sulfur and selenium share close chemical and physical qualities and their absorption by roots is also similar.

Deficiency: Selenium is seldom if ever deficient. No apparent symptoms.

Cause: No selenium in growing medium

Confused with: No deficiency

Solution: No action

Silicon - (Si)—immobile (beneficial)
About: Silicon deserves mention even though I have never seen a diagnosed deficiency. Low levels of silicon can reduce overall yield and vigor of cannabis. Only rushes require silicon to complete their life cycle, but it is beneficial in other plants and accumulates in the endoplasmic reticulum, cell walls, and intercellular spaces as hydrated, amorphous silica. Silicon is found in all soils and it is the only nutrient/element that does not hurt cannabis in excess. Silica (gel) accumulates in epidermal plant cells to form a protective shield that promote stronger leaves, roots, stems, and resistance to diseases, pests, and plant stresses (including drought).

Silica (not silicon) is a mineral sand; hydrated amorphous silica SiO_2-H_2O is what Si is deposited as in the intercellular spaces, converted after take-up.

Deficiency: Lodging (falling over) and fungal infections.

Cause: Silicon deficiency is usually only seen in plants not grown on native or natural soils, or plants grown in water.

Confused with: Nothing

Solution: Add silicon to fertilizer in the form of diatomaceous earth or prepackaged supplements. When applied in a highly soluble form, added silicon takes effect after two weeks or more.

Note: Pests and diseases have a difficult time penetrating plants that are sprayed with a silicon-based repellent/insecticide.

Excess: Evidence suggests that too much silicon can be an issue, but little research has been done.

Sodium - (Na)—mobile
At low levels, sodium appears to bolster yields, possibly acting as a partial substitute to compensate for potassium deficiencies. But in excess of 50 ppm, sodium is toxic and induces deficiencies of other nutrients, primarily potassium, calcium, and magnesium.

About: Very low levels of sodium appear to promote higher yields in cannabis.

Deficiency: Not a problem in C_3 plants like Cannabis

Cause: Not a problem

Confused with: Nothing

Solution: No action

Excess: Sodium excess (above 50 ppm) is relatively common, especially in coastal and rural zones. Sodium in excess is a big problem. Small amounts of sodium are quickly taken up by roots. When sodium levels reach 50 ppm, potassium and other nutrient uptake is blocked, resulting in rapid and severe deficiencies. First signs of toxic sodium levels in plants manifest as a potassium deficiency. When mixed with chlorine, sodium turns into table salt (NaCl), which is the worst possible salt to put on plants.

Sodium excess causes potassium deficiency, which in turn causes the internal temperature of foliage to climb and protein cells to burn or degrade.

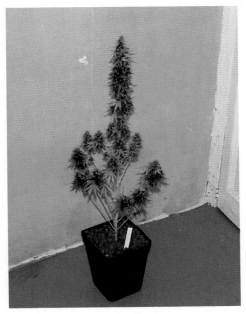

High levels of sodium in tap water will block nutrient uptake and stunt growth.

Evaporation is normally highest on leaf edges, which burn. See Potassium above for more information.

Cause: Overall toxic fertilizer salt condition in growing medium, salts in water from water-softening filters, or sodium in water or soil. Using too much baking soda as a fungicide can also create an excess.

Confused with: Potassium, calcium, or magnesium deficiencies

Solution: Leach growing medium heavily with clean water to wash away toxic sodium. Use reverse osmosis filtration to remove sodium and other dissolved solids from irrigation water.

Note: Use a sodium (Na) meter to check for salt content in all premixed and bulk soils—especially those containing manure fertilizers.

Vanadium
Vanadium is known to be required in certain microbes and algae, but nothing is known about its need in higher plant forms. Some believe it might be required by cannabis in very low concentrations.

Zinc (Zn)—immobile (essential)
About: Zinc works with manganese and magnesium to promote the same enzyme functions. Zinc cooperates with other elements to help form chlorophyll as well as prevent its demise. It is an essential catalyst for most plants' enzymes and auxins, and it is crucial for stem growth. Zinc plays a vital part in sugar and protein production. It is fairly common to find zinc-deficient cannabis. Deficiencies are most common in soils with a pH of 7.0 or more.

Deficiency: Zinc is the most common micronutrient deficiency and is commonly found in arid climates and alkaline soils. The most dynamic evidence of zinc deficiency is when a leaf turns 90 degrees and is combined with some or all of the following symptoms: New and young leaves exhibit interveinal chlorosis, and new leaves and growing tips develop small, thin blades that contort and wrinkle. Some varieties grow pronounced smaller leaves. The leaf tips, and later the margins, discolor and burn. Burned spots

Zn
ZINC

Excess / Deficiency

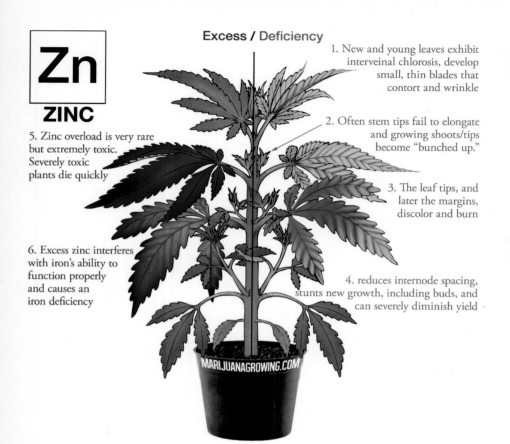

1. New and young leaves exhibit interveinal chlorosis, develop small, thin blades that contort and wrinkle

2. Often stem tips fail to elongate and growing shoots/tips become "bunched up."

3. The leaf tips, and later the margins, discolor and burn

4. reduces internode spacing, stunts new growth, including buds, and can severely diminish yield

5. Zinc overload is very rare but extremely toxic. Severely toxic plants die quickly

6. Excess zinc interferes with iron's ability to function properly and causes an iron deficiency

MARIJUANAGROWING.COM

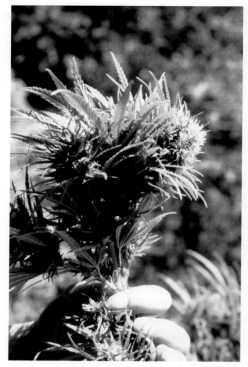

This Colombian bud grown in 1976 is deficient in zinc. The result is bunched-up and contorted growth. (MF)

on the leaves could grow progressively larger. When zinc deficiency is severe, new leaf blades contort horizontally and dry out. Often stem tips fail to elongate and growing shoots/tips become "bunched up." Flower buds also contort into odd shapes, turn crispy dry, and are often hard. A lack of zinc causes reduces internode spacing, stunts new growth—including buds—and can severely diminish yield.

Cause: The pH is too high (above 7.0), which in turn causes iron, manganese, and zinc deficiencies to occur together.

Confused with: Symptoms are often confused with a lack of manganese and iron.

Solution: Treat zinc-deficient plants by leaching the growing medium with a diluted mix of a complete fertilizer containing chelated trace elements, including zinc, iron, and manganese. Or add a quality-brand hydroponic micronutrient mix containing chelated trace elements. Foliar feed if problem is severe.

Be careful; do not overapply chelated micronutrients.

Excess: Zinc overload is very rare but extremely toxic. Severely toxic plants die quickly. Excess zinc interferes with iron's ability to function properly and causes an iron deficiency.

Cause: Oversupply in fertilizer

Confused with: Iron deficiency

Solution: Leach growing medium with a diluted mix of a complete fertilizer.

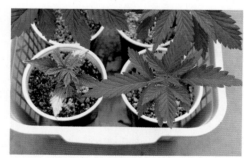

A zinc deficiency on the 'Pakistani' (lower left) is easy to remedy with an application of fritted trace elements (FTE). (MF)

Fertilizers

The selection of fertilizers at hydroponic and cannabis-friendly garden stores can be overwhelming. Local shop personnel generally know which ones work best in the local climate and water. Local hydroponic store staff are often well versed on local water and gardeners' needs.

Nutrients in a fertilizer formula can be classified as inorganic, mineral, natural, organic, and synthetic. Inorganic nutrients have no carbon molecules, mineral elements are inorganic salts; organic substances are animal or vegetable in origin and contain a carbon molecule; synthetic materials are man-made. But mineral elements such as dolomite lime, rock phosphate, and Epsom salts are considered organic. All these terms can be very confusing, and they are often misused!

The main difference between organic fertilizer and mineral fertilizer formulas is the way in which they are taken up by plants. In general, organic fertilizers (mineral and natural) require biological

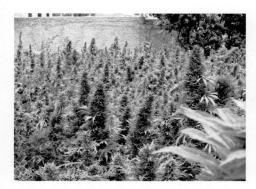

The big buds on these plants were grown in Morocco with the aid of little fertilizer.

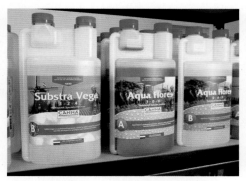

Canna Vega and Aqua formulas are just a few of the many different fertilizers available at hydroponic stores.

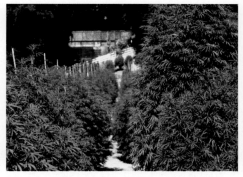

This beautiful field of organically grown cannabis belonged to Eddy Lepp, who is currently serving a 10-year sentence for cultivating cannabis.

life in the soil to break down components and make nutrients available to roots for uptake. Mineral fertilizers (inorganic and synthetic) are taken up by plants exclusively via ionic activity, a chemical bond formed by the attraction of positive and negative soluble ionic fertilizer salts. Virtually all elements, regardless of origin, must be broken down into a single element in order to pass into a cell of a root. Single ionic elements react faster and are easier to control. Of course, the science is much more complex than this simplified explanation. The aim of this book is to give you a basic understanding of fertilizers, so you can efficiently grow a healthy crop of medical cannabis.

Ionic fertilizer salts are separated into two or three different containers so they can be mixed together in a concentrate form and not combine into an insoluble compound. For example, when calcium and sulfur are combined in a concentrated form, they combine into an insoluble compound. This compound (calcium sulfate) settles to the bottom of hydroponic tanks in the form of an insoluble compound (sludge). They may flocculate (form aggregates) or not, depending on agitation. They combine to form an insoluble compound that you may see as crystal growth (flocculation) at the bottom of the tank.

Vegetative and flowering formulas are further separated into different containers.

Nutrients are available for uptake by plant roots within a specific pH range.

In hydroponic gardens this range is from 5.5 to 6.5, and in organic soil gardens the range is a little higher, 6.0 to 6.8. Maintaining a relatively constant pH is essential to nutrient uptake. A common oversight among novice enthusiasts is to forget about pH. For example, iron and manganese deficiencies are rampant when pH climbs beyond 7.0 in hydroponic gardens. No matter how much of each element is in the nutrient solution, they will become available only at a lower pH.

Here is a great site to look up the nutrient percentages in all fertilizers registered in Washington State, the first state to approve recreational use of cannabis. The Washington State Department of Agriculture site is http://agr.wa.gov/PestFert/Fertilizers/FertDB/Product1.aspx

Fertilizers mixed in liquid concentrate form are very convenient to use but are more expensive both in monetary terms and to the environment. Nutrients available in a dry form are much more economical than nutrients mixed with water. Dry fertilizers are also much more eco-friendly because no water/fertilizer concentrate, which is expensive, must be transported. Dry fertilizers are not separated because the elements do not react with one another. Purchase dry fertilizers or concentrated liquid fertilizers that dilute readily in water.

Fertilizers are either water-soluble or partially soluble (gradual-release). Both soluble and gradual-release fertilizers can be organic or chemical. Soluble salt (ionic) fertilizers dissolve in water and are simple to measure and control; they can easily be added or washed (leached) out of the growing medium.

Chemical granular fertilizers work well for perennial shrubs and trees but can easily be overapplied on annual cannabis. Long-lasting granular fertilizers are very difficult to leach out of soil.

Osmocote chemical fertilizers are time-release and are used by many nurseries because they are easy to apply and only require one application every few months. Using this type of fertilizer may be convenient, but exacting control is lost. They are temperature- and moisture-dependent, with release rates calculated at 70°F (21°C) and normal irrigation. I have seen three-month formulations release in total during a month with high soil temps. Also, they release somewhere between 30 percent and 70 percent the first time water is applied. They are best suited for ornamental

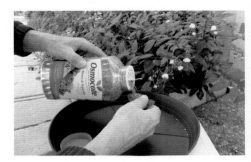

Osmocote time-release fertilizer is perfect for fuchsias and other perennial plants, but it is not a good fertilizer to control a medical cannabis crop grown in containers.

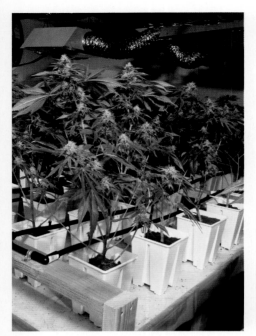

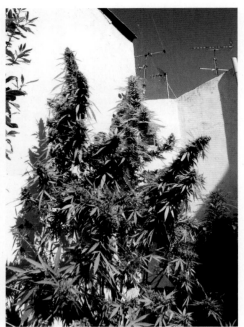

Irrigation hoses with tubing supply a daily dose of properly proportioned nutrient solution to this greenhouse full of plants.

This big plant grown on a patio in downtown Barcelona, Spain, was given a simple fertilizer regimen with plenty of water and sunshine.

containerized plants or perennial plants growing in soil, where labor costs and uniform growth are the main concerns.

Use hydroponic fertilizers designed to supply plants with a specific diet that includes all necessary nutrients at the proper ratio required for strong growth. These formulas must be applied on a regular schedule to achieve the best results. Precisely formulated fertilizers allow much easier dosage control dosage by altering the EC. Less-precise fertilizers provide plants more nutrients than they need and let roots absorb what they need. These formulations tend to build up in growing mediums. Subsequently, plants often suffer an excess of nitrogen or other nutrients that are "overapplied" when the mix is changed and flowering is induced.

Apply the proper nutrient combination at the appropriate stage of life. For example, cannabis absorbs more phosphorus and potassium for a short time early on in the flowering stage. Applying more fertilizer earlier or later causes it to build up in soil, sometimes to toxic levels.

1. Ratio for N-P-K fertilizer: start: 2-1-1, veg.: 1-1-1, finish 1-2-2*

2. http://www.eplantscience.com great site!

3. http://en.wikipedia.org/wiki/Plant_ nutrition

*Remember that, by convention, P and K are confusing on the label, while 1-1-1 is correct, the percentage given on the label for P is only 40 percent of actual P, and K is only 80 percent of actual K.

Do not combine fertilizers from different manufacturers. Each manufacturer designs formulas to function with products in their line. Mixing and matching brands could easily lead to deficiencies or excesses.

Take care when including additives in fertilizer mixes. Use additives designed for specific fertilizers and mix them according to the fertilizer schedule. These products are designed to stimulate specific nutrients and plant process. Adding too much or too little—or at the wrong time—could be futile or even toxic.

Fertilizer is big business, and convenience is expensive. Manufacturers often sell "special mixes" that contain just a few of the necessary nutrients. Be wary when purchasing high-priced specialized fertilizers that are broken down into four or more "essential" products. The

"formulas" often include only one or two different nutrients that could easily be combined into a single product and sold for less. In the end, the goal of such fertilizer companies is to sell a thimbleful of salts mixed in a bottle of water—at astronomical profits.

In the United States, nutrients are measured in parts-per-million (ppm), even though they are expressed as a percentage concentration on the label. The ppm scale is simple and finite—well, almost. The basics are simple: one ppm is one part of 1,000,000. To convert from percentage to ppm, multiply by 10,000 and move the decimal four spaces to the right. For example: 2 percent equals 20,000 ppm. For more information on ppm and electrical conductivity, see chapter 23, *Container Culture & Hydroponics.*

Organic Fertilizers

Patients prefer cannabis that is grown organically because it has a sweeter taste, but contrary to popular belief, organically grown cannabis does contain salts. Fertilizer salts are ions; ions are released by the breakdown of organic molecules, which is the only way a plant will take them up, so salts are there, but the levels are lower. Implementing an organic garden outdoors, in a greenhouse, or indoors usually requires a large mass of rich organic soil with good drainage. Space is limited indoors, so growing with a large mass of living organic soil is impractical for most indoor gardeners.

Most **indoor organic gardens use potting soil** high in worm castings, peat, sand, manure, leaf mold, compost, and fine dolomite lime. In a small container, there is little space to build nutrient-rich soil by mixing compost and organic nutrients that interact. Fill containers with rich organic potting soil that is ready to release nutrients. Add a liquid mix of nutrients periodically if necessary.

Biological activity also takes months of valuable growing time, and it could foster destructive diseases and pests. Tossing out used and depleted soil and then recycling it in the outdoor garden keeps indoor and greenhouse gardens clean.

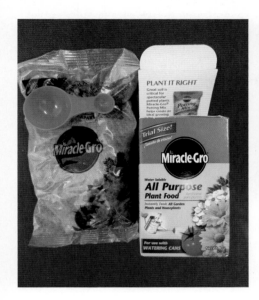

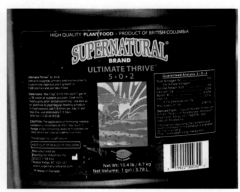

This fertilizer contains N, K₂O, Ca, B, Fe (EDTA), and Mo, which are the major and minor nutrients consumed by cannabis. The mix lacks P, S, Mg, and Z, which are supplied in other products. The nutrients are provided in a readily available form for uptake by roots.

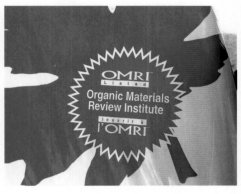

Most countries have an agency that certifies organic materials for gardening. This bale of Canadian peat moss is certified by the Organic Materials Review Institute (OMRI).

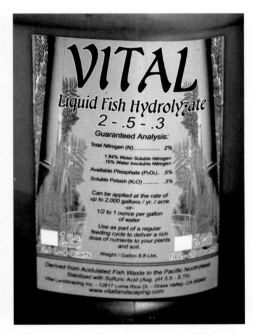

This organic fertilizer lists N, P, and K on the label, showing the chemical composition of each nutrient. At the base of the package is a list of what the nutrients were derived from.

Always read fertilizer labels carefully. Follow mixing and application instructions. Pay special attention to the expiration date, especially on organic nutrient packages. They often contain living organisms that will die or change composition over time. Make sure all necessary nutrients are listed on the label. For example, Miracle-Gro does not contain magnesium!

Miracle-Gro plant food is available everywhere. It is a favorite fertilizer for many flower and vegetable gardeners. The Guaranteed Analysis shows it contains N, P, K, Mn, and Zn. It is derived from urea, potassium chloride, potassium, phosphate, manganese EDTA, and zinc EDTA. But, medical cannabis gardeners prefer a more complete fertilizer that has a complete range of *all* necessary nutrients.

Note the "derived from" part of the label. Using potassium and magnesium carbonate derivatives can cause the pH to climb. If a high pH brings about phosphorus and iron deficiencies, add chelated iron to remedy and to avoid precipitation as well.

Fertilizers must be registered so they can be regulated by governments to ensure content, and protect consumers from illegitimate companies that make false claims. Even when regulated, companies still make false claims not found on labels. The "guaranteed analysis" of nutrients on labels guarantees minimums of specific elements. It does not guarantee that more of these specific elements are in the container. Often lower-quality fertilizers contain other elements as impurities that are not included on the label. All "organic" products should be certified by an independent third party such as the Organic Materials Review Institute (OMRI, www.ormi.org) in North America and the Control Union (www.controlunion.com) in Europe. There are many other organic certification organizations around the world, including, Organic Crop Improvement Association (OCIA, www.ocia.org). Check with these organizations for added information on products that are not allowed.

When using synthetic fertilizers, it is extremely important to carefully read the label and follow the directions. The initials "WSN" and "WIN" that you may see on the label stand for *water-soluble nitrogen* and *water-insoluble nitrogen*. WSN dissolves readily, and it is considered a fast-release nitrogen source. WIN does not dissolve easily. It is often an organic form of nitrogen and is considered a slow-release nitrogen source.

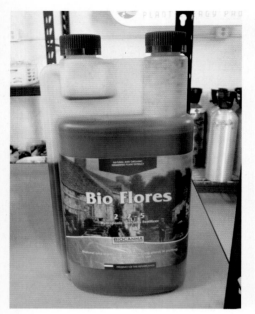

Bio-Canna is one of the many different organic fertilizers available to medical cannabis gardeners.

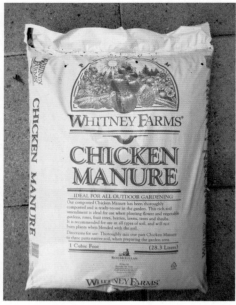

Chicken manure has long been a favorite organic fertilizer for outdoor and greenhouse gardens. It is packed with nitrogen and other soluble nutrients to spur rapid growth.

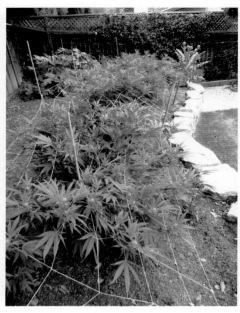

This raised bed is in a suburban backyard garden in California, a medical cannabis state.

Raised beds and very large (50–500-gal [189.3–1892.7 L]) containers with good drainage allow organic soil life to grow in indoor, greenhouse, and outdoor gardens. The raised beds and large containers have enough soil to hold the nutrients, promote soil life, and when managed properly, ensure an available supply of nutrients. There must be enough mass to support healthy soil life. Outdoor organic gardens are much easier to implement and maintain. Using compost tea, manures, compost, and other big, bulky, fragrant fertilizers is much easier outdoors. Gardeners in Northern California are using rich

organic soil mixes to grow big plants, 10 pounds (4.5 kg) plus, with the local nutrient-rich soil mixes, adding about 2 handfuls of bat guano when plants start to flower.

Cannabis plants grow from 2 to 6 months in containers indoors and in greenhouses. Start with rich organic soil and add (soluble) liquid organic nutrients to ensure rapid plant growth. Liquid organic nutrients are often more expensive to manufacture than ionic salt fertilizers. Nutrient-rich organic soil is expensive to build and usually both inexpensive and trouble-free to maintain.*

*Often organic cannabis gardeners get carried away and add too many microbes on a regular basis. Uninformed product producers and retailers may also promote such practices. Consequently microbes are rampantly available, to a fault.

Soil microbes are not all created equal. There are both specific and general decomposers and these different species or types work at differing levels in the soil. Nutrients form what are collectively known as 'pools' (freely available elements locked onto cation exchange capacity (CEC) sites or drifting in the soil solution) in the medium, such as

nitrogen or calcium pools, etc. As organic material decomposes, it adds to these pools when there is more released than is used by the microbes. When mineral fertilizer is used, these same pools collect these elements. The elements are collected in pools over time rather than all at once. Microbes are very much like vacuums and will suck it up faster than plants and will outcompete plants for these elements. Balance in these microbes is essential so the pools stay in place.

For example, a large amount of organic soil starts the breakdown with specific

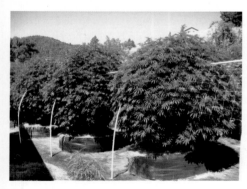

Big pots 2 feet (61 cm) tall and 4 to 6 feet (121.9–182.9 cm) across function like raised beds. They capture extra heat in the spring and carry it through fall. The containers must be shaded if they get too hot in summer.

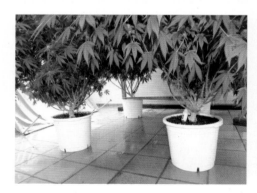

Growing large plants in small containers requires more work. The substrate must receive regular irrigation with nutrient solution and be kept within a good temperature range. These plants have received excellent care!

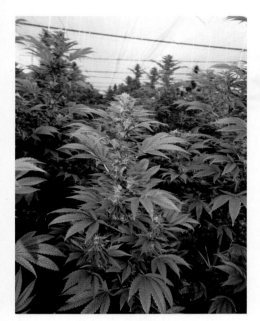

Large plants are growing in 2 × 2-foot (61 × 61 cm) planting holes and the surrounding soil is hard clay. Good organic fertilizer and plenty of water helped these plants grow up to 6 feet (182.9 cm) tall.

microbes, and what they release is broken down by the next type, and so on until it is gone. (For more specific information, check out the book *Teaming with Microbes* by Jeff Lowenfels and Wayne Lewis). When all these general populations of microbes multiply to greater than the available organic material for decomposition, these microbes dip into the pools and outcompete the plants in order to stay alive. Most commercially available microbes are largely made up of general decomposers, and are opportunistic feeders that will eat (take up) anything that is available.

Big issues arise when organic cannabis gardeners apply microbes above and beyond the need (uneducated manufacturers may provide this erroneous information). In turn these microbes take up and use nutrients before the plants can. Proper organic garden maintenance requires constantly supplying new organic matter for all the microbes to enjoy—but not the wrong ones that the nutrient balance.

The organic nutrient content, solubility, and rate of release are characteristically lower than ionic salt-based fertilizer. Organic fertilizers are more dilute and less readily available to plants. They

can change slightly from one batch to another. Testing each batch is necessary to ensure consistent nutrient levels.

Outdoors, organic gardening is easy because all the forces of nature are there for you to seek out and harness. When playing the role of Mother Nature, you must create everything in the environment.

Start with good soil that drains well, and add proper organic nutrients. Organic fertilizers improve soil life and the long-term productivity of soil. Increase soil organisms by providing organic matter and micronutrients to soil life, which aids plants in absorbing nutrients and can drastically reduce pesticides, fertilizer, and energy use, at the cost of decreased yield. Organic fertilizers usually require the use of microbes/bacteria in the soil in order to make the nutrients in the fertilizer bioavailable. That can result in irregular release of phosphorus/calcium. In sterile potting soil, there may be no microbes to release the nutrients.

Note: Nutrients in organic fertilizers may vary greatly depending upon source, age, erosion, and climate. For more precise nutrient content, consult the vendor's specifications. Make sure composts are well-rotted and do not contain pathogens and other disease-causing organisms.

Some commercial liquid organic fertilizers contain living organisms—microbes, bacteria, fungi, etc.—and tend to grow under certain conditions. Do not leave containers of organic fertilizers in warm places. And remember

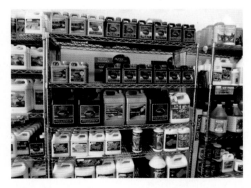

The selection of commercial fertilizers designed specifically for hydroponics and cannabis growth is often overwhelming to gardeners.

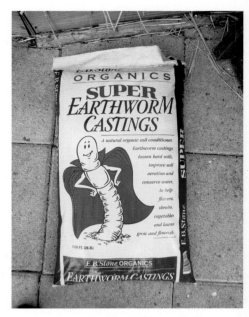

Worm castings supply readily available nitrogen and many other nutrients in an organically available form. Add potent worm castings, and mix well in substrates. They are dense and tend to clump.

to use them before their expiration date! Check labels closely; some companies add preservatives to their mixes.

Organic nutrients (manure, worm castings, blood and bone meal, and so forth) work very well to increase the soil nutrient content, but nutrients are released and available at different rates. The nutrient availability may be tricky to calculate, but it is somewhat difficult to overapply organic fertilizers. Organic nutrients are typically more consistently available when used in combination with one another. Usually, gardeners use a mix of up to 20 percent worm castings with other organic agents to get a strong, readily available nitrogen base.

Organic fertilizers include ground-up and rendered animal and fish products, bird and bat guanos, animal manures, fish, shellfish, kelp, seaweed, rock powders, vegetable meals and extracts, plus coffee grounds, compost and compost teas, ashes, and worm castings. See the "Organic Nutrient List" on page 383 for information about specific organic nutrients.

Brix Mix
Brix Mix Powder is used by many Northern California cannabis gardeners.

GUARANTEED ANALYSIS	PERCENT
available phosphoric acid (P_2O_5)	0.2
soluble potash (K_2O)	18
sulfur (S)	8
copper (Cu)	0.05
iron (Fe)	0.7
zinc (Zn)	0.2

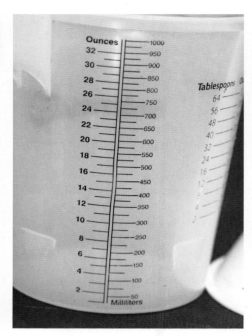

Always use an accurate measuring container.

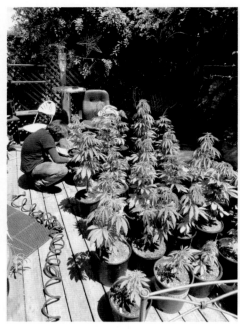

These plants in Dennis Peron's* backyard in San Francisco, California, receive full sun and quite a bit of wind all day long. The pots get too hot and growth is slowed.

*Dennis Peron is coauthor of California Proposition 215, which enacted the first law in the USA allowing patients to purchase cannabis for medicine at dispensaries.

The mix is formulated to increase Brix (sugar content) in plants. The mix is **derived from** *Ascophyllum nodosum* kelp, sulfate of potash, iron lignosulfonate, zinc lignosulfonate, copper lignosulfonate.

Dry Brix Mix contains ratios of Maxicrop, Diamond K sulfate of potash, sugar, and available trace minerals. Brix liquid contains Phytamin 4-3-4, Humax humic acids, pure malt extract, molasses, sulfur, and Therm X70 Yucca Extract. According to the manufacturer, www.peacefulvalleyfarmsupply.com.

Mixing Fertilizers

To mix wettable powder or crystal fertilizers, dissolve into a little warm water. Mix the super concentrate until all powder or crystals have dissolved. Once it has totally dissolved, add the balance of the tepid water. This will ensure that the fertilizer and the water mix evenly. Liquid fertilizers can be mixed directly with water. Always agitate fertilizers before pouring from the container, and keep nutrient solution in tanks agitated.

Unless fortified, soilless mixes require fertilization from the start. I like to start fertilizing fortified soilless mixes after the first week or two of growth. Most commercial soilless mixes are fortified with trace elements.

Mix organic fertilizer components dry. Sprinkle a mist of water overhead to dampen dust. Mix components thoroughly before wetting. Mix large amounts in an electric cement mixer that can be rented for the day. Mix small amounts in a barrel, wheelbarrow, or corner of a basement.

Fertilizer Application

The goal of fertilizing is to supply plants with proper amounts of nutrients for vigorous growth, without creating toxic conditions by overfertilizing. Some varieties of cannabis can withstand high

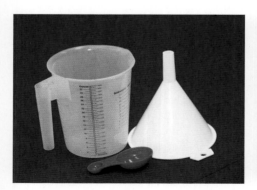

A measuring cup, a measuring spoon, and a funnel are essential to measure and handle accurate doses of nutrients when mixing.

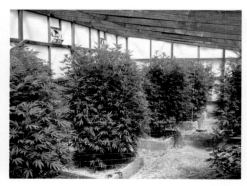

FloraGro and FloraBloom from General Hydroponics are popular hydroponic fertilizers.

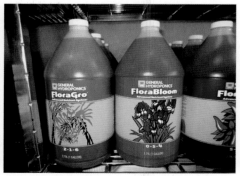

Plants use more nitrogen during the vegetative growth stage. These healthy plants require a spherical trellis to hold up rapid vegetative growth.

doses of nutrients, and other varieties grow best with a minimum of supplemental fertilizer. Every medicinal cannabis variety requires specific fertilizer applications. A blanket application of fertilizer for all varieties is impossible to give. Growing several different varieties in a small garden is common but can lead to underfertilization of some varieties and overfertilization of others.

The metabolism of cannabis changes as it grows and so do its fertilizer needs. During germination and seedling growth, intake of phosphorus is high. The vegetative growth stage requires larger amounts of nitrogen for green-leaf growth, and phosphorus and potassium are also necessary in substantial levels.

During this leafy and vegetative growth stage, use a *general purpose* or a *grow* fertilizer with high nitrogen content. In the flowering stage, nitrogen is still necessary, but potassium and phosphorus intake increases so the N-P-K ratio changes. Using a *super bloom* fertilizer with less nitrogen and more potassium, phosphorus, and calcium promotes fat, heavy, dense flower buds. Cannabis still needs nitrogen during flowering. With no nitrogen, buds do not develop to their full potential.

A 3-gallon (11.4 L) container full of rich, fertile organic potting soil should supply all the necessary nutrients for the first month of growth, but plant development might be slow. After the roots have absorbed most of the available nutrients, more must be added or become available organically to sustain vigorous growth. Medical cannabis growing in small containers will have very little growing medium in which to hold nutrients, and toxic salt buildup may become a problem. Follow fertilizer dosage instructions on the label. Search cannabis cultivation forums for more information on specific fertilizer mixing and application. Adding too much fertilizer will not make the plants grow faster. Too much fertilizer changes the chemical balance of the soil, supplies too much of a nutrient, or locks in other nutrients, making them unavailable to the plant.

Caution! Do not pour nutrients down household drains—or any drain. The nitrates, phosphates, and other contents will pollute the water supply. Use them outdoors in the garden.

Fertilizer/Irrigation Schedule

A regular fertilizing schedule with realistic outcome and known input is the easiest way to ensure that plants receive all the nutrition they need. When choosing a fertilizer, also choose the proper substrate the formula was designed for. Many fertilizer programs are augmented with different additives that expedite nutrient uptake.

If the fertilization schedule does not work, and you have discerned that plant growth is out of whack, check for the following outward signs of nutrient deficiencies.

Determine if the plants need to be fertilized: Make a visual inspection, take an N-P-K soil test, or experiment on test plants. No matter which method is used, remember, plants in small containers use available nutrients quickly and need

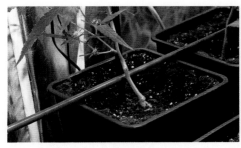

Nutrient solution is delivered at regular intervals via the overhead irrigation tube.

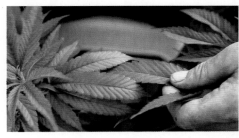

With a little practice it is easy to eyeball plants and tell what they need. The leaf on the right is properly fertilized. The pale plant on the left looks like it is deficient in nitrogen.

frequent fertilizing, while plants in large planters have more soil, supply more nutrients, and can go longer between fertilizing.

Visual Inspection: If the plants are growing well and have deep-green, healthy leaves, they are probably getting all necessary nutrients. The moment growth slows or the leaves begin to turn pale green, it is time to fertilize. Do not confuse yellow leaves caused by a lack of light with yellow leaves caused by a nutrient deficiency. Leaves should be green all the way to the bottom of the plant. But by the time the plant tells you there is an issue, it is too late.

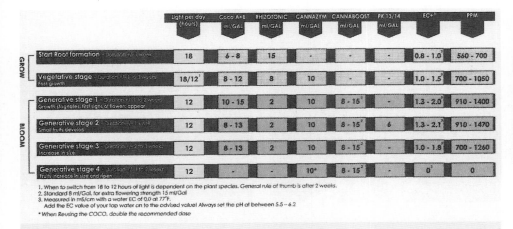

	Light per day (hours)	Coco A+B ml/GAL	RHIZOTONIC ml/GAL	CANNAZYM ml/GAL	CANNABOOST ml/GAL	PK 13/14 ml/GAL	EC*	PPM
GROW Start Root formation - Duration +/- 1 week	18	6 - 8	15	-	-	-	0.8 - 1.0	560 - 700
GROW Vegetative stage - Duration +/- 1 to 3 weeks. Fast growth	18/12¹	8 - 12	8	10	-	-	1.0 - 1.5	700 - 1050
BLOOM Generative stage 1 - Duration +/- 1 to 2 weeks. Growth stagnates, first signs of flowers appear	12	10 - 15	2	10	8 - 15²	-	1.3 - 2.0	910 - 1400
BLOOM Generative stage 2 - Duration +/- 1 week. Small fruits develop	12	8 - 13	2	10	8 - 15²	6	1.3 - 2.1	910 - 1470
BLOOM Generative stage 3 - Duration +/- 2 to 3 weeks. Increase in size	12	8 - 13	2	10	8 - 15²	-	1.0 - 1.8	700 - 1260
BLOOM Generative stage 4 - Duration +/- 1 to 2 weeks. Fruits increase in size and ripen	12	-	-	10*	8 - 15²	-	0	0

1. When to switch from 18 to 12 hours of light is dependent on the plant species. General rule of thumb is after 2 weeks.
2. Standard 8 ml/Gal, for extra flowering strength 15 ml/Gal
3. Measured in mS/cm with a water EC of 0,0 at 77°F.
   Add the EC value of your tap water on to the advised value! Always set the pH at between 5.5 – 6.2
* When Reusing the COCO, double the recommended dose

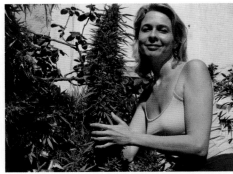

This lovely medical cannabis gardener grew this giant bud in a pot on a patio in Spain. Regular irrigation and fertilization were her keys to gardening success.

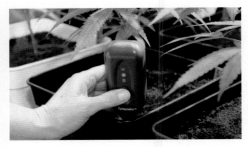

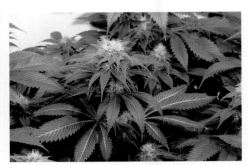

A basic EC meter can tell you if nutrients have built up to toxic salt levels.

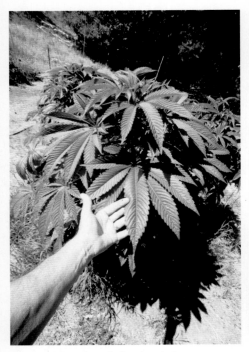

This healthy, properly fertilized plant is growing as fast as naturally possible.

An overall toxic buildup of nutrients is easy to spot in most plants. You can see that these leaves are too dark and shiny. The plant in the center is so overfertilized that leaves have turned dark purple, with the veins remaining green.

The fact is that the relationship between nutrient uptake and plant growth is very subtle. By the time a nutrient deficiency manifests with a discolored leaf or slow growth, the dysfunction has already slowed growth.

To get an idea of which cannabis varieties need a little or a lot of fertilizer, I asked members of my forum on www.marijuangrowing.com. To learn the best way to fertilize specific varieties, you may need to contact the company that sold you the seeds. Start with an EC of 1.6 and build it up as needed. The absolute maximum EC is 2.3.

Varieties that require high doses of fertilizer:

Overall *indica*-dominant clones root well, with the possible exception of 'Hindu Kush' (a landrace, with less vigor and not as nutrient-hungry as hybrid *indicas*). In this case, 'more fertilizer' means using the high end of the recommended dosage, not exceeding it.

A few of the varieties that in general can withstand higher doses of fertilizer include: 'Twilight', 'Green Spirit', 'Khola',

'Hollands Hope', 'Passion#1', 'Shaman' within an EC range of 1.6–2.3.

Varieties that require medium doses of fertilizer:

Many varieties require a standard dose of fertilizer including the varieties below.

'Skunk #1', 'Trance', 'Voodoo', 'Sacra Frasca', 'California Orange', 'Delta 9', 'Skunk Passion', 'Blueberry', 'Durban Poison', 'Purple #1', 'Purple Star', ' Super Haze', 'Ultra Skunk', 'Orange Bud', 'White Widow', 'Power Plant', and 'Euforia'

Varieties that require low doses of fertilizer:

Overall, *sativa*-dominant varieties and hybrids require much less fertilization. There are exceptions, including 'Silver Pearl', 'Marley's Collie', and 'Fruity Juice' (*sativa* hybrids, but with a heavy, *indica*-dominant bud pattern). In this case, less fertilizer means using the low end of the recommended dosage. 'Northern Lights #5 x Haze' has more open buds in its growth pattern but a lot of floral bulk by weight, so may need normal to slightly higher levels of nutrient.

'Isis', 'Flo', 'Dolce Vita', 'Dreamweaver', 'Master Kush', 'Oasis', 'Skywalker' and 'Hempstar' are within an EC range of 1.6 to 2.3. 'Mazar' needs a higher EC during weeks three to five to prevent early yellowing of the leaves.

Take an EC test of runoff water to tell how much nutrient is trapped in the soil. Make a batch of 0.1 EC nutrient solution. Drench plants in containers with one gallon (3.8 L) of solution. Check the EC of the runoff water. If it is above 0.1 EC, there is a toxic buildup of nutrients in the soil. The soil needs to be leached with a mild nutrient solution to purge it of toxic fertilizer salts.

Take an N-P-K soil test to reveal exactly how much of each major nutrient is available to the plant. Test kits mix a soil sample with a chemical. After the soil settles, a color reading is taken from the liquid and matched to a color chart. The appropriate percent of fertilizer is then added. This method is reliable but requires patience. But this test does not measure the amount of each nutrient that plants are actually processing.

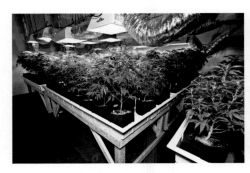

Indoors, regular fertilizer application is essential to ensure rapid growth.

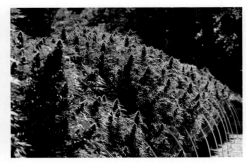

Outdoors, plants can take in virtually all the necessary nutrients from specially mixed soil.

Experimenting on two or three test plants is the best way to gain experience and develop horticultural skills. Start with a fertilization schedule and amend it as needed according to temperature, humidity, and growth stage. Clones (cuttings) are perfect for this type of experiment. A basic premise is to give the test plants a fertilizer schedule and see if they grow better and faster. You should notice a change within three to four days. If it is good for the test plants, it should be good for all plants of the same varieties.

How much fertilizer? Mix the fertilizer as per the instructions and water as normal, or dilute the fertilizer and apply it more often. Many liquid fertilizers are diluted already. Consider using more concentrated fertilizers whenever possible. Remember, small plants use much less fertilizer than large ones. Fertilize early in the day so plants have all day to absorb and process the fertilizer and water. Watering late in the day or at night can lead to waterlogged roots.

Fertilizer programs rely upon soil or substrate drainage. Frequency of irrigation also depends upon drainage. Large plants with a large root system in large containers use more nutrients than small plants in small containers. But small containers must be irrigated more often. The more often the fertilizer is applied, the less concentrated it should be. Frequency of fertilization and dosage are both affected by substrate drainage ability.

The concept in fertilizing is to either apply fertilizer periodically or constantly. Periodic includes dry and liquid fertilizers and is applied at higher ranges (dosages) to get the plant through the use period until the next application. This results in too high a concentration for the first half of the period and too low for the second half. Weekly applications, for example, begin with an ideal range the plant needs to satisfy exactly its requirements. Let's say that this particular plant needs a root zone EC of 1.0 for exactly the right amount of all nutrients to be available. We feed on Monday to bring the level to 1.6, and by the next feeding 7 days later the EC is at 0.4. For 3.5 days the EC is too high and the plant has small issues, from day 4 to day 7 the level is below the ideal level of 1.0 for 3 days as it drops to 0.4 and the plant development also slows. Then feed is again applied, and the plant restarts until the next lag.

The second version is constant feeding. This applies an EC of 1.1 each watering, and by the next watering the EC has fallen to just under 0.9. Then the lag is fixed within a day or a day and a half. The plant never notices and growth goes unabated. All commercial Green Industry producers use constant feeding because the plant is never overfertilized, nor is it ever really underfed. Salt levels remain balanced and the plants do remarkably better.

A pre-fertilized peat-based mix usually has enough calcium and possibly other elements. Coco absorbs large quantities of calcium at the beginning of the growing cycle. Fertilizer schedules need to have this and other details built in to support a successful crop. Choose a substrate and a fertilizer designed for it.

Some varieties can absorb amazing amounts of fertilizer and still grow well. Lots of gardeners add as much as one tablespoon per gallon (14.8 ml per 3.8 L) of a standard dry soluble fertilizer such as Peters (20-20-20) with each watering. This works best with growing mediums that drain readily and are easy to leach. Other gardeners use only rich, organic potting soil. No supplemental fertilizer is applied until a super bloom formula is needed for flowering.

Fertilizing plants in the ground outdoors is much easier than fertilizing containerized plants. In healthy, outdoor organic soil, nutrient uptake is rapid and buffered, and fertilization is not as critical. There are several ways to apply fertilizer. Top-dress a garden bed by applying the fertilizer and working it into the top 2 inches (5.1 cm) of soil. Apply a dilute liquid fertilizer around the bases of plants. Foliar-feed plants by spraying a liquid fertilizer solution on the foliage. The method you choose will depend upon the kind of fertilizer, the needs of the plants, and the convenience of a chosen method.

Use a **siphon (venture pump) applicator**—found at most nurseries—to mix soluble fertilizers with water. The applicator is simply attached to the faucet with the siphon submerged in the concentrated fertilizer solution with the hose attached to the other end. Often, applicators are set at a ratio of 1 to 15. This means that for every single (1) unit of liquid concentrate fertilizer, 15 units of water will be mixed with it. Sufficient water flow is necessary for the suction to work properly. Misting nozzles restrict this flow. When the water is turned on, the fertilizer is siphoned into the system and flows out the hose. The fertilizer is generally applied with each watering, since a small percentage of fertilizer is metered in.

![Containers full of soilless growing medium on Canna Coco slabs in hydroponic garden]

Containers full of soilless growing medium are set on top of Canna Coco slabs in this top-feed hydroponic garden.

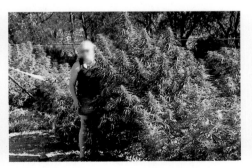

This medical cannabis gardener brings in truckloads of compost and manure. Once in place she uses a tractor to cultivate it into the soil before planting.

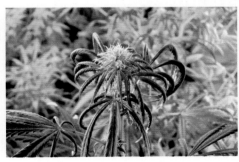

Leaves curl when given a slight fertilizer overdose.

Injector Applicator

A Dosatron fertilizer injection system makes it easy to feed a big indoor, outdoor or greenhouse garden with a consistent pH-balanced fertilizer mix. Fertilizer injectors range in price from $250 to $800 USD depending upon volume injected. Injectors can also meter out pH up and pH down, fungicides, pesticides, etc. When using fertilizer injectors, make sure the nutrient concentrate is completely mixed with water before application in drip emitters.

A garbage can with a garden-hose fitting attached at the bottom that is set 3 to 4 feet (91.4–121.9 cm) off the floor will act as a gravity-flow source for the fertilizer solution. Place the reservoir on the floor of the next level of the house to increase water pressure. The container is then filled with water and fertilizer. Set containers up on a table to gain pressure and flow.

When it comes to fertilization, experience with specific varieties and growing systems will tell gardeners more than anything else. There are hundreds of N-P-K mixes, and they all work, some better than others. When choosing a fertilizer, make sure to read the entire label, and know what the fertilizer claims it can do. Do not be afraid to ask the garden store clerk questions or to contact the manufacturer with questions. Cannabis cultivation forums also help gardeners share their experiences with fertilization of specific varieties.

Once you decide how often to fertilize, put the garden on a regular feeding schedule. Following a schedule usually works very well, but it must be combined with a vigilant, caring eye that looks for overfertilization and signs of nutrient deficiency.

Leach soil with 1 to 2 gallons (3.8–7.6 L) of mild nutrient solution per gallon of soil every month to prevent toxic salt buildup in the soil. Mix the EC 0.2 in soil and peat, 0.5 in coco; Epsom salts are good for soil and peat, but use only nutrients for coco.

Stomata close when there is:

too much CO_2
low humidity
a dry root system

Stomata open when there is:

high light
low CO_2
high humidity

Foliar Feeding

Foliar feeding means to spray nutrients or additives diluted in water onto plant foliage. Foliar sprays can provide a "quick fix" for some nutrient deficiencies. This feeding method is best employed when damaged and stressed roots are not working properly. Some sources claim foliar feeding speeds rooting time of clones (cuttings) when applied sparingly. Easy to overdo, foliar feeding can leach nutrients, especially when plants are young or have few or no roots.

Making complete or general recommendations on foliar feeding is impossible because we do not know everything. Scientists believe that most of the nutrients and stimulants stay in the location they enter unless specifically designed by Mother Nature to translocate, which means that the rest of the plant will not benefit from foliar feeding.

We know that nitrogen (N) and iron (Fe) translocate well, but phosphorus (P) does

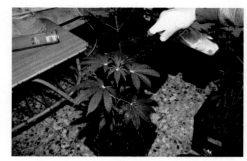

Foliar feeding is a quick fix for some nutrient deficiencies.

not move well within the plant because of its ion size. Using dimethyl sulfoxide (DMSO) or another carrier helps everything move but is also harmful for the consumer, especially medical patients!

Some commercial products, such as Canna's Boost, can be applied as a foliar spray every 3 days but mineral fertilizer should not be applied nearly so often. Furthermore, accumulating nutrient residues will *burn* plant tissue if they are not taken up. Complex organic molecules seldom burn plant tissue or cause problems.

Not all elements are able to translocate across the outer skin (epidermis) of foliage. The waxy (cuticle) surface coating (cystolith hairs and resin) on cannabis foliage makes for very poor water absorption. This barrier wards off pest and disease attacks, but it also slows the penetration of sprays.

Young, supple leaves are more permeable than older leaves. Nutrients and additives penetrate immature leaves faster than tougher, older leaves, and they are easier to damage with strong sprays.

Spraying foliage underneath so the spray is able to penetrate the stomata located on the leaf's underside does not work. Experts seem to agree that application to the stomatal areas is no more effective than application to the leaf surface, because the structure of the stomata will seldom allow intrusion by the liquid.

Plants properly maintained hardly, if ever, need foliar feeding. The roots are designed by Mother Nature for nutrient uptake and are still be best means of

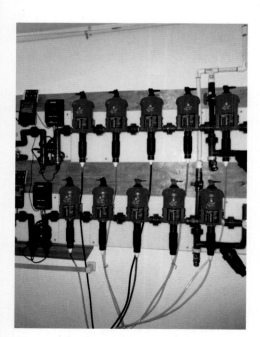

Dosatron fertilizer injection systems are becoming more popular.

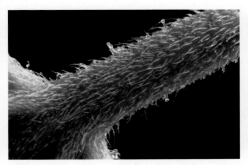

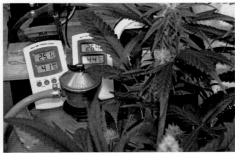

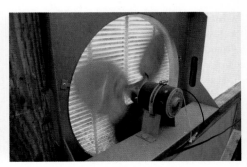

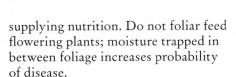

Leaves and stalks have waxy, cystolith hairs that act like feathers on a duck to shed water. See chapter 24, Diseases & Pests, for information on spraying.

Always calibrate thermometers and hygrometers to ensure their accuracy.

Adequate ventilation is essential in greenhouses and in indoor garden rooms.

supplying nutrition. Do not foliar feed flowering plants; moisture trapped in between foliage increases probability of disease.

Foliar feeding should be used only as a supplement. Never spray more than once every 7 to 10 days, if at all, and keep the spray concentration at quarter-strength.

Common "Nutrient" Problems

To help avoid common Problems:

1. Use proper, *complete* nutrient
2. Do not overwater
3. Control pH and EC
4. Leach soil once a month

There is a short list of common problems that often result in nutrient deficiencies and excesses. Unhealthy plants grow slowly, produce poorly, and are susceptible to attacks by pests and diseases. Controlling the critical cultural factors that cannabis needs to grow will help avoid nutrient imbalances. Nutrient imbalances are usually a result of incorrect cultural essentials—air, light, water, growing medium, and nutrient solution. Each of these factors, along with pH and EC, will affect nutrient uptake. When the basic needs of plants are not met, controlling pH and EC will have minimal effect on nutrient uptake.

Nutrient deficiencies are less common when using fresh potting soil fortified with micronutrients, or a hydroponic mix containing all necessary elements. If the soil or water supply is acidic, add dolomite lime to buffer the soil pH and to keep it sweet. Evaluate all factors in enclosed

garden rooms and greenhouses, especially temperature and ventilation, before deciding that plants are nutrient deficient.

Overall, plants in indoor gardens start to show outward stress signs in the sixth to eighth week of growth. Once a plant shows symptoms, it has already undergone severe nutritional stress for one or two weeks. It will take time for the plant to stabilize and demonstrate vigorous growth. To help plants retain vigor, correct identification of each symptom—as soon as it occurs—is essential. Indoor, greenhouse, and some outdoor cannabis crops are harvested so fast that plants do not have time to recover from nutrient imbalances. One small imbalance could cost a week of growth. That could be more than 10 percent of the plant's life. In short, incorrect pH is reflected in stunted growth and lower harvest weight.

Air

Temperature: Both low and high temperatures slow the growth of plants. Large fluctuations in temperature—more than 15 to 20 degrees Fahrenheit (8 to 10 degrees Celsius)—cause slow growth by slowing the plants' processes, including nutrient uptake.

Solution: Lower the temperature by removing as many heat sources from the garden room as possible, or with ventilation or air conditioning indoors. Vent greenhouses, cover them with reflective shade cloth, and install evaporative cooling. Outdoors, install shade cloth above plants. Raise temperatures indoors and in greenhouses by using a heater. Insulate garden rooms and install a heat blanket over greenhouses. Outdoors, cover plants with plastic to raise the temperature.

Humidity: High humidity causes stomata to open wide but slows evaporation, thus reducing water and nutrient movement. Low humidity increases water and nutrient movement, bringing too much to the plant. Low humidity stresses plants because they use too much water and higher nutrient levels.

Solution: Lower the humidity with ventilation, air conditioning, or a dehumidifier in enclosed garden area. Increase humidity by lowering temperature to 70°F (21.1°C) or by placing a humidifier in the garden area.

Carbon dioxide (CO_2): Growth is stifled and slows rapidly when CO_2 is lacking. Nutrient and water consumption slows too. The growing medium is often overwatered, causing soggy roots and growth stagnation.

Solution: Increase air circulation so that all leaves in the garden flutter a little. This will keep CO_2 from stagnating around foliage. Remove dense lower foliage that receives no light. Vent out CO_2-poor air. Install a CO_2 generator or CO_2 emitter to increase CO_2 levels.

Ozone damage: See chapter 16, *Air*, for more information on ozone damage.

Solution: Stop using an ozone generator indoors and in greenhouses.

Indoor air pollution: This causes very difficult-to-solve plant problems. Always be aware of chemicals bleeding or vaporizing from pressboard and other building materials. Such pollution causes plant growth to slow to a crawl. Ozone damage could also affect plant growth.

Solution: Remove problem-causing pressboard. Before reinstalling the re-moved pressboard, wait 6 to 12 months so that harmful chemicals have stopped outgassing. Stop using ozone generators, and switch to carbon filters to clean exhaust air.

Heat Stress

The temperature within the leaves can climb to an excess of 110°F (43.3°C). It happens easily because leaves store heat radiated by lamps and sunlight. At 110°F (43.3°C), the internal chemistry of a cannabis leaf is disrupted. The manu-factured proteins are broken down and become unavailable to the plant. As the internal temperature of the leaves climbs, plants are forced to use and evaporate more water. About 70 percent of the plant's energy is used in this process.

Solution: Leach growing medium to wash out excess fertilizer salts. Increase irrigation frequency, and lower the at-mospheric temperatures with ventilation or other means described above.

High humidity not only causes plants to grow looser but also the florets or indi-vidual flowers* to develop looser so that more water evaporates; this is a survival response. Because they are loose, fewer florets (individual flowers) are produced and overall weight is reduced.

*A bud is a group of flowers, known as an inflorescence, by botanical definition.

Solution: Lower humidity with ventila-tion, a dehumidifier, or an air conditioner that also dehumidifies.

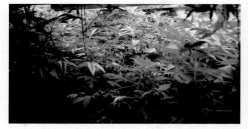

Low light levels cause spindly growth and poor utilization of nutrients. If plants are crowded and have poor air circulation, pests and diseases are more apt to be a problem.

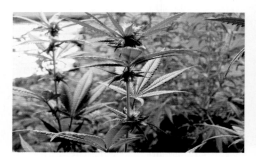

Heat stress causes loose buds.

Light

Lack of light: Nutrients are used poorly, photosynthesis is slow, stems stretch, and growth is scrawny.

Solution: Increase light levels by moving lamp closer to canopy of garden. Bend leggy plants to lower their profile so more light reaches the entire plant.

Too much light: Keep a 600-watt lamp 20 inches (50.8 cm) above plants.

Light burn: Burned foliage is susceptible to attack by pests and diseases.

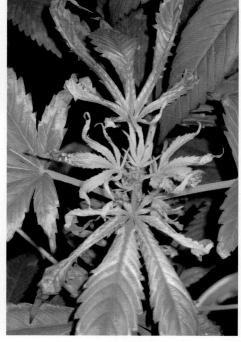

Light-burned plant was too close to the hot HID!

Solution: Indoors, move light further away from plants. Harden-off outdoor plants before placing outdoors so foliage is not soft and prone to burn.

Water

Water quality: Check water quality for excess sodium (more than 50 ppm), and excesses of other dissolved solids such as calcium and heavy metals. Check pH and composition of dissolved solids on a well water analysis or a water analysis from your water district. Compare water analysis to the label of the fertilizer you are using. Add up the total of each ele-

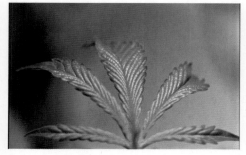

Along with curled leaf fringes, big ridges between veins signify temperature stress. Leaf edges that curl up signify that leaves are trying to dissipate as much moisture as possible. Moisture stress could be caused by toxic salt buildup, lack of water in the growing medium, or high atmospheric temperatures.

Lamp (watts)	Distance (inches)	Distance (centimeters)
250 W	10 in.	25 cm
400 W	15.7 in.	40 cm
600 W	20 in.	50 cm
1000 W	32 in.	80 cm

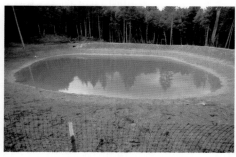

A clean source of water is essential for a healthy garden. Always check the water for dissolved solids with an EC/ppm meter. This pond is full of algae that must be treated and filtered before use.

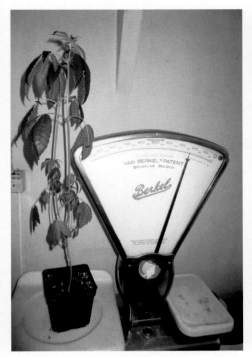

This containerized plant was weighed, dry, at 8.1 ounces (230 gm).

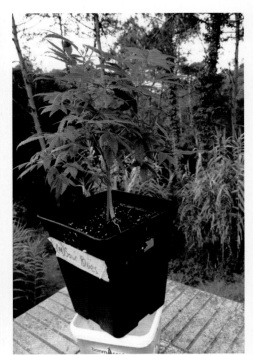

When saturated with water, the same containerized plant weighs 16.6 ounces (470 gm).

Catch runoff water from plants to measure EC and pH.

ment on the fertilizer label and the water analysis to calculate the entire fertilizer dosage plants are receiving.

Irrigation: If the growing medium and root mass are kept saturated with water for 20 minutes or longer, roots will not have adequate oxygen and will die (drown) and start rotting.

Any growing medium that drains *well* can be irrigated or washed (leached) as many times as you want, as long as the soil does not stay saturated (and thus contain no oxygen) for longer than 20 minutes at a time.

Water completely, until a minimum of 20 percent drains from the bottom of the container. Irrigate so that drainage occurs within 20 minutes of starting. Then the 50 percent rule applies before the next watering. See chapter 20, *Water*, "50 Percent Watering Rule," for more information about watering.

pH and EC: Control pH to the desirable soil or hydroponic range. Wash nutrients from soil to lower dissolved salts in growing medium.

Solution: Irrigate using reverse osmosis

(RO) water with fertilizer added. RO water will guarantee that your fertilizer mix will be consistent and easy to control. Manage EC in hydroponic tanks by topping off tanks with water every few days. Change nutrient solution in reservoirs every 7 to 14 days. When running higher EC levels, irrigation frequency must be increased so that plants do not dry down.

Growing Medium
To avoid most common nutrient deficiencies and excesses:

1. Use new store-bought soil indoors and in the greenhouse

2. Use well-composted, amended, or new store-bought soil outdoors

3. Add 1 cup (23.7 cl) of dolomite lime to each cubic foot (28.3 L) of substrate to keep pH "sweet" or in the 6.0 to 7.0 range

4. Measure all bulk soils that tend to change for sodium (Na)

Soil Temperature: Soil over 90°F (32.2°C) will harm the roots. Often, outdoor soil that is used in containers warms up to well over 100°F (37.8°C). I notice that my outdoor garden virtually stops growing when soil temperature reaches about 80°F (26.7°C).

Solution: Cool soil indoors and in greenhouses by lowering the temperature of the garden room and placing containers on concrete or cool floor, if possible. In any container garden, shade containers from light, paint them white to reflect light, and place reflective mulch on soil surface. Outdoors, mulch soil with at least 6 inches (15.2 cm) of straw, hay, or other vegetation, or use any mulch to cool the soil surface.

Roots receiving light: Roots turn green if light shines through the container or the hydroponic system. Roots require a

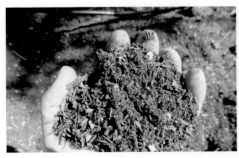

A good growing medium allows good drainage and holds plenty of moisture at the same time. This growing medium is packed with well-composted bark dust and woodchips. Dolomite lime has been added to stabilize pH.

dark environment. Their function slows substantially when they turn green.

Solution: Indoors or out, paint containers an opaque color inside so roots stay in the dark.

pH and EC: Keep both pH and EC at proper levels.

Nutrient Solution

Nutrient balance: Change the nutrient solution in small systems regularly, every 7 to 14 days. This is the easiest way to keep recirculating solutions in balance and avert problems. The nutrient reservoir should also have a top to minimize evaporation and avoid the possibility of pollutants falling into the tank. Topping off the tank every day or two will compensate for water used by plants. Topping off will also keep the nutrient solution from concentrating.

Always use a complete hydroponic fertilizer that contains all necessary nutrients, including micronutrients in a chelated form. Do not use fertilizers designed for soil gardens in a hydroponic system. Use only fertilizers that list all necessary nutrients on the label.

Incorrect pH: Out-of-whack pH level contributes to most serious nutrient disorders in organic-soil gardens. Many complex biological processes occur between organic fertilizers and the soil

during nutrient uptake. The pH can be decisive to the likelihood of these activities. Typically, a pH from 5.2 to 6.0 is acceptable for both vegetative and flowering growth. But a pH range of 5.6 to 6.0 for vegetative growth and 5.4 to 5.8 for flowering is best.

A low-pH, below 5.5, (acidic growing medium and nutrient solution) causes plants to become stunted and fail to reach their potential. A high pH also causes stunted growth, as well as a lack of iron and manganese. With a high pH, plants have very pale green leaves. Either way, adjusting the pH will solve the problem.

Overfertilizing can become one of the biggest problems for indoor gardeners. Too much fertilizer causes a buildup of the nutrients (salts) to toxic levels, and it changes the soil chemistry. When overfertilized, plants' growth is rapid and lush until toxic levels are reached. At this point, things become complicated.

Chance of **overfertilization** is greater in a small amount of soil that can hold only a small amount of nutrients. A large pot or planter can safely hold much more soil and nutrients, but it will take longer to leach if fertilizer is overdone. It is very easy to add too much fertilizer to a small container. Large containers have good nutrient-holding ability.

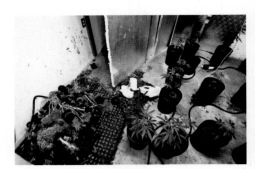

Dirty gardens promote pests and diseases.

Solution: To treat severely overfertilized plants, leach the soil with 2 gallons (7.6 L) of diluted nutrient solution per gallon (3.8 L) of soil to wash out all excess nutrients. The plant should start new growth and look better in one week. If the problem is severe and leaves are curled, the soil may need to be leached several times. After the plant appears to have leveled off to normal growth, apply the diluted fertilizer solution.

Miscellaneous

Spray application damage: Some sprays are phytotoxic, others are very phytotoxic. They can burn foliage if the spray is too concentrated or if it is sprayed during the heat of the day.

Solution: Lower concentration of spray so that it is less phytotoxic. Spray plants early or late in the day when sunlight or artificial light is not shining directly on foliage. The spray should have a chance to dry on foliage before nightfall. Using clean water, wash spray off plants after 24 to 48 hours.

Lazy Practices

One lazy guy mixed Miracle-Gro into the central water system for his house so that he would not have to measure it out and apply. It was always in the water!

A novice grower who purchased a popular fertilizer brand with "A" and "B" nutrients did not read the instructions. He made the error of applying small doses of "A" fertilizer until the bottle was finished. Next he applied "B" nutrient in doses. His crop was a ruin!

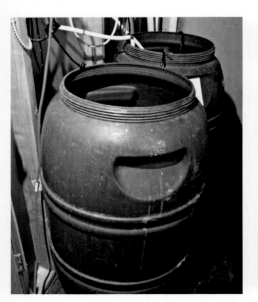

Check the nutrient solution's pH and EC/ppm to ensure that they are in the safe range.

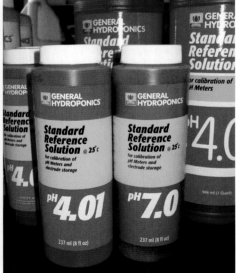

Always keep the pH meter calibrated properly with 7.0 and 4.0 reference solutions.

Organic Nutrients List
Animal-Based Fertilizer Meals
Blood Meal

Blood (dried or meal) is collected at slaughterhouses, dried, and ground into a powder or meal. It's loaded with fast-acting soluble nitrogen (12 to 15 percent by weight), up to 1.2 percent phosphorus, and under 1 percent potash. The proteins are broken down quickly by soil life, and they become immediately available and will last up to 4 months. Blood meal is an ideal nitrogen source for heavy-feeding varieties or to green up a garden. Use as a topdressing and cultivate into soil, or apply up to 1 month before planting. Apply carefully because blood meal is "hot" and can easily burn foliage if overapplied. When blood meal is applied on top of the ground in a band around a garden, it will keep rabbits from eating too much of the crop.

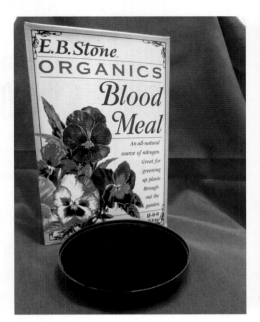

Blood meal

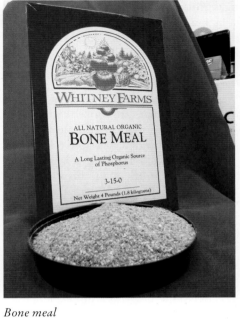

Bone meal

Bone Meal

Bone meal* is an excellent natural source of phosphorus. It increases microbial activity and nutrient uptake to help phosphates become available to plants. The lime found in bones also lowers soil pH. Bone meal also contains calcium and some nitrogen and trace minerals. Finely ground bone meal becomes available more quickly than coarsely ground, and it is faster-acting in well-aerated soil. It is also an excellent supplement for transplants and to promote a strong, extensive root system.

*Bone meal could transport Mad Cow Disease (bovine spongiform encephalopathy). The outbreak of this disease was purportedly contracted by four humans in the UK who *inhaled* bone meal dust while spreading it in their gardens. Now most countries have changed processing standards and do not allow processing of diseased animals, which appears to have curtailed spreading of Mad Cow Disease via bone meal. No outbreaks have been reported in recent history. If you feel uncomfortable using bone meal, please do more research, and post results on www.marijuanagrowing.com.

Bone meal for gardening is available in two main forms: precipitated (unsteamed) and steamed. Avoid raw bone meal because lingering fatty acids slow decomposition. Most often, precipitate bone meal is used for animal feed, and steamed bone meal is used as fertilizer. When sold in animal feed stores, the percentage of phosphorus on precipitated products is shown instead of phosphate (P_2O_5). This means that 12 percent phosphate is equal to 27.5 percent phosphorus. To convert phosphorus to phosphate, multiply phosphorus by 2.29. For example, 12 percent phosphate × 2.29 = 27.5 percent phosphorus.

Precipitated (unsteamed) bone meal is made by grinding and dissolving bones in acid before bathing in lime solution. Calcium and phosphorous from bones bind together and precipitate out; they are extracted from the liquid and then dried. The very fine resulting particles contain 40 percent available phosphate but no nitrogen. The end product is dusty to work with.

Steamed or cooked bone meal is made from fresh animal bones that have been boiled or steamed under pressure to render out fats that slow decomposition. The pressure treatment causes a little nitrogen loss and an increase in phosphorus. Steamed bones are easier to grind into a fine powder, and the process helps nutrients become available sooner. Steamed bone meal contains up to 30 percent phosphorus and about 1.5 percent nitrogen. The finer the bone meal is ground, the faster it becomes available to plants. Till it into soil at the rate of 10 pounds (4.5 kg) per 100 square feet (9.3 m²), or mix it into organic potting soil at the rate of one cup (236.6 cc) per cubic foot (28.3 L). Use as a topdressing and cultivate into soil, or apply up to one month before planting.

Feather Meal

Feather meal consists of feathers that are steamed under pressure, dried, and ground into a powdery feather meal. Feathers are dominated by the protein keratin. This protein occurs in hair, hooves, and horns and is broken down slowly by soil bacteria, making it a good long-term source of nitrogen. The nitrogen level ranges between 7 and 12 percent, depending upon rendering process. Often feathers are cooked with pressurized steam (hydrolysis) that pre-decomposes the meal. It is a good slow-release insoluble fertilizer and compost component that is available after four or more months. Feather meal is often mixed with poultry bedding, which speeds nutrient release. Mixing with bedding other than poultry will not hasten nutrient availability. Use as a supplemental source of nitrogen along with other fertilizers. Till into soil at the rate of 5 pounds (2.3 kg) per 100 square feet (9.3 m²), and add to compost piles and potting soil at the rate of 1 cup (236.6 cc) per 2 cubic feet (56.6 L). Feather meal is available online and sometimes at garden centers.

Hoof and Horn Meal

Hooves and horns collected from cattle at slaughterhouses are cooked, ground, and dehydrated to make this meal. Fine-ground horn meal makes slow-release nitrogen available a little faster. Soil bacteria must break down this slightly alkaline meal before it is available to the roots. Apply it a month before planting, and nitrogen will be available for up to 12 months afterward. It is a good compost activator and improves soil structure, too. This meal contains up to 12 percent nitrogen, 2 percent phosphorus, and no potassium. Use it as a supplemental source of nitrogen along with other fertilizers. Till into soil at the rate of 5 pounds (2.3 kg) per 100 square feet (9.3 m²) and add to compost piles and potting soil at the rate of 1 cup (236.6 cc) per 2 cubic feet (56.6 L). Available online and sometimes at garden centers, or it can be collected from pens for sheep and pigs.

Fish-Based Fertilizers
Fish Emulsion

Fish emulsion, an inexpensive soluble liquid, is high in organic nitrogen, trace elements, and some phosphorus and potassium. This natural fertilizer is difficult to overapply, and it is immediately available to plants. Fish emulsion is available from 1 to 4 months after

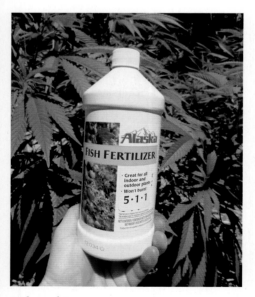

Fish emulsion

LIQUID FISH HYDROLYSATE

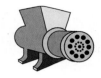

| Fresh fish & fish remains | Fresh fish is ground up | Cold processed natural enzymatic liquidifying | Filtered with fine mesh | Liquid fish hydrolysate |

FISH EMULSIONS

| Saltwater fish | Extract oil & protein with heat | Oil used for cosmetics & other products | Protein removed for animal feed | Depleted liquid concentrated into fish emulsion |

Fish hydroslyate is a better fertilizer than fish emulsion.

application. Inorganic potash is included in some formulas to add potassium to the fish emulsion. Odors from this product can cause real problems with animal pests. Even deodorized fish emulsion smells like dead fish. It contains up to 5 percent nitrogen, 2 percent phosphorus and 2 percent potassium. Apply as a diluted liquid fertilizer at the rate of 6 tablespoons (88.7 cc) per gallon (3.8 L) of water.

Note: Often, fish emulsion is processed after most of the proteins, enzymes, and nutrients have been rendered in previous processes. See "Fish Hydrolysate" below for a more completed fish fertilizer.

Fish Hydrolysate

Fish hydrolysate used as fertilizer is ground-up fish carcasses. It is not rendered nearly as much as fish used in emulsion products. Fish processing factories remove the meat for human consumption, and the rest—bones, cartilage, guts, and scales—are ground up and mixed with water. Enzymes are added to make the mix soluble. Higher-quality fish hydrolysate is ground more finely. Often bones and scales are separated, causing the mix to lack calcium,

minerals and proteins. Oil is rendered from dried products cutting out much of the plant food.

Although more expensive, the highest quality liquid fish hydrolysate processes whole fish, digests them with enzymes before liquefying the product. The cold-processed offal putrefies rapidly and is stabilized with sulfuric acidic at a low pH. The process uses enzyme-digested hydrolyzed liquid fish wastes instead of using heat and acids. This process retains more of the proteins, enzymes, vitamins and micronutrients than fish emulsions. Heated hydrolysate is moderately heated to render and concentrate oils into less complex plant food. Overheating can destroy numerous beneficial organisms. Carefully read product labels.

Fish hydrolysate contains up to 2 percent nitrogen, 4 percent phosphorus, and 1 percent potassium, as well as many proteins, vitamins, and micronutrients. It is often difficult to find at retail outlets but is available via online suppliers. Apply as a diluted liquid fertilizer at the rate of 6 tablespoons (88.7 cc) per gallon (3.8 L) of water.

Fish Meal

Fish meal is made from dried fish or rendered fish carcasses that are heated and often treated with acid before being ground into a meal that is rich in nitrogen and trace elements. It contains up to 10 percent nitrogen that is available immediately and lasts up to four months. Some meals also contain phosphorus and potassium. Incorporate fish meal into soil mixes, cultivate it into soil as a fast-acting topdressing, or use as a compost activator. Unless deodorized, this meal can have an unpleasant odor that may linger indoors. Outdoors, control fish meal odors by cultivating it into the soil, covering it with mulch, and diluting (irrigating) after application. Always store it in an airtight container so it will not attract cats, dogs, or flies. Till into soil at the rate of 10 pounds. (4.5 kg) per 100 square feet (9.3 m²) or mix into organic potting soil at the rate of 1 cup (236.6 cc) per cubic foot (28.3 L). Use as a topdressing and cultivate into soil, or apply up to one month before planting.

Fish Powder

Fish power is similar to meal and hydrolysate before processing. The source and treatment of fish dictates the quality of fish powder. It is dried with heat and turned into water-soluble powder. It is a high source of nitrogen, up to 12 percent, with a trace of potassium, 1 percent phosphorus, and many micronutrients. Hydrolysate powder also contains up to 5 percent potassium and 1 percent phosphorus. Most water-soluble fish powders can be mixed in solution and injected into an irrigation system.

High-quality fish powders consist of dehydrated, pulverized whole fish. Some offer enzyme-treated hydrolyzed fish protein (see below) processed products. Make sure to read labels carefully before applying to plants! Till in 1 to 2 ounces per 100 square feet (9.3 m²), or mix 1 tablespoon (14.8 cc) per gallon (3.8 L) of water.

Crab Wastes

Crab wastes contain relatively high levels of phosphorus and calcium. Crab waste is ground and dried to stabilize decomposition. The location, diet, and species of crab will affect the meal content. Waste contains chitin, which promotes organisms that attack pest nematodes.

Crab waste N-P-K runs about 5-2-0.5 and up to 10 percent calcium in this slow release fertilizer. Add crab waste 2 to 4 months before planting. Broadcast 10 pounds per 100 square feet (4.5 kg per 9.3 m²), and till into topsoil. Add to compost piles and mix into planting holes for seeds or transplants.

Guano
Bat Guano

Bat guano consists of the droppings and remains of bats. It is rich in soluble nitrogen, phosphorus, and trace elements. The limited supply of this fertilizer—known as the soluble organic super bloom—makes it expensive. Mined in sheltered caves, guano dries with minimal decomposition. Bat guano can be thousands of years old. Newer deposits contain higher levels of nitrogen and can burn foliage if applied too heavily. Older deposits are higher in phosphorus and make an excellent flowering fertilizer. Bat guano is usually powdery and is used any time of year as topdressing or diluted in a tea, also a great compost activator. Do not breathe the dust when handling it, because it can cause nausea and irritation in the lungs. Guano superphosphate is also available. Water-soluble bat guano runs about 3-10-1 for N-P-K and is packed with growth-stimulating bacteria and microbes. Nutrients are available immediately for up to 4 months. Add before planting at the rate of 5 pounds per 100 square feet (2.3 kg per 9.3 m²). Add 3 teaspoons per gallon (14.8 ml per 3.8 L) of water and start fertilizing 1 to 2 weeks before flowering. Bat guano also functions as a mild fungicide when applied as a foliar spray.

Seabird Guano

Seabird guano is high in nitrogen and other nutrients. The Humboldt Current, along the coast of Peru and northern Chile, keeps rain from falling, and decomposition of the guano is therefore minimal. South American guano is the world's best and most accessible guano. The guano is scraped off rocks of arid

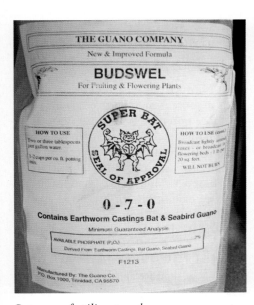

Bat guano fertilizer powder

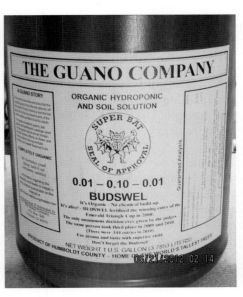

Bat guano fertilizer liquid

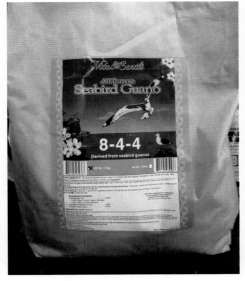

Seabird guano

ocean islands and is often mixed with seal droppings. Sea bird guano is also collected from many coastlines around the world, so its nutrient content varies. The average N-P-K of this soluble fertilizer is 10-3-1 is also packed with organic life. Apply before planting for nutrients that are available for more than four months. Till in 5 pounds per 100 square feet (2.3 kg per 9.3 m²) or as a tea at 3 teaspoons per gallon (14.8 ml per 3.8 L) of water, applied directly to the soil or made into a tea and applied as a foliar spray or injected into an irrigation system. Seabird guano also makes a good compost activator.

Manures
Manure and Bedding
Sometimes manures are collected, packaged, and sold pure. Most often, manures, each of which has specific biological, chemical, and physical characteristics, is packaged or collected with varying degrees of bedding—straw, sawdust, newspaper, chopped hemp fiber*, and cardboard. Livestock diet, weather, cleaning schedules, location, and so forth, dictate manure availability and consistency. Often manure can be delivered in bulk. At least 50 percent of the nitrogen and up to 70 percent of the potassium are found in urine mixed with manures and bedding.

*HempFlax from The Netherlands produces very popular BioBase Bedding for livestock from hemp stalks.

Manures are considered either "hot" or "cold." Hot manures will burn plants, cold manures won't. Poultry and swine manures, and fresh wet manures are "hot" and will burn plants. Most other manures are considered "cold" and seldom burn plants unless fresh. Well-composted manures do not burn plants or contain excessive salts. Fresh manures contain 60 to 70 percent more moisture than dry. Dried manures contain much higher levels of nutrients.

Cow and horse manure mixed with bedding make great additions to the compost pile and as an outdoor soil amendment. Swine manure is very wet and should be mixed with straw. Poultry manure also performs best when mixed with sawdust, straw, or other bedding.

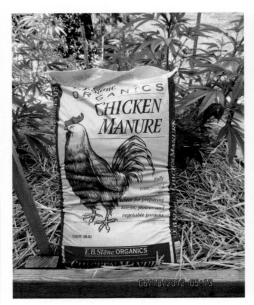

Chicken manure

But be careful: too much straw and sawdust bedding can use much of the available nitrogen and decrease yields.

Chicken (Poultry) Manure
Chicken (poultry) manure is probably the richest single organic fertilizer in relation to available nitrogen, phosphorus, potassium, and trace elements. Purchase dry, composted chicken manure in bags for convenience, or buy it in bulk. Use it as a topdressing or mix it into soil before planting.

Often chicken manure collected from farms is packed with decomposing feathers, which contain as much as 17 percent nitrogen; this is an added bonus. I used chicken manure in bulk and in bags. If you can find it locally at an organic chicken farm, it is the best! Make sure the chicken manure is composted for an extended period before use or it will burn anything because of the high uric acid content. Also weed seeds will be a giant problem.

The N-P-K runs low for chicken manure—about 1.5-1.5-0.5 wet, and 1.1-0.8-0.5 dry—and it is packed with trace elements. Don't let the low nutrient readings fool you; it is available immediately for up to 4 months. It can be heavy and bulky when wet, and bulky when dry. Add chicken manure up to a month before planting. Follow mixing instructions found on the bag label.

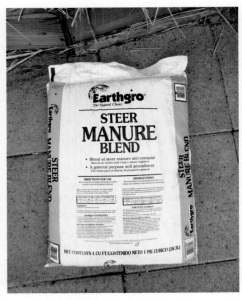

Cow manure

Cow Manure
Cow manure is often sold as steer manure but is sometimes collected from dairy herds. Cannabis gardeners have used cow manure for centuries. It is a fair fertilizer and good soil amendment. Steer manure is most valuable as mulch and as a soil amendment. It holds water well and maintains fertility for a long time. The nutrient value is low, and it should not be relied upon for the main source of nitrogen. Let it compost for several months if salt content is high, which is often the case with feedlot cow manure. Washed dairy manure from healthy cows is an excellent soil amendment. The N-P-K runs very low—about 0.7-0.3-0.4—and it is full of trace elements. Add cow manure to soil a month or two before planting. Best used as a soil amendment and secondary fertilizer.

Goat Manure
Goat manure is much like horse manure but more potent. The uniformly sized "nanny nuggets" are easy to "handle" and apply. They are most effective when broken up while incorporating with soil and compost. This manure increases soil's water-holding ability and microbial activity, and does not attract flies or animals when dry or mixed with soil. Quality of the product depends upon goat feed. N-P-K runs about 1.3-1.5-0.5. Apply goat manure as an amendment or fertilizer.

Horse Manure

Horse manure is readily available from horse stables and racetracks. Use horse manure that has straw, hemp straw, or peat for bedding. Wood shavings could be a source of plant disease. Compost fresh horse manure and bedding for two months or longer before adding it to the outdoor garden. The composting process kills weed seeds, and it will make better use of the nutrients. Hot composting above 140°F (60°C) kills pests and diseases. Many recipes are available on the Internet for horse manure compost.

New straw bedding often uses much of the available nitrogen. The N-P-K runs about 0.6-0.6-0.4, with a full range of trace elements. Add horse manure a month or two before planting. It is best as an amendment and secondary source of nutrients.

Rabbit Manure

Rabbit manure is an excellent fertilizer that is high in available nitrogen and phosphorus. It can be difficult to find locally, except in Spain and via the Internet. Use rabbit manure as you would chicken manure. It breaks down and becomes available quickly. The N-P-K runs about 2.4-1.4-0.6 in this very soluble fertilizer with some trace elements. According to Dr. John McPartland, rabbit poop is the best. Bunnies rule!

Sheep Manure

Sheep manure nutrient content is limited but it makes a wonderful manure tea. Sheep manures contain little water and lots of air. They heat up readily and make an excellent addition to compost piles. They add bulk, air, and nutrients. Use this inexpensive, low-odor manure as mulch, too. The N-P-K runs about 0.8-0.5-0.4, with a full range of trace elements. Add this slow-release soil amendment/fertilizer to planting mixes and compost piles more than a month before planting.

Swine Manure

Swine manure has a high nutrient content but is slower-acting and wetter (more anaerobic) than cow and horse manure. Difficult to find in a bag, most swine manure is available directly from the farm. Ask farmers for details on contents and use. Fresh, anaerobic lagoon sludge or liquid swine manure has an N-P-K of about 0.6-0.6-0.4. It also contains substantial ammonium and many secondary and trace elements. Add this hot manure to compost piles and to soil mixes. Be sparing with this manure because it is usually anaerobic in nature.

Urine

Urine is mixed with barnyard manure. It adds readily available nitrogen and is good for organic cannabis gardens. Urine contains mainly water and urea. The odor of fresh urine dissipates quickly, especially when diluted. It does not attract flies and contains few pathogens. Urine is okay to use in an organic garden but synthetic urea is not. See "Haber process" at right.

Be careful: It is easy to overfertilize with urine! Urine is packed with ammonia plants can't assimilate and it acidifies the soil. Use with caution when applying in liquid form. Human urine can also be used as fertilizer and added to compost.

If your dog, horse, or goat urinates in the same place in the green grass yard, its urine will often burn grass if it contains too much urea. Burn patches are common when urea is repeatedly applied in the same place. I have seen "popular"

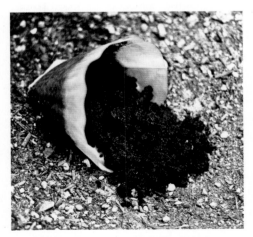

Caution: Urine is loaded with ammonia that cannabis plants cannot assimilate, and it acidifies the soil. Use with care.

The Haber Process

The Haber process, also know as the Haber–Bosch process, is the chemical process used to extract nitrogen in the form of ammonia from the atmosphere. Ammonia is oxidized to make nitrates and nitrites for use in fertilizers and explosives. Synthetic fertilizer generated from the Haber process is believed to help generate one-third of the food in the world!

metal streetlamp poles completely eaten through by dog urine. The N-P-K of urine runs about 12-1-2, and this soluble fertilizer is readily available. Normally it is mixed with animal bedding and manure so it is not as hot.

Miscellaneous
Coffee Grounds

Coffee grounds are slightly acidic—pH 6.0 to 6.2—and fine in texture. The high carbon-to-nitrogen ratio encourages acetic bacteria in the soil. Phosphorus, potassium, magnesium and copper in coffee grounds are readily available. The availability of nitrogen, calcium, zinc, manganese, and iron are low and sometimes deficient. Even though available nitrogen appears deficient, there are 10 pounds (4.5 kg) of total nitrogen per cubic yard (90 cm²) of coffee grounds. The nitrogen becomes available with microorganisms activity. In this way coffee grounds function as a slow release nitrogen fertilizer.

Collect coffee grounds only. Remove paper that uses nitrogen to decompose. Keep coffee grounds in a covered container. This will preserve moisture and nutrients. Mix coffee grounds into soil surface and soil mixes before planting. Add no more than 5 percent coffee grounds to any soil mix or when sprinkling on soil surface.

Sugar

Molasses, honey, and other sugars can increase soil microbial life, enhance regrowth, and make the plants' use of nitrogen more effective. Molasses is the "secret ingredient" in many organic fertilizers and the natural sugar best for organic medical cannabis crops. Sucrose (corn) syrup is the most economical way to buy sugar. However, it lacks many of the qualities found in molasses.

Plants manufacture sugars. Plant roots do not absorb sugars, raw or refined. Bacteria and other soil life consume sugars as food or fuel. Adding organic sugar in the form of molasses to the soil increases soil life and biological processes around the rhizosphere or root zone. Decomposing sugars release CO_2 and increase mineralization of organic elements. Molasses is practically useless in mineral-fed crops for mineralization.

Any sweet taste or flavor that vendors attribute to coming from sugars, does not come directly from adding sugars or flavorings to the nutrient solution. I would like to see vendors scientifically prove this cause-and-effect. Please have them contact me.

Molasses

Unsulphured molasses is top quality and is used in cooking. This grade is made from ripe sugar cane juice that is clarified and concentrated. It can be used in the garden.

Sulphured molasses is made from unripe (green) sugar. Sulfur fumes are applied during sugar extraction. Afterward it is boiled repeatedly. First-boil molasses is of the highest quality because only a small amount of sugar is removed. Second and any subsequent boils turn the molasses dark in color and extract more sugar. It can be used in the garden.

Blackstrap molasses has been boiled three times to extract even more sugar. Mainly used as cattle feed, it is packed with iron. It can also be used in the garden.

Overall, the average N-P-K analysis of molasses is 1-0-5 and it contains potash, sulfur, and many trace minerals in a chelated form. It is also loaded with carbohydrates and a balance of consumables, which are a quick source of energy and food for microorganisms. Molasses can be purchased at hydroponic, grocery, health food, and livestock feed stores. Dilute it at the rate of one

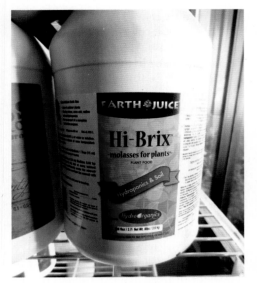

There are three main types of molasses: unsulphured, sulphured, and blackstrap.

tablespoon per gallon (1.5 cl per 3.8 L) of water. Irrigate plants to feed organic life in soil. Start feeding soil life when plants are growing.

Wood and Paper Ash

Wood ash (hardwood) supplies up to 10 percent potash. Softwood ashes contain about 5 percent. Potash washes out of wood ash quickly and can cause compacted, sticky soil. Avoid using high-pH alkaline wood ashes in soil with a pH above 6.5. Collect wood ash soon after burning, and store it in a dry place. Be careful when collecting fireplace ashes. Often such ashes are full of burned garbage that contains heavy metals and undesirable things. Collect and use only wood ashes from fireplaces, and apply sparingly.

Paper ash contains about 5 percent phosphorus and over 2 percent potash. Most inks are now soy-based or non-oil-based. I like to avoid paper ash due to the possible heavy metal content, but when clean and void of heavy metals found in some inks, paper ash is an excellent water-soluble fertilizer. Because the pH is quite high, do not apply paper ash in large doses.

Worm Castings

Vermicast (aka worm castings, worm humus, and worm manure) are excreted, digested humus and other (decomposing) organic matter, the end product in the breakdown of organic matter by

earthworms. Pure worm castings look like coarse graphite powder and are heavy and dense.

Worm castings are an excellent source of non-burning soluble nitrogen and many other elements. Vermicast is also an excellent soil amendment that promotes fertility and structure. Mix with potting soil to form a rich, fertile blend, but do not add more than 20 percent to any mix; vermicast is so heavy that root growth can be impaired. Vermicast is very popular and easier to obtain at commercial nurseries.

Vermicomposting can be done indoors, outdoors, or in a greenhouse. Red Wigglers (*Eisenia fetida* and *Eisenia andrei*) are the most active and commonly used worms in vermicomposting. Check the Internet for vermicomposting setups to turn your vegetable food wastes into rich fertilizer.

Rock (Mineral) Powders
Aragonite
Aragonite is biological and physical marine and freshwater precipitation-formed crystalline deposits of such shells as mollusk and oyster, which contain about 95 percent calcium carbonate. Use Aragonite to restore soil balance after applications of magnesium-rich lime that tie up other nutrients. Mined in Molina de Aragón, Spain, Aragonite is difficult to find in North America.

Ground into a fine powder, aragonite is used to adjust pH and raise calcium levels in the soil. It lowers acidity without increasing magnesium content. Avoid using aragonite with gypsum.

Azomite
This naturally occurring mineral contains micronutrients. Azomite consists of hydrated sodium calcium aluminosilicate derived from a natural volcanic mineral deposit. Add to compost or other fertilizer at the rate of 2 pounds (0.9 kg) per 10 square feet (.9 m²) and mix into soil up to a month before planting. Use in a 1 percent dilution in water.

Biotite
Biotite $[K(Mg,Fe)_3AlSi_3O_{10}(F,OH)_2]$ is a dark mica sheet silicate. It contains available iron, magnesium, aluminum, silicon, oxygen, and hydrogen to form

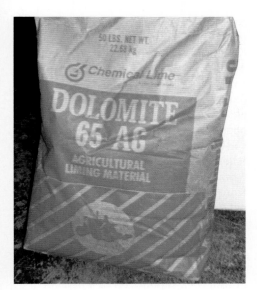

Dolomite lime

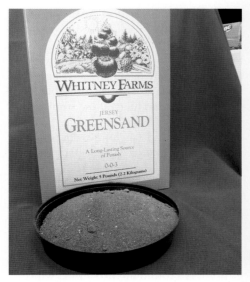

Greensand

sheets that are weakly bound together by potassium ions. This is vermiculite and a source/concern for asbestos. Even though it also increases CEC of the medium, since even though the K is washed out, the bind sites remain. Biotite is also known as "iron mica" and black mica." Phosphorus rock powders are available only when soil pH is below 7.0.

Diatomaceous Earth

Diatomaceous earth (DE), the fossilized skeletal remains of fresh and saltwater diatoms, contains a full range of trace elements. DE is a good insecticide. Apply DE to the soil when cultivating or use it as a topdressing. It is more commonly used as an insecticide than as a source of calcium.

Dolomite Lime

Dolomite lime adjusts and balances the pH and makes phosphates more available. It is generally applied to sweeten or deacidify the soil. It consists of calcium and magnesium, and is sometimes listed as a primary nutrient, though it is generally referred to as a secondary nutrient. Add dolomite lime to acidic soils and potting soils. Purchase flour or fine grades of dolomite that are available a little faster in the soil. Add dolomite a month or more before planting, at the rate of 0.5 cup per cubic foot (11.8 cl per 28.3 L) of soil. Use agricultural calcium if soil magnesium content is high.

Granite Meal

Soft, fine granite rock powders contain trace elements in a water-insoluble, slow-release form. Granite forms naturally in many different chemical structures. Softer granite from the southeastern USA breaks down more easily than granite from the Northeast. Granite dust or granite stone meal contains up to 5 percent potash and several trace elements. Releasing nutrients slowly over several years, granite dust is an inexpensive source of potash and does not affect soil pH. Not recommended indoors because it is too slow acting.

Epsom Salt

Hydrated magnesium sulfate ($MgSO_4$), Epsom salts, is a fast-acting soluble source of magnesium and sulfur. Use Epsom salts in alkaline soils to overcome magnesium deficiencies. Avoid using to raise pH in acidic soils; dolomite lime is a better choice. Apply Epsom salts (9 percent magnesium, 2 percent calcium, and 13 percent sulfur) when plants show a deficiency of magnesium. Continue adding weekly until symptoms disappear. Soluble magnesium sulfate washes out of soil quickly.

Applying Epsom salts is also an outstanding way to leach out excess salts that accumulate in CEC mediums, especially sodium.

Greensand

Greensand (glaucomite) is an iron-potassium silicate sandstone rock. The minerals in which it occurs give it a pale olive-green tint. Greensand is a great source of potassium and trace elements and is used in many organic mixes. It is able to absorb ten times more moisture, making it an exceptional soil conditioner

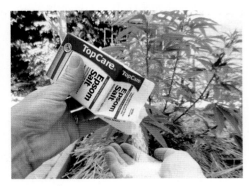

Epsom salts

in potting mixes. It slowly releases its treasures in about four years. It is too slow-acting for indoor gardens but is a good long-term fertilizer outdoors.

Greensand contains potassium, iron, magnesium, calcium, and phosphorus, plus as many as 30 other trace minerals. It is said to mineralize soil, improving plant and soil health by increasing populations of beneficial bacteria that make insoluble mineral nutrients available. Greensand is quite heavy and dense, with the consistency of sand, but can hold one-third its weight in water and has the ability to open tight soils and bind loose soils.

In the USA, greensand is mined from ancient New Jersey–seabed deposits of shells and organic material rich in iron, phosphorus, potash (5 to 7 percent), and numerous micronutrients. Some organic gardeners do not use greensand because it is such a limited resource, yet at the same time it is used to make garden walls in parts of the UK.

Greensand in the UK is often called "Upper" and "Lower" Greensand, which refers to two different deposits separated by Gault Clay. Lower Greensand (aka Woburn Sand) consists of a few deposits that contain of varying degrees of Atherfield (marine) Clay. Upper Greensand is a sand-based deposit within Gault Clay. Both greensands are found in the hills surrounding the London Basin and other sites in the UK.

Stay away from greensand coated with manganese oxide (aka manganese greensand). It is used to remove insoluble oxidized iron and manganese from pipes.

Apply greensand as a long-term source of potassium and to correct potash-deficient soils. Apply up to 100 pounds (45 kg) per 1000 square feet (92.9 m²).

Gypsum

Gypsum, hydrated calcium sulfate, $CaSO_4 \cdot 2(H_2O)$, is similar to plasterboard used in construction. Granular gypsum is ground up into a fine, white powder that is more rapidly available to plants and soils. It contains 23 percent calcium, 19 percent sulfur, and trace amounts of potassium and magnesium. Gypsum converts (ties up) salts, including magnesium in soils, prevents crusty soil, breaks up and aerates clay soils, and regulates micronutrient uptake—copper, iron, manganese, and zinc in cannabis.

Gypsum works by pulling together clay particles in the soil to make bigger particles, creating porous spaces for air, water, and plant roots. For example, in saline-infused soil, gypsum removes sodium and replaces it with calcium. Gypsum adds calcium and sulfur to all soils. It also helps soil retain water and helps decrease soil erosion.

Calcium sulfate ($CaSO_4$), aka Gypsite, is used to lower soil pH and improve drainage and aeration. It is also used to hold or slow the rapid decomposition of nitrogen. The formula carries calcium and sulfur in sulfate form. Cannabis is a major user of sulfur, and this is a great nutrient to add to any planting mix or compost pile.

Gypsite is unrefined gypsum that contains the clays and other minerals from the location it was mined. It is mined in arid areas, not typically wetter areas; it is not usually hydrated gypsum, $CaSO_4 \cdot 2(H_2O)$.

Many states and provinces in the USA, Mexico, Thailand, and Spain have large deposits of calcium sulfate. Gypsum ($CaSO_4 \cdot 2H_2O$) is one of the most common natural minerals and is really a type of rock.

Natural Nitrate of Soda

Natural Nitrate of Soda (NNS) aka Chilean Nitrate of Soda, is highly soluble, quick-acting granular fertilizer with 16 percent nitrogen in **nitrate** form, which is used directly by plants. This form of nitrogen is available to cannabis in cold soils. Temperature-sensitive microorganisms also use this source of nitrogen. But NNS is high in sodium too! Do not use NNS on arid soils where salt buildup is common. It is mined from a desert in northern Chile, where the only known deposit of this mineral salt exists. Mix this nitrate with cocoa meal, peanut meal, compost, and other organic amendments to buffer sodium content. Applying NNS with organic compost increases efficiency of both amendments. The high sodium content makes NNS a poor choice for the main nitrogen source. N-P-K is 16-0-0 and 26 percent sodium in this very soluble fertilizer. Add with an organic amendment and do not rely on NNS for a sole source of nitrogen. NNS is **not** compatible with high-sodium contents found in arid and semi-arid regions.

Rock Phosphate

Rock phosphate (hard) is a calcium or lime-based phosphate rock that is finely ground to the consistency of talcum powder. The rock powder contains over 30 percent phosphate and a menagerie of trace elements, but nutrients are very slow to become available.

Colloidal Phosphate

Colloidal phosphate (powdered or soft phosphate) is a natural clay phosphate deposit that contains just over 20 percent phosphorus (P_2O_5), calcium, and many trace elements. It yields only 2 percent phosphates by weight the first few months. Apply colloidal phosphate to outdoor gardens for uptake of slow-acting potassium during the next four years. The rock powder contains 18 percent total phosphate (2 percent available), 19 percent calcium (27 percent CaO), and 18 trace minerals.

Potash

Potash is also the common name for several mined and manufactured salts that contain a water-soluble form of potassium. Typically measured in fertilizer as K_2O, there are many chemical formulas depending on the source, collection, and form of potash. Occasionally potash will form with traces of organic plant remains. Potash was principally obtained by leaching the ashes of land and sea plants. It was refined from the ashes of broadleaved trees. Most potassium mines are in ancient deposits from inland oceans that evaporated. The potassium salts crystallized into beds of potash ore. The deposits are a mixture of potassium chloride (KCl) and sodium chloride (NaCl), aka table salt.

Potash rock supplies up to 8 percent potassium, and some deposits contain many trace elements. This slow-release fertilizer is not practical indoors but is a good long-term outdoor fertilizer and compost component. Potash is found in several different fertilizers, among them wood ashes and seaweed.

Sulfate of Potash

Sulfate of potash is normally produced chemically by treating rock powders with sulfuric acid, but one company, Great Salt Lake Minerals and Chemicals Company, produces a concentrated natural form. The sulfate of potash is extracted from the Great Salt Lake.

In natural mineral form, sulfate of potash (K_2SO_4) contains more than 50 percent soluble potash and 18 percent sulfur as well as calcium and magnesium. The brands Sul-Po-Mag and K-Mag are natural mineral salts. These water-soluble products are made from langbeinite and contain about 22 percent potash, 11 percent magnesium, and 23 percent sulfur. Apply as a supplement or blend into soil when making organic soil mixes.

Zeolite

The naturally occurring zeolite, clinoptilolite, provides a source of potassium that is slowly released. Some deposits also contain nitrogen that is slowly available over time. Zeolites also function to absorb more than half their weight in water and slowly release it as needed by plants. Incorporating zeolites into desert soils helps them withstand drought during hot dry weather.

Oyster Shells

Oyster shells are ground and normally used as a calcium source for poultry. Garden blends are pulverized to increase assimilation. Calcium formed in this non-crystalline state is more easily dissolved and utilized by the soil and plant. Oyster shells contain up to 55 percent calcium and traces of many other nutrients that release slowly. They are not practical to use indoors because they breakdown too slowly. Outdoors, oyster shells can be used as a long-term steady-release source of calcium and trace elements that raises pH in acidic soils. This is a good additive for compost piles and worm bins. Use 50 pounds (22.7 kg) of Oyster Shell Lime per 1,000 square feet (92.9 m^2), depending on soil analysis and crop.

Seaweed

Seaweed meal and/or kelp meal should be deep-green, fresh, and smell like the ocean. Seaweed contains 60 to 70 trace minerals. Check the label to ensure that all elements are not cooked out. Kelp and seaweed are harvested from the ocean or picked up along beaches, cleansed of salty water, dried, and ground into a powdery meal. Cold-water kelp contains more elements. It is packed with potassium (potash), numerous naturally chelated trace elements, vitamins, amino acids, and plant hormones. It is often combined with fish meal to add N-P-K value. The nutrient content varies according to the type of kelp and its growing conditions. Seaweed meal is easily assimilated by cannabis plants, and it contributes to soil life, structure, and nitrogen fixation. It may also help the plants resist many diseases and withstand light frosts. Kelp meal also eases transplant shock. As an additive, cytokinins are most often derived from the kelp *Ascophyllum nodosum*. Seaweed is expensive to use as a bulk soil amendment unless it is locally available.

Kelp is normally processed three ways, ranked in order of elements available:
(1) enzyme digested (liquid),
(2) cold-processed (usually liquid), and
(3) extracts (meal or powder).

Apply diluted solution to the soil for a quick cure of nutrient deficiencies.

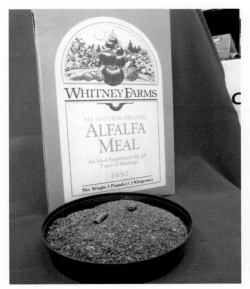

Alfalfa meal

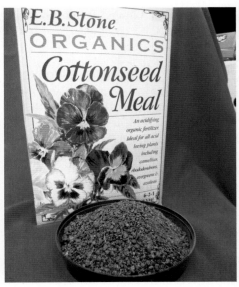

Cottonseed meal

Liquid seaweed is also great for soaking seeds and dipping cuttings and bare roots before planting. Also used as a foliar spray.

Kelp liquid has a negligible N-P-K but is brimming with readily available micronutrients. Add kelp liquid regularly to gardens; it is immediately available and used within a month. Apply 1 to 2 tablespoons (14.8–29.6 ml) per gallon (3.8 L) of water and apply every 2 to 4 weeks.

Kelp meal releases its cache of numerous trace elements 2 to 6 months after mixing it into the soil. Even with an insignificant N-P-K value, kelp meal is an excellent ingredient in potting soils.

Kelp powder has an N-P-K of about 1-0-4 plus many micronutrients. It is an excellent ingredient as a soluble plant nutrient and source of micronutrients. Mix one-half teaspoon per gallon (2.5 ml per 3.8 L) of water and apply to containers once or twice monthly.

Vegetable Meals
Alfalfa Meal

Alfalfa meal is an alternative to blood meal for nitrogen. It is balanced with phosphorus and potassium. It is available in meal or pellets that are commonly livestock feed, which has 17 percent crude protein content equivalent to 2.75 percent nitrogen. Meal and pellets,

available in different sizes, are used to increase organic matter in the soil and also provide soluble nutrients, including trace minerals as well as triacontanol, a natural fatty-acid growth stimulant.

Indoor, outdoor, and greenhouse gardeners use the pelletized livestock feed as a slow-release fertilizer. Alfalfa meal contains fiber and other substrates that feed populations of soil organisms. The carbon-to nitrogen ratio also speeds availability. Alfalfa meal is a great compost activator.

Apply half a cup (11.8 cl) per plant for new plantings; one-half to a full cup (11.8–23.7 cl) to a depth of 4 to 6 inches (10.2–15.2 cm) deep around each plant. Medical cannabis garden beds need 2 to 5 pounds (0.9–2.3 kg) to 100 square feet (9.3 m^2). Do not overapply. Rapid decomposition of alfalfa in the root zone generates heat, which can damage roots. The average N-P-K analysis is 2-1-2 that releases in one to four months. Find alfalfa pellets at feed stores.

Corn Gluten Meal

Corn gluten meal materials have a high percentage of nitrogen. Allow at least one to four months of decomposition in the soil prior to seeding. The allopathic properties inhibit seed germination, but do not affect established and transplanted plants. This product is also marketed as a pre-emergent weed control for annual grasses. Remember, most corn is grown with GMO (genetically modified organism) seeds.

The typical N-P-K analysis is 9-0-0 with a release time of 1 to 4 months. Apply 20 to 40 pounds (9.1–18.1 kg) per 1000 square feet (92.9 m²).

Cottonseed Meal

Cottonseed meal is the by-product of oil extraction and is a rich source of nitrogen. Many pesticides are applied to cotton crops, and residue remains in the seeds. According to the manufacturers, pesticide-free cottonseed is available. They say that virtually all chemical residues from commercial cotton production are dissolved in the oil and are not found in the meal.

Cottonseed meal can be combined with steamed bone meal and seaweed to form a balanced fertilizer blend.

Cottonseed meal is often sold as livestock feed. It contains almost 85 percent water-insoluble nitrogen, and it will acidify soil. Nine pounds (4.1 kg) of lime will neutralize the acidity caused by 100 pounds (45.4 kg) of cottonseed meal. Remember, most cotton is grown with GMO seeds.

The N-P-K is approximately 6-0.4-1.5, and the nutrients are released in 1 to 4 months. Till in 10 pounds (4.5 kg) per 100 square feet (9.3 m²) of regular garden soil.

Peanut Meal

Peanut meal is available in southern states where peanuts are grown. It is high in nitrogen, but water-soluble nitrogen is limited. The average N-P-K is 8-1-2, and the meal is available long term.

Soybean Meal

Soybean meal is the by-product after milling and extracting oil from soybeans. The meal is loaded in protein and is normally sold as a livestock feed. When mixed with soil, the microorganisms change proteins into amino acids and then break down the acids to make ammonium ions and nitrate ions, which are available for roots. Soybean meal acidifies the soil, lowering pH. The average N-P-K analysis is 7-2-1,

and the nutrients are available in one to four months. Purchase soybean meal at livestock feed stores. Remember, most soybeans are grown with GMO seeds. Apply 8 pounds (3.6 kg) per 100 square feet (9.3 m²) of garden soil.

Compost and Compost Teas
Compost

Compost and compost teas are used by many organic gardeners as the only source of fertilizer. Outdoor gardeners love compost. It is inexpensive, abundant, and works wonders to increase water retention and drainage. Biological activity within the pile also increases nutrient uptake in plants. Indoors, compost is not as practical to use in containers unless it has been hot composted and is free of pests and diseases. Unfinished compost could have unwanted guests. If using compost indoors, make sure it is well-rotted and screened.

Compost piles need a mix of elements rich in nitrogen (N) and carbon (C). To ensure proper aerobic composting, the mix should be at the ratio of one part N and three parts C.

Nitrogen-rich elements include:

- Algae blood meal
- Coffee grounds
- Cottonseed meal
- Fish meal

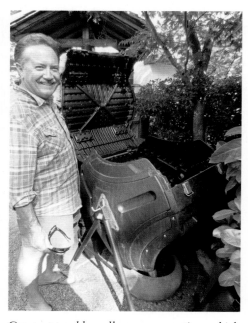
Compost tumblers allow more aeration, which speeds decomposition.

- Green garden clippings: grass clippings, weeds, leaves, etc. (Clippings must not contain chemical fertilizers or other chemicals, including weed-and-feed products used on grass.)
- Legumes: alfalfa, clover, etc.
- Manures: chicken*, cow, goat, horse, pig, rabbit, etc.*
- Seaweed
- Vegetable kitchen scraps

*Salts are commonly found in uncomposted manures (chicken, cow, pig, horse, etc.) Decompose salts by letting them compost for at least 3 months. Bacteria, fungi, and other compost biology will dismantle, bind, and immobilize salts in the compost pile. Use a salt (Na) meter to measure salt levels in manures and composts.

Note: Chicken litter is often packed with different types of weed seed that are very difficult to kill with composting.

Carbon-rich materials include:

- Cardboard, shredded
- Corn stalks, including cobs
- Dried (brown) leaves
- Eggshells
- Needles (fir, pine, etc.)
- Newspaper, shredded
- Paper, with soy-based ink if printed
- Sawdust, in very small amounts and from wood not chemically treated
- Straw
- Woodchips, best if small or pulverized

Do not add:

- Animal meat, fat, or grease
- Ashes from chemically treated wood
- Ashes from coal or charcoal
- Bones
- Cat, dog, or human feces
- Dairy, cheese, milk, yogurt
- Fish scraps
- Meat
- Oils
- Potatoes

The pile will also need:

Air circulation, oxygen is essential to microbial growth in compost piles

Volume of at least 3 feet (0.3 m²) square (any less and heat dissipates faster than it is generated).

Fast, high-maintenance compost:
Compost will be ready in 60 to 90 days, depending upon size and consistency of ingredients. Apply the list below to making compost for outstanding results.

1. Confine the compost in a compost bin or use a freestanding compost pile. Cover or enclose the pile to protect from varmints.

2. The volume of the pile must be at least 3 feet (0.3 m²) square.

3. Lay out a 2-to-4-inch layer of bark chips or twigs. This will provide aeration from below.

4. Combine materials at the rate of 1 part nitrogen to 3 parts carbon. Layer materials or mix thoroughly. Make sure all materials are in small pieces, which will speed decomposition.

5. Add enough water to wet ingredients, but do not saturate. Pile should be like a wrung-out sponge.

6. Cover pile with tarp to protect from excess rainwater or sunlight, which dries the pile quickly.

7. Turn or stir the pile with a fork every 2 to 4 days. Check for even consistency of moisture. Stirring adds oxygen and moves cold outside particles to the inside and cooked particles to the outside. Pile will heat to between 100°F and 160°F (37.8°C–71.1°C) within a few days—even in cold weather. Temperatures above 131°F (55°C) kill most disease-causing pathogens along with seeds and weeds.

8. Add water as needed to keep the pile the consistency of a wrung-out sponge.

9. Compost is finished when the particles are small, uniform, dark brown and smell earthy.

Slow, low-maintenance compost:
This compost will take a few months longer than the recipe above. This recipe is perfect for gardeners who have a little more time to compost. Use the recipe above and add ingredients as they become available. Piles with a volume less than 3 feet (0.3 m²) square will compost much more slowly.

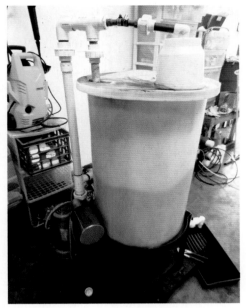
Retail organic garden outlets often make actively aerated compost tea for their clients. This brewer makes tea 24/7.

1. Turn or stir the pile when it is convenient to do so.

2. Do not add weeds or diseased plant residue, because pile will probably not get hot enough to kill pathogens, seeds, and weeds.

3. Solarize used soil to kill pests and diseases. Compost piles must be at least three feet (91.4 cm) square to retain more heat than they give off.

Compost Extracts, Leachates, and Teas
The aim of compost extracts, leachates, and teas is to complement and improve compost/soil mixes rather than replace them. Outdoors the enhanced soil biology continues to improve soil for months after application.

Compost leachate is the dark-colored liquid that leaches out of the bottom of compost piles and worm bins. The solution is most likely rich with soluble nutrients, but it could also contain pathogens early on. The leachate works well to increase soil biology but in general is not a good foliar spray.

Compost extract is made from compost suspended in a permeable bag (burlap, nylon stocking, etc.) in a container of water for one or two weeks. The

extracted liquid fertilizer from this centuries-old technique is usually full of soluble nutrients and soil biology. The volume, richness, and brewing time of the compost determine the potency of the final extract

Non-aerated compost teas are a mix of compost that serves as a source of biology and water. The mix is left to sit for a week or two and stirred occasionally. Anaerobic conditions created in the mix help plant pathogens flourish. Non-aerated compost tea could be detrimental to plants. Most pathogens that attack plants are anaerobic, living in low- and no-oxygen environments. It is easy to eliminate up to three-fourths of potential pathogens by aerating the solution.

Actively aerated compost tea (also called AACT or ACT) is actively brewed using compost, microbial foods, and catalysts added to the solution, which is aerated with a pump to infuse oxygen. The goal is to extract beneficial microbes from the compost and grow (and multiply!) populations of microbes during a 24-to-36-hour brewing period. Compost is the source of microbes. Microbial food (molasses, kelp and fish powders, etc.) and catalysts (humic acid, rock dust, yucca extract, etc.) encourage growth and multiplication of the microbes. Homemade ACTs are as potent as commercial natural or organic fertilizers or amendments. Under optimal conditions, the biology in the tea can increase more than 10,000-fold!

A growing number of farmers, gardeners, and horticulturists love aerated compost tea. It helps suppress pathogens such as *Fusarium*, *Pythium*, *Phytopthora*, and powdery mildew. Aerated compost tea also helps break down soil toxins and those found on plants by inhabiting the space around wounds and infections, thus denying entry to pathogens.

Properly brewed natural organic aerated compost tea cannot be overapplied. Food and oxygen levels are decisive as to the ability of microorganisms to reproduce and multiply. The aim is to maximize beneficial microbe growth without over-replicating, which uses all the available oxygen and causes the tea to become anaerobic. Low- and no-oxygen teas can contain bad stuff including *E. coli* and root-feeding nematodes. Achieve this goal by keeping dissolved oxygen levels above 6 mg/L during all brewing.

Two kinds of aerated compost tea (ACT) include bacterially dominated compost, which is made with humus, vermicompost, and other sources of bacteria. This type of tea is best for annual cannabis. Fungal ACT is promoted and brewed with compost comprised of woody materials and is best for woody perennial plants.

Less oxygen is available at higher elevations, and ACTs require longer brewing times. Brews made at temperatures above 90°F (32.2°C) need a shorter brewing time and often less food. Cold temperatures require a longer brewing time. The water's mineral and chemical content will affect the final tea. Remove bacteria-killing chlorine and chloramines from water before adding compost.

Manure tea is made by placing manure in a permeable bag (burlap or nylon stocking) and suspending it in a container of water. The tea is left to steep for a few days to two weeks. Manure tea is dominated by anaerobic bacteria and other organisms. Pathogens and other bad things are most often present and can burn foliage or cause other problems when applied.

Take a look at the super-compost tea makers at www.soilsoup.com. There is a good "Organic Fertilizer and Amendment Guide" at: http://www.extremelygreen.com/fertilizerguide.cfm.

Recipes for Five Gallons of Compost Tea

Compost tea: Add a shovelful of finished, screened organic compost to a 5-gallon (18.9 L) bucket of clean water. Let soak for 7 days, stirring several times daily to add oxygen. Add a cup or two of alfalfa (pellets) to increase nitrogen if desired. Remove and apply one-quarter strength to full strength to outdoor containers or plants growing in soil.

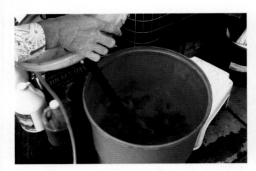

This 30-gallon (113.6 L) compost-brewing barrel makes enough compost tea to cover a 2,000 square foot (185 m²) garden.

Aerated compost tea: Use the above mix and add an air pump. Include an inexpensive aquarium air stone to make bubbles smaller and more dispersed, which will aerate the solution better. This will increase aerobic microbial growth. Add an eighth to a quarter cup of molasses (1 to 2 tablespoons (14.8–29.6 ml) for every 3 days of brewing) to maximize microbial activity. This will boost soluble nutrient levels substantially. Further enhance the mix with catalysts, humic acid, yucca extract, and so forth.

Aerobic tea is ready to use when it has either an earthy or "yeasty" smell or a foamy layer on top of the tea.

Excellent Ingredients for the Compost Pile

Alfalfa meal or pellets: add extra nitrogen, proteins and bacteria

Apple cider vinegar: adds about 30 trace minerals and acidifies the solution a little

Brown sugar and corn syrup: are not as good as molasses

Complex sugars, starches, and carbohydrates: rotten fruit, canned fish, etc., are best for fungal mixes

Corn meal: adds nitrogen, proteins, bacteria, and has fungicidal properties

Epsom salts: a tablespoon or three increases magnesium and sulfur levels

Fulvic acid: increases trace elements and soil fertility

Green weeds: Grind them up to quickly supply more food for bacteria

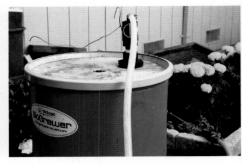

Once set up, air is injected into the active compost mix for several hours.

Humic acid: adds organic matter and water-holding ability to soils

Molasses: available in liquid or powder; an outstanding sugar source for bacteria-rich teas

Organic garden soil: packed with aerobic bacteria, fungi, and other microbes

Seaweed: supplies all trace elements and many growth hormones. But, after a short time they become inactive or break down entirely and add nothing to growth.

Urine water: a potent organic nitrogen source

Yucca extract: great soap-like spreader-sticker and also used as a human health-food supplement

Do not keep compost tea for more than a day or two so that it does not turn aerobic or lose potency. Apply as a soil drench to increase microbial activities and supply soluble N-P-K and trace elements to soil. Foliar feed in conjunction with soil drench as a quick fix to nutrient deficiencies and to protect plants and control diseases.

Do not use harmful liquid soaps or spreader-sticker agents when applying compost teas. Use molasses, fish oil, or yucca extract instead.

22
ADDITIVES

THE TERMS *additives, boosters,* and *supplements* describe the hormones, bacteria, fungi, sugars, vitamins, nutrients, and other substances medical cannabis gardeners use to improve plant growth. Until recently, most additives were a product of the greenhouse industry or developed by organic gardeners.* Today many additives are being developed and popularized by medical cannabis gardeners and hydroponics manufacturers.

*See "Organic Soil" in chapter 18, *Soil,* for more information on the contents of organic supplements or additives.

Many of these substances are effective and true to their claims. Some work quickly, while others require a week or longer to affect growth when applied properly. Application and timing are often very important. Be wary of scientifically undocumented claims about products that promise unrealistic results. Manufacturers of such products are more concerned with taking your money than telling the truth. Read advertising carefully and with a critical eye. Go to medical cannabis forums to see how other gardeners fared with the product. Remember that plant growth regulators cannot correct poor gardening practices. Use additives very carefully or not at all when plants are sick. Also, be wary of different "scientific" websites, and know that most blogs are prowled by charlatans. Beware of shills!

Some additives, such as gibberellic acid, ethylene, and fulvic acid, are available in pure form, but most often they are packaged together with other additives in products to perform specific tasks—to promote rooting, setting more buds, growing bigger flower buds, and increasing overall vigor. Again, read labels; be sure you know what all the ingredients are before giving any additives to plants.

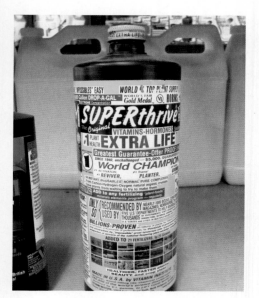

Superthrive was one of the first additives available at garden centers.

Study instructions for additives and carefully determine the correct dosage and application timetable. Additives may be available as liquids, powders, crystals, granules, and more. They are also available in various concentrations. Check with manufacturers and retailers. Most additive manufacturers have a website that provides additional information on their products. As with any additive, make sure the effects of one do not counter the effects of another.

Caution! Additives, especially those containing hormonal products, can be and often are dangerous for the end user. Plant growth regulators (PGRs) are regulated by most governments for a reason— some are proven carcinogens, even at very low rates. Residuals from growth regulators also tend to remain in the plant and in the harvested parts, and are thus passed on to the consumer. The intent of medicinal growing is the same as the intent of a medical doctor—to do no harm. Use of PGR products outside of their specific safety registration is not wise and should be confined entirely to the person or persons that decide to use them, and not passed along to unsuspecting patients or other consumers.

This chapter will give you an overview of additives and how they complement medical cannabis growth.

Hormones

Plant hormones are chemical messengers that control or regulate germination, growth, metabolism, or other physiological activities such as root growth and flowering. Environmental conditions cause plants to release appropriate hormones that will elicit changes in growth.

These organic compounds are generally effective even at very low concentrations. They interact with target tissues to guide cell growth and development. Each response is often the result of 2 or more hormones acting together. Plant hormones can be naturally occurring within plants, and many can be synthesized in the laboratory, increasing the quantity of hormones available for commercial applications.

Hormones are also called plant growth regulators. The successful use of PGRs is often by trial and error, not an exact science. Understanding cannabis growth and development will diminish the learning curve. Hormones are most effective when applied at specific times, in the proper conditions and dosage, and when integrated into regular growth schedules.

To achieve desired results when experimenting with hormones, pay very close attention to dosage concentration and application time, taking into consideration the time of day and the growth phase of plants. Often, plants being treated with hormones must be isolated. For example, a dilute concentration of auxins encourages cuttings to grow roots. But when overdone, the same hormone (auxin) spurs more of another hormone (ethylene) to be produced. Ethylene, the "death hormone," causes plants to grow smaller and have thicker stems and smaller flower buds that ripen earlier.

Two valuable hormone classes, cytokinins and gibberellins, can be used to change plant sex, which is very handy when making plant crosses with a single male or female plant. Cytokinins cause female flowers to form on male plants, and gibberellins cause male flowers to grow on female plants. Colloidal silver, which is not a hormone, also makes male flowers grow on female plants.

Abscisin (Abscisic Acid [ABA])

Abscisin maintains dormancy in seeds and can cause dormancy in developed plants. Its primary effect is to inhibit cell growth. Water stress caused by high temperature, low humidity, or a high EC in the growing medium triggers increases in abscisin synthesis, causing stomata to close. It inhibits shoot growth and may stimulate root growth. It may also help defend from pathogens. During winter, abscisin accumulates to slow or stop cell division to protect plants from cold damage or dehydration. In case of an early spring, abscisin will also prolong dormancy, preventing premature sprouts that could be damaged by frost. Abscisin is a gibberellin inhibitor.

Abscisin II is extracted from cotton as the abscission-inducing chemical. Dormin was extracted from sycamore leaves for the same purpose. ABA does induce dormancy in a few species of plants. Mainly it seems to inhibit the gibberellic acid enzyme production pathways.

Applied in the garden, ABA may help plants resist drought and unseasonable conditions, as well as improve plants' productivity, strength, and performance.

ProTone SL is an example of a product that contains abscisin.

Brassinolide (BR)

Brassinolide is one of the hormones from the brassinosteroid class (plant steroids) that regulate plant development and growth. It promotes stem elongation, root mass, and cell division. It is also involved in other plant processes including drought resistance, stress response, cold resistance, pollen growth, and aging. A deficiency causes stunted growth and infertility. It is a naturally occurring plant hormone that was the first brassinosteroid to be isolated, in 1979. Since then more than 70 BRs have been isolated from plants. Little is known about how BRs relate to cannabinoids. Brassinolide also appears to work with all other hormones to heighten effects or as integral parts of the pathways. They also mimic human steroids and can be anabolic.

MaximaGro is an example of a product that contains brassinolide.

Auxins

Auxins represent a group of plant hormones that regulate growth and phototropism. Auxins affect many processes, including water assimilation, cell division, and cell stretching—often softening cell walls. Top branches grow vertically taller where auxins are concentrated and inhibit lateral buds in the phenomena known as "apical dominance." "Pinching off" branch tips or pruning branches will reduce the auxin level and encourage bushy, lateral growth as well as inducing new root formation.

Auxins are ingredients in many rooting products because they encourage roots to form on stems. Medical cannabis gardeners use various auxins to encourage root growth. Synthetic auxins are more stable and last longer than natural solutions. In high concentrations, auxins are sometimes used as potent herbicides.

One of the many examples of auxin hormonal action is seen in phototropism, the movement of plants in response to a light source. Light causes auxins to be transported to the shaded side of the shoot. Auxins cause the cells on the shaded side to elongate more than the cells on the lit side. The shoot or leaf bends toward the light and hopefully improves its exposure.

Experiments by Canna proved that weak concentrations of auxins slightly stimulated flower formation but flowers took longer to ripen. High concentrations inhibited growth and caused deformities and tumor-like symptoms.

Indole-3-acetic acid (IAA) is the most potent naturally occurring plant auxin. It is manufactured primarily in young leaf shoot tips, in embryos, and in developing flowers. It suppresses leaf drop and flowering in cannabis. However, IAA is unstable and therefore not used as a commercial plant growth regulator.

1-naphthaleneacetic acid (NAA) is a synthetic organic compound similar to IAA but with a longer shelf life. This man-made plant hormone is included in many commercial rooting products.

This PGR improves cell division and expansion. As a rooting agent, NAA is used for vegetative propagation of cannabis stem cuttings (clones). NAA tends to be counterproductive to seedling root development, as it inhibits taproot growth and enhances horizontal root growth. NAA also suppresses growth tip development, which redirects growing energy to the roots.

4-chloroindole-3-acetic acid (4-Cl-IAA) is a chlorinated derivative of the IAA auxin. Commonly found in legume seeds and believed to be a "death hormone," maturing seeds use 4-Cl-IAA to induce death of the parent plant and activate nutrients to be stored in the seed.

Indole-3-butyric acid (IBA) is the main rooting plant hormone in many commercial products. It is naturally occurring in small amounts, but most sources are synthetic. Applications of IBA help generate roots, build larger root masses, and improve plant growth and yield.

Many commercial formulas are available in the form of water-soluble salts. Cuttings can be dipped or immersed in IBA before planting, and roots can be dipped, sprayed, or drenched during transplanting. Once established, plants should be treated at 3- to 5-week intervals during the growing season.

There is very little written to support the theory that IBA can be used to encourage regeneration of flowers. However, auxins' effects are many and wide, including floral production, delaying dormancy, and synergistic effects with many other hormones, especially cytokinins and ABA. We do know that it is a required hormone for proper floral development and that it might be the key in producing another batch of flowers, but regeneration of the plant and plant flowers is doubtful. Commercial auxins such as IBA have many other effects that might be categorized as causing a breaking (growth) of any dormant lateral vegetative buds. This may be more of a cytokinin response as it allows previously differentiated cells to begin division again. IBA's possible role in the regeneration of flowers remains in

controversial, and nothing definitive can be stated at this time.

2-Phenylacetic acid (PAA) is primarily found in fruits. Its effects are much weaker than the effect of the IBA. It is also an ingredient in methamphetamines and is a controlled substance in most countries.

The auxin family also contains man-made synthesized herbicides. The infamous Monsanto-Dow product "Agent Orange" included a 1:1 ratio of the synthetic auxins dichlorophenoxyacetic acid (2,4-D) and 2,4,5-trichlorophenoxyacetic acid (2,4,5-T). The illnesses caused by Agent Orange are thought to be a result of contaminated 2,3,7,8-tetrachlorodibenzo-p-dioxin (TCDD) as a result of the manufacturing process, and not a result of the auxins.

Products that contain root-inducing hormones are available in liquid, powder, and gel forms. Examples of such products are Rootone (NAA), Hormex (IBA), Clonex (IBA), Schultz TakeRoot (IBA). Many of these products are available in a generic form that costs much less than the name brand.

Caution! IBA and other hormones are hazardous to humans and animals. Some can cause moderate eye injury and are harmful if inhaled or absorbed through the skin. Read the entire label and follow directions!

Cytokinins (CK)

Cytokinins (aka cell division hormones) are plant hormones that promote cell division in root tips and growing shoots. Cytokinins also affects leaf senescence (aging). Naturally found in coconut milk, cytokinins encourage metabolism by stimulating the transport of sugars and bud development on side shoots. Concentrations are highest in young leaves, root tips, and seeds. Cytokinins also stimulate female flowers to form on male plants.

Added to the soil or sprayed on plants, cytokinins help plants make efficient use of existing nutrients and water in drought conditions. Leaf surfaces are larger and flower formation is faster in cytokinin-treated plants, but harvest time is the same as if cannabis plants were untreated.

Take extra care when using or experimenting with cytokinins mixed with other plant hormones. Many commercial formulas contain hormone cocktails that may include both auxins and cytokinins, which can work in opposition to each another. A high ratio of auxins to cytokinins stimulates root formation. A low ratio promotes shoot formation.

Derivatives of the adenine-type include 6-benzylaminopurine, kinetin, and zeatin. The most active and common is zeatin, isolated from corn (*Zea mays*). Cytokinins are synthesized in the roots, promoting cell division, chloroplast development, and leaf development, and delaying leaf aging. As an additive, cytokinins are most often derived from the kelp *Ascophyllum nodosum*. Look for seaweed products that contain this seaweed. Kelp meal is also added to many organic fertilizers.

6-benzylaminopurine (BAP) is a synthetic cytokinin used to encourage growth, flower setting, and cell division. Pure BAP does not dissolve directly into water; it is first combined with alcohol or another solvent and then diluted with water. BAP is commercially available as the product Configure.

According to some gardeners, a concentration spray of 6-Benzylaminopurine at 300 ppm halfway through flowering will increase flower bud growth and weight.

Kinetin is a cytokinin often used in plant-tissue culture combined with an auxin to induce callus formation. Cytokinin derivatives have been synthesized and many are as effective as kinetin. Different cytokinin:auxin ratios affect growth rate of plants. For example, if kinetin is high and auxin is low, shoots are formed; if kinetin is low and auxin high, roots are formed. Kinetin suppresses ethylene production. Many antiaging skincare cosmetics use kinetin.

Zeatin is a cytokinin growth hormone used to encourage lateral plant growth. Upon germination, zeatin moves from the endosperm to the root tip where it stimulates mitosis. It encourages auxil-iary stem growth that sets more buds. Coconut milk is a naturally occurring source of zeatin. Zeatin is also commonly used in skincare products. It is available as a white crystal powder and in an aqueous solution.

Products that contain cytokinins include Maxicrop, Dr. Earth Kelp Meal, Neptune's Seaweed, Alg-A-Mic, and Bushmaster.

Ethylene (Ethene)

Ethylene is a naturally occurring hormone that activates the aging and ripening of flowers and fruit, prevents the development of flower buds, and retards plant growth. Roots, senescing flowers, and green growth tips contain the largest amounts of ethylene. It is the primary hormone responsible for chlorophyll destruction, leaf detachment, flower senescence, and fruit ripening. This growth regulator is called the "ripening," "post-harvest," or "death" hormone.

Ethylene concentrates in plant tissues when plants suffer stress. Production will increase in roots when necessary to add girth so they can penetrate hard, impairing surfaces. In windy areas outdoors or indoors where a fan is blowing too much air, plants produce more ethylene to increase stem diameter and counteract effects from the wind. The result is thicker stems on smaller plants with small buds that ripen prematurely.

Soggy, waterlogged growing mediums cause ethylene to accumulate in the root zone and migrate up the stem as severity increases. Symptoms include leaf yellowing (chlorosis), thickening of stems, leaf margins curving downward, and greater vulnerability to diseases and pests.

Avoid infusing ethylene where young plants are present, or you will risk dwarfed growth, premature flowering, and small flower buds. Stressed and flowering plants release ethylene that must be vented and removed daily when they are around young plants, to prevent the risk of premature ripening.

Ethylene is also a by-product of fossil fuel combustion in CO_2 generators. High concentrations will cause leaves to yellow very quickly. Adequate ventilation will evacuate "toxic" levels of ethylene. Minute concentrations as low as 10 parts per billion (ppb) in the air can cause abnormal growth and susceptibility to diseases and pests. Excess ethylene can also be a major issue with improperly vented or unvented gas heaters as well as leaking heat exhaust systems, and is normally seen in colder months when plants are grown indoors.

In a sealed environment, natural ethylene production levels increase over time. A closed refrigerator allows ethylene to build up. Any closed environment— a paper bag, room, or jar—will have a similar effect. Placing fruit, tomatoes, or avocados in a sealed paper bag will speed ripening. Ripe fruit will emit ethylene and impact harvested cannabis flower buds in the vicinity. Storage areas should have adequate ventilation to evacuate built-up ethylene.

Sealing dry cannabis in a vacuum will decrease ethylene production by lowering temperature and available oxygen. Ventilation will carry away ethylene and reduce levels to tolerable concentrations.

Seed treatment with carbon dioxide or ethylene before sowing has a positive influence on growth, budding, flowering, and ripening of hemp. Root development, seed production, and total yields also are increased by treatment.

Products that contain ethylene include Ethephon, Etacelasil, Glyoxime, and Sensa-Spray, and are most often available in a liquid (foliar spray). Be careful using Ethephon and Etacelasil or any other systemic plant regulator. Once sprayed with a PGR, plants should not be consumed.

Caution! Ethylene can be phytotoxic if applied during hot weather or when improperly diluted. Isolate plants so that nontarget plants are not affected.

Gibberellins

Gibberellins are natural plant growth hormones that act with auxins to break dormancy and increase seed germination, stem diameter, fiber content, and vertical growth. Found naturally in seeds and young shoots, they stimulate cell division and elongation. At least 75 plant-based gibberellins have been isolated. They are referred to as GA1, GA2, GA3, and so on. Gibberellic acid (GA3) is the most common.

Gibberellic acid is an ingredient in commercial products and is used to extend the garden season and force larger blooms in some agricultural crops. It is widely used in the grape-growing industry to increase production of larger fruit bundles and bigger grapes, and to produce grapes on seedless varieties. GA3's primary use in cannabis gardens is to increase plant height and encourage male flower development on female plants. Be very cautious with application rates; plant stems can grow, stretching up to 4 inches (10 cm) a day! Application during vegetative growth delays flowering.

Pollen from male flowers that were induced with GA3 on female plants is used to pollinate female flowers. Resulting seeds from this union *always* produce female (feminized) plants. Low doses (25–100 ppm) of GA3 sprayed on female plants for 7 to 10 days immediately before flowering will cause up to 80 percent of treated plants to grow male flowers. Use this pollen to pollinate "feminized" seeds. For more information, see chapter 25, *Breeding*.

Environmental factors also cause extra gibberellin production. Low light levels cause gibberellin production that results in lanky growth. Too much light causes buds to shoot up, creating tall, narrow flower tops. A rule of thumb is to keep a 600-watt lamp a minimum of 20 inches (50 cm) above the plant canopy.

When seeds absorb water, gibberellins develop in the embryo and activate plant metabolism to initiate sprouting. GA3 helps difficult-to-germinate seeds sprout. However, I advise to use scarification (see chapter 5, *Seeds & Seedlings*) rather than GA3.

GibGro is an example of a product that contains gibberellic acid. It is available in 5 percent, 10 percent, and 20 percent wettable powder packages, as well as the 4 percent liquid solution.

Caution! If misapplied, gibberellic acid can cause very tall, lanky cannabis plants.

Jasmonate (JA)

Jasmonate is, by definition, a hormone, although it arises from linolenic acid as either jasmonic acid, a response to insect attack primarily involved in gene activation and expression, and jasmonate, which activates resistance, as well as pollen and anther development.

Salicylates (Aspirin) [ASA]

Aspirin, or salicylic acid, is effective in preventing pathogens (bacteria, fungi, and viruses) by speeding up the natural "systemic acquired resistance (SAR)" and thereby reducing the need for pesticides. It is a naturally occurring plant hormone associated with willow tree bark. Often, plants do not produce enough on their own to be effective. Salicylic acid (SA) will block abscisic acid (ABA), allowing the plant to return to normal after a period of stress—something to consider if ABA is being used to strengthen plants. It is added to a vase of water to prolong the life of cut flowers.

Aspirin can be ground up and diluted in water to be used as a spray or soak, or it can be added to compost and rooting compounds. A 1:10,000 solution used as a spray will stimulate the SAR response, and the effects will last weeks to months. "Willow water" also makes a popular rooting bath. See "Willow Water" in chapter 7, *Clones & Cloning*.

Many forms of salicylic acid are available in the form of aspirin.

Caution! Some people have an allergic reaction to salicylic acid, which is responsible for numerous deaths in the world every year.

Enzymes

Enzymes are biological protein catalysts that accelerate rates of reaction but do not change themselves as a result of this action. They are added to fertilizers and growth additives to accelerate biological activity and speed nutrient uptake by roots. For example, the enzyme nitrate reductase reduces nitrates and steals electrons for energy, breaking them down into the nitrite form. This is the first step in assimilating N into organic compounds. Nitrite reductase assimilates nitrite into the ammonium ion.

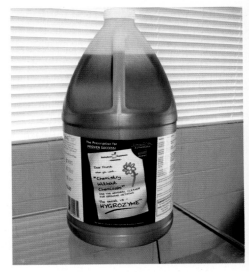

Some products that include enzymes are Sensizym, Hygrozyme, Power Zyme, and Cannazym. Many organic compost products contain beneficial enzymes.

Ammonium is then transferred to the vacuole if high levels are present of 2 other enzymes: glutamine synthetase, which reduces ammonium to glutamine, or glutamate synthase on its way to being converted into amino acids.

More than 1,500 different enzymes have been identified. Enzymes are grouped into 6 main classes: oxidoreductases, transferases, hydrolases, lyases, isomerases, and ligases.

Enzymes are a naturally occurring by-product of composting. Many seaweed extracts are brimming with enzymes (along with many trace elements, hormones, etc.). However, as their function tends to be isolated to cellular function outside of soil or medium function, I am unaware of any beneficial use in applying enzymes.

Most enzymatic reactions occur within a temperature range of 85°F to 105°F (29.4°C–40.6°C), and each enzyme has an optimal pH range for activity. Most enzymes react with only a small group of closely related chemical compounds. Enzymes are highly specific and only function on their matching substrate. For instance, cellulose only breaks the bonds of cellulose, pectinase only breaks down pectin, and individual molecules are usually used over and over until they lose their form, or denature. Also, soil enzymes work at standard soil temperatures of 70°F to 80°F (21°C–26°C]) even though they can speed up, with elevated chemical reactions coming at higher temperatures.

Cellulase is a group of enzymes that act in the root zone to break down organic material that may rot and cause disease. Dead materials are converted into glucose and returned to the substrate to be absorbed by the plant. Cellulase breaks down cellulose fiber. For example, the enzyme contained in the product Cannazym breaks down dead root cellulose and hemicelluloses into simple sugar compounds. Cellulase is used throughout production as roots are constantly shed. It also functions against the cell wall that contains cellulase of several classes of fungi including the water molds (*Pythium, Phytophthora*) and *Rhizoctonia* (decreases the availability of its parent material before its populations get to plant-affecting levels), providing some protection from these pathogens.

Amino Acids

Plants produce biosynthesize amino acids naturally. Applying *specific* supplemental amino acids as a foliar spray or soil drench can increase crop yield and quality. Amino acids can directly or indirectly contribute to a plant's physiological activities. Apply *specific* amino acids as a soil drench or foliar spray to help improve soil life, which in turn facilitates nutrient uptake.

Note: A complete discussion of the many, many amino acids is beyond the scope of this book. This is an isomer form known as an optical isomer that occurs in two states, the L and D forms effectively doubling. Also, plants' amino acid uptake is species dependent, and ectomycorrhizal roots expand this. For instance, the Scot's pine is known to take up 13 types of amino acids, all L isomer and all basically containing 15 nitrogen and 13 carbon atoms. However their function seems to be relatively the same in that they are used for the ammonium ions and the carbon they contain…the only direct uptake and utilization of carbon.

Plants absorb amino acids best through foliar spraying. There is a soil life benefit

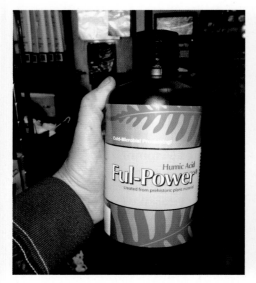
Humic acid is available in liquid form

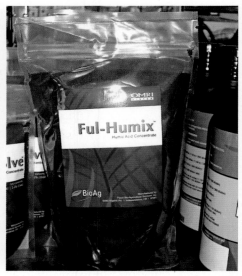
Humic acid is also available in powder form to dilute in water

from exposure, and at least partial soil application is recommended.

Colchicine

Colchicine, an alkaloid, is prepared from the dried corms and seeds of the autumn crocus (*Colchicum autumnale*) that produces saffron; it is available in the form of a pale-yellow, water-soluble powder.

Caution! Colchicine is a very dangerous, poisonous compound. Colchicine poisoning is similar to arsenic poisoning. Cannabis breeders have used it to induce polyploid mutations, and more than 30 years ago started producing polyploid varieties with colchicines. None of the varieties showed outstanding characteristics, and their cannabinoid levels were unaffected.

Colchicine can also be used to induce female chromosomes in female plants that produce seeds. However, many of the resulting seeds may not sprout, and a large percentage of them could have intersex (hermaphrodite) tendencies.

Rather than explain how to use colchicine, I will advise not to use it. It is very toxic and produces no change in potency. I do not know any seed breeders that use it today. If you are not convinced, search the Internet for "colchicine poisoning." For more information, see *Marijuana Botany* by Robert Connell Clarke.

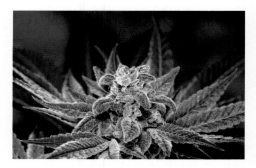
Beautiful 'Mom Booey' × 'Kona Sunset' bud!

Humic Acids

Humic acids are carbons formed by the decomposition of organic matter, primarily vegetation. It is not a single acid; rather, it is a complex mixture of many different acids. Often humic acids are "talked up" by vendors making outrageous claims. Scientific research proves that humic acids do 4 basic things: (1) act as a colloid in providing structure in the soil, (2) act as chelating agents to facilitate nutrient availability to the plant, (3) act like a docking station by attaching to a single cation-exchange site and providing space for many elements to bind, and (4) increase cell permeability, which would also allow for better nutrient uptake. Cannabis roots and plant tissue do not take in humates. Humates act in the soil and help nutrients become more available. Canada does not allow "humates" on fertilizer labels, and neither does the Association of American Plant Control Officials.

Humates Chelate

Organic humic and fulvic acids chelate semisoluble metallic ions (nutrients), making them readily transportable by water. This ability is dependent upon the water pH level. Copper, iron, manganese, and zinc are difficult to dissolve. When mixed in a chelated form, they become readily available for absorption.

Humus is formed from compost that has matured to the point of stability. It is so stable and so mature that it can remain unchanged for thousands of years in that state. Humic acid, fulvic acid, and humin are all humus extracts. Humic acid is made from finely grinding humus and then adding a low-pH water solution so humic acid can be separated from the fulvic acid. Humic acid helps free nutrients from the soil so they become available to the plants.

Humin is the fraction of the soil's organic matter that is not dissolved when the soil is treated with this alkali. Colors range from yellow (fulvic acid) to brown (humic acid) and black (humin).

Fulvic Acid

Fulvic acid is a humic acid that has a lower molecular weight and higher oxygen content than other humic acids. Fulvic acid is commonly used as a soil supplement. Contrary to popular belief, fulvic acid is not able to be absorbed into plant tissue and is not an antioxidant.

Fulvic acid is the fraction of humic substances that is water soluble under all pH conditions. Fulvic acid stays in solution after humic acid dissipates due to acidification. Fulvic acids are polyelectrolytes, unique colloids that easily diffuse through membranes.

Gardeners can create fulvic acid by composting, or it can be purchased from a retailer. It is available in forms that are suitable for hydroponic or soil mediums. See "Organic Soil" in chapter 18, *Soil*, for more information on fulvic acid.

Fungi
Mycorrhizal Fungi

Mycorrhizal refers to a class of fungi that forms a symbiotic relationship

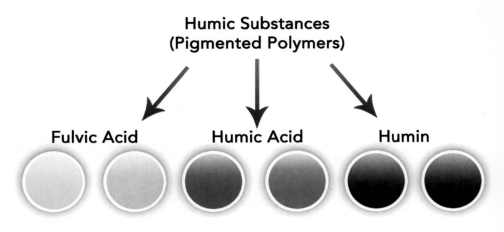

Humic Substances
(Pigmented Polymers)

Fulvic Acid　　**Humic Acid**　　**Humin**

Distinguish fulvic and humic acids and humin by color.

between mycelium of specific fungi and roots of plants. The ectomycorrhizal fungal hyphae (microscopic strands that grow from fungal spores) surround and encapsulate roots and exchange nutrients because they are so close together. Endomycorrhizal fungal hyphae actually enter the cells of roots to exchange nutrients. Mycorrhizal fungi grow around and even penetrate root tissue and grow out into the soil to find more water and nutrients than roots could find on their own. This is essentially a second root system that improves water and nutrient uptake and contributes to the overall health of the plant.

The two fungi species that are known to colonize the roots of cannabis are *Glomus intraradices* and *Glomus mosseae*. Make sure these species are included in any mycorrhizal fungi product you purchase. These species have the maximum potential to colonize cannabis roots. However, there are many mycorrhizal fungi that have yet to be discovered and studied.

Mycorrhizal fungi naturally occur in areas where plants are not disturbed by human activity, but these beneficial fungi are often lacking in urban and indoor environments.

Mycorrhizal fungi take time to become established enough to be of assistance to the plant, so they should be introduced

early in a plant's life cycle. Apply spores to seeds or a cutting's roots when planting. It can take 6 weeks or longer for full mycorrhizae colonization to occur. Plants that grow for 3 months or more receive the most benefit from mycorrhizae colonization.

Apply fungal spores to the seeds or prepared cuttings' roots when planting or transplanting. For best results, inoculate the root zone with a high spore (propagule) count per gram. Typically, *G. intraradices* powder-based products

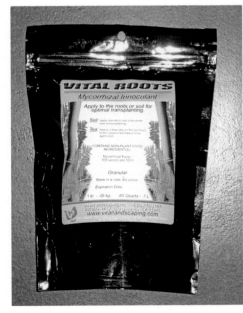

Mycorrhizal fungi, available in powder form

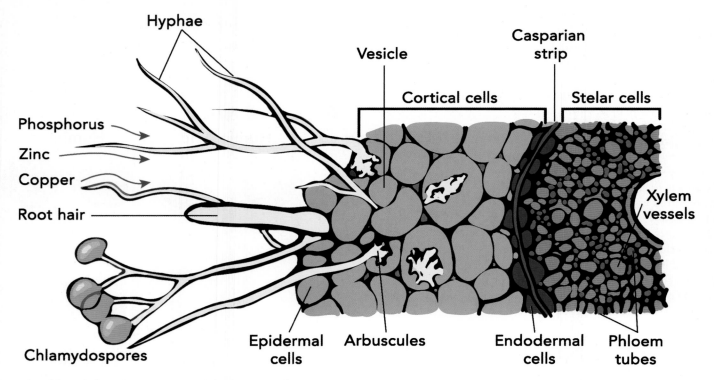

Mycorrhizal fungi help make nutrients in the soil more readily available for uptake. Most organic molecules, especially long-chain types derived from humates breaking down to form humic and fulvic acids, are not taken up by the roots or through the leaves, and the same is true for the fungi.

have about 3,200 spores per gram, and liquid products have about 2 million spores per gram. *G. mosseae* is typically available at 200 spores per gram. Most mixes don't contain both *G. intraradices* and *G. mosseae*. You may have to purchase them separately in bulk. Here is a good resource for products: www.usemykepro.com.

Encourage mycorrhizae by inoculating soil. Compost tea, fulvic acid, humic acid, and carbohydrates are used to promote healthy mycorrhizae growth. Add as a soil amendment or mix with a nutrient solution and use as a drench. Incorporate mycorrhizal fungi into the top 4 inches of soil, or mix with potting soil when planting.

Here is an example of a mycorrhizal fungi mix that comes from my friend Sannie in the Netherlands: www.sanniesshop.com/symbiosis-mycorrhiza.html.

Analysis:
93 endomycorrhizae spores / gram
Glomus intraradices
Glomus clarum
Entrophospora colombiana

Glomus sp.
Glomus geosporum
Glomus mosseae
Glomus etunicatum

Rhizobacteria:
Bacillus subtillus
Paenibacillus azotofixans
Bacillus pumilus
Bacillus polymixa
Bacillus megaterium
Bacillus licheniformis

Trichoderma

Trichoderma are fungi that colonize in the root zone, crowding out negative fungi and microorganisms while stimulating root development and resistance to environmental stress. The result is a stronger, more vibrant plant. *Trichoderma* are naturally present in coconut fiber and growing medium. Note that sterilizing coco growing medium with steam or other means kills *Trichoderma*.

There are 89 species in the *Trichoderma* genus. Several varieties of *Trichoderma* have been developed as biocontrol agents against fungal diseases of plants. The various mechanisms include antibiosis,

parasitism, inducing host-plant resistance, and competition. Most biocontrol agents are from the species *Trichoderma harzianum, T. viride,* and *T. hamatum.* The biocontrol agent generally grows in its natural habitat in the rhizosphere on the root surface, and affects root disease in particular but can also be effective against foliar diseases. *Trichoderma* is also effective in suppressing pathogenic fungi that cause damping-off—rot in the seeds, roots, and stems. Some strains of *T. harzianum* have an antagonistic effect on *Botrytis cinerea* development in some crops.

Canna was the first company to popularize a commercial product as a growth promoter that contains *Trichoderma* fungi. Now there are many similar products available. *Trichoderma* products can be applied to seeds, used during transplanting, mixed with liquid fertilizer or via drip irrigation, and/or watered in. Quality *Trichoderma* products contain living organisms that will reproduce after application, so a small amount will do a lot. Most all are nontoxic and environmentally safe. There is one documented case of a human *Trichoderma*-related death in South America; the species invaded the digestive system and blocked it.

Products that include *Trichoderma* species include Promot Plus and Canna Trichoderma Powder. *Trichoderma* are naturally present in coconut fiber, compost, and compost tea.

Bacteria

Bacteria, considered the earliest form of life, are found in virtually every environment on earth. For at least 3 million years they have managed to adapt to most environments and avoid extinction. Single-celled bacteria are so small that 250,000 to 500,000 of the little single-celled organism could fit on the period to a sentence. More than a billion bacteria, constituting hundreds of species, are found in a single gram of soil. Overall, microscopic bacteria are beneficial to plant growth.

Bacteria are one of the main decomposers of fresh green organic garden matter. Different bacteria eat diverse organic matter. Beneficial bacteria travel short distances and promote good health in medical cannabis. Once food and nutrients are inside bacteria, they are "locked up" until the bacteria are consumed. There are 2 groups of bacteria: aerobic and anaerobic.

Anaerobic bacteria do not need oxygen to survive. In fact, O_2 is poisonous to them. In general, anaerobic bacteria are to be avoided and not promoted. By-products of some anaerobic organic decomposition include hydrogen sulfide and butyric acid, both of which smell like vomit, and ammonia, which smells like vinegar. If you know these odors, you know the smell of anaerobic decomposition. Conditions that promote anaerobic bacteria include standing water or compacted soil with little pore space.

A few species of anaerobic bacteria attack plants. They launch their assault on sick plants with few defenses, or ones that are suffering from diseases or pest wounds. Bacteria colonize, entering through weak tissue and wounds. However, healthy plants are very resistant to bacteria attacks.

Aerobic bacteria need oxygen to live and, overall, are the ones we want in the garden. For the most part, aerobic bacteria are beneficial, but parasitic varieties do exist. Aerobic, organic decomposition does not cause unpleasant odors; instead, it has a sweet, earthy fragrance.

Bacteria recycle 3 basic elements: carbon, nitrogen, and sulfur. Sulfur-oxidizing bacteria make water-soluble sulfates available to plants. Bacteria convert inert atmospheric nitrogen into "fixed" nitrogen—ammonium, nitrate, or nitrite ions. Bacterial slime (biofilm—DNA, proteins and sugars) also buffers the rhizosphere so the pH remains reasonably constant. Bacteria attach to particles of soil and lock up nutrients. The nutrients stay in the same place in the soil and are not leached out. When other organisms eat the bacteria, nitrogen is released in their poop—right next to the rhizosphere where it is readily available to roots. Bacteria act as living containers of organic fertilizer and also serve as food to members of the soil food web.

Beneficial bacteria need decomposing plant material to thrive, and a pH around 7.0. Bacteria are naturally occurring worldwide and will form in the correct environment.

Healthy compost teas are rich in beneficial bacteria.

Rhizobia

Nitrogen in the air becomes "fixed" by rhizobia—bio-fertilizing bacteria. Naturally occurring bacteria such as rhizobia live in the roots of legumes (beans, clover, peas, peanuts, etc.). Once colonized with the bacteria, legumes will create nodules that act in symbiosis with the plant. Because of this symbiotic relationship with nitrogen-fixing bacteria; legumes can be planted as companion plants to cannabis. They are often referred to as "plant growth promoting rhizobacteria" (PGPRs).

Rhizobia are host-specific according to their type and will not work with all crops. With the proper host, however, rhizobia fix atmospheric nitrogen while simultaneously providing an additional source of available nitrogen. Rhizobacteria are added with legume cover crops

to improve nitrogen levels in depleted garden soil. The product Azopar contains nitrogen-fixing *Azospirillum inoculum* for non-leguminous plants.

Miscellaneous Additives
Alginic Acid

Alginic Acid (aka algin or alginate) is an anionic polysaccharide found in cell walls of brown algae. When it binds with water, it forms a viscous gum that holds vast quantities of water. The extracted form soaks up water quickly and can absorb 200 to 300 times its own weight in water. Its color ranges from white to yellowish-brown.

Products that include Alginic acid include: B52, Dr. Earth Kelp Meal, Neptune's Seaweed, Alg A Mic. Many seaweeds and kelps include alginic acid.

Carbohydrates and Sugars

Carbohydrate is a hydrate of carbon. Carbohydrates provide energy to living cells, such as soil life. They are compounds containing carbon, hydrogen, and oxygen with a ratio of 2 hydrogen atoms for every oxygen atom. Carbohydrates are known as sugars, starches, saccharides, and polysaccharides.

Sugars are carbohydrates that can be used immediately to supply energy to living organisms. Molasses, honey, and other sugars can increase soil microbial life, enhance growth, and make the plant's use of nitrogen more effective. Molasses is the "secret ingredient" in many organic fertilizers, and the natural sugar best for organic medical cannabis crops. Sucrose (corn) syrup is the most economical way to buy sugar, but it lacks many of molasses' qualities.

Plants manufacture sugars. Plant roots do not absorb sugars, raw or refined. Bacteria and other soil life consume sugars as food or fuel. Adding organic sugar in the form of molasses to the soil increases soil life and biological processes in and around the root zone. The extra life allows roots to absorb nutrients more quickly and efficiently, which increases plant growth. In fact, flower buds can gain up to 20 percent more weight when a regular regimen of molasses is added to irrigation water.

Buds grow bigger because there was more microbial activity in the soil. Sugars feed the soil life, and more healthy microbial activity makes more nutrients available that are taken in faster. And the soil life releases the carbon as CO_2 that moves up through the plant canopy, enhancing CO_2 uptake and subsequent carbohydrate production by the plant.

Add sugar (molasses) at the rate of 2 tablespoons per gallon (4 ml/L) to soil, starting during vegetative growth and continuing through flowering. Adding more will not increase plant growth; instead it will imbalance soil life and attract scavengers.

NOTE: Any sweet taste or flavor that vendors attribute to coming from sugars, does not come directly from adding sugars or flavorings to the nutrient solution. If they insist that it does, I would like to see scientific proof. Please have them contact me immediately.

Molasses
Molasses is available in 3 main types: unsulphured, sulphured, and blackstrap. One of the ingredients in some compost and potting soil is molasses waste. Molasses is made from several sources, including corn, sugar beets, and sugar cane.

Unsulphured molasses is top quality and is used in cooking. This grade is made from ripe sugar cane juice that is clarified and concentrated. It can be used in the garden.

Sulphured molasses is made from unripe (green) sugar. Sulfur fumes are applied during sugar extraction. Afterward it is boiled repeatedly. First-boil molasses is of the highest quality because only a small amount of sugar is removed. Second and any subsequent boils turn the molasses dark in color and extract more sugar. It can be used in the garden.

Blackstrap molasses has been boiled three times to extract ever more sugar. Mainly used as cattle feed, it is heavy with iron. It can also be used in the garden.

Overall, the average N-P-K analysis of molasses is 1-0-5, and it contains potash, sulfur, and many trace minerals in a chelated form. It is also packed with carbohydrates and a balance of consumables, which are a quick source of energy and food for microorganisms. Molasses can be purchased at grocery, health food, and livestock feed stores.

Products that contain molasses include Hi-Brix, Bud Candy, FloraNectar, and Sweet. It is also available in bulk form for livestock or human consumption. Most molasses is applied at the rate of 1 to 2 tablespoons per gallon.

Caution! Molasses and products that contain it attract large and small scavengers. I have visited more than one garden where molasses-based products attracted bears.

Colloidal Silver (CS)
Colloidal silver is made of particles of metallic silver suspended in distilled water. It is sprayed on female cannabis plants to encourage male flower development. Seeds from a plant using the pollen from these male flowers will be "feminized." Silver ions also inhibit the (female) hormone ethylene. Many commercial cannabis seed producers use colloidal silver to create feminized seeds. A few ounces (ml) of colloidal silver can be purchased online, at many health food stores, and at some drugstores for $30 to $40 USD. It can be made at home by connecting leads to each terminal of a 9-volt battery and a piece of pure silver, which may be hard to find. Each lead (– and +) is connected to a piece of pure (0.999%) silver, usually a coin. The pieces of silver, attached to the battery via clips, are submerged in a small quantity of distilled water and left for several hours. The coins are not allowed to touch one another. The electrical current will deposit minute silver particles into the water, creating colloidal silver. Detailed instructions are available on the Internet.

To apply, mist target branches with a 30 to 40 ppm solution of colloidal silver solution every day, starting a week before flowers emerge. Spray at the same time early in the day, and continue spraying daily until male flowers clearly appear. Pollen from these male flowers is used to fertilize female flowers. The resulting "feminized" seeds will grow female plants.

Caution! Health risks! Do not consume plants that have been treated with colloidal silver. However, it is considered safe to consume cannabis that was grown from seeds that were produced from a mother treated with colloidal silver. Some gardeners spray only one branch with colloidal silver and consume the balance of the plant. They shield the nontarget foliage when spraying. I advise against this practice.

Many products contain emulsified colloidal silver.

Caution! Store colloidal silver in a light-proof container. It kills beneficial bacteria and fungus, so avoid soil contact. It may also be toxic to humans.

Hydrogen Peroxide (H_2O_2)
Hydrogen peroxide (H_2O_2) is similar to water but carries an extra, unstable oxygen atom. This extra atom will either attach itself to another oxygen atom or attack an organic molecule. In medical cannabis gardens, hydrogen peroxide can provide a host of benefits by cleansing water of harmful substances such as spores, dead organic material, and disease-causing organisms while preventing new infections from occurring. It also suppresses algae growth. It removes the methane and organic sulfates often found in well water, as well as removing chlorine from city tap water.

Hydrogen peroxide is often mistakenly used in soil and hydroponic gardens to provide oxygen in substrates with poor soil biology, compaction, and overwatering. Purveyors mistakenly believe that it prevents oxygen depletion in the water around the roots. The free radicle O_2- will rapidly combine with anything but other oxygen molecules. Oxygen is only useful to any life form in the diatomic format O_2. Saturating the medium or water with hydrogen peroxide may clean the water, but it will kill roots as well. There is no oxidative value in this product, and it should be employed only as a last ditch attempt to save a crop from disease issues.

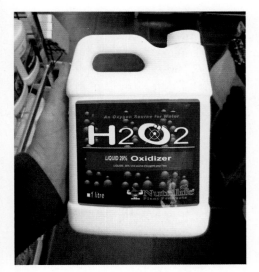
Hydrogen peroxide (H_2O_2)

Hydrogen peroxide also kills other soil life and retards root growth. Small root hairs are very delicate and so is much soil life. Adding H_2O_2 will impair or kill some of the soil life and disrupt soil chemistry. Be extremely careful and sparing when using H_2O_2. Do not use it as a regular constituent of a nutrient or additive program.

Hydrogen peroxide is dangerous at high concentrations and will damage skin, clothing, and most anything else it contacts. Find low-concentrate H_2O_2 (3%, 5%, and 8%) at drugstores or supermarkets. "Food grade" hydrogen peroxide (35%) will need to be diluted before use. Higher strength H_2O_2 formulations are more economical but should be diluted (to 3%) before use.

Wear rubber gloves when using any concentrations above 3%. Hydrogen peroxide concentrations higher than 3% cause bleaching and damage to skin and other surfaces. Clean up splatters and spills to avoid problems. Store hydrogen peroxide in a dark container that holds pressure to preserve potency.

Hydrogen peroxide is best purchased as a generic product in a 3% solution. Stronger 35 percent solutions are available but require more care in handling.

Caution! Use gloves when handling; concentrations above 3 percent can burn skin. Keep away from eyes. Keep out of children's reach. Avoid spilling; it can bleach and damage fabrics or surfaces.

Propolis

Propolis is a resinous mixture that honey bees collect and use as a sealant in hives. It is collected from tree bark and other plant saps. It is sticky above room temperature and hard-to-brittle at lower temperatures. It is used as a local antibiotic and antifungal agent. Propolis is an ingredient in some additives. Propolis can be used as part of a treatment regimen for infected or sick plants.

Propolis may be available from local beekeepers.

Triacontanol

Triacontanol (aka melissyl alcohol or myricyl alcohol) is a naturally occurring fatty acid and growth stimulant. It speeds cell growth and increases cell division, which in turn boosts overall flower yield. Triacontanol is readily available and abundant in alfalfa meal. See "Alfalfa Meal" in chapter 21, *Nutrients*, for more information.

Some products that include Triacontanol include AlfaGrow, Final, Nirvana, and Bloom. Alternatives include Alfalfa meal and pellets.

Caution! Triacontanol can be toxic. It is a saturated fat, and, in some eyes, a plant growth regulator, although there is still some debate on the issue. Triacontanol is not taken up by the plant.

Vitamins

Vitamins C and B_1 as aids may be myths. B_9, a growth inhibitor, is the only one I've found that appears to actually have any use to medical cannabis gardeners.

Ascorbic Acid (Vitamin C)

Vitamin C is thought to build tighter, heavier buds and act as an antioxidant. It is often combined with fructose, molasses, or sugar, and added to the nutrient solution during the last 2 weeks before harvest. However, some botanists believe that although vitamin C is very important in fighting the free radical by-products of photosynthesis, plants make their own vitamin C and are unlikely to recognize any benefit from its addition to the nutrient mix.

Vitamin C tablets sold at grocery stores and drugstores contain ascorbic acid but may contain other things too. Purchase it in the pure form, L-ascorbic acid or L-ascorbate. Ascorbic acid is a better supplement for gardeners than it is for cannabis!

B Vitamins

B_1, aka Thiamin, thiamine, and aneurine hydrochloride, is the term for a family of molecules sharing a common structural feature responsible for its activity as a vitamin. Applying vitamin B_1 to root systems of plants does not stimulate root growth. This common misconception has been repeatedly refuted in scientific trials.

B_3 Niacin is used as a root growth factor. There is no concrete evidence proving that it helps plant growth.

B_9 (folic acid, folinic acid) appears to serve in energy transfer within the plant and inhibits the enzyme that makes gibberellic acid, resulting in a bushier, dwarf-type plant without pruning. B_9

APPLICATION GUIDELINES FOR 3 PERCENT H_2O_2 SOLUTION

Task	teaspoon/gallon	ml/L
irrigation	1.5–3.8 tsp/gal	2–5 ml/L
seed soak	7.5–11.5 tsp/gal	10–15 ml/L
antifungal and anti–root rot	15 tsp/gal	20 ml/L

Apply *only* once per week, and apply *only* when needed!

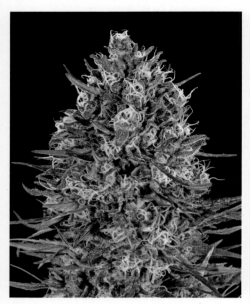

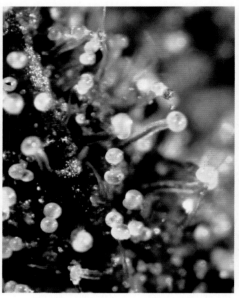

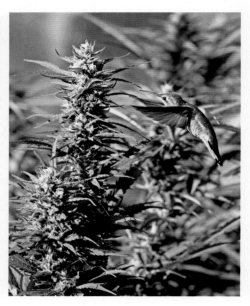

'Cripple Creek' bud a week from harvest

'Cocoa' macro close up showing capitate-stalked resin glands

Hummingbird inspecting a 'Jolly Bud'

can be applied as a spray or as a soil drench. It effectively suppresses growth when applied frequently at low concentrations. Flowering onset and harvest are progressively delayed with increased applications, but flower buds tend to all ripen simultaneously.

Folic acid is also used to increase vase life in cut flower buds and branches. A few branches of a male plant can be kept "fresh" for several days. Dilute B₉ in water and store cut branches of flower-producing male plants to keep them "fresh" for longer periods. B₉ is considered to be a safe, short-term growth retardant with few phytotoxicity problems.

Products that include B vitamins include Ortho Vitamin B Blend and B-52.

Growth Retardants

Caution! Do not use growth regulators on cannabis! NO GROWTH REGU-

LATOR IS LABELED FOR HUMAN CONSUMPTION. All growth retardants leave residues in the plant, and some, like paclobutrazol (aka Bonzi or Bushmaster, among others) remain in the plant for years and will show up in the buds and other foliage. The use of some PGRs will show up in the seeds.

In the USA and Canada, none of these products is allowed on the shelf or for use without a license to sell and apply. One company, Dutch Master, almost went out of business because their formula contained growth regulators. Growth regulators CAUSE CANCER and immune system problems, and have very low mammalian toxicity values and even lower primate values. Ethylene (the gas) and Ethephon (the liquid that converts to ethylene on heating) are about the safest alternatives.

Ill-informed cannabis growers apply growth retardants to inhibit vertical

growth and increase internodal branching. Leaves are supposed to remain the same size but internode length is retarded. Deadly toxic growth retardants are often called "chemical pinchers."

Outside of the use of PGRs for root induction in cuttings, and maybe working with seed production, I would not knowingly consume any plant or plant part that PGRs have been used on. There is a level of risk here that is unacceptable. It makes zero sense to use PGRs in commercial grows and even less in medical gardens.

23
CONTAINER CULTURE & HYDROPONICS

HYDROPONIC GARDENING IS cultivating plants without soil, typically in an *inert* growing medium. "Container culture" is very similar to hydroponics but uses soil, soilless mix, or some other growing medium that is *not* inert, that is, the growing medium *reacts* chemically. Hydroponic and container culture gardening are often confused; container culture is often called hydroponics. I believe that the confusion arises for two simple reasons: gardeners who use the term do not understand the difference, and "hydroponics" sounds so much cooler than "container culture"!

Hydroponics has been a buzzword that alludes to higher production and scientific superiority, something special that is new—bigger and better. The misused word *hydroponic* has also spawned other terms that are invented to distinguish one "unique" product from another. My current favorite terms are *ultraponics* and *fishponics*.

Hydroponic gardens are more technical in nature and require precise measurements and monitoring for high performance. Setting up a hydroponic garden is often more expensive and relies most often on man-made, processed chemicals and electrical power.

Hydroponics and container culture are practical for gardeners who cannot grow outdoors and are limited to an indoor or greenhouse space. Changing and working with soil is inconvenient for many apartment and home dwellers. Household electricity seldom fails, and the small gardens can be monitored easily. Indoor gardens are full of life and provide a "breath of fresh air" during long winter months, too.

Greenhouse setups range from inexpensive to expensive, depending upon the degree of sophistication. Greenhouse dynamics—size, heating, cooling, and so forth—can also be more demanding than growing indoors. Outdoor hydroponic gardens are less common and not practical because dirt and dust can easily pollute the garden. Where electricity is not readily available, container gardens can be maintained with battery-powered irrigation controllers and dust and pollutants filtered easily.

Mother plants grow longer and are best suited to large hydroponics or container culture container gardens, which allow room for root development. The mother plant's root system is easier to control in individual containers, and she is able to produce hundreds of clones during her lifetime. Mother plants need a large root system to take in nutrients in order to keep up with the demanding growth and clone-production schedule.

Hydroponics is not as forgiving as container gardens using soil, soilless mix, coco, and so forth. Soil and soilless mixes not only provide "terra firma" to anchor plants, they also buffer water imbalances and hold air and nutrients well.

Gardens with more components have more to go wrong. Complicated high-tech gardens often require more time and management. Even simple gardens rely on electricity to operate a pump and timer. If the electricity goes out and the pump stops, or even if it only malfunctions, plant growth is impaired. A lack of water for a few hours is long enough to cause damage to plants. Irrigation emitters can clog; pH can climb or plunge, and EC levels can change rapidly. All of these "hydroponic" variables can cause more problems than when growing in container gardens using soil or soilless mix, etc., that provide a buffer or safety zone to hold water and oxygen.

Rule of Thumb: The more parts in a garden, the more there is to malfunction.

Environmentally conscious gardeners select hydroponic fertilizers with an eye on their budgets. Manufacturers consistently dilute nutrient formulas in water to increase profits—often exponentially. Shipping excess water is expensive, costing more fossil fuel and increasing the garden's carbon footprint. Purchasing nutrients in a dry form is less expensive and lowers the environmental impact.

Advantages

- no soil necessary
- water can be reused
- complete control of nutrient levels
- clean environment—no dirt!

Disadvantages

- no soil in hydroponics to buffer problems
- disease can spread through entire crop quickly

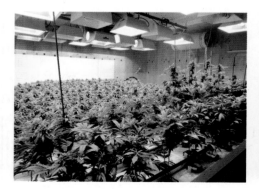

A properly managed rockwool top-feed garden such as this one, from Trichome Technologies, is super productive.

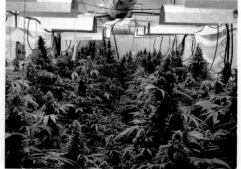

Healthy container gardens like this one are irrigated automatically. Penetrating the foliage in this garden is difficult and could break branches.

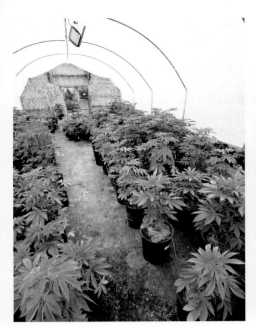

A small hoop greenhouse like this is easy to manage when growing medical cannabis in individual containers.

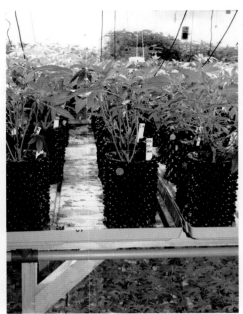

Air root–pruning containers are available that encourage more dense root growth.

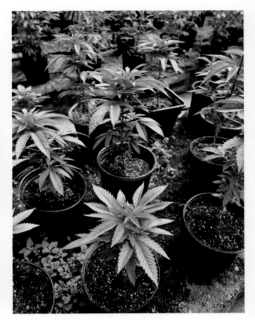

These little seedlings are being hardened-off to transplant outdoors. They are watered from the top with a water wand that has an aerating nozzle.

- large carbon footprint from manufacturing of components and transport to stores
- water can be recirculated with the wastes of the plant

Contrary to popular belief, hydroponically grown cannabis does not grow faster or produce heavier harvests. Scientific research (not funded by commercial interests) since the mid-1950s shows no significant difference between container-grown crops in soil, soilless mix, etc., and hydroponically grown crops. Work by D. R. Hoagland and D. I. Arnon in the first half of last century failed to prove that there was an increase in potential yields from growing hydroponically. They described the first nutrient solution to use for hydroponics, still in use today. To date no one has been able to refute this, and it remains a referenced work.

Container Culture and Hydroponics

Solution Culture

Cannabis grown in hydroponic solution culture gardens does not use growing medium. However, plants in some gardens are started in a small net pot in a handful of substrate. Examples of solution culture include aeroponics, bubbleponics, deep water culture (DWC), deep flow technique (DFT), nutrient film technique (NFT), and raft solution culture. These gardens require an electric pump that must function 24 hours a day to operate nutrient-solution drippers, emitters, air (oxygen) diffusers, misting nozzles, often with a good filter to ensure debris-free solution.

Media Culture

Media-based hydroponics uses an inert substrate such as rockwool or expanded clay pellets. The inert substrate does not react chemically with nutrients. Container culture employs substrate such as soilless mix, or coco coir that is not inert and will react chemically with the nutrient solution. The substrate, whether inert or not, serves multiple functions—to anchor plants and to hold air, water, and nutrients for root uptake. The media also holds precious oxygen that is essential for rapid nutrient uptake. Ideal growing mediums hold plenty of air (oxygen) and nutrient solution at the same time. Soilless mix and coconut coir are two of the most popular growing mediums used in container culture. Rockwool and expanded clay are the most common substrates found in hydroponics. Nutrient solution is delivered to the media via flood-and-drain, top-feed, or passive wicking that relies on capillary action.

In container culture and many types of hydroponics, the supply of oxygen in growing media can be maximized, which in turn allows properly grown plants with healthy roots to take in peak levels of nutrients. However, in "solution culture" it is very difficult, if not impossible, to consistently achieve the same oxygen levels as in properly aerated growing media. Fine-tuned nutrient solutions can steer plants to grow less leafy vegetative foliage and more dense flower buds.

Properly mixed and applied hydroponic nutrients—chemical salts diluted in water—are able to supply exact element levels so that roots have access to them and the possibility of taking them in at maximum capacity. Aerated nutrient solution is absorbed, wicked up from the growing medium, or it passes over roots, later draining off. The oxygen in solution, around roots or trapped in the soilless medium, speeds nutrient uptake. Organic nutrients—natural elements and compounds—are more difficult to control in container culture than their chemical counterparts. In nature these nutrients are often bound in complex

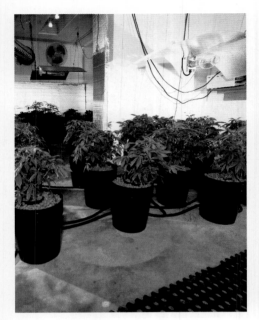

This hydroponic garden is made from 5-gallon (18.9 L) containers connected together with half-inch (1.3 cm) tubing.

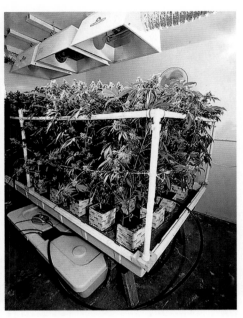

Nutrient solution floods into the garden bed to irrigate. The nutrient solution pulls more oxygen into the moist rockwool cubes when it drains.

growing in deep water that covers roots all the time, but by allowing dry time for the roots; because at this time, the solution on the root surface is still dissolving O_2 at higher levels when the air moves in and the water is gone. No extra aeration is needed other than stirring the nutrient reservoir. The amounts of oxygen needed by the root system will be absorbed at the root surface as well.

Solution Culture
aeroponics
bubbleponics
deep water culture (DWC)
deep flow technique (DFT)
nutrient film technique (NFT)
raft solution culture—passive

Media Culture
ebb-and-flow (flood-and-drain)
hydro-organic
top-feed—containers and slabs
run-to-waste (RTW)
wick—passive

Aeroponic Gardens
Aeroponic gardens are true to their name. Plants grow in a chamber of air and nutrients. Roots are suspended in a dark growth chamber without growing medium and continually or at regular intervals misted with a fine oxygen-rich nutrient solution. Medical cannabis gardeners use efficient aeroponic gardens to root cuttings, but seldom for vegetative or flowering. Since cuttings grow with no media attached, they can be transplanted into solution or media hydroponic gardens as well as soil. However, damage to minuscule root hairs is impossible to avoid.

The origin of aeroponics dates back to the first half of the 20th century; the first patent was issued in 1985 to Richard Stoner. In fact, the first cannabis aeroponic clone garden that I saw was in the mid-1980s, and it was very similar to Stoner's. It was homemade. Aeroponics makes control of conditions in the root zone much easier in hot climates than with conventional hydroponics. Often fatal nutrient-solution stagnation, waterlogging, and oxygen starvation are easier to control with aeroponics. The temperature inside the root chamber is easy to control, which is essential for

living chemical compounds that are difficult to measure accurately.

Regardless of the nutrient-solution application method, nutrient solutions are either run-to-waste (RTW) and not reused, or they are recirculated and used again and again rather than being discarded after one use. Recirculating systems have the added complication of concentrating the nutrient solution and the accumulation of plant wastes— broken roots, leaves, and so forth.

Nutrients are diluted in water in a "soil solution" or in an inert medium "hydroponic solution." In soil, soilless mix, coco coir, etc., there is a naturally occurring ratio of oxygen to nutrient solution. However in hydroponics using rockwool, expanded clay pellets, or other inert ingredients, this ratio must be "manufactured." And in any hydroponic garden where roots are covered with nutrient solution all the time, oxygen is contingent upon oxygenating the solution artificially, and it is very easy to screw it up.

Oxygen is pulled or moves into the soil, soilless mix, etc., or dissolves hydroponic solution where it can move into the roots. If the roots dry out, oxygen movement

becomes restricted, especially if it drops below the critical oxygen pressure (COP) (amount of O_2 dissolved into solution). In cannabis, COP is the point where respiration is first slowed from a lack of oxygen at about 20 mg/L*. The root tips are very active and have relatively high energy requirements, almost as high as humans but below the COP this activity slows.

*Plant Physiology, 3rd ed., by Lincoln Taiz and Eduardo Zeiger, (Sunderland, MA: Sinauer Associates, Inc., 2002).

At maximum levels of stirring, the amount of dissolved oxygen will be barely enough to keep up with O_2 utilization, and to get as close to 60 ppm as possible, oxygen must be diffused into the solution, typically with an electric air pump.

In the older root zones this lack of oxygen becomes an issue earlier at lower rates. Since their uptake is reduced to 10 percent of the tips' uptake, the cores can become anoxic (severely deficient in oxygen) or hypoxic (oxygen deficiency causing a very strong drive to correct the deficiency), killing the roots or affecting performance. The best way to achieve maximum aeration is not by avoiding pathogens and keeping adequate oxygen available. Properly designed and maintained, an aeroponic clone garden will yield a profuse, strong, and healthy root system.

Root systems of small seedlings and clones thrive in net pots specifically designed for aeroponic gardens. Clone roots strike (initiate) and seedling roots grow down from net pots into the dark, humid, nutrient-and-oxygen-rich environment. Regular misting in the 100 percent humid atmosphere prevents tender clones from drying out, all the while speeding root development. The totally dark chamber stops algae growth as root growth thrives.

Solution droplets of less than 30 microns tend to form a fog that humidifies the air but is not easily absorbed by roots. Larger, 30- to 100-micron droplets are more readily absorbed by roots. Droplets of greater than 100 microns

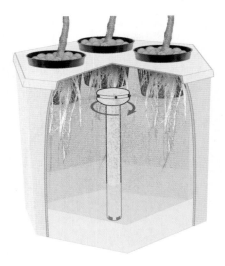

Aeroponic gardens that throw 30- to 50-micron droplets promote fast root growth.

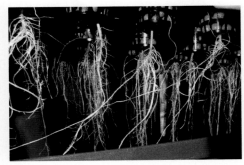

Root growth is phenomenal in an aeroponic clone machine.

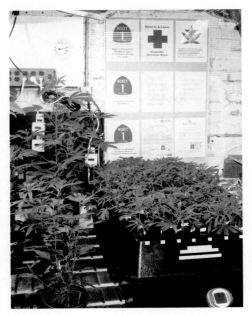

The aeroponic clone garden on the right is in front of medical cannabis prescriptions that certify patients.

precipitate from the air too quickly for root absorption.

The opening on a 30-micron (0.018 inch [0.046 mm]) nozzle is very small, clogs easily, and must be kept super clean. Use reverse osmosis water and low nutrient levels (about 10 percent strength), and maintain pump pressure to keep nozzles free of debris. Using a pre-pump filter and inline filter helps to remove debris and keep nozzles clean. Avoid or heavily filter any additives or nutrients containing organic matter.

Both continual and intermittent operation work well and achieve the same results—as long as the proper environment is maintained. Forcing solution through a 30-micron nozzle requires more pressure and a stronger, more expensive fitting and pump, which are also more costly to operate. If growing in large aeroponic gardens, electricity consumption becomes expensive; intermittent misting will save money. Use a timer that will cycle mist for one to two minutes, and then turn off for up to five minutes, 24 hours a day, to save resources.

Temperatures are easy to control in any climate in an insulated root chamber.

Simply heat or cool the nutrient solution before misting roots to bring the root zone temperature to the desired level. Avoid disease by keeping temperatures below 72°F (22°C) and regularly inspect roots for signs of discoloration, rot, and lack of fine root hairs.

Simple, small aeroponic gardens that pump nutrient solution up from the reservoir located below the root chamber are best suited to clone rooting and seedling growth. These gardens are less expensive than larger gardens with a separate reservoir and rooting chamber designed to grow mature plants. Gardens with a separate reservoir are less likely to clog as mature roots grow into the nutrient solution.

Aeroponic gardens are easy to construct, but fine-tuning a homemade unit could kill a few crops of clones before success is achieved. The basics are simple: the unit must be light- and watertight, and mist from nozzles must be of the proper size and delivered under adequate pressure. For information on readily available aeroponic gardens, visit www. marijuanagrowing.com

EC and pH considerations for aeroponic gardens are the same as for any hydroponic garden. But aeroponic gardens require greater attention to detail. There is no growing medium to act as a water/nutrient bank, and if the electricity goes out, the pump fails, or the nozzles clog, roots will soon dry out, killing tender root hairs. The whole root begins to die, starting at the tip.

There are several variations of aeroponic gardens including the Ein Gedi method, aero-hydroponics, and air-dynaponics.

Deep Water Culture (DWC)

Deep water culture (DWC) is simple and inexpensive. This low-maintenance method is typically employed by casual medical gardeners who want to grow a few plants in a small area. Seedlings and clones are held in net pots full of expanded clay pellets, rockwool, or a similar growing medium. Six-inch (15.3 cm) net pots are most common for single 5-gallon (18.9 L) containers. Smaller 2-inch (5.1 cm) net pots are

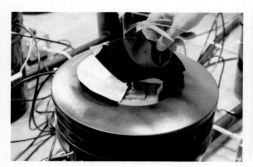

This plant is irrigated from above. The rockwool holds the plant, and the roots grow down into the water about an inch (2.5 cm) below the rockwool. (MF)

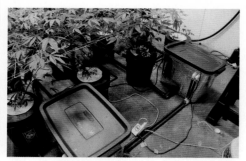

Roots are bathed in nutrient-rich aerated solution in DWC. (MF)

often used for multiple plants in the same container. The net pots are nestled in a plastic lid that covers the reservoir. Roots dangle into a somewhat dilute (75 percent concentration) nutrient solution that is aerated with an air stone and pump. Feeder roots absorb nutrients

and water from the solution in the oxygenated environment. The simple design requires no timer for the air pump that runs 24 hours a day.

Closed or self-contained, recirculating DWC gardens stand alone with

the reservoir directly under the net pot containing the plant. Closed gardens are perfect for gardeners who want to grow a few plants. The gardens also work well for large mother plants and to contain any waterborne diseases. The pH, EC, and solution must be checked for each individual reservoir. Nutrients, pH up, pH down, and any other additives must also be added to each container.

Multi-unit recirculating gardens are more complex, with a central reservoir connected by tubing to several container/reservoirs. A central air pump aerates nutrient solution in each container via a manifold connected to air tubes that are in turn connected to an oxygen diffuser in each container. Although the garden has more complex plumbing, the pH, EC, nutrients, and other additives can be controlled from a central reservoir.

Bubbleponics and Raft or Pond Culture

Bubbleponics and raft or pond culture, are a variation of DWC. In bubbleponics the nutrient solution is delivered via top-feed nozzles or spaghetti tubes to a small amount of growing medium that holds the plant in place. The nutrient solution is allowed to percolate down through the growing medium before falling back into the aerated reservoir and recirculated. Bubbleponic gardens require two pumps, one to deliver nutrient solution, and an air pump attached to an air stone or other diffuser to aerate the nutrient solution. A (submersible) pump lifts nutrient

solution to the top of a discharge tube connected to a top-feed irrigation system. Nutrient solution is delivered to individual plants and cascades down, wetting roots and splashing into the (self-contained) reservoir below, which in turn increases dissolved oxygen in the solution.

In **raft or pond solution culture**, plants are placed in a sheet of buoyant plastic that is floated on the surface of the nutrient solution. Roots are always submerged in artificially aerated nutrient solution.

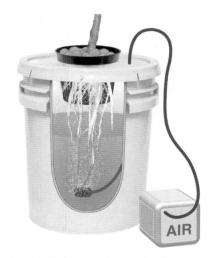

A closed DWC system is completely self-contained.

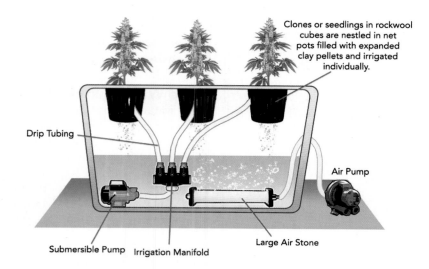

Clones or seedlings in rockwool cubes are nestled in net pots filled with expanded clay pellets and irrigated individually.

Drip Tubing

Air Pump

Submersible Pump   Irrigation Manifold

Large Air Stone

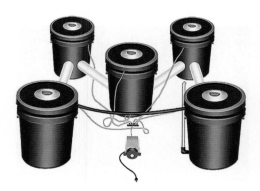

The nutrient solution flows to all containers in this recirculating DWC garden.

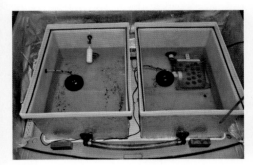
The grow tanks are set up and filled with nutrient solution.

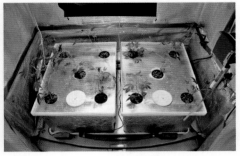
The little plants are set in the beds on top in net pots full of expanded clay pellets. Roots hang down into the aerated solution.

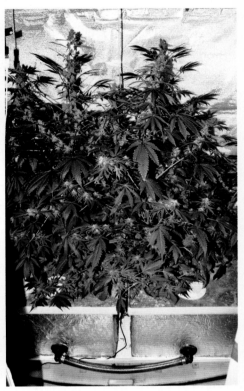

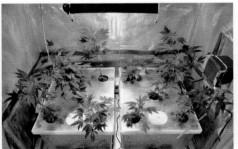
One week later, the same clones look a lot stronger and healthier, but they have not completely recovered from the transplanting.

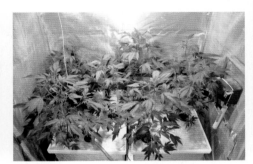
Two weeks later, the garden looks like it is thriving, and plants have put on growth.

The harvest from a small garden is small but enough to sustain many medical cannabis gardeners until the next crop.

The levels of all reservoirs—central and all container/reservoirs—seeks the same solution level. Simply check the reservoir level to learn the level of all the others. Use a Mariotte's bottle or a float valve to automatically maintain the solution level.

The **air pump** must supply each 5-gallon (18.9 L) reservoir with at least 1.3 gallons per minute (4.9 LPM) to ensure that adequate oxygen is available to roots. Less than this amount will deprive roots of oxygen, slow nutrient uptake, and open the door to cultural problems, pests, and diseases.

Set the air pump above the reservoir so that water will not siphon back through the air pump and destroy it if electricity goes out or the pump malfunctions.

Caution! Do not keep air pumps inside CO_2-rich garden rooms or greenhouses, or the extra CO_2 will drive the pH downward as the conjugate acid of the carbonate base or upward as the conjugate base of the carboxyl acid. (It really depends on many factors.)

Transplant Clones or Seedlings

Fill with nutrient solution until the bottom inch of the 6-inch (15.2 cm) net pot is covered. Avoid filling to the level of the stem to prevent stem rot and other diseases. Hand irrigation may be necessary for the first few days if capillary action does not wick nutrients upward to roots. After the roots grow through the net pot, lower the level of the nutrient solution to about 2 inches (5.1 cm) below the net pot. An external dark-green translucent "drain tube" on reservoirs will indicate solution level.

The nutrient solution tends to stay the same temperature as the room unless it is cooled slightly. Insulating and placing it on a cold floor will help keep solution cool. Always aim for the ideal nutrient temperature range 55°F–65°F (12.8°C–18.3°C) to prevent disease and increase dissolved oxygen (DO) in solution. Change nutrient solution at the first sign or suspicion of problems—solution discoloration, pH fluctuation, or a change in EC.

Top off nutrient solution with plain water daily. Change the reservoir every week to ensure proper nutrient levels. Changing the solution can be a bit of a job. If the reservoir has a drain plug, the solution can be drained and replaced weekly without removing the plant. This will help minimize salt buildup too. With no drain plug, the plant has to be removed from the container/reservoir and placed in another container. The air stone must be removed and the solution dumped. Dump old nutrient solution that is full of nitrates, sulfates, phosphates, and so forth, in the outdoor garden rather than down household drains. The container/reservoir must be completely cleaned and refilled with fresh nutrient solution. Many deep water culturists dilute nutrient solution to 75 percent strength to safeguard against overdose. Always run EC at lower levels in DWC gardens. Check with fertilizer manufacturers for recommendations.

Outdoors, the container/reservoir must be shielded or insulated so that direct

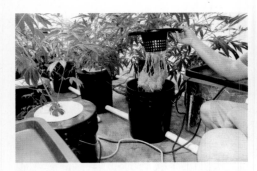

A big, healthy, white root system is a sign that there is enough dissolved oxygen in solution. Note that some of these roots are discolored and only a few roots are strong and white. This root system does not receive enough dissolved oxygen. (MF)

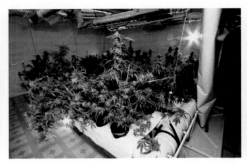

Nutrient solution in the tubes is kept about 6 inches (15.2 cm) deep. The nutrient solution is constantly moving and being aerated as it moves around roots.

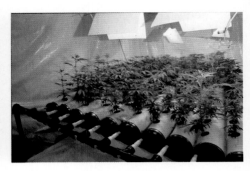

NFT gardens were more popular 15 years ago than they are today.

sunlight does not cause the temperature inside to climb beyond 70°F (21.1°C). Outdoor gardens also need an overflow drainage hole in the side of the reservoir to prevent rainwater from diluting solution or causing it to overflow.

Nutrient Film Technique (NFT)
Deep Flow Technique (DFT)

Deep flow technique is similar to NFT except roots in gulleys are submerged with 1 to 2 inches (2.5–5.1 cm) of nutrient solution. Make sure nutrient solution is well aerated and flows quickly enough through tubes and gulleys to maintain adequate oxygen levels for roots. Check the temperature in different parts of the tubes to ensure that it does not climb above 70°F (21.1°C) and holds at least 8 ppm of dissolved oxygen.

The nutrient film technique (NFT) was developed by Allen Cooper from England in the 1960s. Cooper introduced the garden to the world in his book, *The ABC of NFT*. NFT hydroponic gardens are most suitable for short-term crops with a compact root system including predominantly *indica* and *ruderalis* varieties that are harvested in 3 to 4 months. When grown too long, extensive cannabis root systems tend to block solution flow in gulleys.

The system supplies aerated nutrient solution to plants with roots held in gulleys. Seedlings or cuttings in small net pots full of substrate with strong root systems are placed on capillary matting located on the bottom of a covered channel or gulley. Capillary matting takes the place of a growing medium,

stabilizes nutrient-solution flow, and holds roots in place. The nutrient flow can also be intermittent when used with a base like sand or perlite. Plastic tubes or sleeves are available that can be filled and laid on the ground as well. Well-aerated nutrient solution flows down the gulley, over and around the roots, and back to the reservoir. Irrigation is constant—24 hours a day. Roots receive plenty of oxygen and are able to absorb a maximum of nutrient solution. Gulleys must have the proper incline, volume, and flow of nutrient solution for a successful crop. NFT gardens must be fine-tuned to perform well.

Gulleys or channels are covered to keep humidity high in the root zone. A white exterior reflects light and the interior can be painted black to keep roots in the dark and stop algae growth. Roots that are completely submerged have less access to oxygen in the air compared to oxygen available in the nutrient solution. Maintain a thin layer, 0.4 to 0.8 inches (10.2–20.3 mm) of nutrient solution to

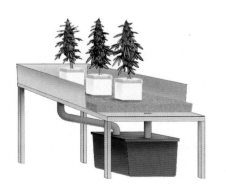

Capillary matting under rockwool cubes holds roots, air, and nutrient solution.

allow for adequate air absorption. Roots submerged in turbulently flowing nutrient solution are intermittently exposed to humid air.

Nutrient solution is pumped from the reservoir into gulleys via a manifold and tubing at the upper end. The table is set up on a slope with a 1:50 fall in 12 feet. For example, if the bed is 50 inches (127 cm) long, the fall is 1 inch in 50 inches, or 1 centimeter in 50 centimeters. The incline helps solution flow that in turn compensates for surface, while avoiding both accumulation and waterlogging the roots. As a general guide, flow rate should be 0.5 GPM (1.9 LPM) at planting. After plants are established, flow rates for each gulley should be at least 0.25 GPM (0.9 LPM) and can be a maximum of twice this amount. Beyond this, extreme nutrient uptake problems can occur.

Gulley length should be less than 40 feet (12.2 m) to avoid slow growth. Oxygen in solution is frequently adequate, but nitrogen can become depleted at the low end of gulleys. Longer runs require meticulous leveling of gulleys to avoid high and low spots that expose roots too much or cause puddles. Double reinforced bottoms make gulleys durable and rigid when supporting large plants, large root systems, and large volumes of nutrient solution. Some NFT gulleys have ribs below to provide support and prevent warping and movement. The ribs also function as drainage channels and direct nutrient solution evenly along the bottom of the gulley.

A good filter will prevent debris from blocking gulleys, supply tubes, and pumps. NFT gardens have very little buffering against interruptions in the flow caused by plumbing blockages, power outages, and so on. In the absence of a growing medium, roots must be kept perfectly moist by the nutrient solution at all times. If a pump fails, roots dry and die. If the garden dries out for a day or longer, small feeder roots will die and grave consequences will result. Problems occur quickly in NFT gardens, and decisive corrective action is necessary. This garden is not recommended for new growers.

Place a filter on the pipe that returns nutrient solution to keep the reservoir clean. Organic garden filters may clog and need cleaning more often. Use 0.25-inch (6.35 mm) microtube feeders so that small chunks of debris pass right through. Filters on pressurized lines create backpressure, which causes pumps to strain and pump efficiency to diminish, consequently a more powerful pump is necessary.

NFT gardens are very easy to clean and lay out after each crop. However, only gardeners with several years of experience should try an NFT garden.

Transplant Clones or Seedlings, and Grow

Start clones and seedlings in small 2-inch (5.1 cm) net pots full of rockwool or substrate that does not shed debris to clog the irrigation system. Or cut large holes in small pots for an inexpensive alternative to net pots. The small pots must permit unrestricted root expansion when growing into gulleys. Do not grow clones and seedlings in soil or media that will shed debris. And do not try to wash media from root mass with cold water. This will severely damage roots, compound transplant shock, and slow their establishment in gulleys. Plants started in soil or messy substrate should be lightly shaken to remove "debris" and then be transplanted. This will lessen damage from the move substantially. Install a temporary filter such as a nylon stocking or something similar at the end of channels to catch debris.

Set small pots in gulleys so that they remain stable while roots are establishing. Keeping clones and seedlings firmly in channels with no vertical movement will

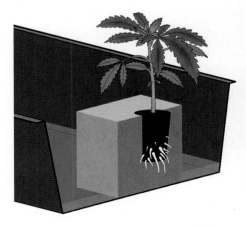

Roots quickly grow into the main growing medium.

reduce transplant shock and speed root growth. Movement of plants can cause damage to roots, which causes stress and possible root disease. Often the first signs include leaf tip burn and slow growth. Even minimal transplant shock will slow growth for several days.

Problems

Most hydroponic garden problems are solved by keeping the garden and surrounding area clean, and by controlling the nutrient solution's dissolved oxygen levels, EC, and pH, and temperature in the reservoir and gulleys. See sections on each for specific information.

Broken or discolored roots found in reservoirs and filters indicate problems from disease, pests, oxygenation, heat, nutrients, and so on. More broken and discolored roots signify a bigger problem. Check for slow nutrient flow and stagnation. Both conditions can cause waterlogged roots. Make sure that gulleys and the entire system are as light-tight as possible to discourage algae growth.

An excellent troubleshooting guide can be found at www.amhydro.com.

Hydro-Organic

Hydro-organic (aka organoponic) is growing in an inert medium fertigated with a soluble organic nutrient solution. When somebody talks about hydro-organics, they probably mean organic container culture. Organic fertilizers are most often defined as containing substances with a carbon molecule or a natural unaltered substance such

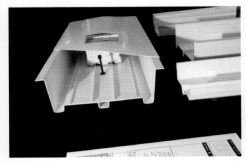

The ridges in each gulley bottom direct water and help add rigidity and stability.

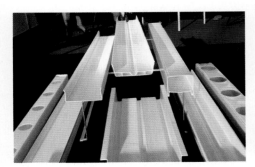

There are many different styles of gulleys for NFT gardens.

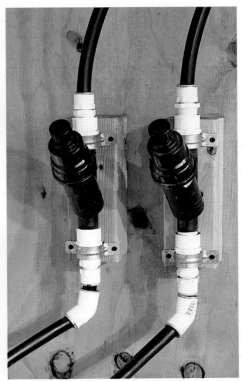

Good filters that are easy to access and clean are essential for NFT gardens.

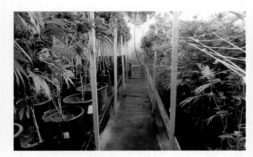

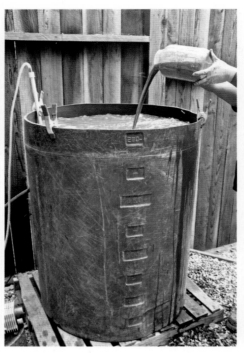

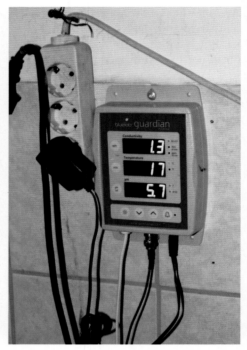

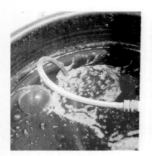

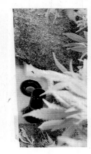

Hydro-organic gardens combine principles of hydroponics and organic gardening.

A dirty reservoir causes nonstop problems!

Hydro-organic nutrient mixes are heavier, requiring a stronger pump and heavy-duty filters.

A constant-readout monitor/controller for nutrient solution takes the guesswork out of nutrient formula delivery.

as ground-up minerals. Many of the nutrients must be "processed" by micro-organisms and be chelated before they are available to plants. These gardens can be top-feed, flood-and-drain, or wick. Refer to those specific sections in this chapter for more information.

Organic nutrients require places to collect. The concept is similar to buffering a video online. Without a place to accumulate, the rate of mineralization will not keep up with need. Much of the released nutrients would be used up by the microlife in the soil, or "volatized." Other major issues arise with macro-nutrients—most notably, P and Ca. It is impossible to grow 100 percent organic cannabis in hydroponics. There must be sources and pools where nutrients accumulate at appropriate levels. Oxygen is also required to break down organic complexes as well as the appropriate varieties and numbers of microflora to be effective.

Dedicated gardeners spend the time and trouble it takes to grow organically because the natural nutrients bring out a sweet organic taste in flower buds. Indoor and outdoor crops grown in less

than 90 days do not have time to wait for organic nutrients to be broken down. Organic nutrients must be soluble and readily available for short-term cannabis crops to benefit.

An exact balance of organic nutrients can be achieved with experimentation and attention to details. Even when you buy ready-mixed commercial fertilizers like BioCanna or Earth Juice, you will need to try different feeding amounts and schedules to get the exact combination to grow a top-quality harvest. Always check with manufacturers for recommendations.

Taking an accurate EC reading or mixing the exact amount of a specific nutrient is very difficult in organic hydroponics. Chemical fertilizers are easy to measure out and apply, and it is easy to give plants the specific amount of fertilizer in each stage of growth.

Organic nutrients have a complex structure, and measuring content is difficult. Organics are difficult to keep stable, too. Some manufacturers with products such as BioCanna have managed to stabilize their fertilizers. When buying organic

nutrients, always buy from the same supplier, and find out as much as possible about the source from which the fertilizers were derived. Always use fertilizers well before the expiration date.

Combine premixed soluble organic fertilizers with other organic ingredients to make your own blend. Experiment to find the perfect mix for the cannabis varieties being grown. Adding too much fertilizer can make the substrate toxic, binding nutrients to the point that they become unavailable. Foliage and roots burn when buildup is severe.

Soluble organic fertilizers are more difficult to overapply, yet they are also difficult to leach from the growing medium. And when overapplied, soluble organic fertilizers are more likely to cause symptoms that are hard to read. For example, too much bone meal causes a pH imbalance of the growing medium that manifests as leaf burn. Fertilizer recirculating systems are the trickiest to control. When the microbial life is off balance by a *small* amount and the conversion of released ammonium to nitrate is slowed, it causes a buildup to toxic levels.

Chelates and Nutrients

Mix seaweed with macronutrients and secondary nutrients to make a hydro-organic fertilizer. The amount of primary and secondary nutrients is not as important as the mélange of trace elements that are in an available form in the seaweed. Major nutrients can be applied via soluble fish emulsion for nitrogen, while phosphorous and potassium can be supplied by bat guano, bone meal, and manures. More and more organic gardeners are adding growth stimulators such as humic acid, *Trichoderma*, bacteria, and various hormones.

Minerals such as silica, nickel, cobalt, and selenium are not essential for plant growth but have the ability to enhance growth and development. They are needed in minute quantities and are provided via the contaminants in the water supply and fertilizer. Add humic and fulvic acids (available in mineral soils) to the hydroponic garden and soilless container gardens. Fulvic acid, a humic acid, is yellow in color and soluble. Humic acids are most effective as additives to the soil to help build soil and stimulate plant growth.

Humic acids have an important ability as chelating agents—they are, in fact, excellent in this role as they are strong enough to protect micronutrients but weak enough to release the microelements to plants when required. Fulvic acid is particularly good for this role of natural chelation, because it has the ability to enter the plant and move throughout its tissue. In organic production gardens where synthetic chelation agents

such as EDTA cannot be used, addition of humic acid appears to be the ideal way of ensuring that micronutrients remain available to the plant through a more natural form of chelation.

Organic nutrients are typically processed by microorganisms before plants can take them up. Humic acids promote the conversion of many elements into a form available to plants. Adding humic acids promotes microbial growth, helps decompose minerals and organic matter, and makes different elements available to plants. Iron would usually be supplied in a chelated compound. In an organic garden, fulvic acid is used instead. Humic and fulvic acids accelerate cell division and increase the rate of development and the length of root systems.

Ebb-and-Flow Gardens

Ebb-and-flow (aka flood-and-drain) gardens are low-maintenance, simple, and inherently efficient by design. This is often the easiest and most cost effective hydroponic or container culture garden for indoor and greenhouse cannabis cultivation, whether growing just a few plants in a small area or a large garden.

Individual plants in pots or rockwool cubes are set on a special table with drainage channels and sides, a growing bed that can hold up to 4 inches (10.2 cm) of solution. The nutrient solution is pumped into the table or growing bed. The rockwool blocks or containers are flooded up through an inlet from the bottom, which *pushes the old, oxygen-poor air out.* Once the nutrient solution reaches a set level, an

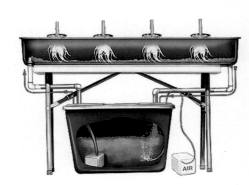

This ebb-and-flow garden has an air stone to increase nutrient-solution aeration.

overflow pipe drains the excess back to the reservoir. At the end of the irrigation cycle, the pump is turned off and the solution drains and *draws new, oxygen-rich air into the growing medium.* The aerated substrate is just what roots need to take in nutrients at a rapid rate. A maze of drainage channels in the bottom of the table directs runoff solution back to the catchment tank or reservoir. This cycle is repeated several times a day. Ebb-and-flow gardens are ideal for growing clones, seedlings, and short plants in a sea of green (SOG) garden.

Ebb-and-Flow Tables

Nutrient solution is pumped up into the bed via an inlet fixture and evacuated out the same inlet/drain. There is only one entrance and exit to clog, leak, or otherwise malfunction. Delivering nutrient solution via more than one outlet compounds problems every time a new emitter is added. An overflow fitting guarantees the nutrient solution will reach a specific level and not spill

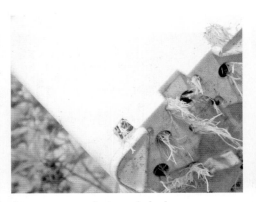

Roots grow out drainage holes but stop growing when they come in contact with air between irrigation cycles.

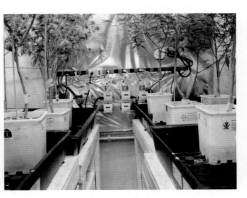

Each bed in this flood-and-drain garden is controlled by timers that can be seen at the end of the aisle.

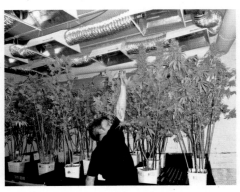

These plants grew for about a week too long and needed to be pruned from below. But as you can see, the buds on the top of the plant are at least 2 feet (61 cm) long.

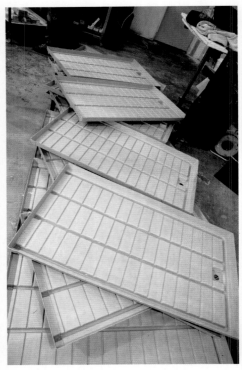

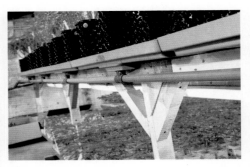

Plants wick up nutrient solution in the ebb-and-flow tables.

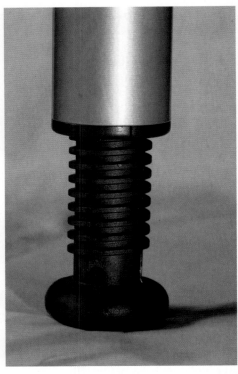

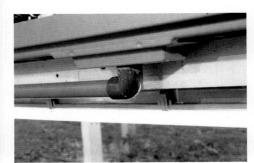

Drains should be efficient and simple to clean.

Adjustable legs make it easy to level and add an incline to a growing table.

Flood-and-drain tables are scrubbed down by hand and disinfected between crops.

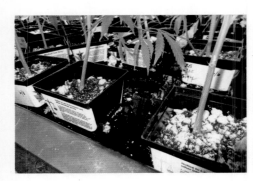

Flooding garden beds is the easiest and most efficient form of irrigation.

over the top of the table. Excess solution drains back into the reservoir via the overflow fitting. The solution is aerated when it cascades from the drain hole in the table into the reservoir below.

Ebb-and-flow tables or growing beds are designed to hold up to 4 inches (10.2 cm) of solution and let excess water flow freely away from the growing medium and roots. Nutrient solution is pumped up into the bed, filling it in 5 to 10 minutes. It should take about 8 minutes for a 350 GPH pump to fill a 4 × 8-foot (1.2 × 2.4 m) table with 40

gallons (151.4 L) of solution 2 inches (5.1 cm) deep. The solution is moved relatively slowly, and a low-volume 350 GPH (1325 LPH) pump is adequate (see "Nutrient-Solution Pumps," on page 434.) These gardens are fairly quiet and use less power than some other setups.

The bed should drain faster than it takes to fill. Total fill-and-drain time cannot exceed 20 minutes or roots will be deprived of oxygen too long and will drown, rot, and attract problems. Passive drainage requires a large tube (at least 2 inches [5.1 cm]) to allow solution to drain rapidly. Complete and speedy drainage is essential so that the growing medium *pulls* fresh air into the growing medium and root zone. Excess solution sitting in substrates after irrigation does *not* allow adequate oxygen to enter. Slow suffocation occurs when nutrient solution does not drain completely. The surface of the growing media must also dry out completely to help prevent algae growth and fungus gnat infestations. Avoid algae growth on substrate surface by covering to exclude light. Remove any debris—dead leaves, organic matter, and so forth—from the surface of the

growing medium to deter pests and diseases. Keep clean, pest-and-disease-free medium enclosed in plastic until it is used.

The table must be sturdy enough to hold a volume of water. For example, a 4 × 8-foot (1.2 × 2.4 m) table that is 2 inches (5.1 cm) full holds 40 gallons (151.4 L) of solution that weighs 240 pounds (108.9 kg).

When flooded with 1 to 2 inches (2.5–5.1 cm) or more of nutrient solution, the growing medium wicks up the solution

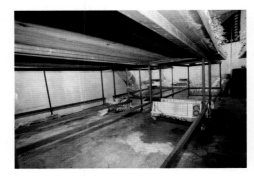

Steel tables with wooden supports bear all the weight of the growing table. The tables are equipped with wheels so an aisle can be opened between them.

into the freshly aerated medium. Tables with drain channels require deeper flooding, up to 4 inches (10.1 cm), to compensate for channels. Homemade tables with no drain channels require shallower levels. But such tables could also allow pools of stagnant water if not perfectly flat and with an adequate incline.

Adjustable-height legs, similar to those found on a washing machine, work well to support ebb-and-flow garden beds. Individual legs can be adjusted to dial in the slope of a garden bed table. Allow enough incline so that solution drains readily but not so much slope that plants at the high end do not receive enough solution. An 8-foot-long table should have a slope of about 0.5 to 0.75 inch (about 1.3–1.9 cm). Growing beds longer than 10 feet (3 m) drain slowly, and solution stays on the beds longer than roots are able to use it.

Growing Mediums

Growing medium must wick solution up and must also hold plenty of air. For example, a 4-inch (10.2 cm) rockwool cube flooded with 1 inch (2.5 cm) of solution wicks up about 3 inches (7.6 cm) into the cube. Growing mediums must provide adequate capillary action for water uptake and movement. Rockwool, soilless mix, and coco are the preferred growing mediums for ebb-and-flow gardens. However, some people do use expanded clay pellets and irrigate deeper and more often.

Irrigation

Flood the table with 1 to 2 inches (2.5–5.1 cm) of solution to ensure even nutrient-solution distribution. Avoid lightweight mediums such as perlite that may cause containers to float and fall over. A large volume of water is necessary to fill the entire table. Make sure the reservoir has enough solution to flood the reservoir and still retain an absolute minimum of 50 percent extra to allow for daily evaporation. Before introducing plants, calculate the amount of solution needed to flood the table. Also calculate the size of reservoir needed. Use the tables at right as a guideline.

TABLE	GALLONS FOR	RESERVOIR	GALLONS FOR	RESERVOIR
Size (ft)	1-inch Depth	Size (gal)	2-inch Depth	Size (gal)
1 × 2	1.25	2.5	2.5	5
2 × 2	2.5	5	5	10
2 × 3	3.75	7.5	7.5	15
2 × 4	5	10	10	20
3 × 3	5.62	11.24	11.24	22.48
3 × 4	7.5	15	15	30
3 × 5	9.4	18.8	18.8	37.6
3 × 6	11.3	22.6	22.6	45.2
4 × 4	10	20	20	40
4 × 5	12.5	25	25	50
4 × 6	15.6	31.2	31.2	62.4
4 × 7	17.5	35	35	70
4 × 8	20	40	40	80
4 × 9	22.5	45	45	90
4 × 10	25	50	50	100

TABLE	CUBIC LITERS FOR	RESERVOIR	CUBIC LITERS FOR	RESERVOIR
Size (cm)	3-cm Depth	Size (L)	6-cm Depth	Size (L)
30 × 60	5400	5.4	10.8	21.6
60 × 60	10800	10.8	21.6	43.2
60 × 90	16200	16.2	32.4	64.8
60 × 120	21600	21.6	43.2	86.4
90 × 90	24300	24.3	48.6	97.2
90 × 120	32400	32.4	64.8	129.6
90 × 150	40500	40.5	81	162
90 × 180	48600	48.6	97.2	194.4
120 × 120	43200	43.2	86.4	172.8
120 × 150	54000	54	108	216
120 × 180	64800	64.8	129.6	259.2
120 × 210	75600	75.6	151.2	302.4
120 × 240	86400	86.4	172.8	345.6
120 × 270	97200	97.2	194.4	388.8
120 × 300	108000	108	216	432

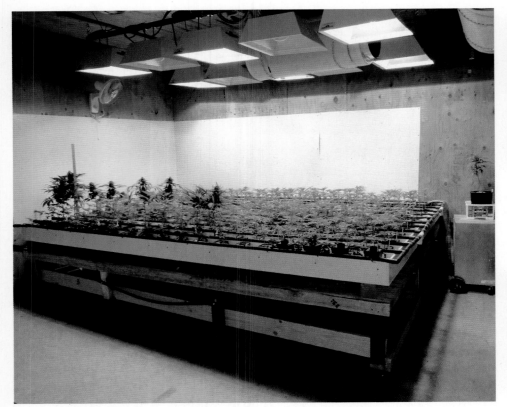

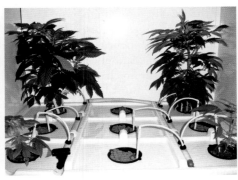

Each clone in this top-feed garden is fed via a spaghetti tube attached to an emitter.

This rockwool hydroponic garden by Trichome Technologies is completely automated.

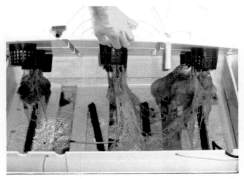

Roots hang in the moist air below the garden bed. Irrigation water is recirculated back to the reservoir.

To check the moisture level, saturate substrate with nutrient solution. Weigh rockwool containers or blocks when saturated, and weigh them again a few hours to a day later to check the amount or percentage of water used. For example, a block that weighs 4 ounces (11.8 cl) when saturated will weigh 2 ounces (5.9 cl) when 50 percent of the nutrient solution has been used. Check with the grow medium or substrate manufacturer for recommendations on moisture content and irrigation frequency. To learn the amount of solution a grow medium contains, weigh it when saturated and after squeezing lightly. Water rockwool when it is 50 percent dry. Remember, rockwool holds a lot of moisture and air, even when saturated. Irrigation frequency and volume change substantially when temperatures go down and light is lacking. Overwatering is much more likely when temperatures cool. Do not let nutrient solution stand on the table for more than 20 minutes. Submerged roots drown in the depleted oxygen environment.

Ebb-and-Flow Irrigation Guidelines

1. Rockwool cubes: 3 times @ 10 minutes
2. Soilless mix: 3 times @ 10 minutes
3. Expanded clay: 6 times @ 10 minutes
4. Lava rock: 12 times @ 10 minutes

Note: Lower the EC to between 600 and 800 ppm when increasing feeding frequency. It is easy to burn plants when irrigation frequency increases.

The first cycle should start first thing in the morning and be followed by cycles 2 to 4 hours apart. The irrigation schedule will fluctuate depending upon variables such as temperature, humidity, plant age, and growth rate. No watering is necessary at night. The entire irrigation cycle must be completed in no more than 20 minutes total, or roots will drown. The fill time is important and should occur relatively quickly, preferably in ten minutes or less. Drain time should be relatively quick so that the draining solution sucks new, oxygen-

rich air into the container or cube. This is an essential principle of irrigation in any flood-and-drain garden.

A large amount of nutrient solution is required to fill garden beds. For example a 4 × 8-foot (1.2 × 2.4 m) table requires 40 gallons (151.4 L) of solution to reach a depth of 2 inches (5.1 cm). Consequently a large reservoir is necessary. Garden beds are flooded in sequence or will have individual reservoirs when more than one such table is set up in a growing area.

The entire table floods and is exposed to air, causing a huge volume of water from the solution to evaporate into the air. This creates more humid atmospheric conditions. Extra ventilation will be necessary to whisk away moist air. The balance of the nutrient solution is also affected and must be compensated.

Since all plants are in the same bed and are irrigated together, pests and diseases can also run through an entire garden

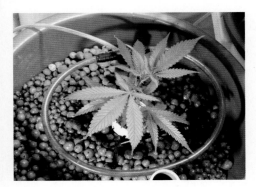

This top-feed container is irrigated by a spaghetti tube that circles the plant. Nutrient solution is delivered around the circle so it penetrates growing medium evenly.

quickly. Keeping garden rooms clean is essential to avoid the spread of pests and diseases.

Variations of Ebb-and-Flow

A few gardeners place a capillary mat between the table and containers to hold nutrient solution and promote root growth. I do not recommend this practice. Once plant roots have anchored into the capillary matting, they cannot be moved without damaging roots. Excessive algae growth and waterlogged roots that leads to root rot are inherent problems with this practice. After irrigation, the water under matting takes a very long time to dry.

Top-Feed Gardens

Top-feed hydroponics and container culture gardens are efficient and productive, and once set up, they are easy to control and maintain. The nutrient solution is metered out in specific doses at intervals over time and delivered to individual plants via spaghetti tubing or an emitter placed near the base of the stem. Aerated nutrient solution flows down into the growing medium. Roots take in some of the nutrient solution and the balance drains out the bottom. The runoff solution is directed back to the reservoir as soon as it drains from the growing medium. Rockwool and expanded clay pellets are the most common growing mediums in hydroponics, and container culture gardens commonly use such mediums as soilless mix, coco coir, and soil. Versatile top-feed gardens can be used with individual containers slabs in individual beds or lined up on tables.

Top-feed 5-gallon (18.9 L) containers of growing medium work well to grow large plants that may require support. Small 1- to 3-gallon (3.8–11.4 L) containers work well for smaller plants.

Top-Feed Containers

Individual self-contained recirculating top-feed container gardens consist of a net pot or pots nested in the lid of a container/reservoir containing a pump. Popular setups include a single net pot suspended in the lid of a 5-gallon container/reservoir or multiple net pots suspended in the lid of a larger container. A submersible pump in the bottom of the container lifts nutrient solution to irrigate individual plants via spaghetti tubing and emitters around the stems. Expanded clay pellets are the preferred growing medium for continuous irrigation, and rockwool for intermittent application. Nutrient solution drips down through the growing medium and runs to waste or falls back into the reservoir before recirculating. The solution is aerated every time drops fall and splash down into the self-contained reservoir below. The pump must cycle nutrient solution 24 hours a day to ensure that water is aerated. This garden does not need a timer.

Roots grow down into the nutrient solution and, over time, form a mass on the bottom. Irrigation from the top circulates aerated nutrient solution and

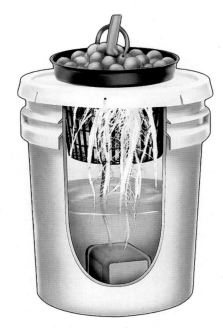

This top-feed container has a reservoir and a pump.

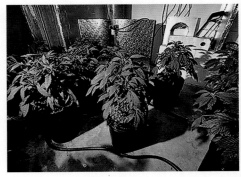

Multiple containers are connected to the same drainage tubing. The containers are irrigated from the top and all drain back into the same reservoir.

flushes out old, oxygen-poor solution. Some containers have a 1-inch (2.5 cm) pipe to draw air directly down into the root zone. Nutrient-solution aeration in the bottom of the container can become a constant problem. Place a grate or platform in the bottom of the container so roots do not sit in water and drown. If the nutrient solution is more than an inch (2.5 cm) deep, an air stone attached to an external air pump must be added to the bottom of the reservoir to ensure that roots receive enough oxygen. At this point the garden changes names. (See "Deep Water Culture" in this chapter.)

Individual top-feed 5-gallon (18.9 L) containers are easy to move and perfect for growing 1 or 2 large plants, including mothers. Culling out and replacing a slow-growing or diseased plant is also quick and easy. Controlling each container's nutrient solution pH, EC, and temperature are the tradeoffs for versatility.

Top-feed gardens cycle for 5 minutes or longer and should be irrigated at least 3 times daily. Often gardeners cycle the nutrient solution 24 hours a day, especially when growing in fast-draining expanded clay or similar mediums. In fast-draining mediums, overhead irrigation is continual. Microirrigation in coco coir is generally 4 to 5 times daily.

Multiple-container, recirculating, top-feed gardens employ several containers that are connected to a main reservoir. A flexible drain hose is attached near the bottom of the container/reservoir. The hose is connected to a drainage manifold

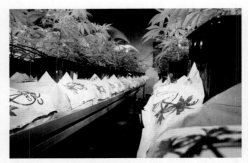

At transplanting, the bottoms are cut out of containers full of coco. Roots grow down into the coco slabs. Individual plants are watered with spaghetti tubing from above.

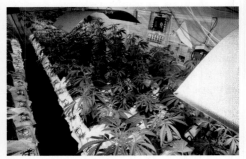

Many plants can fit in a small area when growing in coco slabs.

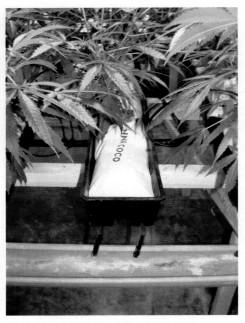

Individual trays with drainage channels can also hold slabs. The trays are connected by a manifold of tubes or troughs that drain runoff to waste or back to the catchment tank. Versatile individual trays are easy to configure for different-sized gardens, but algae growth is common when directing runoff back to the reservoir via an open-faced trough.

ing medium. They deliver a measured dose of nutrient solution. The nutrient solution is aerated as it is applied, before being absorbed by the growing medium and draining back to the reservoir.

In recirculating gardens, slabs should be set on tables that have drainage channels to carry runoff nutrient solution back to the reservoir. Elevated tables are not necessary in run-to-waste gardens. Tables with a flat surface do not allow adequate drainage, and solution tends to puddle and stagnate, quickly leading to problems with root rot, pests, and diseases. Excess nutrient solution drains from pots onto the table with drainage channels and is carried back to the reservoir. Make sure the table is set up on an incline so it drains evenly. Pockets of standing water on the table contain less oxygen and promote rot.

Transplanting Rockwool Cubes onto Slabs

Root clones and grow seedlings in 1- to 2-inch (2.5–5.1 cm) rockwool cubes. When roots are established and just starting to grow through the sides, transplant into larger 3- to 4-inch (7.6–10.2 cm) rockwool blocks. Avoid root damage and minimize shock by not letting roots grow more than a quarter inch (0.6 cm) beyond the sides of cubes before transplanting into blocks.

that shuttles runoff nutrient solution between reservoirs. A central pump distributes solution from a central reservoir to individual containers via an irrigation manifold and spaghetti tubing. Once delivered, the nutrient solution flows and percolates through the growing medium. Roots take in the aerated nutrient solution before it drains onto the tray and back to the central reservoir.

Each reservoir below the growing container can hold an inch (2.5 cm) or more of water. It is important to regularly cycle irrigation in these gardens, so the solution in the bottom of the container does not stagnate and drown roots—remember the 20 minute rule! Top-feed containers can also be lined up on a drainage table. Square containers make most efficient use of space.

More extensive plumbing allows nutrient pH, EC, and temperature to be controlled via the central reservoir. The reservoir must be located below growing containers to avoid high levels of solution stagnating in the bottom of

containers. A reservoir located at the same level or plane as growing containers causes the levels of all reservoirs—central and all container/reservoirs—to seek the same solution level.

Individual containers in top-feed gardens can be easily arranged to fit into the allotted garden space. Plants can also be transplanted or removed from pots and cared for individually.

Top-Feed Slabs

Top-feed rockwool and coco coir slabs (bats) that are covered with plastic serve as growing containers. Clones and seedlings are grown in individual containers, most often rockwool blocks, and set on top of slabs (transplanted). See "Transplanting Rockwool Cubes onto Slabs," at right.

An irrigation tube is attached to a short manifold with spaghetti tubes fed by a pump submerged in a reservoir in a recirculating garden. Spaghetti tubes with or without emitters are attached to thin stakes that are anchored in the grow-

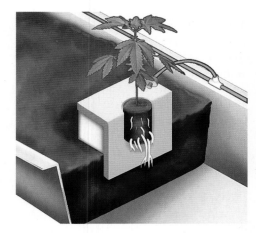

This cutaway drawing shows that nutrient delivery is simple and easy with a top-feed slab garden. Aerated nutrient solution is metered via emitters onto a growing cube. Aerated solution percolates down through the medium. Channels in the bottom of the tray speed drainage back to the reservoir.

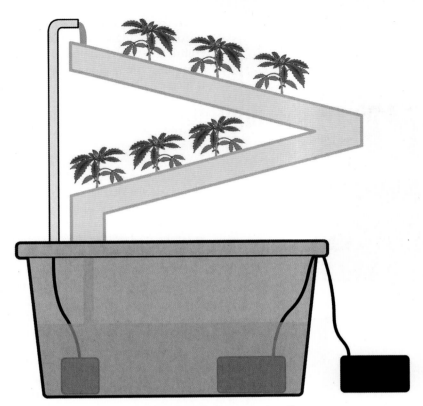

DFT gardens are ideal for growing along a well-illuminated wall.

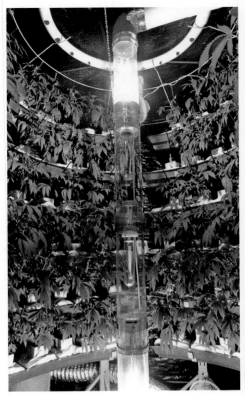

Vertical gardens take advantage of all available HID light.

Transplant blocks onto slabs when the first roots start to show out the bottom of blocks. A 40-inch (101.6 cm) slab can easily support three individual plants. Transplant each of three individual blocks onto a slab by cutting an "X" that corresponds to the corners of the block on top of the slab. Peel the plastic covering back and set block on top of conditioned slab. Hold block in place with toothpicks or thin stakes until established.

Vertical Top-Feed Gardens

Growing small plants in a vertical garden saves space and increases yield per square foot. Fences, sunny garden walls, and bare but well-illuminated walls around garden rooms are usable garden space. Side light in garden rooms is often underutilized or wasted. Backyard fences and walls—sunny, partially shady, and even shady—are also excellent locations for vertical gardens.

DFT gardens and top-feed irrigation can be mounted on a fence or garden wall. Containers can be placed in a trough along the walls of indoor garden rooms to take advantage of lost side light. An automated top-feed spaghetti-tubing manifold can deliver nutrient-solution. Or a sunny backyard fence or wall can be fitted with 4-inch (10.2 cm) tubing to make a DFT garden. Extra heat is absorbed and emitted from fences and walls. Take care to shade nutrient tubes to keep solution cool and prevent roots from baking. Fences and garden walls heat up to beyond 100°F (37.8°C) in direct sunlight. (The fence in my backyard reaches temperatures of about 130°F (54.4°C) during the summer.) In such hot conditions, it would be almost impossible to succeed with this type of garden. Protect gardens and plants by spacing tubes and containers away from excessive heat, and shade all garden beds and tubes. Cool nutrient solution by setting reservoir on cool ground in a shady location. Artificially cooling nutrient solution is expensive, impractical, and environmentally unsound.

A vertical garden that consists of shelves stocked with a layer of cannabis plants in 1- to 3-gallon (3.8–11.4 L) containers is another growing option. Plants are stacked on shelves and trained to grow out and up toward lights located in the center of the room. Shelving can be placed all the way around the lamps. Containers are irrigated with spaghetti-tubing connected to individual emitters. A trough or plumbing tubes below containers carry nutrient solution back to the reservoir.

The light can be either fixed in the center of the room with shelves surrounding it, or mobile and able to move out of the way for maintenance. The latter arrangement is a lot of work to set up and maintain. Few gardeners have the time and energy to make it work properly. Several commercial, vertical, space-saving gardens are still on the market; others have been short lived. Search "vertical marijuana garden" online for more information.

An A-frame structure having growing containers on walls of both sides and a reservoir below will save space. Orient

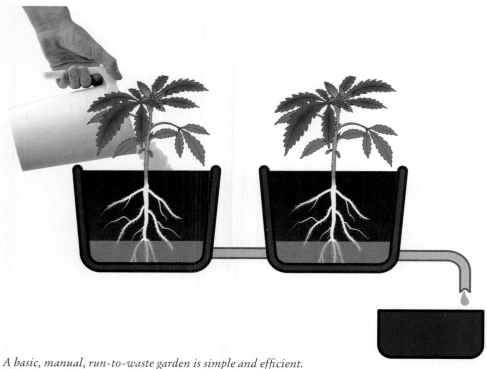

A basic, manual, run-to-waste garden is simple and efficient.

Ideal growing mediums for RTW gardens retain moisture and air well. Substrates that retain moisture and air for a long time require less-frequent watering. Often watering once a day or every few days is all that is necessary. In such gardens, simple manual irrigation is possible. A runoff of at least 20 percent is necessary to ensure a healthy root zone.

There are several inherent benefits to a RTW garden that lend themselves to hot climates and avoiding the spread of diseases. Roots are easier to keep cool on hot days because the nutrient solution is applied only once and not given a chance to recirculate and heat up. The nutrient solution can also be kept in a cool location. Keeping the root zone cool during very hot days can make an incredible difference in plant growth.

Plants can be easily isolated with a run-to-waste garden. Since the nutrient solution is applied only once and not recaptured, it can be applied to individual plants and not be recirculated and applied to all plants. In a recirculating garden, if one plant has a disease, all plants will be affected by the same disease.

Run-to-Waste (RTW) Gardens

Run-to-waste hydroponics and container gardens are among the least expensive, simplest to construct, and easiest to maintain. Many commercial flower and vegetable growers use RTW gardens. Once the nutrient solution is applied, it is absorbed by the growing medium and roots; the excess drains to waste. Used nutrient solution is not recirculated and recycled. Gardeners fertilize perennial the sides of the frame so that they receive the most light possible.

plants, lawns, and flower or vegetable gardens with the runoff nutrient solution.

A run-to-waste garden uses about the same amount of fertilizer as a recirculating garden uses. The nutrient solution is more dilute in a RTW garden. In most recirculating gardens, the nutrient solution is dumped out and changed every 5 to 7 days or the plants' waste products will overwhelm the chemistry of the solution. The solution is concentrated and imbalanced when thrown out. A run-to-waste garden expels a small amount of nutrient solution with every irrigation cycle. Regardless of origin, the "used" nutrient can be recycled to fertilize the outdoor garden. Please *do not* send the used solution down household drains! Dump it in different places outdoors in order to avoid a buildup of fertilizer salts.

A nutrient solution is applied in a run-to-waste garden, and there is reduced chance of problems with pH fluctuations, nutrient buildups, and imbalances. A consistent formula with the proper pH is applied regularly. The formula is dilute so the extra water in the solution will wash away excess salts. Fertilizer residues do not have a chance to build to toxic levels.

Manual Run-to-Waste Gardens

Manual RTW gardens with containers full of substrate will hold moisture longer and requires less-frequent irrigation. Favorite mediums for low-tech manual RTW gardens include a mix of perlite/vermiculite, horticultural-grade coco coir, and soilless mix such as Pro-Mix. Avoid low-quality coir as it tends to harbor sodium and requires heavy pre-soaking, washing, and pH correction.

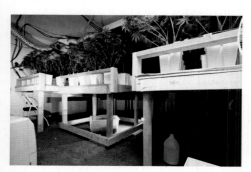

This gardener waters plants by hand so that 20 percent runs out the bottom of each container. Individual containers drain into a larger container that is lifted out and dumped in the outdoor garden.

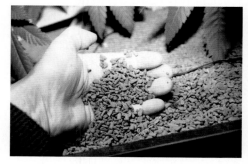

These expanded clay pellets are of different sizes and are irregular in shape. This fine grade of expanded clay pellets holds more nutrient solution for longer periods of time. It also holds plenty of air.

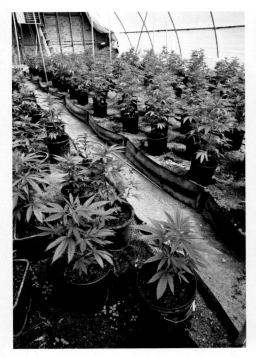

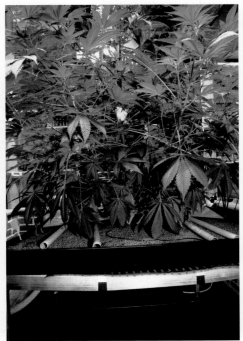

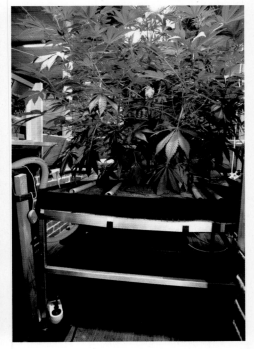

This simple run-to-waste system holds runoff water in the soil below.

This amazing run-to-waste garden is filled with small expanded clay pellets to a depth of 3 inches (7.6 cm).

These plants receive plenty of light and are irrigated with nutrient solution several times a day. As you can see, they are strong and healthy.

Five-gallon (18.9 L) containers are excellent for a low-maintenance garden. To make containers into growing containers, drill a hole as close to the bottom of the container as possible so that very little water sits on the bottom. Insert a thru-hull fitting and attach a drainage hose to the fitting or simply let the irrigation solution run out the fitting or hole into another container. Run the hose down into another container to catch the runoff that will be used in the outdoor garden. Put a screen in front of the drainage hole to keep it free of blockage.

Automated Run-to-Waste Gardens

Automated RTW gardens use a pump and timer to apply nutrient solutions more frequently at regular intervals. The gardens can be set up using the "Top-Feed Gardens" or "Ebb-and-Flow Gardens" above as a guideline. Mediums that work well with more frequent irrigations include expanded clay, coco coir, and rockwool. Algae grow on any uncovered medium with a moist surface, attracting fungus gnats, stem rot, and other problems. Rockwool, coco coir, and peat tend to stay too wet in the upper parts and too wet toward the

bottom when using large volumes in *tall* containers. But when in a low profile, slabs and cubes are much easier to keep moisture and air retention near ideal levels. Regardless of how often plants are watered, there must be at least 20 percent runoff every time.

Wick Gardens

Low-tech wick gardens have no moving parts to break or malfunction. Low initial cost and little maintenance are other positive points. These gardens consist of a container full of an absorbent growing medium such as coco coir, rockwool, or

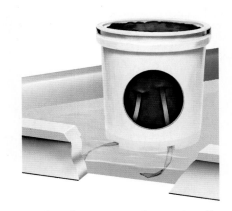

The wick in this passive garden continually draws nutrient solution up to roots.

soilless mix containing more absorbent and air-holding mediums such as peat. A wick made from cotton rope, yarn, or other absorbent material transfers nutrient solution from a reservoir to the growing medium via capillary action.

Simple low-tech wick gardens may not be well suited to the demands of fast-growing cannabis plants. If the growing medium stays too wet and soggy, it can fail to supply enough oxygen for rapid nutrient uptake.

Flood Wick Gardens

High-tech flood wick gardens rely on nutrient solution delivered manually or via a pump. These advanced wick gardens are actually half of a flood-and-drain garden. The difference is that they do not drain; nutrient solution is flooded into a growing table or area with sides to contain the liquid. The liquid is slowly absorbed by plants in containers for one to several days afterward.

Setting up a flood garden is relatively easy and inexpensive. The growing bed can be set up on a table or directly on the floor. The bed must be flat and level so that nutrient formula is available to be wicked up by all plants at the same rate. Unleveled growing beds cause plants on the low end of the table to receive more solution than those on the high end.

These flood wick gardens work best with 1- to 3-gallon (3.8–11.4 L) containers somewhat wider than they are deep. Larger containers tend to hold too much solution, which promotes soggy substrate, low oxygen levels, and root disease. Containers with holes around the bottom rim work better than pots with holes in the bottom only. Containers can be set on capillary mats.

An absorbent substrate such as rockwool or coco coir that holds plenty of air and solution is preferable for these gardens. Substrates can also be mixed together to achieve the desired ratio of air to nutrient solution. There are many variables in substrates, and giving ratios is difficult. Consult other gardeners in your area or check www.marijuanagrowing.com.

Irrigation cycles depend upon plant size, growth habit, humidity, and temperature of the growing area and substrate, as well as the depth of the irrigation solution. When plants are small and growing slowly they consume less water and nutrients and need less-frequent irrigation. In general, irrigate with enough solution to cover the bottom of the table to a depth of 0.5-inch (1.3 cm) so that all the solution is wicked up in a few hours. Increase the frequency and depth of nutrient-solution irrigation as

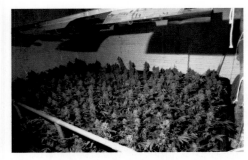

This flood garden is so crowded with plants that watering any other way is impossible.

plants' needs grow. Small plants should use the nutrient solution in 5 days or less. Medium to large plants commonly need irrigation every 2 to 5 days.

Mix nutrient solutions with a low EC and use very clean (low EC or reverse osmosis) water. Since the nutrient solution does not drain away from roots, mineral salts have a big opportunity to build up to toxic proportions. Prevent possible fertilizer salt buildup in the root zone by applying low EC solutions so that plants use nutrients before they build to toxic levels.

I have seen such gardens work quite well even though the substrate appears to stay too wet. Here is why: the higher the salinity, the moister the medium needs to be. Allowing the medium to dry out even a little bit causes ions to come out of solution and onto the medium. When water is reapplied, all the ions go back into solution, even the ones that normally are there, so noth-

ing is on the particle and the EC for a short time spikes causing damage. With proper care, this type of garden can be successful.

If porosity is correct, the medium only appears to stay wet. The reality is that water stays in the small pores and weeps to the larger ones with air. The air pores never fill up; air does not really need suction to get into the root zone with correct pores. The results are a better-watered plant than most, with a steady supply of nutrients, and the roots do not drown. However, salts can accumulate in the medium's topmost layer. The roots cannot fill the total column of medium because of this layer. The level of O_2 is not as high as it would be with suction. The ratio of available ions is skewed to reflect the leftovers.

The feeding schedule should include low EC values to avoid salt accumulation, and a fertilizer would really need to be calibrated to do better than average. This is to allow for irrigation water, plant types, life stage, and seasons.

Under high-salinity conditions it becomes critical to (1) never allow a dry-down, and (2) allow for evaporation between irrigations, which forces us to water more and more often (or further decrease the feed EC) until the roots drown or we can put nothing else in the supply water. Periodic leaching of the medium is essential.

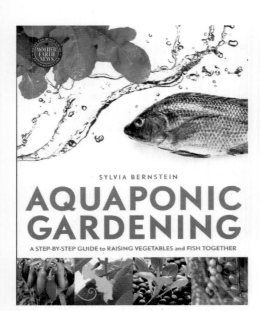

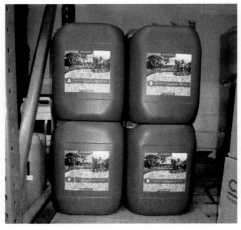

Canna A and Canna B are designed specifically for the coco that Canna sells. Designing nutrient for proprietary products has given this company a big edge for research and development.

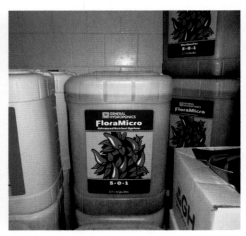

General Hydroponics produces several different formulas that are very popular among medical cannabis gardeners.

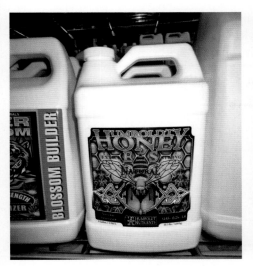

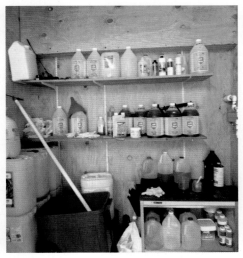

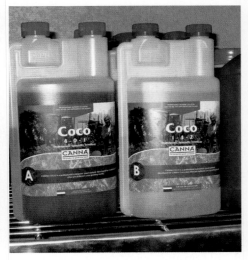

Humboldt Honey from Humboldt Nutrients is a good example of an organic-based fertilizer company that gives medical cannabis gardeners in California the mixes they want.

A clean garden area is essential. Trichome Technologies' gardeners keep all their containers organized and labeled.

Canna produces one of the many fertilizer formulas that are packaged in two parts.

Aquaponics

Aquaponics combines traditional aquaculture (raising aquatic animals) with hydroponics in a symbiotic sustainable environment. The toxic by-products in solution generated by aquatic animals are directed into a hydroponic garden. These toxins, many of which are nutrients, are filtered out and used by plants to grow. Once cleansed of toxins, the water is recirculated back to the fish, shellfish, mollusks, and so on.

Aquaponic gardens are not yet common among cannabis gardeners. The closest thing to an aquaponic garden I have seen was in the mid-1990s in Vancouver, Canada, where an eccentric grower was filtering wastes from his freshwater predatory fish tank into his container culture nutrient tank. Technically, this was only half of an aquaponic garden.

Aquaponic gardens are more complex than standalone hydroponic or container culture gardens and are beyond the scope of this book. For more current information, see *Aquaponic Gardening* by Sylvia Bernstein and check the forum on www.marijuanagrowing.com.

Hydroponic Nutrients

Nutrients are necessary for cannabis to grow. These nutrients must be broken down chemically within the plant, regardless of origin, organic or mineral.

The nutrients could be derived from natural organic bases, or they could be simple chemical elements and compounds, man-made or naturally occurring. When properly applied, each type of fertilizer, organic or chemical, theoretically produces the same results.

Soluble complete nutrients properly applied under the right conditions are immediately available for uptake. Fertilizer designed for use in soil is unsuitable for hydroponics or container gardens because it is not "complete" and does not contain all nutrients a plant needs to grow. Low-quality fertilizers contain impure components that often leave residue and sediments. These impurities build up in reservoirs, containers, and irrigation tubes and nozzles, causing extra maintenance and other problems.

Caution! These impurities will build up in the plant faster than in the soil.

Premium complete fertilizers designed for cannabis container culture and hydroponics are soluble and mixed in the proper ratios to form a balanced formula that includes all the necessary nutrients. Commercial premixed solutions are diluted or dissolved in water before use. These fertilizers come in 1, 2, 3, 4, or more parts. There is a "base" formula that separates calcium from other nutrients, all of which are soluble and dissolve in solution, but calcium will combine with

many other elements when at the right level. When united in a concentrate, the two (calcium and any other nutrient) combine, precipitating and falling to the bottom of the reservoir, unavailable to plants.* It is easy to change the ratio of the mineral elements by mixing other components of the formula to tailor the mix to the native water limitations or the plant growth stage—seedling, vegetative, and flowering. Special nutrient formulations are available for people with "hard water" that contains large amounts of calcium. For more specific information, check the fertilizer application chart provided by manufacturers.

*__Note:__ Be wary of fertilizers that separate out many nutrients into many parts. This is often done to simply increase the product line and make more income!

Purchase 1- and 2-part nutrients in powder or liquid form

Purchase 1, 2, 3+ formulations in liquid form

Soluble complete "hydroponic" fertilizers (nutrient formulas or recipes) are diverse combinations of chemical salts. Mix a predetermined amount of fertilizer concentrate with water to make a nutrient solution. The most frequently used macronutrient chemicals include potassium nitrate, calcium nitrate, potassium phosphate, and magnesium sulfate. Plant nutrients (inorganic and ionic form) are the dissolved cations (positively charged ions) Ca_2^+, Mg_2^+, and K^+. The major nutrient anions (negatively charged ions) in nutrient solutions are NO_3^- (nitrate), SO_4^{2-} (sulfate), and $H_2O_4P^-$ (dihydrogen phosphate). Micronutrients used in hydroponic formulas are Fe (iron), Mn (manganese), Cu (copper), Zn (zinc), B (boron), Cl (chlorine), and Ni (nickel). Chelating agents are regularly added so that Fe stays soluble. Plants use water and some nutrients faster than others; this changes the composition of the nutrient solution and alters the pH. Plants also give off ions such as hydrogen, which will drive the pH up and down, depending upon circumstances, as well making elements such as phosphates more soluble.

Nutrient-solution Composition

The table below is a guideline of acceptable nutrient limits for cannabis expressed in parts per million. To avert nutrient deficiencies and excesses, do not deviate too far from these ranges.

[The table below is a guideline of acceptable nutrient limits for cannabis expressed in parts per million. To avert nutrient deficiencies and excesses, do not deviate too far from these ranges.]

Solution	Vegetative Formula	Weight in Grams	
A	$CaNO_3$	3	calcium nitrate
A	KNO_3	1.044	potassium nitrate
A	TE	0.2	trace elements
B	K_2SO_4	0.23	potassium phosphate
B	KH_2PO_4	0.696	monopotassium phosphate
B	$MgSO_4$	2.24	magnesium sulfate

Main reasons nutrient deficiencies occur:

1. Low nutrient strength—not enough nutrients for plant growth

2. Imbalanced formula that lacks one or more elements

3. Missing fertilizer element or wrong element in mix

4. Balanced solution, but reactions with growing media prevent nutrient uptake

5. Balanced solution, but conditions inside plant prevent nutrient uptake

Homemade Nutrients

Gardeners who mix their own nutrients from dry components save hundreds,

EXPRESSED IN PPM	CHEMICAL	LIMITS	LIMITS	LIMITS	LIMITS
Element	Symbol	Low	Medium	High	Average
nitrogen	N	150	650	1000	250
potassium	P	100	300	400	300
phosphorus	K	50	100	100	80
calcium	Ca	100	350	500	200
magnesium	Mg	50	100	100	75
sulfur	S	200	700	1000	400
iron	Fe	2	7	10	5
manganese	Mn	0.5	3	5	2
copper	Cu	0.1	0.35	0.5	0.05
zinc	Zn	0.5	1	1	0.5
molybdenum	Mo molybdate	0.01	0.035	0.05	0.02
boron	B	0.5	3	5	1

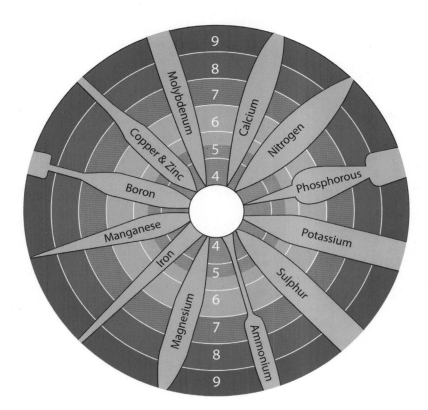

The numbers from 4 to 9 signify pH value of the nutrient solution. Nutrient availability is shown for various nutrients in different pH ranges.

Nutrient-solution pH

When grown hydroponically or when using soilless media, nutrients are available to plants within a narrow band of the pH scale; it is a slightly lower pH than for soil-grown plants. The pH is a measure of positive hydrogen ions. Plants feed via an exchange of ions. The pH changes as ions are removed from solution. Ions are taken up by roots as plants grow, which in turn causes pH to rise. Typically the ideal hydroponics and soilless media pH range is 5.5 to 6.0. Nutrient uptake diminishes quickly beyond this limited range of pH. The pH of the nutrient solution controls the availability of chemical ions that cannabis needs in order to assimilate nutrients.

The nutrient-solution pH in hydroponics is a little lower than for soil and the nutrients' availability is somewhat different too.

Check the input water before mixing hydroponic nutrients into solution. Stabilize the pH of the water before adding fertilizer. If water is "soft" with a low EC (ppm), the pH will climb, sometimes for several days after mixing in nutrients. Adding a stabilizing agent such as Cal Mag (Ca and Mg) will minimize fluctuation. "Hard" water usually contains high levels of calcium and magnesium ions, which in turn can limit availability of other nutrients.

Add fertilizer before altering pH of nutrient solution. Fertilizer salts tend to be acidic and cause the pH of the nutrient solution to fall. Follow the directions on the container for raising and lowering pH. Mix pH adjusters into the reservoir slowly and completely.

Roots take in more water than chemical salts and use the nutrients at different rates, which causes their ratios in solution to change, which in turn causes the pH to climb. When the pH is above 7.0 or below 5.5, some nutrients are not absorbed as fast as possible. Check the pH every day or two and correct with an acid or base to make sure it is within the desired range of 5.5 to 6.0.

Check the pH of the nutrient solution, growing medium, and runoff every few

often thousands, of dollars every year. Most small-scale cannabis gardeners opt to purchase expensive premade formulas from hydroponic stores. Preformulated nutrients are usually the best option for small-scale gardeners. The commercial formulas usually contains all necessary nutrients, and they are available to plants for uptake.

Look forward to at least an eightfold savings when mixing nutrients from scratch. For example, a gallon (3.8 L) of store-bought dilute nutrient (EC 2.0) costs about $0.25 USD a gallon (3.8 L). The same gallon (3.8 L) of nutrient mixed at home costs $0.03 USD a gallon (3.8 L) for two-part soluble powders.

Mix pH Up or pH Down in water for a 10 percent solution, and then use this dilute solution to adjust the nutrient solution in the reservoir. This will avoid the pH "bounce," which causes too much change followed by more change. Such dynamic change or "bouncing" is not good for the ions in solution, as it will cause issues such as precipitation and ion lockup.

Mixing and making hydroponic nutrients is relatively easy. Many variations of the nutrient formulas developed at University of California, Berkeley, by Dr. D. I. Arnon and Dr. D. R. Hoagland have been modified and are widely used today. Here is a base formula you can use and modify to fit your needs.

Working with a concentrated nutrient solution is most convenient. Make a 100X concentrate by mixing 10 times the amount for each "A" and "B" nutrient formulas in 2 separate containers.

For information on where you can buy all-in-one packs of these mix-it-yourself nutrients, visit www.homegrown.ca.

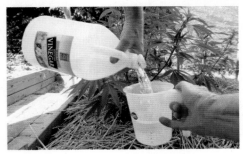

Vinegar can also be used to lower pH, but it is not as stable as phosphoric acid.

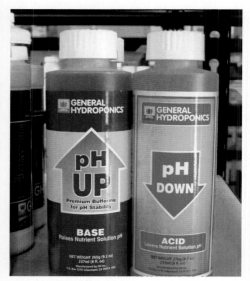

pH Up and pH Down

days, or daily if necessary. Growing medium measurements reveal the pH in the root zone. Runoff pH measurements disclose possible toxic conditions of substrate. For example, if the EC is higher in runoff water than in the nutrient solution or media, you know there is a toxic fertilizer salt buildup in the media. Correct the toxic conditions by leaching media thoroughly with diluted nutrient solution, and replace with new solution. See chapter 21, *Nutrients*, for more information on specific nutrients.

The pH of organic hydroponic gardens is the same as for any hydroponic garden. The ion availability works the same; however ideal pH range may vary because of the need for the product to morph or mineralize for availability.

Correct pH if readings vary ± half of a point. Chemical concentration to move the pH up or down varies. Consult the label on the product for dosage instructions. Use rubber gloves when handling products that alter pH. Small-scale gardeners find that purchasing pH Up and pH Down is more expensive but easier than making it yourself from concentrated acids or bases. Commercial mixes are usually buffered and safe to use.

The pH is influenced by many factors including water quality, growing medium, nutrient content, etc. Please see www.marijuanagrowing.com for more information.

pH Up

potassium hydroxide

(Do not use dangerous and caustic sodium hydroxide to raise pH!)

pH Down

nitric acid

phosphoric acid

citric acid

vinegar

Nutrient-solution EC

The concentration of the nutrient solution has an enormous effect on plant development and growth. Measuring the overall concentration or strength of a "balanced" solution is essential. Focus on nutrient balance and concentration in the solution to head off deficiencies before they cause big problems.

Fertilizers (dissolved ionic salts) conduct electrical current when in solution. The ions in an ionic compound are held together by ionic bonds. These ions "cation" (+ positive) and "anion" (– negative) have positive and negative charges that attract one another and bond. Nutrient (salts) concentrations are measured by their ability to conduct electricity through a solution. A dissolved salts meter measures the overall concentration or strength of a nutrient solution. For example, pure distilled water has no resistance and conducts virtually no electrical current. When nutrients (dissolved ionic salts) are added to pure distilled water it conducts electricity. A greater concentration of nutrients in solution conducts more electricity.

Several scales are currently used to measure how much electricity is con-

ducted by nutrients including: electrical conductivity (EC), conductivity factor (CF), parts per million (ppm), total dissolved solids (TDS), and dissolved solids (DS). Most US gardeners use ppm to measure overall fertilizer concentration. European, Australian, and New Zealand gardeners use EC, however they still use CF in parts of Australia and New Zealand.

The difference between EC, CF, ppm, TDS, and DS is more complex than originally meets the eye. See chapter 15, *Meters*, for a more detailed explanation.

Each variety of cannabis has an ideal EC range for optimum growth. Some varieties are incredibly heavy feeders while others are easy to overfertilize. Check with seed and clone vendors for details. A high EC leads to "water stress," causing plant cells to lose water. The water moves via osmotic pressure into the more concentrated solution surrounding roots. Wilting foliage is the first sign of an EC that is too high. When a mild EC overdose occurs, plants compensate and foliage growth becomes tough or hard, with brittleness to it. Foliage is often darker green, and plants are shorter and have smaller leaves.

Many commercial cannabis gardeners give their flowering crops progressively higher EC concentration. Flower buds plump up and put on weight but this practice tends to make flower buds develop a very harsh taste when smoked or vaporized due to the excess salts left in plant tissues. The residual ash is also very dark and abundant.

EC is also affected by water uptake. On hot days when more water is taken up

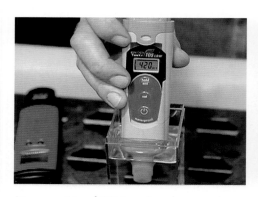

Measure pH and EC (ppm) at the same time on each testing day.

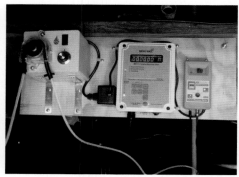

A constant readout pH meter makes keeping track of the nutrient solution much easier.

from the solution, nutrients concentrate and EC climbs. A low EC also causes more water uptake and foliage soon becomes weak and soft, often lighter green too. However, lowering EC during hot spells is essential to avoid problems. Measure EC daily and adjust accordingly in relation to growing conditions.

To check the EC of the nutrient solution, collect samples from the reservoir, growing medium, and runoff. Save time and effort: collect EC and pH samples simultaneously. Collect samples with a syringe or turkey baster used for cooking by inserting it at least two inches (5.1 cm) deep into the rockwool or growing medium. Collect separate samples of runoff and solution from the reservoir. Place each sample in a clean jar—washed and triple rinsed with double-distilled water. Use a calibrated EC meter to measure each of the samples, and record measurement on a piece of paper.

Measure the EC and pH of:
- nutrient reservoir
- substrate
- runoff

Under normal conditions, the EC in the growing medium and the runoff should be a little higher than that of the nutrient solution in the reservoir. If the EC of the solution drawn from the growing medium is substantially higher than the one from the reservoir, there is a fertilizer salt buildup in the substrate. Correct the imbalance by leaching substrate thoroughly with diluted nutrient solution, and replace with new solution. Regularly check the EC of your water, slab, and runoff.

EC Guidelines:

Growth Stage	EC Range
seedling	0.8–1.3
clone	0.5–1.3
vegetative	1.3–1.7
flowering	1.2–2

Note: These guidelines are recommendations only. Some varieties of cannabis require higher or lower EC values than listed above.

Let a minimum of 20 percent of the nutrient solution drain from growing medium after each irrigation cycle to help maintain EC stability. The runoff carries away any excess fertilizer salt buildup in the growing medium. If the EC level of a solution is too high, increase the amount of runoff so that 30 percent of the solution drains out the bottom of containers. To raise the EC, add more fertilizer to the solution, or change the nutrient solution.

Many factors can alter the EC balance of a solution, such as irrigation, evaporation, and nutrient uptake by roots. For example, if the substrate is underwatered or allowed to dry completely, the EC reading will rise. In fact, the EC may increase to two or three times as high as the input solution when too little water is applied to rockwool. This increase in slab EC causes some nutrients to build up faster than others. When the EC doubles, the amount of sodium can increase as much as four to six times under the right conditions! There should not be any sodium present in your garden unless it is in the water supply, and it should not be in excess of 50 ppm.

Nutrient-solution concentration levels are also affected by roots' nutrient absorption and by water evaporation. The solution weakens as plants use nutrients, but water also evaporates from the solution, which increases the nutrient concentration. Counteract the concentration of fertilizer salts by regularly adding plain water to the nutrient solution to replace what has been used by plants.

Dissolved Oxygen

Dissolved oxygen (DO) in solution is essential for nutrient uptake by the root system. Nutrient solutions hold more dissolved oxygen at lower temperatures, and the solutions ability to carry oxygen diminishes as temperatures rise. For example, well-aerated nutrient solution holds 8 to 10 ppm of oxygen between 60°F and 80°F (15.6°C–26.7°C). At 60°F (15.6°C) 10 milligrams per liter (MPL) or 10 ppm is held in solution. But at 80°F (26.7°C) only 8 MPL (8 ppm) of oxygen is available—20 percent less. Deadly *Pythium* loves temperatures above 60°F (15.6°C). *Pythium* is always present but only deadly when it gets out of hand.

Large flowering cannabis plants growing under optimal conditions require 10 ppm of dissolved oxygen. Maintaining high DO levels in solution requires close vigilance of temperature and constant replenishment of oxygen.

Keep nutrient-solution temperature between 60°F and 70°F (15.6°C–21.1°C) to help ensure adequate dissolved oxygen. Never let nutrient-solution temperature climb above 85°F (29.4°C), because its oxygen-holding ability plummets. Once roots weaken, they are easily damaged and susceptible to rot, wilts, and fungus gnat attacks at above 85°F (29.4°C).

The respiration rate of roots doubles between 68°F and 86°F (20°C–30°C). But the ability of the solution to hold dissolved oxygen will drop within this temperature range by more than 25 percent. This causes DO in solution to become depleted at a much higher rate and oxygen starvation then occurs. Organic microbial life also requires oxygen to sustain life and grow. Conversely an increase in nutrient-solution temperature lowers the availability of oxygen. Roots suffocate in low-oxygen environments, causing growth to slow and eventually stop.

When air is cooler than water, moisture rapidly evaporates into the air; the greater the temperature differential, the higher the relative humidity. Maintaining the nutrient-solution temperature around 60°F (15.6°C) will help control transpiration and humidity.

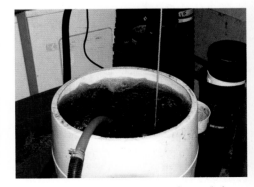

Aerating this organic nutrient solution helps keep microbes and other life flourishing.

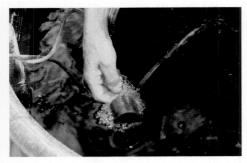

An air pump submerged in the reservoir not only aerates the solution, it will help level out the temperature differential between ambient air and the reservoir.

Solution-based gardens such as NFT, wick, and aeroponic, are extremely sensitive to DO depletion. The air-holding ability of the substrate in media-based gardens offers another source of oxygen, but these gardens are not immune to rapid DO depletion.

Oxygen depletion and starvation symptoms are often general and difficult to diagnose. The first sign is often wilting when midday temperatures climb. Roots' ability to draw in water and nutrients diminishes, slowing the rate of photosynthesis and growth. As malnourishment continues, nutrient deficiencies surface, roots die back and plants become stunted. When severe, anaerobic conditions occur and plants

start producing the hormone ethylene in reaction to stress.

Oxygen starvation causes leaf epinasty, a downward curving of leaf edges. The leaves yellow prematurely when severe. Avoid *Pythium* and other problems associated with lack of oxygen in the root zone by aerating the solution and keeping it in the proper temperature range.

Increase Dissolved Oxygen

Let runoff solution cascade or fall back into the reservoir to introduce more oxygen into solution. The higher the waterfalls to the reservoir, the more oxygen is introduced. Fountains, air pumps, and diffusers (including air stones) break air into smaller bubbles to oxygenate irrigation water more. Use an air pump to add extra oxygen to the nutrient solution. Attach an air stone diffuser to the outlet to break up and multiply bubbles.

Save energy and money by heating cold nutrient solution instead of the air in a room. Use a submersible aquarium heater or grounded propagation heating cables. The heaters might take a day or longer to raise the temperature of a large volume of solution. Do not leave heaters in an empty reservoir. They will soon overheat and burn out. Aquarium heaters seldom have ground wires, a seemingly obvious oversight. But I have yet

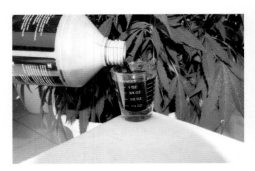

Use an accurate, easy-to-read container to measure out nutrient dosage.

to learn of an electrocution by aquarium heater. Avoid submersible heaters that give off harmful residues.

Solution Mixing and Maintenance

If possible, get a water analysis before water is mixed with hydroponic nutrients. A water analysis will indicate the dissolved ionic salts already in solution. Hard water contains elevated levels of calcium and magnesium. Both elements should be added sparingly to nutrient solutions. Soft water has very few impurities (ionic salts) that cause pH to fluctuate, requiring chemical buffers, usually calcium and calcium compounds, to be added to solution. If no water analysis is available from your local water district, a simple EC reading will measure

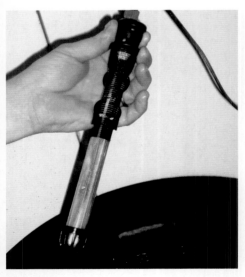

An inexpensive aquarium heater will warm a reservoir by a few degrees in 24 hours. Always purchase a heater that is big enough for the reservoir. Do not let the reservoir run dry when the heater is on, or the heater will burn out!

PERCENTAGE OF OXYGEN IN WATER		FRESH WATER MG/L	
Temperature Fahrenheit	Temperature Celsius	Sea Level	2,000 ft Elevation
50°F	10°C	11.3	10.5
59°F	15°C	10.1	9.4
68°F	20°C	9.1	8.4
72°F	22°C	8.7	8.1
75°F	24°C	8.4	7.8
79°F	26°C	8.1	7.5
83°F	28°C	7.8	7.3
86°F	30°C	7.5	7

Note: Milligrams per liter (mg/L) is approximately equivalent (~) to parts per million (ppm).
(10 mg/L ~ 10 ppm)

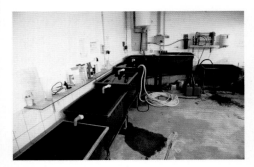

Small reservoirs are easier to manage than large tanks. This ingenious series of reservoirs along a wall uses gravity to keep them all full. Individual reservoirs can be bypassed, drained, and cleaned.

MINIMUM RESERVOIR SIZE

Garden	Size in feet	Size in meters	Gallons	Liters
flood-and-drain	4 × 8	1.2 × 2.4	100	400
top-feed	4 × 8	1.2 × 2.4	100	400
wick	4 × 8	1.2 × 2.4	50	200
DWC	4 × 8	1.2 × 2.4	200	800
NFT	4 × 8	1.2 × 2.4	100	400

the overall concentration of dissolved solids (ionic salts) in native water. If growing hydroponically and EC is 0.3 or higher, treat water with reverse osmosis before adding nutrients. See chapter 20, *Water*, for more information.

Plants use so much water in relation to nutrients that nutrient solutions need to be replenished regularly. Casually topping off the reservoir with pH-balanced water daily will keep the solution relatively balanced for a week, maybe two. Use an electronic EC pen to monitor the level of dissolved solids in the solution. Occasionally you will need to add more fertilizer concentrate to maintain the EC level in the reservoir during topping off. Keep the reservoir full at all times. The smaller the reservoir, the more rapid the depletion and the more critical it is to keep it full. Employing an automatic filling function for smaller reservoirs will help ensure a balanced nutrient solution. A few gardeners top off the nutrient solution with 500- to 600-ppm-strength nutrient solution every 2 to 3 days. If topping off with nutrient solution, keep the EC within safe limits. Avoid problems by draining the reservoir and adding fresh solution regularly.

Most gardeners leach the entire system with weak nutrient solution for an hour or more between changes of the reservoir. Leaching with a mild fertilizer solution avoids an absence of nutrients for any amount of time. But, the EC will still drop to the levels the medium is leached with which removes all the excess, resets the ratio, and ensures that the plant has nutrients at all times.

Check EC of reservoir, growing medium, and runoff nutrient solution at the same time every day. Check solution temperature to ensure that adequate dissolved oxygen is available to plants.

Reservoirs

Reservoirs should be opaque, as large as possible, and have a lid to lessen evaporation, prevent algae growth, and keep debris out of the system. Paint the exterior of reservoirs black or an opaque color to exclude light and stop algae growth. Spray paints are packed with plant-unfriendly chemicals; make sure to keep paint on the outside of the reservoir.

A fast-growing flowering plant in an ideal indoor garden can process a gallon (3.8 L) or more of nutrient solution daily. Ten maturing plants need at least 10 gallons (38 L) of water or more daily. Cannabis consumes a greater percentage of water than the percentage of nutrients from the solution. Simple arithmetic tells us that a 100-gallon (380 L) reservoir depletes at least 10 percent, 10 gallons (38 L) daily, which concentrates nutrients. Measuring EC daily will give a closer estimate of the solution's overall concentration.

A large reservoir and volume of nutrient solution will minimize nutrient imbalances and help ensure that plenty of oxygen is available to roots. A large volume of nutrient solution tends to have a more stable temperature, which in turn helps keep the dissolved oxygen

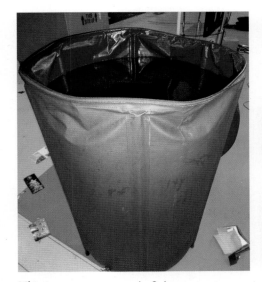

This is a pop-up reservoir. It is easy to store and holds a large volume of solution.

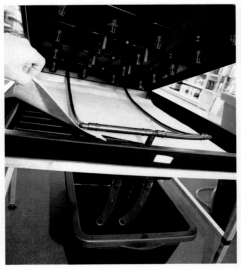

A capillary mat is set under the net pots in this garden. The capillary mat will hold moisture longer so roots will not dry out. Drain holes in the bottom of the table allow excess solution to drain freely.

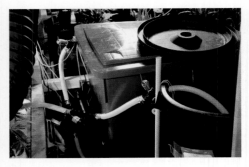

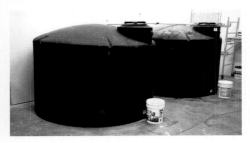

Both feeding hoses in this automated irrigation system have easy-to-clean filters.

Big preformed reservoirs make large amounts of nutrient solution available. They also make it easy to mix and control the chemistry of the solution. These reservoirs require more space to transport and subsequently house in the garden.

in the solution more constant. As plants use water, the concentration of elements in the solution increases; there is less water in the solution and nearly the same amount of nutrients. Add water daily or when the solution level drops more than 5 percent. The reservoir should contain at least 50 percent more nutrient solution than it takes to fill flood-and-drain beds to compensate for daily use and evaporation. The greater the volume of nutrient solution, the more forgiving the system and the easier it is to control.

Install a float valve to automatically replenish reservoirs with water. A float valve or Mariotte's bottle will turn water on to fill the reservoir when the level drops. Check the level of the reservoir daily and replenish if necessary. Forgetting to replenish the water supply and nutrient solution as necessary will cause slow growth and could result in crop failure.

A 2-part nutrient solution is mixed before application. Each reservoir holds 1 part of the solution. However, many professional growers avoid such systems, citing that both parts of the nutrient solution should be present together for a while to stabilize pH and overall chemistry of the mix. Typically, mixing an hour before use provides enough time for stabilization.

If the reservoir does not have graduated measurements to denote liquid volume, use an indelible marker to make a "full" line and the number of gallons or liters contained at that point on the inside of the reservoir tank. Use this volume measure when mixing nutrients.

Set reservoirs below growing beds so recycled nutrient solution can use gravity-flow or be siphoned into a receptacle or the outdoor garden. Drains and pumps should be as big as possible. Most hydroponic reservoirs are built of plastic, but other materials have been used, including concrete, glass, metal, vegetable solids, and wood. Nonreactive plastic is still the preferred choice because other materials could react with the solution.

Clean reservoirs completely after harvesting each crop. Add 1 cup of household vinegar per 5 gallons (23.7 cl per 18.9 L) and let the solution sit overnight to dissolve built-up salts and scum. Drain solution, and scrub reservoir with soap and water. Rinse with plain water to remove residues before refilling. Apple cider vinegar is the least expensive

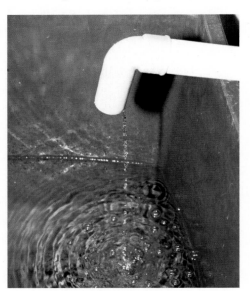

Nutrient solution is aerated when falling through the air while returning to the reservoir.

but there are also commercial products available.

Aeration

Extra aeration is always good for nutrient solutions, especially when gravity gives it to us for free. Nutrient solution is aerated by falling through the air when it returns to the reservoir. Hydroponic and container culture gardens can use the

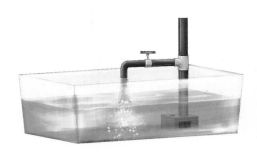

Attach a recirculating pipe with an on/off valve to the pump outlet pipe. This is a convenient, inexpensive, and easy-to-control method of aerating the nutrient solution. Add a water breaker head, similar to a showerhead, with many small holes to increase aeration.

fall of a return solution or fountain, to take advantage of this simple and free aeration principle.

Reservoir aeration is essential in solution culture. Simple gravity and recirculating pipes are not enough to ensure adequate oxygenation of nutrient solution. Make use of an air pump to diffuse air and subsequently guarantee adequate levels of oxygen.

Nutrient-Solution Pumps

Pumps are either submersible or non-submersible. Submersible pumps pump solution from inside a reservoir. Non-submersible pumps are either platform or external, located outside the reservoir. The base of a platform pump stands in the water; the motor and pump stand above the solution and remain dry. Platform pumps are usually inexpensive, and many are not designed specifically to pump nutrient solution.

Always purchase high-quality sealed pumps, especially if they are to be submerged in a nutrient reservoir. Submersible pumps must run cool so they

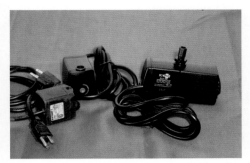

Inexpensive hydroponic pumps can be found at garden centers and aquarium stores.

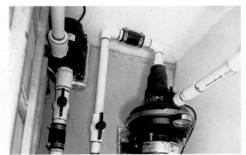

This one-horsepower high-pressure pump supplies the pressure to move nutrient solution through a warehouse garden.

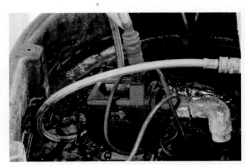

Pumps and plumbing often collect residues when pumping organic fertilizers. Make sure to use a pump that is strong enough to handle the extra weight and volume from the organic fertilizer.

BASIC GUIDELINES FOR PUMP SIZE

GPH	LPH	Plants Watered	USD
30	115	1	$15
70	265	2	$15
90	340	2	$20
190	720	4	$45
240	910	6	$50
350	1325	8	$60
500	1890	10	$100
700	2650	12	$115
950	3600	16	$140
1250	4800	20	$130

do not heat the nutrient solution. They also must be reliable and hermetically sealed so that no internal lubricants leak and contaminate the solution.

The pump needs to be large enough to supply all the demand necessary. The nutrient solution must be lifted a few feet from the reservoir to the growing bed or table. The pump must create enough flow to fill flood-and-drain tables within a few minutes. Microirrigation systems also need adequate flow and pressure through the delivery manifold, spaghetti-tubing drippers, and nozzles. A more powerful pump is also required to lift the nutrient solution, which is heavier and thicker than water.

Caution! Overdriving and burning out a pump is easy when there is no head (backpressure caused by height or restrictions against flow) or when solution viscosity is too high. Most pumps used in hydroponic gardens are fountain or water garden pumps designed to move pure water against a small head. The

more fertilizer added, especially heavy organic nutrients, the higher the viscosity and the harder the pump works. Overcome this obstacle by using a larger pump than "normally" necessary.

Pumps that run on 12-volt direct current (DC) batteries need 12-volt timers and wiring. Deep cell batteries used in golf carts and for power outboard boat motors or marine motors are designed to hold electricity for a long time. Use a solar charger to charge batteries in remote gardens.

Remember the following when installing a new irrigation system. All plumbing pipes and tubes should be opaque or dark in color to stop light from entering and thus prevent algae growth. A handle and stand on larger pumps make them easy to move and mount into a fixed position. A removable foam filter on the intake of submersible pumps removes particles that could clog the impeller and feeder tubes.

AIR PUMPS

Air/GPH	Reservoir/Gallons
320	20
340	20
600	40
800	50

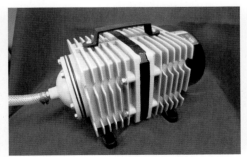

An air pump is easy to set up, but it will make a bit of noise.

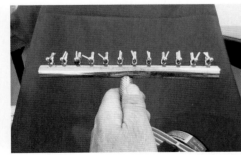

Attach a manifold to the air pump so that air can be dispersed via many different tubes.

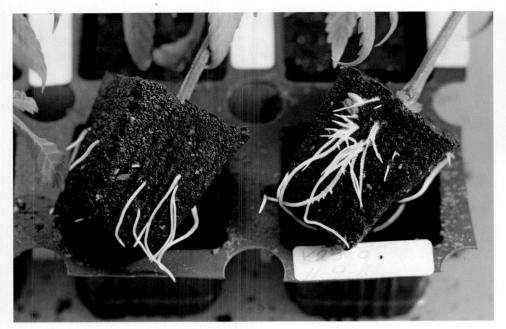

These plants are ready to be transplanted into larger containers. (MF)

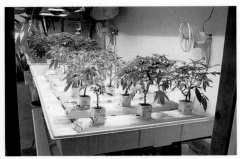

This substrate (rockwool cubes and slabs) has excellent texture, holding both air and nutrient solution.

Air Pumps

Use an air pump when simple gravity aeration does not supply enough oxygen to solution. Air pumps inject air into the nutrient solution, increasing the dissolved oxygen (DO) level. The outlet to the air pump is often attached to an air stone to diffuse or break the air into tiny bubbles. Or air is separated into many small tubes via a manifold before being injected into the solution.

Caution! Air in such gardens should be drawn from outside CO_2-enriched areas to avoid CO_2 combining with Ca to form carbonates and drive the pH up. This is a problem in all air diffusion systems because CO_2 dissolves more readily in water and will drive out O_2 as it competes for available dissolution space in the water, which is limited by pressure and temperature.

Growing Mediums

Hydroponic and container culture substrates provide support for root systems, and they hold oxygen, water, and nutrients. The ratio of oxygen to nutrient solution is a key factor in determining nutrient uptake by roots. Three main factors contribute to cannabis roots' ability to grow and absorb nutrients in a substrate: pH, texture, and nutrient content.

Substrate pH must be within the desired range of 5.5 to 6.0 for optimum nutrient uptake. For best results, monitor pH daily or perpetually and control with pH Up and pH Down. See "Nutrient-solution pH" in this chapter for related information. Substrates such as rockwool must be treated (soaked) in a determined pH solution in order to fall within proper pH parameters. See "Popular Substrates" for more specific information.

Texture

The texture of any substrate is governed by the size and physical structure of the particles that constitute it. Proper texture promotes strong root penetration, oxygen retention, nutrient uptake, and drainage. Growing mediums that consist of large particles permit good aeration and drainage. Increased irrigation frequency is necessary to compensate for low water retention. Water- and air-holding ability and root penetration are a function of texture. The smaller the particles, the closer they pack together and the slower they drain. Larger particles drain faster and retain more air in between.

Irregularly shaped substrates such as perlite and some expanded clays have more surface area and hold more water than round substrates. Avoid crushed

gravel with sharp edges that cut into roots if the plant falls or is jostled around. Round pea gravel; smooth, washed gravel; and lava rocks are excellent mediums to grow cannabis in an active recovery garden. Thoroughly wash clay and rock growing mediums to get out all the dust that will turn to sediment in the system. Fibrous materials like vermiculite, peat moss, rockwool, and coconut coir retain large amounts of moisture within their cells. Such substrates also work well in passive gardens that operate via capillary action.

Mineral growing mediums such as coco coir and peat moss (and rockwool*) are not inert; often they are mistakenly classified as inert growing mediums. They react in solution and supply minerals as they break down, which in turn affects the CEC and moves the pH.

*Rockwool is *not* inert until it is *treated*.

Non-inert growing mediums (mineral and organic) are not hydroponic substrates, and may cause unforeseen problems when minerals and organic substances react chemically with water and supplemental nutrients. Two examples: gravel from a limestone quarry is full of calcium carbonate, and old concrete is full of lime. When mixed with water, calcium carbonate will raise the pH, and it is very difficult to make it go down. Growing mediums made of reconstituted concrete bleed out so much lime that they soon kill the garden. Substrates composed of organic material that is still decomposing will interact with nutrient solutions, altering nutrient availability and pH. These substrates also compact, which eliminates many of the air-filled pores. Even substrates designed to hold air and absorb moisture lose effectiveness when overwatered.

Avoid substrates found within a few miles (km) of an ocean, sea, or large body of salt water. Most likely, such mediums are laden with toxic salts. Rather than washing and leaching salts from the medium, it is easier and more economical to find another source of substrate.

Oxygen is contained in the pores of growing media. Fresh air is drawn into the root zone as nutrient solution drains from the growing medium; that is if the medium is not overwatered or saturated. Oxygen must be replenished habitually to keep up with root tissue needs. The oxygen content in a substrate is essential to a healthy root zone and nutrient uptake. But "oxygen use" is probably the most difficult concept for many container culture and hydroponic gardeners to master.

One of the best ways to maintain high oxygen levels in the root zone is by using proper irrigation techniques. Make sure air-filled pores in substrates are allowed to drain completely between irrigation cycles. Overwatering is one of the main reasons for lack of oxygen to roots.

The duration that nutrient solution is held in a substrate is dependent upon the cation exchange capacity (CEC). Substrates with a high CEC hold nutrient solutions in their ionic form longer than substrates with a low CEC. Nutrient solution is more difficult to leach from substrates with a high CEC rating. Hydroponic mediums with a low CEC offer more exacting control because nutrients can be leached quickly and replaced with new nutrient solution with a different formula. See chapter 18, *Soil*, for more information on CEC.

Buyer beware! There are many over-priced hydroponic growing mediums with "special" qualities. I have seen more than one "new" grow medium hit and miss the marketplace. My best advice is to properly use a tried-and-true medium.

The best way to buy substrate is to go to the manufacturer. It is impossible to ascertain what the values of a soil or soilless mix are by simple written description.

For example, peat vermiculite will depend on the grade and type of peat as well as the vermiculite used by size and age. You need to physically examine the product, like Pro Mix BX or a 3:1 peat perlite mix. The manufacturer will include airspace as well, based on the medium. Usually they list values based on size of the particle. Pro-Mix BX is the typical mix (www.pthorticulture.com).

Popular Substrates

Expanded clay pellets and rockwool are the most common substrates in hydroponics. Soilless mixes and coconut coir are the most popular growing mediums used to grow cannabis in container culture. Peat (Jiffy pellets), Oasis, and small rockwool cubes are the most popular growing mediums used to start clones and seedlings.

Brick shards (not inert) have similar properties to gravel. They have the added disadvantages of possibly altering the pH and requiring extra cleaning before reuse.

Caution! They can cause heavy metal contamination due to poor sources of clay.

Coconut fiber (not inert) also called coco peat, palm peat, coir, coco(s), and kokos is coconut pith, the fiber part just under the heavy husk of a coconut. It is the by-product after the fibrous shell (bolster) has been removed from the coconut. Pith is soaked in water for up to 9 months to remove salts, natural resins, and gums in a process called retting. The retted, straw-brown fiber is beaten to extract the husk. Low-quality, poorly processed coconut fiber may contain undesirable elements (primarily salts) that have not been extracted. Quality coconut coir is guaranteed to have sodium content of less than 50 ppm. Some of the best coconut coir

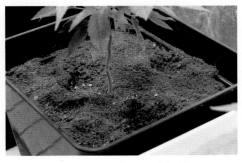
Coco substrate is absorbent and holds air.

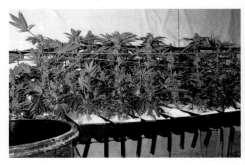
Coco is available in slabs.

is from the interior of the Philippines, where the environment is not heavy with coastal salts.

Darker coco is typically mature at harvest and contains tough, durable lignins and cellulose. It degrades slowly and provides good aeration and solution-holding ability. Coco that is lighter in color generally signifies immature fibers with poor structure that break down quicker and provide less aeration.

To test coco for salts, see Canna's "Coco Infopaper," available for download at http://other.canna.com/media. The "Coco InfoPaper" is outstanding and tells you everything you need to know and do to measure coco root environment for EC and pH.

Quality coir has an appearance and texture similar to peat moss, but coco fiber is tougher and coarser than peat moss and difficult to overwater. The nearly perfect air-to-water ratio of coir compacts very little during the course of a single crop.

Horticultural grade coco is available loose in bags, pressed into bricks, or compressed into slabs and covered in plastic. The fibers can be found in long strands, coarse chopped, and fine chopped, all of which can also be mixed together to provide different air- and solution-holding abilities.

Use coir in containers by itself or mix 50/50 with perlite, expanded clay pellets, or other mediums to add air and drainage to the mix. Coarse, fast-draining coco is often used in lieu of peat moss. Containers full of coco should be low profile because coir holds so much solution that gravity will concentrate liquids in the lower portion of the medium. This creates an uneven ratio of solution to air within the container. Low-profile plastic-covered slabs are very popular and easy to use. See "Top-Feed Gardens" on page 421 for more information.

Washed and pressed blocks or bricks are easy to store and transport and are very popular among outdoor gardeners. Bricks weigh about 1.3 to 2.2 pounds (0.6–1 kg) and typically the pH is between 5.5 and 7.0. To wet, flake dry bricks of coconut coir apart by hand or soak the bricks in a bucket of water for 15 minutes. One brick will expand to about 9 times its original size.

Treating Coco

Often coconut coir must be "conditioned" or "treated" before use. Conditioning usually requires soaking coir in a pH altering solution for a length of time to bring the pH to a neutral 7.0. Check with coir manufacturers or suppliers for more information about specific products.

Unlike most coco, coco sold by Canna and some other companies is colonized with *Trichoderma* fungi that protect

roots and stimulate their growth. It also teams with naturally occurring growth hormones and other biostimulants.

The low cation exchange capacity (CEC) of the coir fiber also helps to reduce incidence of salt burn. The minerals stored in spongelike particles are released over time when roots are able to readily absorb them. However, it does store some anions such as phosphates and sulfates. Coco also offers some buffering against positively charged ions such as sodium.

Coir has a good anion exchange capacity (AEC) and holds onto negatively charged particles. AEC is related to CEC, the measurement of the positive charges in soils that affects the amount of negative charges a soil is able to absorb. Few anions are restrictive in cannabis cultivation, but they are important. For example it will hold phosphate well but not more common nutrients such as calcium, magnesium, etc. This bit of chemistry makes fertilizers containing much phosphorus an issue when overapplied, especially early on during the growth cycle. The AEC usually drops when pH decreases, and rises when pH increases.

Coco fiber can be reused, but it may compact a little. It should also be sterilized or treated to remove any signs of pests and diseases it might be harboring. When reusing any growing media, impurities such as sodium tend to accumulate over time. Check with manufacturers and suppliers for specific guidelines for reusing coco fiber products.

Visit the Canna site (www.canna.com) for detailed information about growing cannabis in coco. See "Coconut Fiber" under "Soil Amendments" in chapter 18, *Soil*, for more information.

Expanded clay pellets (inert) are sold under different names, including expanded clay aggregate, Hydroton, GroRocks, Hydrokorrels, Geolite, and LECHA. Expanded clay pellets are inert and typically pH neutral. They are environmentally friendly, made from naturally occurring clay. Fired and sometimes tumbled in a rotary kiln at 2,190°F (1,198.9°C), clay expands like porous popcorn with a protective shell. Many little catacomb-like pockets form inside each pellet; these pockets hold air and nutrient solution. Shapes are irregular or uniform, and size ranges from 0.8 to 2 inches (20.3–50.8 mm) depending upon the manufacturing process.

This lightweight substrate does not compact over a long lifetime, and it can be reused. Once used, separate the clay pellets from roots and other substrate. Pour expanded clay pellets into a container and soak them in a sterilizing solution of 0.3 ounces (10 ml) hydrogen peroxide per 1.1 gallon (4 L) of water, or 5 percent chlorine bleach or white vinegar. Soak for 20 to 30 minutes. Remove expanded clay and place on a screen of hardware cloth. Wash clay pellets thoroughly with clean water and separate them from remaining dead roots and dust. Let pellets dry and then reuse them. Always reuse!

Caution! Avoid using expanded clay made for the construction of tall buildings, which is not inert and is often full of undesirable substances. This expanded clay also tends to bleed a lot of heavy clay dust that collects in the garden and could contain pollutants.

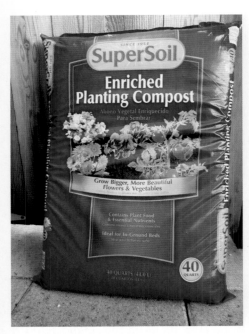

Store-bought compost is available at most garden centers.

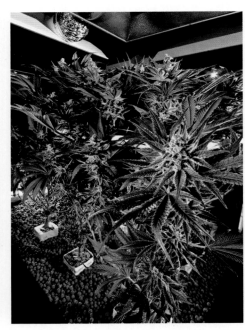

Expanded clay pellets are an excellent medium to mix with Peat-Lite and other soilless mixes in container culture. I like the way it drains so well yet still retains nutrient solution while holding lots of oxygen.

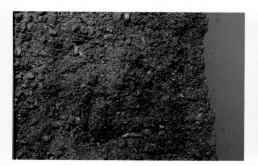
Fine-grade peat moss

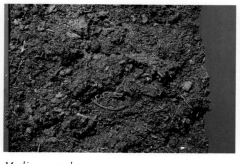
Medium-grade peat moss

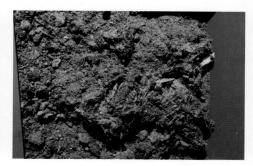
Coarse-grade peat moss

Gravel (not inert) is heavy but inexpensive and easy to keep clean. It holds plenty of air and drains well. Gravel has low water retention and low buffering ability. But it is difficult to overwater and is suited to continuous irrigation. It holds moisture, nutrients, and oxygen on its outer surfaces. Use pea gravel or washed river gravel with round edges that do not cut roots when jostled about. Avoid using crushed rock with sharp edges. Gravel should be 0.125 to 0.375 inches (3.2–9.5 mm) in diameter, with more than half of the medium about 0.25 inches (6 mm) across. Presoak and adjust pH before use.

To reuse, follow guidelines outlined under "Expanded Clay."

Oasis is rigid, open-celled, water-absorbing, phenolic foam. It is designed for optimum callus formation and rapid root growth of clones and seedlings. Oasis rooting cubes have a neutral pH and hold more than 40 times their weight in water. Plus, the water is drawn into the foam by wicking action. Transplant versatile Oasis cubes into any hydroponic medium.

Once used, Oasis cubes lose structure and cannot be cleaned, disinfected, and reused.

Peat moss (not inert) is partially decomposed vegetation. Its decay has been slowed by the cold, wet conditions and low pH of the northern latitudes where it is found in vast bogs. It consists of long strands of highly adsorbent, spongelike material that holds water while simultaneously having good aeration. Water adsorbs onto a peat particle and is not spongelike. Peats are harvested and used to amend soil or soilless mix; they can be used as a growing medium.

There are three common kinds of peat moss: sphagnum, hypnum, and reed/sedge. Sphagnum peat, the most commonly used peat moss, is light-brown and is about 75 percent fiber with a pH of 3.0 to 4.0. This bulky peat gives soil body and retains water well, absorbing 15 to 30 times its own weight. It contains essentially no nutrients of its own, and its pH ranges from 3.0 to 5.0.

After sphagnum moss decomposes for several months, pH could continue to drop and become very acidic. Counter this propensity for acidity and stabilize the pH by adding fine dolomite lime to the mix. Peat adsorbs water by its clinging to the outer portions of the very small stem and leaves and does not absorb it into the tissues of the plant parts.

Hypnum peat is more decomposed and darker in color, with about 50 percent fiber and a pH of about 6.0. This peat moss is less common and contains some nutrients. Hypnum peat is a good soil amendment even though it cannot hold as much water as sphagnum moss can.

Reed/sedge peat is about 35 percent fiber with a pH of 6.0 or more. This peat holds less water and air and is more difficult to find commercially.

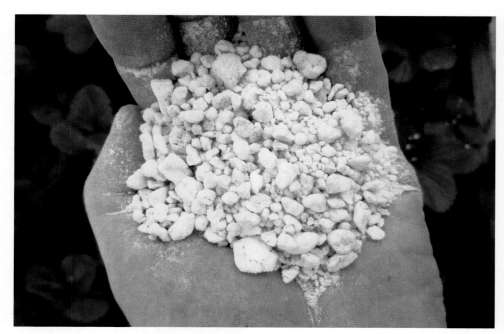
Perlite is available in three main grades: fine, medium, and coarse. Most gardeners prefer the coarse grade as a soil amendment for container planting and outdoor planting. The fine grade is best to use when making a seedling mix. To keep it from floating and stratifying, lightweight perlite should make up less than one third of any mix.

Peat moss is typically bone dry and difficult to wet the first time. Wet peat is heavy and awkward to transport. When adding peat moss as a soil amendment, cut your workload by dry-mixing all of the components before wetting. Lightly sprinkle with water to quell dust, and use a wetting agent.

Another trick to mixing peat moss is to kick the sack a few times to break up the bale before opening.

Purchase peat in dry, compressed blocks, or bails. Peat moss must be soaked in water for approximately an hour to become completely wet before use. Two drops of natural liquid dish soap per gallon (3.8 L) will ensure thorough wetting.

Peat mixed half and half with perlite is one of the all-time favorite growing mediums. It is also an excellent soil amendment. Sphagnum peat moss is a major ingredient in many potting soils and soilless mixes.

Avoid reusing peat, because it compacts. Also, it decomposes over time and sheds small particles that can plug pumps, irrigation lines, and emitters. For more information, see "Soil Amendments" in chapter 18, *Soil*.

Perlite (inert) is sand or volcanic glass that has been superheated and expanded by heat. It holds water and nutrients on its many irregular surfaces, and it drains fast, but it's very light and tends to float when flooded with water. Perlite has no buffering capacity and is best used to aerate soil or soilless mix.

Perlite can be reused once sterilized, but it tends to disintegrate and become smaller.

Caution! Perlite may contain high levels of fluoride (F), which is toxic to plant foliage. See "Soil Amendments" in chapter 18.

Polyurethane grow slabs (inert) have approximately 75 to 80 percent airspace and 15 percent water-holding capacity. As this substrate is so new, very little information is available about it. Cannabis is an accumulator plant that may absorb petroleum-based styrene and pass it to the consumer. Few gardeners use it to cultivate medicinal cannabis.

Polystyrene packaging peanuts are inexpensive, readily available, and have excellent drainage. They are very lightweight and float when mixed with other elements. The same health precautions are applicable to peanuts as to polyurethane slabs.

Do not use biodegradable packing peanuts. They will decompose into sludge.

Rice hulls (not inert) are underutilized by cannabis gardeners even though they are as effective as perlite. A by-product of rice production is commonly used in compost mixes, rice hulls can be very inexpensive through a good source. This free-draining medium has low to moderate water-holding capacity, a slow rate of decomposition, and a low level of nutrients.

Check the origin and storage condition for rice hulls. They are often stored outdoors and, when uncovered, rice hulls are subject to the forces of nature and pollution. They also have a tendency toward salt buildup. Make sure to sterilize rice hulls before use. They decompose

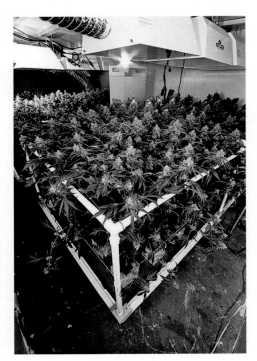

Rockwool cubes

after one or two crops, so avoid reusing rice hulls.

Rockwool, also called stonewool or mineral wool (inert once treated), is an exceptional growing medium and popular among indoor cannabis gardeners. It is a sterile, fibrous, porous, nondegradable growing medium that provides firm root support. Rockwool has the ability to hold adequate levels of both water and air for roots. Roots are able to draw in most of the water stored in the rockwool, but it has no buffering capacity and a naturally high pH. To become inert, rockwool must be treated—soaked in a low pH solution prior to use. Popular brand names in horticulture include Grodan, HydroGro, and Vacrok.

Rockwool is made from molten rock, basalt or 'slag' that is spun into bundles of single filament fibers and bonded into a medium capable of capillary action. It has proven its efficiency and effectiveness as a commercial hydroponic substrate. Fibers run vertically on blocks and horizontally on slabs. Fiber orientation affects air- and solution retention.

Check with specific manufacturers and suppliers for reuse guidelines.

Caution! Use rockwool designed for horticulture only! Do not use rockwool that is designed for insulation, sound-proofing, or filtration, since these typically have all kinds of bad stuff in them, including metals that can bleed into the nutrient solution and accumulate in cannabis plant tissue.

Pumice (not inert) is a naturally occurring, porous, lightweight volcanic rock that holds moisture and air in catacomb-like surfaces. Light and easy to work with, some lava rock is so light that it floats. Be careful that sharp edges on the rocks do not damage roots. Lava rock acts similarly to expanded clay. See "Pumice" in chapter 18, *Soil*.

To reuse follow guidelines outlined in the "Expanded Clay" section.

Sand (not inert) is heavy, inexpensive and readily available. It has no buffering ability. Some sand has a high pH. The best sand to use is a grade known as

#2 mortar in the USA. If it or a similar type is not available, use sharp river sand. These sands have irregular and sharper edges that avoid compacting, thereby creating better airspace. Do not use ocean, sea, or salty beach sand. Sand drains quickly, retains some moisture, and is very slow to decompose. Sterilize it between uses. Sand is best used as a soil amendment in volumes of less than 10 percent. Be sparing when adding sand in order to break up clay soil. Coarse sand has the tendency to wash upward and accumulate on the soil surface.

Sawdust (not inert) is a popular and inexpensive growing medium among many commercial vegetable growers. But it holds too much water for cannabis growth and is usually too acidic, and new or fresh sawdust robs the medium of its nitrogen reserves.

Soilless mixes (not inert) are very popular, inexpensive, lightweight, and clean growing mediums. Commercial greenhouse growers have been using them for decades. Soilless mixes are available in different grades including small, medium, and coarse.

Premixed commercial soilless mixes retain moisture and air while allowing strong root penetration and even growth. The fertilizer concentration, moisture level, and pH are very easy to control with precision in soilless mix. Soilless mixes have good texture, hold water, and drain well. Unless fortified with nutrients, soilless mixes contain no nutrients and are pH balanced near 6.0 to 7.0. Fortified elements supply nutrients for up to a month, but follow directions on the package.

Coarse soilless mixes drain well and are an easy choice to push plants into growing faster with heavy fertilization. The fast-draining mixes can be leached efficiently so soluble nutrients have little chance of building up to toxic levels. Look for ready-mixed bags of fortified soilless mixes such as Jiffy Mix, Ortho Mix, Sunshine Mix, Terra- Lite, Pro-Mix, and Terra Professional Plus (Canna). To improve drainage, mix 10 to 30 percent coarse perlite before planting.

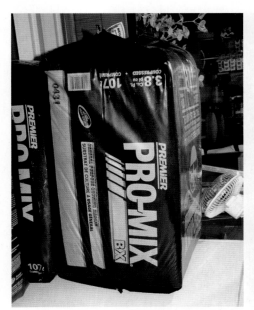

Pro-Mix is a favorite of professional nurseries and medical cannabis gardeners alike.

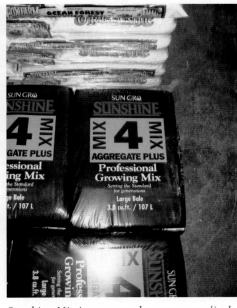

Sunshine Mix is very popular among medical cannabis gardeners from British Colombia, Canada, and western USA.

Add dolomite lime (1 cup per cubic foot [24 cl per 28 L]) to all heavily irrigated soil and soilless mixes when growing cannabis, unless a given mix already contains it. Regular heavy irrigation tends to leach out both calcium and magnesium in most any soil or soilless mix. Add a little calcium carbonate for immediate pH control.

Pro-Mix contains Canadian sphagnum peat moss, perlite, macro- and micro-nutrients, and dolomite and calcitic limestone. At least one product is fortified with beneficial endomycorrhizal fungus to strengthen roots and increase plants' ability to completely utilize available nutrients. One version of Pro-Mix contains MX fungus. Inoculants are often short-lived; some have a shelf life of *only* 30 days.

Sunshine Mix consists of Canadian sphagnum peat, perlite, dolomitic limestone, gypsum, and a wetting agent to provide plants a growing environment with abundant oxygen and quick drainage. This mix comes in different formulas and textures to suit needs of seedlings and clones, vegetative and flowering.

Soilless components can be purchased separately and mixed to the desired consistency. Ingredients always blend to-

gether best when mixed dry and wetted afterward using a commercial wetting agent or organic liquid dish soap to make water more adhesive. Mix small amounts right in the bag. Larger batches should be mixed in a wheelbarrow, concrete slab, or in a cement mixer. Blending your own soil or soilless mix is a dusty, messy job. To cut down on dust, lightly mist the pile with water several times when mixing. Always wear a respirator to avoid inhaling dust.

The texture of soilless mixes—for rapid-growing cannabis—should be coarse, light, and spongy. Such texture allows drainage with sufficient moisture and air retention, as well as providing good root penetration qualities. Fine soilless mix holds more moisture and works best in smaller containers. Soilless mixes that contain more perlite and sand drain faster, making them easier to fertilize heavily without excessive fertilizer-salt buildup. Vermiculite and peat hold water longer and are best used in small pots that require more water retention.
The pH is generally 6.5 to 7.0 in soilless mixes, which are peat-based as a rule but could include coco and other organic products. As the organic components decompose, especially when pH is adjusted to correct more neutral values, the chemistry of the soilless mix

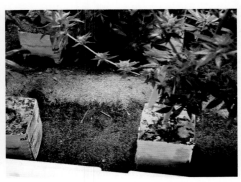

Green algae grow anywhere there is a moisture and light. Algae completely cover this mat!

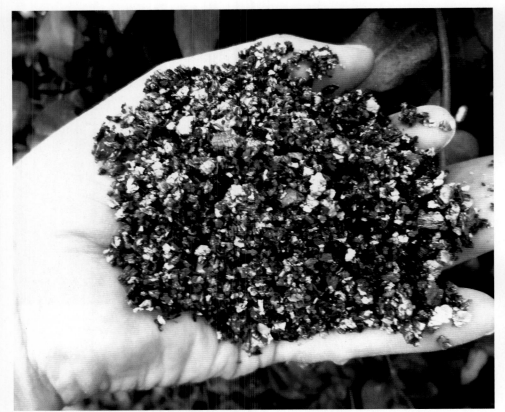

Vermiculite is mica superheated until it expands into small, lightweight pebbles. Its natural wicking ability draws in nutrient solution in passive hydroponic gardens. Vermiculite holds so much water that it is typically mixed with perlite to improve drainage.

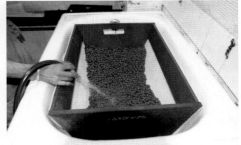

Expanded clay pellets are an easy substrate to wash and reuse. This gardener set a plastic grate inside a container. This allows him to rinse the clay pellets efficiently.

changes. Added lime makes changing the pH of soilless mix very difficult and tends to bring the pH back to adjusted levels in spite of water pH. The acidic quality of basic elements with a large pH capacity like sulfur or lime can alter the pH permanently.

Check the pH of soilless mix regularly—a minimum of once a week. Check the pH of the runoff water to ensure that the pH in the medium is not too acidic.

Avoid reusing soilless mixes. They tend to compact, and they have issues with salts, pests, and diseases. If you do reuse, add 20 to 30 percent used medium to 70 to 80 percent new medium.

Vermiculite (inert) holds a lot of water and is best suited for rooting cuttings when it is mixed with sand or perlite. With excellent buffering qualities, vermiculite holds lots of water and contains traces of magnesium (Mg), phosphorus (P), aluminum (Al), and silicon (Si).

Used in hydroponic wick gardens, vermiculite holds and wicks much moisture. Vermiculite comes in three grades: fine, medium, and coarse. Use fine vermiculite as an ingredient in seedling and cloning mixes. If fine is not available, crush coarse or medium vermiculite between your hands, rubbing palms back and forth. Coarse is the best overall choice as a soil amendment. Use finer vermiculite in seedling and clone mixes.

Do not reuse vermiculite; it breaks down substantially after a single crop.

Caution! Do not use construction-grade vermiculite, which is treated with phytotoxic chemicals.

Caution! Vermiculite has also been a source of asbestos. Most manufacturers test for asbestos at mines. Nonetheless, I am always leery of cheap imports.

See "Soil Amendments" in chapter 18, *Soil*, for more information.

Sterilizing Substrates

Properly sterilizing a growing medium after use ensures that destructive microorganisms, including bacteria, fungi and pests and their eggs, will be eliminated. For most gardeners, sterilizing is easier and less costly, both economically and environmentally, than replacing the growing medium. The most popular ways to sterilize substrates include bathing them in an antiseptic liquid such as laundry bleach, (hydrochloric) acid, or, my favorite, hydrogen peroxide (H_2O_2). Steam sterilization is also an option, but it is too much work for small gardens. Heating in an oven or with natural sunlight also cooks all the bad stuff out of a growing medium. Ultraviolet (UVC) light has limited applications and is seldom used to sterilize growing mediums.

Sterilizing works best on rigid (aggregate) growing mediums such as gravel and expanded clay, which do not

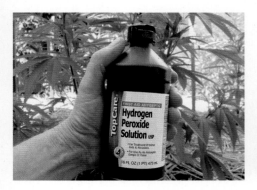

Hydrogen peroxide (H_2O_2) is one of the safest sterilants to use. But do not use H_2O_2 on or around live roots.

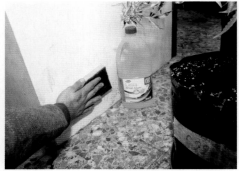

Wash garden room walls, floor, and other surfaces with a mild bleach solution to kill any bacteria, fungus, or insect eggs.

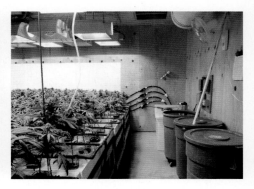

Beds in this garden are irrigated from the 300-gallon nutrient tank at the end of the room, on the right.

lose their shape. Sterilizing and reusing substrates such as rockwool, coconut coir, peat, perlite, or vermiculite may cause them to compact and lose structure. Replace "spent" growing mediums to avoid problems caused by compaction.

Take the growing medium out of the hydroponic garden. Remove all dangling and easy-to-eliminate roots by hand before sterilizing. A 3- to 4-month-old cannabis plant can have a gallon (3.8 L) or more of root mass. Manually remove the mats of roots that are entwined near the bottom of the bed, and shake loose any attached growing medium. Pour growing mediums such as expanded clay and gravel through a screen placed over a large bucket. Most of the roots will stay on the screen. Latent, dead and decaying roots cause pest and disease problems and clog irrigation systems and drains. Substrates can also be washed in a large container such as a bucket, barrel, or bathtub. Washing works best with rigid substrates such as expanded clay. Roots float to the top and are readily skimmed off with a screen or by hand.

Once excess roots are manually removed, submerge the substrate in a sterilant such as a 10 percent laundry bleach (calcium or sodium hypochlorite), or mix a 5 percent solution of hydrochloric acid, the kind used in hot tubs and swimming pools. Place the substrate in a barrel or bathtub and soak for at least an hour. Pour, drain, or pump off the sterilant, and leach the medium with plenty of fresh water. Make sure to wash the harsh chemicals away so no future crops are damaged. It may be necessary to fill the

bathtub with fresh water and drain it several times to rinse any residual sterilants from the substrate.

Hydrogen peroxide (H_2O_2) is an excellent sterilant for aggregate media. H_2O_2 solution breaks down naturally when exposed to air. It does not need to be rinsed out unless you are planting immediately.

Mix the solution at a 9:1 ratio, 16 ounces (47.3 cl) of 3 percent concentration H_2O_2 to 5 gallons (19 L) of water. Or dilute more powerful 35 percent hydrogen peroxide. Mix 4 ounces (12 cl) per 10 gallons (38 L). Wear gloves and protective clothing so 35 percent H_2O_2 does not touch skin.

Place the substrate in the bathtub, bucket, or barrel. Set a screen over the drain, and use the showerhead or a hose to wash the medium. The media must sit in the H_2O_2 solution for at least one hour to be sterilized.

Mix a bucket of dilute bleach solution to scrub walls, tables, pots, and floors. Use a 5 percent bleach solution to scrub down the garden room including the inside of growing beds, reservoirs, and system plumbing. Fill the reservoir with the dilute bleach mix, and cycle it through the irrigation system to sterilize. Pump the solution off. Avoid sending bleach solution down household drains, and definitely do not pump it into a septic tank; the nutrients will disrupt the chemistry. Fill the reservoir again and flush for at least an hour with plenty of fresh water to wash away any trace of bleach.

Once sterilized, lay out growing medium on the floor, and train an oscillating fan on it to dry.

Sterilizing substrates in the oven works for small amounts that are able to fit in the oven. First, roots must be removed and the medium rinsed with plenty of water. Next the medium is set on a baking sheet and placed in an oven at 250°F (121°C). Allow the substrates to bake for 2 hours. Check the temperature inside the substrate to ensure that it has reached 250°F (121°C).

The sun can also be used as a source of heat. Set growing media in the sun in a sealed plastic bag for several days. Place the media-filled bag in full sun, up off the ground. The temperature inside the bag and the growing medium will climb to 140°F (60°C) or more, enough to kill most all harmful pests and diseases.

Irrigation

Irrigation volume and frequency depend on the crop, plant size, climate conditions, type of garden, kind of medium, and the root environment. Each one is as important as the next, and one functioning below optimum levels will drag others to the same level of malfunction. The type of medium is determined by needs of the crop and gardener. Roots need the correct ratio of air, water, and nutrients. Large, round, smooth particles of substrate drain rapidly and need to be irrigated more often, 4 to 12 times daily for 5- to 15-minute cycles. Fibrous mediums with irregular surfaces, such as vermiculite, drain slowly and require less frequent watering, often once per day or less.

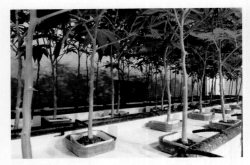

Short spaghetti tubes that come off a larger manifold supply nutrient solution to individual plants.

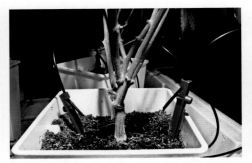

This plant is irrigated with two separate spaghetti tubes so that the entire growing medium will be evenly moist.

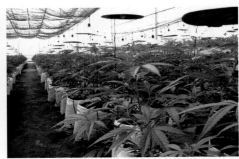

Keep containers in straight rows and arrange rows in a matrix when growing and watering. It is much easier to keep track of watered and fertilized pots when they are lined up in rows.

Cannabis root systems require 100 percent humidity to keep tiny root tips from dying back. The minute tips are responsible for absorbing most of the minerals and water. Further up, root surfaces are more rigid and absorb much less nutrient solution. If root tips die, they must regenerate before being able to push forward into the medium.

During and soon after irrigation, the nutrient content of the bed and reservoir are the same concentration. As time passes between irrigations, the EC and the pH gradually change. If enough time passes between irrigations, the nutrient concentration might change so much that the plant is not able to draw it in.

When minerals are depleted, root tips grow to find and take in more nutrients. When minerals and water are abundant, root systems do not grow and spread out. They do not develop a balanced relationship with green foliage aboveground. When this balance is disrupted and plants do not receive adequate nourishment, they become weak. Small containers must be irrigated more often than large containers, and the oxygen-to-solution balance is more difficult to maintain. Big root systems in large containers make it easier to maintain the oxygen-to-nutrient solution balance. Overall *sativa* and *sativa*-dominant varieties have a more extensive root system and use more water than *indica* and *indica*-dominant varieties.

Growing mediums that drain well can be watered for longer periods because excess water drains away quickly. Poor-draining mediums must be watered for shorter periods. As long as the drainage is good, it is difficult to overwater fast-growing cannabis. When the proper environment is maintained, virtually the only way to overwater is by saturating the medium for 20 minutes or longer, which drives out air and oxygen and drowns roots.

Rule of Thumb: 1 square meter (39.4 in per side) of indoor or greenhouse growing bed covered with foliage will use 4 to 7 quarts (3.8–6.6 L) of water a day. New plants in the same square meter that don't cover table completely with foliage

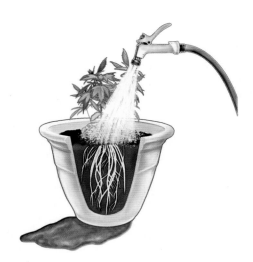

Leach growing medium as per "Leaching Growing Mediums" in chapter 21, Nutrients. Leaching must be completed in 20 minutes or less so that water does not displace oxygen in the substrate and drown roots. Leaching the growing medium monthly helps avoid nutrient excesses and deficiencies.

will use about 3 quarts (2.8 L) of water a day. This rule of thumb holds true whether there are 4 or 40 plants in the square meter quadrant.

Rule of Thumb: Irrigate soilless mixes when they are dry one-half inch below the surface. Stick your finger into the soilless medium to the first knuckle. If it is dry, plants need water.

Small plants with a small root system in small containers or rockwool cubes must be watered often. Water frequently—as soon as the surface dries out.

Flowering cannabis uses high levels of water to carry on rapid floral formation. Withholding water stunts flower formation. Plants that are exposed to wind dry out quickly.

Start irrigation cycles first thing in the morning; plants have used much of the solution during the dark of night. Even slow-draining media dry a little at night. Growing mediums that remain moist enough during the day may need irrigation only in the morning. Avoid watering growing mediums within a few hours of lights-out or nighttime. Excess solution in the growing medium at night displaces oxygen. A soggy medium that lacks air is cooler, and both conditions slow growth, weaken plants, and invite attacks by pests and diseases.

Irrigate mineral soils, soilless mixes, coco, etc., when about 50 percent of the total volume of water in the container is gone. To figure when the moisture level

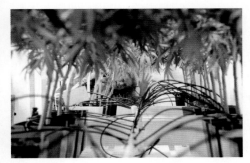

Spaghetti tubes direct nutrient solution to the base of each plant, ensuring complete wetting of the rockwool growing medium.

is at 50 percent, weigh the container when it is bone dry. Water it until saturated, let it sit for 10 minutes, and then weigh it again. The difference in weight is how much water the growing medium and container will hold. When half of this weight is reached, moisture levels are at 50 percent. For example, a 3-gallon (11.4 L) container full of growing medium weighs 10 ounces (29.6 cl) when bone dry and 60 ounces (177.4) when saturated with water. We know the container can hold 50 ounces (147.9 cl) of water. When the plant has used 25 ounces (73.9 cl) of water the growing medium is at 50 percent moisture level.

Once you have an idea of when and how much the plants need to be watered, it is a simple matter of picking up the containers to "weigh" them. When they are about 50 percent full, they need water. After experimenting with this "heft the pot" method for a while, you will have a feel for it and will soon be able to tip each pot to access its moisture level.

You can estimate the water needs of entire gardens can by weighing several containers and figuring the average weight. But the crop must all be the same age, size, light, and ventilation exposure, and so on.

Irrigate containers and let *at least* 20 percent of the solution flow out the bottom as runoff. The runoff solution will carry away any nutrients that build up in the growing medium.

Vertical Gardens: Indoors, grow bags, pots, tubes, or slabs can be positioned vertically around an HID to form a vertical garden. Short plants are usually placed at a 30-degree angle in the medium and fed individually with microirrigation. The runoff drains through the growing medium and back to the reservoir to be reused, or it drains to waste. Plants at the top of slabs receive less irrigation solution than those below. Solution dosage to individual containers should be controlled

by individual emitters. When using DFT, solution depth is controlled by their degree of incline.

Water Supply

A readily accessible water source is essential. If a water tap or outlet is not located in or near the garden room, it is a good idea to plumb one into the area. Water weighs 8 pounds (3.6 kg) per gallon (3.8 L). It is much easier to transport water via a hose than it is to schlep it by hand.

If you are growing hydroponically and your water contains more than 300 ppm of dissolved solids (salts), it should be demineralized with reverse osmosis (RO) before using. If growing in mediums like coco, peat, or mineral soil, the tolerances for salts in the water are higher, and watering is more frequent.

Even Solution Penetration

Use a moisture meter to test growing mediums for even nutrient-solution penetration. Insert the probe into the medium at several different points and levels to check for consistent readings. Dry pockets in growing medium will lead to dead roots. Direct top-feed emitters so that solution will percolate evenly down through mediums, ensuring even penetration to the entire root zone.

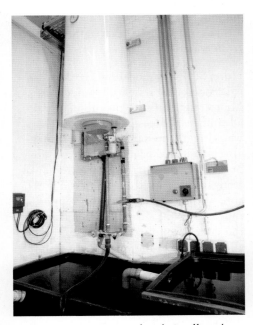

Hot water comes in very handy in all garden rooms. This large room is equipped with an electric water heater.

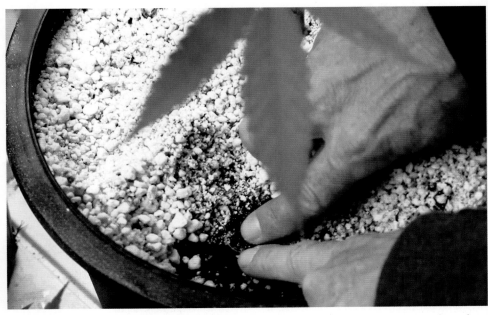

Spread a layer of perlite, expanded clay pellets, or plastic mulch across the substrate surface of hydroponic and container gardens to discourage algae growth. The mulch also protects surface roots from temperature extremes and the force of pelting water.

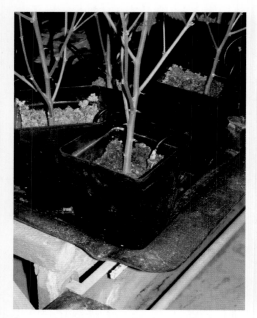

Using a spike, anchor spaghetti tubing in the growing medium. Drops, a spray, or a stream of nutrient solution will be emitted and will percolate down through the growing medium.

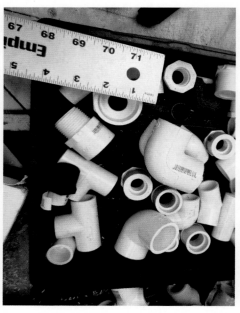

PVC pipe is simple to work with and relatively inexpensive. PVC pipe can be easily plumbed into the garden room from an outside source of water.

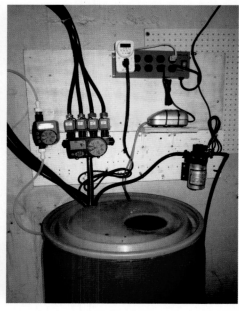

Solenoid valves and a small timer control nutrient supply to 4 different garden beds, as shown here.

Cultivate the surface of soilless mixes to allow the water to penetrate evenly and guard against dry pockets. It also keeps water from running down the crack between the inside of the pot and the medium and then out the drain holes. Using soft-sided containers that conform to the shape of the contracting growing medium will also solve this problem. Gently break up and cultivate the top half-inch (1.3 cm) of the mix with your fingers or a salad fork, being careful not to disturb the tiny surface roots. Another option would be to apply a layer of mulch, which is my preference.

Microirrigation

Microirrigation delivers water or nutrient solution one drop at a time (drip irrigation), as a spray, or in a stream to individual plants. Such systems often deliver low volume and require low-pressure plastic pipe with friction fittings. When under high-pressure, irrigation fittings must be able to withstand the added stress. Microirrigation systems can be used with RTW or recirculating systems.

Automatic microirrigation systems require a pump, reservoir, and delivery system. Top-feed systems require a main feeder tube or manifold and individual spaghetti tubes and emitters. Nutrient solution is pumped through a pipe and out the emitter one drop at a time or at a fixed rate. The emitters that are attached to the main hose are spaghetti tubes, nozzles, or drippers that meter out a specific volume of solution. Microirrigation kits are available at garden stores and building centers. You can also construct your own microirrigation system from component parts.

Note: See "Ebb-and-flow Gardens" in this chapter for irrigation guidelines. Microirrigation systems offer several advantages. Once set up, they lower watering maintenance. Fertilizer may also be injected or nutrient solution pumped into the irrigation system (aka fertigation). Pay attention to the pressure of the water in the main supply tube, and make sure all the emitters have the same amount of pressure so they all deliver the same volume of solution. When setting up a microirrigation system, make sure the growing medium drains freely to prevent soggy substrate or salt buildup. If you are growing many different varieties of plants, , they may have different water and fertilizer needs. If you are growing plants that are all the

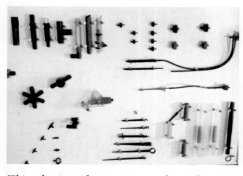

This selection of irrigation nozzles and supplies is outstanding. Always choose nozzles and emitters that are difficult to plug and easy to clean. And always use a filter!

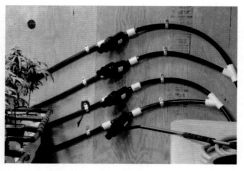

Each irrigation supply line has its own filter. The filters are easy to monitor and access. A clean filter will help you avoid wasting time troubleshooting irrigation emitters and subsequently unplugging them.

same variety, age, and size, an automatic microirrigation system works very well.

Microirrigation systems cost a few more dollars to set up, but with the consistency they add to a garden, their expense is often paid off by a bountiful yield. Vigilantly monitor all vital signs: moisture, pH, ventilation, humidity, and so on. Everything still needs to be checked and adjusted daily. Automation, when applied properly and monitored, adds consistency, uniformity, and usually a higher yield.

A microirrigation system attached to a timer disperses nutrient solution at regular intervals. If using such a system, check emitters and substrate daily to ensure that plants are watered and that all the substrate receives solution evenly. Microirrigation systems are very convenient—often indispensable when you have to be away from the garden for a few days. Avoid leaving automatic irrigation systems unattended for more than 3 to 4 consecutive days, or you could return to a surprise!

Container Culture and Hydroponic Nutrient Disorders

Hydroponic and container culture nutrient disorders show the same signs in plants grown in soilless or soil gardens. But the causes are often specific to hydroponics or container culture. A regular maintenance schedule and adhering to "Guidelines for Success," (on the next page), will help avoid nutrient deficiencies and associated cultural problems.

If nutrient deficiencies or excesses affect more than a few plants, check irrigation fittings to ensure that all plants are receiving a full dose of solution. Check substrate around affected plants to ensure that nutrient solution is penetrating the entire medium and all roots are moist. Check the root zone to ensure that roots have not plugged drainage conduits and are not standing in stagnant solution.

Nutrient disorders most often affect plants of a given variety of cannabis at the same time when they are receiving the same nutrient solution. Different varieties often react differently to the same nutrient solution. Check with seed purveyors for the fertilization recommendations of specific varieties.

Overfertilizing during vegetative growth is a common error. Typically, signs of overfertilization and toxic nutrient lockup appear between the sixth and eighth weeks of growth. It can cause excessive lush leafy growth and can result in overdoses and deficiencies of different nutrients. Flower formation is then often slow and weak.

Hydroponics and container culture provide the means to supply the maximum amount of nutrients a plant needs but can also starve plants to death or rapidly overfertilize them. Many automated gardens are designed for high performance. If something malfunctions—the electricity goes off, the pump breaks, a drain gets clogged with roots, or there is a rapid fluctuation in the pH—major problems could result. A mistake could kill plants or stunt them so seriously that they cannot recover before harvest.

Run-to-waste (RTW) gardens tend to have fewer problems—toxic substrate, pH and EC imbalances, temperature issues, and so on—than recirculating systems do. RTW gardens also use about the same volume of nutrient as recirculating systems use.

Plants absorb different nutrients at different rates, and some nutrients become unavailable before others, creating an imbalanced solution. The best form of preventive maintenance is to change the solution often. Avoid nutrient problems in recirculating systems by changing the solution in small and medium-sized reservoirs every week, and remember to top off reservoirs with fresh water to compensate for water used by plants. Large reservoirs can be changed less often when monitoring nutrient content very carefully.

Nutrient imbalances also cause pH to fluctuate, usually to drop. Avert problems by using pure nutrients and leaching the substrate with fresh water between nutrient-solution changes.

Change the nutrient solution if there is a good flow of nutrient solution through the root zone but plants still appear sickly. Make sure the pH of the water is within the acceptable 5.5 to 6.5 range before adding new nutrients.

Hydroponic gardens have no soil or soilless mix to buffer the uptake of nutrients. This causes nutrient disorders to rapidly manifest as problems like discolored foliage, slow growth, or spotting. Novice gardeners must learn to recognize nutrient problems in their early stages in order to avoid serious problems that cost valuable time for plants to recover. Treatment for a nutrient deficiency or excess must be quick and certain. Once treated, plants take several days to respond to the remedy. For a fast fix of some nutrients, foliar feed plants. See "Foliar Feeding" in chapter 21, *Nutrients*, for more information on nutrient disorders.

Diagnosis of nutrient deficiency or excess becomes difficult when two or more elements are deficient or in excess at the same time. Symptoms might not point directly at the cause. The easiest way to solve most unknown nutrient deficiency syndromes is to change the nutrient solution.

Plants do not always need an accurate diagnosis when the nutrient solution is changed. Overfertilization, once diagnosed, is easy to remedy. Drain the nutrient solution. Flush the system at least 3 times with fresh, dilute (5–10 percent) nutrient solution to remove small amounts of lingering sediment and salt buildup in the reservoir. Replace with properly mixed solution.

The proper balance of nutrients in a solution does not guarantee that all nutrients are available to roots for assimilation. Inside plant tissue, deficiencies occur even when plants have the proper balance of nutrients. Calcium is the most common nutrient found deficient. It results from transport problems within the plant. Leaf tip burn and dry burnt leaf margins are the most common symptoms of calcium deficiency. This sort of calcium deficiency in plant tissue is difficult to diagnose when calcium is abundant in the nutrient solution. Frequently misdiagnosed, calcium deficiency within plant tissue is often confused with damage resulting from chemical salt burn, temperature, or wind.

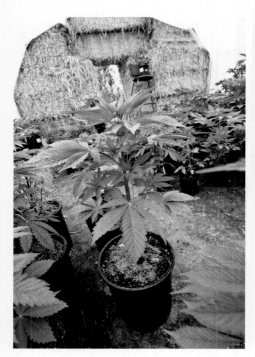

Keeping plants strong and healthy is the first defense against nutrient and culture disorders.

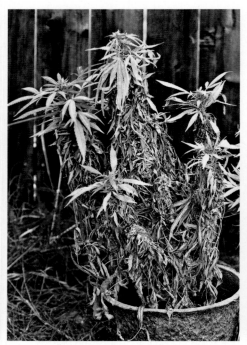

This sad plant is far from strong and healthy!

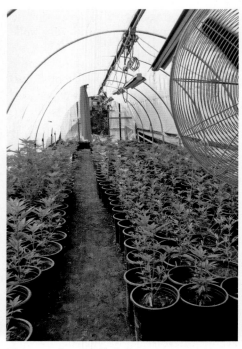

This greenhouse full of clones is growing in a perfect environment.

Tip burn starts on younger inner leaves. At first leaf tissue looks water-soaked, but then it turns brown and ultimately black. Cells break in affected areas causing cell fluid to leak out. The ruptured area is an excellent place for diseases like rot to start growing.

Coco coir contains large amounts of potassium. Calcium and magnesium uptake are affected by high levels of potassium. A nutrient solution that is formulated specifically for coco coir will ensure that cannabis receives the exact balanced blend of nutrients it needs.

The symptoms of calcium deficiencies show as contorted leaves early in older foliage. Tip burn on new growth is caused by the buildup of potassium. Calcium becomes less available and potassium accumulates at tips causing interior salt burn. This is not the normal salt burn that is caused when EC levels are too high in the medium. However, the issue can replicate if potassium is in excess and calcium is being applied correctly. In other words, potassium toxicity is the actual problem in coco.

Do not confuse other problems such as windburn, lack of light, temperature stress, or fungi and pest damage with nutrient deficiencies. But these cultural issues could very well be the cause of nutrient deficiencies. Such problems usually appear on individual plants that are most affected. For example, foliage next to a heat vent might show signs of heat scorch, while the rest of the garden looks healthy. Or a plant on the edge of the garden might be small and leggy because it receives less light or a lower temperature.

Guidelines for Success

- Mix nutrients with low-EC or RO water.
- Keep solution temperature about 60°F (15.6°C).
- Use sterile growing medium.
- Calibrate electronic DO, EC, and pH meters before use.
- Regularly measure and rectify DO, EC, and pH in reservoir, media, and runoff.
- Use high-quality hydroponic nutrients designed to grow cannabis.
- Keep growing area clean.

- Use a black or opaque reservoir with a lid.
- Aerate nutrient solutions continually (24/7) in solution culture gardens.
- Aerate nutrient solutions in hydroponic and container culture gardens during daytime hours.
- Change nutrient solution and clean the reservoir weekly in recirculating systems.
- Regularly check the irrigation system for blockages and leaks.

Main Reasons Nutrient Solutions Create Problems

1. Imbalanced pH
2. Inaccurate pH or EC meter
3. Nutrient solution is too concentrated or imbalanced
4. Input water has too many dissolved solids
5. Nutrients combine and precipitate, becoming locked out
6. Temperature is too high and lacks dissolved oxygen
7. Temperature is too cold and slows root system functions, including water and nutrient uptake

24 DISEASES & PESTS

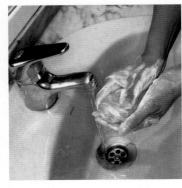

To prevent transmission of diseases, wash hands before and after entering or exiting the garden room.

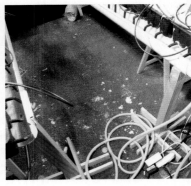

Keeping the garden room clean helps prevent cultural and maintenance problems.

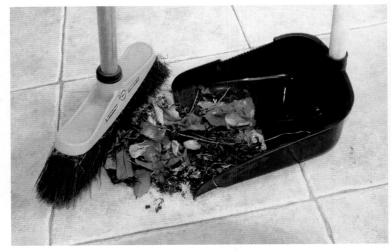

Immediately sweep up any debris on the garden room floor.

THE CANNABIS PLANT is plagued by more than 200 diseases and pests. Diseases are caused by bacteria, fungi, nematodes, viruses, other plants, environmental stress, genetics, and pollutants. Pest insects, mites, mollusks, animals, and many diseases are ushered in by poor sanitation procedures in the garden or garden area.

The most common diseases include powdery mildew, bud rot, and damping-off. Spider mites are by far the most common pest found indoors, and fungus gnats are second. Outdoors and in greenhouses, corn earworms are most destructive. However, other large pests such as mice, squirrels, and wild pigs can cause serious damage.

Most diseases and pests can be avoided by using simple sanitary precautions in the garden. Constant monitoring of foliage and garden area is essential to catch any infestations in their infancy.

Cleanliness and Prevention

Diseases and pests of all kinds can sneak into garden rooms, greenhouses, and outdoor gardens. Some are airborne, others hitch a ride on plants, tools, or gardeners. They will come in and make themselves at home if you let them.

Insects, mites, and maggots slither into garden rooms to eat and reproduce—wasting cannabis. Outdoors, they live everywhere they can. Indoors, they live anywhere you let them. Fungi are present in the air at all times. They may be introduced by an infected plant or from air containing fungus spores. Fungi will settle down and grow if climatic conditions are right. Pests, fungi, and diseases can be prevented, but if allowed to grow unchecked, extreme control measures are often necessary to eradicate them.

Garden Cleanliness Guidelines

Wear latex gloves, and regularly dip into a sanitizing agent.

Use disinfectant-filled footbaths to prevent carrying pathogens on boots and shoes into the garden room.

Disinfect pruning tools and knives.

Do not smoke in the garden.

Do not work in the garden if foliage is wet.

Keep garden room and greenhouse floors clean. Keep outdoor gardens tidy, and always remove debris from soil surface. Insects and fungi like nice hideaway homes found in dirty, dank corners and under decaying leaves or rotting mulch. Indoors and in greenhouses, use clean mulch such as expanded clay pellets or plastic. Outdoors, straw is the best all-around mulch.

Gardeners and their tools often transport microscopic pests, diseases, and fungi into the cannabis garden. To prevent problems, take regular sanitary precautions. Wearing clean clothes and using clean tools reduces problems considerably. A separate set of indoor and greenhouse tools are easy to keep clean. Pests, diseases, and fungi habitually ride from plant to plant on dirty tools. Disinfect tools by dipping in rubbing alcohol or washing with soap and hot water after using them on a diseased plant. Another quick way to sterilize pruners is with a handheld torch. A quick heating with the torch will sterilize metal tools immediately.

Personal cleanliness is fundamental to preventing diseases and pests. Wash your hands before touching foliage and after handling diseased plants. Smart growers do not walk around the buggy outdoor garden and then visit the indoor garden without taking precautions. Think before entering the indoor garden or greenhouse and possibly contaminating it. Stay away from outdoor diseases and pests such as a rust-covered lawn, and indoors stay away from spider mite–infested houseplants. Avoid problems by washing your hands and changing shirt, pants, and shoes before entering a clean indoor cannabis garden. Smokers should be especially careful to clean up and change clothes before entering gardens.

Once a crop has been grown in potting soil or soilless mix, throw out the used growing medium. Some growers brag about using the same old potting soil over and over, unaware that this savings is repaid with a diminished harvest. Used soil may harbor harmful diseases and pests that have developed immunity to sprays. Starting a new crop in new potting soil will cost more up front but will eliminate many potential problems. Used soil makes excellent outdoor garden soil.

Once potting soil is used, it loses much of the fluff in its texture, and compaction becomes a problem. Roots penetrate

compacted soil slowly, and there is little room for oxygen, which restricts nutrient uptake. Used potting soil is depleted of nutrients. A plant with a slow start is a perfect target for disease, and worst of all, it will yield less! Companion planting helps discourage insects outdoors. Pests have nowhere to go indoors, so companion planting is not viable in garden rooms.

Plant insect- and fungus-resistant varieties of cannabis. If buying seeds from one of the many seed companies, always check for disease resistance. If you live in one of the medical cannabis states, you can actually ask local gardeners and other medical patients without being subject to legal penalties.

In general, *Cannabis indica* is the most resistant to pests, and *C. sativa* is more resistant to fungal attacks. Choose mother plants that you know are resistant to diseases and pests. Keep plants healthy and growing fast at all times. Disease attacks sick plants first. Strong plants tend to grow faster than diseases and pests can spread. However, a balance must be struck in order to avoid the excess nitrogen and softer tissue due to fast growth.

Carefully remove and destroy dead leaves. Wash your hands after handling diseased foliage. If the problem attacks one or a few plants, isolate and treat them separately. Diseases can spread like wildfire if the conditions are right. If disease gets a good start even after all preventive measures are taken, extreme control methods may be necessary, perhaps even spraying the entire garden with the proper fungicide.

Disease and Pest Prevention

prevention

healthy atmosphere for plants

cleanliness

low humidity

ventilation

removal

copper, lime sulfur sprays

specific fungicide

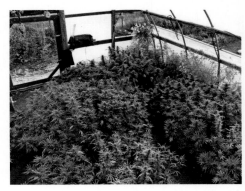

The best approach to disease and pest control is a healthy garden that is easy to maintain and offers a pleasant working environment.

Diseases
This chapter approaches disease and pest control by first encouraging gardeners to grow strong, healthy gardens and to keep all medical cannabis paperwork in order.

Fungi do not produce green chlorophyll, and they reproduce by spreading tiny microscopic spores rather than seeds. Countless fungal spores are present in the air at all times. When these microscopic airborne spores find the proper conditions, they will settle, take hold, and start growing. Some fungi, such as bud-rotting gray mold (*Botrytis*), are so prolific that they can spread through an entire crop in a matter of days!

Unsterile, soggy soil coupled with humid, stagnant air provides the environment most fungi need to thrive. Although there are many different types of fungi and related diseases, they are usually prevented with similar methods.

Anthracnose
Fungus

Common names: anthracnose, leaf blight, leaf shoot, brown blight

Specific diseases that cause anthracnose include: anthracnose (*Colletotrichum coccodes = C. atramentarium Taubenhaus = C. dematium*)

Threat to garden: low to medium

Identify: Leaves show first symptoms when they turn light green. Soon, sunken water-soaked spots that grow into irregular shapes develop grayish centers with dark borders. Stems develop white

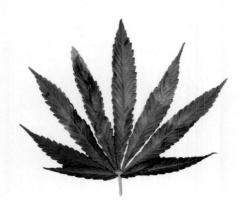

Anthracnose

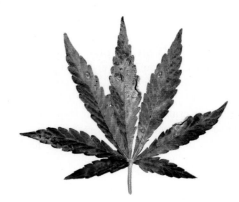

Blight

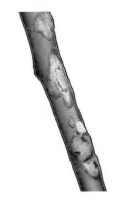

Canker

wounds that turn black. Little black and white dots soon develop in wounds. Stems may develop cankers. This disease is worst during cool, damp weather (especially in clay and bog soils) and when plants are stressed (especially in hydroponic systems). Anthracnose is not transmitted in seeds but can be found on seed surfaces.

Damage: Anthracnose slows growth and diminishes harvest. It is occasionally fatal.

Cause: Anthracnose is caused in cannabis by three species of *Colletotrichum* fungi. *Colletotrichum atramentarium* also causes anthracnose. Brown blight (anthracnose) is caused by *Alternaria* and *Stemphylium*. Fungi overwinter in plant debris or soil, and start to grow in the spring.

Prevention: Sanitation is the best prevention. Remove plant residues. When pruning, make clean cuts with sharp, sterile tools to keep wounds clean. Use new soil, and avoid underwatering or overwatering. Avoid planting in clay soils, or amend clay soils to improve drainage. Do not wet foliage and stems when watering.

Control: *Trichoderma harzianum* (Trichodex) controls anthracnose. Sulfur or copper powders or sprays applied weekly as soon as the disease is identified will keep spores from spreading, but they will not kill the disease. Look for contact fungicides that contain chlorothalonil. There are many systemic fungicides that kill anthracnose.

Blights
Fungal disease
Common names: brown blight, southern blight, twig blight

Specific diseases that cause blight include: bacterial blight (*Pseudomonas syringae* pv. *cannabina*) *Cylindrosporium* blight (*Cylindrosporium* spp., *C. cannabinum* Ibrahimov) *Leptosphaeria* blight (*Leptosphaeria cannabina, L. woroninii, L. acuta*) brown blight (*Alterneria alternata* = *A. tenuis*) southern blight (*Sclerotium rolfsii*), *Sclerotium* root and stem rot (*Athelia rolfsii* [teleomorph]) twig blight (*Dendrophoma marconii, Botryosphaeria marconii* [teleomorph])

Threat to garden: low to medium

Identify: *Blight* is a general term that describes many plant diseases that are caused by fungus, most often a few weeks before harvest. Signs of blight include discolored leaf tips; dark, blotchy spots on foliage; slow growth; sudden yellowing; wilting; and plant death. Most blights spread quickly through large areas of plants.

Damage: kills leaves, slows growth, and kills plants

Cause: unsanitary garden room conditions; infected soil, air or plant tissue is introduced into the garden

Prevention: Cleanliness! Use fresh, sterile growing medium. Avoid excess nitrogen fertilization. Avoid blights by keeping plants healthy with the proper nutrient balance and good drainage to prevent nutrient buildup.

Biological: Use Serenade (*Bacillus subtilis*) against brown blight. Use Binab, Bio- Fungus, RootShield, Supresivit, Trichopel, (*Trichoderma harzianum*) or SoilGuard (*Trichoderma virens*). Use a Bordeaux mixture to stop fungal blights. Stopping blights in advanced stages is difficult; the best solution is to remove diseased plants and destroy them.

Control: Once blight takes over plant tissue, little can be done. Remove plants from the garden and sterilize the area to avoid contamination.

Canker
Fungal disease

Common names: stem canker, hemp canker

Specific diseases that cause canker include: *Cladosporium* stem canker (*Cladosporium cladosporioides, C. herbarum, Mycosphaerella tassiana* [teleomorph])hemp canker (*Sclerotinia sclerotiorum*)*Ophiobolus* stem canker (*Ophiobolus cannabinus, O. anguillidus*) *Phoma* stem canker (*Phoma herbarum, P. exigua*) *Phomopsis* stem canker (*Phomopsis cannabina, P. achilleae, Diaporthe arctii* var. *achilleae* [teleomorph])

Threat to garden: low

Identify: The first water-soaked wounds appear on maturing stems and branches. They develop into dark cankers that continue to deepen, and fungus invades the plant. Finally, the black-hearted disease continues to grow on dead stems.

Damage: Hemp canker, mainly a fiber hemp disease, occasionally affects medicinal cannabis.

Cause: present in soil or unsterile, tainted soil

Prevention: Use fresh soil or growing medium for each crop. Keep garden and garden area clean. Remove all plant residues from soil surface. Compost by

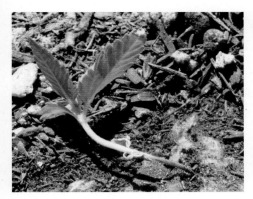

Damping-off hit this seedling before it developed true leaves. (MF)

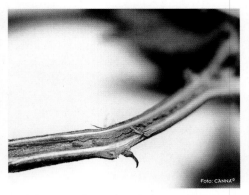

Cut the stem of an infected plant to find evidence of Fusarium

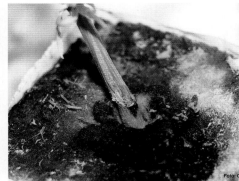

Fusarium wilt destroyed this plant.

using a big pile and high temperatures.

Control: Best to prevent hemp canker. All chemical controls are systemic. Once disease takes over, it is often too late. Contans WG contains *Coniothyrium minitans* bacteria, a parasite to *S. sclerotiorum*.

Damping-Off

Fungus: kills seeds, seedlings, and clones

Common names: damping-off, stem rot, moldy germination, young plant disease

Specific diseases that cause damping-off include: (*Botrytis cinerea, Botryotinia fuckeliana* [teleomorph], *Fusarium oxysporum, F. solani, Nectria haematococca* [teleomorph], *Macrophomina phaseolina, Pythium aphanidermatum, P. debaryanum auct., P. ultimum, Rhizoctonia solani, Thanatophorus cucumeris* [teleomorph] = *Pellicularia filamentosa*).

Threat to garden: High threat to seedlings! See "Gray Mold (*Botrytis cinerea,* aka Bud Mold): Stems, Flower Buds."

About: *Damping-off* is a catchall term; the disease has many causes.

Identify: There are two kinds of damping-off: one kills seeds when they germinate and before they break through the soil; the second type, post/emergence damping-off, is the rotting or wilting of seedlings soon after they emerge from the soil. Succulent stems have become water-soaked and then necrotic and develop a sunken, zone at ground level. The little herbaceous plants fall over on the ground. Root decay follows.

Damage: Damping-off attacks rooting cuttings at the soil line if present in growing medium. As the fungi invade stem tissue, the stem loses girth at the soil line, weakens, and then discolors with a brown, watery soft rot. Finally, fluid circulation is cut, killing the seedling or cutting. Damping-off prevents newly sprouted seeds from emerging and attacks seedlings, causing them to rot at the soil line; it yellows foliage and rots older plants at the soil line.

Cause: Various fungal species, including *Botrytis, Pythium,* and *Fusarium,* are present in the air, growing medium, plant, or seed. This disease breeds in humid conditions and in poorly aerated, overwatered growing mediums. It attacks weak plants.

Prevention: Control soil moisture. Overwatering is the main precursor to damping-off. Careful daily scrutiny of soil will ensure that the proper amount of moisture is available to seeds or cuttings. Germinate seeds between clean, fresh, moistened paper towels and move seeds to soil once sprouted. Do not plant seeds too deeply; cover with soil one and a half times the width of the seed. Use fresh, sterile growing medium and clean pots to guard against harmful fungus in the soil. Start seeds and root cuttings in a fast-draining, sterile coarse sand, rockwool, Oasis, or Jiffy cubes, which are difficult to overwater. Set them on a grate or surface that readily drains. Do not place a humidity tent over sprouted seedlings—a tent can lead to excessive humidity and damping-off. Damping-off is inhibited by bright light; grow seedlings under the HID rather than fluorescent bulbs. Keep fertilization to

a minimum during the first couple of weeks of growth.

Seeds: Coating the seed with protective dust is a form of insurance. Seed disinfection is used to kill organisms of anthracnose and other diseases carried on seed. Damping-off organisms are in the soil, not on the seed. The coating is intended to kill or inhibit fungi in the soil immediately surrounding the seed and so provide temporary protection during germination.

Cuttings: Cuttings are less susceptible to damping-off and love a humidity tent to promote rooting. Keep germination temperatures between 70°F and 85°F (21.1°C–29.4°C).

Control
Biological: Apply Polygangron (*Pythium oligandrum*) granules to soil and seed. Bak Pak or Intercept is applied to the soil and Deny or Dagger—forms of the bacterium *Burkholderia cepacia*—is put on the seeds. Epic, Kodiac, Quantum 4000, Rhizo-Plus, System 3, and Serenade also suppress many causes of damping-off.

Chemical: Dust the seeds with Captan. Avoid benomyl fungicide soil drench because it kills beneficial organisms.

Fusarium Wilt
Fungal root disease

Common names: *Fusarium,* stem canker, *Fusarium* wilt

Specific diseases that cause *Fusarium* wilt include: *Fusarium* foot rot and root rot (*Fusarium solani*)
Fusarium stem canker (*Fusarium sulphureum, Gibberella cyanogena* [teleomorph], = *G. saubinetii*)

Fusarium wilt (*Fusarium oxysporum* f.sp. *cannabis*, *F. oxysporum* f.sp. *vasinfectum*)

Threat to garden: medium to high

Identify: *Fusarium* wilt is most common in warm garden rooms and greenhouses. *Fusarium* starts as small spots on older, lower leaves. Interveinal leaf chlorosis appears swiftly. Leaf tips may curl before wilting and suddenly drying to a crisp. Portions of the plant or the entire plant will wilt. The entire process happens so fast that yellow, dead leaves dangle from branches.

Damage: This disease starts in the plant's xylem, the base of the fluid transport system. Plants wilt when fungi plug the fluid flow in plant tissue. Cut one of the main stems in two, and look for the telltale reddish-brown color.

Cause: The water and nutrient solution carries this disease with it when contaminated. The disease is present in the room, growing medium, or plants. Recirculating nutrient solutions above 75°F (24°C) creates perfect conditions for *Fusarium*. It is also spread by contaminated plants, cuttings, etc. *Fusarium* can also enter via the root system.

Prevention: Cleanliness! Use fresh, clean growing medium. Avoid nitrogen overfertilization. Preventive action is necessary. Keep nutrient solution below 75°F (23.9°C). Hydrogen peroxide kills bacteria and will also arrest *Fusarium*. Always remove and destroy infested plants.

Biological: Mycostop (*Streptomyces griseoviridis*), or Deny, or Dagger (*Burkholderia cepacia*) and *Trichoderma*.

Control

Sprays: Treat seeds with chemical fungicides to eradicate the seed-borne infection. Chemical fungicides are not effective on foliage. A metal spray such as copper or zinc helps by making the leaf environment more difficult to penetrate.

If there is any root rot, do not spray vitamins onto the plants. Vitamins around roots may strengthen the fungus that is attacking your plant. If mold or fungal attacks appear on leaves discontinue sprays and foliar feedings.

Aboveground indications of root rots are difficult to distinguish from wilt diseases. The three most important wilt diseases include *Fusarium* wilt that is caused by two forms of *Fusarium* oxysporum, *Verticillium* wilt that is caused by two *Verticillium* species, and premature wilt (aka charcoal rot) caused by *Macrophomina phaseolina*.

Note: *Fusarium oxysporum* has been studied and genetically modified to create a "mycoherbicide" or an "attack" fungus that preys on cannabis. To the best of my knowledge, the attack fungus has not been released.

Gray Mold (*Botrytis cinerea*, aka Bud Mold)

Fungal disease

Disease/fungi/bacteria/microbe/virus/pathogen/contaminant

Common names: bud mold, stem rot, bud rot

Specific disease that causes damping-off: *Botrytis cinerea*

Threat to garden: very high

Identify: Gray mold is the most common fungus that attacks indoor plants and flourishes in moist, temperate climates common to many garden rooms. It attacks seedlings, clones, stems, buds, and stored cannabis.

Seeds/seedlings, clones: see "Damping-Off"

Stems: Gray mold arises as a gray-brown to blackish mat of fungus and fungal spores. Stems yellow at margins of infection. Soft cankers develop that may cause stems to snap. When advanced, the entire stem dies above the infection.

Damage: Gray mold slows growth, diminishes harvest, could cause plant death, and infects other plants.

Prevention and control: the same as for flower buds

Flower buds: Bud leaflets yellow and wilt, and pistils brown. Inside the bud—where it is difficult to see at the onset, and is grayish-whitish to bluish-green in color—*Botrytis* appears hairlike and similar to laundry lint in moist climates. Entire buds become enveloped in a fuzzy gray mold that morphs into gray-brown slime. Damage can also appear as dark, brownish spots on buds in less humid environments. Dry to the touch, the *Botrytis*-affected area often crumbles if rubbed. Constant observation, especially during the last two weeks before harvest, is necessary to keep this disease out of the garden.

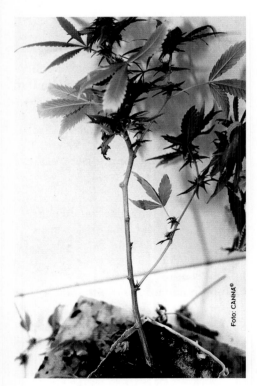

Cut the stem of an infected plant to find evidence of Fusarium

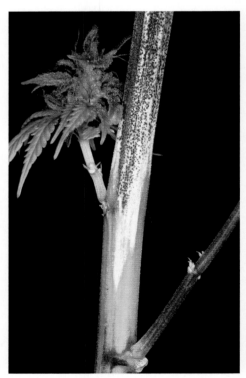

Botrytis *is visible on this stem. It is killing all the growth.*

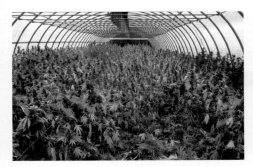
Botrytis cinerea *spread through this entire greenhouse in about two weeks.*

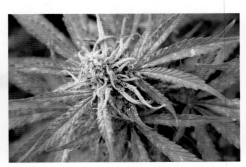
Botrytis cinerea *attacked this flower bud.*

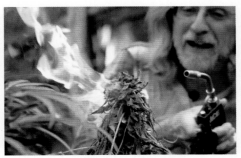
Flaming flowers is one of many ways to kill Botrytis *in the garden. This method is very rewarding and also kills fungus spores.*

Damage: Single leaves that mysteriously dry out on the buds. They could be the telltale signs of a *Botrytis* attack inside the bud. Flower buds are quickly reduced to slime in cool, humid conditions or unsmokable powder in warm, dry rooms. *Botrytis* can destroy an entire crop in seven to ten days if left unchecked. Stem damage—*Botrytis* starts on stems and not buds—is less common indoors. First, stems turn yellow, and cankerous growths develop. The damage causes growth above the wound to wilt and can cause stems to fold over. Transported by air, contaminated hands, and tools, gray mold spreads very quickly indoors, infecting an entire garden room in less than a week when conditions are right.

I saw *Botrytis* destroy an entire greenhouse in Switzerland in two weeks.

Cause: Caterpillars, wounds, humidity, and dense flowers all factor as causes of gray mold. Airborne spores are present virtually everywhere as gray mold attacks many plants. It is also transmitted via seeds. *Botrytis* damage is compounded by humid (above 50 percent) climates. In temperate regions with high humidity (60 to 70 percent) and low temperatures, *Botrytis* can completely destroy a hemp crop within a week.

Prevention: Keep the garden room, tools, and yourself clean. Do yourself a favor and start with clean growing medium! Buy clean medium or treat with steam or electricity. Remove lower leaves and improve air circulation between plants. Grow disease-resistant varieties. Dense, tightly packed, moisture-retaining buds of *Cannabis afghanica* are the most susceptible to gray mold. Some *afghanica* varieties

came from arid climates and have no resistance to gray mold.

Minimize *Botrytis* attack incidence with low humidity (50 percent or less), ample air circulation, and ventilation. Grow varieties that do not produce heavy, tightly packed buds that provide a perfect place for this fungus to flourish. Cool (below 70°F [21.1°C]), moist climates with humidity above 50 percent are perfect for rampant gray mold growth. Many crosses are more resistant to gray mold than pure indica varieties.

Remove dead leaf stems, petioles, from stalks when removing damaged leaves to avoid *Botrytis* outbreaks, which is often harbored by dead, rotting foliage. Increase plant spacing, and air circulation between plants. Increase ventilation, keep humidity below 60 percent, and keep the garden room clean! Use fresh, sterile growing medium for each crop. Water when the lights go on so water does not sit all night. Mulch plants to avoid water splashing from soil onto leaves.

Excessive nitrogen and phosphorus levels make foliage tender, letting *Botrytis* can get a foothold. But higher levels of calcium lower the incidence of *Botrytis*. Make sure pH is around 6.0 to facilitate calcium uptake. Low light levels also encourage weak growth and gray mold attack. Keep the light levels bright. *Botrytis* needs UV light to complete its life cycle; without UV light it cannot live.

Control
Cultural and physical control: As soon as *Botrytis* symptoms appear, use

alcohol-sterilized pruners to remove *Botrytis*-infected buds at least one inch (2.5 cm) below the infected area. Do not let the bud or anything that touches it contaminate other foliage. Remove it from the garden and destroy it. Wash hands and tools after removing infected buds. Increase temperature to 80°F (26.7°C) and decrease humidity to below 50 percent.

Biological: Spray plants with *Gliocladium roseum* and *Trichoderma* species. Prevent damping-off with a soil application of *Gliocladium* and *Trichoderma* species. The *Hemp Diseases and Pests* book suggests experimenting with the yeasts *Pichia guilliermondii* and *Candida oleophila* or the bacterium *Pseudomonas syringae*.

Sprays: Fixed copper (copper hydroxide, copper oxide, copper oxychloride), copper sulfate, hydrated lime, lime sulfur, and elemental sulfur keep early stages of *Botrytis* in check as long as it is present on the foliage. Preventive spraying is advised if in a high-risk area, but spraying buds near harvest time is not advised. Seeds are protected from *Botrytis* with a coating of Captan. Check with your local nursery or hydroponic store for product recommendations.

Sprays of calcium silicate (*Ca-silicate*, 2,000 ppm, a sealant for concrete and egg shells), (California) *calcium bentonite (Ca-bentonite)*, and *calcium formate (Ca-formate*, 2,000 ppm) provide effective control of fungi and are safe alternatives to highly toxic fungicides. Potassium bicarbonate, baking soda, changes the pH of the surface of the foliage it contacts. *Botrytis* cannot grow there.

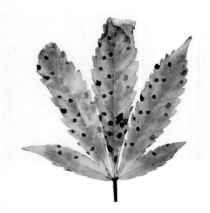

Leaf spot can be caused by many different problems. Once dead tissue appears on leaves, mold and fungus can take hold and grow.

AQ10, a microbial biofungicide that parasitizes powdery mildew, can control and even eliminate the disease. AQ10 will actually eliminate *Botrytis* when plants are no more than 3 percent infected.

See "Sulfur Burners and Pests" under "Sulfur" in this chapter.

Leaf Spot
Fungal and bacterial disease

Common names: brown blight, brown leaf spot, leaf spot root disease, *Curvularia* leaf spot, olive leaf spot, pink rot, tar spot, *Stemphylium* leaf and stem spot, white leaf spot, yellow leaf spot

Specific diseases that cause leaf spot include: brown leaf spot and stem canker (*Ascochyta* spp., *A. prasadii*, *Phoma* spp., *Didymella* spp. [teleomorph], *P. exigua, P. glomerata, P. herbarum*). *Curvularia* leaf spot (*Curvularia cymbopogonis, C. lunata, Cochliobolus lunatus* [teleomorph]
olive leaf spot (*Cercospora cannabis, Pseudocercospora cannabina*)
pink rot (*Trichothecium roseum*)
Stemphylium leaf and stem spot (*Stemphylium botryosum, Pleospora tarda* [teleomorph], *S. cannabinum*)
white leaf spot (*Phomopsis ganjae*)
yellow leaf spot (*Septoria cannabis, S. cannabina* Peck)

Alternaria alternata Keissler is a common fungal pathogen of some 380 different plants and seeds. The opportunistic pathogen causes leaf spot and other diseases.

Caution: Alternaria alternate Keissler also causes upper respiratory tract infections and asthma in people who are sensitive.

Threat to garden: These diseases rarely kill plants, but they do sharply reduce crop yields.

Identify: Leaf and stem fungi, including leaf spot, attack the foliage. Brown, gray, black, or yellow to white spots or blotches develop on leaves and stems.

Damage: Leaves and stems discolor and develop spots that impair plant fluid flow and other life processes. Spots expand over leaves, causing them to yellow and drop. Growth is slowed, harvest prolonged, and in severe cases, death results. Leaf spot is the symptomatic name given to many diseases.

Cause: Bacteria, fungus, and nematodes carry (vector) this disease. Spots or lesions caused by fungi often develop different colors as fruiting bodies grow. Leaf spots are often caused by cold water that was sprayed on plants under a hot HID. Temperature stress causes the spots that often develop into a disease. Viral pathogens are also a major cause of some leaf spots.

Cause: Leaf spot can be caused by

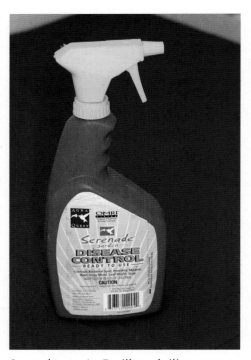

Serenade contains Bacillus subtilis, *a powerful natural fungicide.*

(1) fungi already present in an unsterile rooting medium, (2) overwatering and maintaining a soggy growing medium, or (3) excessive humidity.

Prevention: Cleanliness! Use fresh, sterile growing medium with each crop. Move HIDs away from the garden canopy about 30 minutes before spraying, so plants won't be too hot. Do not spray within four hours of turning the lights off, as excess moisture sits on the foliage and fosters fungal growth. Do not wet foliage when watering, avoid overwatering, and lower garden room humidity to 50 percent or less. Check the humidity both day and night. Employ dry heat to raise the nighttime temperature to five or ten degrees below daytime levels, and keep humidity more constant. Allow adequate spacing between plants to provide air circulation. Remove damaged foliage. Avoid excessive nitrogen application.

Control
Biological: Copper- and sulfur-based sprays may help keep leaf spots in check, but they are often phytotoxic when applied regularly indoors.

Sprays: Copper- and sulfur-based sprays. Many bacterial and fungal diseases can be controlled with *Bacillus subtilis* (Serenade).

Mildews
Fungal disease

Common names: black mildew, downy mildew, powdery mildew

Specific diseases that cause mildew include: downy mildew (*Pseudoperonospora cannabina, P. humuli*)
black mildew (*Schiffnerula cannabis*)
powdery mildew (*Leveillula taurica, Oidiopsis taurica* [anamorph], *Sphaerotheca macularis, = S. humuli, Oidium* sp. [anamorph])

Threat to garden: medium to very high

About: Mildews are called "powdery mildew" among cannabis growers. This term encompasses all mildews. Mildew grows on foliage, leaves, and buds. Most look like foliage was sprinkled with fine flour or talcum powder. Mildews drain the vigor of plants, and pose a health risk for some people when smoked.

Identify: The first indication of infection is small spots on the tops of leaves. Next,

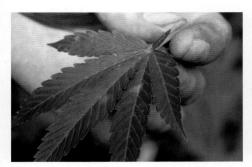

Mildews appear as a little bit of white powder on leaf suface.

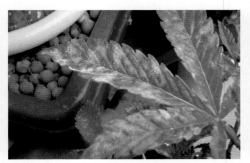

Soon powdery mildew enters plant tissue and spreads.

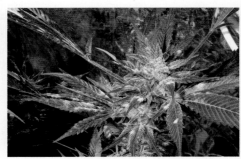

Powdery mildew has taken over this plant.

a powdery looking substance (flowering fungus) appears on foliage. At this point, the systemic disease has been inside the plant a week or more, and the disease can be only arrested by external treatments—but not eliminated. Spots progress to a fine, pale, gray-white powdery coating on growing shoots, leaves, and stems.

Damage: Powdery mildew is not always limited to the upper surface of foliage. Growth slows, leaves yellow, and plants die as the disease advances. Occasionally fatal indoors, this disease is at its worst when roots dry out and foliage is moist. Plants are infected for weeks before they show the first symptoms.

Cause: Mildew is caused by one of the many different species of fungi from the order Erysiphales. Spores are present in the air all the time. They find cool, moist garden rooms with poor circulation the perfect place to live.

Prevention: Once established, mildews must be eliminated from an empty garden room. They cannot be eliminated from plant tissue without the help of a systemic chemical. Cleanliness! Prevent this mildew by avoiding cool, damp, humid, dim conditions in the garden room, as well as fluctuating temperatures and humidity. Low light levels and stale air affect this disease. Increase air circulation and ventilation, and make sure light intensity is high. Space containers far enough apart so air freely flows between plants. Allow foliage to dry before turning off lights. Remove and destroy foliage more than 50 percent infected. Avoid excess nitrogen. Copper, sulfur-lime, and potassium bicarbonate sprays are good prophylactics.

Clones: If buying clones at a dispensary or if acquiring from friends, quarantine or isolate the clones for a week to see if they have powdery mildew and other diseases or pests before introducing them to the main plant population.

Sulfur products such as Safer's Defender prevent powdery mildew on contact with foliage, but the disease is still inside the plant. Applying sulfur make the cannabis taste bad when smoked. It appears to concentrate on resins. Chimera, a cannabis breeder, does not recommend using sulfur on vegetative or flowering plants. He recommends using a sulfur burner in a room to kill all mildew when no plants are in the room.

Apply Serenade (*Bacillus subtilis*) or spray with a saturation mix of baking soda and water to kill surface contamination to keep the disease in check. Copper-based sprays may keep this mold in check. A saturation of baking soda spray dries to a fine powder on the leaf; the baking soda changes the surface pH of the leaf to 7.0, and powdery mildew cannot grow. An organic "systemic" called AquaShield is available from Botanicare, and it has had very favorable reports. A mixture of 10 to 20 percent milk and 80 to 90 percent water is also effective, but it smells bad.

Control: None. Destroy damaged plant material.

Root Rot
Fungal disease

Common names: root rot, soil rot

Specific diseases that cause root rot include: *Phymatotrichum* root rot aka cotton root rot (*Phymatotrichopsis*

omnivore = *Phymatotrichum omnivorum*)
pink rot (*Trichothecium roseum = Cephalothecium roseum Corda*)
Rhizoctonia soreshin and root rot (*Rhizoctonia solani Kühn*)
tropical rot (*Lasiodiplodia theobromae = Botryodiplodia theobromae* Pat)

Threat to garden: medium

Identify: Root rot disease is a catchall term for different fungal and pathogen root infections (see *Pythium* below). These rots cause roots to turn from a healthy white to light brown. As the rot progresses, roots turn darker and become slimy. Growth aboveground is slow. Leaf chlorosis is followed by wilting of the older leaves on the entire plant. When severe, rot progresses up to the base of the plant stock, turning it dark. Root rot is most common when roots are deprived of oxygen and allowed to stand in unaerated water. Soil pests that cut, suck, and chew roots create openings for rotting diseases to enter. Inspect roots with a 10× magnifying glass for signs of pest damage.

Damage: brown slimy roots, slow growth, damaged foliage, and a low yield

Cause: Many fungi cause root rot in cannabis including charcoal rot (*Macrophomina phaseolina*), tropical rot (*Lasiodiplodia theobromae = Botryodiplodia theobromae*), *Rhizoctonia soreshin*, and root rot (*Rhizoctonia solani*).

Prevention: Cleanliness! Use fresh, sterile growing medium. Make sure calcium levels are adequate, and do not overfertilize with nitrogen. Keep pH above 6.5 in soil and about 6.0 in hydroponic mediums to lower disease occurrence, except cotton rot, which likes a

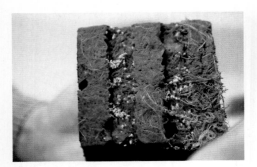

Root rot killed these roots.

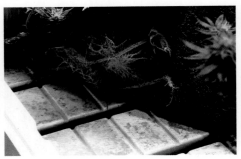

Pythium *attacks roots in the entire garden.*

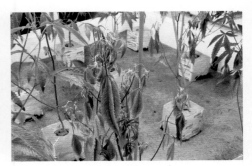

Phytophthora *is killing this garden.*

high pH. Control any insects, fungi, or bacteria that eat roots.

Biological: Binab, Bio-Fungi, RootShield, Supresivit, Trichopel (*Trichoderma harzianum*), or SoilGuard (*Trichoderma virens*).

Control: Once roots are more than half covered with rot, recovery will be very slow if at all. The best control is to toss out the plants. Completely sterilize and sanitize the garden after a bout with root rot.

Sprays: Sprays are not effective for root rot once damage is done.

Pythium
Plant parasites

Common names: *Pythium* wilt, *Pythium*, root rot, damping-off,

Specific diseases that cause root rot in cannabis include: *Pythium irregulare*, *Pythium ultimum*, and *Pythium aphanidermatum*

Threat to garden: high

Identify: *Pythium* can be everywhere and it spreads easily. Infestations can wipe out an entire crop in a greenhouse or indoor garden. *Pythium* is a fungus-like organism that grows and colonizes a plant by producing hyphae (threadlike, filamentous cells) that suck nutrients from host cannabis plants and release enzymes that destroy root tissue. *Pythium* attacks cannabis roots, causes cutting rot, stem rot, and foliar blight under the right conditions. *P. ultimum*, has a very wide range of hosts. *P. ultimum* diseases occur most often at temperatures below 68°F (20°C). *P. aphanidermatum* infections occur more often at temperatures above 77°F (25°C).

Damage: First plants appear stunted and if you look at the root carefully you will see the tips are dead. The roots appear water-soaked and slimy. Seeds may be infested at germination. Stems of seedlings and cuttings may appear soft and watery. Root rot symptoms, regardless of the cause, are surprisingly similar. Accurate diagnosis of *Pythium* is essential because fungicides labeled for other root rot pathogens will not control *Pythium* root rot.

Cause: *Pythium* that attacks cannabis loves wet substrates with high EC. Sometimes they even contaminate soil-less potting mixes. Poor sanitation—using dirty tools and containers or keeping dead infected plants in the garden—are some of the main causes. Fungus gnats and shore flies vector *Pythium* in cannabis gardens.

Prevention: Clean everything! Disinfect everything—walls floor, benches, containers, tools, everything! Use high-quality cuttings—remove any cuttings that show signs of disease. Use clean potting mix. Keep potting soil covered and dry when stored. Growing media, especially peat that holds more than 70 percent moisture is predisposed to P. ultimum damage. Highly decomposed (dark) peat is more susceptible to *Pythium* root rot than a nondecomposed medium or light peat that holds less moisture.

Overwatering and overfertilizing, poorly draining media and roots in standing water all increase *Pythium* infection rates. When overfertilized, excess nitrogen suppresses natural plant defenses. Toxic salt buildup in the substrate damages root tips which provides an easy wound for *Pythium* to infect.

Control
Biological: The commercial products Mycostop and Actino-Iron (*Streptomyces griseoviridis*) are available to protect cannabis and suppress *Pythium*. Applications of Activated Aerated Compost Tea (AACT) will help prevent infection. *Pseudomonas fluorescens*, *Streptomyces griseoviridis*, *S. lydicus*, *Streptomycin lydicus*, *Gliocladium virens*, *Pythium oligandrum* and *Trichoderma harzianum* may be available in commercial substrate mixes to prevent and combat *Pythium*.

Sprays: *Pythium* becomes resistant to sprays after repeated applications. Make sure to rotate sprays to avoid disease resistance. Once *Pythium* infests a plant, sprays do little good. They are best used as a preventative measure. Apply Alude, Biophos, Rampart (phosphorous acid), Banol (propamocarb) and Segway (cyazofamid) as per instructions.

Phytophthora
Fungal disease/host-specific parasite

Common names: water mold, plant destroyer, blight, *Phytophthora* blight

Specific diseases that cause root rot in cannabis include: *Phytophthora* species

Threat to garden: medium to high

Identify: The *Phytophthora* genus, referred to as water molds (Oomycetes), contains an estimated 500 species that damage cannabis. An infestation can wipe out an entire cannabis crop. These pathogens are usually host-specific parasites.

They thrive, grow, reproduce, and infect plant roots in water and saturated soil. *Phytophthora* produces swimming spores (zoospores) are attracted to the roots and infect them. Symptoms are often misdiagnosed.

Damage: This disease attacks the entire plant—roots, stems and foliage—often causing sudden wilting and death. It can infect plants in different growth stages. When plants are infected early in life they die quickly. For example, when clones and seedlings dampen-off they rot at soil line. Infected older plants wilt irreversibly. When you see lesions that girdle the stem, it is too late to save the plant.

First, small dark green spots develop that later get bigger and look scalded. The fungal disease infests and penetrates plant tissue with long threadlike structures (sporangiophores). It causes blights, damping-off and rots. This disease cuts fluid flow within plants and causes leaf yellowing, browning and premature fall and death. These symptoms are worst in hot weather. Plants often wilt and collapse in less than a week.

Belowground you will find rotten roots and few or no feeder roots. The zone between phloem and xylem are dark and discolored. The cambium layer is often reddish brown in color. But conclusive diagnosis requires laboratory analysis of irrigation water or plant material.

Cause: Occurs naturally in most soils and is promoted by excessive substrate moisture and warm wet humid weather. Rain and water spread the disease from plant to plant and throughout garden. *Phytophthora* also survives on and in infested seed. Wind also disseminates the disease.

Prevention: Disinfect all tools, containers, water, soil and garden area with bleach, peroxide or another disinfectant. Keep garden temperatures cool when possible. Avoid overwatering and standing water in garden. Use clean growing media. Avoid excessive nitrogen fertilization.

Biological: Plant resistant cannabis varieties. Composted bark added to soil mixes kills *Phytophthora* as do organic materials that release ammonia and nitrous acid and sulfur-based fertilizers Add composted hardwood or fir bark in potting mixes. They help aerate media, release inhibitors and promote antagonistic soil fungi such as *Trichoderma* sp. to build up

Control: *Phytophthora* is difficult to control with sprays. Fungicides—maneb, mancozeb, zineb and Bravo (Chlorothalonil) are contact fungicides that prevent the disease from entering the seed and plant. Treat water with disinfectant or ozone system. Sterilize growing medium. Keep everything clean!

Sprays: They have limited success. Phosphorous acid (Allude) and the cinnamic acid group (dimethomorph (Acrobat, Forum)) inhibit but do not kill *Phytophthora*. Read label carefully and follow directions because application timing is essential.

Rust
Fungal disease

Common names: rust, hemp rust

Specific diseases that cause rust include: rust (*Aecidium cannabis, Uredo kriegeriana, Uromyces inconspicuus*)

hemp rust (*Melampsora cannabina*)

Threat to garden: very low

Identify: Rust appears as orange blotches on both sides of leaves, mainly on industrial hemp. Tiny yet visible yellow spores fall to infest more foliage.

Damage: Rust discolors and kills foliage but is not fatal.

Cause: Rust is caused by unsterile growing conditions, infested soil, and another host. Sometimes controlling the second plant, the host, will control the rust. In the end, rusts have two separate forms that must have both hosts to propagate.

Prevention: clean growing conditions

Control: It can be controlled by spraying with thiocarbamate (the same stuff they put in Odor Eaters shoe insoles). Thiocarbamate (Zineb-Maneb), is systemic and restricted. DO NOT USE on consumable cannabis.

Verticillium Wilt
Fungal disease

Common names: wilt, *Verticillium* wilt

Specific diseases that cause *Verticillium* wilt include: *Verticillium* wilt (*Verticillium albo-atrum, Verticillium dahliae*)

Threat to garden: low to medium

Identify: Lower older leaves develop chlorotic yellowing on margins and between veins before turning dingy brown. Plants often wilt during the day and recoup when the light goes off. Wilt soon overcomes parts of the plant or the entire plant. Disease starts in the roots and progresses upward, plugging the vascular system. Cut the stem in two and look for the telltale brownish xylem tissue. The fungus blocks the flow of plant fluids, causing wilt and death.

Damage: Blocks the flow of fluids in plants causing wilt and eventual death.

Cause: This fungus is present in unsterile soils and growing mediums. It can be transmitted via cuttings and seeds. *Verticillium* can persist in soils for long periods, and once activated can quickly overtake your garden. It is sensitive to moist soil and moderate temperatures: 75°F (23.9°C) is optimum with 55°F (12.8°C) minimum and 86°F (30°C) maximum for infection to occur.

Prevention: Cleanliness is critical. Use sterile tools. Use fresh, sterile soil with good drainage. Keep plants growing

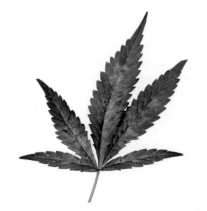

Rust is a fungal disease that is easy to mistake for cultural problems.

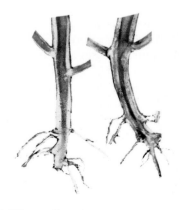

Verticillium *wilt*

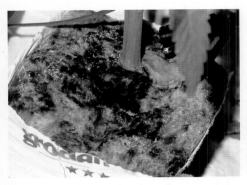

Algae on the surface of rockwool

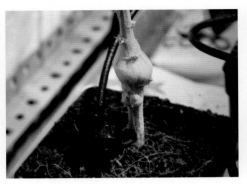

Crown gall on the stem of a cannabis plant

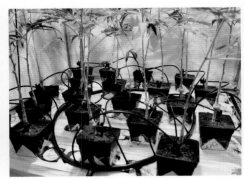

Crown gall infected this entire garden.

strong and vigorous. Avoid wounding plants. Use ammoniacal nitrogen as a source of nitrogen and less overall nitrogen and higher levels of potassium. Do not overfertilize. Make sure to remove infected plants, and keep everything clean!

Biological: Bio-Fungus (*Trichoderma* species), Rhizo Plus (*Bacillus subtilis*)

Control: None. Once *Verticillium* is in the plant, the end is near. Sterilize the entire room if this disease appears.

Sprays: No chemical spray is effective on *Verticillium* wilt.

Algae

Common names: algae, green algae, blue-green algae, green slime

Threat to garden: medium

Identify: Earthy/moldy smelling algae, most often green, can also be brown, reddish, or black. Slimy green algae need nutrients, light, and a moist surface on which to grow. These algae are found growing on moist rockwool and other growing mediums exposed to light. They cause little damage but attract fungus gnats and other critters that damage roots. Once roots have lesions and abrasions, diseases enter easily.

Damage: Algae grow anywhere—growing media; hydroponic, gulleys, pumps, and reservoirs—blocking feeder nozzles and blocking the flow of nutrients in the garden. Algae also attract root-destroying fungus gnats and nematodes. See "Fungus Gnats" and "Nematodes" for more information.

Cause: The earthy/moldy smell comes from decomposition in the growing medium and nutrient solution. Algae

use nutrients and remove oxygen from the nutrient solution, which suffocates roots. Decomposing algae also release toxins that make roots more susceptible to disease attacks.

Prevention: Algae grow when water and nutrients combine under a light source. Remove the light and algae cannot grow. All containers, reservoirs, tubing, channels, and so forth must be lightproof. Prevention of algae is vital. Algae attract fungus gnats and their larvae, as well as nematode infestations. Because control options for these problems and pests once present are limited, the best method of algae control is to prevent the problem. Cover the moist rockwool and growing mediums to exclude light. Run an algaecide in the nutrient solution or water with an algaecide.

Control: A little bit of algae causes few problems, but thick, earthy growth requires action. Clean the system and add an algaecide in the proper proportions. Algae quickly regrow after the algaecide wears off, and the next application must be heavier to be effective. Most often, algaecides are not effective and actually more phytotoxic to roots than damage caused by algae. Unestablished and weak plants will suffer most.

Sprays/drenches: Diazinon, Endosulfan, Propiconazole, Thiram, Ziram, Quinomanid, Irgarol 1051 and hydrogen peroxide. Some grapefruit seed extracts kill algae without harming the plants.

Bacterial Diseases
Crown Gall
Common names: crown gall

Specific disease that causes crown and

stem gall: crown gall (*Agrobacterium tumefaciens*)

Threat to garden: low

Identify: Crown gall (*Agrobacterium tumefaciens*) causes galls or tumorlike growths on stems and the root crown. Plant growth is stunted.

Damage: Large galls form on stems and root crown. Although usually not fatal, once crown gall invades plant tissue, the plant cannot be saved.

Cause: Crown gall is caused by *Agrobacterium tumefaciens* bacteria that live in the soil as well as on root surfaces. It enters and infects plants via a fresh wound.

Prevention: Practice good garden and tool sanitation. Clones are most susceptible to crown gall disease. Take all sanitary precautions when taking clones. Prevent crown gall with applications of *Agrobacterium radiobacter* strain K1026 or strain K84, sold under the brand names Galltrol and Gallex).

Control: None. If crown gall is found in the garden, isolate and destroy affected plants immediately. Disinfect entire garden.

Viruses
Viral disease
Common names: hemp mosaic virus, hemp streak virus (HSV)

Specific viruses include: alfalfa mosaic and Lucerne mosaic (genus *Alfamovirus*, alfalfa mosaic virus [AMV])
arabis mosaic (genus *Nepovirus*, arabis mosaic virus (ArMV))
cucumber mosaic (genus *Cucumovirus*, cucumber mosaic virus (CMV))
hemp mosaic (hemp mosaic virus)

hemp streak (hemp streak virus)

Threat to garden: low to medium-high

Identify: Classic virus infection symptoms include sickly growth, leaf spots, stem spots, yellowing, interveinal yellow streaks, and diminished harvest. Sometimes leaf margins darken sporadically.

Damage: Viruses inhabit the fluid distribution system in plants and impair it. Telltale signs of many viruses include some or all of the following: discolored spots, mottling, chlorosis, streaking, and sometimes margins and leaf tips roll upward. Once a plant gets a virus, little can be done to kill the virus. Viruses seldom kill cannabis, but a viral infection can seriously reduce yields.

Cause: Viruses enter plants via (insect) wounds, pollen, and seed infections. They invade every part of a plant. Once established, viruses multiply in plant cells where they can completely take over the plant. They seldom kill but can severely reduce cannabis yields. Once taking hold in a plant, viruses are almost impossible to exterminate.

Vectors: Viruses are spread by insects, mites, plants, animals, and human vectors. Aphids, whiteflies, seeds, and cuttings are the worst. Infected tools also transport viruses from one plant to another.

Prevention: Cleanliness! Always use fresh, sterile growing medium. Disinfect tools before cutting foliage on different plants. Do not wound plants, and keep other diseases and pests from wounding plants. If you smoke, wash your hands with disinfectant before handling plants. DO NOT SMOKE TOBACCO products around cannabis plants.

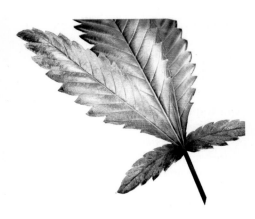

Leaf infected by a mosaic virus

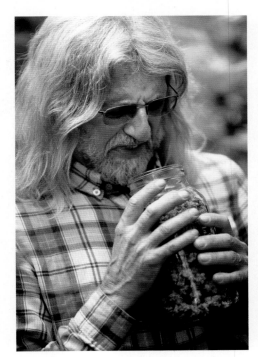

Poorly dried and cured cannabis can smell like ammonia.

Control: Destroy all plants infected with virus.

Biological: none

Sprays: No chemical sprays are effective against viruses.

Storage Fungi and Bacteria Disease

Common names: bacteria, fungi, viruses, gray mold, hemp cancer, brown blight

Specific diseases that cause damping-off include: gray mold (*Botrytis cinerea*)
Sclerotinia sclerotiorum, Alternaria alternata

Bacteria pathogenic to humans found on cannabis include:
Salmonella muenchen, Klebsiella pneumoniae, Enterobacter cloacae, E. agglomerans, Streptococcus (Group D), *Thermoactinomyces candidus, T. vulgaris, Micropolyspora faeni, Aspergillus fumigatus, A. niger, A. flavus, A. tamarii, A. sulphureus, A. repens, Penicillium chrysogenum, P. italicum, Rhizopus stolonifer, Alternaria alternata, Curvularia lunata, and Histoplasma capsulatum.*

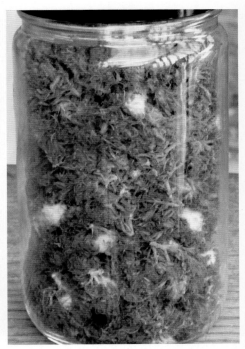

Mold soon becomes a problem when cannabis is improperly dried and cured. These buds were infected with mold, and the jar made a perfect environment for growth. (MF)

Aspergillus can be killed by baking cannabis at 150°C for 15 minutes, but only about 15 percent is destroyed by smoking through a water pipe.

Threat to Dried Buds: high

Identify: Contaminated stored cannabis is often darker, and the texture is changed by the whitish, light-gray fungus that becomes visible. Fungi often appear fuzzy and you may see shades of bluish-green and dark-green. A stale musty "locker room" odor is often apparent. Other times it could exude an ammonia-like odor. If decomposition is rapid, biological activity makes the cannabis warm to the touch.

Damage: Storage molds and bacteria degrade and decompose dry cannabis. Most of the bacteria and fungi that attack dry cannabis are only pathogens and do not infect humans unless they suffer from infections, allergies, or immune system problems. When you light a joint, burning cannabis does not kill fungus. The fungus actually precedes the smoke entering the body. Other contaminants are pet hair, human hair, dust, insect feces, residues, and so on; some of them are highly infectious and others give off toxins.

If any of the above screening tests is positive, the suspect cannabis is discarded without identifying the contaminant.

Cause: Enclosing and storing buds before they are completely dry can give rise to storage fungi and bacteria. Unsanitary contaminated tools, garden rooms, and plants carry pests and diseases.

Prevention: Carefully cultivated and harvested cannabis harbors a minimum of hazardous microorganisms. Thoroughly dry buds and leaves before storage. Available vacuum packing machines are, and will inject inert nitrogen into the storage bag when sealing. Inert nitrogen gas takes the place of all oxygen and prevents further decomposition.

Control: Screen for contamination before packaging for use as medical cannabis. Opportunistic infections pose the greatest danger to immune-suppressed consumers. Sterilize medical cannabis, preferably by gamma irradiation. Baking at low temperatures, gas-sterilizing, even Cobalt 60 irradiation do not kill microbes and are therefore not acceptable methods of decontaminating dry cannabis.

Drying: Dry cannabis contains about 10 percent moisture. Storage fungi cannot live in an environment below 15 percent. Once dry, keep it dry. Avoid damaging dry and drying cannabis. Do not place apple or citrus peels in the drying container; they decompose and attract diseases.

Store dry cannabis in vacuum-sealed containers. Opening sealed containers reexposes cannabis to contaminants and moisture. Be careful avoid letting the dried cannabis absorb more moisture.

Making hash from contaminated cannabis is common—and a bad idea. The contaminants remain in the hash but in a concentrated form, and microbial pathogens and toxins are not always destroyed by heating or other methods of sterilization.

There is no truth to the rumor that moldy cannabis is more psychotropic. Unlike moldy grapes, moldy cannabis is not more potent!

Check out "What to do with a moldy crop?" in chapter 9, *Harvest, Drying & Curing.*

Contaminants

Contaminants adulterate almost all consumed cannabis. Most of these contaminants are harmless, such as dust, but many of the contaminants may be harmful especially to medical patients with a compromised immune system. At best, contaminants taint the taste of cannabis. Contaminants include but are not limited to fungi, bug bodies and feces, sprays, pet hair, dirt and grime, and metal flakes.

In Hayward, California, a well-known cannabis patient with an unusual immune disease died from repeated exposure to the miticide called Avid. Avid is still registered for use in the USA on lawn and garden ornamentals and flowers only.

Caution! DO NOT USE AVID ON MEDICAL OR ANY CANNABIS CROPS. It is derived from the soil microorganism *Streptomyces avermitilis.* Translaminar insecticides and miticides penetrate the leaf tissue and remain in the plant's system. Avid is illegal to sell in the USA, but it is available in Canada. It is for ornamentals only. Avid contains a powerful neurotoxin that is absorbed and accumulates over time.

In the late 1970s, the US government sprayed the herbicide Paraquat on cannabis crops in Mexico, and more recently in Hawaii. Paraquat and other Drug War pesticides permeate vegetative growth. They cause serious health problems in humans.

Fungal or bacterial infections can result from sloppy cultivation techniques. A small number of plant pathogens remain in poorly dried and stored cannabis. Some of these pathogens can infect humans. Individuals with a depressed immune system are most at risk.

Aspergillus, a bacterial contaminant, is found in some improperly stored cannabis. It has been cited by organ transplant experts as a risk to exclude a candidate from receiving a transplant. Tim Garon from Washington state was denied a liver transplant due to these consequences; he passed away in 2008.

Controlling all cannabis for *Aspergillus* and preventing its occurrence with clean gardening and proper drying and storage are essential. See chapter 9, *Harvest, Drying & Curing*, for more information.

Gritweed is cannabis buds covered in tiny, glasslike particles that are actually silica. Gritweed was a big problem in the Netherlands for a few years. It started when the number of coffee shops was cut in half by government policies. Find references to gritweed in old issues of *Soft Secrets* (www.softsecrets.nl).

Pest Insects and Mites
Ants
Common names: ants, piss ants, red ants, big-headed ants, little black ants, pavement ants

Latin names: order *Hymenoptera*

Garden threat: low

Identify: ants

Damage: Ants are annoying; they spread diseases from the outdoor garden to the indoor garden and from plant to plant. Some species of ants "farm" aphids, moving them from source to source for the honeydew aphids give off.

Cause: Ants can enter a garden room that is not sealed shut. They may be drawn by a food source inside the garden room.

Prevention: If ants are entering from outside the garden room, block their entry with a small barrier of cinnamon, Tanglefoot, etc.

Control: Apply as per directions for sweet bait traps: Terro, Pic, Drax Ant Kill Gel (sugar-feeding ants), Drax-FP (grease and sugar-feeding ants), MAXFORCE, (cockroach and Pharaoh ant killer—hydramethylnon). See "Ant Bait" on page 486.

Aphids
Common names: peach aphid, black bean aphid, bhang aphid, hops aphid

Aphid species that attack cannabis include: green peach aphid (*Myzus persicae*, Homoptera: Aphididae. = *Phorodon persicae*)
black bean aphid (*Aphis fabae*, Momoptera: Aphididae)
bhang aphid aka hemp louse (*Phorodon cannabis*, Homoptera: Aphididae. = *Aphis cannabis* = *Mysus cannabis*, =

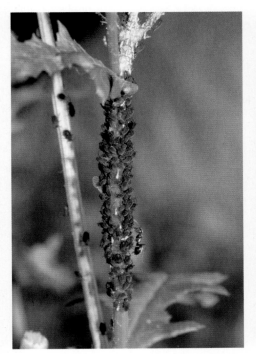

Ants farm aphids, spreading them to other plants.

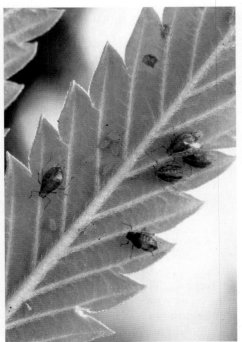

Young adult aphids, translucent with green and brown (MF)

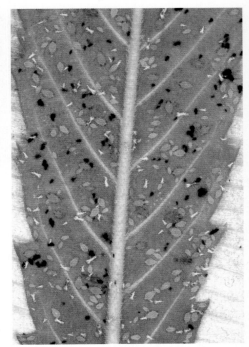

Aphids, spider mite,s and thrips are on this leaf.

Paraphorodon cannabis, = Diphorodon cannabis, = Aphis sativae, = Phorodon asacola, = Capitophorus cannabifoliae, = Semiaphoides cannabiarum) hops aphid (*Phorodon humuli*)

Garden threat: Low. Aphids seldom attack indoor plants and occasionally infest outdoor plants.

Identify: Aphids, also called plant lice, are about the size of a pinhead. They are easy to spot with the naked eye, but use a 10X magnifying glass for positive identification. Aphids are found on leaf undersides, branches, and buds.

Normally grayish to black, aphids can be green to pink. In any color, aphids exude sticky honeydew as they feed. Most aphids have no wings, but for those that do, their wings are about four times the size of their bodies. Aphids give birth to mainly live female larvae, without mating, and can produce 3 to 100 hungry larvae every day. Each female reproduces between 40 and 100 offspring that start reproducing soon after birth. Aphids are most commonly found indoors when they are plentiful outdoors.

Install yellow sticky traps near the base of several plants and near the tops of other plants to monitor invasions of winged aphids, often the first to enter the garden. As they feed, aphids exude sticky honeydew that attracts ants that feed on it. Ants like honeydew so much that they take the aphids hostage and make them produce honeydew. Look for columns of ants marching around plants, and you will find aphids.

Damage: Aphids suck the life-giving sap from foliage, causing leaves to wilt and yellow. Aphids prefer to attack weak, stressed plants. Some species prefer succulent, new growth, and other aphids like older foliage or even flower buds. Look for aphids under leaves or huddled around branch nodes and growing tips. This pest transports (vectors) bacterium, fungi, and viruses. Aphids vector more viruses than any other source. Destructive sooty mold also grows on honeydew. Any aphid control must also control ants, if they are present. Some aphids infest flower tops, causing buds to distort. Aphids can cause entire plants to wilt, be stunted, and die.

Cause: Aphids enter garden rooms and greenhouses on dirty tools, clothes, etc. Or they are naturally present in the garden area outdoors.

Prevention: Grow strong, healthy plants. Inspect plants regularly for aphids. Blast off any sign of aphids with a heavy spray of water.

Control: Manually remove small numbers of aphids. Spot-spray small infestations, and control ants. Introduce predators if problem is persistent.

Cultural and physical control: Manual removal is easy and works well to kill aphids. When affixed to foliage—sucking out fluid—aphids are unable to move and easy to crush with fingers or sponges dipped in an insecticidal solution.

Biological: Lacewings, Chrysoperla species, are the most effective and available predators for aphids. Release one to 20 lacewings per plant, depending on infestation level, as soon as aphids appear. Repeat every month. Eggs take a few days to hatch into larvae that exterminate aphids. Gall midge Aphidoletes aphidimyza is available under the trade name Aphidend; parasitic wasp Aphidius matricariae is available commercially.

Ladybugs also work well to exterminate aphids. Adults are easily obtained at many retail nurseries during the summer months. The only drawback to ladybugs is their attraction to the HID lamp—release about 50 ladybugs per plant, and at least half of them will fly directly into the HID, hit the hot bulb, and buzz to their death. Within one or two weeks, all the ladybugs will fall victim to the lamp, requiring frequent replenishment. *Verticillium lecanii* (fungus)—available under the trade name of Vertalec—is aphid-specific and effective.

Control ants with borax. See "Boric Acid" on page 488.

Sprays: Homemade and insecticidal soap sprays are very effective. Apply two or three times at five- to ten-day intervals. Pyrethrum (aerosol) applied two to three times at five- to ten-day intervals.

Root Aphids

Common name: root aphid

Garden threat: very high

Root aphid species that attack cannabis include: grape phylloxera

Identify: Root aphids (grape phylloxera) are tiny aphid-like insects that feed on a number of plant roots. They are often confused with fungus gnats. Oval- to pear-shaped, phylloxera are small (0.04 inch [1 mm] long) and from yellow/ yellowish green/olive green to light- to dark-brown or orange in color. Oval-shaped eggs are yellow. Nymphs are small versions of adults. The majority of grape phylloxera adults are wingless females.

Root aphids, in the genus *Phemigus*, are increasingly feeding on cannabis root systems and have become a major pest in parts of the USA and other parts of the world. Inspect roots by sliding the root ball out of the container. Root aphids are super tiny insects with legs. Aphids colonize roots on the outside of the root ball especially near drainage holes. They are about the size and color of coco fiber grains.

Damage: Phylloxera feed on roots and rootlets, causing them to yellow from the bottom up, swell, and turn hard. Dead (necrotic) spots develop where pests feed. Secondary fungi infect wounds and often girdle roots, killing large sections. Plants become stunt-ed, and yield diminishes substantially. Infestations can kill plants. Damage is easily confused with disorders caused by nutrients, water, and so forth.

Cause: Root aphids can be introduced

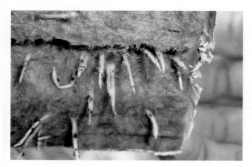

Root aphids

to the garden by infested soil clones or seedlings. They can also be carried in on dirty tools, or fly or crawl into unfil-tered rooms. They overwinter as small nymphs on roots. In spring when soil temperatures exceed 60°F (15°C), they start feeding and growing. Indoors, root aphids are very active 24/7. When soil temperatures fall below 60°F (15°C), all life stages die except the small nymphs. There are three to five generations each year. First instar nymphs are active crawlers and may move from plant to plant in the ground, on the soil surface, or by blowing in the wind. They may also be moved between vineyards on cuttings, boots, or equipment. Grape phylloxera is more common near vine-yards, where they infest grape vines.

Prevention: Avoid cool, heavy clay soils and soils in grape-growing regions that are infested with grape phylloxera. Avoid overfertilization with nitrogen.

Use sticky yellow traps to monitor flying adults.

Pesticide treatment will not eradicate phylloxera populations; even if much of the phylloxera is killed, populations often rebound quickly.

Control: Once the garden is infested, root aphids are hard to dispatch. A multipronged approach may be necessary to completely break their life cycle. A strong drench such as BotaniGard slows root aphids down, followed by releases of predatory nematodes (*Heterorhabditis bacteriophora*), which helps ensure that they are all killed and eaten!

BotaniGard is an insecticide that is composed of a living fungus, Beauveria bassiana. This fungus seeks out aphids

and infects them, causing death. Then it releases spores, waiting for more victims. It also works to control whiteflies and thrips. You can order it at many garden stores or through garden websites on the Internet.

Neem oil and citrus oil have also been used to kill aphids, but they sometimes affect plant roots. Test them on a sample plant before using either of them in the garden.

The aphids should be treated every other day with a minimum of six treatments. Rotate the insecticides.

BotaniGard can be combined with pyrethrum. The neem and citrus oils can be mixed with each other as well as with pyrethrum. The idea is to totally eliminate the pests.

Predatory nematodes (*Heterorhabditis bacteriophora*) are super effective and easy to use. The best part about using the nematodes is that they will kill all of the little root aphids!

Once aphids are gone, it is difficult for them to re-infect the garden. They were probably introduced to the garden by a new element such as a clone or infected planting mix.

Bees and Wasps

Garden threat: none

Bees (*Anthophila*, more than 20,000 known species)

Wasps (order *Hymenoptera* and suborder Apocrita)

Hornets (order *Hymenoptera*, family *Vespidae*, genus *Vespa*)

Identify: Bees and wasps that sting are usually from a half-inch (1.3 cm) to more than an inch (2.5 cm) long. Many have yellow stripes around their bodies; others have none. They are especially attracted to indoor gardens when weather cools outdoors. They move right in.

They have many names and manifesta-tions. For example, in Alabama there are four wasps that sting: red, red-faced, small red, and black. Also, there are two hornets, one that builds big nests and has a bald or white face. European wasps also make appearances.

Note: Many beelike insects are beneficial. See "Beneficial Insects" in this chapter.

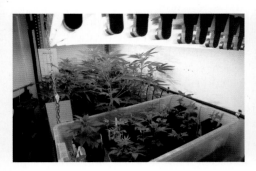

Sticky yellow traps are kept in place to monitor insect populations.

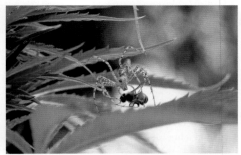

Green lynx spider attacking a bee (MF)

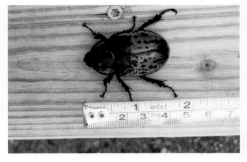

This unknown beetle was captured in Alabama and measures nearly two inches (5 cm) in length!

Damage: No damage to plants but can become a nuisance in garden rooms—they hurt like hell when they sting!

Cause: Bees and wasps occur in garden areas during spring, summer, and autumn in most climates but can be active in winter in warm climates.

Prevention: Exclude from garden rooms and greenhouses with screens and traps.

Control: Bees and wasps are occasionally a problem indoors and are most efficiently controlled with sprays.

Cultural and physical control: They enter garden rooms through vents and cracks, and are attracted by the growing plants, a valuable commodity in the middle of a cold winter! Screen all entrances to the room. Install more circulation fans to make flying difficult. Wasp traps, sweet flypaper, and Tanglefoot impair these pests. Bees and wasps are also attracted to the hot HID and fly into it and die.

Biological: unnecessary

Sprays: Pyrethrum is recommended. Stuff small nests into a wide-mouthed jar—do it at night when the wasps are quiet—and place the jar in a freezer for a few hours. Use Sevin (carbaryl) only if there is a problem with a wasp nest. Use wasp and hornet sprays to control as well, but DO NOT allow the spray to get on plants, as it will damage the plant tissue.

Beetles

Common names: beetles, black beetles, ground beetle, stink beetles, flea beetles

Beetle species that attack cannabis include: beetle (order Coleoptera) hemp flea beetle (*Psylliodes attenuata*, Coleoptera: Chrysomelidae. = *Haltica attenuata*, = *Phylliodes japonica*, = *Psylliodes apicalis*)
tarnished plant bug (*Lygus lineolaris*, Hemiptera: Miridae)
click beetle (family Elateridae)
Japanese beetle (*Popillia japonica*, Coloptera: Scarabaeidae)

Garden threat: low

Identify: Beetles are a large family, and their larvae and grubs often act as borers. Typically, beetles have two pairs of wings: the front pair is hard and shell-like to protect the wings below, which are used to fly. A ladybug (ladybird beetle) is a good example.

Damage: Beetles larvae infest soil and eat roots. They also eat tender plant tips. This mutilates, deforms, and stunts plants. Diseases enter the wounds. Hemp flea beetles feed on seedling and clone foliage. Stalks and stems can be infested by European corn borers and hemp borers, weevils, and an assortment of grubs and borers that love stems.

Cause: Contaminated tools and plant material and an unsterile indoor garden or garden area can lead to beetle infestations. Outdoors, borers' eggs could be present in the soil or could come from adjacent plants.

Prevention: Keep indoor garden area clean. Use sterile growing medium. Exclude beetles from garden. Outdoors, till soil and keep adjacent garden area clean.

Control

Biological: Control wireworms with beneficial nematodes (*Heterorhabidis* and *Steinernema* spp.). Control tarnished plant bugs with predatory spined soldier bug (*Podisus* spp.).

Borers

Garden threat: outdoors medium, seldom seen indoors

Borer species that attack cannabis include: European corn borer (*Ostrinia nubilalis*, Lepidoptera: Pyralidae. = *Pyrausta nubilalis*, = *Botys silacealis*) hemp borer (*Grapholita delineana*,

Wasp traps keep wasps in check and work well to monitor activity

Lepidoptera: Olethreutidae. = *Cydia delineana*, = *Laspeyresia delineana*, = *Grapholita sinana*, = *Cydia sinana*) common stalk borer (*Papaipema nebris*, Lepidoptera: Noctuidae. = *P. nieta*)

Identify: Many boring insects are members of several families that include boring larvae, grubs, minors, maggots, and so forth that tunnel or bore into stems, foliage, and roots. At one stage in their lives they could turn into beetles, caterpillars, or moths of many shapes, colors, and sizes. Look for their entry hole and dead growth on either side of the entry hole along the main stem, often discolored and accompanied by sawdust. Borers are more common outdoors than indoors. Borers are more common in areas where industrial hemp is growing. Borers have accounted for serious crop loss in Europe.

Many borers are able to produce three to five generations per year that flourish in temperatures above 60°F (15.6°C). Borers overwinter in the soil and emerge the following year. Disrupting the life cycle is the best long-term control. Some borers spin cocoons.

Damage: Tunnels and burrows inside stems, foliage, and roots curtail fluid flow and cause plant parts to wilt. If borer damages the main stem severely,

fluid flow to the entire plant could stop, causing death. Wounds and feces attract moisture, disease, and infections. Hemp borers have a ravenous appetite and can destroy flowering tops and cannabis seeds.

Cause: Outdoors, borers are in the soil and in agricultural crops and roses, among other ornamentals and vegetables. Though seldom a problem indoors, borers occasionally attack outdoor crops.

Prevention: Seldom a problem indoors. Bait with *Bt* (*Bacillus thuringiensis*) to prevent and kill borers. Watch for beetles and moths that lay borer eggs.

Controls: Borers can be fought with 50 percent methyl parathion (0.5 oz [14.8 ml]) for 1,000 square feet (9.3 m²). After harvesting, the stubble and waste stalks should be burned, and the field plowed.

Cultural and physical control: Hand-pick all beetle grubs. Borers often cause so much damage on a particular stem that it has to be removed and destroyed.

Sprays: *Bacillus popilliae* is specific to beetles or rotenone individually injected into stems.

Biological: Several mixes of beneficial nematodes control these borers in soil.

Biological Control: The wasp *Trichogramma evanescens* Westwood, Hymenoptera species of parasites and predators prey on *Grapholita delineana*.

Caterpillars and Loopers
Caterpillar species that attack cannabis include: silver moth (*Autographa gamma*, Lepidoptera: Noctuidae. = *Plusia gamma*, = *Phytometra gamma*) dot moth (*Melanchra persicariae*, Lepidoptera: Noctuidae. = *Polia persicariae*, = *Mamestra persicariae*) cabbage moth (*Mamestra brassicae*, Lepidoptera: Noctuidae. = *Barathra brassicae*) garden tiger moth (*Arctia caja*, Lepidoptera: Arctiidae) common hairy caterpillar (*Spilosoma obliqua*, Lepidoptera: Arctiidae. = *Diacrisia obliqua*) beet webworm (*Loxostege sticticalis*, Lepidoptera: Pyraustinae. = *Phlyctaenodes sticticalis*) corn earworm moth (*Helicoverpa zea*) chrysanthemum webworm (*Cnephasia interjectana*, Lepidoptera; Tortricidae. = *Cnephasia virgaureana*) death's-head moth (*Acherontia atropos*, Lepidoptera: Sphingidae. = *Sphinx atropos*)

Garden threat: low indoors, high outdoors and greenhouses

Caterpillars and loopers leave plenty of droppings on the plant. The droppings accumulate between buds. Droppings fall out when the buds are hung to dry; inspect

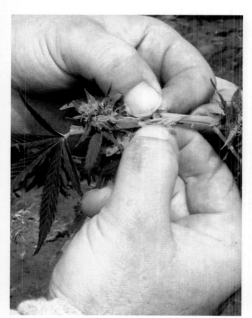

Sticky yellow traps are kept in place to monitor insect populations.

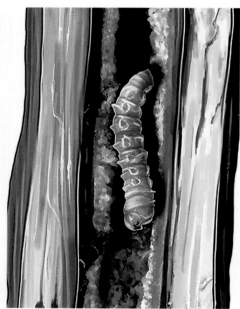

Borers live inside stems.

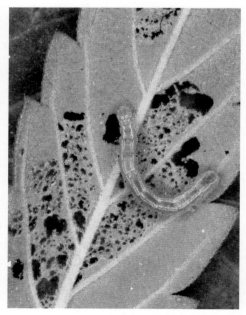

Caterpillar populations can explode. The little worms eat more than their body weight in foliage every day.

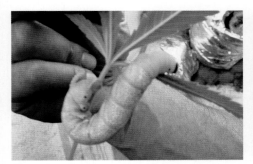

This beautiful caterpillar is able to munch down many leaves in a single day!

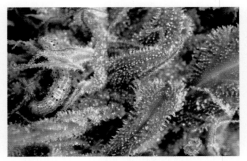

Look closely at the left side of the photo and you will see a corn earworm disguised as part of the resinous foliage. (MF)

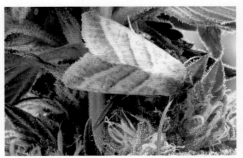

This moth lays the eggs that hatch into the (cannabis) corn earworms. Always keep an eye out for this moth in your garden! (MF)

below the hung buds to find the droppings.

Caterpillars turn into moths or butterflies and fly away. Some transform quickly and fly; others take longer to migrate. Caterpillars have a peak occurrence and can be planned for, in most instances. They may complete a life cycle and do it again, but most typically they develop slower and pupate or lay eggs that overwinter. Some do so as a larva. They will also move like armyworms.

Identify: From a half-inch to four inches long (1.3–10.2 cm), caterpillars and loopers are cylindrical with feet, often green, but can be virtually any color from white to black. Caterpillars have sets of feet the entire length of the body, while loopers have two sets of feet at either end of the body. Loopers place their front feet forward, arch their body upward in the middle, and pull their rear set of legs forward. Some have stripes, spots, and other designs that provide camouflage. Seldom a problem indoors, caterpillars and loopers are in a life stage—between a larva and a flying moth or butterfly—and are most common when prevalent outdoors. One way to check for caterpillars and loopers is to spray one plant with pyrethrum aerosol spray and shake the plant afterward. The spray has a quick knockout effect, and most caterpillars will fall from the plant.

Caterpillars are problems primarily for outdoor growers. Caterpillars eat floral clusters from the inside out, and their activities provide a vector for a pervasive cannabis fungal disease.

Leaf-eating caterpillars spend most of their time on leaves. They often manipulate leaves before eating them; their feeding habits include eating small sections of leaf in between leaf veins, or eating large chunks of leaf outright.

Damage: These munching critters chew and eat pieces of foliage and leave telltale bites in leaves. Some caterpillars will roll themselves inside leaves. An infestation of caterpillars or leafhoppers will damage foliage and slow growth, eventually defoliating, stunting, and killing a plant.

Cause: Untilled soil outdoors around and in garden area. Eggs overwinter in soil and are often killed by tilling. Adjacent plants attract or have caterpillars and their eggs.

Prevention: Bait with *Bt* (*Bacillus thuringiensis*) before caterpillars are normally out.

Control: Shake plants several times a day to dislodge the insects. Preventive sprays containing insecticidal soaps and organic toxins can be used selectively during vegetative cycle, but extreme care must be taken during floral cycle.

Cultural and physical control: Manually remove.

Biological: *Trichogramma* wasps, spined soldier bug (*Podisus maculiventris*, Podibug).

Sprays: Pyrethrum aerosol works great! Homemade spray/repellent, hot pepper and garlic, *Bt*, pyrethrum, rotenone, and neem products.

Crickets
Common names: crickets, field crickets, house crickets, mole crickets, tree crickets

Cricket species that attack cannabis include: family Gryllidae (*Gryllus desertus*, *Gryllus chinensis*) mole cricket (*Gryllotalpa gryllotalpa*, *Gryllotalpa hexadactyla*) tree cricket (*Oecanthus indicus*)

Garden threat: low

Identify: There are more than 900 species of crickets. They range in size from 0.6 to 1 inch (15–25.4 mm). Crickets have somewhat flattened bodies and long antennae. Generally nocturnal, crickets may be confused with grasshoppers that have similar (jumping) hind legs and body structure. The familiar chirp (stridulation) of crickets is produced predominately by males. Crickets are found in moist areas and climates and are known to frequent gardens, especially around water sources, singing their song on warm summer nights.

Crickets are omnivorous scavengers. They eat decaying plant material, fungi, and tender seedling plants. Crickets lay eggs in the fall that hatch in the spring. A single female can lay up to 200 eggs.

Damage: Crickets eat young seedlings and emerging plants.

Cause: Crickets are common in humid conditions in (tropical) warm weather and during hot summers.

Prevention: Keep crickets outdoors! Drive them away from greenhouses by cleaning the perimeter. They have many food sources and seldom attack cannabis.

Cutworms
Common names: beet armyworm, black cutworm, cabbage moth, common cutworm, paddy cutworm

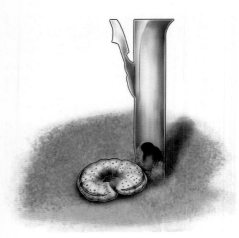

Cutworms live near the base of a plant.

Cutworm species that attack cannabis include: black cutworm (*Agrotis ipsilon* Lepidoptera: Noctuidae. = *Euxoa ypsilon*)
paddy cutworm (*Spodoptera litura Fabricius*, Lepidoptera: Noctuidae. = *Prodenia litura Fabricius*)
beet armyworm (*Spodoptera exigua*, Lepidoptera: Noctuidae. = *Laphygma exigua*)
claybacked cutworm (*Agrotis gladiaria*, Lepidoptera: Noctuidae)
common cutworm (*Agrotis segetum*, Lepidoptera: Noctuidae. = *Euxoa segetum*)
Bertha armyworm (*Mamestra configurata*, Lepidoptera: Noctuidae)

Garden threat: low

Identify: Cutworms are larvae of other pests that are in the soil during a stage of their life. Cutworms are larvae that eat the base of the stem and cut off the plant. They come in many shapes and sizes. Cutworm larvae have a big appetite and will devour seeds, sprouted seeds, and seedlings. They must become strong to transform into moths or butterflies. Once plant roots and stems are stronger and tougher, cutworms are less of a threat. Cutworms rarely find their way into an indoor garden. Outdoors they are most common in backyard gardens and in greenhouses where plants grow in the ground.

Damage: Cutworms dine on emerging plants and seedlings, ultimately killing them. Often small plants emerge for a few days and the roots are eaten by a cutworm.

Cause: untilled soil that contains cutworm eggs

Prevention: Till soil or use new soil.

Control: *Bt* bait mixed in soil

Grasshoppers
Common names: two-spotted grasshopper, clear-winged grasshopper, citrus locust. (I always call them *saltamontes*, Spanish for grasshopper.)

Grasshopper species that attack cannabis include: *Melanoplus bivittatus, Chloealtis conspersa, Camnula pellucida, Zonocerus elegans, Chondracris rosea*

Garden threat: low

Identify: Grasshoppers and locusts pose little threat to cannabis crops unless large swarms of the pests arrive. Some years there are plagues of grasshoppers, and locusts swarm and migrate, eating all plants in sight. They are easy to identify and come in many sizes. With long, folded legs, grasshoppers are built to bound long distances. They are occasionally problematic outdoors. Grasshoppers stay around only for a short period of time and move on. Grasshoppers are best handpicked from your plants if you wish to control them. Birds also eat grasshoppers.

Damage: Very little damage to leaves. Seldom will swarms of locusts appear and eat all foliage in sight.

Cause: You let them into your indoor garden room. Outdoors, grasshoppers have a free range and cause little damage.

Prevention: none needed

Control
Biological: Encourage birds in your garden. Handpick grasshoppers with nimble fingers.

Leafhoppers
Common names: Leafhopper, greenhouse leafhopper, spittlebug,

Leafhopper species that attack cannabis include: (family Cicadellidae) *Zygina (Erythroneura) pallidifrons, Graphocephala coccinea, Empoasca fabae, Empoasca flavescens, Philaenus spumarius, Bothrogonia ferruginea, Stictocephala bubalus*

Garden threat: low indoors, high outdoors and greenhouses

Identify: Leafhoppers include many small, 0.125 inch (3.2 mm) long, wedge-shaped insects that are usually green, white, or yellow, but some are larger and look like green grasshoppers with leafs for wings. They can move very fast. Many species have minute stripes on wings and bodies. Their wings peak like roof rafters when not in use. Leafhoppers suck plant sap for food and exude sticky honeydew as a by-product. Spittlebug and leafhopper larvae wrap themselves in foliage and envelop themselves in a saliva-like liquid, plant sap. They can be serious pests, especially the glasshouse leafhopper (*Zygina pallidifrons*).

Damage: Leafhoppers cause stippling

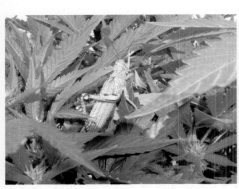

Grasshoppers are normally not attracted to cannabis. But if they get hungry, grasshoppers will eat anything! (MF)

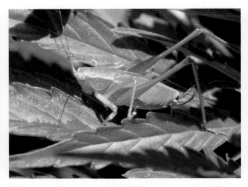

There are many, many different species of grasshoppers. (MF)

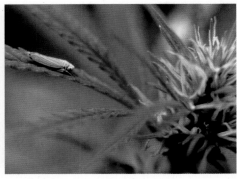

The leafhopper on the left-hand side of the photo blends in with the foliage. (MF)

(spotting) on foliage, similar to that caused by spider mites and thrips. Leaves and plant lose vigor, and in severe cases death could result.

Cause: Eggs come in via unclean garden practices. Adults enter via the front door, cracks, or holes in garden rooms. Outdoors, this pest has free range.

Prevention: Cleanliness! Screen windows and use hygienic control.

Cultural and physical control: Blacklight traps are attractive to potato beetles.

Biological: The fungus *Metarhizium anisopliae* is commercially available under the trade name Metaquino.

Sprays: pyrethrum, rotenone, sabadilla

Leaf Miner

Common name: leaf miner

Leaf miner species that attack cannabis include: (family Agromyzidae) *Liriomyza (Agromyza) strigata, Phytomyza horticola, Agromyza reptans, Liriomyza eupatorii, Liriomyza cannabis*

Garden threat: very low

Identify: Adult leaf miner flies lay eggs that hatch into one-eighth-inch (0.25 mm) long green or black maggots. You seldom see the maggots before you see the leaf damage they create when they tunnel through leaf tissue. Leaf miners are more common in greenhouses and outdoors than indoors.

Damage: The tiny maggots burrow between leaf surfaces, leaving a telltale whitish-tunnel outline. The damage usually occurs on or in young supple growth. It is seldom fatal, unless left unchecked. Damage causes plant growth to slow, and if left unchecked, flowering is prolonged and buds are small. In rare cases the damage is fatal. Wound damage encourages disease.

Cause: These little pests fly in through the door and are often abundant outdoors.

Prevention: Little prevention is necessary because they pose little threat to the garden.

Controls: Leaf miners cause little problems for indoor crops. The most efficient and effective control is to remove and dispose of damaged foliage, which includes the rogue maggot, or to use

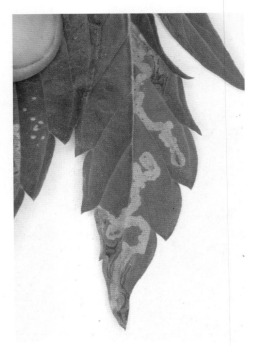

Leaf miners burrow between the surfaces of foliage, leaving telltale channels.

the cultural and physical control listed below.

Cultural and physical control: Smash the little maggot trapped within the leaf with your fingers. If the infestation is severe, smash all larvae possible and remove severely infested leaves. Compost or burn infested leaves. Install yellow sticky traps to capture adults.

Biological: braconid wasp (*Dacnusa sibirica*), chalcid wasp (*Diglyphus isaea*), parasitic wasp (*Opius pallipes*)

Sprays: Repel with neem oil and pyrethrum sprays. Maggots are protected within tunnels, and sprays are often ineffective. *Hemp Diseases and Pests* suggests to water plants with a 0.5 percent solution of neem. This solution works fast and stays on plants for four weeks after application.

Fungus Gnats

Fungus gnat species that attack cannabis are from two families: Mycetophilidae and Sciaridae.

Garden threat: medium

Identify: Winged adult gnats are gray to black, long-legged flies with wings. Related to crane flies that also infest soil and root zones, fungus gnats are also called "sciarid flies" or "sciarids."

Adults measure 0.06 to 0.125 inches (1.5–3.2 mm) long. Spot flies scurrying near plant bases and on growing media or foliage. Females deposit eggs in moist growing media.

White to transparent larva with black heads feed on both dead and living plant tissue, including roots. Maggots (larvae) grow to 0.16 or 0.2 inches (4 or 5 mm) long. Fungus gnats are long with long legs. Look for them around the base of plants in soil and soilless gardens. They love the moist, dank environments in rockwool and the environment created in NFT-type hydroponic gardens. Adult females lay about 200 eggs every week to ten days.

Fungus gnats are believed to spread plant disease pathogens in the media, so good control is important.

Damage: Fungus gnats infest growing mediums and roots near the surface. They can eat fine root hairs and scar larger roots when in large numbers and food is scarce, causing plants to lose vigor and foliage to turn pale. Fungus gnat damage can penetrate roots and stems when severe. Root wounds invite wilt fungi like *Fusarium* or *Pythium*, especially if plants are nutrient-stressed and growing in soggy conditions. Maggots prefer to consume dead or decaying, soggy plant material; they also eat green algae growing in soggy conditions. Adults and larvae can get out of control quickly, especially in hydroponic systems with very moist growing mediums. The adult gnats stick to resinous buds like flypaper! The gnats are very difficult to clean from the buds.

Cause: Overly moist overfertilized soil or growing medium rich in organic nitrogen and green algae growth attract fungus gnats.

Prevention: Keep garden room, tools, supplies, and yourself clean. Do not overwater or overfertilize. Do not let green algae grow on substrate surface. Lower the humidity in the room. Cover air intakes with fine screens. Monitor for fungus gnat presence with yellow sticky traps set out at the base of plants.

Controls: The easiest control for these pests is with Vectobac, Gnatrol, or Bactimos—all contain *Bacillus thuringiensis*

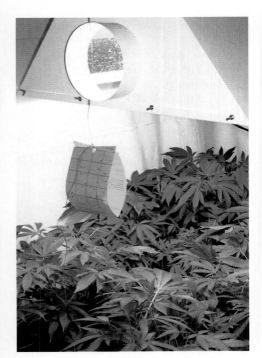

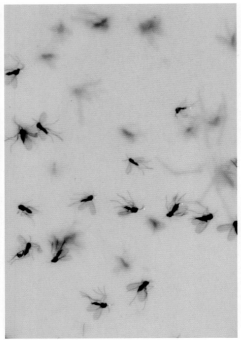

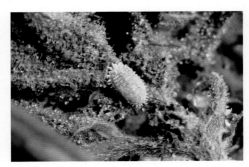

Mealybug (MF)

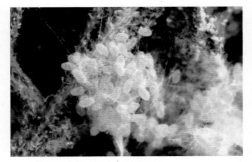

Mealybug eggs (MF)

Fungus gnats often go unnoticed. A yellow sticky trap placed near substrate or above plant canopy helps monitor their presence.

A close-up view of this yellow sticky trap reveals a fungus gnat infestation.

var. *israelensis* (*Bt-i*). This strain of *Bt* controls the maggots; unfortunately, it is available only in one-gallon (3.8 L) containers. It is difficult to find at garden centers; check hydroponic stores.

Azadirachta (neem tree) kinoprene, difubenzuron, or cyromazine can also be effective.
Gnatrol controls larvae, but it must be specific to gnats and not for caterpillar control.

Cultural and physical control: Do not overwater. Keep ambient humidity low. Do not let growing medium remain soggy. Cover growing medium so green algae will not grow. Yellow sticky traps placed horizontally one to two inches (2.5–5.1 cm) over growing medium catch adults.

Biological: *Bt-i* works best. Alternatives include the predatory soil mite Hypoaspis (Geolaelaps mites) and the nematode *Steinernema feltiae*.

Heavy-duty chemical controls include heavy soil drenches with malathion, acephate, or diazinon.

Pyrethrum (pyrethroids) works somewhat effectively, but repeat applications are necessary.

Gnats can be killed by disturbing or heating soil, by predatory wasps, and by applying insecticidal soap, neem, rotenone, or garlic oil to gnat infestations. It is best to control gnats proactively.

Sprays: Apply neem or insecticidal soap as a soil drench.

Mealybugs
Garden threat: medium

Mealybug species that attack cannabis include: long-tailed mealybug *Pseudococcus longispinus*

Identify: Somewhat common indoors, these 0.08 to 0.2 inch (2–5 mm) oblong, waxy-white insects move very little, mature slowly, and live in colonies that are usually located at stem joints. Like aphids, mealybugs excrete sticky honeydew.

Damage: Mealybugs suck sap from plants, slowing plant growth. They leave sticky honeydew in their wake, which attracts sooty mold and draws ants that eat the honeydew.

Cause: Mealybugs can be brought into the garden on contaminated plants or as the result of an unclean garden and surrounding garden area. Humans and animals transfer this pest at the crawler stage.

Prevention: Little damage is caused by these pests, and they are seldom present in clean garden rooms. Outdoor and greenhouse growers must keep gardens clean and tidy to avoid infestations. They are most problematic during mid to late summer.

Control: Manual removal is tedious but very effective. Wet a Q-Tip in rubbing alcohol and wash scale away. A small knife, fingernails, or tweezers may also be necessary to scrape and pluck the tightly affixed mealybugs and scales after they are treated with alcohol.

Biological: There are numerous species of mealybugs. Each has natural predators, including species of ladybeetles

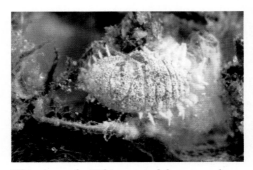

This photo of a Hibiscus mealybug was taken on an infested 'Haze' plant. Males have wings and are not stationary. Nymphs move and are known as crawlers. An immature female, pictured above, reaches maturity in a few weeks. (MF)

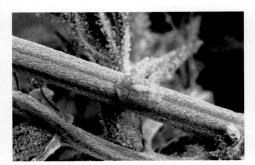

Scale on cannabis stem (MF)

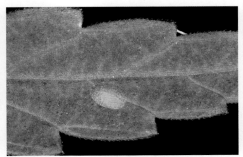

This little scale is living on the surface of a leaf.

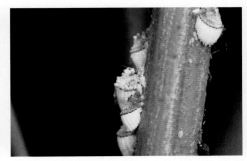

This colony of scale is living on the plant stem. They spread fast!

(ladybugs) and parasitic and predatory wasps. There are so many species of each that it would be exhaustive to list them here. For more specific information, see *Hemp Diseases and Pests*.

Sprays: Homemade sprays that contain rubbing alcohol, nicotine, and soaps all kill these pests. Insecticidal soap, pyrethrum, and neem oil are all recommended.

Scale

Common names: Scale

Scale species that attack cannabis include: cottonycushion scale (*Icerya purchasi*)
European fruit lecanium (*Parthenolecanium corni*)
hemispherical scale (*Saissetia coffeae*)
white peach scale (*Pseudaulacaspis pentagona*)

Garden threat: low to medium

Identify: Scale looks and acts similar to mealybugs but is usually more round than oblong. Scales may be white, yellow, brown, gray, or black. Their hard protective shell is 0.08 to 0.15 inch (2–3.8 mm) across. Once established, mealybugs and scale rarely or never move. Check for them around stem joints where they live in colonies. Scales sometimes excrete sticky honeydew.

Damage: These pests suck sap from plants, which causes growth to slow. They also exude sticky honeydew as a by-product of their diet, which encourages sooty mold and draws ants that eat the honeydew.

Cause: Scale can be brought into the garden on contaminated plants or as the result of an unclean garden and surrounding garden area. Humans and animals transfer this pest on dirty tools, clothes, and so on.

Prevention: Keep garden and surrounding area clean. Do not bring in infested plants.

Controls: These pests present little problem to indoor growers. The easiest and most efficient control is listed under "Cultural and physical control" below.

Cultural and physical control: Manual removal is somewhat tedious but very effective. Wet a Q-Tip in rubbing alcohol and wash scale away. A small knife, fingernails, or tweezers may also be necessary to scrape and pluck tightly affixed mealybugs and scales after they are treated with alcohol.

Biological: There are numerous species of mealybugs and scales. Each has natural predators, including species of ladybeetles (ladybugs) and parasitic and predatory wasps. There are so many species of each that it would be exhaustive to list them here. For specific information, see *Hemp Diseases and Pests*.

Sprays: Homemade sprays that contain rubbing alcohol, nicotine, and soaps all kill these pests. Insecticidal soap, pyrethrum, and neem oil are all recommended.

Nematodes

Common names: root-knot nematode, stem nematode, nematodes, needle worm, eelworm

Nematode species that attack cannabis include: cyst (*Heterodera humuli Filipjev, H. schachtii Schmidt*)
needle (*Paralongidorus maximus* (Butschli) Siddiqi = *Longidorus maximus* (Butschli) Th. et Swang)
root-knot (*Meloidogyne incognita* (Kofoid &White) Chitwood, *M. javanica* (Treub) Chitwood) stem (*Ditylenchus dipsaci* (Kühn) Filipjev)

Garden threat: low to medium

Identify: Of the 15,000 of species of microscopic nematodes, only a few are destructive to plants, including cannabis. Most often nematodes attack roots and are found in the soil; however, a few nematodes attack stems and foliage. Big ones are sometimes called eelworms. Others, called needle worms, can be seen only under a microscope. Root nematodes can often be seen in and around roots with the help of a 30X microscope. Often growers just diagnose the damage caused by destructive nematodes rather than actually seeing them. Do not confuse nematode symptoms with nematode attacks. If plants already have adequate water and nutrients, be sure to check for nematodes.

Damage: Slow growth, leaf chlorosis, wilting for several hours during daylight hours from lack of fluid flow—symptoms can be difficult to discern from nitrogen deficiency. Root-knot nematodes are some of the worst. Root damage is evidenced by swollen knots and galls. Lesion nematodes make reddish brown wounds and cause leaf yellowing when they scrape stems. Cut and scraped roots are compounded by fungal, viral, and bacterial attacks. Roots turn soft and mushy. Bad nematodes attack both hydroponic and soil gardens. Stem nematodes live aboveground, attacking foliage that then swells and yellows. Foliage later distorts and plants are stunted.

Cause: Nematodes spread from soil to hydroponic gardens in the wind and on

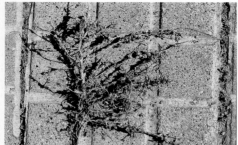

Root-knot nematodes cause growth to slow dramatically. Roots develop nodules and have a difficult time drawing in water and nutrients.

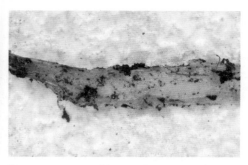

Root maggots ate this root down to a point. The little maggots consumed all the tender root hairs.

equipment, pets, and people. Fungus gnats and their larvae also transport and spread nematodes. Unsterile, infected soil and water also carry nematodes.

Prevention: Do not raise seedlings in soil and transplant to hydroponics.

Control: In soil, control with fumigation; in hydroponics, clean the system. Remove and destroy all plant material and growing medium. Disinfect and sterilize garden room with bleach.

Cultural and physical control: Cleanliness! Use new, sterilized potting soil or soilless mix to exclude nematodes' entrance. Nematodes rarely cause problems indoors in clean garden rooms.

Biological: French marigolds (*Tagetes patula*) repel soil nematodes, as does the fungus *Myrothecium verrucaria*, trade name DiTera ES).

Sprays: Neem used as a soil drench.

Root Maggots

Common names: Root maggots, seedcorn maggot

Root maggot species that attack cannabis include: seedcorn maggot (*Delia platura*)
cabbage maggot (*Delia radicum*)

Garden threat: low to medium

Identify: Both the seedcorn maggot and the cabbage maggot attack cannabis roots. The seedcorn maggot is 1.5 to 2 inches (3.8–5 cm) long. The seedcorn maggot converts into a fly that is a bit smaller than a common housefly. Cabbage maggots are 0.3 inch (0.8 cm) long, and the adult fly is bigger than a housefly. These pests winter over in unclean soil. In the spring they emerge as adult flies and soon lay eggs in the soil at the base of young plants. The squirmy, whitish larvae hatch several days later with a ravenous appetite.

Damage: Root maggots chew and burrow into stems and roots. The seedcorn maggot attacks seeds and seedling roots. Cabbage maggots attack roots, leaving hollowed-out channels and holes in larger roots. Both maggots destroy small, hairlike feeder roots. Wounds made by

root maggots also foster soft rot and fungal diseases.

Cause: unsterile soil or growing medium

Prevention: Cleanliness! Use fresh, new, store-bought soil when planting in containers. Cover seedlings with Agronet to exclude flies, and plant late in the year to avoid most adult flies. Place an 18-inch (45.7 cm) collar of foam rubber around the base of the plant to exclude flies.

Cultural and physical control:
Biological: Control with nematodes *Steinernema feltiae* or *Heterorhabditis bacteriophora*.

Sprays: Kill root maggots with neem and horticultural oil used as a soil drench.

Seed Maggots

Common names: seed maggots, seed worms

Species that attack cannabis seeds include: *Delia platura*

Garden threat: low to medium

Identify: Several species of mites, (fly) maggots, and weevils attack stored seed. Once established, these pests are difficult to destroy.

Damage: Pests burrow into seeds and eat seeds and sprouted seeds.

Cause: contaminated seeds, pests already in the storage container, or pests allowed to enter seed storage area

Prevention: Mechanical damage of hempseed stimulates the breeding of mites.

Control: fungitoxic preparations (i.e., Panogen and Aldogen)

The miticide Cinnamite (cinnamalde-

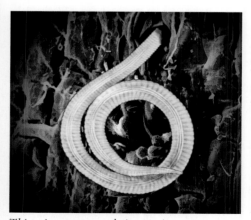

This minute nematode is entering a root to suck the life from the plant!

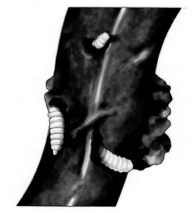

Root maggots are found in and around roots

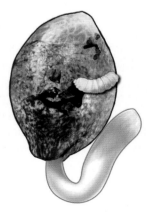

Seed maggots are relatively uncommon in cannabis seeds.

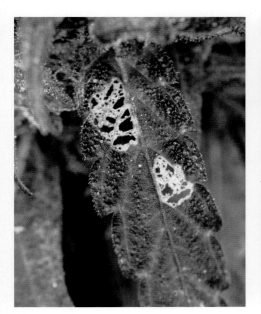

Snail damage

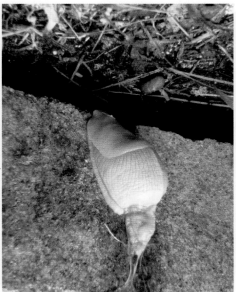

Slugs leave a slimy trail and can be a big problem in moist climates.

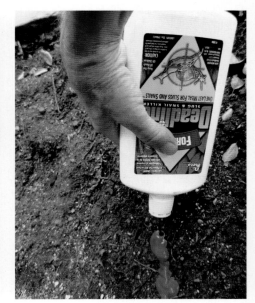

Deadline stays on the soil for weeks.

hyde), produced by Mycogen, is very effective.

Tyrophagus mites can be controlled by seed treatment.

See "Cutworms" and "Crickets" in this chapter.

Slugs and Snails

Slug and snail species that attack cannabis include: (gastropods from the Mollusk phylum) *Agriolimax* species, *Arion* species, *Helix aspersa*, *Deroceras reticulatum*

Garden threat: high for tender seedlings, low as plants mature

Identify: Slugs and snails are soft and slimy white, dark, or yellow, occasionally striped. They are 0.25 to 3 inches (0.6–7.6 cm) long. Snails live in a circular shell; slugs do not. Slugs and snails hide by day and feed at night, leaving a slimy, silvery trail of mucus in their wake. They lay translucent eggs that hatch in about a month. Slugs and snails reproduce prolifically, and the young mollusks often eat relatively more than adults.

Damage: Slugs and snails make holes in leaves, often with a weblike appearance. They will eat almost any vegetation, roots included. These creatures winter over in warm, damp locations in most climates. Slugs and snails especially like tender seedlings. They will migrate to adjacent gardens in quest of food.

Cause: Snails and slugs overwinter in the soil and garden debris. They are distributed in unsterile soil and garden residue.

Prevention: Till garden soil and soil around garden perimeter to disrupt life cycle. Use clean tools and soil.

Control

Cultural and physical control: A clean, dry perimeter around the garden will make it difficult for slugs and snails to pass. Spotlight and handpick them at night. A thin layer of lime, diatomaceous earth, or salty beach sand about two to six inches (5–15 cm) wide around individual plants, beds, or the entire garden will present an impassable barrier. The lime is not thick enough to alter soil pH, yet it will repel or dissolve pests. To trap, attach short one-inch (2.5 cm) feet on a wide board and leave it in the garden. The pests will seek refuge under the board. Pick up the board every day or two, and shake the slugs off and step on them. Poisonous baits usually have metaldehyde as a base. Confine the bait to a slug hotel. Cut a 1 × 2-inch (2.5–5 cm) slot in a covered plastic container to make a slug and snail hotel. Place slug and snail bait inside the hotel. The hotel must keep the bait dry and off the soil. In a slug hotel, none of the poison bait touches the soil, and the bait is inaccessible to children, pets, and birds. Place slug and snail hotels in out-of-the-way

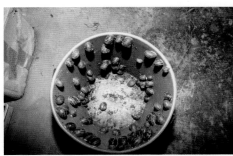

This gardener tossed snails into a bucket every time he found one. He fed the snails cornmeal for a week and sautéed them in garlic cannabis butter.

places. Natural baits include a mix of jam and water and beer. If using beer, it must be deep enough to drown mollusks.

Biological: The predatory snail *Rumina decollata*—available commercially—is yet another way to combat plant-eating slugs and snails.

Sprays: Young slugs and snails are not attracted to bait; spray for young at night or early morning with a 50 percent ammonia-water solution. After an hour, rinse off solution with water.

Spider Mites

Spider mite species that attack cannabis include: two-spotted spider mite (*Tetranychus urticae*, Acari: Tetranychidae. = *Tetranychus bimaculatus*, = *Tetranychus telarius* = *Epitetranychus althaea*)

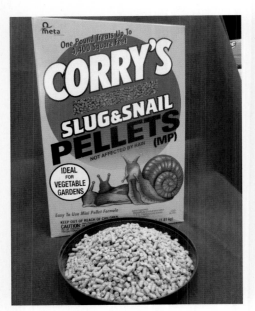

Slug and snail bait is an option for outdoor gardens.

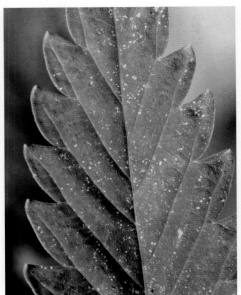

Spider mites stippled this leaf.

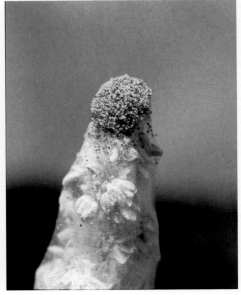

Spider mites have covered this male branch of flowers with webbing. They are congregating at the top of the plant because it is dead, and they do not know where to go!

carmine spider mite (*Tetranychus cinnabarinus*, Acari: Tetranychidae. = *Tetranychus telarius*)
hemp russet mite (*Aculops cannabicola, A. (Vasates) cannabicola*, Acari: Eriophyidae)
oriental mite (*Eutetranychus orientalis*)
privet mite (*Brevipalpus obovatus*, Acari: Tenuipalpidae, *Brevipalpus rugulosus*)
ta ma mite (*Typhlodromus cannabis*, Acari: Phytoseiidae)

Garden threat: common in all garden rooms, especially untidy rooms

Identify: Find microscopic spider mites on leaf undersides, sucking away life-giving fluids. To an untrained naked eye, the 0.04-inch (1 mm) mites are hard to spot. Early infestations produce little visible evidence. Spider mites appear as tiny specks on leaf undersides; however, their telltale signs of feeding—yellowish-white spots, stippling on the tops of leaves—are easy to see. Stippling is virtually identical to damage caused by thrips. A magnifying glass or low-power microscope (10X to 30X) helps to identify the yellow-white, two-spotted brown or red mites and their translucent eggs. Indoors, the most common is the two-spotted spider mite, but many other mites attack cannabis.

After a single mating, females are fertilized for life. Females lay up to 20 eggs

per day during a lifespan of two to four weeks. Eggs hatch in three days at 80°F (26.7°C). A single female can spawn a million mites a month in ideal conditions!

Accelerated reproduction allows mites to quickly adapt and become resistant to pesticides. Effective control measures must incorporate many different methods and products.

Damage: Mites suck life-giving sap from plants, causing overall vigor loss and stunting. Leaves are pocked with suck-hole marks and are yellow from failure to produce chlorophyll. Leaves lose partial to full function, and then turn yellow and drop. Once a plant is overrun with spider mites, tiny webs can easily be seen when misted with water. Spray water mist on suspect stems and under leaves as infestations progress. Severe cases cause plant death. Spider mites also function as vectors, spreading diseases as they mutilate foliage. Some estimates claim 60 percent of British Colombia, Canada, garden rooms are infested with spider mites.

Cause: Mites enter a garden on infested clones, plants, clothes, pets, etc., or they can blow in with the wind. Unclean growing conditions are the main cause of mites.

Prevention: Cleanliness is the most important first step to spider mite

control. Keep the garden room and tools spotless and disinfected. Mother plants often have spider mites. Spray mothers regularly with miticides, including once just three days before taking cuttings. Dip cuttings in a miticide after roots have formed and before they are moved out of the clone room. Dip small plants again one week later.

If spider mites become established in a garden room, they are nearly impossible to exterminate. You must remove all grow equipment and plants and clean the entire garden room with a 5 percent bleach solution. You can also rent a wallpaper steamer to steam/sterilize cracks in the room.

Cultural and physical control: Spider mites thrive in a dry, 70°F to 80°F (21.1°C–26.7°C) climate, and reproduce every five days in temperatures above 80°F (26.7°C). Create a hostile environment by lowering the temperature to 60°F (15.6°C) and spray foliage, especially under leaves, with a jet of cold water. Spraying literally blasts mites off the leaves, as well as increases humidity. Manual removal works for small populations. Smash all mites in sight between the thumb and index finger, or wash leaves individually in between two sponges. Avoid infecting other plants with contaminated hands or sponges.

Remove leaves with more than 50 percent damage and securely destroy them, making sure insects and eggs do not reenter the garden. If mites have attacked only one or two plants, isolate the infected plants and treat them separately. Take care when removing foliage not to spread mites to other plants. Severely damaged plants should be carefully removed from the garden and destroyed.

Smear a layer of Tanglefoot around the lip of containers and at the base of stems to create barriers spider mites have a difficult time crossing. Spider mites can also stream a web strand and float to the next branch or plant. Avoid overcrowding. This will help isolate them to specific plants.

Note: To contain spider mites, smear a layer of Tanglefoot at each end of drying lines when hanging buds. Once foliage is dead, mites try to migrate down drying lines to find live foliage with fresh, flowing sap.

Biological: *Neoseiulus (Amblyseius) californicus and Mesoseiulus Phytoseiulus) longipes*, are the two most common and effective predators. *Phytoseiulus persimilis, Neoseiulus (Amblyseius) fallacius, Galendromus (Metaseiulus) occidentalis, and Galendromus (Typhlodromus) pyri* predators are also available commercially. When properly applied and reared, predatory spider mites work very well. Read the section "Beneficial Insects" in this chapter before ordering. There are many suppliers; just type "spider mite predator" into a web browser such as Google.

About predators: First, predators can eat only a limited number of mites a day; the average predator can eat 20 eggs or 5 adults daily. As soon as the predators'

source of food is gone, some mites die of starvation while others survive on other insects or pollen. Check with suppliers for release instructions related to specific species. A general dosage of 20 predators per plant is a good place to start. Predatory mites have a difficult time traveling from plant to plant, so setting them out on each plant is necessary. Temperature and humidity levels must be at the proper levels to give the predators the best possible chance to thrive. When spider mites have infested a garden, the predatory mites cannot eat them fast enough to solve the problem. Predatory mites work best when there are only a few spider mites. Introduce predators as soon as spider mites are seen on vegetative growth, and release them every month thereafter. This gives predators a chance to keep up with mites. Before releasing predators, rinse plants thoroughly to ensure that toxic-spray residues from insecticides and fungicides are gone.

Persimilis (Phytoseiulus persimilis) will destroy spider mites

Progressive control measures for spider mites

Cleanliness: Clean the garden room daily and disinfect tools. Do not introduce new pests into the garden on clothes. No animal visits, etc.

Create hostile environment: humidity, temperature, water spray

Create barriers: Smear Tanglefoot around pot lips, at the base of stems, and on the ends of drying lines.

Dip cuttings and vegetative plants: Dip small plants in pyrethrum, horticultural oil, or neem oil.

Remove damaged foliage: Removefoliage that is more than 50 percent damaged.

Introduce predatory mites: Release predators before infestations get out of hand.

Homemade sprays often lack the strength to kill infestations, but they work as a deterrent by repelling mites. Popular homemade sprays include Dr. Bronner's soap, garlic, hot pepper, citrus oil, and liquid seaweed combinations. If these sprays do not deter spider mites after four to five applications, switch to a stronger spray such as neem oil, pyrethrum, horticultural oil, nicotine sulfate, or cinnamaldehyde. Insecticidal soap does a fair job of controlling mites. Usually two or three applications at five- to ten-day intervals will do the trick.

Horticultural oil smothers eggs and can be mixed with pyrethrum and homemade sprays to improve extermination.

Rotate sprays so mites do not develop immunity.

Spray: Pyrethrum (aerosol) is the best natural miticide! Apply two to three applications at five- to ten-day intervals. Pyrethrum is the best control for spider mites. Spider mites should be gone after two or three applications at five- to ten-day intervals, providing that sanitary preventative conditions are maintained. Eggs hatch in five to ten days. The second spraying will kill the newly hatched eggs and the remaining adults. The third and subsequent applications will kill any new spider mites, but mites soon develop a resistance to synthetic pyrethrum.

There are no pesticides registered for hemp growing. This is a bridge that will be crossed as cannabis becomes legal.

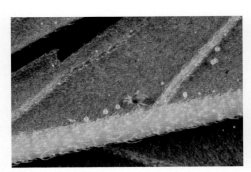

Spider mite adults, juveniles, and eggs on a leaf underside (MF)

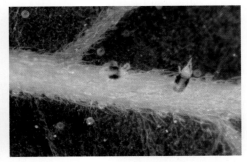

Close-up of spider mite adults and eggs (MF)

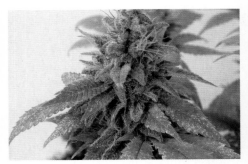

Stippling on leaves is the clue that spider mites live on the undersides.

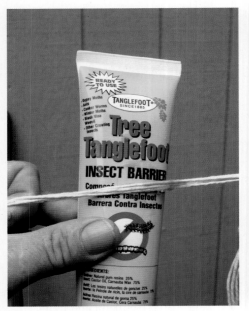

Tanglefoot is an excellent product to help contain spider mites. Smear it around the lip of containers, the base of stems, and at the end of drying lines.

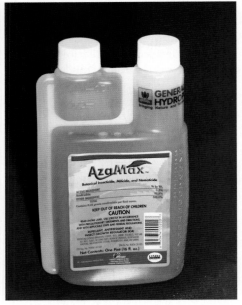

AzaMax is developed from neem seed and very potent.

Neem Oil

Heavy-duty chemical miticides are available but are not recommended for use on plants that will be consumed by humans. If using any chemical miticide, be sure it is a contact poison and not systemic. Use Stirrup M (cinnamaldehyde) extracted from *Cinnamomum zeylanicum*. The synthetic hormone attracts spider mites, and is used very successfully to enhance miticides.

Miticides: acaricides
Miticides: The organotins are a group of acaricides that double as fungicides. Of particular interest is Plictran (cyhexatin).

Floramite is a contact miticide, and thorough coverage is essential. This miticide is active on all mite life stages, including eggs. Do not apply less than a week before harvest.

TetraSan is a growth regulator for mites, inhibiting the molting process to control mites in greenhouses and on outdoor ornamentals. It is a contact and translaminar miticide that leaves four weeks' residual control after one application. It is effective on all stages of life; even adult females become sterile.

Vendex: This product is a restricted-use pesticide

Broad/Cyclamen Mites

Garden Threat: low to high
Common Names: Broad mite, yellow tea mite, citrus silver mite, tropical mite, chilli mite, jute white mite, rubber leaf mite. Cyclamen mite, *Stenotarsonemus pallidus*

Broad Mite Species that Attack Cannabis include: *Polyphagotarsonemus latus*, Acari species

Common names: broad mite, yellow tea mite, citrus silver mite, tropical mite, chilli mite, jute white mite, rubber leaf mite, cyclamen mite (*Stenotarsonemus pallidus*)

Broad mite species that attack cannabis include: *Polyphagotarsonemus latus*, *Acari* species
Broad mites (*Polyphagotarsonemus latus*) and cyclamen mites (*Stenotarsonemus pallidus*) are very similar in their life cycle and the damage they cause, so they are together in this section. First

they are distinguished, and then symptoms and control measures are lumped together.

Broad mites and cyclamen mites live and breed on many plants, including cannabis. They migrate to lower leaves and infest plants quickly. The symptoms can easily be confused with nitrogen deficiency. They do not make spiderwebs.

Garden threat: low to high
Identify broad mites: Aggressive adult mites are microscopic, about 0.1 mm long with eight legs. Larvae have six legs and are hungry at hatch. They are less than half the size of the red spider mite. Soft-bodied nymphs move fast. Color is translucent white and yellowish and other light tones. Broad mites reproduce most prolifically at temperatures between 70°F to 80°F (21.1°C–26.7°C). The long eggs (0.08 mm) have a series of about 30 whitish bumps, an oval shape with protruding circular surface, and they stick hard to the leaves. The adult has a dark dorsal band. Each female can produce 40 to 50 eggs in a lifetime. They hatch in two to three days—with an appetite. After eating for two to three days, they start the pupal stage en route to adulthood.

Identify cyclamen mites: Less than 0.2 mm long, these waxy looking mites have four pairs of legs and range from colorless to green or brownish. Cyclamen mites share many characteristics with broad mites. Male cyclamen mites have a very strong claw mounted at the end of each fourth leg.

These mites avoid light and prefer high humidity and cool 60°F (15.6°C) temperatures. They hide inside buds, under leaves, and in any protected place on foliage. Eggs are smooth and hatch in about 11 days when deposited in dark, moist locations.

Damage: Mites secrete a plant growth regulator or toxin as they feed. And a

BRAND NAME	ACTIVE INGREDIENT	SAFETY	RESIDUAL DAYS
Avid	*Streptomyces avermitilis*	DO NOT USE	28
TetraSan	etoxazole	DO NOT USE	28

CHEMICAL INSECTICIDES AND MITICIDES

Trade Name*	Active Ingredient	Safe for Cannabis	Notes
Akari SC	tert-butyl	No	Do not use in successive applications.
Avid	abamectin	No	Produced by soil fungi, *Streptomyces* species
Brigade	bifenthrin	No	Systemic miticide/insecticide, DO NOT USE
Floramite	bifenazate	Limited	Apply only once then rotate to another miticide.
Forbid 4F	spiromesifen	No	Systemic miticide/insecticide, DO NOT USE
Hexygon W	hexythiazox	No	Systemic miticide/insecticide, DO NOT USE
Judo	spiromesifen	No	Systemic miticide/insecticide, DO NOT USE
Kelthane	dicofol	No	Selective miticide, DDT relative, DO NOT USE
Mavrik	tau-fluvalinate	No	Systemic miticide/insecticide, DO NOT USE
Orthene	acephate	No	Systemic miticide/insecticide, DO NOT USE
Ovation SC	clofentezine	No	Systemic miticide/insecticide, DO NOT USE
Pentac	**dienochlor**	**No**	**Canceled!**
ProMITE	fenbutatin-oxide	No	Systemic miticide/insecticide, DO NOT USE
Pylon	chlorfenapyr	No	Systemic miticide/insecticide, DO NOT USE
Pyramite	pyridaben	No	Systemic miticide DO NOT USE
Sanmite SC	pyridaben	No	Systemic miticide DO NOT USE
Savey	hexythiazox	No	Systemic miticide/insecticide, DO NOT USE
Shuttle O	acequinocyl	No	Systemic miticide/insecticide, DO NOT USE
Sirocco	bifenazate/abamectin	No	Systemic miticide/insecticide, DO NOT USE
Temik	aldicarb	No	Systemic miticide DO NOT USE
TetraSan	diphenyloxzoline	No	Do not apply more than twice per crop
Ultiflora	milbemectin	Yes	Derived from soil microorganisms and fermentation
Vendex	fenbutatin-oxide	No	Systemic miticide/insecticide, DO NOT USE
Whitmire Beethoven	etoxazole	No	Toxic to fish and aquatic organisms
Zeal	etoxazole	No	Systemic miticide DO NOT USE

*Not all trade names are included. Check insecticides and miticides for chemical names.

few mites can cause a lot of damage fast! Feeding damage deforms and distorts young buds and leaves. Leaf edges can curl up or entire leaves can cup down, pucker, crinkle, become brittle, and show signs of scarring. Internodes shorten, growing tips are stunted, and overall growth is underdeveloped. New growth can blacken and die. Damage resembles herbicide damage and can also be confused with viral disease, micronutrient deficiency, or herbicide injury. Damage may appear for weeks after the mites have been controlled.

Damage is usually not detected until significant damage is incurred. Damaged foliage will not recover. A microscope will be necessary to detect the actual mites; a handheld loupe is not powerful enough to see them.

Cause: Microscopic or micro-mites are able to walk short distances and are dispersed long distances by wind or by attaching themselves to people, tools, or a winged insect (aphid, whitefly, etc.) and hitching a ride. Male mites actually transport eggs to new foliage. They migrate to cannabis from many plants, including but not limited to houseplants, African violets, cyclamen, begonias, snapdragons, impatiens, gerbera daisies, fuchsias, daisies, azaleas, ivy, camellias, jasmine, lantana, marigolds, grapes, and vegetable hosts—beets, beans, cucumbers, eggplants, peppers, potatoes, and tomato plants. Mites are also common greenhouse pests in some crops.

Prevention: Cyclamen mites cannot take temperatures above 92°F (33.3°C) but the spider mite will. If you drop the

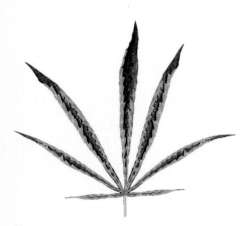

This leaf shows signs of a severe infestation of hemp russet mites.

humidity to 30 percent, they cannot develop into adults. But the conditions in most garden rooms are perfect for spider mites to thrive.

Do not let broad mites enter the garden room or greenhouse. They are more difficult to prevent, and they thrive in hot conditions. Use certified pest-free growing mediums. Keep the garden room very clean. Wear clean clothes and shoes into the garden room and greenhouse. Do not grow ornamental or food plants that attract cyclamen or broad mites.

It is important to eliminate broad mites before flowering because plants cannot recuperate if they go into flowering with broad mite damage.

Control
Biological: Locally occurring mite predators give satisfactory control in many areas. Two natural enemies—*Euseius stipulatus* and *Typhlodromus* ovalis are being evaluated as biocontrol agents of these mites.

Amblyseius californicus eats red spider mites and broad mites Polyphagotarsonemus latus. If there is no food for the predators, they leave or die. Amblyseius californicus can also eat pollen to maintain themselves. The strawberry (*Ricinus communis L.*) and *margaritas* (genebra) are some of the foods with pollen.

Sprays: Broad mites and cyclamen mites are not susceptible to some dinitrophenol compounds and synthetic pyrethroids. Submerging plants completely in a miticide dip is very effective to treat small plants. Fenbutatin, diazinon, and dicofol (Kelthane)—all very harsh chemicals that I do not recommend—have been effective in the control of mites.

Hemp Russet Mites
Garden Threat: low to high

Common Names: hemp russet mite, mites

Hemp Russet Mite species that attack cannabis include: *Aculops cannabicola*

Identify: Hemp russet mites are not well-known but this appalling pest is growing in infamy because it is so hard to control. The mites are very small reaching only 0.2 mm in length and

they have just two pairs of legs attached to their pale beige bodies. Even though hemp russet mites are virtually impossible to see with the naked eye, they are easy to distinguish from other destructive mites because they leave no webbing. At 80°F (27°C) hemp russet mites achieve a 30-day life cycle.

Damage: Feeds on all types of cannabis plants. They live and feed mainly on leaves, petioles, and meristems. Feeding damage causes leaflets to curl at edges followed by chlorosis and necrosis. Leaves and petioles become brittle. Infestations turn leaves beige with hemp russet mite bodies! Mites feed on female stigmas rendering them sterile. They also consume resin glands which can reduce resin production severely. Hemp russet mites feed on cannabis plants until host is dead. They congregate on the upper part of the plant as it dies. Hemp russet mites vector viruses.

Cause: Introduced to gardens by unsanitary practices, contaminated stock and bad luck. Hemp russet mites hide on plants indoors and in greenhouses. They are believed to overwinter on contaminated seed indoors and outdoors. The minute mites spread easily to nearby plants by splashing water. Wind also carries them greater distances.

Prevention: Keep garden area clean and disinfected. Introduce only pest-free stock into gardens. Disinfect seeds. Keep the garden below 70°F (21°C) and below 50% humidity to slow reproductive process. Remove seriously damaged foliage and plants from garden.

Control
Biological: The fungus, *Hirsutella thompsonii*, is a pathogen to hemp russet mites, but I have not seen it available commercially.

Sprays: Miticides and sulfur sprays are somewhat effective. Make sure to get complete foliage coverage when spraying.

Termites
Common names: termites, wood termites

Termite species that attack cannabis include: *Odontotermes obesus* (Isoptera: Termitidae)

Garden threat: low indoors moderately high outdoors

Identify: Termites can be a big problem

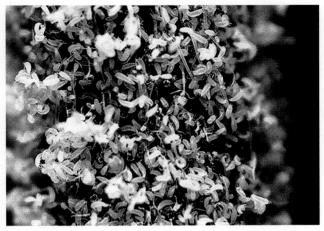
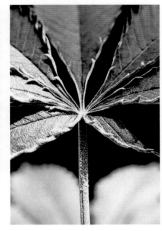

These microscopic hemp russet mites (Aculops cannabicola) infested Cannabis *plants in a secure greenhouse at Indiana University. This picture by Karl Hilling shows them on a leaf petiole that was about 2 mm wide.*

in outdoor gardens. They are worse near wooded areas, and they have been a big problem in California and warm states in the southern USA and similar climates. They live entirely underground or in elevated tubes.

Damage: Termites like weak and dead plants more than they like wood. Weak, diseased plants will attract termites. Termites eat roots and gnaw away at stems. In fact, they can even burrow through the center of stems and kill plants. Termites are seldom noticed until damage occurs.

Cause: Termites are present in rotten wood or decaying plant matter near the garden.

Prevention: Spray termite insecticide around the perimeter of the garden. Set termite bait in the garden and outside garden structures. Paint exposed wood in garden with a borate to disrupt termite life cycle. Avoid mulching plants with woodchips.

Replace the wood with a slow-acting pesticide available at your local home and garden store. The pesticide will be spread through the colony when the termite returns home.

Control: Locate termite colonies in attics, walls, and in underground burrows under and near buildings. Spray each colony and the surrounding area.

Control requires that termites are physically prevented from entry, which is very difficult, or the colony must be eradicated.

Biological: Add natural predators to your environment. Encouraging ants, flies, and spiders around your home is one way to keep termites out—they'll eat them! Frogs are also good predators.

Sprays: Terminix or Spectracide stakes are often used to control termites. They come in a box of 20 ($70 USD) with a drill bit to put them in the soil. The active ingredient is 0.1 percent and is slow-acting bait so the termites can take it back to the mound. The bait does not release into the soil nor does the plant pick it up.

Thrips

Common names: greenhouse thrips, western flower thrips, onion thrips

Thrip species that attack cannabis include: greenhouse thrips (*Heliothrips haemorrhoidalis*)
onion (tobacco) thrips (*Thrips tabaci*)
marijuana thrips (*Oxythrips cannabensis*)

Indian bean thrips (*Caliothrips indicus*)
western flower thrips (*Frankliniella occidentalis*)

Attacks: foliage

Attacks: roots

Garden threat: low to high both indoors and outdoors

Identify: These tiny, winged, fast-moving critters are hard to see but not hard to spot. From 0.04 to 0.05 inch (1–1.3 mm) long, thrips can be different colors, including white, gray, and dark colors, often with petite stripes. Check for them under leaves by shaking parts of the plant. If there are many thrips present, they choose to jump and run rather than fly to safety. But often you will see them as a herd of specks thundering across foliage. Females make holes in soft plant tissue where they deposit eggs that are virtually invisible to the naked eye. Winged thrips easily migrate from infested plants to the entire garden. Several different thrips attack cannabis; some, known as marijuana thrips, are specific to cannabis. Thrips are more common in greenhouses than indoors.

Damage: Thrips rasp and scrape tissue from leaves and buds, and then suck out the sap for food. Stipples—whitish-yellowish to silvery specks—appear on top of leaves; chlorophyll production diminishes and leaves become brittle. You will also see black specks of thrip feces and little thrips. Many times thrips feed inside flower buds or wrap up and distort leaves. Thrips prefer succulent young leaves and flowering tops. Common thrips often eat female calyxes, causing deformed flower tops.

Cause: Thrips enter the garden on contaminated plant stock and on

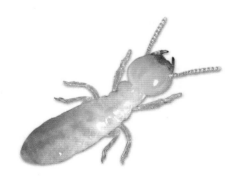

Termites are most common in wooded areas.

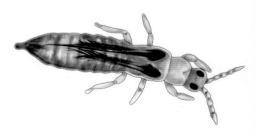

Thrip

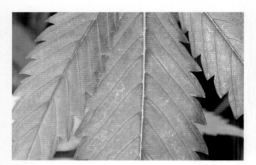

Thrips rasp the top of leaves.

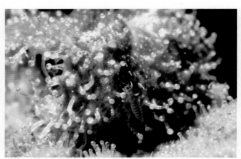

Thrips will attack cannabis in all stages of life. (MF)

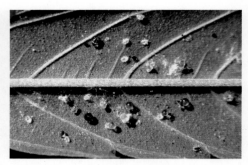

Whiteflies in all stages of growth can be seen on this leaf. (MF)

gardeners, tools, and pets as a result of an unclean garden and garden area.

Prevention: Cleanliness! Use yellow sticky traps, which attract thrips, to monitor populations and impair movement. Misting plants with water impairs thrips. Manual removal works okay if only a few thrips are present, but they are hard to catch. Thrips can be very vexing to control once they become established.

Thrips migrate daily. They hide in soil and foliage and feed actively in the mornings. The best time to kill them is during feeding. Soil treatments work well too.

Control
Biological: Predatory mites (*Amblyseius cucumeris* and *Amblyseius barkeri, Neoseiulus cucumeris, Iphiseius degenerans, Neoseiulus barkeri, Euseius hibisci*), parasitic wasps (*Thripobius semiluteus, Ceranisus menes, Goetheana shakespearei*), pirate bugs (*Orius* species). The fungus *Verticillium lecanii* is effective.

Sprays: Homemade sprays such as tobacco/nicotine (nicotinic acid) base; commercial pyrethrum, synthetic pyrethrum, insecticidal soap, and garlic. Apply two to four times at five- to ten-day intervals.

Whiteflies
Common names: greenhouse whitefly, sweet potato whitefly, tobacco whitefly, silverleaf whitefly

Whitefly species that attack cannabis include: greenhouse whitefly (*Trialeurodes vaporiorum*, Homoptera: Aleyrodidae)
sweet potato aka tobacco whitefly

(*Bemisia tabaci*, Homoptera: Aleyrodidae, = *Bemisia gossypiperda*) silverleaf whitefly (*Bemisia argentifolii*, Homoptera: Aleyrodidae, = *Bemisia tabaci* (strain B)

Garden threat: low to high, worse in hot climates

Identify: The easiest way to check for the little buggers is to grab a limb and shake it. If there are any whiteflies, they will fly from underneath leaves. Whiteflies are easily spotted with the naked eye. Whiteflies look like a small, white moth about 0.04 inches (about 1 mm) long, approximately the size of the tip of a pencil lead. Adult whiteflies have wings. They usually appear near the top of the weakest plant first. They will move downward on the plant or fly off to infest another plant. Eggs are also found on leaf undersides, where they are connected with a small hook. Whiteflies behave very much like spider mites do.

Damage: Whiteflies hide underneath leaves and suck sap from them. Like mites, whiteflies may cause white speckles known as stipples on the tops of leaves. Chlorophyll production and plant vigor diminish as the infestation

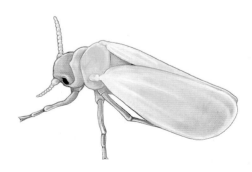

Whitefly

progresses. Whiteflies leave residue on foliage that attracts harmful fungi and diseases.

Cause: unclean garden room, sloppy hygiene

Prevention: Cleanliness! Screen the incoming air.

Control
Cultural and physical control: Adults are attracted to the color yellow. To build a whitefly trap similar to flypaper, cover a bright, yellow object with a sticky substance like Tanglefoot. Place the traps on tops of pots among the plants. Traps work very well. When they are full of insects, toss them out.

Biological: The (assassinator) wasp *Encarsia formosa*, released before an infestation of whiteflies, is the most effective parasitic control. These small wasps only attack whiteflies; they do not sting people. Set new wasps in the garden every two weeks. All toxic sprays must be completely washed off plants before introducing parasites and predators. Since *Encarsia formosa* is a parasite about 0.125 inch (about 3 mm) long—smaller than the whitefly—it takes them much longer to control or even keep the whitefly population in check. The parasitic wasp lays an egg in the whitefly larva that later hatches and eats the larva alive, from the inside out—death is slow. If you use *Encarsia formosa*, set them out at the rate of two or more parasites per plant as soon as the first whitefly is detected. Repeat every two to four weeks throughout the life of the plants.

The fungus *Verticillium lecanii* aka *Cephalosporium lecanii*, trade name Mycotal, is also very effective as whitefly control.

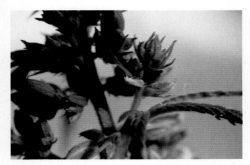

You can see the winged whitefly trying to hide under the male flower cluster! (MF)

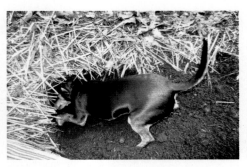

I love dogs—especially cute, little ones. But my little dog loves to dig and chase moles! The moles do enough damage. So far moles one, little dog zero.

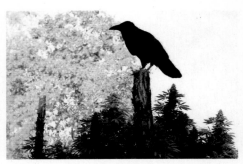

Edgar, a raven friend from Northern California, provided endless amusement as he bullied the dogs, cats, and other animals around the cannabis farm.

Sprays: Easily eradicated with natural sprays, pyrethrum works great to kill whiteflies when they are airborne. Before spraying, remove any leaves that have been over 50 percent damaged and cure with heat or else burn infested foliage. Homemade sprays applied at five- to ten-day intervals work well. Insecticidal soap applied at five- to ten-day intervals. Pyrethrum (aerosol) applied at five- to ten-day intervals.

Pest Mammals

Once your plants are in the ground, well fed and watered, check them weekly (if possible) for pest and fungal damage. Inspect the top and bottom of leaves for stippling (small spots) from mites or damage from chewing insects and slugs and snails. First identify the pest, and then determine a course of action. Properly grown outdoor cannabis has few problems with pests.

Low-tech, natural approaches to pest control work well. A few large pests like caterpillars and snails can be handpicked from the foliage. Caterpillar populations can be reduced at the source by installing bat houses. Resident bats will eat moths and decrease the number of chewing caterpillars. Birds will eat caterpillars too, as well as aphids and other insects. Attract birds with suet, birdhouses, birdbaths, and feeders, but cover tender seedlings and clones with wire or nylon mesh to protect from birds, too! Ladybugs and praying mantis are good options for insect control and can be purchased from nursery supply stores.

Barn owls eat mice, gophers, and voles but are hard to come by in the city. If you are lucky enough to have barn owls nearby, take advantage of their ability to eat plant pests. On the other hand, rodents such as moles and shrews help your garden by dining on slugs, insects, and larvae.

Marigold cultivars of the *Tagetes erecta* and *T. patula* species will repel nematodes (aka eelworms) from the soil for two to three years if planted in an infested area and then tilled under. Just planting these marigolds in an area doesn't accomplish anything. Numerous tests indicate that they do not have an effect on insects above the ground.

Bears

Bears present the biggest problems in gardens where there is a food source. If bears are common in your area, do not plant other garden fruits and vegetables nearby. Remove or secure all containerized garden fertilizers, especially ones containing molasses or sugars. Bears may appear out of nowhere if they are in the area, but normally they avoid contact with humans.

Birds

Insect- and pest-eating birds are welcome guests in most gardens, but the bad birds eat cannabis seeds and young tender plants.

Common names: birds, flying pigs, doves, hemp linnet, magpies, nuthatch, pheasants, pigeons, quail, sparrows, starling, crows, blue jays, cardinals

Garden threat: Low to medium. Seeds, tender seedlings, and clones are most vulnerable.

Damage: Birds eat seeds and young plants.

Cause: Birds are in the area and hungry, with little else to eat.

Prevention: Cover young plants with plastic or wire netting. Make sure the netting is securely attached around the perimeter of the garden to keep birds from sneaking underneath. Remove netting when plants are one to two feet (30.5–61 cm) tall. Inflatable plastic snakes and owls often scare birds, but not for long!

Control: scarecrow, sonic boom machine, shotgun or rifle (only in hunting season)

Boar (Wild Pigs)

Common names: wild pigs, wild boar, *javali* (Spain)

Garden threat: medium, but could be devastating

Identify: wild pigs, mostly nocturnal and travel in packs

Damage: uproot plants and eat lower foliage and roots

Cause: Wild pigs run loose in many rural areas and along the perimeters of urban areas.

Prevention: Install a battery-operated electric fence around outdoor plants. Keep a big, protective dog near the plants to scare off pigs. Do not leave out anything that will attract them; securely stow fertilizer and safely dispose of garbage.

Control: Shoot pigs with a gun (only in hunting season), and keep a big dog to protect garden from pigs. Big box traps are also available for pigs.

Sprays: none

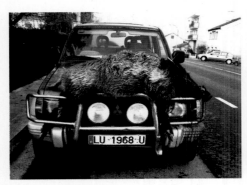

Wild pigs from Northwest Spain have uprooted many gardens.

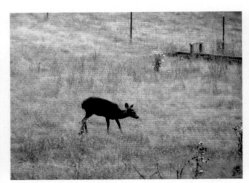

Deer stop by and munch a few tender buds every night.

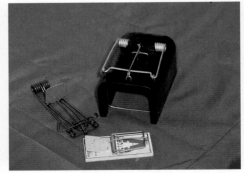

Gopher traps (pictured at top of image) and a mouse trap (pictured at bottom of image) are very important means of rodent control in outdoor medical cannabis gardens.

Deer

Common names: deer (buck, doe, fawn), elk (cow, bull, calf)

Garden threat: low to medium

Damage: Deer are browsers and eat the tender new growth first, but they can devour buds too! They take a bite (or maybe several bites) of a plant and move to another plant. Damage ranges from sporadic bites to large parts of plants being eaten.

Cause: Deer are in the area and have few food sources, of which cannabis is one. Prevention: A proper fence or a cage around plants will help keep deer away from plants. Deer are afraid to jump into a small, enclosed area. Set up the fence a few feet around plants so they cannot reach over or through it to get to foliage. The ideal deer fence for large rural gardens is eight feet (2.4 m) tall with the top foot (30.5 cm) sloping outward, away from the garden at a 45-degree angle. Electric fences and large dogs are also good deterrents.

If a fence is too conspicuous or difficult to construct, use repellents. Place handfuls of dried blood in cloth sacks and dip in water to activate the smell. Hang sacks from a tree to discourage dogs and other predators from eating them. Scented soaps have repelled deer from some gardens, but soap has also been known to attract rodents.

Predator urine, most often coyote urine, keeps deer away well when applied regularly. It is available at garden centers and many hunting stores. Some guerilla growers say that to deter deer damage, they urinate in several locations around the perimeter of the garden so animals take their human presence seriously. Some growers save urine all week and disperse it during regular visits to their patch.

Control: It is best to prevent damage. Shooting deer out of season or in populated areas is illegal and dangerous.

Elk are somewhat of a problem, and deer *are* a problem!

Gophers

Common names: pocket gopher

Identify: herbivorous rodents

Garden threat: low to medium

Damage: Gophers eat roots and foliage and disrupt soil with tunnels. Annually, females bear four to five litters of up to eight offspring. That's a lot of hungry mouths to feed!

Cause: Gophers may just stop by for a meal and like the way the plants taste.

Prevention: Line planting holes with hardware cloth or fine chicken wire 12 to 18 inches (30.5–45.7 cm) deep and 3 feet (91.4 cm) aboveground to exclude gophers. The gopher plant (Euphorbia lathyris) and castor beans/plants are said to repel gophers when stuffed in holes, but they have not worked for me.

Control: Traps are difficult to use and require experience and skill to actually catch gophers. Avoid getting any human scent on the trap. If human scent is apparent, gophers simply push dirt onto the trap, making it harmless.

Mice, Rats, and Voles

Gopher Granola is available for areas such as the Northern California mountains, where wood rats and gophers will eat your crop if given any opportunity to do so. The best fence in the world will not keep rats away from your plants! (If rats are a problem in your area, do not use soap to keep deer away; the fat in soap is edible for rats.) Put the poison grain in a feeder only small rodents can enter, so that birds and deer can't eat it. Set out poison early, before actual planting begins. Rats must eat the grain for several days before it will have any effect on them. Ultimately, you may find it's easier to grow in a greenhouse shed in your own backyard rather than try to keep the rats from eating your outdoor plot.

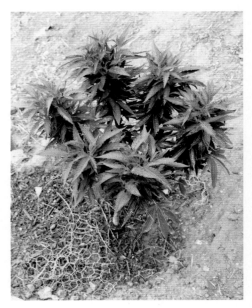

The root system of this 'Jack Herer' female is protected with chicken wire. (MF)

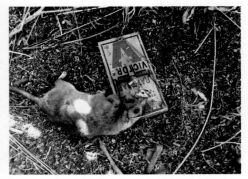

Mice populations can skyrocket outdoors in the late summer. Setting traps around plants helps monitor rodent populations and keep them in check.

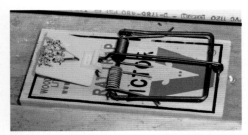

A mousetrap properly set and baited is one of the most effective means of mouse control.

Common names: mice, voles, rats, kangaroo rats, vermin

Garden threat: low indoors; medium to high outdoors and in greenhouses

Damage: Mice and voles can chew bark from around the base of cannabis plants (girdling).

Cause: Rodents have a nearby food source and are expanding their territory.

Prevention: Keep mulch a foot away from plants, and install wire mesh around the trunks. Mice and voles make nests in large piles of mulch, and they are attracted to stored water. Cover all water sources to exclude them, but keep in mind that they might chew through the container if water is super scarce. The best mouse deterrent is a cat that is serious about hunting.

Control

Physical: Mousetraps work well on small populations. Removing a large number of mice with traps can be tedious and unpleasant.

Caution! DO NOT USE POISON! Scavenger animals will eat the dead rodents and may become poisoned themselves.

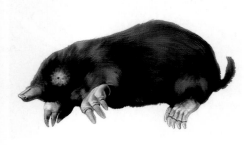

Moles are generally not a problem unless the soil is chock-full of worms and insects.

Moles

Common names: mole

Garden threat: low

Damage: Moles are minor pests. They are primarily insectivores that eat cutworms and other soil grubs, but their tunnels may dislodge cannabis roots. Moles dig tunnels a few inches below the soil surface, creating a maze of tunnel mounds in the garden.

Cause: Moles are living nearby and looking for a new food source.

Prevention: Repel moles with castor plants or gopher (mole) plants (*Euphorbia lathyris*). Castor bean leaves and castor oil, as well as applications of tobacco and red pepper, will repel moles if put into their main runs.

Mixing: Blend two tablespoons (30 ml) of castor oil with three tablespoons of dish soap concentrate and ten tablespoons (148 ml) of water. Mix in a blender. Use this as a concentrate at the rate of two tablespoons per gallon (4 ml/L) of water.

Application: Apply as a soil drench directly over mole holes.

Control

Physical: Barrel traps, scissor traps, and guillotine traps are effective and kill moles instantly.

Rabbits

Common names: Cottontail, bunny rabbit, rabbit, hare

Garden threat: very low

Rabbits are burrowing, plant-eating mammals of the Leporidae family. They can be recognized by their long ears and short, fluffy tails. Rabbits are voracious eaters and can reduce a crop to nothing in a couple of days. They will continue to feed from the same patch until they are done or the patch is destroyed. The best way to keep rabbits from your garden is to use predator urine. Rabbits also shy away from cats and dogs.

Identify: Long-eared rabbits (Bugs Bunny!) are plant-eating mammals. Most often cottontails, little "bunny rabbits" inhabit outdoor gardens. They multiply quickly and often eat from the same patch until it is destroyed.

Damage: Rabbits eat cannabis plants.

Cause: Rabbits have the opportunity to enter the cannabis garden and eat cannabis plants.

Prevention: Repel rabbits with a light dusting of rock phosphate on young leaves or dried blood sprinkled around the base of plants. Manure tea sprayed on leaves and soil may keep rabbits from dining on your plants. They also find plants dusted with hot pepper or a spray of dilute fish emulsion and bone meal repulsive. A dog will help keep rabbits in check, but the only surefire way to keep rabbits out of the garden is to fence them out with one-inch (2.5 cm) poultry wire. The poultry wire should be buried at least six inches (15.2 cm) in the ground to prevent burrowing and should rise two or three feet (61–91.4 cm) aboveground. Wrap trunks with wire mesh

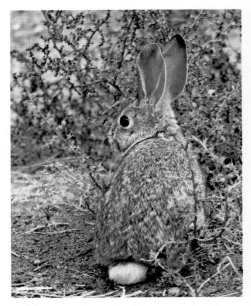

Rabbits may be cute in the country, but they can be extremely destructive in a garden.

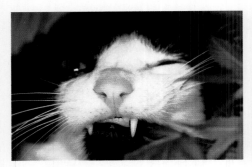

Cats are particularly fond of cannabis.

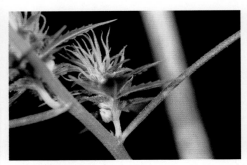

Rogue pollen is a big problem in some parts of the world when growing outdoors. Indoors, an occasional male flower can pollinate an entire roomful of plants. Always be on the lookout for spontaneous male flowers on female plants.

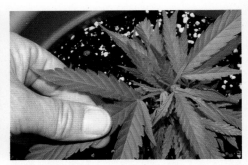

Manually remove small populations of insects and pests by smashing them between your thumb and index finger or between two sponges. Smash all pests (and their eggs).

or aluminum foil to keep rabbits from chewing bark in winter or early spring.

Control: Rabbit baits and traps are difficult to use. Pull out the shotgun or rifle as a last resort. Observe local gun laws and hunting regulations.

Other Large Pests

Domestic and wild animals that can be a problem in cannabis gardens include: cats, cows, chipmunks, dogs, groundhogs ("woodchucks"), hamsters, horses, monkeys, raccoons, rats, squirrels, and voles.

Rogue Pollen

Common names: rogue pollen, pollen from the neighbor

Garden threat: low to medium

Identify: Female plants develop seeds, yet there are no male flowers in the garden.

Damage: Once pollinated, female plants spend all their energy developing seeds and bud growth stops. Such plants produce less consumable harvest.

Cause: Male plants are within a few inches to several hundred miles, depending on wind patterns, from receptive female plants.

Prevention: Indoors, if neighbors are growing cannabis from seed and do not cull out male plants, or if your garden is near an industrial hemp farm, you will have to cover intake air ducts with fine mesh screen and wet it occasionally to keep rogue pollen outside. Outdoors, inspect plants continually and pick off all developing seeds. Once plants are seed-

ed, they stop putting on flower weight.

Control: Keep female plants out of the path of male pollen. Remove all male plants from the garden.

Disease and Pest Controls

Prevention and cleanliness are at the top of the control list. Problems first establish on weak plants, but even when all prevention measures are taken, disease and pest problems can arise. The first measures of control include identifying the problem. The next step is to use the least-toxic means of solving the problem. Remove pests manually, if possible, or spray them off with water. Next use organic sprays. Fungus can be stopped with many surface sprays that are not harmful to plants or the environment.

I do not recommend using chemical fungicides, fungistats, insecticides, or miticides on plants that are destined for human consumption. Most contact sprays that do not enter the plant system are approved for edible fruits and vegetables.

Read all labels thoroughly before using control measures. Use only contact sprays that are approved for edible plants. Avoid spraying seedlings and tender unrooted cuttings. Wait until cuttings are rooted and seedlings are at least a month old before spraying.

Common chemicals with their trade names and the insects they control:

Note: Do *not* apply these substances to edible plants.

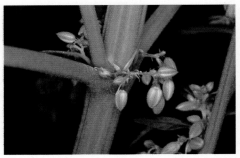

Minute grains of pollen can escape from male flowers and pollinate females. Be careful when working with male plants!

Note: This list is not all-inclusive. The basic rule is to *not* use systemic products. Organic contact pesticide, miticide

Controls: russet and spider mites, fire ants, leaf miners, and nematodes.

Brand names: Abba, Affirm, Agri-Mek, Avid, Dynamec, Epi-Mek, Genesis Horse Wormer, Reaper, Vertimec, Zephyr, and Cure 1.8 EC.

About: Abamectin derivatives include emamectin and milbemectin. It does not bioaccumulate. Not truly systemic, abamectin is absorbed from the exterior of foliage to other leaf parts, especially young leaves, in the process of translaminar activity.

Forms: liquid

Mixing: DO NOT USE!

Application: DO NOT USE! DO NOT APPLY!

Persistence: DO NOT USE!

Safety: DO NOT USE! Toxic to mammals, fish, and honeybees in high concentrations. Sucking insects are subject

GENERIC NAME	PURPOSE	ENTER SYSTEM	DO NOT USE
griseofulvin	fungicide	systemic	Do NOT Use
streptomycin	bactericide	systemic–registered for various food crops	Do NOT Use
carbaryl	fungicide	systemic	Do NOT Use
tetracycline	bactericide	semisynthetic	Do NOT Use
nitrates	foliar fertilizers	systemic	Do NOT Use
abamectin	insecticide not a true insecticide	translaminar	Do NOT Use
dienchlor	miticide	systemic	Do NOT Use
aldicarb	insecticide	systemic	Do NOT Use
neem	insecticide	systemic	Do NOT Use
triforine	fungicide	systemic	Do NOT Use
carboxin	fungicide	systemic	Do NOT Use
acephate	insecticide	systemic	Do NOT Use

NATURAL REMEDY TABLE

Active Ingredient	EPA Class
Bacillus species	G, D, WP *Bt*, DiPel, M-Trak, IV Match, Javelin, etc.
copper sulfate	D, WP, Brscop III
copper sulfate/lime	D, WP, Bordeaux mixture III
diatomaceous earth	D, Celite IV
neem	O, EL Neem, BioNEEM IV
nicotine sulfate	L, D, Black Leaf 40 II
oil, dormant horticultural	O, Sunspray IV
pyrethrin	A, L, WP Many trade names III, IV
quassia	WP, bitterwood IV
rotenone	D, WP, EC Derris, Cubé II, III
ryania	D, WP Dyna 50 IV
sabadilla	D, Red Devil IV
soap, insecticidal	L, M-Pede, Safer's IV
sodium bicarbonate	P, baking soda IV
sodium hypochlorite	L, bleach II, III
sulfur	D, WP, Cosan V

Caution! We do not recommend using any products in any form in a manner inconsistent with their label. Note that no pesticide, fungicide, or any other product is approved by any government for use on cannabis.

If you should decide to use any of the products mentioned in this book, please FOLLOW THE LABEL DIRECTIONS!

Medicinal cannabis is to be consumed by sick patients, and a pesticide-and-fungicide-free crop must be ensured.

Many fungicides and pesticides are SYSTEMIC and FOR USE ON ORNAMENTAL PLANTS ONLY! Do not use such dangerous products on consumable cannabis. PLANT GROWTH REGULATORS, SYSTEMIC PESTICIDES, AND FUNGICIDES CAN BE FATAL TO HUMANS!

Legend

L	liquid	O	oil
A	aerosol	EL	emulsifiable liquid
WP	wettable powder	G	glandular
D	dust		

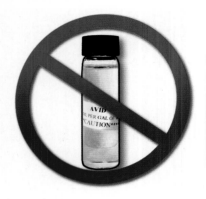

DO NOT USE Avid on cannabis!

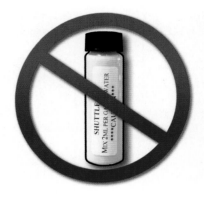

DO NOT USE Shuttle on cannabis!

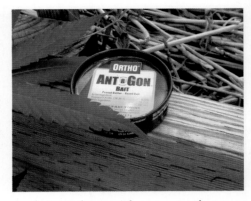

Ant baits work great. The ants enter the container and do not leave.

to control, while beneficials are not hurt. Wear gloves, mask, and safety glasses.

In one example from Hayward, California, a well-known cannabis patient with an unusual immune disease died from repeated exposure to the miticide Avid. Avid is now illegal to sell in the US, though it remains available from Canadian sources. Directed for used on ornamentals only.

SHUTTLE 15 SC: Do Not Use!

Systemic pesticide, miticide

Controls: Two-spotted spider mite (*Tetranychus urticae*) and spruce spider mite (*Oligonychus ununguis*). SHUTTLE destroys damaging mites at every life stage, from eggs to adults.

Brand names: SHUTTLE (For ornamentals only)

About: SHUTTLE Miticide developed by Arvesta Corporation is for use on ornamentals only. SHUTTLE provides excellent control of two-spotted mite, red mite, and related species. It does not demonstrate cross-resistance to miticide resistant mite species. A reduced risk compound, it has no impact on most predacious species. Some growers use this chemical on mother plants and wait one month before taking clones.

Safety: Do Not Use! Kills fish and water life, although it is not carcinogenic. Wear protective clothing, goggles, and gloves. Read label carefully. Do not use on cannabis that will be consumed!

Ampelomyces quisqualis
Fungicide

Controls: powdery mildew

Trade name: AQ-10

Caution! This product registration that was started in 1994 was canceled in 2004. This product is no longer available in the USA. For more information see http://www.pesticideinfo. org/Detail_Product.jsp?REG_ NR=05563800016&DIST_NR=071771

Ant Baits
Organic contact pesticide

Controls: ants

Brand names: Terro, Pic, Drax Ant Kill Gel (sugar-feeding ants)
Drax-FP (grease and sugar-feeding ants)
MAXFORCE, (cockroach and Pharaoh ant killer—hydramethylnon)

About: Sweet-loving ants are easy to attract and control with sweet baits mixed with ant-specific poison. They return to the nest and distribute the poison, killing the nest in a matter of days. Ants start feeding on bait within two hours.

Forms: store-bought containers or homemade

Mixing: homemade

Application: Set out or lay a barrier where ants are prevalent.

Persistence: Poison stays in container and is good for several months. We recommend baits with boric acid or hydramethylnon as their active ingredient. Big-headed ants, little black ants, and pavement ants are attracted to animal grease, protein, and fruits. A plastic squeeze bottle with a pointed tip is a great applicator. Make a protein/grease bait with:

- 4 tablespoons peanut butter
- 6 tablespoons honey
- 3/4 teaspoon boric acid

Sweet Baits
- Argentine ants
- carpenter Ants
- odorous house ants
- small honey ants

Grease and Sweet Baits
- big-headed ants
- little black ants
- pavement ants

Safety: Read label carefully and follow directions.
Bacillus thuringiensis (Bt) **and**
Bacillus **Species**
Bacillus pumilus: QST 2808

Organic beneficial fungus

Controls: *Fusarium*

Name: *Bacillus pumilus* strain QST 2808

About: *Bacillus pumilus* strain QST 2808, commonly found in soil, is sprayed on crops to control many fungal, mildews, blights and rusts pests. It forms a barrier between leaves and bad fungal spores, and *B. pumilus* strain QST 2808 actually colonizes the spores. Like several other varieties of *B. pumilus*, this strain may also stimulate the plant's own resistance system by inducing systemic acquired resistance (SAR).

Forms: Wettable powder

Mixing: Follow instructions on label for tomatoes and vegetables.

Application: Ground, aerial, or chemical spray; follow instructions on label for tomatoes and vegetables.

Persistence: Stays around until weathered or washed away.

Safety: No adverse environmental effects and *Bacillus pumilus* strain QST 2808 is NOT harmful to insects, birds, mammals, plants, or marine species when used as directed.

Bacillus thuringiensis (Bt) Species
Organic contact pesticide, miticide

Controls: caterpillars, larvae, and maggots

Pesticide: insecticide

About: *Bacillus thuringiensis (Bt)* is a well-known bacterium. There are several varieties, each with special qualities that are listed below. *Bt* kills pests a few days after it is eaten by pests. But they stop eating soon after ingesting *Bt*. Commercial *Bt* products do not reproduce within insect bodies, so several applications may be necessary to control an infestation. Commercial *Bt* products do not contain living *Bt* bacteria, but the *Bt* toxin is extremely perishable. *Bt* is most effective on young caterpillars, larvae, and maggots, so apply as soon as they are spotted.

Forms: powder, granules

Mixing: as per instructions on label

Application: Spray, dust, or granules. Inject liquid *Bt* into stalks to kill borers. Keep within prescribed temperature range, and apply according to the directions. Get the most out of *Bt* applications by adding a UV inhibitor, spreader-sticker, and a feeding stimulant such as Entice, Konsume or Pheast. *Bt* is completely broken down by UV light in one to three days.

Controls: fatal to caterpillars' larvae and maggots, cabbage loopers, cabbageworms, corn earworms, cutworms, gypsy moth larvae, and hornworms

Safety: Microbial *Bt* bacteria are nontoxic to animals, humans, beneficial insects, and plants; however, some people do develop an allergic reaction to it.

Bacillus thuringiensis var. *kurstaki (Btk)* is the most popular *Bt*. *Bacillus thuringiensis* var. *aizawai (Bta)* is effective against hard-to-kill budworms, borers, armyworms, and pests that have built up a resistance to *Btk*.

Controls: moth and caterpillar larvae, including most of the species that feed on cannabis

Brand names: DiPel, BioBit, Javelin, etc., *Btk* is also available in a microencapsulated form, M-Trak, Mattch, etc. The encapsulation extends the effective life on foliage to more than a week.

B. thuringiensis var. *israelensis (Bt-i)* kills mosquito and fungus gnat larvae. Use *Bt-i* to get rid of them as soon as they are identified. *B. thuringiensis* var. *morrisoni* is a new strain of *Bt* under development for insect larvae with a high pH in their guts.

Controls: larvae of mosquitoes, blackflies, and fungus gnats

Brand names: Gnatrol, Vectobac, and Bactimos. All are lethal to larvae. Adults do not feed on plants and are not affected.

B. thuringiensis var. *san diego (Btsd)*

Controls: larvae of Colorado potato beetles, elm beetle adults, and other leaf beetles

Bacillus thuringiensis var. *tenebrionis (Btt)* is lethal to the Colorado potato beetle

Bacillus cereus helps control damping-off and root-knot fungus. It flourishes in water-saturated mediums and promotes beneficial fungus that attacks the diseases.

Controls: Colorado potato beetle larvae

Bacillus subtilis is a soil-dwelling bacterium that curbs damping-off. Soak

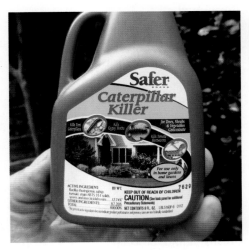

Bacillus thuringiensis is one of the most versatile and safe pesticides in the garden.

seeds and apply as a soil drench.

Controls: *Fusarium, Pythium,* and *Rhizoctonia* that cause damping-off

Brand names: Epic, Kodiac, Rhizo-Plus, Serenade, etc.

Bacillus popilliae colonize larvae and grub bodies that consume it, causing them to turn milky-white before dying. It is often called milky spore disease.

Controls: It is most effective against Japanese beetle grubs.

Beauveria bassiana (Beneficial Fungi)
Pesticide: pesticide/miticide

Controls: mites and insects—broad-spectrum kills ALL

Controls: whiteflies, thrips, aphids, and other soft-bodied sucking insects

Brand names: Naturalis H&G, BotaniGard, Mycotrol

About: Spores of Beauveria bassiana germinate upon contact with insects. The fungus grows directly into the pest/host. The fungus kills the insect in a week or two, and in doing so multiplies to infest new pest/host insects!

Forms: beneficial fungi wettable powder, liquid

Mixing: Follow instructions on label.

Application: Follow instructions on label.

Safety: kills beneficial insects

Baking Soda
Fungistat controls: powdery mildew and other surface fungus

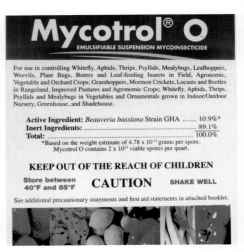

Beauveria bassiana is a broad-spectrum pesticide/miticide. It kills all insects and mites, good and bad!

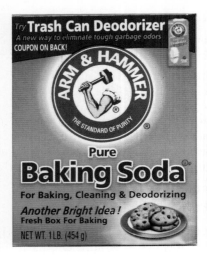

Baking soda

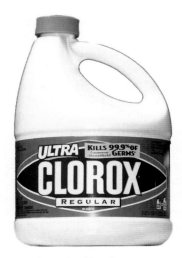

Laundry bleach

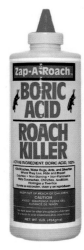

Boric acid

Brand names: Arm & Hammer

About: Baking soda (sodium bicarbonate, $NaHCO_3$) acts as a fungistat to change the pH of foliage surface so that fungal diseases cannot grow there.

Forms: powder, wettable powder

Mixing: dilute 2 tablespoons (30 ml) per quart (liter)

Application: Use as a duster or spray. Baking soda will persist on foliage one to three days and is easily washed off. Wash off with plain water after three days.

Safety: Baking soda is not toxic to mammals, fish, or beneficial insects. Wear a mask to avoid inhaling dust.

Bleach, Laundry
Germicide and disinfectant

Controls: numerous bacteria, fungi, and pests

Brand names: Clorox and many generic brands

About: Liquid bleach (sodium hypochlorite, NaClO) is a strong disinfectant for pots, walls, tools, and more when mixed in 10 percent solution with water. Apply with a brush, mop, or rag, or use as a dip.

Forms: liquid

Mixing: dilute in water at rate of 1 part bleach to 10 parts water.

Application: Spray, wipe on with rag or mop, or submerge seeds. To control stripping (seed virus), dilute a 25 percent solution of bleach and water, adjust to

9.0 pH. Soak seeds for ten minutes, and then rinse with fresh water. Residues linger a day or two.

Safety: Diluted bleach solution evaporates, leaving a slight residual in a couple of days. It is toxic to fish, beneficials, animals, and humans if swallowed or comes in contact with the eyes. Wear a mask and gloves when handling concentrate. Avoid respiration and skin contact. The concentrate burns skin and stains clothes.

The Bordeaux and Burgundy mixtures are too strong for indoor and outdoor cannabis plants in most conditions. You can find many recipes for them on the Internet. I have decided not to include them in this book.

Boric Acid
Pesticide: insecticide

Controls: earwigs, cockroaches, crickets, termites, fleas, silverfish, and ants.

About: Boric acid (also called boracic acid, orthoboric acid, or Acidum boricum (H_3BO_3)) is a lethal stomach poison for earwigs, cockroaches, crickets, termites, fleas, silverfish, and ants. Purchase ready-to-use products or mix borax soap powder or crystals in equal parts with powdered sugar to make toxic bait. Do not wet the bait or it will disperse quickly. Set bait on soil near plant base.

Forms: liquid, powder, crystals

Mixing: Follow instructions on label. Boric acid dissolves in water.

Application: Follow instructions on label.

Safety: Phytotoxic when applied to foliage. Not toxic to honeybees and birds. Avoid breathing boric acid dust.

Bug Bombs

Pesticide controls: everything in the room

Brand names: Look for brands with the highest concentration of pyrethrins—0.5 percent.

About: Single-application aerosol bombs are usually packed with strong insecticides and miticides, including synthetic pyrethrins that exterminate every pest in the room. Piperonyl butoxide and N-Octyl bicycloheptene dicarboximide are often added to pyrethrums to inhibit pest life processes. Propellants are also added to distribute the insecticide/miticide. Bug bombs were developed to kill fleas, roaches, and their eggs that hide in furniture and in carpets. Place the bug bomb in the empty garden room, turn it on, and leave the room.

Forms: single-use aerosol can

Mixing: none required

Application: Set the bug bomb in the middle of the clean garden room with all equipment removed, turn it on, and leave the room.

Safety: Be careful; read the entire label before using a bug bomb. Even though they have a low residual and persist for only a day or two, use these products as a last resort. Wear a mask and gloves, and cover exposed skin and hair.

Castor Oil

Pesticide: said to control moles

Brand names: Mole-Med, Mole-Go, Mole Repel

About: Castor oil plant or castor bean plant, Ricinus communis, is the same one that yields castor oil. We used to stuff bean pods and leaves down gopher holes, but I have never seen it work.

Forms: oil

Mixing: Follow instructions on label.

Application: Follow instructions on label.

Safety: Raw castor beans are toxic to humans if ingested Avoid contact with skin. A lethal dose in adults is four to eight seeds, although reports of poisonings are unusual.

Compost Tea

Compost teas, especially the "fast teas," are teaming with beneficial microbes that protect roots and foliage from disease and pest attacks.

See chapter 18, *Soil*, for more information.

Copper
Fungistat

Fungicide controls: gray mold, foliar fungus, anthracnose, blights, mildews, and a number of bacterial diseases.

Brand names: There are many manufacturers of copper fungicide.

About: Common ingredients—copper sulfate, copper oxychloride, cupric hydroxide, and cuprous oxide—are forms of fixed copper and are less phytotoxic than unfixed (pure) copper. Mix powder or liquid as per instructions and apply immediately after preparing. Agitate the mixture often while spraying, so ingredients do not settle out. Be careful when applying, and make sure the temperature is not too hot. The temperature range for application is 65°F to 85°F (18.3°C–29.4°C). It is best to stay nearer the bottom end of the temperature range.

Forms: liquid, powder

Mixing: Follow instructions on label for tomatoes and vegetables.

Application: Follow instructions on label for tomatoes and vegetables.

Safety: Easy to overapply and burn foliage or create a copper excess in plants. Copper fungicide lasts two weeks or longer indoors if not washed off. It is

toxic to fish. Not toxic to birds, bees, or mammals. Wear a mask and gloves, and cover exposed skin and hair.

Coriander Oil

Pesticide: insecticide, miticide

Controls: spider mites and soft-bodied insects

Brand names: SM-90, Brigade 2EC

About: Plant coriander seed and harvest cilantro plants. Although not a mainstream miticide and insecticide, coriander oil is at the base of a few popular products. This contact poison kills by drying out pest insects. SM-90 is made from coriander oil, sulfonated canola oil, and an acidic emulsifier.

Forms: emulsifiable liquid, liquid

Mixing: Follow instructions on label.

Application: Follow instructions on label.

Safety: Use protective clothing when handling and spraying.

Diatomaceous Earth (DE)

Pesticide: insecticide, miticide

Controls: Diatomaceous earth (DE) abrades the waxy coating on the shells and skin of pests, including aphids and slugs, causing body fluids to leak out.

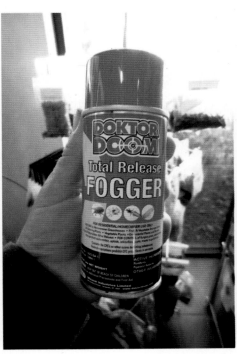

A bug bomb is designed to be set in the middle of the room and disperse the entire contents of the can at one time.

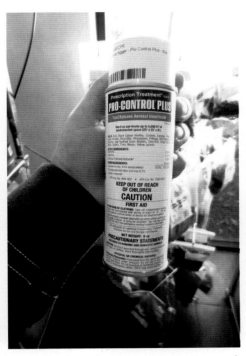

This aerosol pyrethrum (0.5 percent) is one of the best sprays for spider mites and insects.

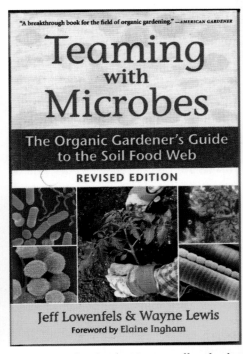

Teaming with Microbes *is an excellent book to learn about life in soil, compost, and compost teas.*

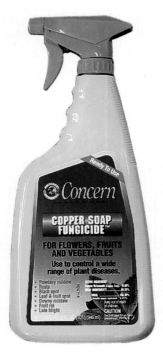
Copper fungicide

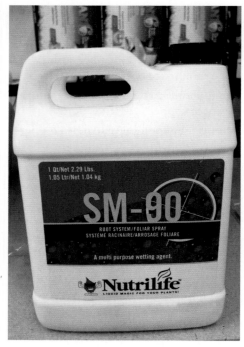
SM-90 was developed in Canada more than 20 years ago as a natural miticide.

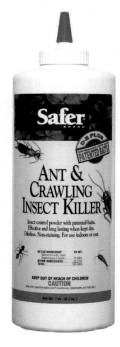
Diatomaceous earth is safe and works very well as a pesticide in many cases.

Once ingested, the razor-sharp particles in DE rip tiny holes in the pest's guts, causing death.

Brand names: There are many.

About: Naturally occurring DE includes fossilized silica-shell—remains of the tiny one-celled or colonial creatures called diatoms. It also contains 14 trace minerals in a chelated (available) form. Apply powder on soil, dust it onto foliage, or create a barrier around plants. Dilute DE in water as per instructions for spray. Apply weekly as soon as pests are apparent.

Forms: powder, wettable powder, liquid

Mixing: Follow instructions on label.

Application: Follow instructions on label. DE is swept away by wind and rain.

Safety: Use only horticultural-grade DE. Do not use chemically treated DE meant for swimming pools. DE stays on foliage for a few days or until washed off. Earthworms, animals, birds, and humans can digest diatomaceous earth with no ill effects. Avoid contact with skin and eyes. To guard against respiratory and eye irritations, wear a protective mask and goggles when handling this fine powder.

Homemade Sprays for Diseases and Pests
Organic pesticide/miticide controls: diseases and pests

Brand names: Homemade, however, many store-bought controls include the same elements as active ingredients, most often in a concentrated form.

About: A strong hot taste, smelly odor, and a desiccating powder or liquid are the main components in home-brewed pesticide and fungicide potions. Homemade sprays discourage and control pests such as aphids, thrips, spider mites, scale, and many others. Be careful when testing a new spray; apply it to a single plant and wait for a few days to learn the outcome before applying it to all plants.

Forms: liquid, powder, emulsifiable liquid, plant matter

Mixing: To make organic pesticide/ miticide spray concentrates, mix repellent substances with a little water in a blender. Strain the resulting slurry concentrate through a nylon stocking or fine cheesecloth before diluting it with water for application.

Application: Spray foliage until it drips from both sides of leaves.

Safety: Safe. In fact, ingredients can be found in most kitchens.

Toxicity: Homemade organic pesticide/ miticide usually is not toxic to humans in dosages lethal to pests.

Safety: Wear a mask and gloves, and cover skin and hair. Avoid contact with eyes, nose, lips, and ears.

Homemade Recipes and Controls
Alcohol: Add isopropyl (rubbing) alcohol to sprays to dry out pests.

Bleach: Use a 5 percent solution as a general disinfectant. Use 10 percent for a sure kill. Use a 25 percent solution when treating seeds. Wash off residual bleach with plenty of fresh water.

Cinnamon: Dilute cinnamon oil with water. Use two teaspoons per quart of water, or a few drops per pint as a fungicide or pesticide. It is relatively effective to slow powdery mildew and control a host of insects.

Citrus: Citrus oils are great ingredients that kill insects.

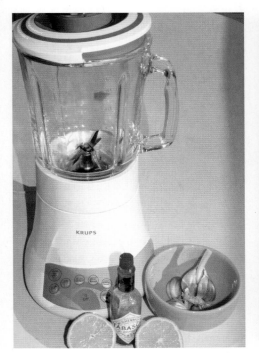

Making your own organic insecticide, miticide, or fungicide is as easy as blending the ingredients together with water.

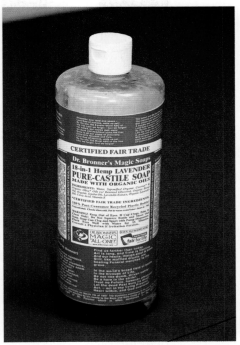

Dr. Bronner's Pure-Castile Soap is natural soap that is a great insecticide, miticide, fungicide, and cleaning agent. Also, mix Dr. Bronner's soap with garlic, hot pepper, citrus oil, and liquid seaweed combinations.

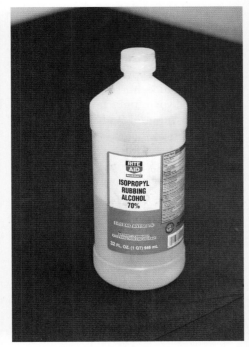

Isopropyl alcohol is widely available.

Clove: Clove oil is aromatic and repels pests.

Garlic: Use a garlic press to squeeze garlic juice into a homemade mix. Use liberal amounts.

Horseradish: Add as you would garlic. Best to use fresh root.

Hot pepper: Dilute Tabasco or any store-bought hot pepper concentrate in water.

Capsaicin: hot pepper spray; Bonide Hot Pepper Wax; Repellex mole, vole and gopher repellent; BrowseBan, and Liquid Fence for deer

Hydrated lime: Saturate in water to form a fungicide.

Mint: Mint oil drives insects away. Dilute in water; measure several drops per pint.

Oregano: Grind up fresh herb and use as a repellent. Mix with water.

Rosemary: The predatory mite

Phytoseiulus persimilis is less susceptible to rosemary oil and ECOTROL than spider mites, both in the laboratory and in the greenhouse. The parasitic wasp *Encarsia formosa* is more susceptible to rosemary oil than whiteflies.

Sesame: Use sesame oil or any other light oil sparingly to kill pests.

Soap: I like Ivory or Dr. Bronner's Pure-Castile soap. Use as an insecticide and wetting agent. Mix a few drops with water.

Tobacco: Mix tobacco with hot water to extract the poisonous alkaloid. Do not boil. Dilute concentrate with water.

Vegetable oil: Mix vegetable oil (comprised mainly of fatty acids and glycerides) with rubbing alcohol to emulsify in water. See "Oils" in this chapter.

Recipes for Homemade Mixes to Control Diseases and Pests
Cooking or heating preparations can destroy active ingredients. To draw out (extract) ingredients, mince plant

material and soak in mineral oil for a couple of days. Add this oil to the water, including a little detergent or soap to emulsify the oil droplets in water. Biodegradable detergents and soaps are good wetting-sticking agents for these preparations. Soap dissolves best if a teaspoon (5 ml) of alcohol is also added to each quart (0.9 L) of mix.

Chrysanthemum, marigold, and nasturtium blossoms; pennyroyal; garlic; chive; onion; hot pepper; insect juice (target insects mixed in a blender); horseradish; mint; oregano; tomato; and tobacco residues will all repel insects such as aphids, caterpillars, mites, and whiteflies. Spray made from pests ground up in a blender and emulsified in water will reputedly repel related pests. Best used on large pests! The insecticidal qualities in the dead bug parts will degrade quickly if combined with other things; do not include insects mixed in a blender with other ingredients besides water. Mixes that include tobacco may kill these pests if the mix is strong enough. These mixes can vary in proportions, but always filter the blended slurry before combining with water for the final spray. Straining avoids clogging spray nozzles and plumbing.

Recipe One: Mix three tablespoons (44 ml) each of isopropyl alcohol, lemon juice, garlic juice, horseradish juice, Ivory liquid soap, and a few drops each of Tabasco, mint oil, and cinnamon oil. Mix all the ingredients in a small bowl to form a slurry. Dilute the slurry at the rate of one teaspoon per pint (5 ml per 470 ml) of water and mix in a blender. Potent mix!

Recipe Two: Place one teaspoon (5 ml) of hot pepper or Tabasco sauce and four cloves of garlic in a blender with one pint of water. Liquefy, then strain the mix through a nylon stocking or cheese-cloth before using it in a sprayer.

Recipe Three: A mix of one-eighth to one-quarter cup (30–60 ml) of hydrated lime combined with a quart (0.9 L) of water makes an effective insect and mite spray. Mix a non-detergent soap with lime. The soap acts as both a sticking agent and an insecticide. Lime can be phytotoxic to plants in large doses. Always try the spray on a test plant and wait a few days to check for adverse effects to the plant before applying to similar plants.

Recipe Four: Liquid laundry bleach (sodium hypochlorite) is a good fungicide for non-plant surfaces. Mix as a 5 or 10 percent solution. It is an eye and skin irritant, so wear goggles and gloves when using it. Mix 1 part bleach to 9 parts water for a 5 percent solution. Mix 1 part bleach to 4 parts water for a 10 percent solution. Use this solution as a general disinfectant for garden room equipment, tools, and plant wounds. The bleach solution breaks down rapidly and has little, if any, residual effect.

This mix is an antifeedant when eaten by pests. It performs best in rooms with 60+ percent humidity.

Hydrogen Peroxide (H$_2$O$_2$)
Germicide: disinfectant

Controls: algae and slime

Fungistat: It is said to be helpful in controlling bacterial wilt, *Pythium* and *Fusarium* wilts.

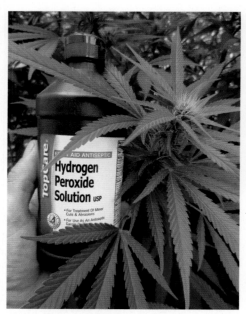

Hydrogen peroxide (H$_2$O$_2$) is readily available and best used to disinfect branches of flower buds after harvest. H$_2$O$_2$ can be destructive if used on live roots, even if diluted in solution.

Brand names: generic product

About: Hydrogen peroxide acts as an algaecide and disinfectant in water. Although effects are short-lived, they can be devastating to small feeder roots. Do not use H$_2$O$_2$ in hydroponic systems or as a soil drench. Use only to sterilize and clean. It will kill diseases, but not after they have entered the plant's system. All municipal water systems and old plumbing pipes contain slime mold. H$_2$O$_2$ kills slime mold and lots of other stuff, including algae.

Forms: liquid

Application: Use to kill diseases and pests on harvested cannabis and to clean garden containers, tool, and so forth. H$_2$O$_2$ dissipates quickly when not kept in an airtight container. H$_2$O$_2$ controls diseases on surface for three to five days but can destroy tender feeder roots.

Safety: H$_2$O$_2$ is safe for humans. On contact, it kills pathogens that cause infections. It kills tiny feeder roots on plants.

Limonene
Pesticide: insecticide, miticide

Fungistat: Limonene controls some fungus on the surface of foliage.

Brand names: Concern Citrus Home Pest Control, Clean Green

CONCENTRATIONS

0.5-1 cup (118–237 ml)	6 gallons (22.7 L) water
8 tablespoons (11 ml)	2 gallons (7.6 L) water
4 tablespoons (59 ml)	1 gallon (3.8 L) water

500 to 1,000 ppm is the recommended concentration of 3 percent H$_2$O$_2$ solution. MAKE SURE you are using 3 percent H$_2$O$_2$, NOT a higher concentration. Higher concentrations burn plants and skin.

About: Limonene occurs naturally in citrus fruits, a few vegetables, meats, and spices. It is normally an extract from orange peels (D-limonene). Limonene has insecticidal, miticidal, and fungicidal properties. It is antimicrobial and also a dog and cat repellent. Limonene can be used as a wetting and dispersing agent. It is often used as a solvent in household and industrial cleaners and degreasers. It is very flammable and can be used as a fire starter. It destroys an insect's system. Effective contact spray.

Mealybug and scale control
Forms: liquid

Mixing: Insoluble in water, must emulsify in water. Read instructions on label for tomatoes and vegetables. Corrosive—clean equipment after use.

Application: Follow instructions on label for tomatoes and vegetables.

Safety: can produce localized skin, mucus membrane, and lung irritation on contact. It has a very low toxicity in humans. Keep away from kittens and puppies. Leaves an oily film on water and can be toxic to aquatic life. Corrosive.

Neem and Neem Oil
Pesticide: insecticide, miticide

Germicide: sterilant, disinfectant

Fungistat: controls some fungi on the surface of foliage

Pesticide/miticide controls: many diseases and pests

Brand names: There are many.

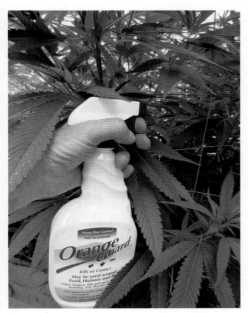

Limonene is found as the base of many natural insecticides.

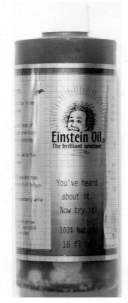

Einstein Oil is a popular brands of neem oil.

About: The Indian neem tree, *Azadirachta indica*, and the chinaberry tree, Melia azedarach, have spawned a host of insecticides and miticides. The active ingredient, azadirachtin, is most effective against young insects and is available in various concentrations. It is an antifeedant and disrupts insect life cycles. Neem is available in powders, liquids, oils (always use cold pressed oil), and cakes. Different parts of the tree and fruit, including the seeds, are used to make pesticides. Neem also contains nitrogen, phosphorus, potassium, and trace elements. Neem is used for a host of other things too.

Neem's traditional use is based on its detoxifying benefits that help maintain healthy circulatory, digestive, respiratory, and urinary systems. It is used for external applications in skin diseases. Neem extracts possess antibacterial and antiviral properties. Its principle constituents are nimbin, nimbinin, and nimbidin. All parts of the plant yield B-sitosterol.

Forms: oil, concentrate, liquid

Different products control different insects

Neem controls: Neem is most effective against caterpillars and other immature insects, including larvae of whiteflies, fungus gnats, mealybugs, and leaf miners.

Mixing: Neem is often mixed with vegetable (canola) oil. Just before using, add neem to water with a pH below 7.0, and use a spreader-sticker. Agitate constantly while using to keep the mix emulsified. Throw out excess.

Application: Use as a soil drench or add neem to the nutrient solution. This allows neem to enter the plant's tissue and become systemic. Used in a sprayer, neem becomes a contact spray.

Toxicity: Toxicity to beneficial insects has been reported, but neem is not toxic to humans.

Safety: Neem irritates eyes and skin; wear a mask and gloves. Neem products have numerous other applications. For additional product and safety information, check out the Neem Foundation, www.neemfoundation.org and www. einsteinoil.com.

Pesticide organic

Neem oil controls: Neem oil is effective against spider mites, fungus gnats, and aphids. It is also a fungistat against powdery mildew and rust.

Brand names: NeemGuard, Triact, Einstein Oil

Mixing: Just before using, mix emulsifiable concentrate in water with a pH below 7.0, and use a spreader-sticker. Agitate constantly while using to keep the mix emulsified. Throw out excess.

Application: Spray on foliage, especially under leaves, where mites live. Apply every few days so hatching larvae will eat it immediately. Spray heavily so mites have little choice but to eat it. Avoid spraying the last few days before harvest. Some growers report a foul taste when applied just before harvest.

Persistence: Contact neem stays on foliage for up to a month or until it is washed off. Stays in plant system up to a month when absorbed via roots.

Toxicity: Toxicity to beneficial insects has been reported, but neem is not toxic to humans.

Safety: Neem irritates eyes and skin; wear a mask and gloves. Neem products have numerous other applications. For additional product and safety information, check out the Neem Foundation, www.neemfoundation.org and www. einsteinoil.com.

Botanical insecticide, miticide, and nematicide

AzaMax controls: spider mites, thrips, fungus gnats, aphids, whiteflies, leaf miners, worms, beetles, leafhoppers, scales, mealybugs, nematodes, and other soilborne pests.

AzaMax is a natural (neem tree) product with a broad spectrum of pest control and broad plant applications. Contains azadirachtin A and B as active ingredients and more than 100 food-grade limonoids.

Application: AzaMax can be applied up to the time or day of harvest. It leaves no harmful residue on foliage and buds.

Nicotine and Tobacco Sprays

Pesticide: insecticide, miticide

Pesticide organic: sucking and chewing insects

Brand names: There are many brands available.

About: This nonpersistent pesticide is derived from tobacco, *Nicotiana tabacum*. It is a stomach poison, contact poison, and respiratory poison. This very poisonous compound affects the neuromuscular system, causing pests to go into convulsions and die. Nicotine sulfate is the most common form. Use a spreader-sticker when mixing this liquid. Seldom phytotoxic when used as directed. Combine with insecticidal soap to increase killing ability.

The nicotinoids are new (nicotine-based) systemic insecticides. The active ingredient, imidacloprid, could sell more than all pesticides, but it has no effect on mites or nematodes.

Forms: liquid

Mixing: Follow instructions on label for tomatoes and vegetables.

Application: Follow instructions on label for tomatoes and vegetables.

Safety: Nicotine and tobacco sprays are very toxic to most insects (including beneficials), honeybees, fish, and humans for a week to ten days after application. If concentrate is ingested or built up over years, humans may develop lung cancer and other cancers. Wear a mask and gloves; avoid skin and eye contact. Do not swallow any of this vile poison. Do not use around nightshade family—eggplants, tomatoes, peppers, and potatoes—because they may contract tobacco mosaic virus (TMV) from exposure to tobacco-based substances.

Oil, Horticultural
Organic contact pesticide insecticide, miticide

Controls: Virtually invisible, horticultural oil kills slow-moving and immobile sucking insects, spider mites, and their eggs by smothering them.

Brand names: There are many brands available.

About: Similar to medicinal mineral oil, horticultural oils are made from animal (fish) oils, plant seed oils, and petroleum oils refined by removing most of the portion that is toxic to plants. Lighter-weight oil (viscosity 60–70) is less phytotoxic. Vegetable oil is also horticultural oil. Mix ¾ teaspoon (75 ml) of oil liquid spray—no more than a 1 percent solution—per quart (0.9 L) of water. More than a few drops could burn tender growing shoots. Spray foliage thoroughly, including the undersides of leaves. Apply oil sprays up until two weeks before harvest. Repeat applications as needed. Usually three applications, one every five to ten days, will put insects and mites in check. Lightweight-oil residue evaporates into the air in a short time.

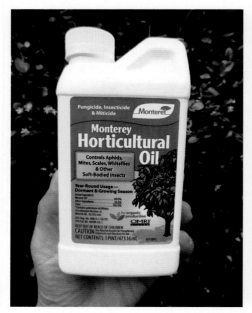

Horticultural oil should be lightweight and organic.

Forms: oil

Mixing: Follow instructions on label for tomatoes and vegetables.

Application: Follow instructions on label for tomatoes and vegetables.

Safety: Residuals disappear in one to three days under normal growing conditions. Horticultural oil is a safe, nonpoisonous, and nonpolluting insecticide. It can become phytotoxic if too heavy (viscosity), if applied too heavily, or when temperatures are below 70°F (21.1°C), or when very humid; this slows evaporation, increasing phytotoxicity. Wear a mask and gloves. Do not use lubricating oils such as 3-in-1 or motor oil!

Vegetable Oil
Pesticide: insecticide, miticide

Pesticide organic controls: Vegetable oil is virtually invisible. Like horticultural oil, it kills slow-moving and immobile sucking insects, spider mites, and their eggs by smothering them.

Brand names: There are many brands available at the grocery store.

About: Comprised of fatty acids and glycerides, lightweight vegetable oil smothers slow-moving and immobile sucking insects, spider mites, and their eggs. Mix two drops of oil—no more

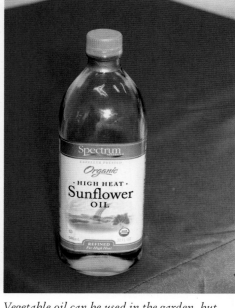

Vegetable oil can be used in the garden, but its use should be limited. Do not add too much vegetable oil in sprays, or the spray will disperse unevenly across leaves.

than a 1 percent solution—per quart of water. Spray foliage thoroughly, including the undersides of leaves. Stop spraying two weeks before harvest.

Forms: oil

Mixing: 1 tablespoon per gallon (15 ml /L)

Application: Mix sparingly in sprays because it tends to decompose and leave a residual that lasts several days.

Safety: Not toxic to mammals or fish. Wear a mask and gloves.

Predator Urine
Discourages: rabbits, mice, voles, deer, and other animals

Brand names: Piss Off!

About: Predators eat herbivores (plant-eating animals), and predators' urine scares away cannabis-munching varmints. Create a predator (coyote) urine barrier to frighten off rabbits, mice, voles, deer, and more by applying predator urine around problematic gardens. Note that the urine washes off in a few days. This is why coyotes continually pass by to mark their territory.

There are also numerous products containing hot peppers, citrus, eggs, salts, soaps, garlic, and so on that work in

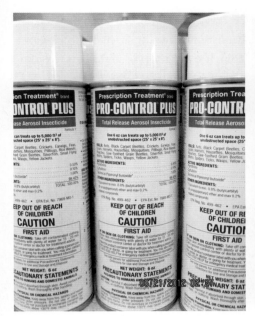

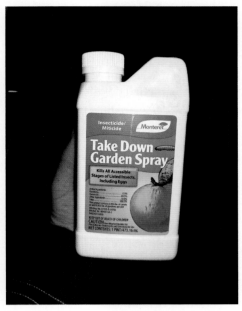

Pro-Control Plus *is one of many brands of encapsulated pyrethrum available. Whitmire's X-clude is another brand-name product with encapsulated pyrethrum that lasts several hours after application.*

Liquid pyrethrum can be as effective as aerosol brands if it covers foliage completely.

varying degrees as repellents. They must be applied properly to be effective.

Use also: fine plastic netting, wire fence

Forms: liquid

Mixing: Follow instructions on label.

Application: Products are often applied via weatherproof applicators or "scent rags" hanging around the garden. Follow instructions on label for tomatoes and vegetables.

Safety: Do not let any spill on you!

Pyrethrum

Pesticide: insecticide, miticide (broad spectrum)

Controls: Pyrethrum kills aphids, whiteflies, spider mites, and insects—including beneficials. It is very effective to control flying insects, but they must receive a killing knockdown dose.

Brand names: Whitmire's X-clude is encapsulated and lasts longer

About: Natural pyrethrum is extracted from the flowers of the pyrethrum chrysanthemum, *Chrysanthemum coccineum* and *C. cinerariifolium*. Pyrethrins—pyrethrins, cinerins, and jasmolins—are the active ingredients in natural pyrethrum and kill insects and mites on contact. Pyrethroids are axonic poisons that affect nervous system of

insects and mites, eventually causing paralysis.

Synthetic pyrethroids act as broad-spectrum, nonselective contact insecticides and miticides. There are more than 30 synthetic pyrethroids available in different formulations. Deltamethrin is available as a sticky paint that is used as a trap when applied to stems and colored objects. Many insects and mites are resistant to pyrethroids.

Natural pyrethrum is expensive and decomposes rapidly in sunlight, with a short effective life. Synthetic pyrethrin-like materials, pyrethroids are stable in sunlight and are effective against insect and mites.

Pyrethrums have gone through four evolving generations:

1. Pyrethrum, naturally occurring
2. Tetramethrin, resmethrin (Synthrin, 20 times as effective as pyrethrum), bioresmethrin (50 times as effective as pyrethrum)
3. Permethrin is virtually unaffected by ultraviolet light in sunlight, lasting four to seven days on crops.
4. Current generation, bifenthrin, cypermethrin, cyfluthrin, deltame-

thrin, esfenvalerate, fenpropathrin, flucythrinate, prallethrin, tau-fluvalinate, tefluthrin, tralomethrin, zeta-cypermethrin. All are photostable. They do not degrade in sunlight, and the residual effectiveness is up to ten days.

Pyrethrum is often combined with other botanical pesticides—rotenone, ryania, etc.—to ensure effectiveness. Aerosol forms contain synergists. (See "Application" below.) Pest insects and mites become immune to pyrethrins; alternating with other sprays works best.

Synthetic Pyrethroids

Nonselective pyrethroids: kill all insects and mites, including beneficials and bees

Forms: powder, liquid, aerosol

Mixing: Follow instructions on label.

Application: Follow instructions on label. Make sure to spray undersides of leaves so spray contacts pest insects and mites.

Persistence: 30 minutes to several hours

Toxicity: Toxic to all insects. Synthetic pyrethroids are somewhat toxic to mammals.

Safety: Wear a mask and protective clothing when applying sprays or breathing in any form of pyrethrum, especially aerosols. Aerosols contain toxic piperonyl butoxide (PBO) and MGK 464—possible carcinogens that are easily inhaled.

Caution: Do not mix with sulfur, lime, copper, or soaps. The high pH of these substances render the mix ineffective. Wash these substances off foliage with plain water (pH below 7.0) before applying pyrethrum.

Application: Spot spray infested plants. Aerosol sprays are most effective on spider mites. This can burn foliage—spray is ice-cold when it exits the nozzle—if applied closer than one foot. Aerosol spray contains a synergist, PBO or MGK 264. Both are toxic to people. Pyrethrum dissipates within a few hours in the presence of air, HID light, and sunlight. Overcome this limitation by applying just before turning off the lights, the circulation, and vent fans for the night. Use encapsulated aerosol pyrethrum.

Persistence: Effective several hours after application when the lights are on, longer when applied after lights-out and the fan is turned off.

Forms: wettable powder, dust, liquid, granular bait, and aerosol

Toxicity: Synthetic pyrethroids are not toxic to animals and humans when eaten but become toxic to people when inhaled. Toxic to fish and beneficials.

Safety: Wear a mask and protective clothing when applying sprays or breathing in any form of pyrethrum, especially aerosols. Aerosols contain toxic PBO and MGK 464 (possible carcinogens), which are easily inhaled. The pyrethroids have a low-to-moderate acute toxicity to mammals and may be irritating to the skin.

Quassia, Rotenone, Ryania, and Sabadilla

This "group" of pesticides—quassia, rotenone, ryania, and sabadilla—is often combined to improve pest kill rate.

Quassia

Pesticide: insecticide, miticide

Controls: Soft-bodied insects including aphids, leaf miners, and some caterpillars.

About: Quassia is made from a subtropical South American tree, *Quassia amara*, and the tree-of-heaven, *Ailanthus altissima*. It is most often combined with rotenone, ryania, and sabadilla because it is difficult to extract.

Mixing: Follow instructions on label for tomatoes and vegetables.

Application: Follow instructions on label for tomatoes and vegetables. Quassia stays active for two to five days on the surface of plants.

Safety: Wear a mask and gloves; cover exposed skin and hair. Avoid skin contact.

Toxicity: Quassia is safe for mammals and (possibly) beneficials.

Rotenone

Pesticide: insecticide

About: Rotenone is an extract from roots of several plants, including Derris species, *Lonchocarpus* species, and *Tephrosia* species. Rotenone is a nonselective contact insecticide, stomach poison, and slow-acting nerve poison.

Controls: Nonselective control of beetles, caterpillars, flies, mosquitos, thrips, weevils, and beneficial insects, but death is slow. According to *Hemp Diseases and Pests*, target insects can consume up to 30 times their lethal dose before dying!

Forms: powder, wettable powder, liquid

Mixing: Follow the manufacturer's instructions.

Application: Rotenone breaks down in three to ten days.

Toxicity: This insecticide kills beneficials, birds, and fish; the effect on mammals is undetermined. Chronic exposure may cause Parkinson's disease.

Safety: Wear a mask and gloves; cover exposed skin and hair. Avoid skin contact.

Ryania

Pesticide: insecticide

Controls: Ryania is toxic to aphids, thrips, European corn borers, hemp borers, flea beetles, leaf rollers, and many caterpillars. Once pests consume ryania, they stop feeding immediately and die within 24 hours.

Forms: powder, wettable powder

Mixing: Follow instructions on label for tomatoes and vegetables.

Application: Follow instructions on label for tomatoes and vegetables. Stays for active two weeks or longer.

Safety: Wear a mask and gloves; cover exposed skin and hair. Avoid skin contact.

Toxicity: somewhat toxic to mammals, birds, fish, and beneficials

Sabadilla

Pesticide: insecticide, miticide

About: This alkaloid pesticide is made from the seeds of a tropical lily, *Schoenocaulon officinale*, native to Central and South America, and a European hellebore, *Veratrum album*.

Controls: A contact and stomach poison, this centuries-old poison controls aphids, beetles, cabbage loopers, chinch bugs, grasshoppers, and squash bugs.

Forms: powder, liquid

Mixing: Follow instructions on label for tomatoes and vegetables.

Application: Sabadilla is most potent when applied at 75°F to 80°F (23.9°C–26.7°C). Follow directions on package.

Persistence: two or three days

Toxicity: Sabadilla is somewhat toxic to mammals, toxic to honeybees.

Safety: Wear a mask and gloves; cover exposed skin and hair. Avoid skin contact.

Seaweed

Pesticide: insecticide, miticide organic

Brand names: There are many brands; check with your local hydroponic store or retail nursery for a recommendation.

About: Seaweed contains numerous elements, including nutrients, bacteria, and hormones.

Controls: Suspended particles in seaweed impair and even kill insects and spider mites by causing lesions. The particles cut and penetrate soft-bodied pest insects and mites, causing their body fluids to leak out.

Forms: powder and liquid

Mixing: Dilute as per instructions for soil application.

Application: Spray on foliage, especially under leaves where mites live. Stays active up to two weeks when a spreader-sticker is used.

Toxicity: Seaweed is not toxic to mammals, birds, or fish, but it is nonselective and kills beneficials.

Safety: Wear a mask and gloves.

Sevin, carbaryl

Pesticide: insecticide, miticide

Controls: Sevin is often used to kill bees and wasps; it kills all insects, good and bad!

Brand names: Sevin

About: The development of carbamate insecticides in the 1950s was a major breakthrough because they do not persist as long as chlorinated pesticides.

Carbaryl is broad spectrum, killing both targeted and beneficial insects and crustaceans. Carbaryl is detoxified and eliminated rapidly in vertebrates. It does not concentrate in fat and milk.

Forms: liquid, powder

Mixing: Follow instructions on label for tomatoes and vegetables.

Application: Follow instructions on label for tomatoes and vegetables.

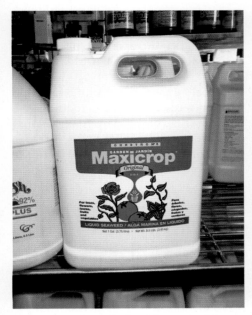

Seaweed can be applied to foliage in a dilute spray to kill insects and mites.

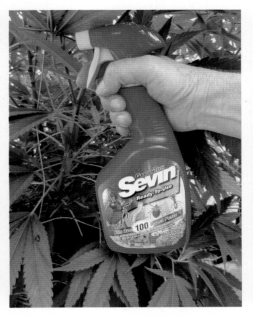

Sevin is a very strong insecticide often used to kill wasps.

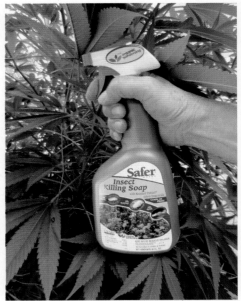

Applying insecticidal soap is one of the first control measures in the garden.

Safety: Carbaryl is toxic to humans and is considered a likely human carcinogen by the EPA. Carbaryl is illegal in several countries, including the United Kingdom, Austria, Denmark, Sweden, Iran, Germany, and Angola.

Soap, Insecticidal
Pesticide: insecticide, miticide

Brand names: There are many brands available

About: Insecticidal soaps are contact insecticides made from fatty acids of animals and plants and are considered organic. A variety of soaps are available in potassium-salt-based liquid concentrates. Soft soaps such as Ivory liquid dish soap, Castile soap, and Murphy's Oil soap are biodegradable and kill insects in a similar manner to commercial insecticidal soaps, but they are not as potent or effective.

Controls: Insecticidal soaps control soft-bodied insects such as aphids and mealybugs, spider mites, thrips, and whiteflies by penetrating and clogging body membranes.

Caution: Do not use detergent soaps, because they may be caustic.

Forms: liquid

Mixing: Add a few capfuls of soap to a quart of water to make a spray. Ivory or Castile soap can also be used as a spreader-sticker to mix with other sprays. The soap helps the spray stick to the foliage better.

Application: Spray at the first appearance of insect pests. Follow directions on commercial preparations. Spray homemade mixes every four to five days. Soft soaps will last only for about a day before dissipating.

Toxicity: These soaps are safe for bees, animals, and humans.

Safety: Wear a mask and gloves.

Spinosad
Pesticide: insecticide, miticide organic

Brand names: Spinosad

About: Spinosad (spinosyn A and spinosyn D) is a new chemical class of insecticides. The active ingredient is derived from the rare species bacterium *Saccharopolyspora spinosa* actinomycete. Spinosad kills susceptible species by exciting the nervous system after being ingested by the insect. Spinosad must be ingested by the insect, therefore it has little effect on sucking insects and nontarget predatory insects.

Spinosad is relatively fast-acting. The pest insect dies within one to two days after ingesting the active ingredient. It is classified as an organic substance by the USDA National Organic Standards Board. The Organic Materials Review Institute (OMRI) listed Spinosad for use in organic production.

Controls: Fruit flies, caterpillars, leaf miners, thrips, sawflies, spider mites, fire ants, and leaf beetle larvae. It kills caterpillars, fire ants, fruit flies, leaf beetle larvae, leaf miners, sawflies, spider mites, and thrips.

Forms: liquid

Mixing: Mix 4 tablespoons per gallon of water.

Application: Follow instructions on label.

Toxicity: Spinosad has low mammal

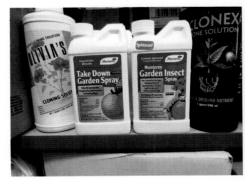

Spinosad is a great natural pesticide against caterpillars, thrips, and leaf miners.

toxicity when ingested and no adverse effects from chronic exposure. There is a slight toxicity to birds, moderate toxicity to fish, and moderate toxicity to aquatic invertebrates. It is highly toxic to bees and to oysters and other marine mollusks. Avoid application where it is toxic.

There is little or no phytotoxicity for cannabis. To prevent insect pesticide resistance, do not spray Spinosad more than 10 times in 12 months in a garden room or greenhouse.

Safety: Always wear protective clothing when spraying Spinosad.

Streptomyces griseoviridis
Fungicide
Beneficial bacteria organic controls: fungi that cause seed rot, root and stem rot, wilt, and damping-off diseases

Brand names: MycoStop, RootShield, Microgrow

About: More than 500 species of *Streptomyces* bacteria are known. *Streptomyces griseoviridis* strain K61 is a naturally occurring soil bacterium that was isolated from decaying peat in Finland. It produces spores that cause it to have an earthy odor. It works to prevent fungal attacks and must be applied before fungi invade. *Streptomyces griseoviridis* colonizes plant roots before the disease organisms arrive, displacing the bad guys taking their food. It also makes other chemicals that attack harmful fungi. This fungicide is effective against *Alternaria, Botrytis, Fusarium, Phomopsis,* and *Pythium. Streptomyces* bacteria also produce secondary chemicals, root-stimulating hormones that increase germination, as well as root growth and overall plant vigor. Applying *S. griseoviridis* is an excellent prevention measure to use in Integrated Pest Management (IPM) programs.

Apply fungicide as a preventative measure before any sign of harmful fungus so *S. griseoviridis* has a chance to colonize and get established to prevent harmful fungal attacks. Apply to seeds, soil, or roots, and to transplants as a dip or spray.

Forms: wettable powder (dried spores and mycelium)

Mixing: Follow instructions on label for tomatoes and vegetables.

Application: Follow instructions on label for warm weather crops—tomatoes, peppers, etc.

Safety: OMRI Listed for use in organic production. Wear protective gear including a respirator that filters dust and mist when handling. Mild skin, eye and lung irritation is possible. Watch for possible side effects on pH and EC.

Sulfur
Sulfur Burners and Pests
Fungicide
Beneficial bacteria organic controls: Sulfur protects against fungi that cause seed rot, root and stem rot, wilt, and damping-off diseases.

Brand names: MycoStop, RootShield, Microgrow

About: *Streptomyces griseoviridis* strain K61, a naturally occurring soil bacterium, colonizes plant roots before the disease organisms arrive, displacing the bad guys taking their food. It also makes other chemicals that attack harmful fungi. This fungicide is effective against *Alternaria, Botrytis, Fusarium,*

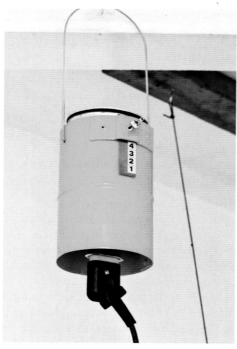

A thin coat of sulfur on foliage will kill many insects, mites, and eggs. It also makes an inhospitable environment for newly germinating fungal spores. Vaporized sulfur is not labeled for insect control even though it is toxic to insects, as well as desiccating.

Phomopsis, and *Pythium. Streptomyces* bacteria also produce root-stimulating hormones that increase germination, as well as root and plant vigor.

Apply before any sign of harmful fungus. Apply to seeds, to the soil, to roots, to transplants as a dip or spray. Apply before diseases start so the *Streptomyces griseoviridis* has a chance to get established and can prevent harmful fungal attacks.

Forms: powder

Mixing: Follow instructions on label for tomatoes and vegetables.

Application: Follow instructions on label for warm weather crops—tomatoes, peppers, etc..

Safety: OMRI Listed for use in organic production. Watch for possible side effects on pH and EC.

Pesticide: insecticide

Pesticide/miticide/fungicide

Brand names: many

About: Sulfur is a centuries-old fungicide that is toxic to insects and controls fungus but is also quite phytotoxic to plants if overdone. Application temperatures should be about 60°F (about 15°C). Sulfur can be applied directly to foliage or evaporated into the air in an enclosed area when using a sulfur burner.

Sulfur is easiest and most economical to apply in a liquid spray. Sulfur mixed with liquid must not stay on foliage or it will burn and damage it. Follow instructions on the product label.

Sulfur evaporated in a garden room stops *Botrytis cinerea* and powdery mildew from growing on surfaces and plants, but it does not enter the system of the plant. Use only high-grade refined sulfur. Sulfur burners heat sulfur to evaporate it into the atmosphere of gardenrooms and greenhouses. Evaporated or volatized sulfur hangs in the air and coats surfaces when it falls.

Controls: Sulfur can kill mildews, *Botrytis,* and more diseases and pests such as spider mites.

Caution: Do not apply in temperatures above 90°F (32°C) and less than 50 percent humidity. It will burn foliage.

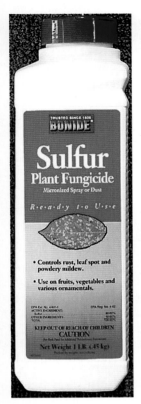

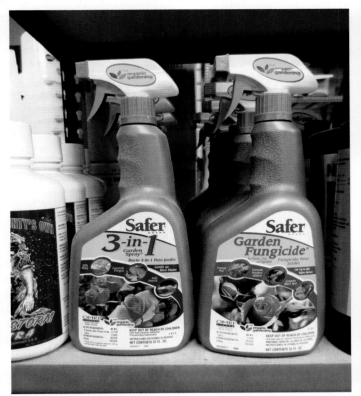

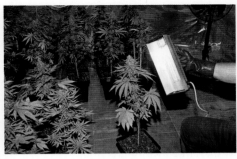

Regular applications of UVC light with a small handheld lamp will help keep pathogens and pests out of your garden.

Sulfur fungicides are very strong and can burn foliage if applied when temperatures are too hot. Sulfur is a common ingredient in many fungicides.

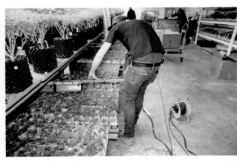

Ultraviolet light works incredibly well to kill molds and mildews. The gardener passes the UVC lamp briefly over the tender little clones every day to kill any new mold spores. You can also spot mold in the garden with a UVB or green light. I put my headlamp on and walk around the garden at night looking for signs of iridescent mold on foliage.

Forms: powder

Mixing: Follow directions on package.

Application: Apply in light concentration. It is phytotoxic during hot, arid weather. Follow instructions on label for tomatoes and vegetables.

Evaporated sulfur: Turn off the vent fans and lights when using evaporated sulfur. Apply one hour after lights go off. Apply for at least two hours to be effective. Exhaust for three hours before lights come back on. Apply weekly, biweekly, or more often. Do not apply two weeks before harvest.

Sulfur dusted on the floor of garden rooms volatilizes in arid climates to provide long-term protection from infection. Phytotoxicity can be a problem during high temperatures. Sulfur stays on foliage several days or until washed off.

Toxicity: Too much sulfur results in burned pistils in the buds closest to the evaporator. Way too much sulfur turns the leaves yellow in the margins between the veins. Sulfur is toxic to insects but phytotoxic to plants. It is not toxic to honeybees, birds, and fish.

Safety: Wear a mask, gloves, and safety goggles; cover exposed skin and hair. Avoid skin, eye, ear, and nose contact. Sulfur irritates eyes, lungs, and skin.

Trichoderma
Beneficial fungi organic controls
Brand names: *Trichoderma* is sold under many brand names; look for the word *trichoderma* on the label or ingredients list.

About: *Trichoderma* is added to many soil mixes and hydroponic growing mediums to protect plants from diseases and pests and increase plant vigor. *Trichoderma* spp. are common free-living fungi found in soil and root ecosystems. Some varieties colonize roots and release antifungal antibiotic compounds that induce resistance to diseases and pests. *Trichoderma* enhances root growth and development, crop productivity, resistance to abiotic stresses, and the uptake and use of nutrients.

Forms: *Trichoderma* is mixed in various products.

Mixing: Follow instructions on label for tomatoes and vegetables.

Application: Follow instructions on label for tomatoes and vegetables.

Safety: safe

UVC Light
Disinfectant, germicide, miticide, insecticide
Brand names: Big Blue, Turbo Twist, Air Probe Sanitizer

About: Germicidal UVC light deactivates the DNA of mites, bacteria, viruses, and other diseases in air, liquids, on surfaces, and on plants. The diseases die or try to reproduce and then die. This natural purifier also kills allergy- and disease-causing microbes. Special UVC lamps are available and produce no residual contamination. Low-level mercury lamps made from special glass emanate 253.7 nanometers, precisely the bandwidth to kill diseases.

UVC light is a sterilant and germicide. It destroys any microorganisms that may be directly exposed to it. UV light has little penetrating ability and is unable to pass through opaque material, glass, or water. Quartz is transparent to UV light. UV rays from sunlight are filtered off by the time the sun's light reaches earth's surface.

Application: UVC light is used to sterilize medical cannabis in The Netherlands. Run buds under UVC light for a few seconds to kill bad stuff such as mold, mold spores, and *Botrytis*.

Forms: artificial light

Safety: UV light is damaging to the skin and eyes. Avoid all contact!

Vinegar
Pesticide: insecticide

Germicide: disinfectant

Fungistat: kills many fungi on contact

Pesticide/miticide

Controls: Vinegar helps with many garden problems. See "Application" below.

Brand names: generic

About: Table vinegar ranges in concentration from 4 percent to 8 percent by volume. Pickling vinegar can be up to 18 percent. Any type of vinegar can be distilled into a white (colorless) solution of about 4 percent to 8 percent acetic acid in water. White vinegar is used for cleaning and sterilizing. Find white distilled vinegar at your local grocery store.

Forms: liquid

Mixing: Dilute in water.

Application: To preserve cut flower buds, add 2 tablespoons (30 ml) white distilled vinegar and 1 teaspoon sugar (5 ml) to a quart of water in a glass.

Clean pots with a 50 percent solution of white distilled vinegar.

Remove rust on spigots and tools by soaking overnight in undiluted white distilled vinegar.

Neutralize garden lime by adding white distilled vinegar to the area.

Increase the acidity of soil by adding white distilled vinegar to your watering can.

Eliminate anthills by pouring white distilled vinegar into them.

Kill slugs by spraying them with a 1:1 vinegar:water mix using white distilled vinegar.

Catch moths with a mixture composed

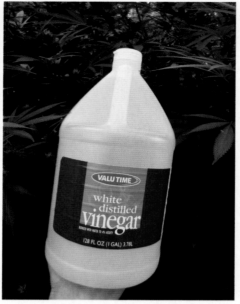

Vinegar has a low pH and can be used as a disinfectant and to decalcify plumbing and reservoirs. It is inexpensive and smells bad.

of 2 parts white distilled vinegar and 1 part molasses. Dangle the mix in a tree.

Cats, dogs, and rabbits are repelled by vinegar-soaked cotton balls. Put them in a small container with a few holes in it to let the smell out.

Remove mold from terra cotta pots by soaking in a solution of 1 cup white distilled vinegar, 1 cup chlorine bleach, and 1 gallon of warm water before scrubbing with a steel wool pad.

Safety: Vinegar has a low pH and is corrosive. It also smells bad!

Traps
Pesticide: insecticide, miticide

Brand names: Tanglefoot

About: Sticky traps, such as Tanglefoot resins, can be smeared on attractive yellow or red cards to simulate ripe fruit. When pests land on the "fruit," they are stuck forever!

Controls: Traps help contain spider mites and nonflying insects within the bounds of the barriers. Traps monitor fungus gnat populations and help control thrips. Other insects get stuck haphazardly to the sticky stuff. Black-light traps catch egg-laying moths and other flying insects, most of which are not plant pests. Light and fan traps attract many insects including beneficials, and

their use may do more harm than good. Sex-lure traps exude specific insect pheromones, sexual scents, of females that are ready to mate. These traps are most effective to monitor insect populations for large farms.

Caution: Do not touch sticky substance. It is difficult to remove!

Forms: sticky, thick paint

Mixing: Follow directions on container. Smear on desired objects.

Application: Smear Tanglefoot around the edges of pots, base of stems, and at the end of drying lines to form an impenetrable barrier-trap against mites and insects. This simple precaution helps keep mites isolated. However, resourceful spider mites can spin a web above the barrier. The marauding mites also ride from plant to plant on the air currents created by fans! Tanglefoot is persistent until it is wiped off or completely fouled with insect bodies.

Toxicity: Traps are not toxic to mammals or insects. Trapped insects and mites starve to death.

Safety: Wear gloves, and do not breathe fumes. Read and follow directions.

Sticky Yellow Traps
Hang **sticky yellow traps** around your growing area to catch whiteflies, adult fungus gnats, winged aphids, and many other garden pests. They're not only effective pest control, they're also a great early warning system. Pests are much easier to spot against the yellow than on your plants. Place the traps about three feet (about 90 cm) apart within or just above plant foliage.

Sticky blue traps: Similar to the orig-

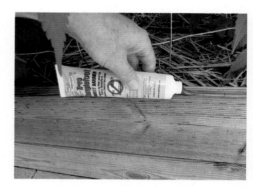

Tanglefoot is an excellent product that keeps pests from crossing a given boundary. Wipe on stems, container lips, drying lines, and more to contain pests.

inal sticky yellow traps, sticky blue traps attract pests to the blue portion of the color spectrum. Customers report success using Sticky Blue Traps against thrips and leaf miners.

Water

Pesticide: insecticide, miticide organic

Brand names: Use tap water or reverse osmosis (RO) water. Bottled water is too expensive.

About: A cold jet of water—preferably with a pH between 6.0 and 7.0—blasts insects, spider mites, and their eggs off leaves, often killing them. Hot water vapor and steam also work as a sterilant.

Controls: A cold jet of water is an excellent first wave of attack against spider mites, aphids, and other sucking insects. Steam controls spider mites, insects, and diseases on pots, growing mediums, and other grow-room surfaces.

Caution: Avoid spraying fully formed buds with water. Standing water in or on buds promotes gray mold. Do not apply hot steam to foliage.

Forms: liquid

Mixing: Use RO or low-EC water when possible.

Application: Spray leaf undersides with a jet of cold water to knock off sucking spider mites and aphids. Apply water as a mist or spray when predatory mites are present. The extra humid conditions impair the pest mite lifecycles and promote predatory mite health. Rent a wallpaper steamer. Get it cooking, and direct a jet of steam at all grow-room cracks and surfaces.

Toxicity: Water is not toxic to mammals, fish, or beneficials.

Safety: Do not spray strong jet of water

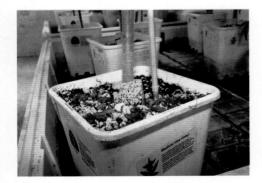
Sticky yellow traps can be used to monitor insect activity and to trap pest insects over time.

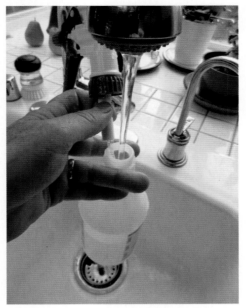
Water is a great pesticide. Spray foliage vigorously with water to dislodge and mutilate insects and their eggs. Often a brisk water spray will be all the insect control necessary on outdoor plants.

in eyes, up nose, or into other body orifices.

Beneficial Insects

The predators for specific insects and mites are listed in the entry after each pest under "Beneficial Insects." This section is about predators, how to identify them, and how to receive, introduce, and apply their help in medical cannabis gardens. Predators and parasitoids are the two types of predators. Most predators are larger than their prey. Parasitoids are typically smaller than hosts. Parasites lay eggs on or inside the host. The eggs hatch into larvae and eat the host from the inside out. Parasites kill one to several hosts. Predators kill many pest prey.

Predator and parasite availability and supply have changed substantially over the last few years. Today many more beneficial insects are available to medical cannabis gardeners than ever before. Shipping, care, cost, and application of each predator or parasite is very specific and detailed instructions should be provided by the supplier. Make sure the supplier answers the following:

1. Latin name of the predator, so there is no confusion as to identity
2. Specific pests attacked by the predator
3. Life cycle information
4. Preferred climate, including temperature Application rate and mode of application

For more information about predators, check out the following web pages:

Nature's Control:
www.naturescontrol.com
Koppert Biological Systems:
www.koppert.nl/english
University of Wisconsin-Madison, Department of Entomology:
www.entomology.wisc.edu/mbcn/mbcn.html

By definition, a predator must eat more than one victim before adulthood. Some predators such as ladybugs (ladybird beetles) and praying mantises have chewing mouthparts to eat their prey whole. But lacewing larvae have piercing-sucking mouthparts to suck the life from victims. Typically adult parasitoids insert a single egg into many hosts. The egg hatches for the larva to eat the host from the inside out, often emerging as adults.

Predators like to be surrounded by prey. When the prey population diminishes, predators look for infestations where food is easy to find. They never completely eradicate the pest insects. Predators are best used for preventive control.

Of all insect species, more than 97 percent of those usually found around the home landscape are beneficial or are not interested in cannabis.

To get the most from predators, get used to a little pest damage on plants. Cannabis is tough and can deal with the damage. Beneficials also need shelter in the form of leaf litter and debris (mulch) to hide and cool down on hot days. Growing other non-cannabis plants helps provide a diverse environment to accommodate other natural enemies of pests.

Most beneficials stay in the garden when there is a constant source of pollen and nectar (available commercially) substitutes available when prey is scarce.

Flowers and plants that attract and maintain beneficials include: aster species, sweet alyssum, pansies, dill,

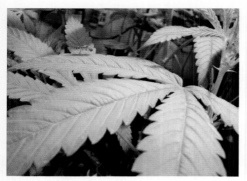
Beneficial wasp hunting for prey

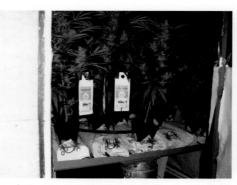
Beneficial insects being released

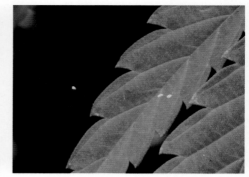
Lacewing eggs on a long stock (MF)

Queen Anne's lace, angelica, fennel, yarrow, sunflowers, coneflowers, daisies, cosmos, lavender, goldenrod, hyssop, evening primrose, and buttercups.

Release as many predators and parasites as possible if you have an infestation. This will get the problem under control quickly. Remember, the good bugs need to outnumber the bad bugs. Predators and parasites outbreed their victims, reproducing faster than pests are able to keep up with.
Stop using all-toxic chemicals at least two weeks before introducing predators to the garden. You can apply pyrethrum and insecticidal soaps up to four days before, but all residues must be washed off with water. No spraying whatsoever after predators and parasites are released.

Sterilize garden rooms and greenhouses between crops for best results. Perpetual crops are perfect for predators because they can live from one crop to the next. Nonflying predators fare best in garden rooms that have an HID; ladybird beetles fly into the lamp and die in a few days.

Do not use "zapper" lights to electrocute insects. Although perhaps amusing to watch, these death trap lamps kill more beneficial insects than pest insects!

It takes a bit of time and patience to introduce predators to the garden, and they need a consistent climate. Once established, predators and parasites will keep problem insects and mites under control.

There are some outstanding commercial sites that sell beneficial insects and controls. I debated whether or not to include a large descriptive section on beneficials and decided to make a quick overview of attracting beneficials and reference some selected commercial websites that specialize in beneficial controls for indoor and greenhouse growers.

Check these websites for more information on beneficial insects:
Nature's Control:
www.naturescontrol.com
Koppert Biological Systems:
www.koppert.nl/english
Arbico Organics:
www.arbico-organics.com
Growquest: www.growquest.com

Predators and parasites are shipped special delivery—usually next day air. Always open the package as soon as it arrives. Do not let predators sit in a sun-baked mailbox. High temperatures will kill the little predators and parasites.

Distribute eggs and insects and integrate them into the garden. Monitor their progress and keep them alive until they get ahead of pest insects and mites. The pests gradually disappear, and the beneficials take over. Overall, beneficials are more active in slightly humid environments.

Green and Brown Lacewings
Lacewings lay their eggs at the end of long stalks, probably to protect them from ants and other lacewing larvae. The larvae of both green and brown lacewings are alligator-like with sickle-shaped mandibles. Adult green

lacewings are approximately 0.75 inches (19 mm) long and pale green, with large copper-colored eyes. They are attracted to lights at night, and can produce a noxious odor when handled. Brown lacewing adults are tan or brown and about half the size of green lacewing adults.

Green lacewing larvae (aka aphid lions) attack and consume large numbers of aphids, mites, lace bugs, and other small insects. Pollen, nectar, and even honeydew sustain the generally more passive adults.

Spiders
Spiders, including the green lynx, have no antennae. They have two body parts, eight legs, eyes, mouth, and an abdomen, which contains the digestive organs, genitals, and spinnerets. More than 3,000 species reside in North America. Most spiders have venom glands but rarely bite people. Brown recluse and black widow spiders and a few others bites can be fatal to humans.

Spiders are the most abundant group of predators found in gardens. They feed on insects typically caught in a web. Jumping spiders and wolf spiders are active hunters. Crab spiders ambush their prey.

There is a long list of predators below that you may find in your outdoor garden. Attract predators by gardening organically. Avoid using pesticides or fungicides. Spot spray if necessary.

praying mantis (*Tenodera sinensis*)
big-eyed bugs

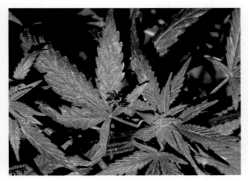
Spider on the prowl for prey

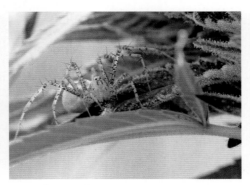
Green lynx spider (MF)

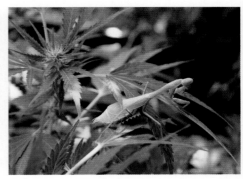
Praying mantis eats all insects and mites (MF)

dustwings

fly parasites (mixed species)

fungus gnat predators (*Hypoaspis* sp.)

green and brown lacewings

ground beetles

hover flies (syrphid flies or flower flies)

lady beetles, ladybird beetles (ladybugs)

mealybug destroyers (*Cryptolaemus montrouzieri*)

minute pirate bugs

parasitic flies

parasitic wasps (*Trichogramma* wasp)

pirate bugs (*Orius* sp.)

predaceous stink bugs

predatory nematodes "Double-Death Mix" (*Steinernema / Heterorhabditis* mix)

predatory spider mites, *Neoseiulus (Amblyseius) californicus, Mesoseiulus (Phytoseiulus) longipes, Phytoseiulus persimilis, Neoseiulus (Amblyseius) fallacius, Galendromus (Metaseiulus) occidentalis*, and *Galendromus (Typhlodromus)* pyri

predatory wasps, Ichneumonoidea wasp

soldier beetles

spider mite destroyers (*Stethorus punctillium*)

tachinid flies

thrips predator mites (*Amblyseius cucumeris*)

whitefly parasites (*Encarsia formosa*)

whitefly predators (*Delphastus pusillus*)

Frogs and Toads

Frogs and toads eat insects and slugs. The frogs will need a water source, while toads are more terrestrial. Large snakes in the garden will eat gophers, squirrels, and mice as well as moles and shrews. Snakes can give you a good scare if you come across one unexpectedly! The snake will also want to eat your frogs. Plan carefully before committing to any mini predator to solve pest infestations.

Frogs, toads, snakes, and other reptiles are extremely sensitive to pesticides, fungicides, and other chemicals. To attract these beneficials, avoid using chemicals and minimize all control sprays the garden.

Troubleshooting

Simple troubleshooting will solve 90 percent of the problems encountered when growing cannabis. The first, keep the growing area clean all the time. Remove all trash and dead foliage on growing medium and in the garden. They are the source of contamination and provide habitat for interlopers.

Is the problem cultural or caused by diseases or pests. Normally cultural problems lead to disease and pest issues. If there is a cultural problem, you can check the symptoms and examples in chapter 21, *Diseases & Pests*, "Common 'Nutrient' Problems."

The disease or pest should be identified. In many cases insects in the garden are beneficial. Once diseases start causing plant damage they become a problem. Look for plant damage carefully. Check foliage for damage, check stems and soil for damage and strange growth. Take a close up photo of the disease or pest and compare it to the images in this chapter for a match. Find the closest match and

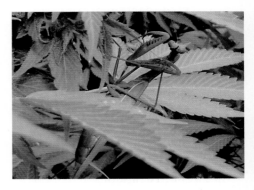

follow control measures outlined in this chapter.

Less disease and pest damaged is suffered when plants are healthy. Diseases and pests always attack weak plants. Check slow-growing plants extra for problems.

Set out yellow and blue sticky traps to monitor flying insect populations.

Most problems occur after plants are two months old.

Always use the least toxic means of control first.

Unexplained Problems
Abiotic diseases

Diseases from abiotic (nonliving) causes often arise suddenly. They usually resemble diseases caused by living organisms. Plants that suffer stress are more susceptible to diseases and pests. Nutrient deficiencies are also a major problem.

Pollutants take their toll. Sulfur dioxide, for example, can cause interveinal leaf chlorosis. Hydrogen fluoride causes chlorosis. Ozone and other air pollutants, nitrous oxides, and so forth all do great damage.

Sprays and Spraying

Spreader-Stickers

Many products already contain a surfactant, surface-active substance (adjuvant), which enhances the effectiveness of foliar fertilization.

Spreaders (wetting agents) reduce the surface tension of sprays and keep them from beading up and rolling off the foliage. Big, bulbous drops on leaves mean you need to use a spreader. Flat drops that slide off the foliage mean there is too much spreader. There are nonionic, anionic, and cationic spreaders. The nonionic spreaders that do not ionize in water are the most common, and they do not react with most pesticides. Anionic and cationic spreaders are not used often.

Stickers are designed to help spray adhere to the leaf, so it does not wash off when it rains or when dew forms. But research proves that direct laminal translocation (through the surface or cuticle of the leaf [lamina]) is the only option. Stickers also have the ability to seal off stomata—not a good idea. They also slow evaporation and impart a waterproof coating. Some stickers are spreaders, too. Organic stickers include yucca extract, fish oil, fatty acid soaps, and emulsified soybean oil.

Extenders (stabilizing agents) protect applied sprays against the UV radiation and heat that degrade sprays. But the nutrient will only move in as long as it is in solution. The amount of time under normal conditions would make the use of extenders pointless, as it will take longer to affect the nutrients by UV than the water will (or should) remain on the leaf.

Liquid soaps make an excellent spreader or water tension breaker (surfactant). I use Ivory or Castille liquid soap at the rate of 2 drops per gallon (3.8 L) and it works perfectly. No need to spend extra money on commercial products! Use only natural soaps with no weird additives. Professional greenhouse commercial growers use Tween 80 because it does not react with other elements in solution.

Application

1. Spray foliage with a fine mist, and do not create droplets on the leaves. Fine mist is electrically attracted by the foliage. Even young cannabis plants have waxy hairs that impair liquid penetration.

2. Do not spray plants that are hot or when the atmosphere is too dry. Spray in low light, either before the lights go off or just as they are coming on. If spraying in hot conditions, first spray everything with plain water until the temperatures of the room and foliage drop, before applying the real spray. Spraying when the plant foliage is hot causes the spray to crystallize on the surface, which stops the penetration. Spraying with water ten minutes afterward often increases the penetration. Mobile nutrients move freely within a plant. Immobile nutrients move slowly, but once deposited, they stay.

3. Apply mobile nutrients sparingly. Immobile nutrients—sulfur, boron, copper, iron, manganese, molybdenum, sulfur, and zinc—often require two or three applications. Calcium and boron are poor candidates for foliar feeding because they translocate poorly. But urea nitrogen applied as a spray in high humidity penetrates almost instantly into leaves. Be careful when spraying urea-based fertilizers, and keep them diluted. Urea also carries other nutrients into the plant and works well for a base to the mix. Foliar feeding should turn the plant around in less than a week. A second spray could be necessary at week's end to ensure that the cure sticks.

4. Boron, calcium, and iron move slowly during flowering. A sup-

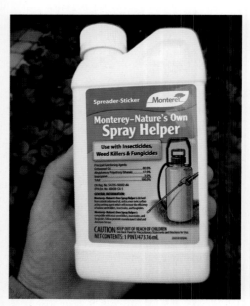

Spreader-stickers help keep sprays in place so they are effective.

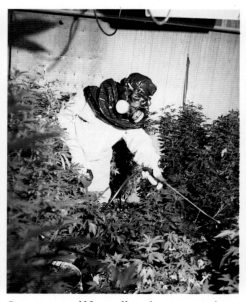

Protect yourself from all garden sprays indoors and outdoors.

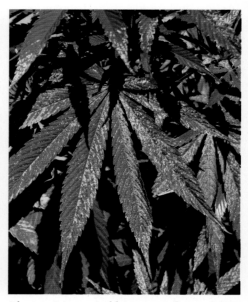

Phytotoxicity caused by spray on leaves (MF)

plemental foliar dose often speeds growth when it slows. A foliar spray of potassium can also help flowering, especially if the temperatures dip below 50°F (10°C) or above 80°F (26.7°C).

5. Always spray new growth. The thin, waxy layer and a few trichomes allow for good penetration.

6. Measure the pH of the spray, and keep it between 7.0 and 8.5. Potassium phosphate (K2HPO4) becomes phytotoxic below pH 4.0 and above 8.5. Stomata are signaled to close within these pH ranges.

7. Use a surfactant with all sprays, and apply these as per the instructions on the label. Add the proper amount of surfactant so droplets do not form on the leaves. Once formed, droplets roll off the foliage, rendering the spray ineffective.

8. Stop the application before droplets form on the leaves. Make a test spray on a mirror to ensure that the spray is even and does not form droplets that roll off the mirror.

Fungicide and Pesticide Application Basics

Use only contact sprays approved for edible fruits and vegetables.

Warning: DO NOT USE TOXIC SYSTEMIC CHEMICALS! Read the entire label on all sprays. The toxic or active life of the spray is listed on the label. Wait twice as long as the label recommends, and thoroughly wash any foliage before ingesting it. Toxic life is many times longer indoors, because sunlight and other natural forces are not able to break down chemicals.

Sprays are beneficial if not overdone. Every time a plant is sprayed, the stomata are clogged and growth slows. At 24 to 28 hours after spraying, rinse leaves on both sides with plain water until it drips from leaves. Avoid sprays that leave a residual during the weeks before harvest. Spraying increases chances of gray (bud) mold once dense buds form.

Phytotoxicity is the injury to plants caused by sprays. Symptoms include burned leaves, slow growth, or sudden wilt. Spray a test plant and wait a few days to see if spray is phytotoxic. Water plants before spraying. Phytotoxicity is diminished when more liquid is in foliage.

Temperatures above 68°F (20°C) make virtually all sprays, even organic ones, phytotoxic and damaging to foliage.

Intense light causes leaves to take in the chemicals too quickly and will often cause leaf damage.

Spray early in the day so ingredients are absorbed and foliage dries. Spraying two hours or less before lights-out can cause foliar fungus when water sits on leaves for too long.

Do not mix two products. It could change the characteristics of both.

Warm temperatures mean spraying twice as often, because bugs breed twice as fast.

Use a clean, accurate measuring cup or spoon. Measure quantities carefully!

Mix pesticides and fungicides just before using them, and safely dispose of leftovers.

With soil active sprays (sprays that leave an active residue in soil), precautions should be taken to avoid overapplication. Spray applications require more attention to detail, because overspray material lands or drips onto the medium.

Remember that dosage equals concentration times volume (dose = concentration × volume).

Spray equipment: To assure proper spray volumes, your compressed air sprayer should be equipped with a pressure gauge and regulator. Your sprayer should be calibrated by determining the output of the chemical with the selected

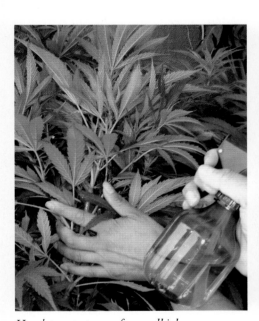

Hand-pump sprayer for small jobs

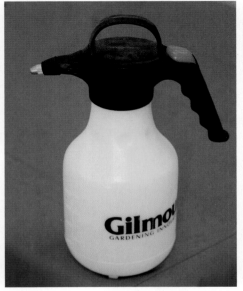

Pump-up hand sprayer for small gardens

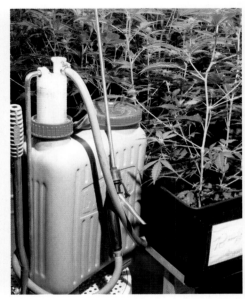

Pump-up sprayer for large gardens

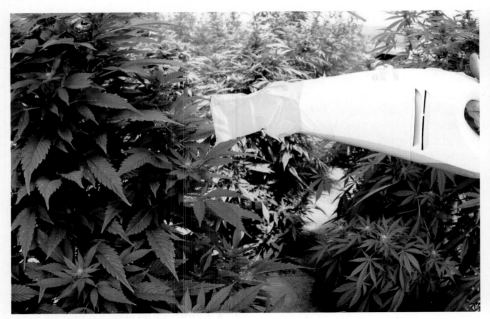

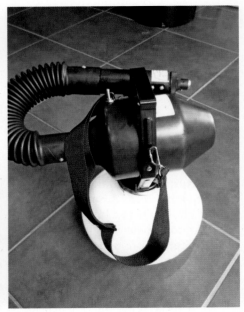

Hand fogger for powders.

Electric fogger for larger gardens

nozzle at the selected pressure within a specified time period. Using this information, you can apply a known amount of material to a known area. Spray droplet size also affects response, with smaller droplet sizes providing better coverage, but only up to a point. Many mist or fog type applicators do not provide adequate volume for coverage of plant stems and have not been effective when used with compounds like Bonzi*. Dramm makes one of the best application systems that is a cold fogger, but be advised that vapor applications such as thermal are also extremely effective and dangerous.

*Caution: DO NOT USE Bonzi on cannabis! Anyone doing so deserves to be arrested and jailed. And I mean any product (Dutch Master) that is sold to this industry is the same—deadly and persistent for years in the plant.

Sprenches are high volume foliar sprays that result in runoff into the media, providing a drench effect. Concentration levels are lower than those recommended for sprays.

Powder applicators require a little more skill to use. The powder is dispersed in a fog around plants so that it adheres to foliage. Powder applicators work best when there is no wind and there is plenty of room around plants to use the device. Always wear a protective mask, goggles, and gloves because the powder tends to go everywhere.

Soil drenches are easier to apply uniformly than sprays because the drench volume is easily measured, and when applied to moist media, it is easy to obtain good distribution in the media. In general, apply four ounces of drench solution to

a six-inch "azalea" pot, and that volume is adjusted up or down with pot size to obtain a volume where about 10 percent of the solution runs out the bottom of the pot when the media is moist.

Chemigation or application through the irrigation system: In flood (subirrigation) or drip irrigation, the nutrient, additive, or organic agent can be added to the nutrient tank like a water-soluble fertilizer. This process is also called "watering in." Many products are recommended to be injected into the irrigation water and can often be applied at very low rates of active ingredient when irrigating.

25
BREEDING

CASUAL AND SERIOUS cannabis breeders working with Mother Nature use selective breeding have transformed a wild plant into countless varieties of medicinal cannabis. New varieties are easy, fun, and satisfying to create. Home cannabis gardeners breed plants for many reasons—to increase yield, cannabinoid profile, disease and pest resistance, and so forth. Most often, modern medicinal cannabis has been bred for high cannabinoid content (specifically THC), for heavy yield, for early harvest indoors, and occasionally for harsh outdoor climates. Today, more attention is being given to other cannabinoids, such as CBD, and cultivation stress—resistance to diseases and pests and tolerance of drought and cold.

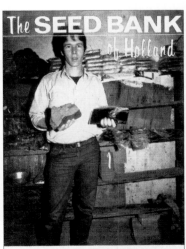

This photo was taken on one of my seed hunting expeditions at the Phyber Pass. This Mazari I Sharif hash is top grade.

Countless cannabis gardeners are patiently applying their imagination and creativity using basic breeding (sexual propagation) techniques to create new generations of seed. Breeding is easy, low-cost, fun, and exciting. It requires minimal time and skill but results in big rewards.

Nevil, founder of the Seed Bank of Holland, traveled the world to find the best cannabis seeds.

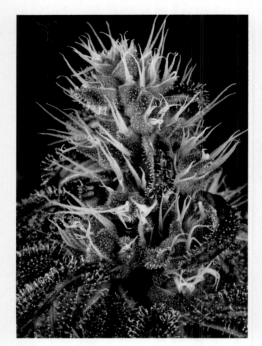

This colorful 'Pakistan Chitral Kush' from CannaBioGen is a pure landrace line from Chitral, Pakistan. It is also on the cover of this book!

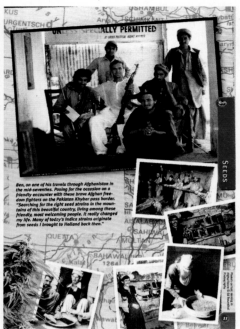

Seated in the center in white, Sensi Seeds owner Ben Dronkers is pictured collecting seeds in Afghanistan.

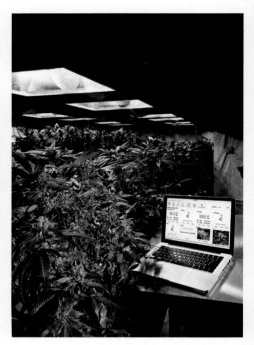

The Internet has changed the availability of genetics (seeds) worldwide.

The basics outlined in this chapter show any gardener how to start breeding and create new generations of viable medicinal cannabis seeds. Indoor, backyard, and greenhouse breeding is essential to acclimate varieties to local climates and to increase resistance to diseases, pests, and stress. Indoor and greenhouse cultivation can expedite outdoor breeding programs. Unfortunately, medical cannabis seeds are not available in some jurisdictions, and indoor breeding is a matter of necessity for patients and caregivers.

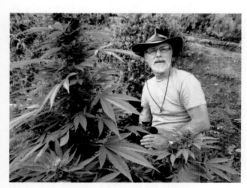

To date, much of the cannabis breeding in the USA has been done by clandestine breeders such as Mel Frank, who introduced varieties such as 'Afghani', 'Nepalese', and 'Mexican', as well as many Colombian varieties.

On the surface, breeding is simple: pollen from a male plant is used to fertilize (pollinate) a female plant, and seeds result. In fact, this is what most cannabis crosses are based upon—crossing a cannabinoid-potent male with a cannabinoid-potent female plant, often referred to as "pollen chucking." However, a few important genetic details are involved.

Crossing cannabis plants can become very complex, and plants take time to grow to express their genes. Modern plant breeders study statistics, chemistry, plant physiology, microbiology, and other disciplines to understand and breed plants. The basic information presented here is in an easy-to-understand format so it is as straightforward to reference as possible. Cannabis breeding is a long-term process, and the possible outcomes of progeny are infinite.

Much more scientific information about plant breeding is available on the Internet, including modern genetic principles by Gregor Mendel and inspiring stories from American breeders such as Luther Burbank. Be sure to read about Dr. Kevin McKernan, who mapped the cannabis genome!

Please continue studying after you have digested this basic chapter. Remember, breeding cannabis is a long-term endeavor—even in an indoor garden room where four generations are possible.

The cannabis world today consists of millions of small gardeners in more than 200 countries around the world*. Many gardens exist in unstable and difficult growing conditions. Adopting new cannabis varieties developed for cultivation in faraway climates and indoor grow rooms does not meet the needs of many outdoor gardeners and their local

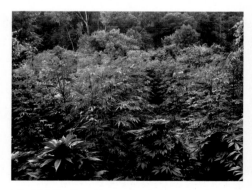

The 'Afghani' × 'Congolese' plants in the foreground are the product of selective breeding. The miscellaneous sativa plants in the background represent wild cannabis plants. (MF)

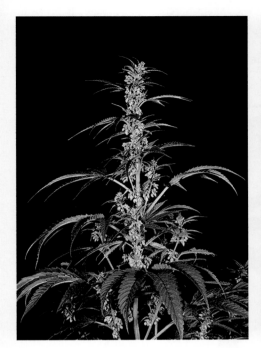

Choosing the proper male breeding stock is half of the equation. Choose the best males possible that exhibit the desirable traits you want.

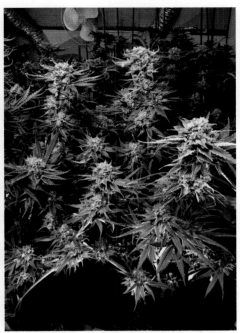

This beautiful garden of 'Sonoma Coma' females is the result of years of selective breeding in a valley full of vineyards in California.

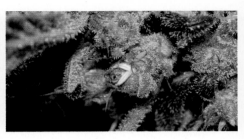

Individual male flowers that appear on a female flower bud are often called "bananas" because they look like little bananas.

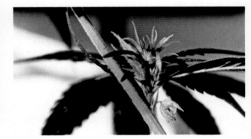

This 'African' grown in 1977 has a small male flower on this predominately female flower bud. This is an intersex male flower.

climates. The Internet* and cannabis gardeners' ingenuity have broken ground for gardeners everywhere to participate in the breeding process. Breeding goals can now be identified and defined by local gardeners instead of large seed companies or fad-driven advertising.

*For example, the following YouTube video has received more than 5 million hits from more than 180 countries: www.youtube.com/user/jorgecervantesmj.

Most gardeners prefer to acquire seeds from a reputable seed company, and too often assume they these seeds are consistently of the highest genetic quality. Often, commercially available seeds are produced by a few large seed makers who wholesale to resellers, many of them with Internet sites and retail store outlets. Other seeds are produced by basement growers, small startups, or small- to medium-sized established companies.

Few small companies can maintain a library of true-breeding stock and breed stable parent stock over time. Stock produced by large companies usually fills demand and maintains standards.

Unforgettable Qualities of Cannabis

Cannabis has a unique set of qualities that influence its life cycle and reproduction. Working with these natural qualities is essential to breeding cannabis. Please remember them when working on all breeding projects.

Cannabis is **photoperiodic reactive**, flowering under 12 hours of uninterrupted darkness and 12 hours of light, which gives breeders the ability to grow up to 6 crops every year. These characteristics facilitate fast-track breeding because 6 years of crosses can be completed in 1 year.

Cannabis is **dioecious**; it produces each of the male (staminate; stamen bearing) and female (pistillate; pistil bearing) sexual organs on different individuals, and it is one of the few annual dioecious plants. This quality makes it very easy to cross an individual male cannabis plant with an individual or population of females.

Male (staminate) and female (pistillate) plants are easy to distinguish. See close-up details of male and female flowers

along with full descriptions below in this chapter.

Monoecious varieties produce both staminate and pistillate flowers on the same plant. Monoecious varieties are mainly used for hemp seed production. Monoecious varieties do not make good medical cannabis breeding stock. Plants with both male and female flowers are often called by the misnomer "hermaphrodite."

Outcrossing plant: Outcrossing cannabis grows best when plants cross with other plants with different genes. Corn, dogs, cannabis, and people are all outcrossers. Backcrossing and inbreeding cannabis for too many generations will be detrimental.

Intersexuality occurs when flowers of a male plant grow on a predominantly female plant, or when female flowers grow on a predominately male plant. It is a trait that can be caused by both genetic and environmental factors. Intersex plants with the inherited gene grow flowers from both sexes on the same plant even in perfect growing conditions. Intersex plants are often called by the misnomer "hermaphrodite."

Indoors, plants are easily exposed to stress—inconsistent or extreme temperature, light cycles, fertilizer, pH, etc.—and this stress can cause female plants to grow an occasional male flower. Breeders prefer not to perpetuate the intersex gene, and when possible they eliminate it. A single male flower on a female plant can pollinate a big part of the female. See "Feminized Seeds," on page 521.

Physiology of Male and Female Flowers

Male Flowers

Male (staminate) cannabis flowers are about 0.25 to 0.5 inches (0.6–1.3 cm) long, and thousands of individual flowers can develop on a large plant. Most of the flowers develop in loose clusters (*cymes* or *cymose panicles*) of about 5 or 10 flowers each, borne on tiny branches and their side (lateral) branches. The clusters can pile atop each other to form dense aggregates of hundreds of individual flowers, particularly at the ends of stems and branches.

Each male flower's calyx consists of 5 tepals (sometimes identified as "sepals")—usually white, yellowish or greenish, but often tinged purple—that might be described as "petals," and 5 pendulous stamens that bear pollen in sacks called anthers. Anthers hang by a thin, threadlike filament and together, filament and anther make up the stamen. Once mature, 2 openings on opposite sides of each anther open zipper-like, starting at their base, to slowly release their pollen into the wind, carrying it (hopefully) to stigmas. It has been estimated that the thousands of flowers on a single male can release more than 500 million pollen grains.

Unopened male flower clusters remind some growers of tiny grape clusters, and fresh anthers look somewhat like bunches of tiny bananas. Male flowers are simply called male flowers or male flower clusters, and the pollen holders are referred to as either stamens or anthers.

Female Flowers

Each female marijuana flower has 2 stigmas that protrude from the single ovule enclosed in the bracts; fresh stigmas are "fuzzy" (hirsute), about

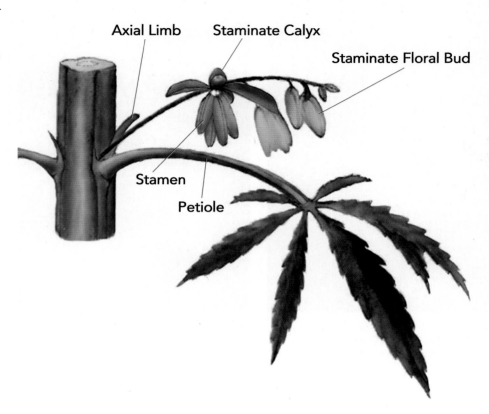

This drawing shows the main parts of a male cannabis plant.

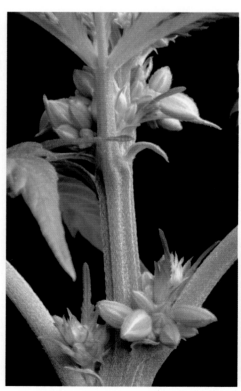

'Jack Herer' male (staminate) flowers fully formed in clusters but not yet open. (MF)

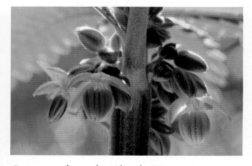

Outer tepals on the 'Skunk #1' staminate calyxes have separated, exposing the pollen-containing anthers. (MF)

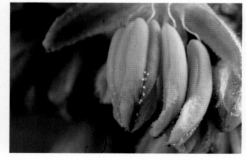

As anthers on this 'Jack Herer' mature, they rupture to disperse superfine grains of pollen into the air. (MF)

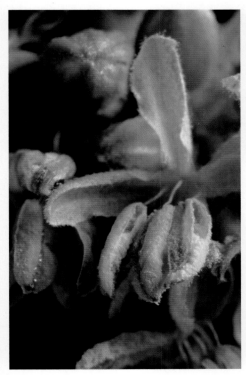

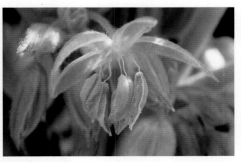

Anthers hang in the wind after dispersing all their pollen throughout several days. (MF)

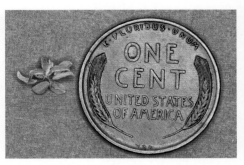

Compare this tiny male flower to the size of a US penny. (MF)

Staminate anthers on this 'Skunk #1' grown in 1987 continue to split open and disperse more and more pollen into the air. (MF)

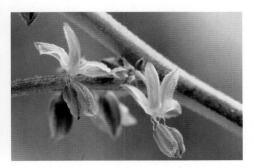

Pollen from this 'Skunk #1' has been dispersed from anthers in the foreground. Staminate calyxes in the background will disperse pollen in the near future. (MF)

0.25 to 0.5 inches (0.6–1.3 cm) long, and usually white, but sometimes they are yellowish or pink to red, and, rarely, lavender to purple. Stigmas (*stigmata* is another botanical plural) are the pollen catchers. Stigmas are often misidentified as pistils. By definition, a pistil is all of the reproductive parts of a flower—2 stigmas and an ovule make up the female pistil. Each flower then has only 1 pistil but has 2 stigmas. The term is misused in much of popular culture, which describes a single cannabis flower as having 2 pistils.

Stigmas begin dying after pollination and begin to turn rust-colored about 3 days later; if not pollinated, as with sinsemilla (seedless buds), stigmas begin to die when they are about 4 or 5 weeks old. Upon landing on a stigma, a pollen grain germinates and begins to grow a pollen tube through the style passage-way to pass its DNA to join the ovule's DNA (the 2 stigmas of each female flower make up a **bifid** style). The fertilized ovule becomes a fruit, essentially a single seed (an achene). The perianth, which includes the calyx, tightly clasps the seed and often contains tannins, which give mature seeds their mottled or spotted coat. Between a thumb and finger you can rub the perianth off of seeds. A well-pollinated single bud develops dozens of seeds, a cola easily holds many hundreds, and even a small, but thoroughly pollinated female can bear thousands of seeds.

Cannabis female flowers do have a calyx, but it is barely perceptible even with a microscope. The female calyx is one part of the perianth, a nearly trans-parent, delicate tissue that partially encloses the ovule, or prospective seed.

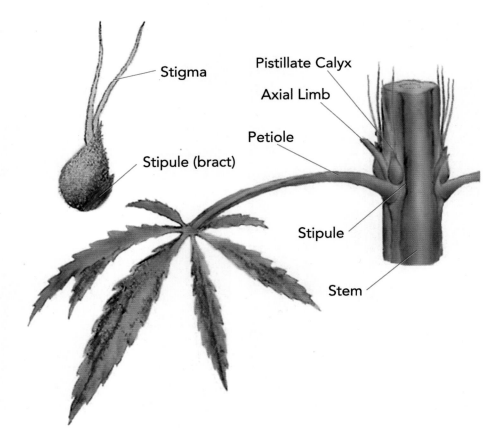

This drawing shows the main parts of a female cannabis plant.

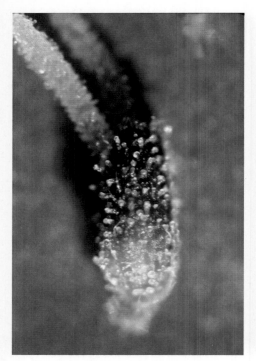

The seed bract still covers the perianth, pistillate calyx, gametes, and ovule connected to a pair of stigmas. (MF)

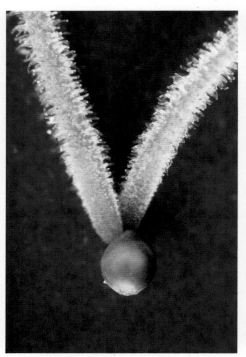

The seed bract has been stripped away to reveal the perianth and pistillate calyx, both of which appear transparent, covering the gametes and ovule. Note the white stigmas have not been pollinated. (MF)

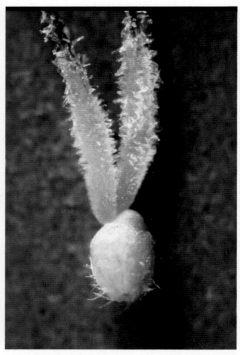

Stigmas start dying back as soon as pollen is ushered down the shaft to unite with the ovule below. (MF)

Each female flower has a single ovule partially enclosed in its perianth, which is encapsulated by bracteoles, which are covered by a whorl of bracts. The bracts and bracteoles are small, modified leaves that enclose and protect the seed in what some growers refer to as the seedpod. Bracts contain the highest concentration of THC and other cannabinoids of any plant part and about 50 percent of a plant's total THC. The perianth and its calyx contain no THC.

By definition, a perianth consists of a corolla and a calyx. In more familiar showy flowers, the corolla is the brightly colored petals we generally appreciate when looking at flowers, and the calyx is the smaller green cup (sepals) at the flower's base. Bright showy colors, large flower sizes, and enticing fragrances have naturally evolved to attract insects such as bees and flies, or animals such as birds and bats that collect and transfer pollen (unintentionally) to other flowers. Cannabis flowers are not brightly colored, large, or enticingly fragrant (at least to most nonhumans); cannabis plants are wind-pollinated with no need to attract insects or animals to carry

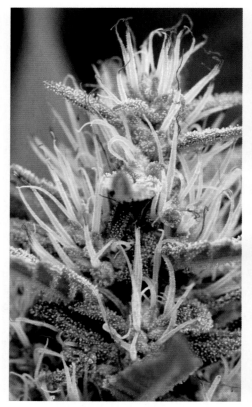

The stigmas on this 'Haze' × 'Northern Lights' × 'Sensi Star' flower top are just starting to turn a rusty color. (MF)

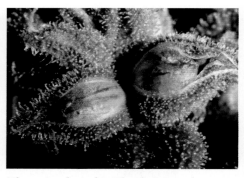

The perianth on this 'Skunk #1' can be seen near the top of the seed on the left. (MF)

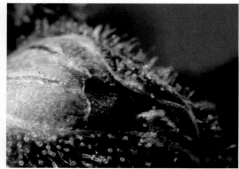

The female perianth is clearly visible as a nearly transparent layer covering the seed. (MF)

males' pollen to female flowers; cannabis plant parts never naturally evolved into colorful, attractive, or showy parts. Cannabis breeders, though, do breed for fragrance and color once cannabinoid content is firmly established.

The cannabis perianth is only about 6 cells thick, so to distinguish calyx cells from corolla cells is best left to botanists. This book uses the botanically correct term *bracts* for the green or purple, resin-gland-studded specialized "leaves" encasing each female flower, and uses *perianth* or *calyx* for the translucent "veil" that clasps and covers about 60 to 90 percent of a mature seed.

Hopefully, when growers use botanical terms such as *calyx, bracts, stigma, pistil, anther* and *stamen*, they will follow this book and use the terms correctly. Since readers will find seed catalogs and Internet sites calling bracts *calyxes* and stigmas *pistils*, it is important for readers to understand this confusion when reading other sources. Hopefully, this chapter will help get us all on the same page.

Sexual Propagation

Sexual propagation is the process in which male and female sex cells (gametes) from separate parents unite in the female plant to form what will eventually mature into a new, genetically distinct individual. This process occurs when pollen from a male (staminate) parent unites with an ovule within the ovary of a female flower to create an embryo. This embryo, when mature and fully developed, will become a seed.

In nature, cannabis is wind-pollinated. Male flowers shed pollen (dehiscence), dispersing millions of grains into the wind. Wind carries the pollen to a "chance" rendezvous and acceptance by a female stigma.

Pollination occurs when male pollen grains land on a female stigma. The evolutionary attraction is both physical and chemical. The grain of pollen, with moisture found in the stigma, germinates. This is the best part: A grain of pollen germinates just like a seed, sending a taproot down, but instead of sending it into the ground, the grain of

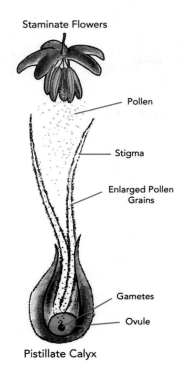

Staminate Flowers

Pollen

Stigma

Enlarged Pollen Grains

Gametes

Ovule

Pistillate Calyx

pollen sends the "root" down the stigma toward the ovary. Once united with the ovary, the pollen fertilizes the ovule. This union creates an embryo that grows within a seed coat. When mature in 4 to 6 weeks, the seed can be planted.

Fertilization occurs when the tiny grain of male pollen sticks to the stigma. Then it develops a tube through the style, and releases 2 gametes, 1 to fertilize the ovule and 1 to fertilize the endosperm (double fertilization). Seeds are the result of this sexual propagation and contain genetic characteristics of both parents. Once fertilized with male pollen, female plants put the bulk of their energy into producing strong, viable seeds.

Actual fertilization takes place when the minute grain of male pollen sticks to the stigma. The successful angiosperm pollen grain (gametophyte) containing the male gametes (sperm) gets transported to the stigma, where it germinates and its pollen tube grows down the style to the ovary. Its 2 gametes travel down the tube to where the gametophyte(s) containing the female gametes are held within the carpel. One nucleus fuses with the polar bodies to produce the endosperm tissues, and the other with the ovum to produce the embryo hence the term *double fertilization*.

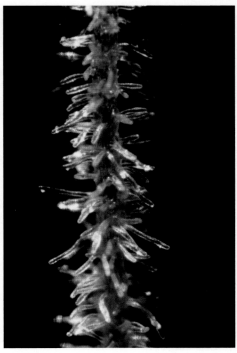

(MF)
Close-up photo of a female stigma shows that no resin glands are located on the entire length. The well-defined protruding growth appears as fuzz on the stalk of the stigma. The stigma is the plant version of a vagina. It is covered with stigmatic fluid that acts like glue when a piece of pollen lands on it. The fluid is packed with sugars that are food for the pollen. When in place, the grains of pollen start growing a new "pollen tube," a long tunnel that pushes through the tissue of the style all the way to the ova, where it fuses with egg cells to create a little baby plant. The ovules go through a series of steps known as meiosis, a type of cell division by which a cell duplicates into 2 genetically identical daughter cells. The chromosomes in the cell nucleus separate into 2 matching sets of chromosomes, each with a nucleus.

Deoxyribonucleic acid (DNA) or "genetic material"* is coiled into long strands or chromosomes. The DNA is located inside the nucleus of each cell. When cannabis is pollinated, each individual seed inherits 10 different chromosomes from the male, and 10 different chromosomes from the seed mother—20 chromosomes total. Each seed has 2 copies of each of the 10 chromosomes, or 1 full genome each. There are 2 copies of every gene in the plant, 1 from the

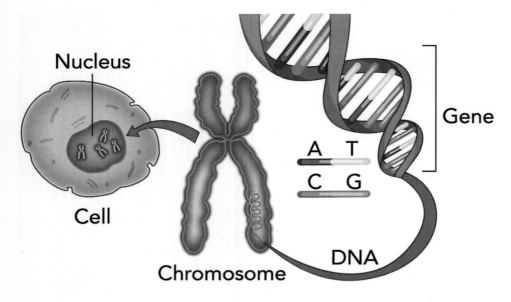

Nucleus

Cell

Chromosome

Gene

A T
C G

DNA

mother and 1 from the father. Every cell in the plant has a copy of this unique DNA. The genetic code of this unique individual is embedded in a specific location along the length of the chromosome strands.

Each seed contains genes from both parents. Progeny grown from seed usually have slightly different traits than other plants from the same seed lot. The same happens in humans; biological children are different from one another in many aspects and at the same time they resemble their parents. In cannabis, the variability is marked, like it is in apples.

Sexual reproduction is used to cross different individuals with a population or family of plants. It can also be used to hybridize unrelated lines and inbreed their offspring. This phenomenon, "recombination of traits," also gives breeders the opportunity to recover individuals with a combination of the positive traits of both parental lines.

Genes are hereditary units that consist of a sequence of DNA that resides in a precise place on a chromosome and it determines a specific trait in cannabis. Little bits of DNA are codes or templates for proteins.

* Proteins are made in the sequence of DNA. Like instructions in a recipe for making brownies, the DNA and sequence of proteins is the recipe or instructions.

Having 2 versions of the same protein, from 2 different genes, is better than having just 1, particularly if the protein plays some vital part in cannabinoid production. This effect is called overdominance. For example, if there are 2 different proteins, and both work well but 1 works a little better under hot conditions and the other works well under cool conditions. Having 2 versions of the same protein gives the plant a wider range of climates where it produces effectively. See "Multiline," on page 531.

The majority of DNA is the same; it deals with basic cell processes, photosynthesis, chlorophyll production, etc. A few or a combination of genes control variables such as height, leaf shape, fragrance, and disease resistance. But we are not sure exactly which genes are responsible for specific traits, even though the cannabis genome has been mapped. These traits are influenced by multigene families (a group of genes that evolved to become a little bit different from each other, even though they started out as copies of the same gene). Knowing the **named genes** would make it easier to find individual plants with your desired traits. But single genes controlling specific traits of cannabis are neither isolated nor well studied.

Multigene traits allow you to fine-tune to your favorite characteristics. For

example, a single gene that controls leaf size would give only 2 leaf sizes, large and small. Many genes influencing the same trait provide many different leaf sizes.

Naturally occurring **mutated cannabis genes** are uncommon. They are abnormal genes that are mutations of normal genes. When a mutated gene combines with a normal gene, there is no detrimental outcome. But when 2 mutated genes join, the result is much different.

For example, in people and animals the number of albinos or dwarfs is minimal. The same is true in cannabis. Growing large populations of cannabis or treating cannabis with stress or chemicals will bring about mutation. Overall, most cannabis plants grow normally with no mutations whatsoever. Many different genes control the desirable traits we care about. Broken recessive genes do not play a role in most breeding programs.

Deleterious recessive genes: The plants most likely to have the same dangerous mutation in the immediate family are inbred. Marry your sister and inbreeding genes take over to start all kinds of problems because recessive deleterious genes appear.

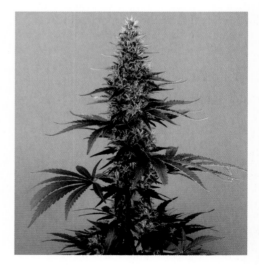

'Royal Moby', *predominately* sativa, *is very THC-potent. This variety is quite similar to 'Moby Dick' from Dinafem Seeds in Spain. Once a good variety reaches the marketplace, many similar varieties appear within a year or two.*

Classical Cannabis Breeding

Classical breeding is an ancient cyclical process that cannabis breeders still use today. Decisions are made based on observation of large numbers of plants; the breeder does not know exactly what genes have been introduced to the new cultivars. All the breeder can do is choose plants based upon visual inspection, smell, and gut-feeling.

Classical cannabis breeding is simple: 2 varieties, a male and a female, are chosen. Each parent has desirable characteristic—fragrance, potency, mold resistance, and so forth. The male pollen fertilizes the female flower and their genes combine into a new genetic mix contained in the seed.

The next step is to choose individual plants with the desirable traits of both parents. A lot of the time you get lucky and the offspring carry the desirable genes and traits. Cannabis breeders often take clones of these desirable individual plants. Too often they do not retain the male plant and have a "clone only" variety.

When a desirable trait has been bred into a plant, crossing other plants to this parent makes new plants similar to the favored parent. For example, to make the mildew-resistant progeny of the cross most like the high-yielding parent, the progeny will be backcrossed to that parent for several generations (see "Backcrossing," page 519). This process removes most of the genetic contribution of the mildew-resistant parent.

To breed for mold resistance, grow out plants in moldy conditions. Remove plants from garden that contract mold easily. Keep plants that do not get mold or are late to get mold. Breed plants that do not mold

It is very difficult to isolate specific genes to guarantee specific qualities such as extreme resistance to powdery mildew or insect and mite attacks. There are recessive genes and dominant genes that are controlled by alleles; this is where breeding becomes much more complex. See "Influence of Alleles."

Other traits, such as acclimatization to a specific climate, are relatively easy because the plants that grow best in the environment are continually selected. Organic gardeners breed plants acclimated to their outdoor climate and achieve much higher yields. For this reason, organic medical gardeners in Northern California are able to grow 10-pound (4.5 kg) plants.

To breed for cold tolerance, grow out plants in cold conditions. Remove plants that suffer cold damage easily. Breed plants that withstand cold temperatures.

Thin-Layer Chromatography

Thin-layer chromatography can be used to take tests and make selections based upon cannabinoid profiles. Cannabinoid profiles are similar throughout a plant's life stages, and breeding decisions can be based upon these profiles. For example, the cannabinoid profile can be tested on 2-month-old seedlings. Plants with desirable profiles are kept, and those with undesirable plants are culled.

See "Modern Cannabis Breeding" at the end of this chapter for an overview of marker-assisted selection (MAS).

Influence of Alleles

The phenotypes seen in a given individual are the result of an interaction between the plant's genotype and the environment. For example, here are 3 phenotypes: short, medium, and tall. Remember, the genotype describes

Phenotypes	Genotypes
short	ss
medium	Ss
tall	SS

the genetic condition responsible for the phenotype, and to represent it in discussion we assign it symbols.

There are always 2 versions of every gene (allele). For example, if there are 2 lower-case "s" plants with "small stature" the plant will be shorter. But if the plant has capital "S" and has the "tall" gene, the phenotype is tall. If both genes are inherited, the plant is medium height.

Homozygous / heterozygous: These are terms used in describing the genotypic condition of a plant, with regard to the similarity of the alleles for a given trait. If a plant is homozygous for a given trait, it has 2 copies of the same allele. If a plant is heterozygous, it has 2 different alleles for a given trait.

The offspring inherits 1 set of alleles from each parent. This inheritance of alleles can be homozygous (both alleles are the same) or heterozygous (each alleles is different). Furthermore recessive alleles do not surface completely for several generations. The influence of alleles makes it impossible to use simple mathematical probability to predict the outcome of offspring.

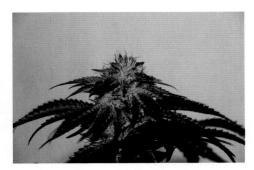

'LA Confidential' from DNA Genetics was the first Cannabis indica *variety to have its genome mapped.*

In August 2011, Dr. Kevin McKernan announced that his company had successfully mapped the genomes (shotgun sequence) for *Cannabis sativa* ('Chemdawg' variety) and later *C. indica* ('LA Confidential'). Medicinal Genomics then publicized its work on *C. sativa* via Amazon's EC2, a cloud-computing service that gives free access to the scientific community. Search "Cannabis genome EC2 cloud" on www.google.com for more information.

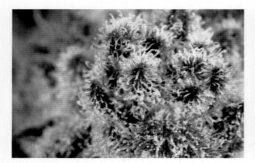

This indica-dominant 'Peyote Purple' was developed by CannaBioGen.

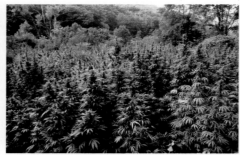

'Afghani'-dominant crosses are in the foreground and sativa-dominant crosses are in the background. (MF)

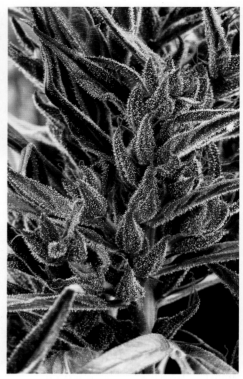

This genetically purple 'Mexican' sativa from 1980 is one of the varieties that added a purple hue to many current varieties. (MF)

Dominant and Recessive Traits

Dominant and recessive traits are dictated by alleles that are inherited from both parents. But, even though the cannabis genome has been decoded, specific gene function has not been deciphered. Consequently, the examples below must be used as guidelines because many traits are driven by a combination of genes.

Dominant: An intra-allelic interaction such that the presence of an allele of 1 parent masks the presence of an allele from another parent plant, in the expression of a given trait in the progeny. Only the dominant trait is shown in the first generation of offspring. Of the F2 generation, 75 percent will also show the dominant condition.

Recessive: An intra-allelic interaction such that an allele of 1 parent is masked by the presence of an allele from the other parent plant, in the expression of a given trait in the progeny. The recessive trait is not shown in the first generation of progeny (F1) but will reappear if siblings are mated, and the F2 progeny will result in 25 percent of plants showing the recessive condition.

Numbers Can Be Misleading

Simplistic math models are often used to explain what happens when male and female cannabis plants are crossed. These models do not take into account dominant and recessive genes, they allow nothing for genotype and phenotype, and they do not consider that specific traits may be controlled by many different genes.

Use the Punnett square to help predict the outcome.

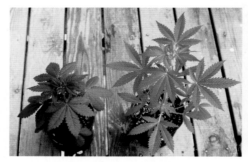

The 'Afghani' seedling on the left demonstrates the dominant traits of short, squat growth and broad leaves. The 'Kush' seedling on the right demonstrates the dominant traits of taller growth, and has much different leaf formation.

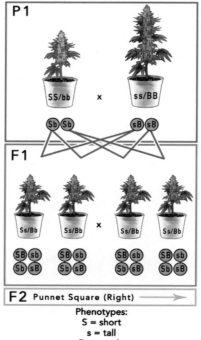

P1 SS/bb × ss/BB

F1 Ss/Bb × Ss/Bb

F2 Punnet Square (Right) →

Phenotypes:
S = short
s = tall
B = purple
b = green
Capital letter represents dominant phenotype.

P1 = original parents
F1 = first generation
F2 = second generation

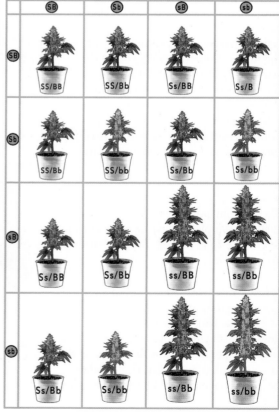

The hypothetical dihybrid cross ratio is demonstrated in the Punnett square.

We can demonstrate Mendel's Laws in a Punnett square to predict the possible outcome of 1 genetic trait (monohybrid). The example below uses Mendel's pea plant experiment. He crossed 2 yellow pea plants, and they produced 3 quarters yellow peas and 1 quarter green peas. The Punnett square accounts for all the possible combinations for 1 gene. Each of the 4 squares in the box represents 1 new offspring.

A **monohybrid** is a genetic cross between 2 parents; 1 parent has 2 dominant alleles for a specific gene and the other 2 recessives for the same gene. The offspring, monohybrids, have 1 dominant and 1 recessive allele for that gene. A cross between the offspring produces a 3:1 ratio when grown out of the following (F2) generation of dominant:recessive phenotypes.*

*This example is based on Mendel's monohybrid pea plant cross. Little information is available to the public about specific gene loci of cannabis. An excellent worksheet is available at BiologyCorner.com (www.biologycorner. com/worksheets/pennygene_key.html).

A **dihybrid** is a genetic cross between parents that have 2 characteristics controlled by genes at different loci.* The example below shows both parents AaBb and AaBb are heterozygous for both traits (color and height). The possible outcome can be predicted with the help of a Punnett square. The example below is based on Mendel's dihybrid cross with pea plants. Note the dihybrid Punnett square has 16 different possibilities. This will yield a genotype ratio of 1:2:1:2:4:2: 1:2:1 and a phenotype ratio of 9:3:3:1.

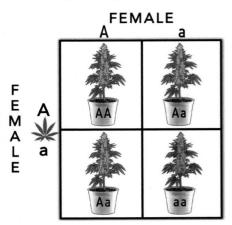

The monohybrid cross ratio is demonstrated in the Punnett square.

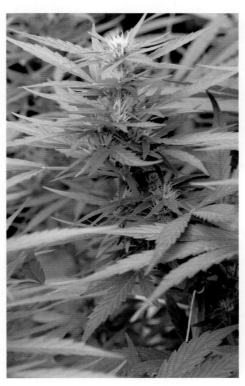

At 4 weeks of flowering, 'Big Bud' is just starting to put on weight. The genetics of 'Big Bud', from northwestern USA, are found in many of today's varieties.

This example is based on Mendel's pea plant cross, and is hypothetical because little information is available to the public about specific gene loci of cannabis.

True Breed
True-breeding (or inbred) **plants make the best breeding stock.** A true-breeding variety (aka inbred line [IBL] and true line) of cannabis is the result of a seed lot that has been bred for generations while selecting repeatedly for specific traits. These plants breed true for the specific traits—cannabinoid content, strong growth, desirable aroma and flavor, and so on. There is little or no variation of traits, growth is uniform, and the outcome of future generations is easier to predict. These plants are said to be stable.

If seed is true breeding (IBL) it should be easy to reproduce by open pollination. See "Making Seeds at Home," page 523, for a list of true-breeding seed varieties. After many generations of repetitive breeding and selecting for the same traits, other genetic traits may deteri-

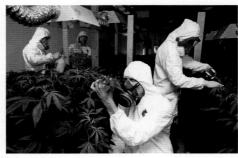

'Purple Urkle' is an Oregon 'Big Bud' hybrid.

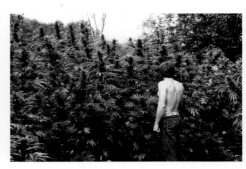

Here is a little more of Mel Frank's breeding handiwork. The cross is between 'Afghani #1' and 'Congolese' and was grown in New York in 1982. (MF)

orate. See "Inbreeding," page 518, for more information.

Hybrids
Hybrids are a product of a cross between genetically distinct parents. Hybrids do not reproduce their parent characteristics completely or reliably when reproduced sexually. Develop hybrid cultivars by using inbred (true-breeding) genetics or by segregating populations, inbreeding them, and selecting for hybrid line production. Various hybrid varieties are described below.

Hybrid Crosses
F1 hybrids ('Northern Lights' × 'Blueberry', 'Northern Lights' × 'Haze') 3-way crosses ('Skunk #1'—a cross of ('Mexican' × 'Colombian') × 'Afghani') 4-way or double cross hybrids (cross of 2 unrelated F1 hybrids 'Haze' ('Afghani' × 'Thai') × ('Mexican' × 'Colombian').

F1 Hybrid Varieties
Achieve an F1 hybrid population by crossing 2 unrelated, true-breeding varieties. F1 hybrids are uniform when

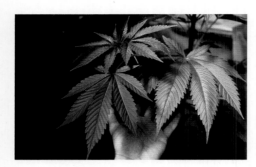

This 'Afghani #1' × 'Mexican #3' was the product of a cross made in 1981 by Mel Frank. (MF)

grown from seed, but, like all hybrids, they are genetically unstable. If reproduced sexually by inbreeding within the F1 population, the subsequent generation will be neither uniform nor similar to the F1 generation. Seeds from F1 hybrids, F2, will all be different; parents are heterozygous and diverse. They average twice as many monozygous genes and will be less vigorous. Seeds lose uniformity and hybrid vigor.

F1 hybrid vigor (heterosis) occurs when 2 true-breeding varieties are crossed. The resulting seed and plant has "hybrid vigor,"—growing more robustly, stronger, faster, and with a heavier harvest than both parents. For example, a ('Skunk#1' × 'Blueberry') F1 hybrid grows faster and yields more than either the pure 'Skunk #1' or 'Blueberry' parent populations.

F1 hybrid seeds grow into strong plants that produce well. Seed companies sell them because they keep clients coming back for more seeds every year. Few seed companies are interested in selling seed that is easy to open pollinate or easy to reproduce. Most seed companies make and release hybrids. Often "true-breeding" (IBL) seeds are not stable. Competitors in the unregulated market continually pirate seed varieties from companies that have developed the seeds.

F1 hybrid is a term used in genetics and selective breeding. *F1* stands for Filial 1, the first filial generation of seeds/plants or animals.

Maintaining strong, reliable F1 hybrid stock requires growing 2 different lines of the same parents. The 2 lines are

crossed to make seed. Deviation is minimized. This is necessary to maintain genetic diversity and avoid recessive trait domination.

For information on F2, F3, etc., generations, see "Filial Breeding," on page 520.

Cross-pollination is the transfer of pollen from an individual male cannabis flower to a stigma of the flower of a female plant. Strive to combine the best qualities of a true-breeding line with other lines to increase desired traits when using cross-pollination in cannabis breeding.

Inbreeding

Inbreeding is crossing a group, family, or variety of plants within themselves with no addition of genetic material from an outside or unrelated population. "True Breed," above, is an example of inbreeding. The most severe form of inbreeding is the self-cross (see "Self-Pollination (Selfing)" on page 520), in which only one individual's genetic material forms the basis of subsequent

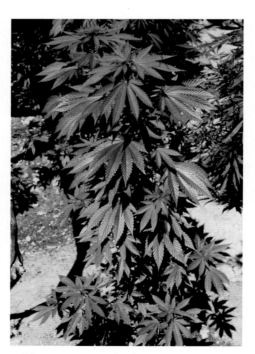

'Afghani #1' is an inbred variety that was developed over years of inbreeding among large populations of cannabis plants. This landrace variety was collected in the mountains of Afghanistan by Sacred Seeds in the 1970s. It was one of the first pure indica *true-breeding strains used in worldwide cannabis breeding programs. (MF)*

generations. And 1:1 hybrid populations are only slightly less narrow, derived from the genetic material of 2 individuals. Such tight or narrow breeding populations lead to a condition called "inbreeding depression" upon repeated self-breeding or inbreeding.

Inbreeding depression is a reduction in vigor (or any other character) due to prolonged inbreeding. This can manifest as a reduction in potency or a decrease in yield or rate of growth. Progress of depression is dependent, in part, on the breeding system of the crop.

Cannabis is an outcrossing or cross-pollinating species. Cross-pollinated cannabis exhibits a higher degree of inbreeding depression when "selfed," or inbred, than do selfing crops such as tomatoes, which can be selfed for 20 generations with no apparent loss in vigor or yield.

In cross-pollinated crops, deleterious genes remain hidden within populations, and the negative attributes of these recessive traits can be revealed when inbred several generations.

Inbreeding depression can be noticeable in S1 (see "Self-Pollinating (Selfing)," on page 520) populations after a single generation of self-fertilization. When breeding cannabis using small populations, as is often the case with continual 1:1 mating schemes, inbreeding depression typically becomes apparent within three to four generations. This 1:1 breeding model is being used today by most commercial seed banks.

Cannabis is naturally an outcrossing or cross-pollinating species and existed in wild breeding populations of hundreds if not thousands of individuals. Within these many individuals lies a wide range of versions of different genes. When only 1 or 2 plants are selected from this vast array as the breeding population, there is a drastic reduction in the genetic variability found in the original population, resulting in a genetic bottleneck. Once this variability is lost from a population, it is gone.

If space is available, overcome this problem is by maintaining 2 separate parallel breeding lines. After generations of inbreeding, when each of the inbred lines or selfed populations start showing inbreeding depression, they are hybridized or outcrossed to each other to restore vigor and eliminate inbreeding depression while preserving the genetic stability of the traits under selection.

Outbreeding

Outbreeding is the process of crossing or hybridizing plants or groups of plants with others to which there is no relation or the relationship is very distant. Any time a breeder is hybridizing using plants that reside outside of the family, group, or variety, hybrid seed is produced.

An F1 hybrid seed is the first generation offspring that results from crossing 2 distinct true-breeding plants or populations. Each of the (true-breeding) parents was hybridized (outcrossed to each other) to produce the new generation, which is now comprised of genetics from both parental populations. Outcrossing results in the introduction of new and different genetic material to each of the pools.

Often there are recessive genes or dominant genes that have not had a chance to fully express themselves until being inbred 3 to 4 times, or being outcrossed several times. It is important to remember that cannabis is naturally outcrossing. Inbreeding plants that are naturally outcrossing too many generations sacrifice the health of offspring. Keep outcrossing plants healthy, and maintain diversity by growing large numbers of plants.

Filial Breeding: Siblings of the same progeny lot and generation are intermated to produce new generations. The first hybrid generation of 2 distinct true-breeding lines is the F1 generation (F, filial). If 2 F1 siblings are bred, or the F1 population is allowed to be open pollinated, the resulting generation is labeled F2, F3, F4, etc. Mating siblings chosen from the F2 results in the F3 population. F4, F5, F6 generations, etc., are produced the same way, by crossing plants of the same generation and progeny lot.

Note: As long as any number of siblings of a generation (F[n]) are mated, the resulting generations is denoted (F[n+1]).

Filial inbreeding with selection for specific traits is the most common method for establishing a pure or a true-breeding population in cannabis. After a few generations, genetic problems will surface.

Backcrossing

Backcrossing is the pollination of a female flower from a male flower on the same plant. Backcross breeding is repeated crossing of progeny with one of the original parental genotypes. It is cross-pollinating 1 generation back to a previous generation; most often the progeny is crossed with the mother plant. The parent is called the "recurrent parent." The nonrecurrent parent is the "donor parent."

Backcross breeding is the most widely used form of breeding cannabis to date. Backcross breeding is simple and can be done with small populations of plants. Most often the goal of backcrossing is to create a population from the genetics of a single parent (the recurrent parent).

Donor parents are chosen based on desirable traits. One parent is backcrossed to another to introgress genetics, to move genes from one variety to another. Repeated backcrossing is the best way to achieve this goal.

Use backcrossing to add desirable traits to a mostly ideal, relatively true-breeding genotype. The recurrent-parent should be an ideal genotype such as an existing inbred line. Look for traits that are easily identified in the progeny of each generation. The best donor parent must possess the desired trait, but should not be seriously deficient in other traits. Backcross line production is repeatable, if the same parents are used.

Simple backcrossing to incorporate a dominant trait is easy and very common among the vast majority of breeders. However, plants come with both dominant and recessive genes. When making selections, it is best to select for one single quality at a time and select the absolute best males possible from each population.

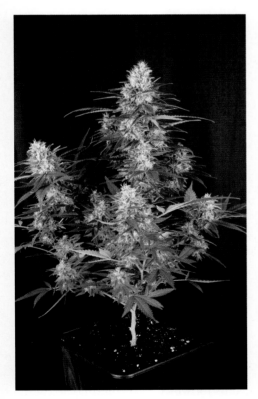

'Super Skunk' from Sensi Seeds is a good example of an outbred variety. It takes the stable 'Skunk #1' and adds a dominant amount of 'Afghani' genetics.

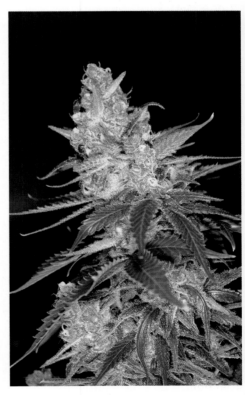

'Apollo 13 BX' (Back Cross) from TGA Genetics is a good example of a backcrossed variety.

Backcrossing also uses the terms *squaring* (to denote the second backcross to the same parent) and *cubing* (to designate the third backcross).

Backcrossing: Incorporating a Dominant Trait

Step One: Cross recurrent parent × donor parent

Step Two: Select desirable plants showing dominant trait, and hybridize selected plants to recurrent parent. The generation produced is denoted BC1 (some cannabis breeders call this generation B×1. [BC1= B×1]).

Step Three: Select plants from BC1 and hybridize with the recurrent parent; the resulting generation is denoted BC2.

Step Four: Select plants from BC2 and hybridize with the recurrent parent; the resulting generation is denoted BC3.

Backcrossing: Incorporating a Recessive Trait

Recessive traits are more difficult to select for in backcross breeding, since their expression is masked by dominance in each backcross to the recurrent parent. An additional round of open pollination or sib-mating is needed after each backcross generation to expose homozygous-recessive plants. Individuals showing the recessive condition are selected from F2 segregating generations and backcrossed to the recurrent parent as in the "Backcrossing: Incorporating a Dominant Trait" above.

Step One: Cross recurrent parent × donor F1 hybrid generation

Step Two: Select desirable plants, and create an F2 population via full cross-pollination.

Step Three: Select plants showing the desired recessive trait in the F2 generation. Hybridize selected F2-recessive plants to the recurrent parent. The generation produced is denoted BC1.

Step Four: Select plants from BC1, and create a generation of F2 plants via sib-mating; the resulting generation can be denoted BC1F2.

Step Five: Select desirable BC1F2 plants showing the recessive condition, and hybridize with the recurrent parent; the resulting generation is denoted BC2.

Step Six: Select plants from BC2, and create an F2 population via sib-mating; denote the resulting generation BC2F2.

Step Seven: Select plants showing the recessive condition from the BC2F2 generation, and hybridize to the recurrent parent; the resulting generation is denoted BC3.

Step Eight: Grow out BC3, select and sib-mate the most ideal candidates to create an F2 population, where plants showing the recessive condition are then selected and used as a basis for a new inbred, or open-pollinated, seed line.

This new generation created from the F2 is a population that consists of, on average, about 93.7 percent of genes from the recurrent parent, and only about 6.3 percent of genes leftover from the donor parent.

Note: Only homozygous-recessives were chosen for mating in the BC3F2 generation; the entire resulting BC3F3 generation is homozygous for the recessive trait, and breeds true for this recessive trait. Our new population meets our breeding objective. It is a population derived mainly from the genetics of the recurrent parent, yet breeds true for our introgressed recessive trait.

Backcross-derived lines are most often well-adapted to the environment in which they will be grown. Indoor garden rooms are easily replicated, and plants grow in a similar environment to that in which they were bred. Progeny therefore need less extensive environmental field-testing.

If 2 or more characters are to be introgressed into a new seed line, these would usually be tracked in separate backcross programs, and the individual products would be combined in a final set of crosses after the new populations have been created by backcrossing.

Backcrossing has drawbacks. If the recurrent parent is not very true-breed-

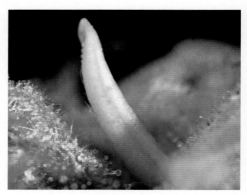

Small male flower appears on this Chemdog inbred female flower. Inbreeding often causes male intersex flowers to form on female plants.

ing, the resulting backcross generations segregate, and many of the traits deemed desirable to the line fail to be reproduced reliably. Another limitation of the backcross is that the "improved" variety differs only slightly from the recurrent parent (e.g., one trait). If multiple traits are to be introgressed into the new population, other techniques, such as inbreeding or recurrent selection, may be more rewarding.

Self-Pollinating (Selfing)

"Clone Only" Varieties

Often, 2 hybrid plants are crossed and the "variety" is given a name, but soon the male plant is lost, and the plant is available only as a clone. In this case the plant must be "selfed" to produce male flowers on a female plant.

Self-pollinating (aka selfing) is the process of creating seed by pollinating a plant with its own pollen. Self-pollinating is a plant having sex with itself. Self-crossing can derive populations of plants from a single individual. The first generation population derived from selfing an individual is called the S1 population. An individual from S1 that is selfed again is called S2. Subsequent generations derived in the same manner are denoted S3, S4, etc.

Traits for which the plant is homozygous remain homozygous upon selfing, whereas heterozygous loci segregate and may demonstrate novel expressions of these characters.

We know homozygous loci remain homozygous in future generations upon selfing. Heterozygous loci are increased by 50 percent. Every subsequent generation will be 50 percent more homozygous than the parent from which it was derived.

Repeated selfing, or single-seed descent, is the fastest way to achieve homozygosity within a group or family. The more plants grown from a selfed population, the better probability a breeder has of finding selfed progeny that show all the desired traits.

Self-Pollinating Breeding

Step One: Identify superior genotypes for the trait under selection.

Step Two: Cross superior genotypes and select improved progeny.

Step Three: Repeat steps One and Two over a series of generations.

Feminized Seeds

Breeders produce all-female or feminized seeds by obtaining pollen from a male flower on an individual female and using this pollen to fertilize another female plant. In order to produce feminized seed, pollen must be collected from male flowers that occur on an otherwise female plant.

As stated in "Sexual Propagation"), there are 20 chromosomes in each plant cell. Female cannabis plants have 2 copies of the X chromosome, and their genotype is expressed as XX. Male plants have 1 copy of the X chromosome and 1 copy of the Y chromosome. The genotype expression of male plants' sex chromosomes is XY. However, the ability to change sex based on external factors is believed to be controlled by X-autosome or X-A.

When pollen is created within the plant, 1 of each of the sets of chromosomes from each parent is packaged into the cells that develop into pollen. This process, mitosis, is the process of a single cell dividing into 2 identical cells. Each cell contains the same chromosomes and genetic content as the parent. Each pollen grain or ovule contains

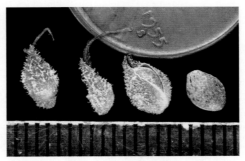

Seeds must develop completely before they are ready to harvest. (MF)

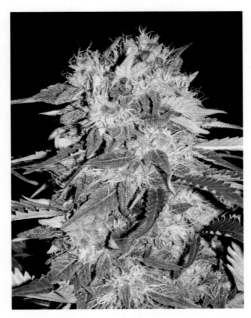

'Sour Bubbly' is one of the many new feminized autoflowering varieties.

10 chromosomes, 1 copy of each pair. When the pollen deposits the genetic material into the ovule, the 10 chromosomes from the pollen and the ovule unite to make a total of 20 chromosomes, a full genetic complement. There are 2 gametes: 1 fertilizes the ovule of the female, the other fertilizes the endosperm of the seed that gives the new plant its initial food source and chemical profile.

Use a Punnett Square to predict the outcome of a breeding cross. It is used to determine the probability of an offspring having a particular genotype. The Punnett square summarizes all possible combinations of 1 maternal allele with 1 paternal allele.

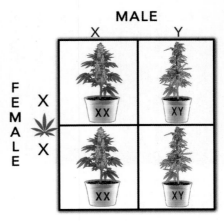

Punnett square view of a simple male:female cross

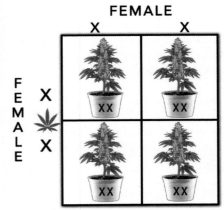

This Punnett square of a female cross demonstrates that female:female breeding crosses produce only female (XX) offspring. Pollen from a few male flowers that appear on a female plant is used to produce female only (XX) offspring.

The next step is to produce male flowers on a female plant. Pollen from the male flowers is used to fertilize the same female plant (selfing) or other female plants (outbreeding). If this female plant is the same self-pollinated plant, it will be a mix of its own genes. If the plant is different and from outside the genetic pool of the first plant, new genes will be introduced to the outbred cross.

There are 2 common ways to induce male flowers on a female plant—inducing environmental stress and altering hormone levels.

Environmental Stress

Pollen from environmentally stressed intersex plants is used to fertilize females that will produce mostly (more than

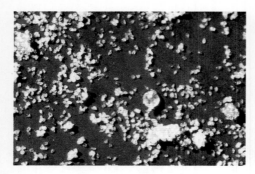

Large, round, capitate-stalked resin gland heads add perspective to minute grains of male pollen. (MF)

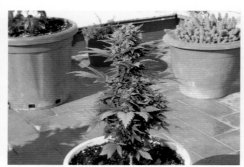

This autoflowering feminized 'Big Low' from Seeds of Life is one example of the many new "auto-fems" available today.

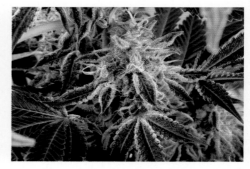

'Jack 47' from Sweet Seeds proves that autoflowering feminized seeds produce plenty of resin.

99%) female seeds. But, the offspring will have intersex tendencies. More pronounced intersex tendencies in parent plants bring about the same traits in offspring. There is no way around this simple genetic fact.

Produce feminized seed by collecting pollen from carefully selected, latent, stress-induced male flowers on a female plant, and use it to pollinate female plants.

One of the easiest stress techniques is to let the plant flower and continue growing. Sooner or later most females will produce a few male flowers. Other stress methods include irregular light cycle or low temperature. The process is time-consuming but yields mostly female plants when grown without stress. As soon as stress is introduced, intersex tendencies can quickly surface.

Remember, genetic weaknesses—including a predisposition for male flowers to appear on female plants—will be passed to offspring. To select against the intersex condition, take female breeding candidates and grow them under stressful conditions such as irregular light cycle or high heat. Only plants that resist intersexuality under stressful conditions should be tested to produce an all-female seed lines. Intersex-resistant plants are called "true females." Always select females that resist changing sex to pass the trait to offspring.

Environmental stress is not the only way to produce male flowers on a female plant.

Alter Hormone Levels

Feminized seeds can also be produced with applications of sprays that alter the hormonal concentration of the plant. There are 2 popular methods of inducing male flowers on a female plant. Both methods require a spray application to the plant.

Colloidal silver (CS) consists of very small silver particles suspended in water. There is quite a bit of disagreement as to the overall safety and efficacy of colloidal silver. Please research safety aspects before using it. In cannabis, CS inhibits female flowering hormones, so male hormones dominate. Male flowers appear on an otherwise female plant.

Purchase high-quality CS at health food stores, natural pharmacies, or via Internet stores. Look for CS that is 15 to 30 ppm concentration. Or you can make it yourself at home, which is a bit more complicated. There are many YouTube videos and Internet methods to follow. They involve using a 9- to 12-volt battery or generator that can produce at least 250 milliamperes, a silver rod or coin, and distilled water. For instructions on colloidal silver, see chapter 22, *Additives*.

Silver thiosulfate is more difficult to find than CS, but it is available on the Internet. It works on the same principles as CS. Check package for spray concentration and application.

Gibberellic acid (GA3) is a very popular hormone used to produce feminized seeds. See chapter 22, *Additives*, for complete information.

Ethylene, a plant hormone, plays a major role in the determination of sex by regulating which flowers should be produced—male or female. High concentrations of ethylene sprayed on male flowering plants causes female flowers to form. See chapter 22, *Additives*, for more information on ethylene.

Applying ethylene-inhibiting agents to pistillate individuals as they enter flowering results in the formation of stamens in place of pistils. Breeders use this technique to create "feminized" seeds (all-female [gynoecious] seed lots).

Day-Neutral (aka Autoflowering) Feminized Varieties

Day-neutral cannabis plants are called autoflowering plants in the popular cannabis industry today. Autoflowering feminized seeds are produced the same way as other seeds, except 1 or both of the parents are autoflowering. These varieties were originally created by cross-pollinating *Cannabis ruderalis* that flowers after 3 to 4 weeks of growth with regular cannabis plants that flower under 11 to 12 hours of darkness after the vegetative growth stage is complete. Autoflowering varieties are relatively easy to create, but they take time to stabilize. Seed companies sell them to you every year so that you do not have to reproduce them.

Breeding new autoflowering varieties is more difficult when making hybrids and incorporating a non-autoflowering variety. A few short-day cannabis varieties are heterogeneous, contain the recessive day-neutral (autoflowering) genes and dominant short-day genes.

Autoflowering plants have homozygous recessive traits for the day-neutral genes. Most short-day varieties and autoflowering crosses produce few autoflowering progeny in the F1 generation. When recrossed, the F2 generation contains approximately 25 percent of homozygous recessive plants that are autoflowering. Once this point is reached, the population requires further stabilization.

Learn to breed with regular seeds before starting to breed autoflowering feminized plants. Once you have a good background with the variety you are breeding, you can start autoflowering breeding. Remember, half the equation is finding a male that fits your needs and is super strong-smelling, resinous from an early age, disease- and pest-resistant, and so on. Such males are often short and squat, with female-like growth and stature characteristics.

Once autoflowering plants are genetically stable, they are feminized via inbreeding pollen from a male flower that occurs on a predominately female plant. The process is fairly simple and is outlined below.

Breeding Basics for Autoflowering Feminized Plants

1. Cross regular seed with an autoflowering variety.
2. Cross F1 seeds together again under a 12/12 photoperiod.
3. The first generation contains recessive autoflowering genes that manifest in the next generation.
4. The next generation has some autoflowering genes.
5. Plant and stabilize over time to get 100 percent autoflowering plants.
6. Feminize 100 percent autoflowering female and produce seeds.

Backcross regular seeds to an autoflowering male to achieve an autoflowering plant too.

Making Seeds at Home
Making seeds at home requires a secure garden area that can be dedicated to breeding. It must be clean and free of male pollen. Indoor garden rooms and greenhouses are best suited to breeding cannabis if there is danger of rogue pollen from neighboring male cannabis plants contaminating faraway seed crops. If growing more than 1 male to produce pollen, measures must be taken to isolate each male once they start producing pollen. Segregate pollen-producing male plants by keeping them in an enclosed area as far away from flowering females as possible.

The basics of breeding cannabis at home are simple:
1. Start with diverse group of plants and know their traits.
2. Cross desirable plants.
3. Select desirable individuals and maintain diversity.

Slow and steady breeding is not dynamic, but it is very effective. Pollinate a few branches on several plants and have more seeds than you can grow. The breeding project is never finished!

Grow small seed crops inside a garden closet or inside a portable wardrobe made from fine cloth or something similar that will block pollen from entering or escaping.

Recordkeeping is the most important aspect of cannabis plant breeding. Accurate written and photographic records with dates help you to make informed decisions.

Naming Varieties
Many varieties have names known only in the local area where they are cultivated. These varieties often bear the name of the region from which they originated or a person with whom they are associated. Other varieties are named for fragrance, bud size, effect, or appearance. The names are often very descriptive and creative!

Making Seeds: Step-by-Step
Step One: What is your goal?
Common goals include making seeds for next year's crop, reproducing new parents just like the old ones, and adding new traits to existing plants. When setting a goal, work with a single trait at a time so that it is easier to control the selection and outcome. Breeding will bring about dominant and recessive genes. Each has its own qualities. Impeccable recordkeeping and a consistent, stable climate are essential. Write out a breeding plan and plot your findings.

Step Two: Select parents—(A) female, (B) male—to breed.
Few varieties commercially available to medical cannabis gardeners are true-breeding and stable. Most often seeds have many different genes and are not stable or uniform. True-breeding seed stock ensures F1 hybrid seeds that have hybrid vigor. Stable true-breeding stock is sometimes difficult to find from seed companies, and gardeners often elect to stabilize their own.

Simply crossing 1 of the stable true-breeding varieties (see list below) with another stable variety will produce an F1 hybrid.

List of relatively stable seeds
'Afghan#1' (IBL)
'Big Bud' (IBL)
'Blackberry' (VISC)
'Burmese' (VISC)
'Durban Poison' (IBL)
'Hash Plant'
'Hindu Kush'
'Island Sweet Skunk'
'KGB' (VISC)
'Malawi Gold' (IBL)
'Master Kush' = stabilized hybrid
'Original Blueberry' = stabilized hybrid
'Original Haze' (IBL)
'Power Plant' (IBL)
'Skunk Passion' (IBL)
'Skunk #1'
More stabilized seed stock is updated at www.marijuanagrowing.com

Step Two A: Select a female that has been flowering for about 4 weeks and has many white stigmas.
Female plants are easy to select. Medical cannabis gardeners and patients know the growth characteristics of each plant in the garden. The most common desirable characteristics include cannabinoid

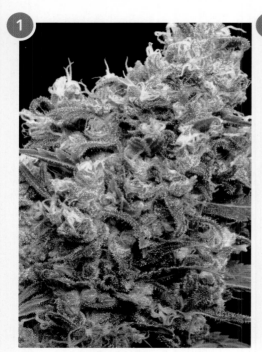

1

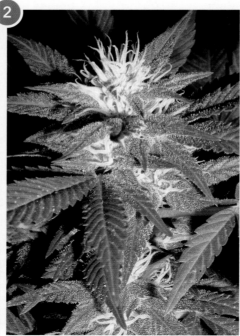

2

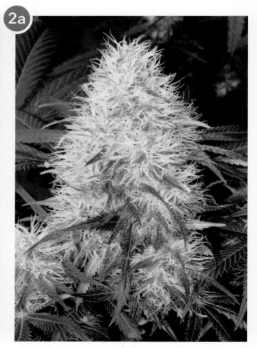

2a

'Skunk #1' is a stable breeding plant and is at the base of many varieties and breeding programs. Choose stable breeding stock whenever possible. (MF)

This beautiful medical 'Chronic' female is an excellent candidate for a breeding program.

'Hash Plant' × 'G13' × 'Chronic' yielded this pistil-heavy female. Although showy, the breeder culled the plant in favor of others with heavier bud development.

profile with quality fragrance and flavor, strong growth habit, heavy yield, and resistance to diseases and pests. Outdoor gardeners in climate-sensitive areas look for strong branching, a big root system, and tolerance of drought, heat, and cold

Take a thin-layer chromatography test to help make correct choices based upon cannabinoid profiles. Cannabinoid profiles are similar throughout different life stages of a plant, and breeding decisions can be based upon these profiles.

Observe plants carefully as they develop during the season. Watch for desirable characteristics. Pay close attention to flower buds and how they fill out and mature. Apart from looking at resin gland development and stigma senescence, take a toke. Vaporize a sample bud from each plant to determine taste, fragrance, effect, and so on. Remember that flower bud flavors and aromas can change over time as they dry and cure. Additional tasting may be necessary.

Step Two B: Select a male with desirable characteristics.
Choosing male plants for breeding is difficult. One basic test is to rub the stem with your finger. If it exudes a

pungent, resinous odor, it *may* be rich in cannabinoids. Look for male plants that are short with dense foliage and that contain other desirable characteristics—cannabinoid profile, strong growth, disease and pest resistance, drought, heat and cold tolerance.

To determine cannabinoid profiles, make thin-layer chromatography tests before males flower. Soon laboratory analysis of the cannabinoid profile and genetic marker (alleles) tests will become more common.

The most reliable way to select the best male breeding stock is to use the pollen from specific males to pollinate chosen females. The plants are grown to maturity and males are then selected. It takes time to stabilize males, and few seed companies put much time into male plant selection. Once selected, a super male and subsequent male lineage can be kept alive for years.

Clone promising male plants and cull the rest to keep stock alive.

Step Three: Collect pollen.
Set up small "plates" of aluminum foil to collect pollen. Once plates are in place,

jiggle branches so pollen is dispersed and falls onto plates for collection.

Carefully collect pollen from male flowers and store it in an airtight container in a cool dry place or in a low-humidity refrigerator or freezer. Or cut a male branch from a plant and store it in a glass of water in subdued light.

Pollen can be stored for several years if kept cool and dry. Viability decreases as time passes. But consider that there are millions of grains of pollen in a single male flower. It takes just a fraction of the pollen to fertilize an entire bud. Even though pollen has lost viability, there is still enough good pollen to fertilize pistils and produce seeds.

One branch of male flowers will supply all the pollen necessary for small-scale breeders to produce many seeds for personal use.

Strip away other branches to guard against accidental random pollination. To avoid premature pollination, isolate the male as soon as anthers show. Be considerate of the fact that airborne pollen can travel miles. Brushing up against a plant jostles and releases

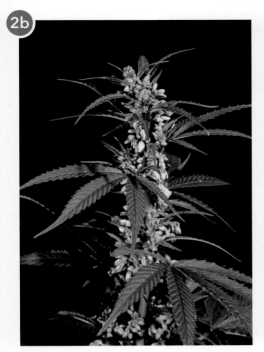

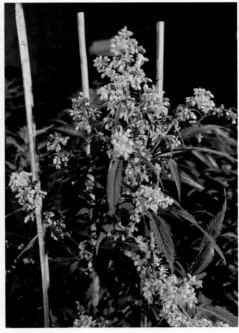

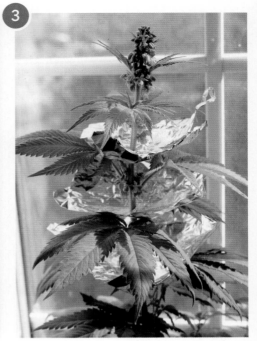

Testing male plants with thin-layer chromatography is a good way to learn much about the cannabinoid profile. Without the test, cannabinoid profile would have to be measured subjectively.

Waiting for a male plant to mature is difficult when growing females in the same vicinity.

Pollen is being collected on lightweight aluminum foil. (MF)

millions of grains of pollen that travel everywhere.

Step Four: Store pollen.

Store small amounts of pollen in aluminum foil, enclosed with silicon to absorb excess moisture so that it does not destroy the pollen. Pollen has a short shelf life in nature. High temperatures and moisture destroy it. Pollen can be stored in the freezer for several months.

Store pollen in an airtight container along with silicon pellets to absorb any moisture in the container. Periodically remove silicon to dry and then be

Carefully remove pollen from the collection bag and pass it through a screen to remove flower remnants. Remember, dead flowers and foliage attract moisture and will contaminate and spoil pollen. Place wax paper under the screen to catch pollen. Pour pollen into a sterile test tube or small container from a craft store. Scrape remaining pollen into tube or container with a sterile instrument. Seal test container. Put test tube in a larger airtight container with several packets of silicon to absorb moisture. Seal pollen with silica gel and leave at room temperature so the silica draws moisture from pollen before putting it in the freezer.

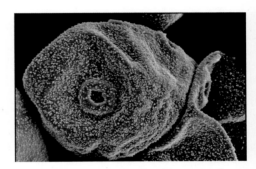

Grains of male pollen such as the one in the photo (magnified 4,000 times) stick to the stigma, develop a tube through the style, and release 2 gametes—1 to fertilize the ovule and 1 to fertilize the endosperm.

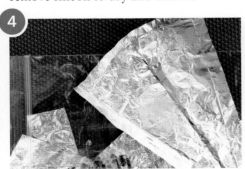

(MF)

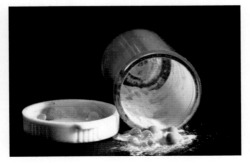

(MF)

returned to the container. Make sure to let container sit at room temperature for several hours to avoid moisture condensation from temperature change.

At pollination time, pull pollen out of freezer and let it warm up to room temperature. Do not open the container when cold or water will condense inside

and kill the pollen. Keep refrigerator at low humidity. Thawing and refreezing pollen will diminish its viability.

Step Five: Pollinate female.

Flowering females grow many ready, receptive stigmas until pollination occurs. Best pollination takes place about 3 to 5 weeks after females show their first flowers. At this point the majority of receptive stigmas are ready for pollination. This is when a few of the stigmas start to curl and slightly discolor, signifying the onset of senescence. Receptive stigmas are turgid and most often are white or off-white in color.

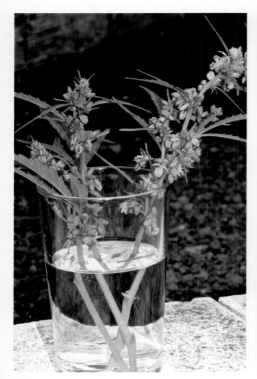

Male flowers can be stored for a few days in a glass of water, but they have a tendency to open prematurely.

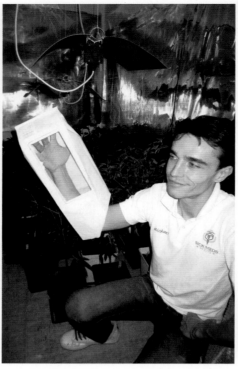

Cannabis is very promiscuous! Michael from www.SickMeds.com demonstrates a special bag with a window to prevent pollination. Paper bags are good indoors and in greenhouses; waterproof plastic may be necessary outdoors.

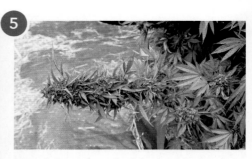

A single lower branch of this big female is fertilized with male pollen. The seeds are left to mature for about 2 weeks after flower buds have been harvested.

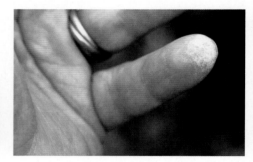

A little dab of pollen is all that is necessary to selectively pollinate a few stigmas.

Senescing and dying stigmas that are brownish are not viable.

Not all pollinations are successful. If in doubt, you may want to pollinate 2 or 3 times to ensure your success.

Once pollinated, the majority of the female's energy is directed toward seed production, and bud formation stops. Pollinate well-formed buds packed with well-formed stigmas to produce the maximum number of viable seeds.

Home breeders need to pollinate a flower bud full of stigmas or a single branch full of buds to make more seeds than they need. Humboldtlocal calls pollinating one branch "planned parenthood." The unpollinated branches are sinsemilla. The sinsemilla tops are harvested when ripe. Seeded branches continue to mature for another week or two until ripe.

A little bit of pollen on your thumb or finger is the best way to pollinate specific sets of stigmas in a flower bud. Human skin is oily and it holds pollen well without altering it. Brush pollen-laden thumb or finger lightly to disseminate countless grains of pollen to fertilize females. Be very careful with remaining pollen on finger. Rinse fingers in water to remove pollen, or quickly lick pollen with your tongue.

Label everything. It is easy to lose track of names. Cross-reference notes or codes on plants with copious notes in a notebook. Color-code pollinated females with small pieces of yarn for easy identification. Some breeders use barcodes to track plants. The barcode is fixed onto the plant tag and attached to the plant.

Put a little pollen into a plastic bag. Carefully cover a single female branch packed with receptive ripe stigmas with the bag. Tie the end of the bag around the stem of the branch to ensure that no pollen escapes. Shake the branch lightly for complete dispersal of pollen to all stigmas. Leave the bag for 2 days and nights to ensure thorough pollination.

Move the target plants to a "safe" area to avoid accidental pollination of other plants. Be careful not to scatter pollen when removing the bag.

Avoid using an artist's paintbrush to pollinate individual buds. Pollen is very fine; a paintbrush tends to hold too much pollen, and it is difficult to contain. Pollen can easily disperse beyond the targeted stigmas.

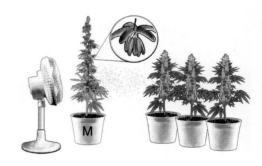

Set a group of females in an enclosed area. Set a single male plant a few feet from an oscillating circulation fan. Turn on the fan to help disperse pollen in the room to pollinate all the females.

Some commercial breeders and seed makers place multiple males or clones of the same male in the **seed production garden room** with their breeding females. Males release pollen in the well-vented room, allowing complete pollination of the crop.

Wash clothes and shower afterward to avoid transporting pollen to nearby plants away from the breeding zone.

Spray pollinated females with water a couple of times before returning them to the normal "sinsemilla" grow-room population.

Clean seed room thoroughly after each seed crop to avoid accidental pollination of future crops.

Step Six: Harvest seeds.

Seeds are ripe when they are mostly dark brown or gray. Many seeds are spotted and mottled; some are even tiger-striped. Green, yellow, or white seeds are almost always immature and not viable. Seeds that are lighter in color or float in water after 24 hours are slow to germinate and often unviable.

When a few seeded buds are mature, remove seeds from the bracts by picking seeds out by hand. This can be done with green buds or dry seeded flower buds. Once dry, rub seeded buds between your fingers and hands over a screen or tray. A little bit of light friction will not damage seeds. However, they are susceptible to heat, cold, and moisture. Avoid all three when harvesting and handling seeds.

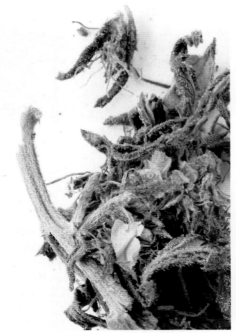

Cleaning seeds by hand can be a laborious task. (MF)

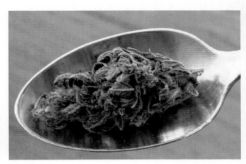

This seeded bud of 'Afghani' × 'Chiba Colombian 60' × 'African 3' was grown as a seed crop in 1980. (MF)

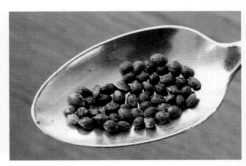

The same bud from above held 50 seeds. (MF)

Note: Do not use excessive heat or a microwave to dry seeded buds.

Collect seeds and foliage on the tray or screen. Move the tray back and forth so that lightweight foliage stays on one side as the tray is tipped and seeds congregate on the other end. Remove excess foliage by hand and repeat the process. Rub separated seeds together gently in your hands to remove traces of seed bracts that still adhere to seeds. If not

collecting resin, use canned air, a fan, or your breath to blow away small amounts of lightweight foliage.

Test for ripeness by pressing a few seeds between your thumb and finger. Seeds that do not crush easily are most often viable.

Under humid and rainy conditions, ripe seeds can actually sprout in place, in flower buds. Once moisture enters

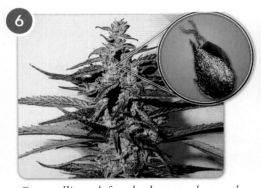

Once pollinated, female plants produce seeds that become ripe in 6 to 8 weeks. (Occasionally they mature later.) As seeds mature they become darker. Eventually the containing seed bract starts to senesce and dry out around the edges to expose the maturing seed within.

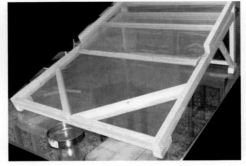

Seed-cleaning devices save hours of work. The seeded buds are placed on top of the upper screen. Human seed cleaners rub buds together between their hands. The friction causes seeds to separate from seed bracts and buds. Cleaned seeds are collected below in a pan.

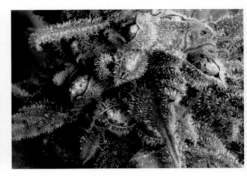

Seeded 'Diesel' female (MF)

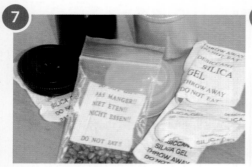
Plenty of silicon desiccant and small containers are needed to store a variety of seeds.

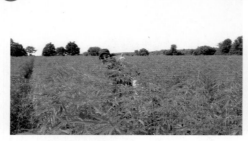
A Canadian friend near Montreal sent me this photo. He was fantasizing about making breeding selections. Unfortunately, this is a field of industrial hemp!

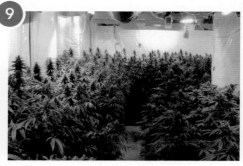
Continue to grow out your crops and make selections, as is being done in this beautiful garden from DNA Genetics.

the outer shell of the seed, it starts to germinate. Or if foliage dries around seeds and they fall to the ground, they often germinate on the soil surface. But most often they are planted outdoors and consumed by birds or many other hungry creatures.

Seeded flower buds can contain as much resin as sinsemilla flower buds. However, much resin is degraded during the harvest process. Resin glands are broken or resin sticks to fingers and is exposed to excessive light and air when seeds are removed. Seeds are often cleaned over a screen so that the resin powder can be collected below.

Step Seven: Store or plant harvested seed.
Seeds are ready to plant immediately after harvest, and will germinate well. Maintain high germination rates by letting seeds dry in a cool, dark, well-ventilated place after harvest. Seeds that dry for a month or longer before planting develop a hard outer cask to protect the embryo inside. See "Storing Seeds" in chapter 5, *Seeds & Seedlings.*

Place harvested seeds in a glass or rigid plastic container with a desiccant. Label and date the container. Store seeds in a cool, dry, dark place. Change desiccant every month or two.

Step Eight: Grow and evaluate.
Growing more plants means greater variation and a bigger pool of individuals. Undesirable plants are easy to cull in order to provide more space for adjacent plants to grow.

Felix from Owls Production, Switzerland, culled all plants that did not meet his requirements for tolerance to cold and mold. This simple technique worked very well. Only the strongest individuals survived the selection process.

Criteria
1. Cannabinoid profile
2. Growth habit
3. Susceptibility to diseases and pests
4. Climatic conditions for acclimatization
5. Genetic stability

Step Nine: Monitor, select, and apply selection pressures.
Post-harvest selection requires either partial seeding of each plant or keeping clone copies of each and every plant for future seed-production use once post-harvest evaluations are done.

Pursue Goals
- Desirable characteristics—cannabinoid profile
- Overall vigor and good health—growth habit, susceptibility to diseases and pests
- Genetic stability
- Acclimatization to your climate and conditions

Varieties for indoor cultivation: These include short, squat, bushy growth; large, densely formed buds; discernible taste or particular flavors and aromas; high content of specific cannabinoids, and quality of the effects (long-lasting, soaring, sedative); and resistance to diseases and pests.

Often, varieties that grow well indoors will also perform well in a greenhouse and outdoors after 2 to 3 years of acclimatization. During the first year in which varieties are moved from an indoor environment to an outdoor garden or greenhouse, some will grow better than others and acclimate more quickly. However, varieties that grow well outdoors often grow poorly indoors, especially pure *sativa* and *sativa*-dominant varieties.

Greenhouse varieties grow well in containers. Both outdoor and indoor varieties often grow well in greenhouses. Look for robust growth habit and early flowering if plants are grown in containers. Plants grown in Mother Earth in the floor of the greenhouse must mature before they consume 75 percent of the space inside the greenhouse. Air circulation and ventilation, as well as diseases and pests become problematic if plants grown in greenhouses become too big.

It is especially important for **outdoor varieties** to be acclimated to local conditions. Heat, humidity, rain, and cold temperatures are the main aspects of concern among outdoor breeders. Outdoor varieties should be acclimated to the local climate before selecting plants. Smart breeders select plants that mature early in their climate. Pragmatic breeders select the earliest plants with a desirable cannabinoid profile. Selecting for an early harvest without considering cannabinoid content is counterproductive.

It is important to balance positive and negative aspects of each plant and future generations. Selecting plants that may

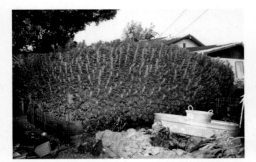

This unknown outdoor variety was developed in Northern California to grow well in a localized climate.

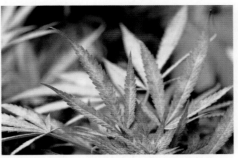

To date, very little breeding has been done to develop disease- and pest-resistant varieties of cannabis. Powdery mildew continues to be one of the main problems among cannabis gardeners.

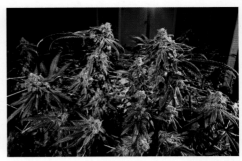

'Granddaddy Purple' is a well-known variety of cannabis.

have some genetic weakness will require that the unwanted negative traits are removed later.

When planting a large number of seeds, some traits of plants differ greatly but in all other respects are virtually identical. For example, some plants are more or less susceptible to fungal infection such as *Botrytis* (gray mold) or powdery mildew.

Plants can be exposed to a particular pathogen or environmental stress as a selection pressure. Growing potential breeding parents in a stressful environment may expose genetic strengths and weaknesses associated with a particular environment. Heat- and cold-tolerant plants may experience excessive predator attacks or be weak and susceptible to pathogens. Very little selective breeding has been done to preserve cannabinoid profiles and tolerance for diseases and pests.

Seed-Crop Care

Cannabis grown for seed production requires a complete balanced diet from seed germination through harvest. Give seeded mother plants a complete fertilizer that supplies *all* nutrients. Often vegetative and flowering fertilizers are mixed together and applied from an early age. I prefer to use complete, balanced, organic-based soil mixes to produce the most healthy, viable seeds.

Breeding Terms

A grasp of basic breeding terms is necessary to full understanding of essential concepts in this chapter. The breeding terms that follow are easy to look over

quickly and decide which ones to study in detail.

A **variety***—is a subdivision of a (cannabis) species comprised of naturally occurring or selectively bred populations or individuals that have distinct characteristics from all other varieties in the species. The variety must be uniform and stable under normal growing conditions. However, minor variations may be apparent.

A **cultivar** (cv)* is a distinguishable plant or group of like plants selected for desirable characteristics, and maintains distinguishing traits when propagated. Most cultivars are selectively bred but

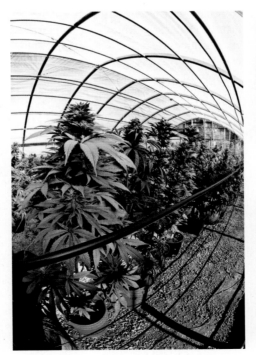

Growing seed crops in a greenhouse is a good way to keep them isolated from other plants.

some are selections from the wild. The terms *cultivar* and *variety* are equivalent.

Unique plants selected from a group or population derived from a cultivar that show enough variation from the parent are considered a different variety and deserve their own name.

*According to some taxonomists, using the term *strain* to define variety or cultivar is botanically incorrect. For more information, see chapter 8, *Flowering*.

Open-pollinated varieties are reproduced by random pollination within the variety. Each female has the potential to mate with any and all male plants. Open pollination ensures genetic diversity and

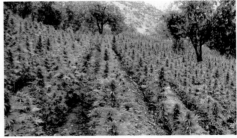

The distinct cultivars of cannabis in this photo were bred in Europe and are shown growing in Morocco.

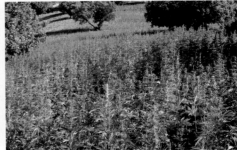

These open-pollinated cannabis plants are growing in the Rif Mountains in Morocco.

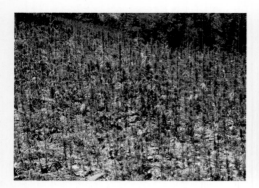

Male and female plants are grown together in this landrace stand of cannabis. The seeded plants are growing in drought conditions.

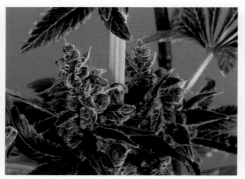

Two different genotypes of 'Blueberry' × 'Sandstorm' grown indoors demonstrate different color and growth habits.

preserves current traits. An open-pollinated crop must be isolated from outside cannabis pollen. Both male and female plants from the same population are grown together. All males have the possibility to pollinate all females. Heirloom and landrace varieties are open pollinated.

Pollen travels outdoors! Industrial hemp breeders plant seed crops a long way away from other fields of cannabis to avoid contamination from airborne rogue pollen.

Heirloom varieties and seeds are cultivars that were grown before 1950 and are not used in modern, large-scale growing. *Heirloom* is a term seldom used when referring to medicinal cannabis varieties, because they were developed after 1950. Heirloom varieties retain their traits via open pollination and breed fairly true, producing plants very similar to the parent plants. Weak and weird plants are culled from the population. Heirloom varieties are still seen in Morocco and other hashish-producing regions in other parts of the world.

A **landrace** is a localized variety of a plant that has developed mainly by natural processes. The plant adapts to the microclimate in which it lives. Landrace varieties are not deliberately or selectively bred to achieve a specific goal. Overall landrace varieties are more genetically and physically diverse than selectively bred plants. Many selectively bred plants started out as landraces and are attempts to improve the gene pool.

Phenotype is the outward physical characteristics or genetic traits expressed that can be observed or measured in cannabis. The phenotype is how the genetic map is expressed as acted on by any environmental factors, internal or external, that occur outside the nuclear envelope.

For example a genotype can be short or tall, but if it grows in a low-light environment, either phenotype could grow tall. If the plant is abused, suffers cold temperatures and heavy winds a plant that would normally grow tall, may be short. Environmental factors can influence the expression of genetic qualities. The same plant grown indoors will look completely different outdoors when given a chance to express traits. Harsh environmental factors also change phenotype expression. For example, cutting the top off a plant changes the genetic expression and the plant grows short and bushy. The genes are the same but the outward appearance of the plant has changed.

All phenotypes are the observable result of genes acting within the cells of the plant. Sometimes a single gene controls one trait (monogenic traits), and sometimes sets of genes operate together and contribute to make what we see as a phenotype (polygenic traits).

Genotype is the inherited set of instructions carried in a plant's genetic code. Not all cannabis plants with the same genotype look the same because appearance is modified by environmental conditions (phenotype). And all cannabis plants that look alike do not necessarily have the same genotype.

Environmental conditions often trigger genotypes to express themselves differently. Green leaves often turn purple when exposed to cold temperatures. But leaves on other plants remain green no matter how cold it gets. The plants possess different versions of the gene(s) that control purple pigment production on leaves. These gene versions, alleles, dictate whether or not purple pigment is produced.

In the beginning, both plants had the green-leaved phenotype; one of the plants developed an altered phenotype (purple leaf) in response to the cold environment. It was caused by the plant's genetic trait interacting with the environment.

A simplistic way to think of this important concept is:

phenotype = genotype + environment

Chemotype was a term coined in 1968 by Dr. Rolf Santesson and his son Johan Santesson. A chemotype is a chemically distinct entity in a plant with differences in the composition of the secondary metabolites. Minor genetic and environmental changes have little or no effect on plant growth or appearance but may produce large changes in the chemical phenotype. Cannabis chemotypes may be indistinguishable in appearance, but differences in chemotypes appear to affect the existence and percentage of cannabinoids and essential oils.

Here is the "Classification of Chemotypes" Mel Frank made in the *Marijuana Grower's Guide* (1982):

Type Cannabinoid Profile
I high THC—low CBD
II high CBD—moderate to high THC
III high CBD—low THC
IV produce propyl cannabinoids in significant amounts (over 5 percent of total cannabinoids) form a fourth group from both type I and II plants

A **multiline** variety is a mixture of 2 or more pure lines of similar phenotype with slightly different genes that are resistant to different qualities such as disease, pest and drought resistance, and early maturity. Multiline varieties of the same or closely similar genotypes are also called isogenic lines. The varieties are grown and bred separately but are later mixed together and sold in the same seed package. The diverse genetics often provide extra disease- and pest-resistance or more acclimatization in inconsistent environment.

In a perfect growing year, a gardener may not reap the highest yield from a multiline as is possible with a single hybrid variety suited to the climate, but the degree of variation present in a multiline helps to ensure that as many plants as possible are harvested. This sophisticated breeding technique is common in vegetable and agricultural crops but has yet to be developed for medicinal cannabis varieties.

A **synthetic variety** is developed by intercrossing several different genotypes that are known to give superior hybrid performance when crossed in all combinations. Synthetic varieties have exceptional hybrid vigor and produce outstanding seed. Synthetic varieties are maintained by open pollination and often recurrent selection in future generations.

(By contrast, a variety developed by mass selection is made up of genotypes bulked together without having undergone preliminary testing to determine their performance in hybrid combination.)

In **single-seed descent,** a plant is self-fertilized and the resulting seed collected. One of these seeds is selected and grown, again self-fertilized, and seed produced. All progeny and future generations have descended from a single ancestor, as long as no pollen from an external family is introduced. Each generation is the result of selfing one individual from the previous generation.

Recurrent selection refers to any breeding program designed to concentrate favorable genes scattered among a number of individuals by repeated cycles of selection for favorable traits.

Ploidy Factor

Cannabis plants are, by nature, diploids with 20 chromosomes. At meiosis, each parent's gamete contributes 10 chromosomes to the zygote they have formed. Cannabis cells may be haploid (have 1 copy of each chromosome set (n) as in gametes, or diploid (2 chromosome sets per cell).

Diploid plants have 1 set of chromosomes ($2n$), which occur in pairs within each plant cell. Diploid plants are considered "normal."

Polyploid plants occur in groups of 3 to 4 instead of in pairs.

Tetraploid plants occur with 4 pairs of chromosomes ($4n$) in each cell.

A few early, poorly researched studies claimed polyploid cannabis as being more THC-potent. To date there have been no studies that prove polyploid plants contain more or higher levels of cannabinoids. I know of no polyploid or tetraploid plants available from any seed supplier.

Polyploid characteristics can be induced with an application of colchicine, a poison. See "Colchicine" in chapter 22, *Additives*, for more information on this poisonous substance.

Applying radiation, alkylating agents, colchicine, or EMS (ethylmethyl-sulfonate) will induce variation, but doing so changes the plant's DNA.

Modern Cannabis Breeding

Modern plant breeding may use techniques of molecular biology to select desirable traits of individual plants or a

Two terminal buds from Mel Frank's 'Kush #4' (1977) demonstrate different phenotypes. The first was grown outdoors under harsh conditions—2,000-foot elevation, very hot days and cold nights, and brutal sun. The second phenotype was grown in his Oakland greenhouse with moderate temperatures and filtered sunlight. (MF)

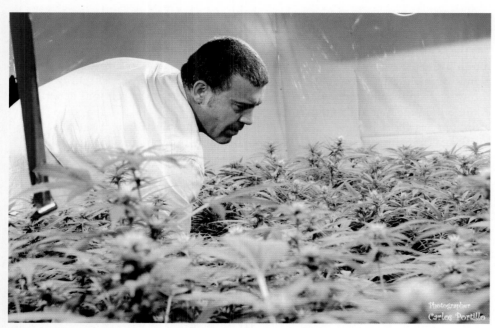

To make breeding selections, Jaime from Resin Seeds uses all of his senses and years of knowledge, along with scientific tests.

population of plants. When biotechnology or **molecular biology** is applied to the plant selection process, it is called molecular breeding.

Molecular markers or DNA fingerprinting can map thousands of genes. Using the process of marker-assisted (or aided) selection (MAS) based on DNA/RNA (deoxyribonucleic acid/ribonucleic acid), variation is used by scientific breeders as an indirect selection tool.

Marker-assisted selection allows breeders to screen large populations of plants for disease resistance, stress tolerance, productivity, and so on. Screening is based on the presence or absence of a specific gene or genes rather than relying on visual observation of a trait in the plant. In MAS, DNA markers are used instead of visual observation to select phenotypes. Marker-assisted selection significantly accelerates the selection process and makes it possible to grow fewer plants for selection. The process can be used at any time in the plant's life cycle. Plants can be tested in the vegetative growth stage and do not need to flower.

Breeding using molecular biology and marker-assisted selection is more complex than first meets the eye. The process allows breeders to measure, select, and cross specific alleles found within the genome. A closer look at MAS reveals that it is the selection of individuals with specific alleles for traits controlled by a limited number of loci (up to 8).

Marker-assisted backcrossing (MABC) is the transfer of a limited number of loci (e.g., transgene, disease resistance loci, etc.) from one genetic background to another.

Marker-assisted recurrent selection (MARS) is the identification and selection of 20 or more genomic regions.

Historically, most of the genetic research for agriculture and commercial flower and vegetable crops has been done in agricultural university laboratories in the USA and other countries. Most all universities in many countries with a good agricultural department are equipped to make all the DNA and RNA tests necessary for a scientific MAS breeding program.

Until the last 10 years, limited marker-assisted selections have been used in cannabis breeding programs. A few years ago only a few large companies such as GW Pharmaceuticals (www.gwpharm.com) were able to use MAS in their breeding programs. They are able to breed for specific cannabinoids. Until recently, molecular biology technology was too expensive, and cannabis cultivation illegal. Today these barriers have been broken and the technology is accessible and legal in various parts of the world. In fact, setting up a small home laboratory is much less expensive than it was a few years ago. For instructions on setting up an inexpensive lab, visit www.marijuanagrowing.com and search "Set Up Cannabis Testing Lab at Home."

Laboratories in medical states and in other countries may be willing to work with medical cannabis breeders to make MAS tests. Agricultural university laboratories may also be receptive to MAS testing of cannabis. There are at least 2 laboratories in the USA that specialize in molecular plant breeding and have worked with cannabis: ACGT, Inc. (www.acgtinc.com/marijuana_genotyping.htm) and Life Technologies (www.invitrogen.com).

Genetic Modification
Genetic modification of plants is achieved by adding a specific gene or genes to a plant, or by knocking down a gene with RNAi (RNA interference) to produce a desirable phenotype. Both processes are expensive and have not been perfected in cannabis.

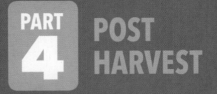

26 MEDICINAL CONCENTRATES & TINCTURES

SEPARATING RESIN GLANDS from foliage concentrates cannabinoids into dry powdered resin glands (kief*); when pressed into blocks the resin concentrate is called hashish or hash. Resin glands can be separated using water. Solvents can be used to separate cannabinoid-rich resin glands from foliage, too. Once separated from foliage, cannabinoids can remain suspended in a solvent such as

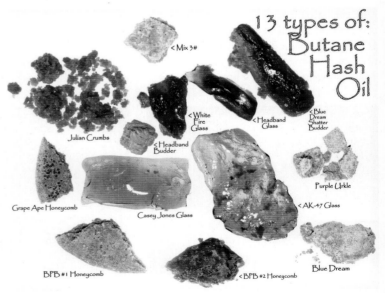

Concentrates come in all shapes, textures, and colors. Todd McCormick of Hempire Media put together this collection of fine hash concentrates that demonstrate different textures and colors.

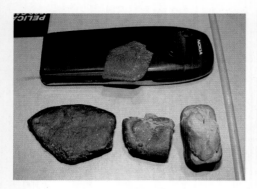

Here are several pieces of pressed resin separated using cold water and sieves.

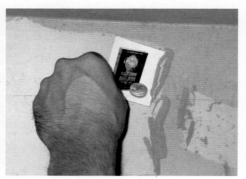

Once separated from buds and leaves, kief is collected.

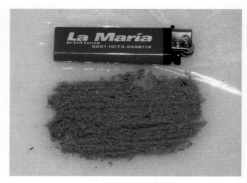

Kief is collected and made ready to press together into hashish.

butter, coconut butter (as a food), or alcohol (as a tincture), or the solvent can be removed so that concentrated oil remains.

Resin glands are oil-based and plant foliage is water-based. The two act differently, and this simple difference has been used for many years to separate resin glands from foliage. The first and most common form of separation is for the oily resin glands to accumulate on fingers and trimming tools. This is commonly referred to as "hand rub" or "finger" hashish.

Resin can be collected by separating it from foliage and letting it fall through a sieve. Or it can be separated from foliage using a combination of cold water and sieves.

Dry cannabis foliage and flower buds can also be sieved to separate resin glands. The resin, bits of foliage, and foreign matter fall through the sieve. The resulting powder below the sieve is

called kief*. Europeans often mistakenly call it "pollen."** This golden-colored resin dust is lightweight. It can easily be collected and pressed lightly together to form a ball. Kief is pressed to form hash.

*Kief** consists of resin glands that are collected after passing through a sieve. Once pressed together it forms hashish, also known as hash. The more resin in the processed cannabis, the more resinous the hashish. This chapter will touch on the basics of making hashish using safe extraction methods. Detailed information on chemical extraction methods using butane, acetate, different alcohols, and toxic dangerous solvents has been omitted because of possible health risks from explosion, fire, and fumes. Chemical damage may result from premature use of the end product before all solvents and residuals have been extracted. You can find much information on these subjects at many Internet sites.

Pollen: In Europe and other parts of the world, sieved resin powder is

called pollen. The term is used because the two look similar, but resin powder is not pollen. When you hear somebody talking about "pollen," you know they are most likely referring to resin powder.

Wet separation uses a similar principle to separate resin from foliage, except cannabis is immersed in cold water before passing through the separation screen. Once separated wet resin is collected and dried.

Resin can also be separated and concentrated with the use of solvents such as petroleum, fats, oils, and CO_2.

When concentrated in an alcohol or oil-based solvent, the solvent is removed and a cannabinoid-potent liquid remains. This liquid, hash, or cannabis oil is usually very dense and increases in viscosity as it warms. The concentrate can also be manipulated with a vacuum to inject air and change the appearance of the end product.

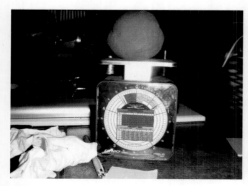

Kief was rolled into a big ball and weighs in at just under 12 ounces (340.2 gm).

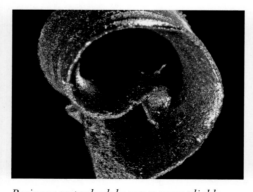

Resinous water hash becomes more pliable when warm.

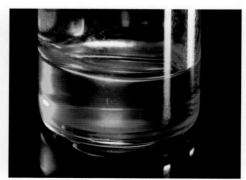

Clear amber denotes purity in concentrated CBD oil.

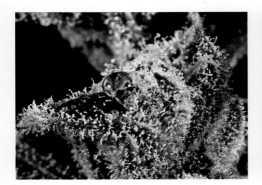

This bud of 'Sour Tsunami' is so resinous that it actually globs together.

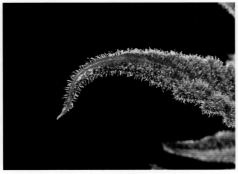

Capture resin glands with small heads by using a smaller mesh sieve.

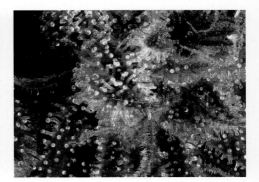

Sativa-dominant varieties often have smaller heads on capitate-stalked resin glands than indica-dominant varieties have. Smaller mesh sieves do a good job of separating smaller resin heads.

Before Making Hashish

Make sure your plants are as clean as possible before you begin to make hashish. Remove all stems and large or damaged leaves. Any oil-based residues on leaves will show up in the separated resin glands. For example, if extracting resin with water, you can see impurity residues as sheen of oil on the surface of the water. During the month before harvest, do not use any harmful chemicals that leave residues. To avoid potential health risks after harvest, I prefer to use only water-based organic products.

Leach growing medium with water for 5 days before harvest to remove built-up fertilizers in the soil and foliage. This will help ensure clean, sweet-tasting hash.

See chapter 9, *Harvest, Drying & Curing*, for more on washing plants with hydrogen peroxide (H_2O_2) at harvest.

Freeze First: Once dry, freeze cannabis to prepare for making kief and pressing it into hashish. Place leaves in a paper bag or cardboard box in the freezer for an hour or longer. Remove them from the freezer, and use a dry or wet sieve to separate gland heads from foliage. Freezing makes it possible to collect more resin by making foliage and resin glands brittle. Cold, brittle resin glands snap off and separate easily from foliage.

The yield from 7 ounces (198.4 gm) of leaves and small buds is between 0.2 and 0.7 ounces (5.7–19.8 gm) with the average around 0.36 ounces (10.2 gm). The quantity of hash produced depends upon the quality of the original material. Clean stems, large leaves with no visible resin, dead material, and any debris from leaves and buds before making kief. Male plants do contain resin with THC but much less overall than is contained by female plants. Outdoor plants are subject to wind, rain, and dust, which may prevent resin growth or cause much of the resin to be knocked off the plant. Plants protected in indoor and greenhouse environments exude as much resin as possible. Such plants with heavy resin are best for kief-making. Great hash also comes from the closely trimmed leaves around buds.

Keep the entire hash operation clean. This is the key to keeping everything separated properly and having minimal contamination.

Yield Per Ounce/Gram of Leaf and Small Buds

Quantity of Leaf
3.53 oz (100 gm)

Dry Sieve
0.14–0.21 oz (4–6 gm)

Water Extraction
0.21–0.283 (6–8 gm)

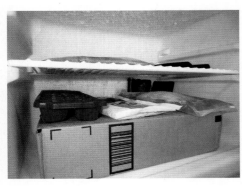

Place cannabis leaves and buds to be made into hash in a cardboard box in the freezer.

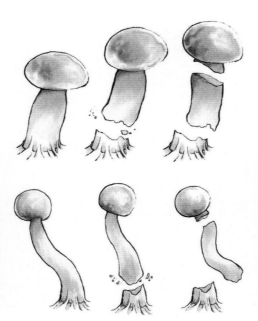

Resin glands generally break off near the bottom of the stalk and just under the round head.

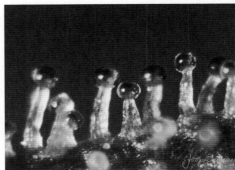

Indica-dominant varieties often have larger resin heads with short, stout stocks.

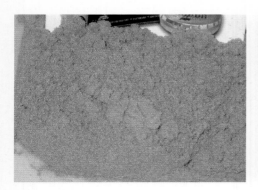

Dry-separated resin is passed through sieves. It retains natural fragrances and flavors.

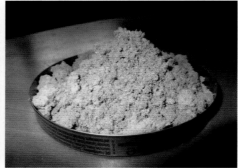

This big batch of resin was collected from leaves. In earlier days it would have been tossed out with the leaves!

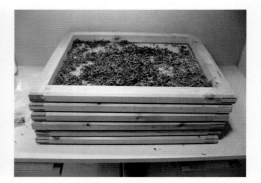

This box of sieves makes dry-sieving cannabis easy. Each sieve below is a different size mesh to collect different grades of resin.

Dry Separation

Many hash-makers prefer dry separation because with this method the natural resin fragrances are retained. Dry-sieve kief is not as concentrated as water-extracted hash. Along with plants' essential fragrances, dry kief retains more contaminants—plant matter, stigmas, insect parts, dirt, and so forth.

The resin is simply sifted through a sieve or a series of fine sieves. Resin heads are different sizes. With the help of different-sized sieves, you can use the differences in resin head sizes to separate them from other plant matter. Typically, a minimum of two sieves is used to make hash. The first one filters out the large plant matter and larger debris, letting the resin glands and small debris pass through to the second sieve.

The first sieve should have approximately 110- to 150-micron pores. The second sieve allows small resin glands to pass, while it holds back large, mature resin glands. The pores on the second sieve should have 60- to 150-micron pores. You can find silkscreens at your local

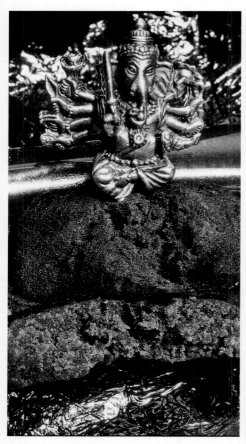

This sieved resin from 1999 has been pressed into hashish.

CONVERSION TABLE FOR SIEVE OPENINGS

US Mesh	Inches	Microns μ	Millimeters
40	0.0165	400	0.400
45	0.0138	354	0.354
50	0.0117	297	0.297
60	0.0098	250	0.250
70	0.0083	210	0.210
80	0.0070	177	0.177
100	0.0059	149	0.149
120	0.0049	125	0.125
140	0.0041	105	0.105
170	0.0035	88	0.088
200	0.0029	74	0.074
230	0.0024	63	0.063
270	0.0021	53	0.053
325	0.0017	44	0.044
400	0.0015	37	0.037

A micron = one millionth of a meter (1/1,000,000 m) or one-thousandth of a millimeter (1/1000 mm) or a micrometer or the symbol for micron "μ" hobby and art supply store. Printing supply stores also sell framed screens.

The sieves can be stretched out flat and fastened to a frame or stretched over a cylinder to form a tumbler. (Tumblers are typically automated.)

Sieves

Sieves are made from woven wire, nylon (silkscreen), and laser-cut metal. Wire screens generally have wider openings and are made from various materials, including stainless steel. Nylon silkscreen is the most common sieve material used for resin separation. It is relatively inexpensive, durable, and the sizes of the small micron holes are relatively consistent. Laser-cut sieves are much more expensive and are not used by skilled hash-makers. Check this link for an example, http://www.precisioneforming.com.

In the USA, the number of openings across 1 inch is the mesh size. For example, a "5 mesh screen" means there are 5 little squares across 1 linear inch (2.5 cm) of screen. A 100 mesh screen has 100 openings.

Mesh size is not precise, relative to particle size. Screens are made with different thicknesses of wire, which causes the holes in the sieve to change size too. Wires are closer on fine-weave mesh. If the weave is too fine there is no space between wires. Sieve mesh is rated with a "–" or "+". For example, –100 mesh aluminum means all particles would pass through a 100 mesh screen. A +100 mesh means all particles are retained on a 100 mesh screen.

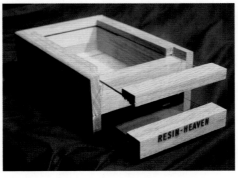

The Resin Heaven from Portland, Oregon, USA, was the first rolling tray equipped with a screen to collect resin. This device has spawned countless similar products.

Make sure sieves are labeled with the micron size. Color-coding helps too.

Flat Sieves

A flat screen can be stretched taut and fastened to the frame. Find nylon silk-screen and frame at your local art supply store. Or you can also buy prefabricated screens and frames at art supply stores for screen-printing. Or you can find one through many retailers on the Internet. Always use monofilament rather than multifilament mesh. Frames of different micron sizes can be stacked on top of one another to render different qualities of kief. Do not use pantyhose or any similar filters.

To sieve, plants should be as dry as possible and cold (about 41°F [5°C]) so resin glands break off easily. Be careful not to force plant material through the sieve. Forcing will break more resin glands and smear their contents on the sieve and other plant material. The contents of these ruptured glands

cannot be recovered. Normally, the largest mature resin glands fall first. They are followed by less-mature glands and debris, including pistillate hairs and plant debris. If you force too much through the sieve, much green matter passes; the resulting hash will be green and of low quality.

Atmospheric relative humidity can slow the sieving process to a halt because it causes the pores of the sieve to clog. High humidity also remoistens dry plants, thus making it more difficult for resin to fall free.

Once prepared, break up buds and foliage over a sieve, and tap the sieve lightly to jostle resin heads through the pores. You can also rub the leaves lightly on the sieve, but this will force through more green foliage and other contaminants. Resin powder will sift through the screen. The more resin on the plant material, the more resin that will fall through the sieve. Use a credit card to move the cannabis back and forth across the sieve. Exert minimal pressure on the cannabis to coax the highest-quality resin through the sieve. The first layer of powder will be the purest. Sieved hash contains more debris than most other methods, but sieving is a simple and inexpensive method to make hash.

Remember, there are several sizes of resin glands. Use the appropriate screen size to collect the most resin powder for the varieties you are processing. Fine *sativa* glands can be collected with a 70-micron sieve. A 110-micron sieve is the best all-around sieve, and

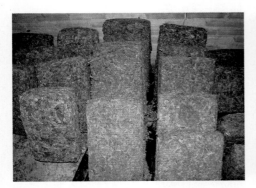

These bails of Mexican cannabis were pressed tightly together and many of the resin glands were compressed and ruptured.

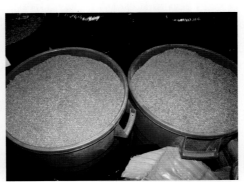

The bails were broken up into a powder, which further broke down the resin glands and mixed them with green matter.

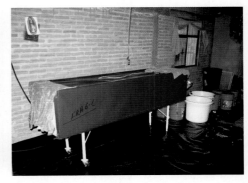

This version of the 6.5-foot-long (2 m) Pollinator works great to make hash.

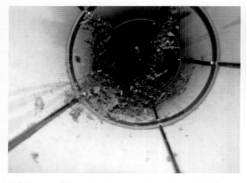

The cannabis spins down a long sloped tube made from fine-mesh sieve material.

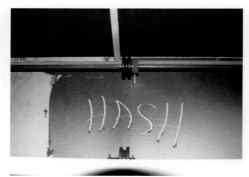

Scrape the resin from the bottom of the box. Collect the dry resin, and press it into hash.

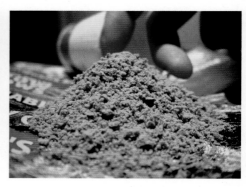

Water-extracted hash after it has been dried

a 150-micron sieve is best for very resinous varieties.

Sift hash through screen. Let drop onto paper with a piece of cardboard below. The dry paper and cardboard will help draw the moisture out of the separated resin glands.

Collect the powder below the sieve. Now the resin powder is ready to press into a piece of hash. Pressing generates a little heat, which also helps the resin glands and debris congeal.

Tumbler Sieves

Mila, owner of the Pollinator in Amsterdam, Holland, and a good friend, has spent much of her life learning and teaching how to extract more resin from cannabis. She invented and popularized the Pollinator, a motorized cylindrical sieve to separate resin powder from leaf and buds.

The Pollinator consists of a drum that turns inside a box. Cold, dried cannabis is placed inside the drum that is made from 150-micron screen. A motor turns the drum, and resin glands fall through the screen as the cannabis tumbles inside. Resin is

collected below the drum. Today there are several other devices that use the same principles.

Highest-quality resin falls through the screen first. Progressively lower-quality resin falls through the mesh the longer the drum turns. More green matter and other adulterants fall through the screen when the Pollinator turns for longer periods of time.

But first the dry cannabis must be prepared. The leaf must be bone-dry so that it does not gum up the sieve. Put super dry cannabis in the freezer for 2 hours, until it freezes. This will make

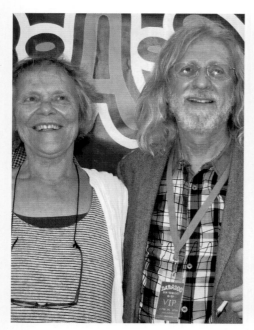

Mila, from the Pollinator in Amsterdam, hosted the Dab-a-Doo celebration in Berkeley, California. Jorge Cervantes is pictured on the right.

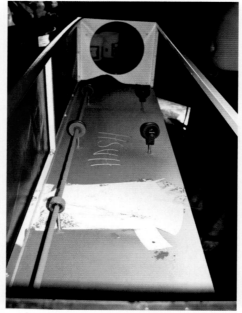

Once the process is complete, the sieve is removed and the hash remains.

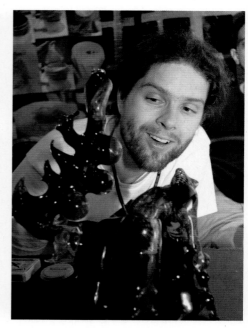

Bubble Man continues to contribute to and innovate in the world of cannabis concentrates.

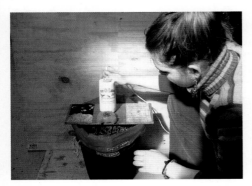

Making hash with one of the original Ice-O-Lator setups

hours. The kief falls through the sieve and is collected afterward.

Water-Extracted Resin

Resin (glands) extracted using cold water is known as water hash, ice hash, or Ice-O-Lator hash. Very pure hash will bubble and release volatile resins when exposed to a flame, hence the name *bubble-hash*. This boiling effect is called "full-melt bubble."

Mila continued to play with the separation method and refined it. Within a short time, she combined the dry sieving process with ice-cold water; the outcome was Ice-O-Lator bags. They are 3 waterproof nylon bags with progressively smaller micron silkscreens sewn into the bottom of each. Clean cannabis is chopped and placed in ice-cold water in the bags. The water is mixed. When the slurry settles, the resin glands pass through the screens, and the foliage and debris are retained in bags. The water is drained, and a few nice clumps of high-quality hash remain.

Bubble Man refined the process by adding more bags with progressively smaller mesh. He uses 7 different screens to sieve resin. He found that each screen separates unique sediments, some of

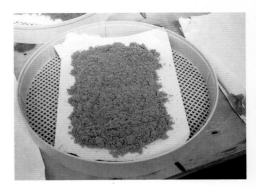

Once processed and separated, residual hash is left to dry.

which contain exceptionally pure THC. This hash is so pure that it bubbles when heated. Bubble Man popularized this saying, "If it don't bubble, it ain't worth the trouble."

Water-soluble terpenoids found in cannabis resin contribute to fragrance and taste. The majority of these soluble terpenoids dissolve and are washed out when extracting resin with water. The result is often hash with little flavor and aroma.

Now the hash is out of the bag! Many manufacturers have jumped

the cannabis resin glands separate more easily from the foliage and make the sieving process much more efficient and productive.

Let the drum turn for 2 to 5 minutes. Use a short-range kitchen timer to avoid running the drum for too long. As the drum turns, the purest cannabinoid-rich resin falls through the screen first, onto the bottom of the box underneath the drum.

Pollinators and similar devices place cannabis in an enclosed drum that spins for a few minutes to several

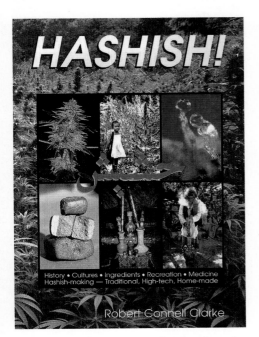

The book HASHISH! *was a landmark work.*

Sadu Sam

Modern water hash extraction started with "Sadu Sam's Secret" that was published in *HASHISH!* by Robert Connell Clarke. Sadu Sam's Secret is simple physics: resin is oil-based, and cannabis foliage is water-based. This difference makes separating the two in aqueous solution easy. Heavy, oil-soluble resin glands will not dissolve in water; they are heavier than water so they will sink. Water-soluble material dissolves in liquid, and foliage is lighter than water, which makes it float!

A passage from *HASHISH!* states, "Sadu Sam's Secret involves stirring a few grams of pulverized flowers or freshly sieved resin powder into a tall container of cool water containing ten to twenty times the volume of water to dry powder. Cool or cold water is essential because warm water softens the resin, which tends to stick together forming an unmanageable lump. The mixture must be stirred vigorously for several minutes until the lumps of the powder disperse. Once stirring ceases, the differing particles in the suspension begin to separate. Plant particles and other light debris (such as plant "hairs") float to the surface. Small, immature resin glands also tend to float. Mature resin glands and any dense debris such as sand and mineral dust sink, settling to the bottom." You can still use this method to separate resin from foliage.

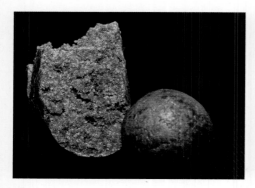

When pressed, Ice-O-Lator resin sticks together into easy-to-manage hash.

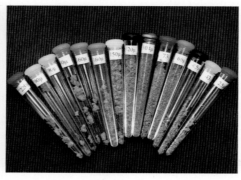

This is the 19 grams (6.7 oz) that my friend Mono separated from 100 grams (3.53 oz) of resinous leaf. There are 14 vials, one for each bag. The 15th bag or "work bag" is not counted because it retains the bulk of the leaf material.

4. 120μ bag – good bubble

5. 160μ bag – best for big-headed *indica* glands. Debris can also settle here.

6. 190μ bag – removes the majority of the big debris from the settling process

7. 220μ bag – is the first filter where all the big stuff stays

Washing Machine Hashish

Using a washing machine rather than a bucket and an egg beater, to separate resin from leaf saves labor. A large machine is necessary to make big runs of water hash. A big machine saves hours of labor. Use a small machine to make runs of up to a half pound (226.8 gm).

For complete examples, please see *Marijuana Horticulture: the Indoor/ Outdoor Medical Grower's Bible*, chapter 15, *Hash and Oil Making*, "Washing Machine Hash."

Carbon Dioxide (CO$_2$) Extraction

In this extraction process, dry CO_2 literally freezes resin glands, making them easy to shake loose from foliage.

Properly set up CO_2 extraction is very efficient. Large-scale extraction would

on the bandwagon. Your time and budget will dictate how many bags you want to use for making water hash.

Use 3 bags and process the mix twice to extract the bulk of the THC-rich resin. Keep the wet plant material from the first water hash extraction. Freeze it and process again to extract more resin. Or you can use 5 or more bags in a single run and harvest different qualities, some of which are very pure.

Use leaves that have visible resin. Using large fan leaves or immature leaves will result in disappointing hash.

This method calls for a mixer with paddles. Note that paddles can bruise resin glands. If you can, find one with long shanks on the paddles for easy, deep mixing in a 5-gallon (18.9 L) bucket. You can cover the bucket when mixing to help contain splashes. However, moving the mixer around the perimeter of the slurry helps mix up any dry or stagnant places.

When you press powder, the resin crystals will break and the oil will be released. The mix will darken as it oxidizes. The resin crystals from very fresh leaf will remain white, a very high quality. For more information see www.pollinator.nl.

For complete examples, please see *Marijuana Horticulture: the Indoor/ Outdoor Medical Grower's Bible*, chapter 15, *Hash and Oil Making*, "Ice-O-Lator Instructions" and "Water Hash with 15 Bags."

More wet sieves separate more and different qualities of cannabis resin. Resin heads are different sizes and therefore fall through different size pores in a sieve. You can separate different sizes of resin glands with wet or dry sieves having progressively smaller sized pores.

The "work bag" is the one that contains the bulk of the processed, resinless leaf. The work bag is usually drained and set aside so the debris inside can be discarded at will. Bags with rigid sides perform better because they retain their shape inside the bucket and are easier to use when only one person is making water hash.

The hash-laden water that is left over after passing through six bags is separated again by running it through eight more bags. The resulting hash is very clean.

When starting with 100 grams (3.53 oz) of pretty good leaf from a resinous variety, using water extraction with 15 sieves you should be able to separate out 10 to 15 grams (0.35-0.53 oz).

This synopsis was adapted from Bubble Man's postings on www.overgrow.com (now closed).

1. 25μ bag – most often full of *sativa* full-melt and physically the smallest bag

2. 45μ bag – nice head hash, most often consistent and yellowish to white in color

3. 73μ bag – full melt all the way

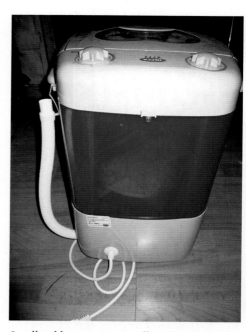

Small, tabletop, 5- to 10-gallon (18.9–37.9 L) washing machines are available at hydroponic and discount stores, and on the Internet. The agitator in these small machines works like a lawn sprinkler and does not rip and tear foliage.

function under high pressure and have precision tolerances to get the most out of the separation process. When CO_2 is used as a solvent, it requires much pressure (73.8 bar [1070.38 psi]), and the initial setup is expensive. Please see www.marijuanagrowing.com for more information on using CO_2 as a solvent to concentrate cannabis resin. Most people are interested in small-scale separation.

Supercritical fluid extraction (SFE) is the most precise way to extract not only cannabinoids, but essential oils as well, and is a means of separating different elements of botanicals. Herbal essential oils, hops for beer, pharmaceutical precursors, and decaffeinated coffee are all processed using SFE.

The supercritical fluid extraction method forces a solvent (CO_2) through plant matter under high pressure. When the solvent is pushed through the plant matter at such a high pressure, it can separate the matter precisely, which allows us to isolate only the purest essence of our botanicals—in this case, cannabis. The result is pure, transparent, amber oil.

Supercritical CO_2* has high diffusion rates which allow it to penetrate solids faster than a liquid solvent. Naturally occurring carbon dioxide leaves no residue. Other popular solvents used to extract resin, such as butane, can leave heavy metal residues in the extracted resin.

*See http://en.wikipedia.org/wiki/ Supercritical_carbon_dioxide

Dry ice is solidified CO_2 gas. When frozen, CO_2 is super cold and must be kept in a special freezer that is even colder. It sublimes (transforms from a solid to a gas) and evaporates into the atmosphere. Dry-ice extraction freezes off resin glands. The frozen glands fall through a 120 to 220 mesh sieve and are collected below.

A 5-pound, solid piece of dry ice costs $15 to $20 USD. If kept in a freezer overnight, dry ice will lose up to half of its weight. For most people, using frozen CO_2 to separate resin is too ex-

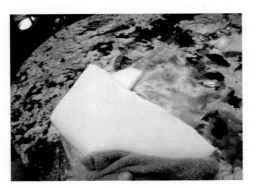

A chunk of dry ice is actually frozen CO_2 gas.

pensive to be practical. And it is so cold that it can burn skin on contact. Always handle with gloves.

Dry ice is easy to use. Cover a 5-gallon plastic bucket with a 120 to 220 mesh sieve Bubble Bag normally used to make water hash.

The final product can be of many grades. The first few shakes will yield the highest quality. The smaller sieves (120, 160, etc.) let less green matter through. Larger mesh (200, 220, etc.) lets a lot through!

Always shake over a large, flat mirror or large, smooth surface. Such an area makes it easy to scrape up kief.

Dry Ice Kief: Step-by-Step
Step One: Place a few chunks of dry ice in a can or container. Add about 3 times as much leaf and small buds to the container with the dry ice. Let the pieces of dry ice mix with the pre-chilled cannabis so that it freezes resin glands. The cannabis should be as intact as possible. Do not grind it up.

Step Two: Place a Bubble Bag (or something similar) with a 160 mesh sieve at the bottom over the container. The sieve end of the bag should cover the container opening. The bag may fit completely over the container. Secure the bubble bag so its screen is taut over the opening.

Step Three: Shake the CO_2 cannabis mixture in the can so the chunks of dry ice break up and freeze the pre-

cooled cannabis.

Step Four: Turn the container upside down so the sieve is facing the mirror below. Shake the container for a few seconds or up to 5 minutes. White vapor emerges from the container as the CO_2 sublimes and resin glands slide through the sieve onto the mirror.

The first couple of shakes you'll get top-quality resin glands. The resulting powder progressively turns to green leaf matter. Shake the container a few times so that the highest-quality kief passes through the sieve. Collect this kief before progressing to the next grade. Repeat process as many times as desired.

Step Five: Remove any remaining pieces of dry ice. Scrape kief from sieve and inside the container onto the mirror. Scrape kief that fell through sieve into a pile. Store the kief in a glass container and use for cooking. The hash is lower quality and contains contaminants. But the cannabinoids are concentrated in the final product.

In simple experiments, this method yields 15 to 18 percent or more final kief. As with any kief, the end product is contingent on the original buds. Resinous buds make the best kief. Lower-quality leaf and buds make lower-quality kief. This process is an easy way to store large quantities of leaf and small buds that might otherwise go to waste.

Storing Separated Resin
Make sure hash is completely dry before storing. Moist hash contracts fungus easily and decomposes quickly. Decomposition decreases THC levels. If you make hash using ice and water, be careful to dry it well. Dry by pressing the water hash into a flat pancake that has much surface area. Leave the pancake out in an arid room for a few days to dry completely. Cover the hash with a paper towel so dust does not contaminate it. If you made hash with a dry method such as sieving, you should not have to take any extra precautions before storing, unless you are working in a humid climate.

My favorite way to store high-quality water hash is to put it in a glass tube. This way all the resin stays intact until it

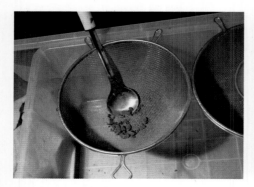
Semidry water hash is passed through a strainer to help remove moisture locked inside larger pieces.

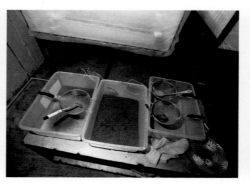
Once resin passes through the large sieve, it is collected and left to dry in containers for a few days.

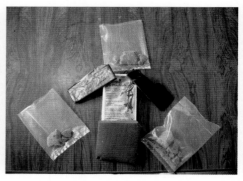
Dry resin is pressed into slabs. The two dark pieces in the middle top contain the most resin.

is consumed. Upon smoking, you should press it a little so it will burn evenly. Store hash in a cool, dark, dry place. Keep in an airtight container with a packet of silica crystals. You can also put hash in the freezer for long-term storage.

For a complete account of the history and detailed methods of production, see *HASHISH!* by Robert Connell Clarke, (Redeye Press, 1998), www.fsbookco. com. If you want to make the best hash and have a springboard to launch into advanced processes, this is the book for you!

Pressing Hashish
Once collected, kief (resin powder) is often pressed into hash to facilitate handling and storage. Bulky resin powder is awkward to handle. It is easily spilled, blown away, or contaminated by dust and dirt. Kief is also more difficult to smoke, especially if no screen is available.

Once pressed into a piece of hash, however, the resin is easy to handle, store, transport, and consume. Proper pressing is essential for easy handling, storage, and to slow decomposition. Pressing determines how hash will burn and also affects taste and smell.

Small amounts of hash can be pressed by hand (hand rub); larger amounts will need to be pressed with an object such as a bottle or rolling pin. Mechanical presses are able to apply more pressure. Hydraulic presses apply the most pressure to make larger pieces.

Pressing hash creates heat that fuses resin glands together. Heating resin with a hair dryer is not necessary with pure resin. If heat is applied, a drop or two of water or alcohol can be added while pressing to make less-pure hash stick together in a block. The idea is to heat the hash a little but not melt it, keeping the heat level constant. This will help the resin bond together.

Regardless of how the resin glands are pressed, they must be contained in cellophane plastic. The cellophane is essential because the resin does not stick to this type of plastic. Do not use more durable plastic found in Ziploc bags or the resin will stick to it. Use inexpensive cellophane.

Mechanical presses must be precise and align well so pressed hash does not ooze out seams of cellophane bags. When pressed, heat and friction cause the outer layer of pressed hash to oxidize and turn darker than the interior. In fact, hash can have a dark exterior and a blonde interior packed with creamy resin glands.

Pressing Small Amounts of Hashish
By hand pressing, you experience the transformation of the resin powder into your very own piece of fragrant, dense hash. To hand press, collect one to four grams of resin powder in the palm of your hand and apply pressure to the

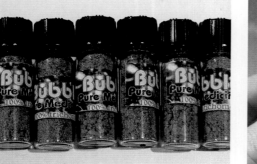
Store dry resin pieces in small containers for easy transport and consumption.

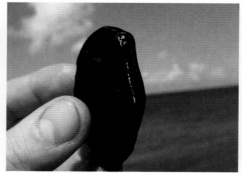
Pressing ruptures resin glands and warms the resin, causing many volatile aromatic terpenoids to release their aromas but many flavors are held in the pressed hashish.

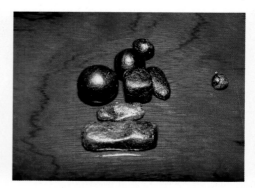
This bubble-hash is so resinous that machine pressing is not necessary. All these pieces have been worked into shapes by hand.

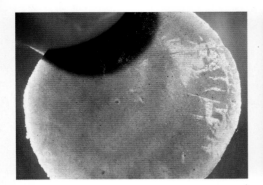

A small hand press makes nice little hash wafers.

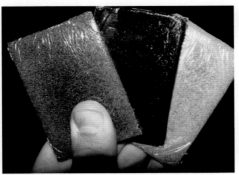

Here are three different kief collections pressed into hash, still in the cellophane bags used for pressing. Make sure to pre-press water-extracted hash in a piece of cellophane to contain it and help get rid of the water. The cellophane will give the pressed hash a shiny skin.

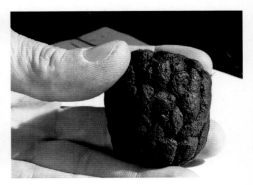

This piece of "finger hash" was scraped from fingers and trimming tools in a single day of trimming!

powder, working it between the palms of your hands. Also push your thumb into your palm full of resin powder to work it into a piece of hash. Continue this process for 10 to 30 minutes until the piece of hash is completely pliable and whole. Heat will be generated and help rupture and meld the resin glands together. Relatively pure resin powder will congeal faster than less-potent powders that contain impurities. But a little vegetable matter and debris gives hash different flavors and more body.

Potent resin powder is a creamy white to gold in color. Pressing the powder together and working it in your hands ruptures and oxidizes resin glands, which makes the mass turn ever darker.

Hand-Rub Hash
Hand-rubbing hash is simple and easy but horridly inefficient and wasteful. All you need to hand-rub are a good pair of hands, adequate cannabis buds,

and desire. Much of the resin falls to the ground or becomes "lost" deep within buds or it sticks to other foliage. Overall, hand-rubbed hash is lower quality and contains more debris than sieved or water-extracted hash.

Hand-rubbing is most common in the Himalayan foothill regions of Nepal, India, and Kashmir where "charas" (the Indian word for [hand-rubbed] hash) is fairly popular. Most small-scale and commercial growers collect the little bit of hash from their hands and tools during manicuring. This is the closest thing to hand-rubbed hash most growers experience.

Plants that are best suited to hand-rubbing have sticky resin that adheres to hands much better than it sticks to other foliage. At the same time, the resin must be relatively easy to roll into little balls to remove from hands.

Collect hand rub from healthy, strong, mature plants with green leaves. Some large leaves may already have started to turn yellow. Remove brown, crisp, and dead foliage before rubbing. Remember, cannabis plants are generally pretty tough and can take vigorous (but not abusive) rubbing.

Once collected on hands, resin must not be allowed to collect other debris or foliage. Any foreign matter that sticks to resin-laden hands should be able to be brushed off easily.

Gather resin by rubbing individual flowering branches firmly between hands. Slowly move hands up from the bud, continually rubbing back and forth.

Rub palms and fingers in between resin-covered flower clusters so they come in contact with as much resin as possible. Each branch should be rubbed for 20 seconds or more. After rubbing

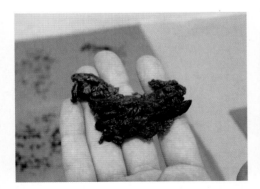

Small pieces of resin accumulate on hands, gloves, and trimming tools. This resin is scraped up and consolidated.

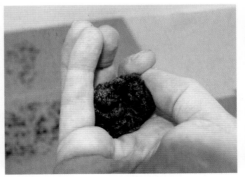

Once in hand, the small pieces of resin are molded together. The body heat generated by the hand and light pressing melds the small pieces together.

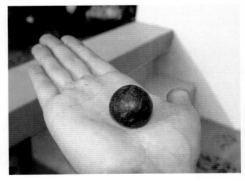

After a few minutes of handwork, the pieces of hand-rub hash form a spherical ball that is easy to store, transport and use.

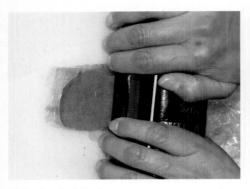

Use a bottle full of warm water to press resin powder between two pieces of cellophane. The heat and pressure from the bottle will heat the resin so that it sticks together. The cellophane keeps the resin in place during pressing and serves to protect the hashish afterward.

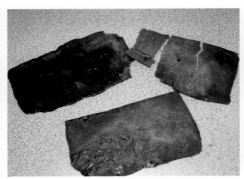

These thin pieces of potent hash were pressed between cellophane using an office laminator.

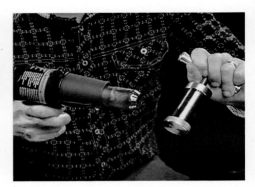

Add a little heat to hard-to-press hash that contains impurities. The heat will help the mass congeal so bricks do not need excessive pressure to stay together. But remember that pressing also increases heat; do not heat the resin too much or it will be damaged.

a few branches, you settle into an intoxicating, hypnotic rhythm. Aromatic fragrances are released as you rub the buds.

The resin sticks to hands slowly at first, but once they are covered with a light sheen of resin, the accumulation process speeds. Brush off any foliage or debris from hands as soon as it sticks so the resin remains reasonably pure.

To remove the resin from hands, rub your palms together so resin clusters together into sticky little balls. At first the resin will ball up relatively quickly. Lump the balls together to form a single piece. Use this piece to rub on resin that is still on your hand to help remove it. If hands are moist or sweaty, soak up moisture with a paper towel before removing hash.

Once collected, knead resin in your hand until it reaches your desired consistency. Hand-rubbed hash is best enjoyed within a few weeks of collection. Collecting hand-rubbed resin is time consuming. An average collector can rub all day and collect a mere 5 to 10 grams!

Bottle Pressing

Press small amounts of resin powder between cellophane to form a pancake. Fill a long cylindrical bottle with warm water and use it as a "rolling pin" to press the pancake of hash. The extra heat from the warm water will help loosen and blend the kief into hashish.

Use a laminator—the kind that overlays photos and documents between 2 sheets of plastic—to press hashish. Sprinkle the best resin powder, kief, you can make onto a piece of cellophane. Lay another piece of cellophane on top. Roll over it with a bottle full of warm water to get it into preliminary shape and make it easy to work. Remove the piece of hash from the cellophane; treat it like you would a document and laminate it. Laminating machines usually have a heat control that helps with pressing hash.

Mechanical Pressing

Place resin powder in a plastic bag or cellophane wrapper to contain it while pressing. All the powder will be pressed within the wrapper into a brick or plaque of hash. Poke a few small pinholes in the bag before pressing to allow trapped air to escape. The bag is placed into a heavy-duty steel mold, and pressure is applied with a hydraulic jack. Hydraulic jacks have a capacity from 10 to 20 tons and are mounted to heavy-

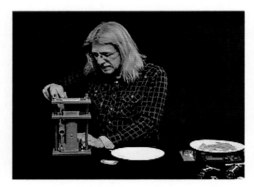

Use a hydraulic press to press larger amounts (50–100 gm) of kief into hashish.

duty steel frames that normally contain a 100-gram mold.

The pressure exerted to form a cohesive block is contingent upon the volume of contaminants in the powder. The more pure the resin powder, the less pressure it takes to form it into a block.

If your hash was made with water, make sure it is totally dry before pressing, to avoid mold. Water hash does not react like dry-sieved hash when pressed. Resin has been melded together in a different way than dry powder. Pressing the resin when it is wet will trap moisture inside the hash. The hash will not dry completely, and it will not properly gel together later. It will retain a powdery consistency.

Dry-sieved resin powder will press easily and stay together under lower pressure when it is relatively pure. If it is adulterated with impurities, more pressure and heat will be necessary to press it into a block.

You can also add a drop of alcohol in the form of brandy, whiskey, bourbon, rum, etc., to help meld the glands together. Spirits with higher alcohol content are favored. Be careful to add only a drop at a time; alcohol takes a few minutes to completely penetrate and act.

Hammering Hashish

Hammering hash is a popular pressing method in Morocco but uncommon elsewhere. Hammering bursts and blends resin glands together into a cohesive mass.

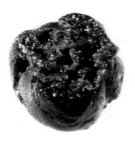

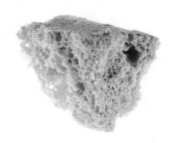

'Granddaddy Purple' (left) and Head Cheese' (right) are two examples of "wax"—concentrated resin containing cannabinoids that have been extracted with solvent, usually butane. Harmful residual chemicals from butane hash oil (BHO) are purged by placing it in a vacuum under controlled conditions. Texture, color, and structure of the wax are governed by the duration and exposure to vacuum pressure and heat.

Often resin glands are hammered before being hydraulically pressed into plaques.

To hammer hash, pour resin powder into an extra-heavy-duty plastic bag. Place the bag on a wooden board and top it with another board. Whack the board with a hammer until the resin powder forms a cohesive pancake. Remove the hash from the bag and fold once or twice to make it smaller and thicker. Repeat hammering and folding until resin glands transform into a sticky piece of hash. Hammering will heat the resin, but apply a little heat if the hash is slow to form.

Online resources: Supplies and equipment for making kief or water hash:
www.GreenHarvest.ca
www.BubbleBag.com
www.IceCold.org

Concentrated Cannabis Resin

Hash oil is a concentrate of hash or cannabis (cannabis oil) that has been dis-solved in a solvent. The ingredients are combined, the mix "cooks" for a time, and the cannabinoids are later separated from the liquid solvent. The solvent is usually removed by evaporation, leaving concentrated cannabis. Impurities can be filtered, but the process takes longer.

More if not all residual butane, other solvents and impurities can be purged in a vacuum chamber. Once purged of impurities, concentrated resin takes on a new texture and is often referred to as wax, earwax, budder, shatter, and crumble.

Nasty hydrocarbon solvents such as ether and alcohol are used to extract cannabinoids. When improperly processed, cannabis, hashish cannabis, and hemp oils retain residues from solvents used to extract cannabinoids. These residual solvents are often locked in chemically. Such solvent residues pose a health risk. The residual is a sludge that contains chlorophyll, plant waxes, other debris, and cannabinoids. These residues are a health risk when inhaled. **I do not recommend volatile solvent extraction because it requires the use of dangerous chemical solvents.**

Explaining in detail how to make solvent-based cannabis concentrates and oils is beyond the scope of this book. **I do not like such concentrates because the residuals are often difficult to remove.** There are numerous videos on YouTube and website forums that explain in detail many of these processes.

Hydrocarbons are released when using petroleum products to extract resin. The process is usually finalized by boiling or evaporating off the solvent. Ventilation must be adequate, and the heat source should be electric. An open flame is out of the question. Fire and explosions are a reality!

Cannabis oils can be very concentrated and potent. Honey oil was popular in America in the early 1970s. The oil was a translucent golden-amber color. The oil transformed from stiff, toffee-like consistency to runny oil when warmed. Today there are many different cannabis and hashish oils.

Cannabis oils that are greenish in color contain chlorophyll; dark colors signify other contaminants. Filtering the oil through charcoal will remove most of the impurities. Hashish oils never became super popular because they are inconvenient to consume, and many people do not want to be exposed to the

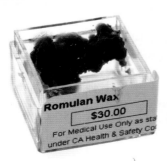

'Romulan' wax

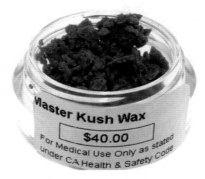

'Master Kush' wax

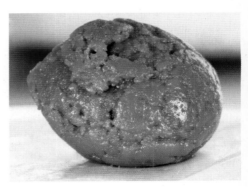

"Maui Wowie" wax

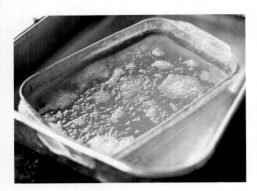

Boiling extract mixes to remove solvents from concentrate almost always leaves solvents locked in residuals.

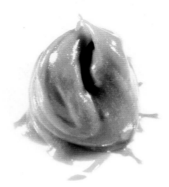

Golden Buddha oil is a popular concentrate at California medical cannabis dispensaries.

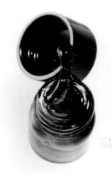

Hash oil has a high concentration of cannabinoids.

health risks associated with the solvents used for processing.

Making cannabis oil is easy, though. First the solvent and cannabis are combined. Next the cannabinoids migrate chemically to the solvent. This could take a few minutes to a couple of months. Later the solvent-laden cannabis mix is placed in an open container to evaporate. Once the solvent is completely evaporated, the concentrated cannabis oil remains.

Solvent efficiency is dictated by its chemical properties and purity. Overall the polarity of a solvent determines what it is able to dissolve. Solvents are polar, nonpolar and semipolar. Extract cannabinoid molecules only with nonpolar solvents. Nonpolar solvents dissolve only oil-based resin and the resulting concentrate is a rich honey color. Polar solvents extract only water-soluble plant

material molecules including chlorophyll. Semipolar solvents extract oil-soluble cannabinoids and water-soluble plant material. The contaminants—water soluble plant material including chlorophyll—cause a green color and taste. Impurities include water and commercial additives combined with the solvent during manufacturing and can be an issue with industrial solvents.

Butane and hexane are non-polarity solvents and extract only cannabinoid molecules. Butane and hexane are the most common solvents used to make concentrated cannabis oil.

Isopropyl alcohol, methanol alcohol, and ethyl alcohol are all semipolar solvents and extract both cannabis resin and plant material. A higher concentration of alcohol with few contaminants will extract the greatest amount of canna-

binoids. For example high-grade ethyl alcohol (95%) has only 5 percent water to dissolve plant matter.

Solvents
Butane (nonpolar)
Severely hazardous

Very flammable

Highly explosive

Boiling point: 31.1°F (-0.5°C)

Flash point: -76°F (-60°C)

Butane is a non-polar solvent that does not dissolve plant material. Butane hash oil (BHO) is made by passing butane gas through chopped cannabis in an enclosed container. Butane dissolves cannabinoids very quickly. The liquefied, butane-laden cannabis resin mix is carried by gravity out the drain on the lower end of the airtight receptacle. The liquid is collected in an open bowl.

Dangers and Safety

The **boiling point** is the temperature at which a liquid boils and turns to vapor.

The **flash point** of a flammable liquid is the lowest temperature at which it can form an ignitable mixture in air. At this temperature the vapor may cease to burn when the source of ignition is removed.

The **fire point**, is defined as the temperature at which the vapor continues to burn after being ignited

Note: The ideal solvent has a high flash point and a low boiling point.

Solvent must have a lower boiling point than the residual cannabis resin (380°F [193°C] and CBD at 320°F–356°F [160°C–180°C]). Solvents with a boiling point greater than the highest temperature achieved will remain in the concentrate! DO NOT USE!

The chemistry of solvent separation is complex. For example butane may refer to either of two structural isomers, n-butane or isobutene (methylpropane)

or a mixture of the two "butanes." The flash point of isobutene (i-butane) is higher than n-butane. As isomers n-butane and i-butane have the same chemical formula but different structures and do not always share the same properties.

Research each chemical you are considering using to extract cannabinoids. Check all chemistry, hazards – flammability, health warnings, etc. Here is a good place to start: www.engineeringtoolbox.com.

The butane is then allowed to evaporate into the air. Setting the bowl in a pan of warm water will speed evaporation. Once the butane has dissipated completely, the residual, honey-colored oil can be scraped from the bottom of the glass collection pan.

Butane lighter fluid refill cans are the most common source of this solvent. It is relatively inexpensive, easy to find, and very fast-acting. Avoid brands that contain additives.

Caution! Butane gas is very flammable. Be extremely careful when using it. Use only in a well-ventilated area and never around an open flame, sparks, or anything that might ignite it. Wear protective gloves and a breathing mask when handling butane. Avoid contact with skin and body parts.

To Make Butane Hash Oil

Step One: Fill a 1-quart (1 L) plastic beverage container with chopped cannabis leaf or flower buds. (Higher-quality cannabis contains more cannabinoids and will render higher-quality hash oil.) Do not pack cannabis too tightly in container. Butane needs airspace to be able to penetrate all the cannabis quickly.

Step Two: Poke a small hole in the bottom of the container and insert the fitting provided with the butane cans.

Step Three: Cut a small hole in the cap of the container. This is where cannabinoid-laden oil will exit into an open bowl below.

Step Four: Move outdoors. Do not stay indoors to complete this project! You will be working with very volatile butane under pressure. It is extremely flammable and requires much ventilation. Do not have any lit cigarettes, barbeques, or any open flames within 50 feet (15.2 m) of the project. Turn the container upside down and start filling it with butane fuel.

A 10-ounce (29.6 cl) container of butane will extract cannabinoids from a half-ounce (14.2 gm) of cannabis buds, trim, or shake. Always use premium-grade pure butane with no additives.

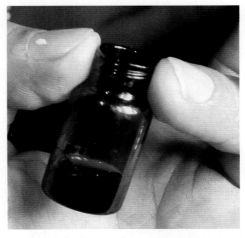

A small vial of butane hash oil (BHO) is very concentrated. Almost all homemade BHO contains unhealthy residuals.

Step Five: Place the cap of the container over an open bowl so that solvent drains out the hole and into the bowl. When the last can of butane has run through the cannabis, the solvent is ready to evaporate.

Step Six: Butane in an open bowl is very volatile and must be kept away from open flames, lit cigarettes, etc. The project should be completed outdoors to provide adequate ventilation to carry away toxic fumes. Evaporation can be natural over time. Set the bowl in a safe, well-ventilated place outdoors, and the solvent will evaporate within a few hours. Or (still outdoors) set the bowl in a pan of water on an electric skillet for faster evaporation.

Step Seven: Once all butane is evaporated, collect the oil by scraping it from the bottom of the glass bowl. A flat-bottomed glass or Pyrex bowl is much easier to scrape than one with a round bottom.

Caution! Making butane hash oil is dangerous. Fumes are toxic, and a small flame or spark will make the butane explode. Butane hash oil **must** be made in a well-ventilated or outdoor location.

Jelly hash is a mix of high-quality hash and cannabis butane oil. The recipe is as follows: 8 parts hash and one part butane hash oil. Dark jelly hash is sticky, oily, and difficult to handle.

Caution! Do not use a pressure cooker to make cannabis oil. Solvents do not react like water under pressure. Solvents under pressure may explode.

Other methods: Bathe cannabis in solvent, then squeeze out the solvent and let it evaporate from the solvent/cannabinoid/plant material mix. Once evaporated, the remaining cannabinoid and plant residue mix can be extracted again with another solvent that will remove water-soluble contaminants.

Hexane (nonpolar)

Hazardous

Flammable

Highly explosive

Boiling point: 177.8°F (81°C)

Flash point: 0.4°F (18°C)

Hexane is made by refining crude oil. It is inexpensive, but it can be hard to find. It is often available in paint stores. Even though it is highly flammable and slow to evaporate, hexane is commonly used to make concentrates.

Petroleum Ether

Petroleum ether is also known as benzene, VM&P Naphtha (varnish makers' & painters'), petroleum naphtha, naphtha ASTM, petroleum spirits, X4, or ligroin (semipolar)

Hazardous

Very flammable

Highly explosive under pressure

Boiling point: 100.4°F (38°C)

Flash point: <0°F (<-17.8°C)

Petroleum ether is a very selective solvent. To minimize danger and cut costs, petroleum is first extracted from the cannabis with alcohol and re-extracted with petroleum ether.

Petroleum ether is available at hardware stores in most countries. Do not confuse petroleum ether with diethyl ether. The term "ether" most often refers to diethyl ether.

Petroleum ether has a specific gravity of between 0.6 and 0.8, depending on its composition.

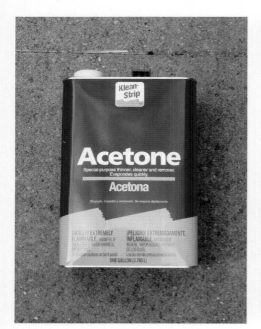

Acetone is an explosive and very flammable chemical mix.

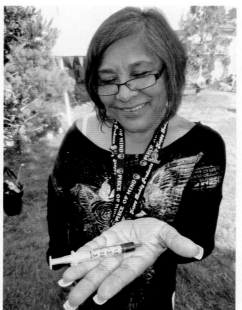

Madeline Martinez, owner of the World Famous Cannabis Café in Portland, Oregon, and Executive Director of Oregon NORML, holds a syringe of Rick Simpson Oil.

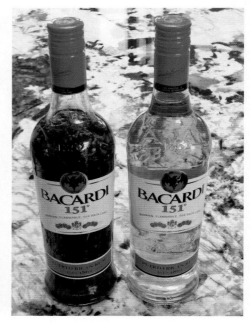

The bottle on the left has been packed with cannabis flower buds.

The following distillation fractions* of petroleum ether are commonly available:

30°C to 40°C

40°C to 60°C

60°C to 80°C

80°C to 100°C

80°C to 120°C

100°C to 120°C

The 60°C to 80°C distillation fraction is often used as a replacement for hexane. Petroleum ether is mostly used by pharmaceutical companies and consists mainly of pentane. It is sometimes used instead of pentane.

*See http://en.wikipedia.org/wiki/Distillation_fraction

Do not confuse petroleum ether (synonym of benzene) with benzene or benzyne. Do not confuse with gasoline. The words *benzin* (German), *benzine* (Dutch), and *benzina* (Italian) are all used to describe gasoline. Petroleum ether is a mixture of alkanes (e.g., pentane, hexane, and heptane), whereas benzene is a cyclic, aromatic hydrocarbon, C_6H_6. Likewise, petroleum ether should not be confused with the class of organic compounds called ethers, which contain the R-O-R' functional group.

For Rick Simpson's "Hemp Oil Recipe" using naphtha, hit our site, www.marijuanagrowing.com.

Acetone

Severely hazardous

Very flammable

Highly explosive under pressure

Boiling point: 132.8°F (56.1°C)

Flash point: -4°F (-20°C)

Acetone is readily available and sold as a solvent or degreaser and as fingernail polish remover. Do not use acetone mixed with other chemicals. It evaporates rapidly and is generally recognized as safe to use. It has low acute and chronic toxicity if ingested or inhaled. It is rated as a GRAS (generally recognized as safe) substance for food use.

Acetone is very flammable. Temperatures above acetone's flash point of -4°F (-20°C) and an air mixture of 2.5 to 12.8 percent acetone by volume, may explode. Vapors can drift for distances to ignition sources and flash back. Acetone is too dangerous for safe use. Acetone's boiling point is 132.8°F (56.1°C).

This solvent has relatively low acute and chronic toxicity if accidently inhaled or ingested.

Ethanol / Ethyl Alcohol / Grain Alcohol

Hazardous

Flammable

Explosive under pressure

Boiling point: 173°F (78.3°C)

Flash point: 53.6°F (12°C)

Purchase high-percentage (high proof) ethyl alcohol at liquor stores. Look for Everclear that is 95 percent alcohol (190-proof). If this is not available, use 151-proof rum (75% alcohol). A higher-proof alcohol means less residual water content. Oil made from ethyl alcohol is dark or greenish in color because it dissolves water-soluble plant material as well as cannabinoids.

The easiest way to infuse cannabis into ethyl alcohol is to place flower buds in bottles of brandy, rum, vodka, gin, or various liqueurs. Always find the most potent alcohol—the highest percentage or "proof," which is half the percentage (i.e., 80-proof is 40% alcohol).

The bottle of 151-proof rum started life as one fifth of a gallon (0.8 qt [757 ml]) and 1.8 ounces (50 gm) of manicured cannabis buds. (Some liquid is displaced as the cannabis is added to the bottle.)

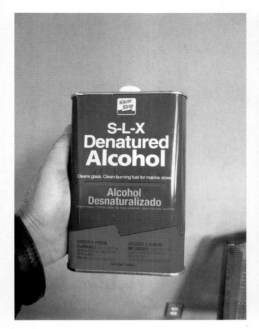

Do not use denatured alcohol!

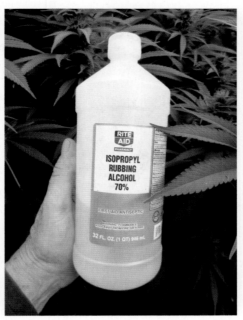

Rubbing alcohol is easy to find at any pharmacy or supermarket.

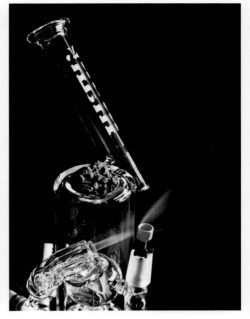

The torch heats the bowl red-hot before a small piece of hashish or oil is dropped or "dabbed" in.

The dry buds suffered being squeezed through the neck of the bottle. Many broke up. The good news is that they are inside the bottle, soaking up the 151-proof alcohol. Buds were as dry as possible, with few stems, all of which contain moisture that dilutes the ability of the alcohol to absorb cannabinoids.

Alcohol can be evaporated so that a potent concentrate remains. However, when using beverage alcohol as a solvent, the alcohol serves to hold the cannabinoids and make a potent elixir.

Isopropyl Alcohol / Isopropanol– Rubbing Alcohol (moderately polar)

Hazardous

Flammable

Explosive under pressure

Boiling point: 180°F (82.2°C)

Flash point: 53.6°F (12°C)

Rubbing (isopropyl) alcohol is easy to find in a 70 to 99 percent concentration. Isopropyl is highly toxic to ingest. When used to extract there is almost always residual solvent in the concentrate. This alcohol dissolves THC, other cannabinoids, and plant fiber. It makes dark-green oil that contains water, and water-soluble substances are also extracted. Cannabis oil extracted with isopropanol is sometimes referred to as "ISO (oil)".

Re-extract the oil later with a more selective solvent to remove impurities. Once most of the alcohol is evaporated, the water and remaining isopropyl alcohol that were in the solvent remain with the oil. Terpenes and aromatics are also destroyed.

This solvent is less toxic and explosive than methanol, but it is flammable! Be careful when handling.

Methanol / Methyl Alcohol / Wood Alcohol (moderately polar)

Hazardous

Flammable

Explosive

Boiling point: 149°F (65°C)

Flash point: 53.6°F (12°C)

This popular solvent evaporates at approximately 149°F (65°C) with a boiling point of 149°F (65°C). It dissolves cannabinoids and plant material to make green-black oil. Methanol (as stove fuel and paint thinner) is easy to find at paint stores and hardware stores.

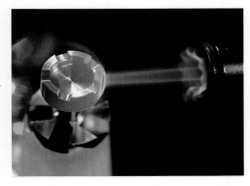

Cannabis concentrates are often consumed in a titanium bowl heated with a torch. A little "dab" of concentrate is placed on the hot metal to immediately smoke and burn.

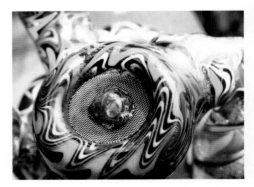

A small amount of concentrated hashish is placed on a stainless steel pipe screen and ignited. Within a second, the concentrated hash melts and bubbles.

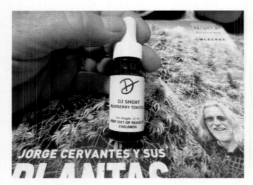

DJ Short Blueberry Tincture is unique in the medical cannabis industry in that it is one of the few tinctures that has the ingredients printed on the label.

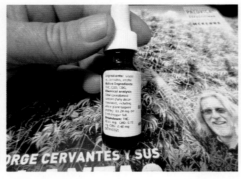

The total cannabinoid content is fully decarboxylated including whole plant terpene profile: 11.24 mb per 1 ml dropper full: THC: 10.11 mg, CBD: 0.73 mg, CBG: 0.40 mg (sCFP/CO$_2$)

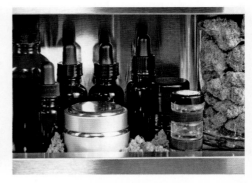

Cannabis tinctures are becoming very popular at medical dispensaries. Avoid products that do not show a "guaranteed analysis."

This solvent is toxic and explosive. Fumes are toxic to inhale. Any traces of methanol in the oil are extremely hazardous to the consumer.

Denatured Alcohol

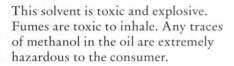

Severely hazardous

Very flammable

Explosive under pressure

Boiling point: 173.3°F (78.5°C)

Flash point: 57°F (13.9°C)

This very toxic solvent has extraction properties similar to methanol. Poison is added to denatured (ethanol) alcohol to lower the beverage alcohol tax and discourage consumption. Do NOT drink denatured alcohol! It is more widely available and is cheaper than poison-free ethanol, but the denaturing agent MUST be removed. Depending on what type of poison is used to create the denatured alcohol, the poisons are impossible to completely remove from the alcohol with evaporation.

Caution: Do NOT use denatured alcohol as a solvent!

Consuming Cannabis Oil

Cannabis oil can be wiped on joint papers, cigarettes, pipe screens, and hot knives. A popular smoking method is to smoke it in an oil pipe—a stem with a glass bubble on one end. A little oil is placed inside the glass bubble. When heat is applied, the THC vaporizes and is inhaled through the stem.

You can find out more about these processes on many Internet cannabis sites.

A new and popular method to consume such high-potency oils and resins is to place them on a piece of titanium and heat it super-hot. The resin or oil volatize immediately at 428°F (220°C); the rest is overkill but looks cool! However, there may be a health risk. Superheating titanium may give off unpleasant chemical substances. More study is necessary.

Cannabis oil can be placed in a vacuum container and over time of turning on and off the vacuum, air is infused into the oil and removed. The process causes oil to turn a golden yellow in color with air holes interspersed. The resulting material is known as "earwax."

Tinctures

11.24 mg per 1 ml dropperful

THC 10.11 mg

CBD 0.73

CBG 0.40 mg

{sCFP/CO$_2$}

Suggested dosage on the DJ Short Blueberry Tincture label is: 5.5 mg or 0.5 dropper every 4 hours Protect from light and heat and store at room temperature

The following text was extracted from "Marijuana Tincture Recipe, How to Make Cannabis Tincture" by Jay R. Cavanaugh. Please check the late Dr. Cavanaugh's Wikipedia entry http://en.wikipedia.org/wiki/Jay_Cavanaugh.

A cannabis tincture is an extraction of active cannabinoids from the cannabis plant. Ethanol alcohol or glycerin is used as a solvent to extract the cannabinoids. Properly extracted cannabinoids do not upset the stomach or taste bad. Cannabinoids are extracted and the vast majority of terpenes and chlorophylls volatilize or are lost in the process.

A tincture delivers medicine quickly with consistent dosing. High-quality tinctures can be applied under the tongue, sublingually. The cannabis

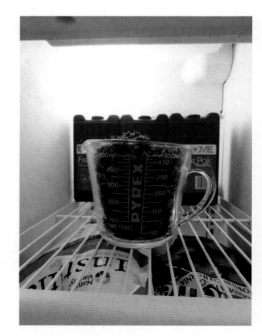

Set buds in freezer for 1 to 2 hours.

tincture is absorbed by the arterial blood supply under the tongue in a few seconds. If tincture is swallowed, absorption is via the gastrointestinal tract, which slows effects by 1 to 2 hours. The dosage is delivered via a medicine dropper, teaspoon, or spray. Dosage depends upon potency of tincture.

While the methods are optimized for purity and potency, ultimately these will be determined by the purity and potency of the cannabis from which the tincture is made.

A rough rule of thumb is to select *indica*-dominant varieties for cramping and muscle spasticity and *sativa*-dominant for pain relief. The reality, though, is that the variety may be unknown or not well characterized. Trial and error is usually required to acquire the appropriate variety and the proper dose level.

There are two main solvents: methanol alcohol and glycerin. The extraction process can be cold, warm, or hot, but always below 173°F (78.3°C), the boiling point of alcohol. Dangerous hot processes are discouraged, and excessive heat degrades cannabinoids.

Common Tincture Processes Include:

Cold extraction with ethanol alcohol

Warm extraction with ethanol alcohol

Hot extraction with ethanol alcohol

Glycerin-based extraction

Sunshine extraction

Cold Extraction with Ethanol
Utensils:

- Grinder or blender
- Freezer
- Strainer
- Cheesecloth
- 1 quart (L) container with lid that can withstand freezing
- Small dark bottles to store tincture

Ingredients:

- 1 oz (28.3 gm) cannabis
- 16 oz (1 pt [47.3 cl]) ethyl alcohol—Everclear (190-proof) or 151-proof rum

Step One: Cold-processing cannabis tinctures preserves the integrity of cannabinoids. Use high-quality flowers or kief made from small leaves and trim. Ensure that the material is dry by placing it in a defrosted, low-humidity freezer at 25°F to 14°F (-3.9°C to -10°C) for 1 to 2 hours.

Step Two: Once frozen, place dried buds in a coffee grinder and grind until thoroughly ground but not powdered. Kief and pre-pressed hashish can be ground as well. This process will open more surface area on the material, allowing cannabinoids to transfer more quickly.

Step Three: More cannabinoids are extracted when using high-percentage or high-proof ethyl alcohol (ethanol). Proof refers to half of the percentage of alcohol. For example, 90-proof is 45 percent alcohol and 150-proof is 75 percent. The highest-proof alcohol available is Everclear at 190-proof or 95 percent ethanol alcohol. Pure 100 percent, 200-proof alcohol is not available. If unable to find Everclear, 151-proof rum is a good substitute. Other spirits that are popular for tinctures include Russian vodka in a lower proof. Some patients prefer lower proof alcohols because they burn less when sprayed under the tongue. Any distilled spirits will work.

Place the high-proof alcohol in the freezer to keep it cold.

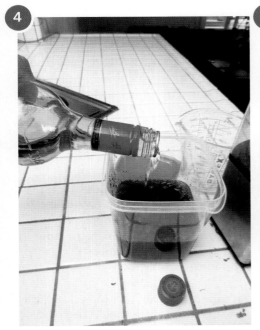

Step Four: Mix one ounce (28.4 grams) ground flowers or kief per pint (16 ounces [47.3 cl]) of ethanol alcohol. Combine in a pre-cooled mixing container with a lid.

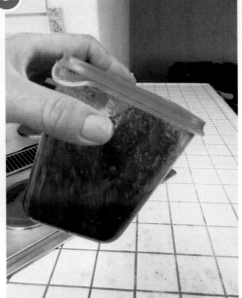

Step Five: Close tightly and shake vigorously for about five minutes.

Step Six: Place in freezer.

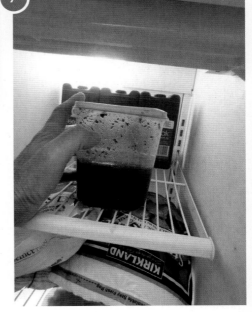

Step Seven: Remove container and shake every two to eight hours and refreeze. Repeat process for 48 to 72 hours. Remove the container from the freezer.

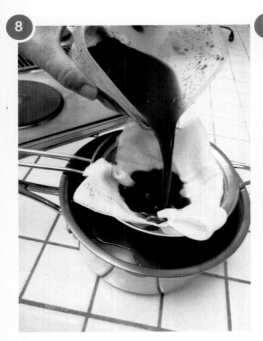

Step Eight: Use rubber gloves throughout the rest of the process. Pour the cold mixture through a kitchen strainer and then pour through a double thickness of sterile cheesecloth. The ball of cheesecloth can be saved in the freezer for topical applications.

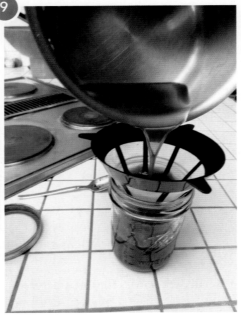

Step Nine: Pour the liquid that was collected through the cheesecloth, through a paper coffee filter—twice. Squeeze the last drops from the cheesecloth and coffee filters into the container. Make sure to wear gloves!

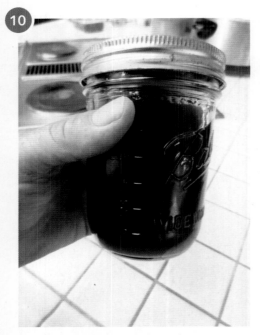

Step Ten: Batches of Everclear or a clear alcohol should yield a pale-green or possibly golden color. Amber-colored alcohol generally stays amber and may darken in color or change hue.

Let the alcohol soak for a few months. A few drops of flavor extract can be added to the alcohol to impart a pleasant taste.

Storage: Both heat and light adversely affect cannabinoids and should be avoided or minimized. Tinctures should be stored in airtight, dark glass containers kept at room temperature or below. Avoid plastic containers if storing for more than a day. The ethanol in the tincture may solubilize some of the free vinyls in the plastic.

Today **Green Dragon** is a popular name for many different cannabis tinctures. Green Dragon is made just like any other alcohol-based tincture using high-quality flower buds, small leaf and trim, or kief and hashish. Some Green Dragon recipes are glycerin-based tinctures. There are several Green Dragon recipes, some of which heat the alcohol to 170°F (76.7°C). Heating alcohol tinctures is dangerous, and excessive heat degrades cannabinoids.

The name "Green Dragon" may have originated among cannabis tincture pioneers before the process was perfected. A green color signifies plant material and other pollutants in the tincture.

Warm Extraction with Ethanol

Warm extraction with ethanol is just like cold extraction, except heat is added to speed the process.

Utensils:

- Grinder or blender
- Strainer
- Cheesecloth
- 1 quart (L) container with lid
- Small dark bottles to store tincture

Ingredients:

- 1 ounce (28.3 gm) cannabis
- 16 ounces (1 pt [47 cl]) ethyl alcohol—190-proof Everclear or 151-proof rum

Step One: Use small leaf trim and large leaves for this recipe. Grind the leaves to expose more surface area. Use a hand grinder for small amounts and a blender for large amounts. Do not pulverize.

Step Two: Use ethanol alcohol for a solvent, as described above in the same proportions. In this preparation the materials are kept warm (not hot). Light must be avoided.

Step Three: Place the ethanol and chopped cannabis in a large glass jar. Shake it vigorously for a few minutes and at least once a day thereafter. Place the jar in a dark-brown bag to exclude light.

Step Four: Place in a warm spot (near a window) for 30 to 60 days. The mixture will turn a very dark green. Strain as through cheesecloth and a coffee filter, as described for cold extraction.

Step Five: Once strained, the tincture is finished. The taste of this powerful cannabis tincture is usually unpleasant and may upset stomachs. Mix the tincture with coffee, cranberry juice, or sugar so it is more palatable.

Save the "shake ball" for topical applications. The shake ball should also be kept in the freezer. For topical applications, just take out the cold shake ball and apply a few drops of fresh tincture to the cloth then hold it on the affected area of skin or wound for a few minutes with gentle rubbing.

Cannabis Glycerin Tincture

Utensils:

- Blender or grinder
- Crock-Pot
- Dark glass jars
- Strainer
- Cheesecloth

Ingredients:

- 100 gm high-quality cannabis flower buds
- 1 qt (94.6 cl) USP food-grade glycerin

Doses: about 100

Estimated Time: 6 hours—5 weeks

Make a glycerin-based tincture with gland-rich cannabis flowers, about 2 cups (47.3 cl). If possible, make your batches of tincture variety-specific.

Soak cannabis in cold water for 15 to 20 minutes to rinse away much chlorophyll; let drain. Put enough trim in your jar to fill it to about three-fourths full. Add vegetable-grade glycerin to within a few inches of the top. Cap and store in a cool, dark place, taking it out at least daily to roll and shake for 5 to 10 minutes. This process should be done for at least 60 days, and can be left even longer for stronger tincture. I then set the jar into a pot of hot water under very low heat for 10 to 15 minutes to help separate more of the trichomes (never getting over 185°F [85°C]), which makes it easier to strain. Then strain and or press to separate trim from glycerin. Some people use coffee filters for final straining; I use silkscreen.

Keep refrigerated.

The recipe below was extrapolated from "Glycerin-based Tincture" by Leanne Barron. The original work appears on the Marijuana Growing forum: http://www.marijuanagrowing.com/showthread.php?1674 Glycerine based Tincture&p=10700#post10700.

Glycerin is vegetable-based and has little impact on blood sugar and insulin levels. Even though it is sweet, it has less than 5 calories per gram and contains no alcohol. Alcohol-based tinctures have a longer life than glycerin-based tinctures. Extend the life of glycerin-based tinctures by keeping them in the refrigerator.

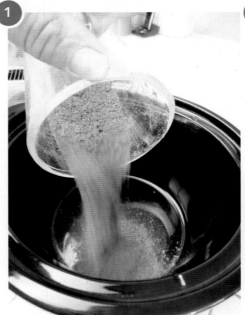

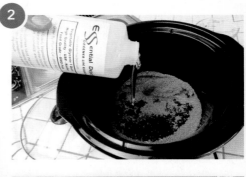

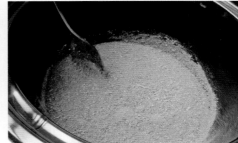

Step One: Place cannabis in a clean coffee grinder or blender, and grind.

Step Two: Pour glycerin and cannabis into a Crock-Pot. Carefully brush residual cannabis out of the grinder. Stir. Set the Crock-Pot on its lowest possible setting. Some Crock-Pots' low settings are too high and cannot be used. If there is a "Keep Warm" setting, that is the best option.

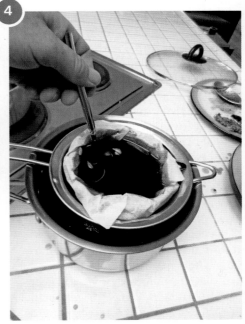

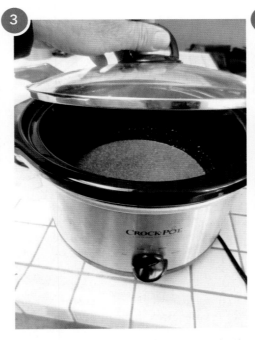

Step Three: Do not let the mixture boil! Keep the temperature below boiling, and let simmer for up to 24 hours.

Step Four: Turn off the Crock-Pot and let mixture cool enough to handle with gloves. Strain the mixture through cheesecloth. It takes longer for glycerin to pass through the process than alcohol. Be patient. Do not use a paper coffee filter that will clog.

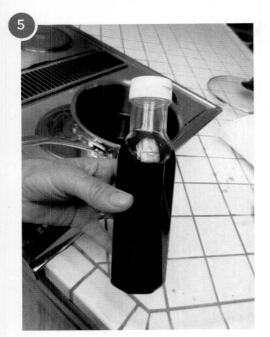

Step Five: Tincture is ready to be bottled in dark glass containers.

If using a clear container to contain the tincture, store in a dark place and minimize contact with sunlight and artificial light.

Lotions and Salves
Cannabis Lotions
The basic recipe for any lotion is incredibly simple: Oil and water are combined and bonded together with an emulsifier. Once the emulsifier is blended in, fragrance and essential oil are added.

There are two types of emulsifiers. Oil-in-water (o/w) emulsifiers keep oil drops packed in water. The other kind, water-in-oil (w/o) emulsifiers keep water drops packed in oil. Use w/o emulsifiers for sun-protection creams. Use o/w emulsifiers for moisturizing body lotions.

Make cannabis body lotion with skin-nourishing cannabis oil and pure water. Add vitamin E oil to the mix as a short-term preservative, and keep natural products in the refrigerator. See http://www.makingcosmetics.com for more information.

Step One: Combine a half cup (11.8 cl) of cannabis oil and 2 tablespoons (28.3 gm) of beeswax, an emulsifier, in a saucepan on the stove. Melt the beeswax and mix with the cannabis oil.

Step Two: Slowly pour distilled water into the warm mixture and stir rapidly with a whisk until well blended. Use a stick blender to add air to the mix and make it fluffy. Be careful when submerging the mixer and keep it on a low speed to avoid splashing.

Step Three: Let lotion cool, during which time it will become thicker, and spoon it into a clean jar with a pump applicator.

Cannabis Salves
Cannabis salves and balms are easy-to-make topical medicinal ointments. First the beneficial properties of cannabis are extracted in oil or glycerin, then beeswax is added to harden the oil. The base to all recipes is either hemp oil or a cannabis tincture mixed with oil. Cannabis salves, ointments, and balms are applied to the skin, and cannabinoids do not transfer to the bloodstream, so the quality and concentration of specific cannabinoids is less important. Low-cannabinoid, clean leaves are ideal for making these topical medicines.

Grape-seed oil is a particular favorite ingredient because it is easily absorbed by the skin. Coconut oil and glycerin are also popular. Olive oil is avoided because it is much slower to be absorbed.

Many other essential oils can be incorporated into the mix. Some mixes such as Tiger Balm can be used as a base to which extracted cannabis is added. The ingredients are usually added near the end of the process, once the mix has cooled. Active ingredients are added and emulsify in the mix. Stirring evenly is important to get an even mix. Popular healing salves today often include menthol crystals, ichthammol, phenyl alcohol, or *Arnica montana*, echinacea, and calendula. There are numerous recipes on the Internet.

Do not use fresh cannabis unless you add a preservative such as Germaben. Balms and lotions made with fresh cannabis should be stored in the refrigerator to prolong life.

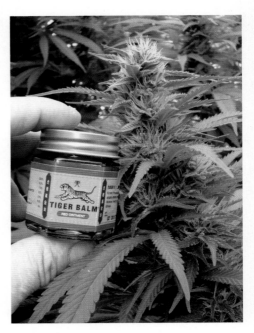

Tiger Balm

RECIPE FOR TIGER BALM

Ingredient	Red	White
menthol	10%	8%
camphor	11%	11%
dementholised mint oil	6%	16%
cajuput oil	7%	13%
clove bud oil	5%	1.5%
cassia oil	5%	0%

The mix is held together with a paraffin base and petroleum jelly.

Cannabis Salve: Step-by-Step
Ingredients:
- 1 pt (47.3 cl) of grape-seed oil
- 1.5 oz (42.5 gm) beeswax
- 1 oz (28.3 gm) cannabis leaf

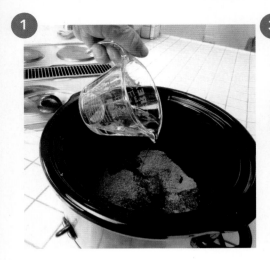

Step One: Add cannabis to a glass, enamel, or stainless steel Crock-Pot. Add one pint (47.3 cl) grape-seed oil.

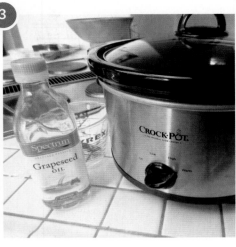

Step Three: Heat the mix on low heat for 2 to 3 hours. Do not let boil. I prefer to use a Crock-Pot because the heat is easy to control and they are lined with a ceramic bowl.

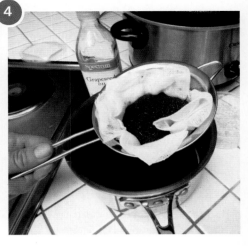

Step Four: After heating, let the oil mix cool before pouring through a cheese-cloth-lined strainer. Once oil has filtered through and cooled enough to handle, pick up cheesecloth containing cannabis and squeeze out residual oil.

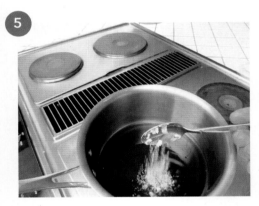

Step Five: Add beeswax to the warm oil mix and heat on low until the wax melts. To test to see if your salve is hard enough, put some on a spoon and set it in a cool place for a few minutes. If your salve is too soft, add more beeswax.

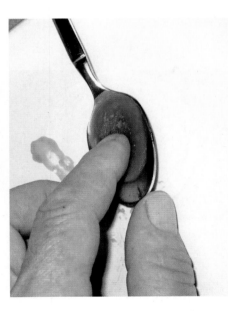

Step Six: If you are using essential oils or vitamin E you can blend them in now. Finally, pour your salve into containers and label.

Glycerin-Based Salve

We have two recipes for glycerin-based salves. The first recipe uses an emulsifying wax and liquid vegetable glycerin along with a couple of preservatives. The second uses beeswax, coconut oil, aloe vera oil, and hemp oil as a base. Note: The coconut oil can consist of cannabis coconut oil.

Ingredients:

- 24 oz (71 cl) distilled water
- 4.0 oz (11.8 cl) strong cannabis oil or fat
- 1.2 oz (3.5 cl) emulsifying wax
- 1.2 oz (3.5 cl) cosmetic grade (benign) stearic acid
- 1 oz (3 cl) liquid vegetable glycerin
- 0.3 oz (0.9 cl) Germaben (a natural preservative that prevents spoilage)
- 0.3 oz (0.9 cl) essential oil of your preference

Step One: Heat all ingredients in a double boiler until melted, and then whisk until creamy.

Step Two: Add the last two ingredients and whisk thoroughly. Add menthol crystals instead of essential oils to make a cooling menthol sunburn salve.

Step Three: While warm, pour into bottles. Makes approximately 32 ounces (94.6 cl)

Alcohol-Based Salve

Utensils:

Crock-Pot

Ingredients:

- 0.5 lb (226.8 gm) beeswax
- 32 oz (94.6 cl) unrefined coconut oil
- 8 oz (23.7 cl) aloe vera oil
- 32 oz (94.6 cl) hemp oil or cannabis tincture
- 0.5 to 1 tsp (0.25–0.5 cl) essential vanilla oil
- 0.5 to 1 tsp (0.25–0.5 cl) vitamin D oil (optional)

Step One: Melt 2 cups of cannabis coconut oil in a Crock-Pot. Set the Crock-Pot to low and simmer. Do not bring to a boil.

Step Two: Melt and measure 1 ounce (28 gm [1/8 cup]) of beeswax into the Crock-Pot. Add 5 ounces (14.8 cl) cannabis (unrefined) coconut oil. Stir until clear. Add aloe vera oil and stir until clear.

Step Three: Turn off the Crock-Pot and put the liner with contents into the refrigerator until a skin develops on the top.

Step Four: Remove mixture from the refrigerator and stir in hemp oil, vanilla oil, and 1 tablespoon vitamin E oil and any drops of fragrance and other oils now. Mix together in Crock-Pot. Stir or whisk until well mixed. An immersion blender can also be used to "fluff" salve, adding air and volume.

Step Five: Scoop salve into small containers with lids for storage, and use.

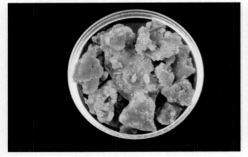

Budder, aka wax, is a super-rich concentration of cannabis resin glands. (MF)

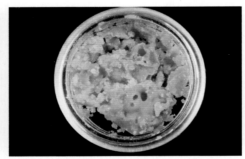

Budder (wax) (MF)

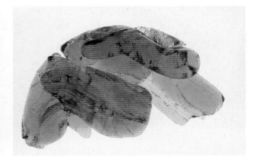

Glass or shatter will burst into countless pieces if dropped on a hard surface. (MF)

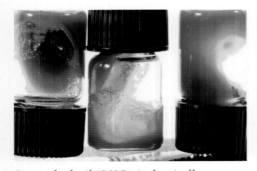

Butane hash oil (BHO) is chemically extracted from dry cannabis. (MF)

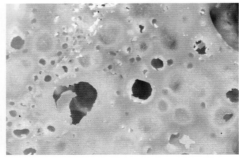

Budder (wax) close-up (MF)

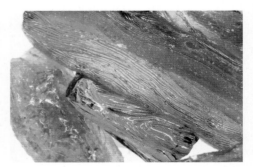

A close-up view of this shatter shows the subtle differences in the extraction. (MF)

27
COOKING WITH MEDICINAL CANNABIS

CANNABIS CAN BE cooked or baked into food for medical consumption. Cannabinoids are liberated and become "active" when mixed with fats, oils, and alcohols. Fats can be saturated or unsaturated. Saturated fats often turn solid at room temperature and are often from animal origin. Unsaturated oils such as avocado, canola, olive, safflower, sesame, and sunflower are preferable. Olive, with a large oleic acid molecular structure, appears to help cannabinoids dissolve and is a good choice.

The recipes in this chapter for cannabis butter, clarified butter, milk, coconut oil, vegetable oil, and so forth are designed to concentrate medicinal cannabinoids in a fat, oil, or alcohol that can be used with other recipes. Concentrating in fats and oils (lipids) converts cannabinoids from the non-psychoactive form to the psychoactive form, preserves them for storage, and makes it easy to include them in many cooking and baking recipes. Cannabis in oils can be added to salads, noodles, and more.

The bulk of cannabinoids in cannabis are located in the resin. Resin is soluble in alcohol, fats, and oils. Combine cannabis leaf, buds, hash, and so on with an oil or alcohol to liberate the cannabinoids into the solvent. Later, separate the green leafy matter from the concentrated resin and solvent.

Cannabis-potent butter, oil, and alcohol are concentrated, which makes them easier and more consistent to measure out into recipes. Keeping dosage consistent is a major concern for cannabis patients. Extraction has already liberated

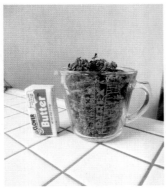

Combine cannabis with butter, vegetable oil, or any fat to liberate cannabinoids.

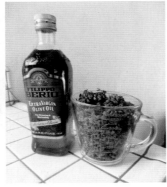

Combine 1 ounce (28 gm) of cannabis with a quart (0.9 L) of vegetable cooking oil to liberate cannabinoids.

cannabinoids. Cooking with concentrates is much easier than using bulky and messy dry or fresh cannabis.

Cannabis used in cooking often retains much of the unpleasant taste associated with green foliage. Soaking cannabis in cold water for two to three hours will leach out much of the chlorophyll and other pollutants. Concentrating resin into kief, hashish, or oil will alleviate most if not all of the "green" taste. Lingering unpleasant tastes and odors can be masked by powerful ingredients such as chocolate, lemon, cinnamon, and mint.

Decarboxylation and Solubilization

Raw cannabis is generally non-intoxicating, but may have some psychoactive effects depending on how much free THC is present versus THCA. Patients report that the therapeutic effects of raw cannabis include providing relief from spasticity and inflammation and some reported no therapeutic effect.

Cannabinoids are found in the form of acids (THCA) and attached to the carboxylic group (COOH). It must first be "liberated"; that is, cannabinoids including THC must change from an acid to a nonacid form to become psychoactive.

The process of decarboxylation converts CBD and non-psychoactive THC acid found in raw cannabis to psychoactive nonacid THC. Decarboxylation converts CBD to its nonacid form, which is extremely therapeutic.

The process of solubilization also converts CBD and THC found in dry cannabis from their acid forms to their nonacid forms. Decarboxylation and solubilization, achieve the same end but through different processes.

Decarboxylation is a chemical reaction that releases carbon dioxide (CO_2). Decarboxylation of cannabis denotes a reaction of carboxylic acids, removing a carbon atom from a carbon chain.

Decarboxylation can be achieved by heating THC-dominant dry canna-

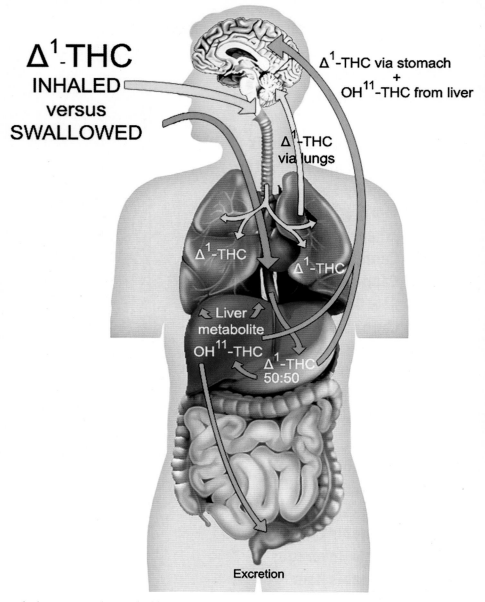

Smoked or vaporized cannabis that enters the lungs passes directly to the brain via the blood system; the effects are usually felt within 30 to 90 seconds. The dose is easy to control. Decarboxylized and solubilized cannabis that is eaten passes through the stomach and liver before entering the blood system. Effects normally appear in 45 to 60 minutes and last up to 12 hours. Dosage is more difficult to control.

bis to above 212°F (100°C) or heating CBD-dominant dry cannabis to above 295°F (146°C) for 60 to 90 minutes. Do not heat cannabis – both THC-dominant and CBD-dominant – to above 320°F (160°C) to prevent boiling off cannabinoids. Heating beyond 320°F (160°C) may cause desirable cannabinoids, CBD and THC, to volatize and be lost when they mix with the air.

Decarboxylation also occurs rapidly during vaporization: heating cannabis

to 370°F to 380°F (187.8°C–193°C), at which point it vaporizes and the conversion to the "active" nonacidic form takes place. Do not heat above 380°F (193°C) or it may cause preliminary burning/charring. This process frees molecules to convert into carbon dioxide (CO_2) and water vapor (H_2O).

Note: THC is liberated rapidly at temperatures between 370°F to 380°F (187.8°C–193°C), and CBD is liberated rapidly at 370°F to 380°F

(187.8°C –193°C). The other 80+ known cannabinoids volatize at different temperatures often lower than 380°F (193°C).

The same decarboxylation process also occurs at a very rapid rate when cannabis combusts (burns). Heat in smoked cannabis causes THC to convert into the psychoactive form. CBD is converted into its nonacid form. Combustion releases many toxic compounds—aromatic hydrocarbons such as benzopyrene and other carcinogens—that are inhaled into the lungs. See www.marijuanagrowing.com for more information.

Cannabinoids are soluble in fats, sugars, and oils (lipids), alcohol, and other oil-based solvents. Once combined, cannabinoids are soluble and convert from the acid to the nonacid form. THC becomes psy-choactive, and CBD becomes much more therapeutic.

Solubilization occurs when cannabis is mixed with fats, sugar, oils, alcohol, and other oil-based solvents. The cannabinoids migrate and concentrate in the solvents.

Combine cannabis with these solvents, and heat at low temperatures (122°F–145°F [50°C –62.8°C]) for 60 to 90 minutes to solubilize (extract) cannabinoids. Simmering and stirring ensures that complete extraction occurs.

Combining cannabis with alcohol (spirits or glycerin) requires no heat, but the process takes much longer. For example, place a bud in a bottle of ethyl alcohol—vodka, rum, or spirits of any kind. Over time the alcohol will take on the flavor and the potency of the cannabis. Or the alcohol can be evaporated to leave a concentrate.

Carbon dioxide (CO_2) can also be used as a solvent to liberate cannabinoids. CO_2 is becoming a popular method to extract CBD and THC from dry cannabis. See chapter 26, *Medicinal Concentrates & Tinctures*, for more information.

Safety – Clean Cannabis

Growing your own medicine or purchas-

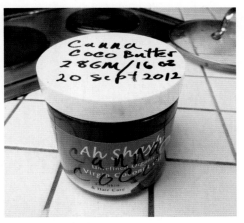

Always label cannabis recipes and cooking concentrates clearly to ensure they are not mistakenly used by others. Keep out of the reach of children!

ing it from a medical cannabis dispensary that tests cannabis for pollutants, molds, and insect residues are excellent options. However, little control is exercised in the marketplace and many dispensaries do not test the cannabis they sell. Wash fresh cannabis with a 0.5 percent solution (see page 122) of hydrogen peroxide (H_2O_2) to remove surface fungi and pest carcasses, eggs, and feces. Washing dry cannabis requires extra care. Concentrating cannabis in tinctures, kief, hashish, or oils also concentrates pollutants such as pesticides, fungus, and insect residues. Dry plants can be sterilized with UVC light before processing. The UVC light will kill pathogens and insects on the surface of the plant. Only short applications are given to avoid damaging resin with UVC radiation.

Patients susceptible to plant fungi should use only cannabis that is certified to be clean, or grow it at home to ensure purity.

Mold, mildew, and many other fungi can be present inside plant tissue and not visible to the human eye, and even when visible, an untrained gardener will not notice. When minor infections are present, small amounts of mold and mildew can slip into drying containers. Take special care to weed out this infected plant tissue. For example, dry flower buds infected with powdery mildew feel mealy and are easy to crush. They are not firm, and have little substance; instead, they are soft, pliable, and easy to compress.

Heat kills potentially dangerous fungi such as Aspergillus, powdery mildew and bud mold (*Botrytis cinerea*). Heating cannabis to 302°F (150°C) for 5 minutes will kill the organisms without degrading THC; other cannabinoids volatize below this temperature. But these temperatures do not degrade or decompose microbial toxins.

Aspergillus, a common household mold, seldom causes harm in humans. However, people with compromised immune systems, AIDS, cancer, asthma, and other diseases can be affected by *Aspergillus*. Powdery mildew is caused by many species of fungi from the order Erysiphales.

Pesticides and fertilizer residues stay longer on indoor and greenhouse plants than on outdoor plants. Wind, natural sunshine, and rain weather away anything that is applied to leaves. Indoors, degradation of pesticides and fertilizers is much slower. Indoor plants should be watered with pure water for 5 to 6 days before harvest. This rinse will help plants use all the fertilizer in their tissue before harvest. Commercial products are also available to expedite the final leaching and make it more efficient.

Microscopic fungus, dead insects, spider mites, and their eggs and feces stay on plants after harvest. Caterpillar and larvae feces attract fungus that must be cleaned from cannabis. Pests stick

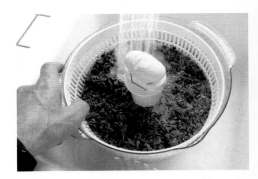

To wash cannabis in H_2O_2 water before drying, fill a large container with a 0.5 percent solution of hydrogen peroxide. Submerge manicured, bud-filled branches in container and agitate for 1 to 5 minutes. Fungus and other debris form a thin layer on the surface of the water or, if heavy, sink to the bottom. Use a sponge to skim off the layer of scum. Remove bud-filled branches, rinse and lightly shake water from foliage. Let branches drip dry for 30 minutes in front of an oscillating fan.

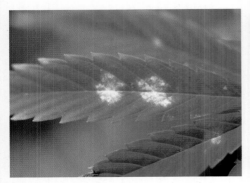

Diseased and desiccated foliage should be removed and discarded. Do not consume it. Foliage with nutrient deficiencies is okay to use, but it may have lower levels of cannabinoids.

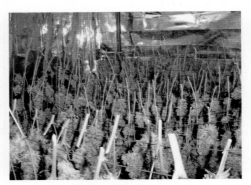

Cannabis roots contain no cannabinoids, but little is known as to their therapeutic effects. Roots are recycled back into the garden or compost.

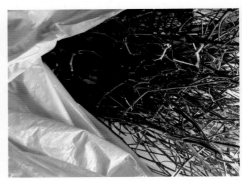

Stems have little or no cannabinoid content. After harvest, small buds and foliage may remain on stems. Separate stems from leaves and small buds. Do not add stems to recipes. Stems make good compost when chopped.

to resinous buds and are consumed by patients. Cooking alone is not enough to destroy bacteria, fungi, pest carcasses, eggs, and feces.

Here is a short list of laboratories that can test for contaminants of medicinal cannabis in California:

Pure Analytics, http://pureanalytics.net/

Steep Hill Halent Laboratories, Inc., http://steephilllab.com/

The Werc Shop, http://thewercshop.com/

Cooking with fresh cannabis is not always possible; dry cannabis is usually all that is available. Keep dry cannabis

in an airtight container in a cool, dark place to maintain minimal preservation of active ingredients, cannabinoids. See "Storage" in chapter 9, *Harvest*.

Grades of Cannabis

Cooking with kief, hash, or oil instead of flower buds or leaf has many benefits.

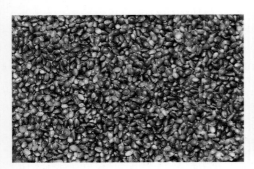

Seeds are rich in oil and omega-3. Find hemp seeds in bulk by searching "hemp seeds bulk" on www.google.com. Sometimes you can find hemp seeds from China, where they grow varieties that produce huge seeds.

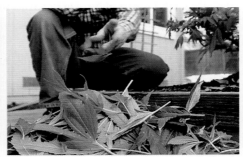

Large leaves contain low levels of potent cannabinoids.

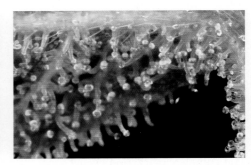

Small leaves around flower buds are often glistening with resin and make excellent hashish and tinctures for cooking. (MF)

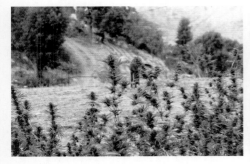

Flower buds, the most resinous part of cannabis plants, are often small and lightweight but still contain high levels of cannabinoids. Chop fresh flower buds. Chop or grind dry flower buds before adding to fats, oils, and alcohols.

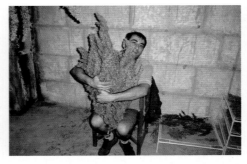

Large flower buds are often loaded with visible cannabinoid-rich resin. We advise people to use high-quality buds for cooking. Large flower buds are often submerged in cooking and salad oils or bottles of spirits.

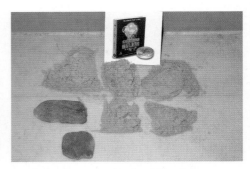

Kief (also known as keef or kif), the raw resin glands that fall from buds and leaves, is collected. It is usually adulterated with small amounts of foliage and debris from the garden. Kief is best used when added directly to fats, oils, and alcohols.

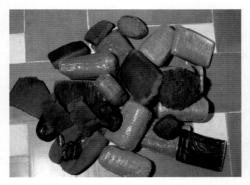

Hashish (aka hash) is concentrated, compressed resin glands (kief). Hashish must be broken into small pieces or ground before adding to fats, oils, and alcohols.

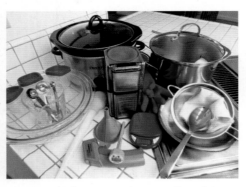

Here are the basic utensils you will need to make most medicinal cannabis concentrates.

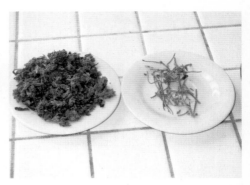

Remove all stems and small leaf debris from manicured buds before making concentrates.

Cannabis leaves and buds are in their acid form and not decarboxylized. The cooking process must perform the decarboxylation, and most often it is inefficient. Consistent dosage and no "green" flakes or taste are other strong reasons to use only cannabis concentrated in fats, oils, and alcohols. Water hash is most economical, and since many terpenes are already gone, heating while cooking does not destroy more flavors.

Hemp is industrial-grade cannabis that is often used for its fiber, seed, and oil. Hemp has low levels of THC and, most often, other cannabinoids. Hemp is an ingredient in many balms, lotions, and soaps. Hemp fiber is used to make clothing and rope along with new products such as cannabis bedding for animals.

Large leaves are separated at harvest. Dry leaves in a paper bag, turning every day by hand. Leaves have low cannabinoid content. Large, older leaves near the bottom of plants contain less cannabinoids than those located further up. Remove leaf stems before grinding or adding to recipes. Often large quantities of large leaves must be added to achieve therapeutic effects. Discard brown or discolored leaves.

Small leaves are located higher on the plant and around flower buds. Resin is often visible on these "trim" leaves that are packed with cannabinoids. Small leaves without visible resin, or recently formed and immature leaves contain fewer cannabinoids. Remove leaf stems. Chop fresh leaves and grind or chop dry leaves before adding to fats, oils, and alcohols.

Temperature and Volatility

THC volatizes into the air at 380°F (193°C), CBD volatizes at 360°F-380°F (182°C-193°C), and the other 80+ known cannabinoids volatize at lower temperatures. See chapter 2, *Measuring Cannabinoids*, for more information on the boiling point of specific cannabinoids.

Baking and cooking require a heat source that is easy to control so that high temperatures do not cook out beneficial elements. Temperatures are easiest to control quickly with a gas stove or oven. Electric burners often heat and cool slowly. However, a hot plate is a convenient source of heat that can be plugged in anywhere. If you use recipes that heat beyond 300°F (148.9°C), calibrate with an accurate thermometer to avoid volatizing cannabinoids.

NOTE: To avoid destroying cannabinoids, do not bake cannabis recipes at more than 350°F (176.7°C).

Low heat = 200°F (93.3°C)

Medium heat = 250°F-275°C (121.1°F-135°C)

High heat = 300°F-350°F (148.9°C-176.7°C)

Utensils

Use Pyrex glass, ceramic, or stainless steel utensils when following these recipes.

A Crock-Pot is a stand-alone electric cooker that supplies low, even heat. A removable ceramic liner is very practical to simmer cannabis recipes for hours. The liner can be removed for cleaning, and it can be placed in the refrigerator or

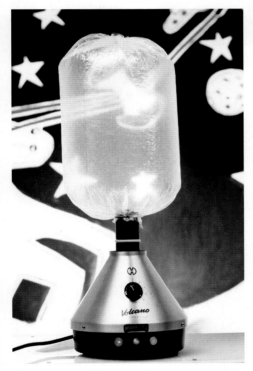

Once vaporized for several minutes, terpenes are volatized into the air and the dried cannabis loses its fragrance. However, vaporized buds still retain more than half their original cannabinoid content. Grind vaporized buds into a powder just before adding to fats, oils, and alcohols.

CONVERSION SCALE

Standard Measurement	Centiliters
1 teaspoon (tsp)	0.5
1 tablespoon (tbsp)	1.5
1 cup (c)	23.7
1 pint (pt)	47.3
1 quart (qt)	94.6
1 ounce (oz)	3

freezer separate from the heating element of the Crock-Pot. This versatility saves the space and hassle of using a separate container.

A double boiler is an alternative to a Crock-Pot. It consists of a small cooking pot suspended inside of a larger container. Water boils in the larger container and heats the contents to be cooked in the smaller container. The temperature is relatively easy to control, and the possibility of burning the recipe is next to nil.

List of utensils for basic recipes:
- 2 large bowls
- measuring cup
- measuring spoons
- scale to weigh dry measure
- blender to pulverize cannabis
- sifter/sieve
- strainer
- saucepans
- large cooking pot with a lid
- Crock-Pot
- cheesecloth
- string or large rubber bands
- large spoon (can be wooden)
- ladle
- thermometer, accurate to within 5°F (3°C)
- funnel
- rubber gloves
- plastic storage containers with lids

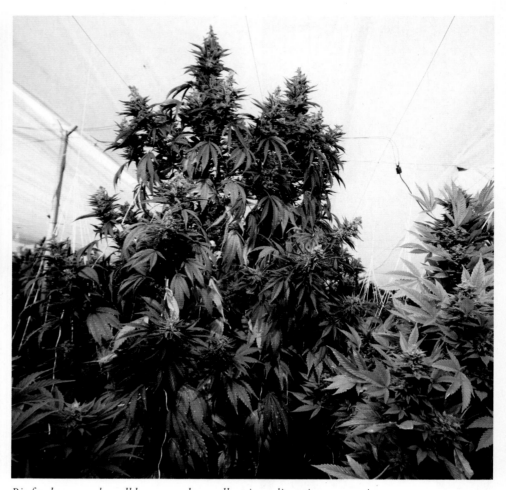

Big fan leaves and small leaves can be excellent ingredients in many recipes.

Cooking with Cannabis
Smoke Points
butter: 250°F–300°F (121.1°C–148.9°C)

olive oil: 375°F–475°F (190.6°C–246.1°C)

peanut oil (refined): 450°F (232.2°C)

sunflower oil (refined): 440°F (226.7°C)

Cannabis butter is a main ingredient in many recipes. It can be used alone, as butter on bread, or mixed into countless recipes. Cannabinoids are bound to milk fats in butter and are preserved as long as butter is safe to consume. Use salted butter for most recipes; it has a higher smoke point than unsalted. Use unsalted butter for baking. Slow, even cooking at a low temperature and adequate stirring are essential to avoid burning when making cannabis butter.

Quick Cannabis Butter
Process small amounts of cannabis butter, less than 2.2 pounds (997.9 gm) of cannabis butter by sautéing it in a pan and adding cannabis. Process larger amounts of cannabis with the recipe that follows:

Utensils
- coffee grinder or food processor
- 2 saucepans
- strainer
- cheesecloth

Ingredients
- 0.25 oz (7.1 gm) finely manicured cannabis flower buds
- 1 stick (0.5 c [23.7 cl]) butter

Quick Cannabis Butter: Step-by-Step

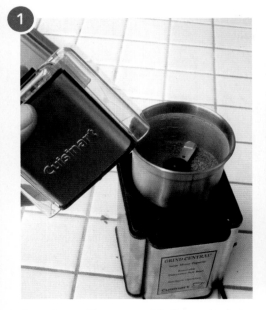

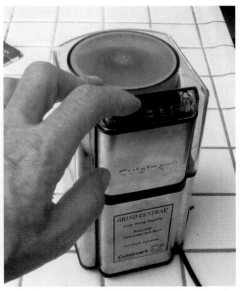

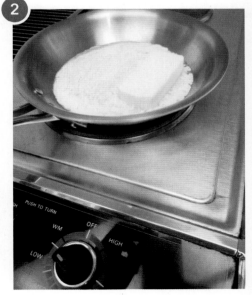

Step One: Chop cannabis flower buds in a small coffee grinder (or food processor). Make sure coffee grinder is clean and used only for cannabis. Chopped flower buds release cannabinoids into the butter faster.

Step Two: Melt the butter on low heat.

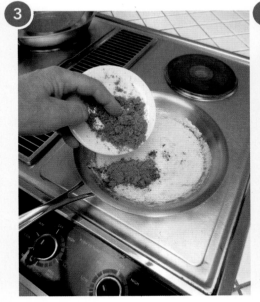

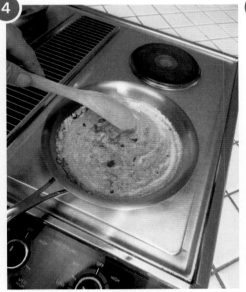

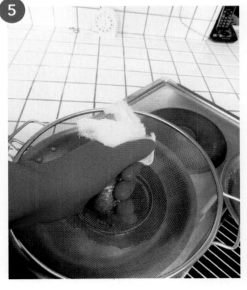

Step Three: Once the butter has melted, add the chopped cannabis.

Step Four: Let the butter and cannabis mix simmer for about 45 minutes, stirring every few minutes, which mixes cannabinoid and butter molecules and speeds, speeding absorption.

Step Five: Filter butter and cannabis through a cheesecloth-lined strainer. Wait until the mix has cooled enough to handle, and then wear rubber gloves to squeeze residual liquid from cheesecloth.

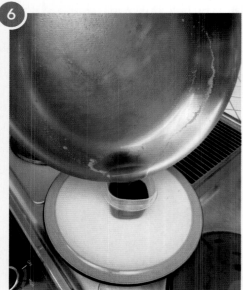

Step Six: Pour the cooled, filtered liquid into a storage container.

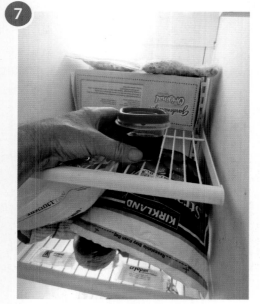

Step Seven: Refrigerate the liquid until solid.

Cannabis butter is green because milk fat takes on green plant molecules and cannabinoid molecules. The taste of green cannabis is objectionable to most people. Here are some quick, easy recipes to disguise the taste of cannabis in butter.

Basil Butter—Add a minced clove of fresh garlic and 0.5 cups (11.8 cl) of fresh chopped basil to every 0.5 cups (11.8 cl) of butter. Great garnish for chicken or fish.

Cilantro Lime Butter—Add 3 tablespoons (4.4 cl) chopped cilantro and two 3 teaspoons (1.5 cl) of lime juice to every 0.5 cups (11.8 cl) of butter. You can spice it up with a dash of hot sauce, too!

Garlic Butter—Mince 1 clove of garlic and combine with 0.5 cups (11.8 cl) butter. Use the butter on garlic bread and meat dishes. Chop up some parsley to add more flavor.

Lemon Butter—Add 1 teaspoon (0.5 cl) fresh lemon juice and 1 tablespoon grated lemon peel to 0.5 cups (11.8 cl) of butter. Pour it on chicken, fish, or my favorite, grilled asparagus.

Blue Cheese Butter—Add 2 ounces (56.7 gm) blue cheese to 0.5 cups (11.8 cl) of butter. Include minced chives or shallots, rosemary, or thyme.

Clarified Cannabis Butter (Ghee)

Clarified butter (aka drawn butter, ghee, or *samna*) has a longer shelf life than cannabis butter and a higher smoke point, which makes it desirable for sautéing, basting seafood, and numerous recipes. A certain percentage of butter is lost to friction, to butter that remains

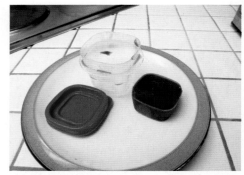

Dark green cannabis butter is ready to use!

in the saucepan, and to contaminants in the clarifying process. However, clarified butter has negligible amounts of lactose and is acceptable for most lactose-intolerant consumers.

Avoid "green" taste by using concentrated cannabis resin that contains little plant material. Clarified butter made from good kief has little objectionable foliage and contaminant residues which helps exclude the foliage taste.

Utensils
- saucepan or double boiler
- spoon
- measuring cup
- scale
- strainer
- cheesecloth
- airtight storage containers

Ingredients
One stick (0.5 c [11.8 cl]) of cannabis butter infused with 0.25 oz (7.1 gm) cannabis flower buds)

Time to prepare: 30 minutes
Cooking time: Cooking time at 150°F to 200°F (65.6°C–93.3°C)

Clarified Cannabis Butter (Ghee): Step-by-Step

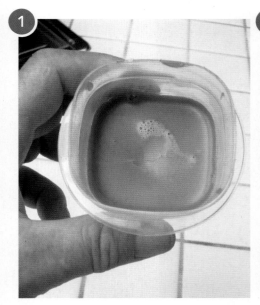

Step One: Follow instructions to make Cannabis Butter, above.

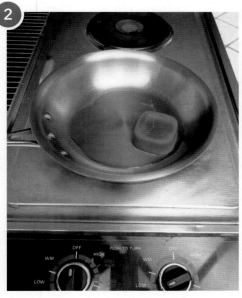

Step Two: Melt cannabis butter in a pan or double boiler at low heat. Do not boil.

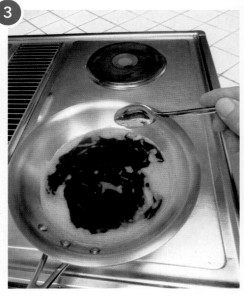

Step Three: Simmer butter for 30 minutes, stirring regularly.

A bubbly froth may come to the top during **Step Three**, but if the butter was filtered with cheesecloth, much less froth develops. Skim froth and scum that forms on surface. It thins slowly and the color of the butter changes to deep green. Continue simmering until butter turns greenish-golden color. The green tint will always remain. Residues settle on the bottom and the clarified cannabis butter is a translucent golden color with a deep, rich fragrance.

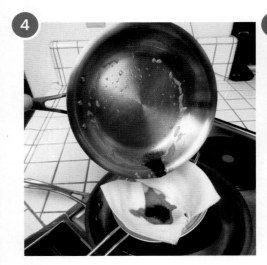

Step Four: Pour the liquid butter through a strainer lined with two layers of cheesecloth. Ball up and push the cheesecloth containing residuals against the strainer to exude all remaining butter into a warmed saucepan below.

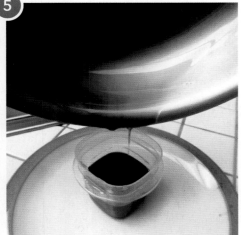

Step Five: Pour the clarified butter into a receptacle.

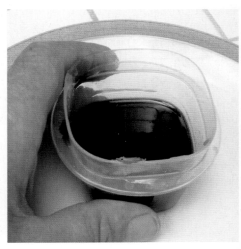

Note that the clarification process removed a volume of butter. The "freeze line" from cannabis butter can be seen above the butter's surface.

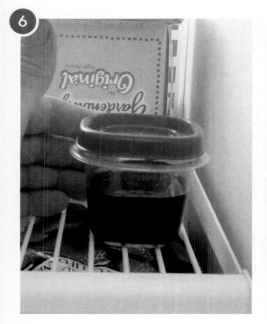

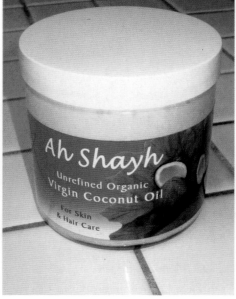

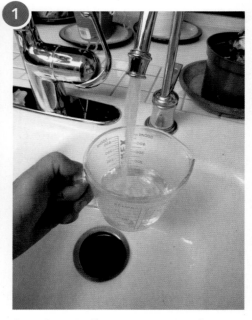

Step Six: Store clarified cannabis butter in airtight containers in the freezer or refrigerator. It will last up to a year or longer in the freezer and several months in a refrigerator. Bathing butter in water extends shelf life.

Cannabis Butter
(2.2 pound [1 kg] plus)
This recipe requires separating water from butter and is best used to process several pounds (kg) or more of cannabis butter.

You will need a couple of days to make this recipe, but the process is low maintenance and easy to follow. In fact, you can follow instructions for making "Cannabis Coconut Oil," at right. Simply substitute the same quantity of butter and cannabis.

Cannabis Coconut Oil
Coconut oil, a healthy saturated fat, absorbs the maximum amount of cannabinoids. Coconut oil is solid at room temperature; if semiliquid, a half hour in the freezer will solidify it. Coconut oil (unrefined) has a higher smoke point (350°F [176.7°C]) than butter. (It can also be used for skin salves and creams, as well as be put into capsules.) Coconut oil can be used in many recipes as a substitute for vegetable oil or butter.

Utensils
- large pot
- 1 qt (1 L) water
- spoon
- container to store cannabis-coco-butter

Ingredients
- 16 oz (453.6 gm) organic coconut oil
- 1oz (28.3 gm) cannabis flower buds

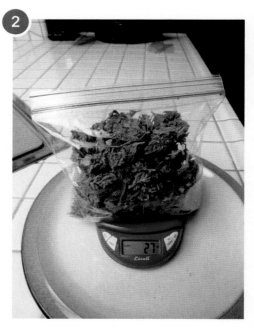

Step One: Boil one quart (1 L) of water in a large pot.

Step Two: Add 1 ounce (28.3 gm) of manicured cannabis flower buds.

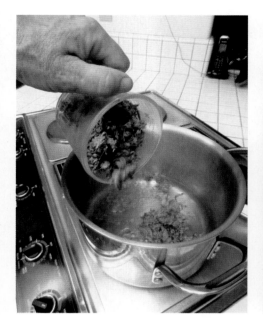

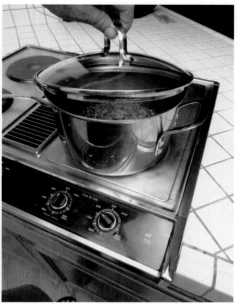

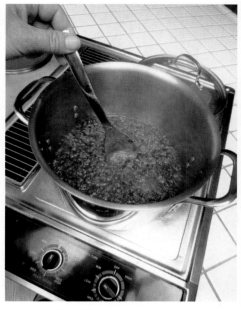

Let simmer and stir during the next hour.   Remove the lid and stir regularly.

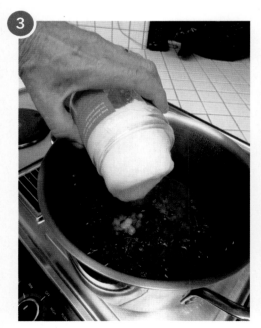

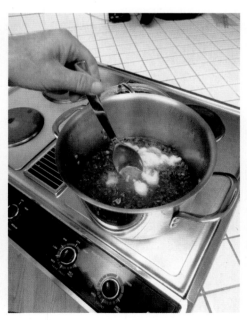

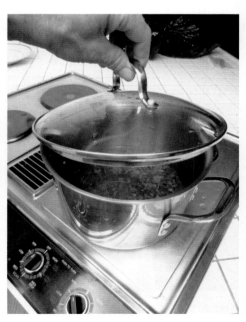

Step Three: Add 16 ounces (47.3 cl) coconut oil kept at room temperature to the hot water/cannabis mix.

Stir in coconut oil for at least a minute to ensure that it is well mixed.

Cover and continue simmering for 10 minutes.

4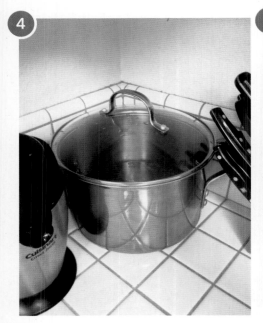

Step Four: Remove from heat. Set aside for two days so that more cannabinoids can be absorbed by the coconut oil.

5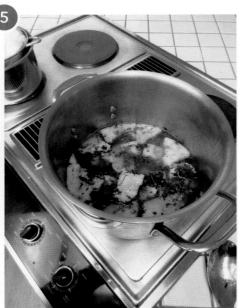

Step Five: Set the pot on the stove and bring to a simmer so that all the coconut oil is dissolved.

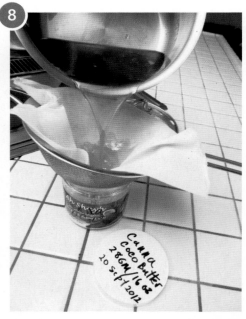

6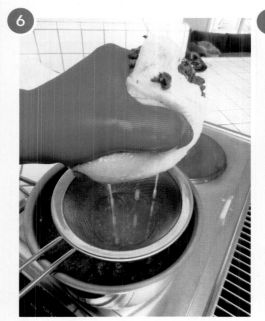

Step Six: Pour the mix through a strainer and cheesecloth. Let cool. Wear rubber gloves and squeeze the cooled cannabis/coconut oil mix so that all the liquid comes out.

7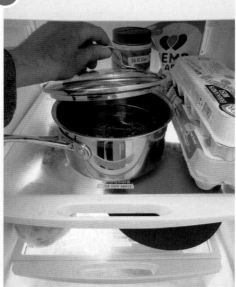

Step Seven: Refrigerate the mix overnight so that the water and coconut oil separate. Remove the pot and pour off water. Retain solidified coconut oil.

8

Step Eight: Heat solidified coconut oil in a saucepan until liquid. Pour into small containers with lids for storage. Place in refrigerator to store.

Cannabis Vegetable Oil: Step-by-Step

Cannabis Vegetable (Olive) Oil

Choose your preferred vegetable oil—olive, canola, sunflower, flaxseed, grape seed, etc.—to use in this recipe. Notice that different oils react differently to heat. For example, the smoke point of olive oil is 375°F–475°F (190.6°C–246.1°C), the smoke point of peanut oil (refined) is 450°F (232.2°C), and the smoke point of sunflower oil (refined) is 440°F (226.7°C). This should make little difference at low heat levels. If using my favorite, olive oil, always purchase extra virgin (first cold press) to ensure the highest quality. Avoid using bland oils such as canola with little taste. Always use gloves to avoid contamination.

Vegetable oils must be placed in the freezer for several hours and frozen to become solid.

The first method is not as efficient as the second, but it is much easier.

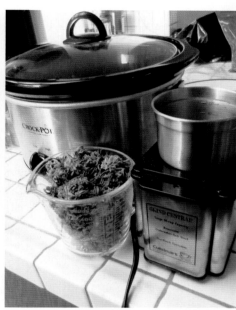
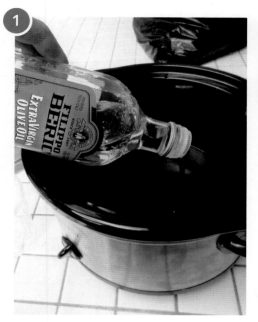

Step One: Use a Crock-Pot to heat 4 cups (94.6 cl) of olive oil. When it reaches 150°F (65.6°C) add 1 ounce (28.3 gm) dry, manicured cannabis flower buds. Add buds slowly so that they are sure to be permeated with hot oil.

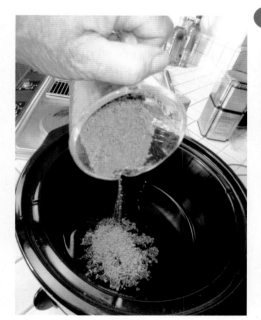
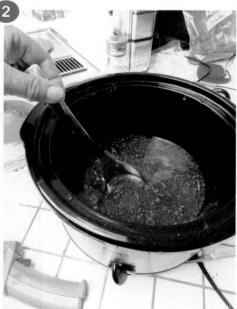
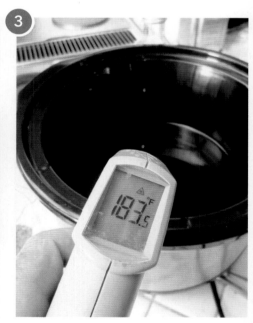

Step Two: Simmer the mix on low heat for 45 minutes and stir regularly.

Step Three: Remove from heat and let cool before handling.

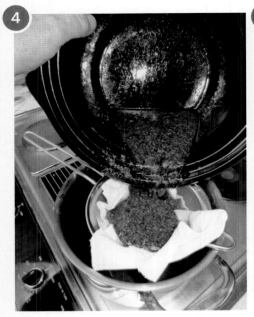

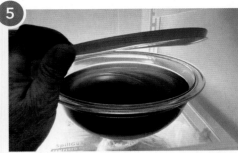

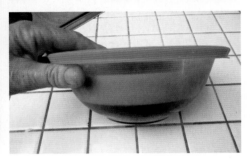

Step Four: Pass mix through a strainer lined with cheesecloth and collect liquid in a receptacle below. Press out residual liquid from cheesecloth using rubber gloves. Compost cheesecloth and cannabis mix.

Step Five: Set in the refrigerator overnight to separate out the water.

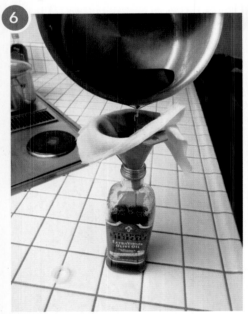

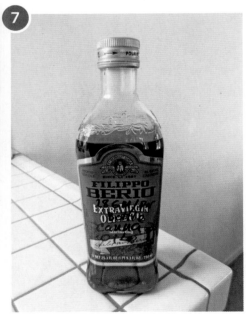

Step Six: Save oil in an airtight container.

Step Seven: Store in the refrigerator for up to 60 days.

Notes: A pressure cooker can be used to reduce cooking times and extract more cannabinoids, but chlorophyll and other contaminants are also extracted.

One half cup of cannabis olive oil is roughly equivalent to one ounce of cannabis.

Raw Cannabis

Dr. William Courtney (http://www.cannabisinternational.org) advises that raw cannabis plants eaten or juiced don't get anyone high. The CBD overpowers the THC. Dr. Courtney believes raw cannabis eaten or juiced prevents more diseases than any other food available. A growing number of doctors are taking notice. For a complete description on YouTube, see http://www.youtube.com/watch?v=qa0nLdVJiIg.

Utensils
wheatgrass juice extractor

Ingredients
raw cannabis leaves

Juicing Raw Cannabis
Raw cannabis leaves are fed into a juicer and deep-green cannabis juice trickles out a nipple while the bulk of the processed leaf is expelled from another outlet.

Juice 15 to 20 cannabis leaves. Juice a carrot or two. Mix 10 parts carrot juice to 1 part cannabis juice. The sweet carrot juice will cut the bitter taste of the cannabis juice.

The juice will keep in the refrigerator about 3 days, but it is best to consume during the first day. Drink in 3 to 4 servings throughout the day. Keep refrigerated.

Avoid using stems and large, damaged, or discolored leaves. Upper foliage and flower buds make the most concentrated juice.

Cannabis (Hemp) Seeds
In spirits, hemp seeds are used to flavor beer, cider, wine, liquors, and other spirits. Toasted cannabis (hemp) seeds instill creamy, earthy, and nutty characteristics in ales. Normally they are soaked in the mix and strained out, however some spirits leave them to swim around in the bottom of bottles. Little is known about the nutritional value of alcohol-marinated seeds. Hemp seeds contain easily digested proteins, essential fats (omega-3 and omega-6), gamma linolenic acid (GLA), antioxidants, amino acids, fiber, iron, zinc, carotene, phospholipids, phytos-

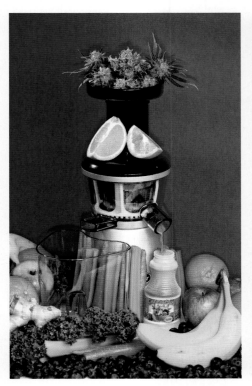

Cannabis buds and leaves are fed into the hopper of this high-quality juicer.

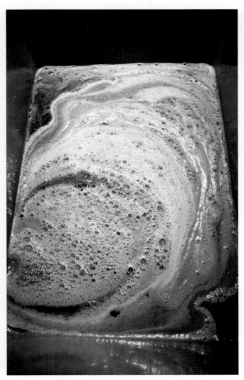

Various vegetables are juiced and the juices blended together.

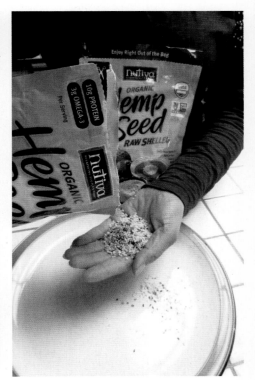

Cannabis seeds contain all the essential amino acids (EAAs) and are rich in essential fatty acids (EFAs), mainly omega-3 and omega-6. Cannabis seeds are also high in magnesium and have the maximum levels of digestible and absorbable globulin protein.

terols, vitamin B_1, vitamin B_2, vitamin B_6, vitamin D, vitamin E, chlorophyll, calcium, magnesium, sulfur, copper, potassium, phosphorus, and enzymes. All amino acids essential to optimum health are found in hemp seeds, including the rarely found gamma linolenic acid.

The recommended minimum daily intake of shelled hemp seeds is 4 heaping tablespoons (42 gm). Larger individuals or those suffering with chronic health conditions such as arthritis, high blood pressure, high cholesterol, cardiovascular disease, acne, eczema, psoriasis, diabetes, circulation problems, intestinal problems, constipation, obesity, or prostate problems (to name a few) may want to consider taking 5 to 6 heaping tablespoons (55 gm) per day.

Hemp seeds contain approximately 25 percent protein, 31 percent fat (in the form of nutritious hemp oil), and 34 percent carbohydrates (mostly from fiber), in addition to an excellent array of vitamins and minerals.

Hemp Flour

Hemp flour is typically sold at health food stores and on the Internet. It is milled from hemp seeds. Hemp flour is an alternative to wheat and corn flour. It is rich in omega-3, omega-6, vitamins B and E, calcium, potassium, and fiber. It is also completely gluten-free. *Make sure to keep hemp flour refrigerated after opening, because it contains no preservatives.*

Hemp Milk

Hemp milk or hemp seed milk is made from hemp seeds. The seeds are soaked in water and ground into creamy milk with a nutty flavor. Health and fitness stores may stock hemp milk, and you can also find it via the Internet.

Cannabis (hemp) seeds contain virtually no THC. The seeds hold a 3:1 ratio of omega-6 and omega-3 essential fatty acids, plus magnesium, phytosterols, ascorbic acid, beta-carotene, calcium, fiber, iron, potassium, phosphorus, riboflavin, niacin, and thiamin. Hemp milk is easy to digest and contains 10 essential amino acids.

Hemp Oil

Hemp oil or **hempseed** oil is made by pressing hempseeds. Cold-pressed, unrefined hemp oil is dark to light-green or clear in color, with a nutty flavor. Darker colored oils have a green, hempy taste. THC and cannabinoid content in seeds is miniscule. Hempseed oil has no psychedelic effects.

Hempseed oil has a three-to-one ratio of omega-6 to omega-3 essential fatty acids—in perfect balance with the human body. The clear, colorless oil is also used for body care products, lubricants, paints, inks, and biofuel.

Do not confuse hempseed oil with hash oil, Rick Simpson Oil (RSO, also known as Phoenix Tears). Hash oil is used for both medicinal and recreational purposes and is made from the mature female flowers and leaves of the drug cannabis, thus having a much higher THC content. Hash oil should not be confused with hemp, as the modern usage of the word *hemp* is reserved for plants that meet the legal requirement of containing 0.3 percent THC or less.

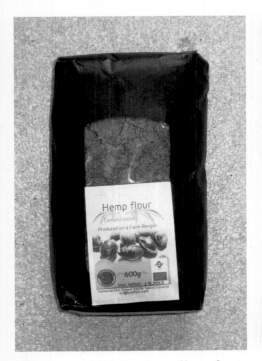

This 2.2-pound (1 kg) package of hemp flour was produced on Farm Renego in Slovenia.

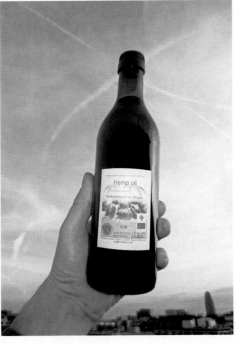

This 16.9 ounce (0.5 L) bottle of hempseed oil was produced on Farm Renego in Slovenia.

Storage

Store cannabis butters and oils in the refrigerator. Cannabis tinctures do not need refrigeration, but it does not hurt them.

Store dry cannabis in a cool, dry, dark location. Sunlight, heat, and air are the biggest enemies of stored cannabis. Store larger amounts of cannabis in airtight containers. Keep airtight packages in cool, dry, dark surroundings.

Recipes

Cannabis Brownies

Utensils
- large mixing bowl
- wooden mixing spoon
- 9 × 13-inch (22.9 × 33 cm) baking pan
- measuring cup
- measuring spoons
- wire cooling rack

Ingredients
- 4 oz (28.3 gm; 4 squares) unsweetened chocolate
- 0.75 c (17.7 cl) cannabis butter (recipe, page 562)
- 2 c (47.3 cl) white (granulated) sugar

- 3 eggs
- 1 tsp (0.5 cl) vanilla extract
- 1 c (23.7 cl) all-purpose flour
- 1 c (23.7 cl) chopped walnuts

Directions

Step One: Preheat oven to 350°F (176.7°C)

Step Two: In a saucepan on low heat, melt chocolate and cannabis butter. Stir the mix as it melts in the pan.

Step Three: When the mix has melted and combined, slowly stir in sugar. Next

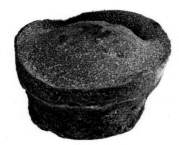

Cannabis brownies are easy to make and very popular among medical cannabis patients. Brownies became famous in North America during the 1960s when it seemed that everybody started making them. Of course, grandma always made the best brownies!

add eggs one at a time while blending into the mix. Add vanilla. Stir in flour and chopped walnuts. Mix until batter is consistent.

Step Four: Spread the batter in a greased 9 × 13-inch (22.9 × 33 cm) baking pan.

Step Five: Bake in preheated oven for 35 minutes at 350°F (176.7°C). Remove from the oven, let cool, and consume!

Cannabis Cookies (Biscotti)

Utensils
- large mixing bowl
- wooden mixing spoon
- cookie sheets
- measuring cup
- measuring spoons
- wire cooling rack

Ingredients
- 0.25 lb (113.4 gm) cannabis butter (recipe, page 562)
- 0.5 c (11.8 cl) white (granulated) sugar
- 0.5 c (11.8 cl) brown sugar
- 2 eggs
- 1 tsp (4.9 ml) vanilla extract
- 2 c (47.3 cl) unbleached all-purpose flour
- 1 tsp (4.9 ml) baking powder
- 0.5 tsp (2.5 ml) salt
- 3 c (71 cl) quick-cooking oats
- 0.5 c (11.8 cl) chocolate chips

Step One: Cream butter and sugar in a large bowl. Beat in eggs separately, and stir in vanilla. Stir in flour, baking powder, and salt. Stir in oats and chocolate chips, mixing to a consistent dough. Cover and chill for 1 hour or more.

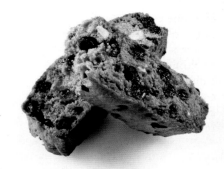

Cannabis chocolate chip biscotti

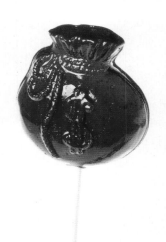

Cannabis lollipop!

Step Two: Preheat oven to 350°F (176.7°C). Grease cookie sheets. Form dough into balls about the size of a walnut, and set on 2-inch centers on the cookie sheets. Use the back of a spoon to flatten each ball a little.

Step Three: Bake for 10 to 12 minutes (8 to 10 minutes if you like chewy cookies). Let cookies cool for 5 to 10 minutes on cookie sheets or transfer to a wire cooling rack for faster cooling.

Cannabis Lollipops
Utensils
- parchment paper or tinfoil or small ice-cube tray or candy mold (Lollipop molds are available at most large stores with a cooking section.)
- cooking spray (nonstick)
- candy thermometer
- cooking pot
- stirring spoon
- measuring spoon

Ingredients
- 0.25 c cannabis butter (recipe, page 562)
- 2 c (47 cl) white (granulated) sugar
- 0.66 c (15.6 cl) corn syrup

- 0.5 c (12 cl) water
- 0.5 tsp (.25 cl) cream of tartar
- 2 tsp (1 cl) flavored dry Jell-O mix
- of your desired color and flavor

Step One: Prepare your molds by spraying them with nonstick cooking spray. Insert lollipop sticks into the molds.

Step Two: Melt cannabis butter in a heavy-bottomed pot over medium heat. Slowly stir in sugar.

Step Three: Add syrup and stir the mixture thoroughly. Stop stirring when it is well blended and starts to boil.

Step Four: Hang candy thermometer on the side of the pot. Be careful! The pot and mixture are very hot!

Step Five: The blended mixture will continue to boil and will ultimately reach 275°F (135°C).

Step Six: Remove from heat and add flavored Jell-O mix. Stir thoroughly. The flavor and color of the Jell-O determines the flavor and color of the lollipops.

Step Seven: Spoon the mix into the mold cavities and make sure to cover the back of the stick. Or set lollipop sticks out on nonstick parchment paper or tinfoil and cover the end of each stick with one tablespoon (1.5 cl) of mix. The candy mix is heavy and forms a circle around the stick.

Step Eight: As they cool to room temperature, lollipops harden. Wrap separately in plastic wrap or consume! Refrigerate wrapped lollipops for up to a month. Makes about 12 lollipops.

Cookbooks
Here is a short list of some of my favorite cookbooks. They are chock-full of recipes and everything you need to know to combine the concentrated cannabis butter, oil, milk, etc. into flavorful dishes.

The Joy of Cooking – This indispensable classic cookbook explains everything about cooking.

The Fannie Farmer Cookbook – This basic American cookbook has nearly 2,000 recipes.

The Official High Times Cannabis Cookbook is outstanding! It is a must-have for all cannabis cooking.

Betty Crocker Cookbook: 1500 Recipes for the Way You Cook Today – Classic cookbook!

The Cook's Illustrated Cookbook: 2,000 Recipes from 20 Years of America's Most Trusted Cooking Magazine – Amazing instructions to prepare great meals!

Jerusalem: A Cookbook – Diverse Muslim, Jewish, and Christian recipes.

The Everything Gluten-Free Cookbook – This book is a great resource for all sufferers of celiac disease (gluten/wheat allergy).

Check our website forum "Cooking with Cannabis" at www.marijuanagrowing.com for more cookbook information and recipes.

Cannabis Beverages
Cannabis Beer
Countless beer recipes can easily incorporate cannabis. This short section will discuss cannabis preparation and when to add it to the brew. Hemp, low-cannabinoid cannabis, can be added to the brew for flavoring. Medicinal cannabis is to be added to beer to impart flavor and/or meter out cannabinoid-rich beer.

Raw cannabis often lends an unpleasant taste to beers, which has made marketing difficult. Avoid the "hempy" taste by using kief, hashish, or oil that does not contain foliage residue. Soak cannabis in cold, low-EC water for 3 to 4 hours

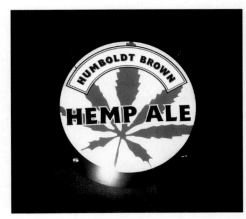

Hemp is used to flavor ale. Cannabis concentrate can also be added for extra effect!

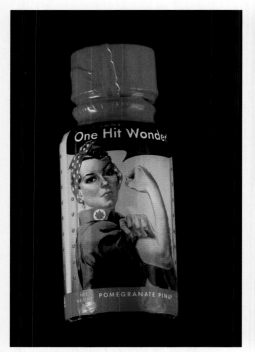

Pomegranate-flavored cannabis drink (MF)

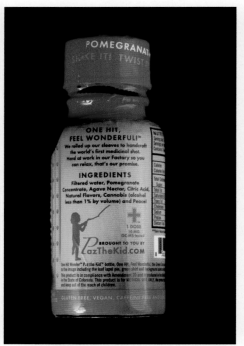

The ingredients in this beverage include cannabis (alcohol less than 1% by volume). (MF)

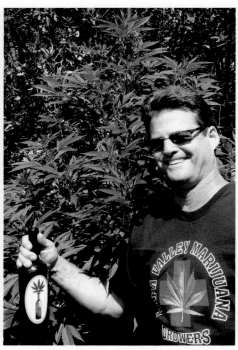

Crane Carter from Napa Valley Marijuana Growers is holding one of their bottles of cannabis wine.

to remove water-soluble chlorophyll and tars responsible for the "green" flavor. This will help purge the hempy taste.

Shake water off and dry cold-water-washed cannabis to the point that it crumbles into a powder before adding it to the brew. Contain ground cannabis in a nylon stocking or similar "tea bag" found at beer brewing stores. Add approximately 01.7 to 0.7 ounces (4.81–19.8 gm) of leaves per 3 ounces (8.9 cl) of finished beer.

Ales and beers can be any style: pilsner, porter, cream, stout, and so on. Strong-flavored brews work best to mask the cannabis taste. Cannabis is put into beer brews when hops are added. Some of the alcohol- or oil-soluble cannabinoids dissolve into the mix as it ferments.

A few hemp beers include Greenleaf (Germany), Hanfblüte (Switzerland), Humboldt Hemp Ale (USA), Liquid Hemp (Austria), and Nirvana (Holland). **Note:** Cannabis and hops (*Humulus*

lupulus) are both from the Cannabinaceae family, but hops grafted to cannabis rootstock does not produce cannabinoids.

Cannabis Drinks

Several companies in the USA and other countries have launched carbonated and concentrated cannabis drinks. Concentrated cannabis syrup is added to different products after the heating process so as to not destroy the active cannabinoid ingredients. The list of new cannabis products is growing rapidly.

Cannabis Wine

"Cannabis wine is becoming popular in the wine country of California. In fact, I believe it is the only original style of wine created in the New World," said Crane Carter, president of Napa Valley Marijuana Growers, and later added, "Cabernet sauvignon from the Stag's Leap district is thought to pair particularly well with pot."

Cannabis wine delivers cannabinoids more quickly than baked foods, and the

combination of alcohol and cannabis produce a different effect.

To make cannabis wine, add 0.05 to 0.1 ounce (1.5–3 gm) of cannabis per bottle (75 cl) of fermenting wine. Cannabinoids are extracted as part of the alcohol fermentation process, but to date little is known about the efficacy of cannabinoids extracted thus. Nonetheless, high-quality cannabis produces more cannabinoid-potent wine. Aging cannabinoid wine for nine or more months before bottling ensures the maximum amount of cannabinoids will be extracted. Aging also mellows cannabis flavor.

Many cannabis wines and spirit drinks are available in Austria, Germany, Holland, and Switzerland.
The scope of this chapter is to introduce subjects and stimulate thought. Please consult our website, www.marijuanagrowing.com, to learn more about cannabis wine.

APPENDIX: MEASURES & ABBREVIATIONS

Light Measurement Scales

fc = foot-candle(s)

K = kelvin(s)

lm = lumen(s)

lx = lux

PAR = photosynthetically active radiation

PPFD = photosynthetic photon flux density

W/cm² = watts per square centimeter

W/m²/nm = watts per square meter per nanometer

μmol m²·sec = micromole per square meter per second

μE·m²·sec = microeinsteins per square meter per second

2,000 μmol·m²·sec ~ intense sunlight

CPW = cost per watt = cost of fixture divided by watts

VPW = value per watt **1 joule of energy per second** = 1 watt

1 lumen = 1 candle from 1 foot away shining on 1 square foot

1 lumen = 10 lux. 1 lux has only 1/10 the photons of a lumen

1 lux = 1 candle from 1 foot away shining on 1 square meter

1 mired = 1 million divided by the color temperature in kelvins

foot-candle = lumens per square foot

illumination = lumens per area = 1 $\cos(a)/r^2$

lux = lumens per square meter

luminous flux = lumen = 1/685 watts @ 555 nm (energy = lumens per sec)

microeinsteins (μE) are occasionally used to indicate 1 mole per square meter per second. 1 μE = 6 x 1023 photons that fall on 1 square meter of leaf surface. Using this system, the amount of radiant flux that initiates photosynthesis can be defined in microeinsteins, μmol-2.-s1 or PAR watts per square meter.

phot = lumens per square centimeter

Plant Nutrients

Al aluminum

B boron

Ca calcium

Cl chlorine

Co cobalt

Cu copper

Fe iron

K potassium

Mg magnesium

Mn manganese

Mo molybdenum

N nitrogen

Na sodium

Ni nickel

N-P-K nitrogen; phosphorus; potassium

P phosphorus

S sulfur

Se selenium

Si silicon

Zn zinc

Other Abbreviations

AACT actively aerated compost tea (aka ACT)

ABA abscisin (abscisic acid)

ABV already been vaporized

AC alternating current

A/C air conditioning

AEA anandamide, aka N arachidonylethanolamine

AIDS acquired immune deficiency syndrome

amp ampere

ASA salicylates (aspirin)

ATC automatic temperature compensation

ATTRA National Sustainable Agriculture Information Service

BAC beaded activated carbon

BAP 6-benzylaminopurine

BC before Christ

BCE before the Christian Era / before the Common Era

BCSR base cation saturation ratio (soil test)

BHO butane hash oil

BLD broad-leaf drug

BR brassinolide

Brix sugar content of plant

***Bt** Bacillus thuringiensis*

Btu British thermal unit

Btu/h Btus per hour

B_1 aka thiamin, thiamine, and aneurine

B_3 niacin

B_9 aka folic acid, folinic acid

C Celsius, centigrade

CBB Calvin-Benson-Bassham cycle (Calvin cycle)

CBC cannabichromene

CBCV cannabichromevarin

CBD cannabidiol

CBDV cannabidivarin

CBE cannabielsoin

CBG cannabigerol

CBGM cannabigerol monomethyl ether

CBGV cannabigerovarin

CBL cannabicyclol

CBT cannabicitran

cc cubic centimeter(s)

CCI chlorophyll content index

CCT color corrected temperature

cd candle or candela

CE Conformance European

CEA controlled environment agriculture

CEC cation exchange capacity

CF conductivity factor

cfh cubic feet per hour

CFL compact fluorescent lamp

cfm cubic feet per minute

CK cytokinin

cl centiliter

cm centimeter

CNN Cable News Network

CO_2 carbon dioxide

COP constable on patrol

COP critical oxygen pressure
CPU central processing unit (microchip)
CRI color rendering index
CS colloidal silver
CSA Canadian Standards Association
C3 plant carbon fixation of most plants
C4 plant carbon fixation of fast-growing plant
CB1 cannabinoid receptor 1
CB2 cannabinoid receptor 2
cm^3/min cubic meters per minute

dB decibel
dc direct current
DEA Drug Intelligence Agency
DFT deep flow technique
DIY do-it-yourself
DMSO dimethyl sulfoxide
DNA deoxyribonucleic acid
DO dissolved oxygen
DPA dichlorophenoxylacetic acid
DS dissolved solids
DWC deep water culture

E einstein(s)
EAC extruded activated carbon
EC electrical conductivity
ECS endocannabinoid system
ERGS energy released per gram of soil
Eye a division of Iwasaki Electric Co.

fc foot-candle(s)
FIM "F%&k, I missed!" pruning technique
FTE fritted trace element(s)

GA/GA3 gibberellic acid
GAC granulatar activated carbon
GE General Electric
GFI ground fault interrupter
GHz gigahertz
GI gastrointestinal
gm gram(s)
GPM gallons per minute
GPS global positioning system
GRAS generally recognized as safe

H hydrogen
H_2O water

H_2O_2 hydrogen peroxide
HEP high-efficiency plasma (lamp)
HEPA high-efficiency particulate air (filter)
HID high-intensity discharge
HIV human immunodeficiency virus
HO high output
HP high-pressure sodium lamp
HSA Homeland Security Act
HVAC heating, ventilating, and air conditioning
Hz hertz

IAA indole-3-acetic acid
IACM International Association for Cannabinoid Medicines
IBA indole-3-butyric acid, 3-indolebutyric
IBL inbred lines
ICRS International Cannabinoid Research Society
ID identification
ISO oil cannabis oil extracted with isopropanol

j joule
JA jasmonate

K kelvin(s), Kelvin-scale temperature
kg kilogram
kmh kilometers per hour
kV kilovolt
kW kilowatt
kWh kilowatt-hour

L liter
lb pound(s)
LCD liquid crystal display
LEAP Law Enforcement Against Prohibition
Leca light expanded clay aggregate
LED light-emitting diode
LEO law enforcement organization
LEP light-emitting plasma
lm/W lumens per watt
LP gas natural gas
LP low-pressure sodium lamp
LPH liters per hour
LPM liters per minute
lx lux

m meter
mA milliampere
MABC marker-assisted backcrossing
MARS marker-assisted recurrent selection
MAS marker-assisted selection
MCPCB metal core printed circuit board
MD medical doctor
mEq milliequivalents
MH metal halide
mired micro reciprocal degrees
MJ marijuana
mL milliliter
MMJ medical marijuana
mph miles per hour
mS millisiemen(s)
mW milliwatt(s)
N-P-K nitrogen; phosphorus; potassium
m^2 square meter
m^3 cubic meter
m^3/h cubic meters per hour

NAA 1-naphthalenaecetic acid
NDIR nondispersive infrared sensor
NFT nutrient film technique
NIDA National Institute on Drug Abuse
NLD narrow-leaf drug
NLD narrow leaflet diameter or narrow-leaf drug
NLDA narrow-leaf drug ancestor
NLH narrow-leaf hemp
nm nanometer
NORML National Organization for the Reform of Marijuana Laws
OCIA Organic Crop Improvement Association
OH hydroxide
OMRI Organic Materials Review Institute
OPD overfill prevention device
ORP oxygen reduction potential
O'S O'Shaughnessy's (publication)
oz ounce(s)
O_2 oxygen
O_3 ozone
PAA 2-phenylacetic acid

PAC powdered activated carbon

PAR photosynthetically active radiation

PCB polychlorinated biphenyl

PE polyethylene plastic

PGR plant growth regulator

ph phot

pH potential hydrogen

PPF photosynthetic photon flux

PPFD photosynthetic photon flux density

ppm parts per million

psi pounds per square inch

PSP phenolsulfonphthalein

PV photovoltaic

PVC polyvinyl chloride

RF radio frequency

RH relative humidity

RICO Racketeer Influenced and Corrupt Organizations (Act)

RNA ribonucleic acid

RNAi RNA interference

RO reverse osmosis

rpm revolutions per minute

RTW run to waste

SCF supercritical fluid

sCF subcritical fluid

SCFP supercritical fluid process

SCROG screen of green

SFE supercritical fluid extraction

SLAN sufficiency level of available nutrients (soil test)

SOG sea of green

sp. / spp. species singular; species plural

ssp. / sspp. subspecies singular; subspecies plural

SRP soft rock phosphate

STC sound transmission class

T5 lamp tube diameter is 0.625 inches

T8 lamp tube diameter is 1 inch

T12 lamp tube diameter is 1.5 inches

TDS total dissolved solids

THC tetrahydrocannabinol

THCA tetrahydrocannabinolic acid

THCV tetrahydrocannabivarin

thm therm

UK United Kingdom

UL Underwriters Laboratories

US / USA United States of America

USD United States dollar

UV ultraviolet light

UVA ultraviolet light A ~ mild

UVB ultraviolet light B ~ somewhat harmful

UVC ultraviolet light C ~ harmful

V volt

VAC volts of alternating current

var. variety

VDC volts of direct current

VHO very high output

VOC volatile organic compound

W watt(s)

W/K watts per kelvin

w/o water-in-oil emulsifier

Wi-Fi Wireless Fidelity, transmission of data over wireless networks

WIN water-insoluble-nitrogen

WLD wild leaflet diameter *or* w

WSN water-soluble-nitrogen

W/ft² watts per square foot

W/m² watts per square meter

XHO extra high output

μE microeinstein(s)

2-AG 2 arachidonoylglycerol

2,4 DPA dichlorophenoxylacetic acid

4-Cl-IAA 4-chloroindole-3-acetic acid

420 (4/20) code word for anything cannabis-related

CONTRIBUTORS

The names below represent most of this book's contributors from around the world. More and more people are proud to see their legal name in print here; others prefer anonymity and the use of a pseudonym.

I have done my best to include everyone who has contributed to this work. To include any names I might have missed, I started a thread at www.marijuanagrowing.com.

10K
2mins4roughing
420USAPride
Aaron (DNA Genetics)
Adam Dunn (T.H.Seeds)
Al (Insta Print)
Alan Dronkers (Sensi Seeds)
Albert (Sensi Seeds)
Aleen (FS Books)
Aleksandr
Alex (Flowery Field)
Alex (Marimberos Seeds)
Alex de Nasario (RIP)
Allen St. Pierre (NORML)
Amadeo (RIP)
Ammiraglio
André Grossman (*High Times*)
Annie Riecken
Apollo11Genius
Arjan (Strain Hunters)
Arno Hazekamp (Bedrocan)
Aurora Avanseña
Badar
Balta
Barbas
Barge
Barry Cooper (LEAP)
Bean (*High Times*)
Belpe
Ben Dronkers (Sensi Seeds)
Bernard Rapaz (Valchanvre)
Bev
Beverly Potter (author)
BigIslandBud
BigSkyBud THC
Bill
Bill Cattterson (RIP)
Bill Drake (author)
Bill Kuffler
Bill R.

Blackdog
Bob Van Patten
BOG (Bushy Older Grower)
Boy Ramsahai (*Soft Secrets*)
Breeder Steve (Spice of Life Seeds)
Brian (SNB)
Bubbasix
Bubble Man
Bud-E
Buddy (Nirvana), Holland
Buddy R.
Buko
Candi Cooper
Carlos
Carlos Hernandez
Cezar Doll (*Cáñamo*)
Charlie
Charlie Frink (author)
Chimera (Chimera Seeds)
Chris Conrad (author)
Chris Ivenson
Chris Payaso
Chris Simunek (*High Times*)
Christopher Valdés
ClassicNugz
Cliff Cremer (*High Life* and *Soft Secrets*)
Clint Werner (author)
Connie (*Hanf*)
Consuelo
Cosmic Jimmy
Crystal (Kind Seeds)
Crystal P. (Green Universe)
Crystalman (Joop Dumay), Holland
Curt, Holland
D. B. Turner
D. C.
D. J. Short (DJ Short Seeds)
DaChronicKing
Dan (Vancouver, BC)
Dana Larsen (*Cannabis Culture*)
Darryll (Kind Seeds)
Daryl
Dave (Sonoma Patients Group)
Dave Bienenstock (author)
David
David (Flowery Field)
David Garcia (translator)
David Strange (*Heads*)
David Tatelman (Homestead Books)
David W.
David Watson (author)
Debbi (Homestead Books)
Debbie Goldsberry (Berkeley Pts. Grp.)

Dennis (*Grass Times*)
Dennis H.
Dennis Peron (coauthor Prop. 215)
Dennis Stovall (author)
Dennos
Derry (Barney's Farm)
Deva
Dieter Hagenbach
Dion (*Nug*)
Dirk Rehahn
Doc Ontario
Doctor Dangerous
Don Collins (Pypes Palace)
Donald Abrams, MD
Donna (OrganiCann)
Donny
DoobieDuck
Doug (Hemp Works)
Dr. John McPartland (author)
Dr. Lester Grinspoon
Drew Bennie
Dutch Grown
Eagle Bill (RIP)
Ed Borg, Holland
Ed Rosenthal (author)
Ed S., Canada
Eddie (Flying Dutchmen)
Eddy Lepp (drug war prisoner)
Eduardo DC
Eirik (photographer)
Elise McDonough (author)
Elizabeth
Elmar (BTT)
Emilio Gómez Reig
Enric
Eric Taylor (California Botanicals)
Ernesto (*Cáñamo*)
Ernesto (Hemp Trading)
Estella Cervantes
Everybody's kids
Evie Hayes
Farmer in the Sky
Fatima
Felipe
Felipe Borallo (*Cáñamo*)
Felix Kautz (Owl's Production)
Feran (Good House Seeds)
Fergetit
Flick Ford (*High Times*)
Fluus
Foz
Fran (Osona Canem)
Franco Casalone (author)

Franco Losa (Strain Hunter)
Frank
Frank (Canna)
Fred Gardner (www.projectcbd.org)
G. I. Joe
Gabbi (Water Spout)
Gaspar Fraga (*Cáñamo*) (RIP)
Gato
George
GIB
Gillis (Canna)
Gisela (worldly woman)
Glass Joe
Gloria (Kind Seed)
Gonz
Gordon
Grant
GrassDaddy
Green Man
Greg (Northern Lights)
Gregorio (Goyo) Fernández
Grey (Humboldt)
Grubbycup
Guido (*Hanfblatt*)
Gurney
GvtCheese
Gypsy Nirvana (drug war prisoner)
Hank Gonzales
Harmon Davidson
Harry (Cultiva)
HashMan
HempHappy
Henk (Dutch Passion)
Henk (HESI)
Hillary Black
Homer
Howard Marks (Double Agent)
Huero
Hugo (*Soft Secrets*)
Humboldtlocal
Ian
Ignaci Peña (author)
Ignacio Acuña
Ivan (Ivanart)
ixnay007
J. D., Spain
Jack Herrer
Jaime Carion (Resin Seeds)
Jaime Prats (*Cáñamo*)
Jan
Jan Sennema (Biker)
Jane (Homestead Books)
Jane Klein (Quick Distribution Co.)
Jason King (author)
Jason Miller (Pure Analytics)
Javi
Javi (The Plant)
Javis

Jay (NGSC)
Jeff Lowenfels (author)
Jeff Raber, PhD (The Werc Shop)
Jeffrey Y. Hergenrather, MD
Jen Matthews
Jerry
Jess
Jim
Jim from Chicago
Jim Gierach (LEAP)
Jim Goodwin (breeder)
Jim R.
Jimmy Chicago
JJ Jackson (Advanced Hydroponics)
JJ Turner (RIP)
Joel, Forestville
Joey
Joey Perez
John
John (Avalon)
John H.
John L.
John S.
John Williams
Johnny Sage, Ocean Beach
Joint Doctor (Low Ryder)
JomJom
Jordi Bricker (*Cáñamo*)
Josete (*Cáñamo*)
Juan
Juan Vaz, Uruguay
Juan, Barcelona
Juaquin (El Conde) Bucati
Justin McIvor
Karen (The Amsterdam)
Karl Hilling
Karulo (l'Interior)
Kees (Super Sativa Seed Club)
Keith Stroop (Founder of NORML)
Kelly
Ken
Ken Morrow (Trichome Technologies)
Kevin
Klaatu
Kristen Nevedal (bud whisperer)
Kyle (Kind Seed)
Kyle Kushman (Veganics)
Larry Armantrout
Larry Turner (photographer)
Lars (Nirvana Seeds)
Laura (Sow What! Association,
    Barcelona)
Laura Blanco, Uruguay
Laurence Cherniac (author)
Laurence Ringo (RIP)
Leaf
Lee Bridges (Cannabis Poet, RIP)
Lennarts

Les
Liam (Pollinator)
Linda
Lock
Lord of the Strains
Lorna (Cannabis College)
Loti, Switzerland
Luc Krol (Paradise Seeds and Cannabis
    Medical Bike Tour)
Lyndon (*CC Newz*)
Madeline Martinez (OR NORML)
Mani, Spain
Manuel Guzmán, PhD
Marc Brown
Marc Emery (*Cannabis Culture*)
Marco Kuhn (CannaTrade)
Marcus Von Bueler
Maria Garcia (translator)
Mario Belandi (Reyna Madre)
Martin Lee (author)
Martin Palmer (Avalon)
Martin Trip
Mary Anderson
Master Haze
Matej (Medical Cannabis Bike Tour)
Matt Stang (*High Times*)
Mauk (Canna founder)
Max Acuña
Max Messerli
Mel Frank (author)
Melani (Sow What! Association,
    Barcelona)
Michael
Michael (SickMeds Seeds)
Michael A.
Michka (Mama Editions)
Mickey
Mieko Perez (Unconventional Founda-
tion for Autism)
Miguel
Miguel Bella
Miguel Gemino
Miguel Torres (Abogado, Barcelona)
Mike
Mike A. S.
Mike Brown
Mike Miller
Mikki Norris (activist)
Mila Jansen (Pollinator)
Moisés Lopéz (*Cáñamo*)
Moño
Mr. Beaner
Mr. Ito
Mr. MaJick
Murphy Stevens (author)
Napoleon (Martin)
Natalia Casado
Nate Bradley (LEAP)

Ned Eduardo
Neil Wilkinson
Nevil (The Seed Bank)
Nick (*Red Eye Express*)
Noel Palmer (Montana Botanical
    Analysis)
Nol Van Schaik (Willie Wortel's)
Nomaad
Noucetta
Oakie
Ocean
Olaf (Greenhouse)
Olde Sonoma Public House
Oli, Switzerland
Oneshot LED
Opti
Oscar (Osona Canem)
Patricia
Patrick (Paradise Seeds)
Patrick, Switzerland
Patty Collins (Pypes Palace)
Paul
Paul (Austrian videographer)
Paula Morris (Medea Labs)
Peace and Medicine
Pete Sargosis (Sargosis Solar & Electric)
Phil (*Weed World*)
Pim (Super Sativa Seed Club)
Podencoid
PREMIER
Psychotropic Nomad
R.C. (founder, overgrow.com)
Raphael Mechoulam, PhD, (Isolated
    THC and CBD)
Ravi Dronkers (Sensi Seeds)
Red (Legend Seeds)
Reeferman
Richard (Plant Photonics)
Richard Lake County
Richard Lee (Oaksterdam University)
Rick
Rick Cusick (*High Times*)
Ringraziamenti
Roach from Spain
Rob
Rob Clarke (author)
Robbie (Agromix)
Robert Melamede, PhD
Robert the ex-COP
Robert W.
Roberto C.
Roger
Roger (Nachtschatten Verlag)
Roger Botlanger (*Hanf*)
Roger Watanabe (RIP)
Rolf
Rollitup.com – BigSkyBud THC
Romulan Joe

Ron Turner (Last Gasp)
Ron Wilks
Ross
Rubio
Salvatore
Salvatore Casano (Phytoplant)
Sam S.
Sam the Skunk Man
Samantha Miller (Pure Analytics)
Sammy
Saskia (Canna)
Saskia from OZ
SC
Scott
Scott (Rare Dankness)
Scott Blakey (Mr. Nice)
Sebastain Orfali (RIP)
Sébastien Béguerie (AlphaCAT)
Sergi Doll (*Cáñamo*)
Simon (Serious Seeds)
Sita Von Wilhelm
Sixfinger
Skip
Skip Stone
Snoofer
Soma (Soma Seeds)
Spanish Hash Guy
Spence (Cannabis College)
Stefan Meyer (Phytoplant)
Steve
Steve Bloom (celebstoner.com)
Steve from Amsterdam
Steve from OZ
Steve Hagar (*High Times*)
Steve Huxley (Steve's Beer)
Steve Rogers
Steve Solomon (author)
Steven DeAngelo (Harborside Health
Center, founder)
Stitch (Super Autos)
Subcool (TGA Genetics)
Sus
Susan (Canna)
Susan LaPolice
T.
Taylor (Kind Seeds)
Tea House Collective
Ted B.
Ted Zitlau (RIP)
The thinker
Theo Tekstra (Gavita Holland)
Tigrane (Mama Editions)
Tim
Tim G.
Tim I.
Tom Alexander (*Sinsemilla Tips*)
Tom Flowers (RIP)
Tom Hill

Toni (Barney´s Farm)
Toni13
Tony (Sagarmatha)
Tony B.
Twenty Three
Twofingered
Uncle Ben
Uncle Stoner
Valdudes
Valerie Corral (WAMM)
Vansterdan
Vic High
Vital Landscaping
Wally Duck
Warlock
Watcha
Wayne Oliver (RIP)
Wendover Brown
Wernard Bruining (author, visionary)
Whirly
Wili
William
William (Grow Room)
William L. Courtney, MD AACM
Willie (*Hanfblatt*)
Wilson (Steep Hill Laboratory)
Wim (Pollinator)
Winnie (*Grow!*)
Wismy (*Yerba*)
Xavier Nadal (Phytoplant)
Xus (RIP)
Yechiel Gaoni, PhD, (Isolated THC
    and CBD)
Yorg, Switzerland
Yorgos
Zeke Van Patten
    (marijuanagrowing.com)
ZtefaN

INDEX

Page numbers in italics indicate pages with pictures.

589

ABOUT JORGE

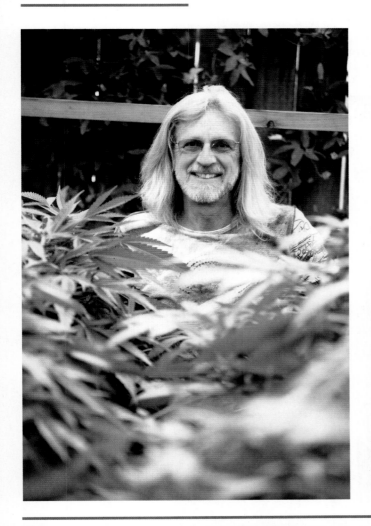

Jorge Cervantes is the nom de plume that George Van Patten took to conceal his identity from 1983 to 2010. Taking the name of his wife, Estella Cervantes, and that of his favorite author, Miguel de Cervantes, Van Patten wore black dreadlocks and a beret to cloak his public identity. Cervantes came "out of the closet" in a 2010 interview on National Public Radio (USA), and continues to research, publish, make videos, and draw a discussion about his favorite plant with an international community on his forum at www.marijuanagrowing.com.

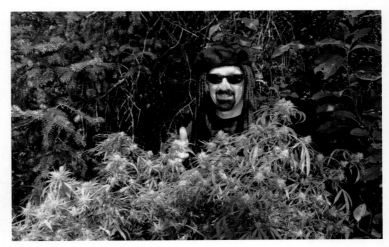

JORGE'S 30-YEAR PUBLISHING HISTORY

The Bible

1983 First edition *Indoor Marijuana Horticulture* is self-published. The 96-page book was dubbed the "Indoor Grower's Bible" by growers.

1985 Second edition *Indoor Marijuana Horticulture*

1993 Third edition *Indoor Marijuana Horticulture.*

2002 Fourth edition *Indoor Marijuana Horticulture.*

2006 Fifth edition *Marijuana Horticulture: The Indoor/Outdoor Medical Grower's Bible.*

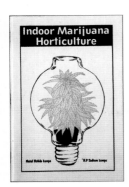 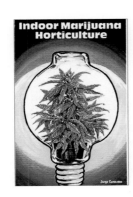 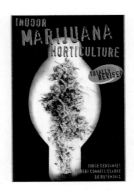 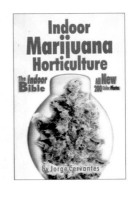 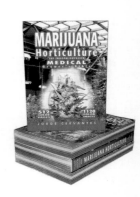

Translated Books

1988 *Marihuana Binnen*, Dutch

1994 *Marihuana Drinnen & Draußen*, German

2001 Jorge contributes to *Pourquoi & comment cultiver du chanvre*, French

2001 *Marihuana en Exterior Cultivo de Guerrilla*, Spanish

2002 *Marihuana Cultivo en Interior*, Spanish

2003 *Marihuana drinnen: Alles über den Anbau im Haus*, German

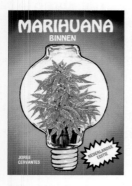 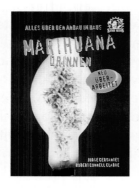 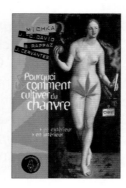 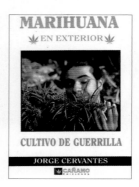 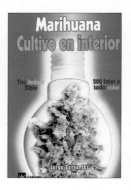

2005 *Culture en intérieur*, French

2007 *Marijuana: horticultura del cannabis La biblia del cultivador Médico de interior y exterior*, Spanish

2007 *Culture en intérieur: Basic Edition*, French

2007 *Culture en intérieur: Master Edition*, French

2008 *Marijuana: Orticoltura Indoor/Outdoor La Bibbia del coltivatore Medico*, Italian

2008 *Hydroponic Basics*, Japan

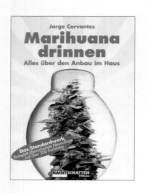 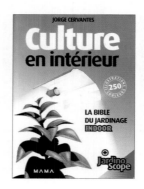 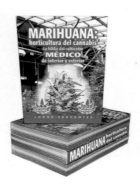 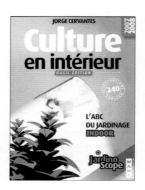 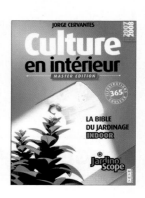

2011 *Marihuana Fundamentos de Cultivo*, Spanish

2011 *Marihuana Anbaugrundlagen*, German

2012 *Marijuana Horticulture*, Russian

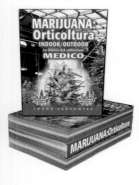 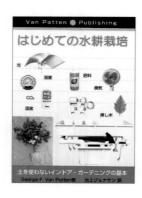 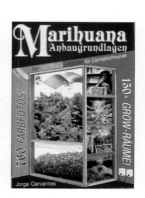 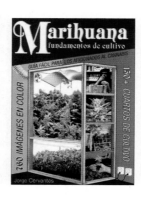 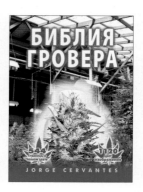

2006 Jorge Cervantes' *Ultimate Grow DVD*

2007 Jorge Cervantes' *Ultimate Grow DVD 2*

2008 Jorge Cervantes' *Ultimate Grow DVD III* (3-box set)

2012 Jorge Cervantes' *Cannabis Expeditions: The Green Giants of California* DVD

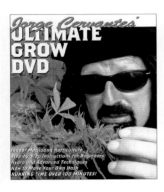 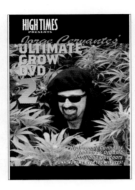 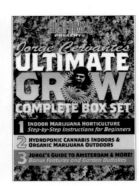 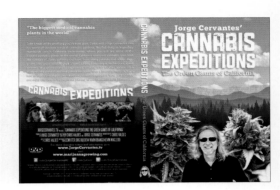

Internet

1997 Started the website www.marijuanagrowing.com

2013 Jorge Cervantes' Channel on YouTube tops 7 million views!

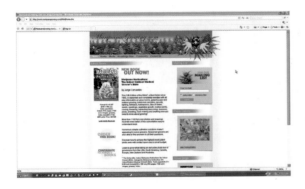 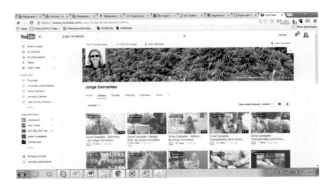

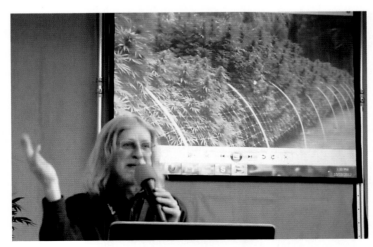

Jorge conducts a seminar to a crowd of hundreds at the Cultiva Cannabis Fair in Vienna, Austria.

Cannabis Fairs Jorge Attends
CannaTrade – Bern, Switzerland
Cultiva – Vienna, Austria
Expo Cannabis – Madrid, Spain
GrowMed – Valencia, Spain
Hemp Fair – London, UK
HighLife – Barcelona, Spain
HighLife – Amsterdam, Netherlands
High Times Cannabis Cup – Amsterdam, Netherlands
High Times Cannabis Cup – San Francisco, CA, USA
Interhanf – Colon, Germany
International Cannabis & Hemp Expo – San Francisco, CA, USA
Spannabis – Barcelona, Spain
THC Expose – Los Angeles, CA, USA

Magazines Jorge Writes For

1984 *Sinsemilla Tips*, USA

1985 *High Times*, USA

1998 *Cannabis Culture*, Canada

1998 *Cañamo*, Spain

2000 First of 10 years of "Jorge's Rx" Q&A column *High Times*, USA

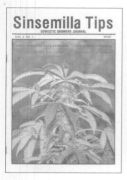

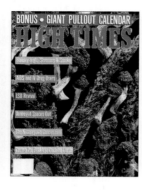

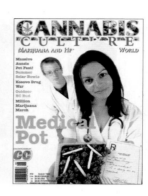

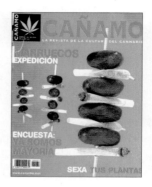

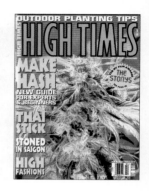

2004 *High Life*, Netherlands

2004 *Weed World*, UK

2005 *Soft Secrets*, UK, France, Italy, Germany, Poland, Czech Republic, Spain, Argentina, Chile

2006 *Dolce Vita*, Italy

2010 *Cannabis Kultusz*, Hungary

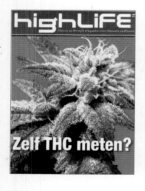

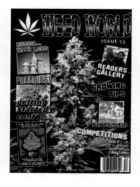

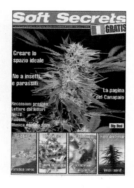

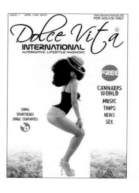

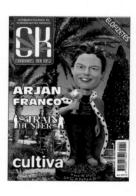

2010 *Canna Habla*, Spain

2012 *THC*, Argentina

2013 *TPABA*, Russia

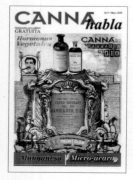

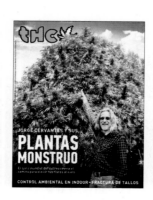

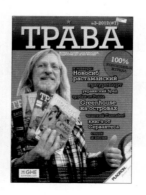

Magazines Not Pictured

Burst High, Japan
CC News, UK
Cânhamo, Portugal
Grass Times, Germany
Grow!, Germany
High Times Medical Marijuana, USA
Il Ligito, Italy
International Cannagraphic, Netherlands
Red Eye Express, UK
THCene, Germany
Yerba, Spain

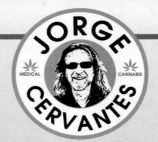

JORGE CERVANTES

MEDICAL CANNABIS

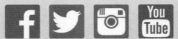

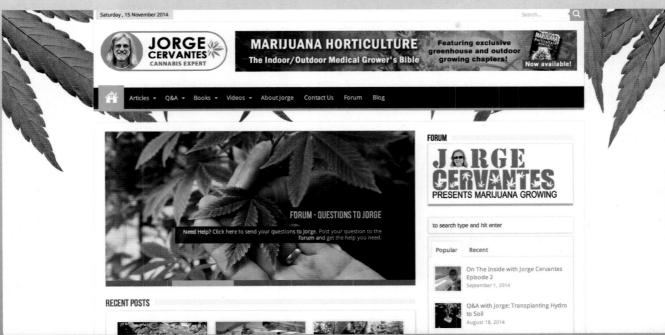

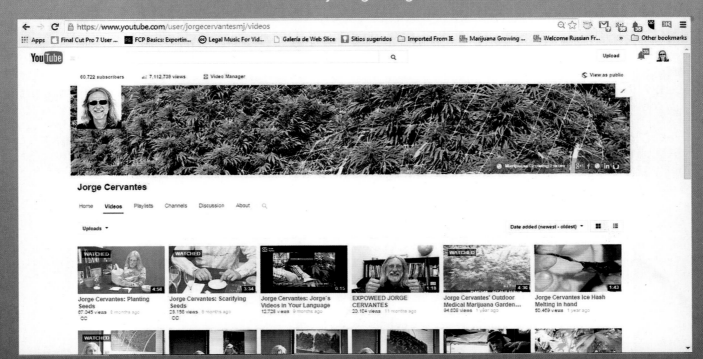

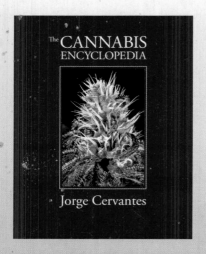
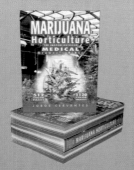
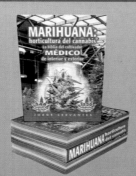
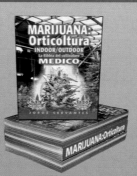
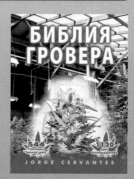
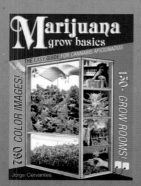
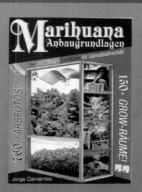
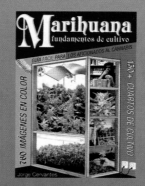